# Pediatric Environmental Health

## 4th Edition

Author: **Council on Environmental Health**
**American Academy of Pediatrics**

**Ruth A. Etzel, MD, PhD; Editor**
**Sophie J. Balk, MD; Associate Editor**

Suggested Citation: American Academy of Pediatrics
Council on Environmental Health. [chapter title].
In: Etzel RA, ed. Pediatric Environmental Health,
4th Edition; Itasca, IL: American Academy of Pediatrics;
2019:[page number]

American Academy
of Pediatrics

DEDICATED TO THE HEALTH OF ALL CHILDREN®

4th Edition
3rd Edition – 2012
2nd Edition – 2003
1st Edition – 1999


Published by the American Academy of Pediatrics
345 Park Blvd
Itasca, IL 60143
Telephone: 630/626-6000
Facsimile: 847/434-8000
www.aap.org

The American Academy of Pediatrics is an organization of 67,000 primary care pediatricians, pediatric medical subspecialists, and pediatric surgical specialists dedicated to the health, safety, and well-being of infants, children, adolescents, and young adults.

The recommendations in this publication do not indicate an exclusive course of treatment or serve as a standard of medical care. Variations, taking into account individual circumstances, may be appropriate.

Inclusion in this publication does not imply an endorsement by the American Academy of Pediatrics (AAP). The AAP is not responsible for the content of the resources mentioned. Addresses, phone numbers, and Web site addresses are as current as possible, but may change at any time.

The publishers have made every effort to trace the copyright holders for borrowed materials. If they have inadvertently overlooked any, they will be pleased to make the necessary arrangements at the first opportunity.

This publication has been developed by the American Academy of Pediatrics. The contributors are expert authorities in the field of pediatrics. No commercial involvement of any kind has been solicited or accepted in development of the content of this publication.

Every effort is made to keep *Pediatric Environmental Health* consistent with the most recent advice and information available from the American Academy of Pediatrics.

Special discounts are available for bulk purchases of this publication.
E-mail Special Sales at aapsales@aap.org for more information.

Printed in the United States of America.

3-334/1018          1 2 3 4 5 6 7 8 9 10


MA0882
ISBN: 978-1-61002-218-7
eBook: 978-1-61002-219-4
Library of Congress Control Number: 2017963888

# 2017–2018
# Council on Environmental Health Executive Committee

Jennifer A. Lowry, MD, FAAP - *Chairperson*
Samantha Ahdoot, MD, FAAP
Carl R. Baum, MD, MSc, FACMT, FAAP
Aaron S. Bernstein, MD, MPH, FAAP
Aparna Bole, MD, FAAP
Lori G. Byron, MD, FAAP
Philip J. Landrigan, MD, MSc, FAAP
Steven M. Marcus, MD, FAAP
Susan E. Pacheco, MD, FAAP
Adam J. Spanier, MD, PhD, MPH, FAAP
Alan D. Woolf, MD, MPH, FAAP

## Liaison Representatives

John M. Balbus, MD, MPH
*National Institute of Environmental Health Sciences*
Nathaniel G. DeNicola, MD, MSc
*American Congress of Obstetricians and Gynecologists*
Ruth A. Etzel, MD, PhD, FAAP
*US Environmental Protection Agency*
Diane E. Hindman, MD, PharmD, FAAP
*AAP Section on Pediatric Trainees*
Mary Ellen Mortensen, MD, MS
*CDC/National Center for Environmental Health*
Mary H. Ward, PhD
*National Cancer Institute*

## AAP Staff

Paul Spire

# Contributors

The American Academy of Pediatrics (AAP) gratefully acknowledges the invaluable assistance provided by the following individuals who contributed to the preparation of this edition of *Pediatric Environmental Health*. Their expertise, critical review, and cooperation were essential to the development of this book.

Every attempt has been made to recognize all those who contributed to this effort; the AAP regrets any omissions that may have occurred. Organizational affiliations are provided for identification purposes only.

John L. Adgate, PhD, MSPH; *Colorado School of Public Health; Aurora, CO*

Terry Adirim, MD, MPH, FAAP; *US Department of Defense; Arlington, VA*

Samantha Ahdoot, MD, FAAP; *Virginia Commonwealth University School of Medicine, Inova Campus; Falls Church, VA*

John M. Balbus, MD, MPH; *National Institute of Environmental Health Sciences; Research Triangle Park, NC*

Sophie J. Balk, MD, FAAP; *Children's Hospital at Montefiore, Albert Einstein College of Medicine; Bronx, NY*

Carl R. Baum, MD, MSc, FACMT, FAAP; *Yale School of Medicine; New Haven, CT*

Nancy Beaudet, MS, CIH; *University of Washington; Seattle, WA*

Aaron S. Bernstein, MD, MPH, FAAP; *Harvard Medical School; Boston, MA*

Linda S. Birnbaum, PhD; *National Institute of Environmental Health Sciences; Research Triangle Park, NC*

Aparna Bole, MD, FAAP; *Case Western Reserve University School of Medicine; Cleveland, OH*

Ashley Brooks-Russell, PhD, MPH; *Colorado School of Public Health; Aurora, CO*

Todd A. Brubaker, DO, FAAP; *Regional West Medical Center; Scottsbluff, NE*

Heather L. Brumberg, MD, MPH, FAAP; *New York Medical College; Valhalla, NY*

Lori G. Byron, MD, FAAP; *Hardin, MT*

Carla C. Campbell, MD, MS, FAAP; *University of Texas at El Paso; El Paso, TX*

Stuart A. Cohen, MD, MPH, FAAP; *Rady Children's Hospital; San Diego, CA*

Nathaniel G. DeNicola, MD, MSc; *George Washington University Hospital; Washington, DC*

Ruth A. Etzel, MD, PhD, FAAP; *Milken Institute School of Public Health, The George Washington University; Washington, DC*

Harold J. Farber, MD, MSPH, FAAP; *Baylor College of Medicine and Texas Children's Hospital; Houston, TX*

Joel A. Forman, MD, FAAP; *Icahn School of Medicine at Mount Sinai; New York, NY*

Mamta Fuloria, MD, FAAP; *Children's Hospital at Montefiore, Albert Einstein College of Medicine; Bronx, NY*

Laurence J. Fuortes, MD, MS; *University of Iowa Carver College of Medicine; Iowa City, IA*

Ami Gadhia; *American Academy of Pediatrics; Washington, DC*

Maida P. Galvez, MD, MPH, FAAP; *Icahn School of Medicine at Mount Sinai; New York, NY*

Robert J. Geller, MD, FAAP; *Emory University School of Medicine; Atlanta, GA*

Benjamin A. Gitterman, MD, FAAP; *The George Washington University; Washington, DC*

Lynn R. Goldman, MD, MS, MPH, FAAP; *Milken Institute School of Public Health, The George Washington University; Washington, DC*

Michael T. Hatcher, DrPH, MPH; *Agency for Toxic Substances and Disease Registry; Atlanta, GA*

Marissa Hauptman, MD, MPH, FAAP; *Harvard Medical School; Boston, MA*

Diane E. Hindman, MD, PharmD, FAAP; *Phoenix Children's Hospital; Phoenix, AZ*

Catherine J. Karr, MD, PhD, MS, FAAP; *University of Washington School of Medicine/School of Public Health; Seattle, WA*

Michele A. La Merrill, PhD, MPH; *University of California at Davis; Davis, CA*

Philip J. Landrigan, MD, MSc, FAAP; *Boston College; Boston, MA*

Zachary Laris, MPH; *American Academy of Pediatrics; Washington, DC*

Lily Lee, BA; *The State University of New York Downstate Medical Center; Brooklyn, NY*

Martha Linet, MD; *National Cancer Institute; Bethesda, MD*

Jennifer A. Lowry, MD, FAAP; *Children's Mercy; Kansas City, MO*

Carmen Amelia Marable, MPH; *Rollins School of Public Health; Atlanta, GA*

Steven M. Marcus, MD, FAAP; *Rutgers New Jersey Medical School; Newark, NJ*

Mark F. Miller, PhD; *National Institute of Environmental Health Sciences; Research Triangle Park, NC*

Mary Ellen Mortensen, MD, MS; *Centers for Disease Control and Prevention; Atlanta, GA*

Nicki Nabavizadeh, MD, FAAP; *Portland, OR*

Nicholas Newman, DO, MS, FAAP; *Cincinnati Children's Hospital Medical Center; Cincinnati, OH*

Sasha Ondusko, MD; *Oregon Health Sciences University; Portland, OR*

Deborah Ort, MD; *The University of Texas Southwestern Medical Center; Dallas, TX*

Susan E. Pacheco, MD, FAAP; *University of Texas McGovern Medical School; Houston, TX*

Jerome A. Paulson, MD, FAAP; *Alexandria, VA*

Devon Payne-Sturges, DrPH; *University of Maryland School of Public Health; College Park, MD*

David B. Resnik, JD, PhD; *National Institute of Environmental Health Sciences; Research Triangle Park, NC*

Steven J. Rippentrop, MD, MPH, MA, MHA; *University of Iowa Carver College of Medicine; Iowa City, IA*

James R. Roberts, MD, MPH, FAAP; *Medical University of South Carolina; Charleston, SC*

Leslie Rubin, MD, FAAP; *Morehouse School of Medicine; Atlanta, GA*

Carol W. Runyan, MPH, PhD; *Colorado School of Public Health; Aurora, CO*

Megan T. Sandel, MD, MPH, FAAP; *Boston University School of Medicine; Boston, MA*

Sheela Sathyanarayana, MD, MPH, FAAP; *University of Washington School of Medicine; Seattle, WA*

Adam J. Spanier, MD, PhD, MPH, FAAP; *University of Maryland School of Medicine; Baltimore, MD*

Paul Spire; *American Academy of Pediatrics; Itasca, IL*

June Tester, MD, MPH, FAAP; *University of California San Francisco Benioff Children's Hospital; Oakland, CA*

Leonardo Trasande, MD, MPP, FAAP; *New York University School of Medicine; New York, NY*

Ian Van Dinther; *American Academy of Pediatrics; Itasca, IL*

Nita Vangeepuram, MD, MPH; *Icahn School of Medicine at Mount Sinai; New York, NY*

Susan C. Walley, MD, FAAP; *University of Alabama at Birmingham; Birmingham, AL*

David Wallinga, MD; *Natural Resources Defense Council; San Francisco, CA*

Mary H. Ward, PhD; *National Cancer Institute; Bethesda, MD*

Michael L. Weitzman, MD, FAAP; *New York University School of Medicine; New York, NY*

Karen M. Wilson, MD, MPH, FAAP; *Icahn School of Medicine at Mount Sinai; New York, NY*

Nsedu Obot Witherspoon, MPH; *Children's Environmental Health Network; Washington, DC*

Alan D. Woolf, MD, MPH, FAAP; *Harvard Medical School; Boston, MA*

Robert O. Wright, MD, MPH, FAAP; *Icahn School of Medicine at Mount Sinai; New York, NY*

Lauren M Zajac, MD, MPH, FAAP; *Icahn School of Medicine at Mount Sinai; New York, NY*

Judith T. Zelikoff, PhD; *New York University School of Medicine; New York, NY*

Marya G. Zlatnik, MD, MMS; *University of California San Francisco; San Francisco, CA*

# Contents

## VII. Appendices

# Preface

The publication of *Pediatric Environmental Health,* 4th Edition, reflects many advances in our understanding of the etiology, identification, management, and prevention of diseases and conditions linked to the environment. The field of environmental health is growing rapidly, and new information becomes available every day. Hardly a week goes by in which parents don't read a blog or hear a story about the effects of the environment on health, and they may ask their pediatrician for advice about this topic. In 2018, stories about the disastrous wildfires in California featured prominently in the news. Dramatic events such as these offer an opportunity to bring focus to environmental issues, to teach children about them, and to bring attention to prevention and remediation. They also highlight the many different "environments" in which a child lives: the bedroom, the home, the school, the neighborhood, the community or town, the state, the country, the world—these are concentric circles. Although large-scale events, such as massive forest fires, heighten our awareness that environmental crises have important physical and psychological effects on children and their families, it is easy to overlook the fact that less visible (or invisible) environmental threats also can have profound physical and psychological effects on children and their families. We as pediatricians must attend to both. This book provides a foundation for understanding where to begin.

First published in 1999, this book is intended for pediatricians and others who are interested in preventing children's exposures to environmental hazards during infancy, childhood, and adolescence. In this edition, we present updated summaries of the evidence that has been published in the scientific literature about environmental hazards to children. Eight new chapters have been introduced in this edition, including topics such as fracking, green offices, community design, and exposures to perfluoroalkyl and polyfluoroalkyl substances. Major modifications have been made to all 59 chapters from the third edition. Knowledge, research, and information relevant to pediatric practice began growing at an exponential pace after the children's environmental health and disease prevention research programs were established by the US Environmental Protection Agency and the National Institute of Environmental Health Sciences. New associations are being discovered and our knowledge of existing ones is constantly being refined and expanded. As the field of pediatric environmental health evolves, appropriate guidance may change with the publication of additional research findings.

Although all of the 72 contributors to this book are from the United States, most of the information presented here should be useful to those in other parts of the world. Children's exposures to some contaminants may be higher in low-income countries; nonetheless, the book can be expected to provide reliable background information for clinicians who are faced with providing practical advice to parents and communities. A chapter about environmental health considerations for children in low- and middle-income countries gives pediatricians in the United States a glimpse of the array of problems facing children growing up in less-privileged settings.

The book is meant to be practical, containing information that is useful in office practice, but that could also be helpful to a clinician preparing a grand rounds presentation for colleagues or providing testimony before a group of state legislators. Throughout the book, we have taken the liberty of combining the contributions of multiple authors in each chapter. Although the fourth edition is 300% longer than the first, there are still many aspects of environmental health that could not be covered. The Council gave priority to those topics that appeared to have the greatest effect on child health or to be of concern to parents. I hope that the information presented in the book will foster an informed understanding of environmental health among those who care for children.

For the purpose of this book, our definition of the environment is limited to those topics under the purview of the AAP Council on Environmental Health, which is to advise the AAP Board of Directors regarding protection of the health of the fetus, infant, and child from debilitating or hazardous environmental agents. We understand that the environment can be defined much more broadly to include injury prevention and prevention of gun violence. These and other high priority pediatric issues are beyond the scope of the Council on Environmental Health and are not addressed in this book.

Parents and guardians of young children are intensely interested in the impact of the environment on their children's health. They may look to their pediatrician for guidance about how to evaluate news reports about potential hazards in the air, water, and food. Yet the history of such well-established hazards as the exposure of children to secondhand smoke shows many years of epidemiologic and laboratory research before the weight of the evidence compels a consensus. While the evidence is accumulating, what should a worried parent do? Prudently avoid exposure after the first study suggesting problems is published? At what point should the pediatrician advocate a specific action? Obviously, there are no easy answers to these questions. Issues of value, scientific understanding, and cost are involved. Each hazardous exposure must be considered in the context of other problems facing the child and the financial, emotional, and intellectual resources available to surmount them. After fully understanding the facts and uncertainties, reasonable pediatricians may choose different ways to respond to the accumulating evidence.

I have many people to thank for their contributions to this book. First, I am grateful to those who contributed the 33 chapters to the first edition, the 43 chapters to the second edition, and the 59 chapters to the third edition; their outstanding work has provided an excellent foundation for this revised and expanded fourth edition. Thirty-nine councils, committees, and sections of the American Academy of Pediatrics (AAP) reviewed and provided comments on new and revised chapters of this edition. I owe special thanks to Paul Spire, who expertly juggled requests from multiple authors and editors with unflagging good humor and worked tremendously hard to keep this book on track, and to Gayle Murray, medical copy editor, and Theresa Wiener, Production Manager, Clinical and Professional Publications, for their invaluable help in its preparation. I am immensely grateful to the associate editor, Sophie J. Balk, MD, FAAP, for her clinical wisdom and careful attention to ensuring that complex topics were clearly explained and key action steps for the clinician were provided. Thanks also to Jennifer A. Lowry, MD, FAAP, Chair of the Council on Environmental Health for her strong leadership and to the hardworking members of the Council, who drafted many new chapters and reviewed and updated the existing chapters of the book. I owe special thanks to Stuart A. Cohen, MD, MPH, FAAP, a member of the AAP Board of Directors for his thoughtful and comprehensive review of the book for consistency with AAP policy.

This edition is dedicated to Herbert L. Needleman, MD, a giant in the field of pediatric environmental health who passed away in 2017. When I first joined it in 1986, Dr. Needleman was a member of the (then) Committee on Environmental Health and he authored the chapter on lead poisoning for the first edition of this book. He taught by example that a pediatrician can persevere and triumph in the face of relentless attacks on emerging environmental health science from powerful special interests. We hope to live with the kind of courage and intellectual integrity he personified. This book is dedicated to the memory of this treasured man.

Ruth A. Etzel, MD, PhD, FAAP
Editor

Chapter 1

# Introduction

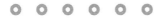

Environmental hazards are among the top health concerns many parents have for their children.[1-3] Little time is spent during medical school and pediatric residency training on environmental hazards and their relationship to illness among children, and many pediatricians report that they are not fully prepared or comfortable taking an environmental history or addressing parents' concerns about the environment in clinical practice.[4-10] When pediatricians receive specific training about environmental hazards, they are better equipped to address parents' concerns in their practices.[11-15] General medical and pediatric textbooks devote scant attention to illness as a result of environmental factors. Information pertinent to pediatric environmental health is widely scattered in epidemiologic, toxicologic, and environmental health journals that may not regularly be read by pediatricians.[16]

Sixty-one years have passed since the American Academy of Pediatrics (AAP) formed its first committee on environmental health. In that time, substantial progress has been made in understanding the role of the environment in the illnesses of childhood and adolescence. Consideration of illnesses traditionally associated with the environment, such as waterborne and foodborne diseases, has expanded to include study of toxic chemicals and other environmental hazards that derive from the rapid expansion of industry and technology.[17]

This is the fourth edition of *Pediatric Environmental Health*, a book written by the AAP Council on Environmental Health and intended to be useful to practicing pediatricians and other clinicians. The first edition was published by the AAP in 1999; the second in 2003, and the third in 2012.[18-20] This book is organized into 7 sections. The first section gives background information. The second, third, and fourth sections focus on specific environments, food and water, and chemical and physical hazards. The fifth section addresses a variety of special topics. The sixth section provides information about public health aspects of environmental health, and the seventh section describes resources for pediatricians and others.

Most chapters on chemical and physical hazards are organized in sections that describe the pollutant, routes of exposure, systems affected, clinical effects, diagnostic methods, treatment, and prevention of exposure and include suggested responses to questions that pediatricians may have or that parents may ask. The Resources section refers readers to additional resources to be considered when further information is needed.

The AAP Council on Environmental Health recognizes that pediatric environmental health is a specialty field in the early stages of development. Knowledge in some areas has evolved rapidly, whereas in other areas, there may be more questions than answers. The Council and the editors have attempted to make readers aware of the controversial areas and gaps in scientific information. The goal of this book is to provide clinicians with the most accurate information needed to prudently advise parents and children about specific pollutants and situations commonly encountered in 21st century life. Such advice is essential as we move to prevent childhood illness linked to the environment.[21]

## References

1. Stickler GB, Simmons PS. Pediatricians' preferences for anticipatory guidance topics compared with parental anxieties. *Clin Pediatr (Phila)*. 1995;34(7):384–387

2. US Environmental Protection Agency. *Public Knowledge and Perceptions of Chemical Risks in Six Communities: Analysis of a Baseline Survey*. 1990. Publication No. EPA 230-01-90-074

3. Garbutt JM, Leege E, Sterkel R, Gentry S, Wallendorf M, Strunk RC. What are parents worried about? Health problems and health concerns for children. *Clin Pediatr (Phila)*. 2012;51(9):840–847

4. Pope AM, Rall DP, eds. *Environmental Medicine: Integrating a Missing Element into Medical Education*. Washington, DC: National Academies Press; 1995

5. Roberts JR, Gitterman BA. Pediatric environmental health education: a survey of US pediatric residency programs. *Ambul Pediatr*. 2003;3(1):57–59

6. Roberts JR, Balk SJ, Forman J, Shannon M. Teaching about pediatric environmental health. *Acad Pediatr*. 2009;9(2):129–130

7. Kilpatrick N, Frumkin H, Trowbridge J, et al. The environmental history in pediatric practice: a study of pediatricians' attitudes, beliefs, and practices. *Environ Health Perspect*. 2002;110(8):823–827

8. Trasande L, Schapiro ML, Falk R, et al. Pediatrician attitudes, clinical activities, and knowledge of environmental health in Wisconsin. *WMJ*. 2006;105(2):45–49

9. Trasande L, Boscarino J, Graber N, et al. The environment in pediatric practice: a study of New York pediatricians' attitudes, beliefs, and practices towards children's environmental health. *J Urban Health*. 2006;83(4):760–772

10. Trasande L, Ziebold C, Schiff JS, Wallinga D, McGovern P, Oberg CN. The role of the environment in pediatric practice in Minnesota: attitudes, beliefs, and practices. *Minn Med*. 2008;91(9):36–39

11. Balk SJ, Gottschlich EA, Holman DM, Watson M. Counseling on sun protection and indoor tanning. *Pediatrics*. 2017;140(6):e20171680

12. Galvez MP, Balk SJ. Environmental risks to children: prioritizing health messages in pediatric practice. *Pediatr Rev*. 2017;38(6):263–279

13. Rogers B, McCurdy LE, Slavin K, Grubb K, Roberts JR. Children's environmental health faculty champions initiative: a successful model for integrating environmental health into pediatric health care. *Environ Health Perspect*. 2009;117(5):850–855

14. McCurdy LE, Roberts J, Rogers B, et al. Incorporating environmental health into pediatric medical and nursing education. *Environ Health Perspect*. 2004;112(17):1755–1760

15. Zickafoose JS, Greenberg S, Dearborn DG. Teaching home environmental health to resident physicians. *Public Health Rep*. 2011;126(Suppl 1):7–13

16. Etzel RA. Introduction. In: *Environmental Health: Report of the 27th Ross Roundtable on Critical Approaches to Common Pediatric Problems*. Columbus, OH: Ross Products Division, Abbott Laboratories; 1996:1

17. Chance GW, Harmsen E. Children are different: environmental contaminants and children's health. *Can J Public Health*. 1998;89(Suppl 1):S9–S13

18. American Academy of Pediatrics, Committee on Environmental Health. *Handbook of Pediatric Environmental Health*. Etzel RA, Balk SJ, eds. Elk Grove Village, IL: American Academy of Pediatrics; 1999

19. American Academy of Pediatrics, Committee on Environmental Health. *Pediatric Environmental Health*. 2nd ed. Etzel RA, Balk SJ, eds. Elk Grove Village, IL: American Academy of Pediatrics; 2003

20. American Academy of Pediatrics, Council on Environmental Health. *Pediatric Environmental Health*. 3rd ed. Etzel RA, Balk SJ, eds. Elk Grove Village, IL: American Academy of Pediatrics; 2012

21. Etzel RA. Children's environmental health: the role of primordial prevention. *Curr Probl Pediatr Adolesc Health Care*. 2016;46(6):202–204

# Chapter 2

# History and Growth of Pediatric Environmental Health

○  ○  ○  ○  ○  ○

## HISTORY OF PEDIATRIC ENVIRONMENTAL HEALTH IN THE AMERICAN ACADEMY OF PEDIATRICS

The origins of the current Council on Environmental Health can be traced back to 1954. That year, the US government tested nuclear weapons on Bikini Island in the Marshall Islands, and acute radiation burns from beta radiation developed in people living on nearby islands. Severe hypothyroidism developed in 2 children after being exposed to radioactive fallout as infants. Thyroid neoplasia and leukemia also were diagnosed in children younger than age 10 who were exposed to this radiation; among 18 children, 1 case of leukemia, 13 benign neoplasms, and 1 malignant thyroid neoplasm were diagnosed.[1] Meanwhile, in the western United States, sheep became sick, apparently as a result of fallout from weapons testing in Nevada, and people living in southwestern Utah became concerned about the later effects of radiation. Because of the population's growing worries about radiation exposure, in 1956 the National Academy of Sciences and the British Medical Research Council convened expert committees that issued reports about the biological effects of ionizing radiation on humans. After these reports were made available, radiotherapy was less often used for noncancerous conditions and the use of fluoroscopy was curtailed. The American Academy of Pediatrics (AAP) responded to these concerns by forming a Committee on Radiation Hazards and Congenital Malformations in 1957. This new Committee was charged with developing policy on exposure of children to ionizing radiation. Years later, it became the current-day Council on Environmental Health.

The Council has had several different names in the interim. In 1961, it became the Committee on Environmental Hazards. In 1966, the Committee organized a Conference on the Pediatric Significance of Peacetime Radioactive Fallout.[2] Among the pediatricians who spoke was Dr. Benjamin Spock, who talked about the psychological effects of radioactive fallout on children. Scientists from government health agencies, radiobiologists, and general pediatricians also participated.

The Committee, recognizing that man-made chemicals were increasingly permeating the environment, organized the Conference on the Susceptibility of the Fetus and Child to Chemical Pollutants, held in 1973 in Brown's Lake, WI.[3] Fresh thinking was sought by bringing together scientists knowledgeable about the effects of chemicals on the environment but not about child health and, conversely, pediatricians who knew about child health but had not given much thought to environmental effects. This meeting led to more interaction between pediatric experts and staff working in federal agencies concerned with the environment to discuss the possible effects of the environment on the health of children.

The Conference on Chemical and Radiation Hazards to Children, held in 1981 and chaired by Drs. Laurence Finberg and Robert W. Miller, was an expert consultation on the topic that enabled the exchange of concerns and information with the pediatric community[4] and led to further interactions between the committee and federal environmental health agencies. The Council on Pediatric Research called for including pediatricians in meetings of government agencies and on other committees that make policy or deliberate on environmental matters of national importance. To foster relations with other groups, the AAP Committee on Environmental Hazards, which met twice a year, held every other meeting at an organization concerned with environmental research, such as the US Environmental Protection Agency (EPA), the National Institute of Environmental Health Sciences (NIEHS), the Kettering Laboratories, and the National Institute of Child Health and Development.

In 1991, the name of the Committee on Environmental Hazards was changed to the Committee on Environmental Health to emphasize prevention. In 2009, the Committee was renamed the Council on Environmental Health, with responsibility for advising the Board of Directors on policy issues involving child health and the environment and also developing educational materials for pediatricians.

## GROWTH OF PEDIATRIC ENVIRONMENTAL HEALTH IN THE UNITED STATES

Over the period of 1981 to 1993, academic and health organizations became more interested in studying the impact of the environment on infant and child health.[5] In 1992, a special interest group on pediatric environmental health was organized in the Ambulatory Pediatric Association, reflecting growing interest in this topic among academic pediatricians. In 1993, the publication of a report by the National Academy of Sciences, titled *Pesticides in the Diets of Infants and Children,*[6] was instrumental in highlighting environmental hazards unique to children and the relative paucity of information relating environmental exposures and child health outcomes. In October 1995, US EPA Administrator Carol Browner directed the agency to formulate a new national policy requiring, for the first time, that the health risks to children and infants from environmental hazards be considered when conducting environmental risk assessments.[7]

In 1996, the Food Quality Protection Act became law. One requirement of this act was that the US EPA use an additional safety factor in risk assessments when risks for children are uncertain.

On April 21, 1997, President Clinton issued Executive Order 13045, Protection of Children from Environmental Health Risks and Safety Risks, which directed agencies to ensure that policies, programs, activities, and standards address disproportionate risks to children that result from environmental health risks or safety risks. In 1997, the US EPA established the Office of Children's Health Protection to make the protection of children's health a fundamental goal of public health and environmental protection in the United States. The President's Task Force on Environmental Health Risks and Safety Risks to Children, co-chaired by the Secretary of the US Department of Health and Human Services and the Administrator of the US EPA, was established to recommend federal environmental health and safety policies, priorities, and activities to protect children.[8,9] Through this Task Force, 17 Federal Departments/Agencies/Offices have worked together for more than 20 years on issues such as reducing childhood lead exposures, combating childhood asthma, and highlighting the effects of climate change on children.

Since 1998, many Centers for Children's Environmental Health and Disease Prevention Research have been funded by the US EPA and the NIEHS. Combining research and outreach, these Centers form a national network to address a range of childhood diseases and outcomes that may result from environmental exposures, including impairments in overall growth and development, impairments in nervous system development, and respiratory dysfunction. Center investigators work closely with communities, health care providers, researchers, and government officials to conduct research with the goal of preventing and reducing childhood diseases in these areas.

Pediatric Environmental Health Specialty Units, established in 1998 and funded by the Agency for Toxic Substances and Disease Registry (ATSDR) and the US EPA, have increased awareness and knowledge of health care providers and health agency officials about pediatric environmental health. They are an important resource for information about children's environmental health issues and for assistance in clinical evaluations, such as guidance on the utility of biological or environmental testing or interpreting test results.

The first edition of the AAP *Handbook of Pediatric Environmental Health* was published in October 1999.[10] It was distributed to more than 27,000 pediatricians and pediatric residents and was widely used in the United States and other countries to teach about the health effects to children when exposed to contaminants in the environment.

In 2000, the Committee on Environmental Health initiated the first in a series of 4 annual workshops on pediatric environmental health for incoming pediatric chief residents held at the annual meetings of the Pediatric Academic Societies. This effort was funded by the Office of Children's Health Protection at the US EPA. That year, the AAP also launched the Environmental Health Nexus, an AAP Section open to pediatricians with an interest in environmental health that was primarily involved in designing and planning educational programming for the AAP. The Nexus was incorporated into the Council on Environmental Health in 2009. In many state AAP chapters, committees on environmental health developed and continue to develop educational activities and programming for chapter meetings.

In March 2001, the Committee on Environmental Health held a workshop, with funding from the ATSDR, to bring together pediatricians from each chapter of the AAP with experts in pediatric environmental health from the regional offices of federal agencies (including the ATSDR and the US EPA). The proceedings of this conference were published in a special supplement to *Pediatrics*.[11] In 2002, through the Ambulatory Pediatric Association (later renamed the Academic Pediatric Association), the first formal fellowship training programs in pediatric environmental health were initiated. These 3-year training programs are designed to provide pediatricians with specific competencies[12] to enable them to undertake environmental health research, teaching, and advocacy. Fellowship training in pediatric environmental health[13] has been available in Boston, New York, San Francisco, Seattle, and Washington, DC.

The second edition of *Pediatric Environmental Health* was published in October 2003.[14] It was distributed to more than 24,000 pediatricians and pediatric residents in the United States and abroad. A book focusing on environmental threats to child health was published by Oxford in 2003.[15]

In 2000, the US Congress authorized the planning and implementation of a National Children's Study. The study planning was led by a consortium of federal partners, including the US Department of Health and Human Services (including the *Eunice Kennedy Shriver* National Institute of Child Health and Human Development, the NIEHS, and the Centers for Disease Control and Prevention), the US EPA, and the US Department of Education.[16]

The National Children's Study was designed to examine the effects of environmental influences on the health and development of more than 100,000 children across the United States, following them from before birth until age 21. The goal of the study was to improve the health and well-being of children. Researchers planned to analyze how environmental exposures, genetic influences, and psychosocial experiences interact with each other and what helpful and/or harmful effects they might have on children's health. By studying children across phases of growth and development, researchers anticipated being better able to understand the role of these factors on health and disease.

The seven initial National Children's Study research sites began recruitment of families into the National Children's Study in 2009.[17] The study was discontinued by the NIH Director in 2014. About 5,000 children were enrolled prior to closure of the study, and their data were made available to researchers after closure.

The third edition of *Pediatric Environmental Health* was published in 2012.[18] The first textbook on children's environmental health was published in 2014.[19]

The AAP became a leader in educating pediatricians about climate change with a meeting in 2015. The meeting convened pediatricians representing each of the major sections, committees, and councils to discuss a campaign to raise the profile of climate change education in the AAP. Table 2-1 lists a brief history of pediatric environmental health.

| Table 2-1. A Brief History of Pediatric Environmental Health | |
|---|---|
| **YEAR** | **EVENT** |
| 1957 | AAP established Committee on Radiation Hazards and Congenital Malformations |
| 1961 | Committee name changed to Committee on Environmental Hazards |
| 1966 | Conference on the Pediatric Significance of Peacetime Radioactive Fallout |
| 1973 | Conference on the Susceptibility of the Fetus and Child to Chemical Pollutants held in Brown's Lake, WI |
| 1981 | Conference on Chemical and Radiation Hazards to Children |
| 1991 | Committee name changed to Committee on Environmental Health |
| 1992 | APA organized Special Interest Group on pediatric environmental health |
| 1993 | National Academy of Sciences published *Pesticides in the Diets of Infants and Children* |
| 1995 | US EPA Administrator Carol Browner released a new national policy requiring that the health risks to children and infants from environmental hazards be considered when conducting environmental risk assessments |
| 1996 | US Food Quality Protection Act became law |
| 1997 | President Clinton issued Executive Order 13045, Protection of Children from Environmental Health Risks and Safety Risks |

*(continued)*

## Table 2-1. A Brief History of Pediatric Environmental Health (*continued*)

| YEAR | EVENT |
|------|-------|
| 1997 | US EPA established the Office of Children's Health Protection |
| 1998 | US EPA and NIEHS funded first Centers for Children's Environmental Health and Disease Prevention Research |
| 1998 | ATSDR established Pediatric Environmental Health Specialty Units |
| 1999 | AAP published the first edition *of Pediatric Environmental Health* |
| 1999 | WHO set up Task Force for the Protection of Children's Environmental Health |
| 2000 | AAP launched Environmental Health Nexus |
| 2000 | US Congress authorized the planning and implementation of a National Children's Study |
| 2000 | AAP launched PAS annual workshops for incoming chief residents |
| 2001 | COEH workshop to bring pediatricians together with federal officials |
| 2002 | APA initiated first fellowships in pediatric environmental health |
| 2002 | First WHO International Conference on Environmental Threats to the Health of Children: Hazards and Vulnerability |
| 2003 | AAP published second edition of *Pediatric Environmental Health* |
| 2003 | Oxford published book focusing on environmental threats to child health |
| 2005 | WHO published *Children's Health and the Environment: A Global Perspective* |
| 2005 | Second WHO International Conference on Children's Environmental Health, Healthy Environments Healthy Children: Increasing Knowledge and Taking Action |
| 2007 | IPA launched International Pediatric Environmental Health Leadership Institute |
| 2007 | IPA gave first qualifying examination in pediatric environmental health |
| 2009 | Committee was renamed the Council on Environmental Health |
| 2009 | Third WHO International Conference on Children's Health and the Environment, From Research to Policy and Action |
| 2012 | AAP published third edition of *Pediatric Environmental Health* |
| 2014 | Oxford published *Textbook of Children's Environmental Health* |
| 2014 | NIH discontinued National Children's Study |

Abbreviations: AAP, American Academy of Pediatrics; APA, Ambulatory Pediatric Association; ATSDR, Agency for Toxic Substances and Disease Registry; COEH, Committee on Environmental Health; EPA, Environmental Protection Agency; IPA, International Pediatric Association; NIEHS, National Institute of Environmental Health Sciences; NIH, National Institutes of Health; PAS, Pediatric Academic Societies; WHO, World Health Organization.

## GROWTH OF INTERNATIONAL PEDIATRIC ENVIRONMENTAL HEALTH

In 1999, the World Health Organization (WHO) set up a Task Force for the Protection of Children's Environmental Health. Its objectives were to prevent disease and disability associated with chemical and physical threats to children, taking into consideration biological risks in the environment and acknowledging the importance of social and psychosocial factors. The Task Force promoted the development of training materials about children's health and the environment and advocated for environmental policies to protect children.[20,21]

In 2002, the first WHO International Conference on Environmental Threats to the Health of Children: Hazards and Vulnerability was held in Bangkok, Thailand. The conference focused on science-oriented issues, research needs, and capacity building while addressing the concrete needs for action and policies at the community, country, regional, and international levels. The major outcome of this conference was the Bangkok Statement, which set priorities for action and a commitment to national and international activities in the area of children's health and the environment.[22] In 2005, the WHO published a book titled *Children's Health and the Environment: A Global Perspective.*[23] The second WHO International Conference on Children's Environmental Health, Healthy Environments Healthy Children: Increasing Knowledge and Taking Action, was held in Buenos Aires, Argentina in November 2005. This conference responded to calls for action concerning children's health and the environment that were made by the preceding Health and Environment Ministerial of the Americas (June 2005) and the Summit of the Americas (November 2005). In June 2009, the third WHO International Conference on Children's Health and the Environment, From Research to Policy and Action, was held in Busan, Republic of Korea. Table 2-2 lists international conventions and resolutions related to children's health and the environment.

A number of countries, including Canada, Mexico, Spain, Uruguay, Chile, the Republic of Korea, and Argentina, set up Children's Environmental Health Units to increase the awareness and knowledge of health care providers about pediatric environmental health.[24]

In 2007, the International Pediatric Association, in collaboration with the WHO, launched the International Pediatric Environmental Health Leadership Institute, with funding from the US EPA Office of Children's Health Protection. As part of this Institute, training courses on children's health and the environment were held in Nairobi, Kenya; New Delhi, India; and Port au Prince, Haiti.[25] The training sessions used the WHO Training Package for Health Care Providers, a set of modules covering the major environmental issues for children.[26] The trainees were expected to complete a community project, give a presentation at their home hospital, and document children's environmental diseases using a "green sheet" in the medical record. Those who did so were eligible to take an examination for special certification. The first qualifying

## Table 2-2. Conventions and Resolutions Relating to Children's Health and the Environment

| 1989 | **UN Convention on the Rights of the Child**<br>www.unicef.org/crc |
|------|------|
| 1990 | **Declaration on the Survival, Protection and Development of Children** (World Summit for Children)<br>www.unicef.org/wsc/declare.htm |
| 1992 | **Agenda 21, Chapter 25** (United Nations Conference on Environment and Development)<br>sustainabledevelopment.un.org/content/documents/Agenda21.pdf |
| 1997 | **Declaration of the Environment Leaders of the Eight on Children's Environmental Health**<br>www.g7.utoronto.ca/environment/1997miami/children.html |
| 1999 | **Declaration of the Third European Ministerial Conference on Environment and Health**<br>www.euro.who.int/document/e69046.pdf |
| 2001 | **UN Millennium Development Goals**<br>www.who.int/mdg |
| 2002 | **United Nations General Assembly Special Session on Children**<br>www.unicef.org/specialsession<br>**The Bangkok Statement (WHO International Conference)**<br>www.who.int/docstore/peh/ceh/Bangkok/bangkstatement.htm<br>**World Summit on Sustainable Development:** Launch of the Healthy Environments for Children Alliance and the Global Initiative of Children's Environmental Health Indicators<br>www.who.int/heca/en<br>www.who.int/ceh/publications/924159188_9/en/index.html |
| 2003 | **IFCS Forum IV Recommendations on Children and Chemicals**<br>www.who.int/ifcs/en |
| 2004 | **Fourth Ministerial Conference on Environment and Health (Europe):** Adoption of the Children's Environment and Health Action Plan for Europe (CEHAPE)<br>www.euro.who.int/__data/assets/pdf_file/0006/78639/E83338.pdf |
| 2005 | **International Conference on Children's Environmental Health: The Buenos Aires Commitment**<br>www.who.int/ceh/news/pastevents/buenosairesdecleng/en/index.html |
| 2006 | **Strategic Approach to International Chemicals Management (SAICM)**<br>www.saicm.org |
| 2007 | **Declaration of the Commemorative High-Level Plenary Meeting Devoted to the Follow-up to the Outcome of the Special Session on Children**<br>www.un.org/ga/62/plenary/children/highlevel.shtml |

| Table 2-2. Conventions and Resolutions Relating to Children's Health and the Environment (*continued*) | |
|---|---|
| 2009 | **G8 Environmental Ministers' Meeting in Siracusa, Italy, April, 2009**<br>g8.utoronto.ca/environment/env090424-summary.pdf<br>**3rd WHO International Conference on Children's Health and the Environment: Busan, Republic of Korea, June, 2009**<br>www.who.int/ceh/3rd_conference/en/ |
| 2012 | **United Nations Conference on Sustainable Development, Rio+20**<br>Document1sustainabledevelopment.un.org/rio20 |
| 2013 | **Jerusalem Statement**<br>www.isde.org/Jerusalem_Statement.pdf |
| 2015 | **Transforming our world: the 2030 Agenda for Sustainable Development**<br>www.un.org/sustainabledevelopment/sustainable-development-goals/ |
| 2016 | **G7 Toyama Environmental Ministers' Meeting, May 2016**<br>www.env.go.jp/press/files/jp/102871.pdf |
| 2018 | **Seoul Pledge of Action for Children's Health and the Environment, June 2018**<br>http://www.inches2018.org/register/2018_09/file/SeoulPledge_English_signed.pdf |

examination in pediatric environmental health was held in Athens, Greece, in August 2007; the second in Johannesburg, South Africa in 2010; the third in Melbourne, Australia in 2013; and the fourth in Vancouver, Canada in 2016. In 2017, the World Health Organization published 2 documents. *Inheriting a Sustainable World: Atlas on Children's Health and the Environment* presented the continuing and emerging challenges to children's environmental health and sought to promote the importance of reducing the exposure of children to modifiable environmental hazards.[27] *Don't Pollute My Future! The Impact of the Environment on Children's Health* was a summary of the burden of disease in children attributable to the environment in 2012. It included respiratory infections; diarrheal disease; malaria; neonatal conditions; protein-energy malnutrition; cancers; mental, behavioral, and neurological disorders; asthma; congenital anomalies; and injuries.[28]

These and other activities should further enhance pediatricians' understanding of the effects of environmental hazards on children's health throughout the world.

## References

1. Merke DP, Miller RW. Age differences in the effects of ionizing radiation. In: Guzelian PS, Henry CJ, Olin SS, eds. *Similarities and Differences Between Children and Adults: Implications for Risk Assessment.* Washington, DC: International Life Sciences Institute; 1992:139–149

2. American Academy of Pediatrics, Committee on Environmental Hazards. Conference on the Pediatric Significance of Peacetime Radioactive Fallout. *Pediatrics.* 1968;41(1):165–378

3. American Academy of Pediatrics, Committee on Environmental Hazards. The susceptibility of the fetus and child to chemical pollutants (special issue). *Pediatrics.* 1974;53(5 Spec Issue):777–862

4. Finberg L. *Chemical and Radiation Hazards to Children: Report of the Eighty-fourth Ross Conference on Pediatric Research.* Columbus, OH: Ross Laboratories; 1982

5. Landrigan PJ. Children's environmental health: a brief history. *Acad Pediatr.* 2016;16(1):1–9

6. National Research Council. *Pesticides in the Diets of Infants and Children.* Washington, DC: National Academies Press; 1993

7. US Environmental Protection Agency. *Environmental Health Threats to Children.* 1996. Publication No. EPA 175-F-96-001

8. Firestone M, Berger M, Foos B, Etzel R. Two decades of enhancing children's environmental health protection at the U.S. Environmental Protection Agency. *Environ Health Perspect.* 2016;124(12):A214–A218

9. Etzel RA, Howard SN. Renewing the federal commitment to advance children's health: The President's Task Force on Environmental Health Risks and Safety Risks to Children. *Environ Health Perspect.* 2016;124(1):A3–A4

10. American Academy of Pediatrics, Committee on Environmental Health. *Handbook of Pediatric Environmental Health.* Etzel RA, Balk SJ, eds. Elk Grove Village, IL: American Academy of Pediatrics; 1999

11. Balk SJ, ed. A partnership to establish an environmental safety net for children. *Pediatrics.* 2003;112(Suppl):209–264

12. Etzel RA, Crain EF, Gitterman BA, Oberg C, Scheidt P, Landrigan PJ. Pediatric environmental health competencies for specialists. *Ambul Pediatr.* 2003;3(1):60–63

13. Landrigan PJ, Woolf AD, Gitterman B, et al. The Ambulatory Pediatric Association fellowship in pediatric environmental health: a 5-year assessment. *Environ Health Perspect.* 2007;115(10):1383–1387

14. American Academy of Pediatrics, Committee on Environmental Health. *Pediatric Environmental Health.* 2nd ed. Etzel RA, Balk SJ, eds. Elk Grove Village, IL: American Academy of Pediatrics; 2003

15. Wigle DT. *Child Health and the Environment.* New York, NY: Oxford; 2003

16. Branum AM, Collman GW, Correa A, et al. The National Children's Study of environmental effects on child health and development. *Environ Health Perspect.* 2003;111(4):642–646

17. Scheidt P, Dellarco M, Dearry A. A major milestone for the National Children's Study. *Environ Health Perspect.* 2009;117(1):A13

18. American Academy of Pediatrics, Council on Environmental Health. *Pediatric Environmental Health.* 3rd ed. Etzel RA, Balk SJ, eds. Elk Grove Village, IL: American Academy of Pediatrics; 2012

19. *Textbook of Children's Environmental Health.* Landrigan PJ, Etzel RA, eds. New York, NY: Oxford University Press; 2014

20. European Environment Agency. *Children's Health and Environment: A Review of Evidence. A Joint Report From the European Environment Agency and the WHO Regional Office for Europe.* Echternach, Luxembourg: Luxembourg Office for Official Publications of the European Communities; 2002. Environmental Issue Report No. 29

21. United Nations Environment Programme, United Nations Children's Fund, World Health Organization. *Children in the New Millenium: Environmental Impact on Health.* Nairobi, Kenya: United Nations Environment Programme; New York, NY: United Nations Children's Fund; and Geneva, Switzerland: World Health Organization; 2002

22. The Bangkok Statement. A Pledge to Promote the Protection of Children's Environmental Health. International Conference on Environmental Threats to the Health of Children: Hazards and Vulnerability, Bangkok, Thailand, 3-7 March 2002. http://apps.who.int/iris/bitstream/10665/67366/1/WHO_SDE_PHE_02.02.pdf. Accessed April 18, 2018

23. World Health Organization. *Children's Health and the Environment: A Global Perspective. A Resource Manual for the Health Sector.* Pronczuk-Garbino J, ed. Geneva, Switzerland: World Health Organization; 2005

24. World Health Organization. Children's Environmental Health Units. Geneva, Switzerland: World Health Organization; 2010. http://www.who.int/ceh/publications/units/en/. Accessed June 27, 2018

25. International Pediatric Association. http://www.ipa-world.org/. Accessed April 18, 2018

26. World Health Organization. Training Package for Health Care Providers. http://www.who.int/ceh/capacity/trainpackage/en/. Accessed June 27, 2018

27. World Health Organization. *Inheriting a Sustainable World: Atlas on Children's Health and the Environment.* Geneva, Switzerland: World Health Organization; 2017

28. World Health Organization. *Don't Pollute My Future! The Impact of the Environment on Children's Health.* Geneva, Switzerland: World Health Organization; 2017

Chapter 3

# Children's Unique Vulnerabilities to Environmental Hazards

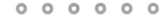

## KEY POINTS

- Children are more vulnerable than adults to environmental hazards because they breathe more air, consume more food, and drink more water than adults do, in proportion to their weight.
- The central nervous, immune, reproductive, and digestive systems of a child are still developing; during certain critical windows of time, exposure to environmental toxicants can lead to irreversible damage.
- Children behave differently from adults and have different patterns of exposure to environmental hazards.
- Children have little control over their environments; they may be both unaware of risks and unable to make choices to protect their health.

## INTRODUCTION

This chapter discusses the scientific basis for children's unique vulnerabilities to environmental hazards. It describes differences between adults and children and among children in different life stages, in physical, biological, and social environments. It explains why children should not be treated as "little adults." Seven developmental stages are considered: fetus (although there are multiple stages of fetal development); newborn (birth to age 2 months); infant/toddler (2 months to age 2 years); preschool child (age 2 to 6 years); school-aged child (age 6 to 12 years); adolescent (age 12 to 18 years); and young adult (age 18 years to early 20s).

## CRITICAL WINDOWS OF VULNERABILITY

The developing fetus and child are uniquely susceptible to toxicities of certain drugs and environmental toxicants (a "toxicant" refers to a chemical agent; "toxin" is appropriately used for a biological agent). Extensive epidemiological evidence supports a causal relationship between prenatal and early childhood exposure to environmental toxicants and a variety of resulting health effects on the fetus and child.[1] Well-known adverse outcomes for the developing fetus attributable to transplacental exposure include the effects of thalidomide on limb development, ethanol on brain development, and diethylstilbestrol on the reproductive system. The neurotoxic effects of lead have been demonstrated repeatedly with prenatal exposure as well as during early childhood.[2] Fetal and childhood development occur rapidly and may be easily deranged. The timing of exposures with regard to developmental outcome is an important concept. In embryonic or fetal stages, some narrow "critical windows of exposure"—highly susceptible periods of organogenesis—have been defined.[3] In contrast, there are very few actual "critical windows" known in childhood. Because data are lacking, there is significant uncertainty about many of the effects of environmental toxicants on children. This area is the subject of intense investigation. Some of the work on "critical windows" was published in a supplement to *Environmental Health Perspectives* (http://ehpnet1.niehs. nih.gov/docs/2000/suppl-3/toc.html). Conducting studies in this area poses special challenges.[4] Genetic and epigenetic factors interact with environmental exposures to contribute to effects on health and development (see Chapter 4).

## HUMAN ENVIRONMENTS

A child's environment can be divided into physical and social components. Both components interact with each individual's unique biology to influence that individual's health. The manner in which a child's body absorbs, distributes, and metabolizes environmental toxicants not only is determined by that child's genetic code but also is heavily affected by developmental stage. The physical environment consists of anything that comes in contact with the body. Air, for example, which is in constant contact with the lungs and skin, is a large part of the physical environment. The physical environment consists of the large geographical environment (a "macro" environment) that is made up of many smaller units ("micro" environments). For example, the macro environment for a child may be Detroit; a micro environment may be the floor of the kitchen of a house on a certain street in Detroit. Micro environments can differ enormously between adults and children. For example, in a room in which the air is contaminated with mercury, the mercury vapor may not be evenly dispersed; because mercury vapor is heavier than air, the air near the floor may have a higher concentration of mercury than air near the ceiling.[5]

The environment of an infant lying on the floor, therefore, would be different from that of a standing adult. The social environment includes the day-to-day circumstances of living as well as regulations that may affect day-to-day living.

## EXPOSURE: THE PHYSICAL ENVIRONMENT

A child's exposure is the sum of the exposures in several environments during the course of a day, including the home, school, child care setting, vehicle(s), and play areas. Adolescents and young adults may be exposed to toxicants present in work environments. Estimates of exposure often are made retro-spectively because it is difficult to study the activities and exposures of young children. Even if the total amount of exposure to a toxicant is the same for 2 children, different patterns of exposure may have different health effects. For example, ingestion of nitrates in well water may cause hemoglobin to become reduced to methemoglobin.[6] If, however, the nitrates are ingested at a slow enough rate for enzymes to oxidize the methemoglobin back to hemoglobin, no deleterious health effects occur. This is an example of a threshold effect; the health problem will not occur until the toxicant reaches a particular level in the body.

## EXPOSURE FROM CONCEPTION TO ADOLESCENCE AND YOUNG ADULTHOOD

In most instances, fetal exposures come from the pregnant woman. Preterm infants who spend weeks or months in the neonatal intensive care unit have very different exposures (ie, noise, light, compressed gases, intravenous solutions, plasticizers, diagnostic radiation) compared with healthy full-term infants.[7,8] Exposures of newborns, infants, toddlers, preschool children, school-aged children, adolescents, and young adults differ with changes in physical location, breathing zones, oxygen consumption, types of foods consumed, amount of food consumed, and normal behavioral development.[9,10]

## PHYSICAL LOCATION

Physical location changes with development. Newborn exposures usually are similar to those experienced by the mother. A newborn, however, frequently spends prolonged periods in a single environment, such as a crib. Because infants and toddlers often are placed on the floor, carpet, or grass, they have greater exposures to chemicals, such as pesticide residues, that may be found on these surfaces. Biomonitoring data often demonstrate greater body burdens of chemicals in young children. For example, residues of metabolites of the pesticide chlorpyrifos were nearly twice as high in children aged 6 to 11 years as in adults.[11] In addition, infants who are unable to walk or crawl may experience sustained exposure to some agents or situations because they cannot remove themselves from their environment (eg, prolonged exposure to the sun or noise). Preschool-aged children may spend part of their day in child care settings with varied environments, including some time outdoors. School-aged children may be exposed to toxicants when schools are built near highways (resulting in exposure to motor vehicle emissions). Adolescents have a school environment and also are beginning to select other physical environments, often misjudging or ignoring risks. For example, listening to loud music may result in permanent hearing loss. Adolescents and young adults may work part-time or full-time in hazardous physical environments.[12,13] Children may participate in after-school sports that often occur outdoors in the mid to late afternoon when levels of ozone peak.[14] This situation poses an increased risk to children with asthma.

## BREATHING ZONES

The breathing zone for an adult is typically 4 to 6 ft (1.2 to 1.8 meters) above the floor. For a child, it is closer to the floor, depending on the height and mobility of the child. Within lower breathing zones, chemicals heavier than air, such as mercury, may concentrate.[15] Chemicals vaporizing from carpet or flooring also will have higher concentrations near the floor.

## OXYGEN CONSUMPTION

Children are smaller than adults, and their metabolic rates are higher. Thus, children consume more oxygen than adults and produce more carbon dioxide ($CO_2$) per kg of body weight. This increased $CO_2$ production requires higher minute ventilation. Minute ventilation for a newborn and adult are approximately 400 mL/min per kg and 150 mL/min per kg, respectively.[16,17] Thus, a child's dose of air pollutants is greater than that of an adult when adjusted for body mass.

## QUANTITY AND QUALITY OF FOOD CONSUMED

The amount of food that children consume per kg of body weight is higher than that of adults, not only because children need more calories to maintain homeostasis than adults do, but also because children are growing. Figure 3-1 shows grams of food consumed daily per kg of body weight. The difference is threefold between a child younger than 1 year and an adult. Additional data on children's food intake at various life stages are available in the US EPA Exposure Factors Handbook.[10]

In addition, children consume different types of food, and the diversity of the foods they eat often is much smaller than it is for adults. The diet of newborn infants is generally limited to human milk or infant formula. The diet of a typical child contains more milk products and certain fruits (ie, apple sauce and apple juice) and vegetables compared with a typical adult diet.[17] Figure 3-2

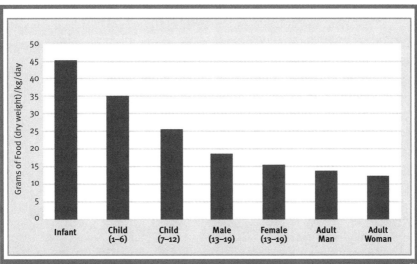

Figure 3-1. Grams of Food (Dry Weight) Per Kilogram of Body Weight Per Day Consumed[17]

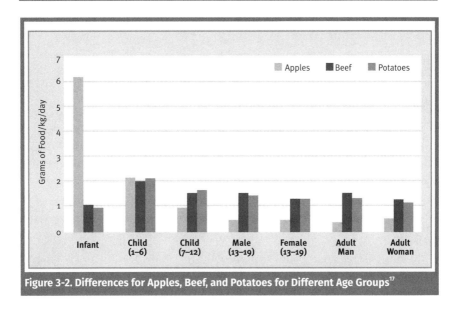

Figure 3-2. Differences for Apples, Beef, and Potatoes for Different Age Groups[17]

shows differences in consumption of apples, beef, and potatoes for different age groups.

## WATER

An average newborn consumes 6 oz (180 mL/kg/day) of human milk or formula per kg of body weight (for an average male adult, this is equivalent to drinking 35 twelve-oz cans [about 12.4 liters] of a beverage per day). If a

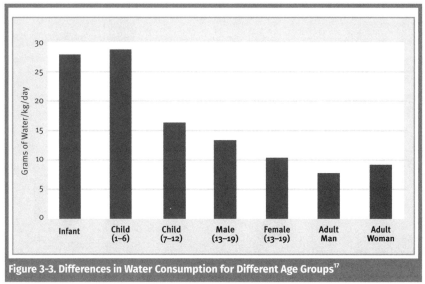

**Figure 3-3. Differences in Water Consumption for Different Age Groups**[17]

Note: The citation of grams of water consumed per kilogram per day in this table is considerably under-estimated because water consumed as breast milk was not included in the analysis. Thus, for total water consumption per kilogram per day, the values in the text are accurate.

newborn drinks reconstituted formula and the water used to reconstitute the formula comes from a single tap water source, the newborn may be exposed to any contaminants in the water (see Chapter 16). Differences in water consumption for different age groups are shown in Figure 3-3. If the water or liquid contains a contaminant, children receive more of it per kilogram of their body weight compared with adults.[17]

## LARGER RATIO OF SURFACE AREA TO BODY MASS

In a newborn, the ratio of surface area to body mass is 3 times larger than in an adult; in a child, the ratio of surface area to body mass is 2 times larger than in an adult. Thus, with regard to a toxicant contained in a substance in contact with skin, children are exposed to more of the toxicant kilogram for kilogram than are adults.[10,17]

## NORMAL BEHAVIORAL DEVELOPMENT

Infants and young children pass through a developmental stage of intense oral exploratory behavior. This normal oral exploration may place children at risk, such as in environments with high levels of lead dust. Wood used in some playground equipment was treated with arsenic (as chromated copper arsenate [CCA], see Chapter 22) and creosote, potentially exposing children when they place their mouths directly on these materials or when they place their hands in their mouths after playing on these materials. In addition, children often lack the experience or cognitive ability to recognize hazardous situations.

School-aged children generally spend more time outside than older children and adults. They therefore may be exposed to excessive ultraviolet radiation (UVR) from sunlight because they may not recognize the hazard and may not protect themselves. Adolescents, as they gain freedom from parental authority, may be less protected from some exposures. Although adolescents are at a stage of development at which physical strength and stamina are at a peak, they are still acquiring abstract reasoning skills. Adolescents often fail to consider cause and effect, particularly delayed effects such as the increased skin cancer risk because of UVR exposure received from indoor tanning facilities. Thus, adolescents may place themselves in situations with greater risk than many adults would.

## ABSORPTION, DISTRIBUTION, METABOLISM, AND TARGET ORGAN SUSCEPTIBILITY: THE BIOLOGICAL ENVIRONMENT

### Absorption

Absorption generally occurs by 1 of 4 routes: transplacental, percutaneous, respiratory, and gastrointestinal. Absorption also may occur via the intravenous route. Absorption through mucosal surfaces, including through the eye, also may occur.

### Transplacental

Many toxicants readily cross the placenta. These include compounds with low molecular weight, such as carbon monoxide; those that are fat soluble; and specific elements, such as calcium and lead. Because carbon monoxide has a higher affinity for fetal hemoglobin than for adult hemoglobin, the concentration of carboxyhemoglobin is higher in the fetus than in the pregnant woman.[18,19] Therefore, the infant may have a reduced level of oxygen delivered to tissues. Lipophilic compounds, such as polycyclic aromatic hydrocarbons (found in cigarette smoke), methylmercury, and ethanol, also readily gain access to the fetal circulation; levels of methylmercury are higher in the fetus than in the mother.[20]

### Percutaneous

With regard to percutaneous absorption, newborns and infants have a larger surface area-to-body mass compared with older children and adults. The skin undergoes enormous changes during development, resulting in changes in absorptive and other properties.

Pathways of absorption through the skin are particularly important for fat-soluble compounds. Chemicals such as nicotine and cotinine have been described in amniotic fluid,[21,22] but absorption through the fetal skin has not been studied. The skin of a fetus lacks the exterior dead keratin layer, one of the major barriers of fully developed skin. The acquisition of keratin occurs over 3 to 5 days following birth. Therefore, a newborn's skin remains particularly absorptive up to about 2 to 3 weeks of life.[23] Epidemics involving absorption of chemicals through the skin in newborns include hypothyroidism from iodine in povidone-iodine scrub solutions,[24] neurotoxicity from hexachlorophene,[25] and hyperbilirubinemia from a phenolic disinfectant used to clean hospital equipment.[26] Scientific consensus has not been reached about when in development the characteristics of newborn and infant skin become similar to those of adult skin. Some researchers assert that the skin continues to develop throughout the infant's first year. Others find that infant skin continues to develop structurally and functionally up to age 3 months, and some researchers believe that the skin barrier function of a full-term infant is similar to adult skin at birth or within 2 to 4 weeks. It has been agreed that the skin of a premature baby has a poor epidermal barrier with few cornified layers, and therefore has increased permeability to exogenous materials.[27-29]

## Respiratory

Lung development proceeds through proliferation of pulmonary alveoli and capillaries until the age of 5 to 8 years. Thereafter, the lungs grow through alveolar expansion.[30] Lung function continues to increase through adolescence and is vulnerable to exposure to air pollutants. Exposure to hazardous air pollutants at currently observed concentrations has been associated with statistically significant deficits in forced expiratory volume in 1 second ($FEV_1$) attained at age 18 years.[31]

## Gastrointestinal

The gastrointestinal tract undergoes numerous changes during development. Certain pesticides as well as chemicals from tobacco smoke are present in amniotic fluid,[22] but it is not known whether the fetus, which actively swallows amniotic fluid, absorbs them. Following birth, stomach acid secretion is relatively low, but adult levels are achieved by several months of age, markedly affecting absorption of chemicals from the stomach. If acidity levels are too low, bacterial overgrowth in the small bowel and stomach may result in the formation of chemicals that can be absorbed. For example, several cases of methemoglobinemia in infants in Iowa were traced to well water contaminated with nitrate that was converted to nitrite by intestinal bacteria.[6]

The small intestine transports certain chemicals to the blood and may respond to increased nutritional needs by increasing absorption of that particular nutrient. For example, the intestines of infants and children absorb more calcium from food sources compared with adults. Lead, which may be absorbed in place of calcium, also may be absorbed to a greater extent: an adult absorbs 5% to 10% of ingested lead, whereas a child aged 1 to 2 years can absorb up to 50%.[32]

## Distribution

The distribution of chemicals varies with body composition, such as fat and water content, which vary with developmental stage. For example, animal models show that lead is retained to a larger degree in the infant animal brain than in the adult animal brain.[33] Lead also may accumulate more rapidly in children's bones.[34]

## Metabolism

Metabolism of a chemical may result in its activation or deactivation.[35] The activity in each step of these metabolic pathways is determined by the child's developmental stage and genetic susceptibility. Therefore, some children are genetically more susceptible to adverse effects from certain exposures. For example, children (and adults) with glucose-6-phosphate dehydrogenase (G6PD) deficiency are at risk of hemolytic anemia if exposed to chemicals such as naphthalene. Large differences also exist in the activity of enzymes at various developmental stages. The same enzyme may be more or less active depending on the age of the child. Two examples are the enzymes involved in the P450 cytochrome family, which metabolize such xenobiotics as theophylline and caffeine,[36] and alcohol dehydrogenase, which converts ethanol to acetaldehyde.[37]

The differences between metabolism in children and adults may harm or protect children from environmental hazards or drugs. Such is the case for acetaminophen. In the adult, high levels of acetaminophen are metabolized to products that may cause hepatic failure. Infants born to women with high blood acetaminophen levels have similar acetaminophen levels but do not sustain liver damage because of several factors: (1) increased glutathione turnover; (2) children's livers are proportionately larger (4% of body weight in a 1-year-old versus 2.4% in an 18-year-old; and (3) their metabolic pathways have not yet developed enough to break down acetaminophen into its harmful metabolites.[38–43]

## Target Organ Susceptibility

During growth and maturation, children's organs may be affected by exposure to harmful chemicals.[43,44] Following cellular proliferation, individual cells undergo 2 further processes to become adult cells: differentiation and migration. Differentiation occurs when cells take on specific tasks within the body. The trigger for differentiation may be hormonal, so chemicals that mimic hormones may alter the differentiation of some tissues. Because children's organ systems, including the reproductive system, continue to differentiate, chemicals that mimic hormones may have effects on the development of those organ systems. For example, a growing body of evidence documents such endocrine-disrupting effects from phthalate exposure in animals and humans.[45]

Cell migration is necessary for certain cells to reach their destination. Neurons, for example, originate in a structure near the center of the brain and then migrate to predestined locations in one of the many layers of the brain. Chemicals may have a profound effect on this process (eg, ethanol exposure resulting in fetal alcohol syndrome).

Synaptogenesis occurs rapidly during the first 2 years.[46] Waves of synapses are formed as learning continues to occur throughout life. Dendritic trimming is the active removal of synapses. The brain of a 2-year-old child contains more synapses than at any other age. These synapses are trimmed back to allow more specificity of the resulting neural network. Data suggest that low-dose lead may interfere with this synapse trimming.[47]

Some organs continue developing for several years, increasing the vulnerability of these organs. For example, brain tumors frequently are treated by radiation therapy in adults resulting in uncomfortable but reversible adverse effects. However, in infants, radiation therapy generally is avoided because of the profound and permanent effects on the developing central nervous system. Similarly, lead and mercury affect the brain and nervous system of children. The brain attains 80% of its adult size by the end of the second year of life.[48] By adolescence, there are no gross changes in brain morphology,[48] but electroencephalographic and other studies demonstrate continued neurodevelopmental maturation.[48] Magnetic resonance imaging data confirm that the brain changes until the late teens and early 20s, with higher-order association cortices maturing after lower-order somatosensory and visual cortices.[49]

Exposure to secondhand smoke (SHS) compromises lung development. The rate of growth of lung function in children exposed to SHS is slower than that of children who are not exposed. $FEV_1$ values of children exposed to SHS are measurably lower than those of children without exposure.[50] Adolescents' increased susceptibility to tobacco dependence (see Chapter 43) illustrates the "critical windows" concept. The adolescent central nervous system is more vulnerable to nicotine dependence compared with that of adults. Adolescents may become dependent easily, often before the onset of daily smoking.[51,52]

Tissues undergoing growth and differentiation are particularly susceptible to cancer because of the shortened period for DNA repair and the changes occurring within the DNA during cell growth. The epidemic of scrotal cancer among adolescent chimney sweeps of Victorian England illustrates the likelihood that the scrotum at this developmental stage has increased susceptibility to the chemicals in soot.[53] Although occupational exposure at that time to cancer-causing chemicals, such as soot, was common in many occupations, scrotal tumors were uncommon except in young male chimney sweeps. Children and adolescents are more susceptible to the effects of ionizing radiation, as was demonstrated by the effects of the 1986 meltdown of the nuclear reactor in Chernobyl, Ukraine. This event resulted in heavy contamination of the area with plutonium, cesium, and radioactive iodine; almost 17 million people were exposed to excess radiation. Four years after exposure, a large excess of cases of thyroid cancers in adolescents and in children began to emerge, underscoring the special vulnerability at young ages to the effects of radioactive iodine.[54,55] The Chernobyl disaster is one example illustrating children's susceptibilities during and after disasters.[56]

## REGULATIONS AND LAWS: THE SOCIAL ENVIRONMENT

Regulatory policies usually do not take into account the unique combinations of developmental characteristics, physical environment, and biological environment that place children at risk. Most laws and regulations are based on studies using adult men weighing an average of 70 kg and, hence, are intended to protect adult men. Advances have been made, however, to change regulations to protect children. For example, the Food Quality Protection Act of 1996 stated that pesticide "tolerances" (the amount of pesticide legally allowed to be left in or on a harvested crop) must be set to protect the health of infants and children. In the United States, rules eliminating cigarette vending machines made cigarettes less available to children compared with countries where these machines are ubiquitous, allowing unfettered access by children. A ban on flavored cigarettes in the United States that took effect in September 2009 is another example of legislation specifically aimed at protecting children from exposure to environmental toxicants. Several US states have increased the minimum age for tobacco purchase from 18 to 21 years. The Consumer Product Safety Improvement Act of 2008 focused specifically on the unique vulnerabilities of children by applying special limitations on toxicants, such as lead, in products intended for children's use.

How can a clinician integrate information about children's developmental susceptibility into his or her daily practice? The roles of educator, investigator, and advocate are extremely important. The most important intervention is educating parents, children, and others about exposures to environmental hazards. Prevention efforts have the most impact when developmentally appropriate[57] (Table 3-1).

| Table 3-1. Special Environmental Health Risks by Developmental Stage | | |
|---|---|---|
| **DEVELOPMENTAL STAGE** | **TIME PERIOD** | **SPECIAL ENVIRONMENTAL AND OTHER EXPOSURE HEALTH RISKS** |
| Embryonic | 8 days to 9 weeks of pregnancy | Thalidomide and phocomelia (day 34 to 50) |
| Fetal | 9 weeks of pregnancy to birth | Microcephaly and mental retardation associated with in utero radiation exposure at 8 to 15 weeks |
| Infancy | Birth to 12 months | Mercury vapor and acrodynia<br>Nitrates and methemoglobinemia<br>Secondhand tobacco smoke and lung diseases<br>Toxigenic molds and pulmonary hemorrhage |
| Young toddlers<br>Older toddlers<br>Preschoolers | 1 to 2 yr<br>2 to 3 yr<br>3 to 5 yr | Radiation and thyroid cancer |
| School-aged | 5 to 12 yr | Nicotine and addiction |
| Adolescence | 12 to 19 yr | Soot exposure and cancer of scrotum |

Parents, children, teachers, community leaders, and policy makers will benefit from additional education from clinicians about the unique vulnerabilities of children to environmental pollution.

The role of the clinician as investigator also is important. Most diseases caused by environmental factors have been diagnosed by alert clinicians, and publication of case studies has enabled further description of these illnesses. Finally, clinicians must advocate for children. In addition to the day-to-day, office-based work advocating for the safety and health of individual patients, clinicians may also have opportunities to ensure that regulatory policies take into account children's unique vulnerabilities.

## References

1. Wigle D, Arbuckle T, Turner M, et al. Epidemiologic evidence of relationships between reproductive and child health outcomes and environmental chemical contaminants. *J Toxicol Environ Health B Crit Rev.* 2008;11(5-6):373–517
2. Bellinger D. Teratogen update: lead and pregnancy. *Birth Defects Res A Clin Mol Teratol.* 2005;73(6):409–420
3. Selevan SG, Kimmel CA, Mendola P. Identifying critical windows of exposure for children's health. *Environ Health Perspect.* 2000;108(Suppl 3):451–455

4. Braun JM, Gray K. Challenges to studying the health effects of early life environmental chemical exposures on children's health. *PLoS Biol.* 2017;15(12):e2002800

5. Agocs MM, Etzel RA, Parrish RG, et al. Mercury exposure from interior latex paint. *N Engl J Med.* 1990;323(16):1096–1101

6. Lukens JN. Landmark perspective: the legacy of well-water methemoglobinemia. *JAMA.* 1987;257(20):2793–2795

7. Lai TT, Bearer CF. Iatrogenic environmental hazards in the neonatal intensive care unit. *Clin Perinatol.* 2008;35(1):163–181

8. Calafat A, Needham L, Silva M, Lambert G. Exposure to di-(2-ethylhexyl) phthalate among premature neonates in a neonatal intensive care unit. *Pediatrics.* 2004;113(5):e429–e434

9. Moya J, Bearer CF, Etzel RA. Children's behavior and physiology and how it affects exposure to environmental contaminants. *Pediatrics.* 2004;113(4 Suppl):996–1006

10. US EPA Exposure Factors Handbook 2011 Edition (Final Report). US Environmental Protection Agency, Washington, DC: EPA/600/R-09/052F; 2011

11. Centers for Disease Control and Prevention. *Fourth National Report on Human Exposure to Environmental Chemicals.* Atlanta, GA: Centers for Disease Control and Prevention; 2009. Updated Tables, March 2018, Volume One. http://www.cdc.gov/exposurereport. Accessed July 6, 2018

12. Runyan CW, Schulman M, Dal Santo J, Bowling JM, Agans R, Ta M. Work-related hazards and workplace safety of US adolescents employed in the retail and service sectors. *Pediatrics.* 2007;119(3):526–534

13. Runyan CW, Dal Santo J, Schulman M, Lipscomb HJ, Harris TA. Work hazards and workplace safety violations experienced by adolescent construction workers. *Arch Pediatr Adolesc Med.* 2006;160(7):721–727

14. McConnell R, Berhane K, Gilliland F, et al. Asthma in exercising children exposed to ozone: a cohort study. *Lancet.* 2002;359(9304):386–391

15. Foote RS. Mercury vapor concentrations inside buildings. *Science.* 1972;177(4048):513–514

16. Snodgrasss WR. Physiological and biochemical differences between children and adults as determinants of toxic response to environmental pollutants. In: Guzelian PS, Henry CJ, Olin SS, eds. *Similarities and Differences Between Children and Adults: Implications for Risk Assessment.* Washington, DC: ILSI Press; 1992:35–42

17. Plunkett LM, Turnbull D, Rodricks JV. Differences between adults and children affecting exposure assessment. In: Guzelian PS, Henry CJ, Olin SS, eds. *Similarities and Differences Between Children and Adults: Implications for Risk Assessment.* Washington, DC: ILSI Press; 1992:79–94

18. Longo LD, Hill EP. Carbon monoxide uptake and elimination in fetal and maternal sheep. *Am J Physiol.* 1977;232(3):H324–H330

19. Longo LD. Carbon monoxide in the pregnant mother and fetus and its exchange across the placenta. *Ann N Y Acad Sci.* 1970;174(1):312–341

20. Sakamoto M, Murata K, Kubota M, Nakai K, Satoh H. Mercury and heavy metal profiles of maternal and umbilical cord RBCs in Japanese population. *Ecotoxicol Environ Saf.* 2010;73(1):1–6

21. Jauniaux E, Gulbis B, Acharya G, Thiry P, Rodeck C. Maternal tobacco exposure and cotinine levels in fetal fluids in the first half of pregnancy. *Obstet Gynecol.* 1999;93(1):25–29

22. VanVunakis H, Langone JJ, Milunsky A. Nicotine and cotinine in the amniotic fluid of smokers in the second trimester of pregnancy. *Am J Obstet Gynecol.* 1974;120(1):64–66

23. Holbrook KA. Structure and biochemical organogenesis of skin and cutaneous appendages in the fetus and newborn. In: Polin RA, Fox WW, eds. *Fetal and Neonatal Physiology.* Philadelphia, PA: WB Saunders; 1998:729–752

24. Clemens PC, Neumann RS. The Wolff-Chaikoff effect: hypothyroidism due to iodine application. *Arch Dermatol.* 1989;125(5):705

25. Shuman RM, Leech RW, Alvord EC Jr. Neurotoxicity of hexachlorophene in the human: I. A clinicopathologic study of 248 children. *Pediatrics.* 1974;54(6):689–695

26. Wysowski DK, Flynt JW Jr, Goldfield M, Altman R, Davis AT. Epidemic neonatal hyperbilirubinemia and use of a phenolic disinfectant detergent. *Pediatrics.* 1978;61(2):165–170

27. Nikolovski J, Stamatas G, Kollias N, Wiegand B. Barrier function and water-holding and transport properties of infant stratum corneum are different from adult and continue to develop through the first year of life. *J Invest Dermatol.* 2008;128(7):1728–1736

28. Giusti F, Martella A, Bertoni L, Seidenari S. Skin barrier, hydration, pH of skin of infants under 2 years of age. *Pediatr Dermatol.* 2001;18(2):93–96

29. Telofski LS, Morello AP, Mack Correa MC, Stamatas GN. The infant skin barrier: can we preserve, protect, and enhance the barrier? *Dermatol Res Pract.* 2012;2012:198789

30. Dietert RR, Etzel RA, Chen D, et al. Workshop to identify critical windows of exposure for children's health: immune and respiratory systems work group summary. *Environ Health Perspect.* 2000;108(Suppl 3):483–490

31. Gauderman W, Avol E, Gilliland F, et al. The effect of air pollution on lung development from 10 to 18 years of age. *N Engl J Med.* 2004;351(11):1057–1067

32. US Environmental Protection Agency. *Review of the National Ambient Air Quality Standards for Lead: Exposure Analysis Methodology and Validation.* Washington, DC: Air Quality Management Division, Office of Air Quality Planning and Standards, US Environmental Protection Agency; 1989

33. Momcilovic B, Kostial K. Kinetics of lead retention and distribution in suckling and adult rats. *Environ Res.* 1974;8(2):214–220

34. Barry PS. A comparison of concentrations of lead in human tissues. *Br J Ind Med.* 1975;32(2):119–139

35. Faustman EM, Silbernagel SM, Fenske RA, Burbacher TM, Ponce RA. Mechanisms underlying children's susceptibility to environmental toxicants. *Environ Health Perspect.* 2000;108 (Suppl 1):13–21

36. Nebert DW, Gonzalez FJ. P450 genes: structure, evolution, and regulation. *Annu Rev Biochem.* 1987;56:945–993

37. Card SE, Tompkins SF, Brien JF. Ontogeny of the activity of alcohol dehydrogenase and aldehyde dehydrogenases in the liver and placenta of the guinea pig. *Biochem Pharmacol.* 1989;38(15):2535–2541

38. Tenenbein M. Acetaminophen: the 150 mg/kg myth. *J Toxicol Clin Toxicol.* 2004;42(2):145–148

39. Byer AJ, Traylor TR, Semmer JR. Acetaminophen overdose in the third trimester of pregnancy. *JAMA.* 1982;247(22):3114–3115

40. Kurzel RB. Can acetaminophen excess result in maternal and fetal toxicity? *South Med J.* 1990;83(8):953–955

41. Rosevear SK, Hope PL. Favourable neonatal outcome following maternal paracetamol overdose and severe fetal distress. Case report. *Br J Obstet Gynaecol.* 1989;96(4):491–493

42. Stokes IM. Paracetamol overdose in the second trimester of pregnancy. Case report. *Br J Obstet Gynaecol.* 1984;91(3):286–288

43. World Health Organization. Environmental Health Criteria 237: *Principles for Evaluating Health Risks in Children Associated with Exposure to Chemicals.* Geneva, Switzerland: World Health Organization; 2006. http://www.inchem.org/documents/ehc/ehc/ehc237.pdf. Accessed July 6, 2018

44. Heyer DB, Meredith RM. Environmental toxicology: sensitive periods of development and neurodevelopmental disorders. *NeuroToxicology.* 2017;58:23–41

45. Swan S. Environmental phthalate exposure in relation to reproductive outcomes and other health endpoints in humans. *Environ Res.* 2008;108(2):177–184

46. Adams J, Barone S Jr, LaMantia A, et al. Workshop to identify critical windows of exposure for children's health: neurobehavioral work group summary. *Environ Health Perspect.* 2000;108(Suppl 3):535–544

47. Goldstein GW. Developmental neurobiology of lead toxicity. In: Needleman HL, ed. *Human Lead Exposure.* Boca Raton, FL: CRC Press; 1992:125–135

48. Behrman RE, Kleigman RM, Jenson HB. *Nelson Textbook of Pediatrics.* 18th ed. Philadelphia, PA: WB Saunders; 2007

49. Gogtay N, Giedd JN, Lusk L, et al. Dynamic mapping of human cortical development during childhood through early adulthood. *Proc Natl Acad Sci U S A.* 2004;101(21):8175–8179

50. Tager IB, Weiss ST, Munoz A, Rosner B, Speizer FE. Longitudinal study of the effects of maternal smoking on pulmonary function in children. *N Engl J Med.* 1983;309(12):699–703

51. DiFranza JR, Savageau JA, Rigotti NA, et al. Development of symptoms of tobacco dependence in youths: 30 month follow up data from the DANDY study. *Tob Control.* 2002;11(3):228–235

52. DiFranza JR, Rigotti NA, McNeill AD, et al. Initial symptoms of nicotine dependence in adolescents. *Tob Control.* 2000;9(3):313–319

53. Nethercott JR. Occupational skin disorders. In: LaDou J, ed. *Occupational Medicine.* Norwalk, CT: Appleton & Lange; 1990

54. Paulson JA, American Academy of Pediatrics Council on Environmental Health. Pediatric considerations before, during, and after radiological/nuclear emergencies. Policy Statement. 2018. *Pediatrics.* In press

55. Linet MS, Kazzi Z, Paulson JA, American Academy of Pediatrics Council on Environmental Health. Pediatric considerations before, during, and after radiological/nuclear emergencies. Technical Report. 2018. *Pediatrics.* In press

56. American Academy of Pediatrics Disaster Preparedness Advisory Council, Committee on Pediatric Emergency Medicine. Ensuring the health of children in disasters. *Pediatrics.* 2015;136(5):e1407–e1417

57. Perlroth NH, Branco CW. Current knowledge of environmental exposure in children during the sensitive developmental periods. *J Pediatr (Rio J).* 2017;93(1):17–27

Chapter 4

# Individual Susceptibility to Environmental Toxicants

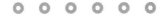

## KEY POINTS

- Except for Mendelian disease (ie, cystic fibrosis, phenylketonuria [PKU], etc), genetics plays a small role in explaining why children become ill.
- Even Mendelian diseases have environmental triggers. Often these triggers can determine the severity of the genetic disease.
- Social environments and nutritional status also affect susceptibility to environmental toxicants.
- Susceptibility often relates to life stage and depends on exposures that occur during the stage when an organ system (eg, brain, lung, kidney, endocrine) is rapidly developing.

## INTRODUCTION

Substantial variation exists among individuals in the effects of a given dose of an environmental toxicant. That variation typically takes on the distribution of a bell-shaped curve. The location of a particular individual on the bell curve is not random; it is determined largely by the factors that constitute that individual's susceptibility. In recent years, the environmental health community has paid increasing attention to the causes of variation in susceptibility to toxic chemicals and physical toxicants, such as air pollution. A better understanding of this variation allows us to appreciate which patients may be at increased risk of a toxicant's ill effects and suggests mitigating factors (ie, potential treatments) that may lessen the burden of a given toxic exposure.

This chapter discusses the concepts essential to understanding variation in susceptibility to toxicants and explores 3 important realms: genetic, social, and nutritional variants that have been shown to specifically modify the relationship between environmental toxicant exposure and health outcomes. An individual's age and developmental stage also are important factors in determining susceptibility (see Chapter 3). Underlying chronic disease may also infer susceptibility; for example, a child with autism is more likely to be exposed (typically from pica) and have heightened effects from exposure. Fetuses and young children are often, but not always, considered to be at increased risk of exposure to environmental hazards compared with older children, adolescents, and adults.

Although these concepts apply to many environmental diseases, the chapter focuses on 2 widely studied and prototypical pediatric environmental health issues: asthma and lead poisoning.

## CONCEPTS AND DEFINITIONS

*Susceptibility* is the condition of having one or more risk factors that can interact with an environmental exposure. As the name implies, a susceptible individual is not ill, but is at higher risk for illness from environmental exposure. He or she is either predisposed to, or at enhanced vulnerability to, the effects of an environmental toxicant. Because susceptibility factors vary in all populations, susceptibility results in variation in the size of effect of a given exposure within a population when the dose is held constant. Epidemiologists use the term "effect modification" to describe this phenomenon, and when statistically modeled, it is often referred to as "interaction." Physicians may be most familiar with the terms "synergy" or "potentiation," biological terms that are conceptually similar.

*Effect modification* is similar to the biological concept of synergism. For example, in patients with chronic infections (such as those with cystic fibrosis), a pathogen may be resistant to 2 individual antibiotics, but when exposed to the 2 antibiotics simultaneously, the pathogen is effectively treated. Together, the effect of the 2 antibiotics is multiplicative or synergistic—ie, it is greater than the sum of the individual effects of each antibiotic. Effect modification can also work antagonistically. For example, the herbal remedy St John's wort induces the metabolism of oral contraceptives, decreasing their action and sometimes resulting in breakthrough bleeding and contraceptive inefficacy.[1] When taken together, oral contraceptives are less effective than if taken without St John's wort. The disorder glucose-6-phosphate dehydrogenase (G6PD) deficiency is fundamentally an example of genetic susceptibility to chemicals—in this case, pro-oxidants. A drug with mild oxidant properties would not produce hemolysis in a male who did not carry the allele for this x-linked disorder, but in someone who does carry this allele, this same drug can cause severe hemolysis.

A critical difference exists between effect modification and the more familiar epidemiologic concept of *confounding*. Confounding refers to a mathematical association that induces an incorrect relationship between an exposure and a health outcome. It occurs when a third factor is independently associated with *both* the outcome and the exposure of interest. Under confounding, the relationship between the exposure and outcome is partly or totally driven by the associations with the confounding factor. For example, a study might find that drinking coffee was associated with attention problems. Smoking is also associated with attention problems and people who smoke tend to drink more coffee. A study that measured coffee consumption and attention, but did not measure smoking, may find an erroneous association between coffee and attention problems. If smoking caused the attention problem but was not measured, one would think that coffee consumption caused the attention problem when, in fact, coffee consumption was only a surrogate measure of smoking, the true cause. In our example, there is no intrinsic biological link between coffee and attention problems, other than the observation that they happen to occur together because both are associated with smoking. The combination of coffee and smoking was not needed to produce attention problems. Effect modifiers, however, are intrinsically (ie, biologically) interrelated in producing the outcome of interest. For example, one must have both the genotype for G6PD deficiency and take an oxidant drug to produce hemolysis. As such, effect modifiers have tremendous importance in understanding health and potentially can even point to treatments or preventive measures because they are biological. Confounders do not have this property (ie, in the previous example, eliminating coffee consumption would not have any impact on attention). Understanding the factors that modify the relationship between environmental exposures and their toxic effects can lead to new insights into mechanisms, can identify individuals who are most severely affected by exposure to environmental toxicants, and can suggest interventions to mitigate the effects of exposures.

## GENETIC SUSCEPTIBILITY

Interactions among genes and the environment are unavoidable. Genes, in and of themselves, do nothing. They must have environmental substrate (nutrients, chemicals, etc) to synthesize hormones and proteins, metabolize chemicals, repair damaged cells, etc. In fact, all genetic diseases have significant environmental components and vice versa. To bring this concept into clinical perspective, phenylketonuria (PKU) is defined as a genetic disease. Specifically, it is an autosomal recessive trait; nearly all cases are associated with mutations in the gene encoding phenylalanine hydroxylase, which has been mapped to human chromosome 12q24.1.[2] The devastating neurodevelopmental effects of PKU are caused *by the environment.* Among children with the PKU genotype, excessive intake and accumulation of phenylalanine, an essential amino acid usually metabolized by phenylalanine hydroxylase, induces the disease. Children with PKU who are identified early and treated with restrictive diets develop normally.[3] In this example, there are 2 factors (one genetic and one environmental) necessary for the development of PKU. For the disease to develop, one must have both the genetic disposition and exposure to phenylalanine. PKU is viewed as a genetic disease because exposure to phenylalanine is nearly universal, and PKU mutations are rare. Consider, however, if the converse were true—ie, if a population evolved in which PKU mutations were common, and that population did not consume unrestricted amounts of phenylalanine. New unrestricted exposures to this amino acid would be devastating to this population. In this scenario, phenylalanine would be considered a neurotoxicant (like lead) and excessive ingestion of foods containing it would be considered poisonous. In other words, PKU would be thought of as an environmental disease. Finally, consider the concept of natural selection in which genetic variation predicts better survival in harsh environments. Does a change in genetics or environment drive natural selection? Perhaps the fundamental problem with our approach to research is that too often we think of each factor as independent (ie, nature vs nurture) when in fact, independence is a fallacy. Without exception, all biological events are an interaction of genes with the host environment. The relative importance of each factor may vary depending on the disease, but all diseases are the end result of gene-environment interactions.

With respect to environmental health, diseases with strong environmental triggers are being shown increasingly to have genetic components. These genetic components are different from the more traditional concept of Mendelian genetics. Non-Mendelian chronic diseases are often referred to as "complex genetic diseases." In these diseases, the genetic factors are not the primary cause of disease, unlike, for example, the alleles for cystic fibrosis. Instead, genetic components confer increased *risk* for the development of the disease. The best known of such genetic risk factors is the E4 allele, a variant in the apolipoprotein E gene. This allele is associated with the risk for the development of Alzheimer disease and carriers are also at increased risk for traumatic brain disorder.[4] Individuals with 1 copy of this allele have a 2- to 5-fold increased risk for the development of Alzheimer disease. If a person has 2 copies of the E4 allele, the risk is increased by approximately 10-fold. However, more than half of people homozygous for this allele will never develop Alzheimer disease.[5] The allele is a risk factor and should not be thought of as causal in the way of Mendelian genetic diseases, such as cystic fibrosis. A more appropriate view is that E4 is a risk factor, similar to, for example, risk factors for heart attacks, such as smoking or dietary cholesterol.

Genetic risk factors also exist for childhood diseases, and many of these genetic factors modify the effects of environmental risk factors. Strong evidence shows that genes and the environment interact in the pathogenesis of asthma. Genome-wide association studies of asthma have identified novel risk alleles and loci but few have consistently been replicated like other complex diseases. Asthma-associated genetic alleles always have small effect sizes and account for little of the prevalence of asthma.[6] There are many reasons why this may occur—one reason is that asthma is not a uniform disease. Regardless of the underlying reasons, it is clear that the development of asthma is not primarily driven by genetics. The common misconception is to think of risk factor genotypes as causative. The danger of doing so would be the over interpretation of risk. The presence of such a genotype is akin to the risk of heart disease from elevated serum cholesterol. The risk is higher compared with someone who has lower serum cholesterol, but the *overall* risk for the development of the disease may still be small. With few exceptions, our genes do not predict our fate. We should consider whether the most likely cause of variation in the genetic risk factors for asthma is the variation in unmeasured environmental triggers.

The relationship between genes and environmental exposure can be quite complex, as demonstrated by the CD14/-159 polymorphism and exposure to house dust endotoxin. Individuals with the T-allele of CD14/-159 have higher atopic response (as measured by serum immunoglobulin IgE concentrations) when exposed to high levels of house dust, but individuals with the C-allele have higher IgE concentrations when exposed to low levels of house dust.[7] Therefore, depending on one's genetic makeup, endotoxins in house dust may predispose a child to asthma and allergies, or paradoxically, exposure to house dust may actually be *protective*. This finding, developed by multiple investigators over the past several years, may provide the key to understanding the complex relationship between genes and environment in atopic disease.[8–11] The protective effect of endotoxins in some individuals is direct evidence in support of the hygiene hypothesis, which proposes that microbial exposure during early life protects against later development of atopic disease. This may be the case among individuals with the appropriate genetic makeup.[12–13] Nonetheless, there remain individuals in whom early life exposure is not protective, and this difference may be attributable to genetic susceptibility. This may explain why the hygiene hypothesis, a theory of environmental risk, has been so difficult to validate. It may apply only to individuals with a particular genetic background.

An additional layer of complexity exists in the relationship between genetics, environment, and disease; environmental toxicants, such as metals, may act to alter gene expression through *epigenetic* mechanisms. Epigenetics (literally "on genes") is a field that investigates heritable changes in gene expression that occur without changes in genetic sequence.[14] The term has also grown to include effects on gene expression that are "programmed" but not necessarily heritable. Epigenetics is a biological link between genetics and environment, and explains in large part how environmental factors turn on and off specific genes. A review relating the role of epigenetics to primary care has been published.[15]

Environmental factors can alter epigenetic "marks" (chemical additions to the gene sequence or to histone-binding proteins around DNA that regulate gene expression and alter the function of a gene without altering the DNA sequence). Gene expression is, in part, controlled by multiple epigenetic marks that can occur on DNA itself or on DNA-binding proteins (histones).

The most studied of epigenetic marks is DNA methylation. Cytosine methylation in the DNA sequence is overrepresented in cytosine-guanine repeat sequences. Such repeats are very common in promoter regions that regulate gene expression. This methylation pattern can alter the 3-dimensional structure of DNA. Methylated cytosines lead to a tightly wound 3-dimensional structure that hides the promoter region of a gene within a coil. "Unmethylated" cytosines lead to a more open structure that allows transcription factors to bind to DNA and initiate gene expression.

The extent to which specific DNA sequences are bound to methyl groups is a principal determinant of cell differentiation. The clinical consequences of altered DNA methylation patterns are becoming more apparent. Altered DNA methylation systems in the brain may lead to clinical syndromes, such as intellectual disabilities and autism spectrum disorders.[16] DNA methylation patterns altered by environmental chemicals may be inherited by offspring if these altered methylation patterns occur in gamete cells. Increasingly, there is evidence that methylation marks on histone-binding proteins are drivers of DNA expression, although site-specific measures for histone marks are not as well developed as for DNA methylation. Thus, the research on histones is less well developed than for DNA-binding proteins.

Widespread interest had been shown in DNA methylation and other epigenetic marks as mechanisms of environmental diseases. Several studies have demonstrated an association between DNA methylation and exposure to environmental metals, including nickel, cadmium, arsenic, and lead.[17–19] The effect may be the result of metal-induced oxidative stress. Exposure to specific metals has been shown to result in global DNA hypomethylation and/or gene-specific DNA hypermethylation.[20] In animal models, DNA hypomethylation alters the function and survival of neurons.[21] DNA methylation and histone marks are not the only forms of epigenetic gene expression regulation but are the best studied because they were the first ones discovered. They may or may not be the most important epigenetic marks. Noncoding RNAs have been described: these turn off sets of related genes at the level of translation (rather than transcription which is where DNA methylation and histone protein marks work). Small RNAs known as microRNA (22-24 base pairs long) circulate in the body from one tissue to another. These microRNAs form protein-bound complexes that "chew up" specific messenger RNA molecules, preventing their translation. This newer form of epigenetic gene regulation may play a major role in regulating gene expression from toxic exposures, such as heavy metals, air pollution, bisphenol A, and cigarette smoking.[22–25]

Together, these findings suggest a novel pathway by which environmental chemicals modify the expression of DNA to result in toxicity. By altering such marks in a targeted fashion, there is the potential that environmentally induced diseases, including certain cancers, could be treated.

## SOCIAL SUSCEPTIBILITY

Social factors, such as socioeconomic status and other factors comprising social determinants of health, are widely known to affect many health outcomes; they are implicated in the prevalence of many diseases and have repeatedly been associated with overall morbidity and mortality. Social determinants of health play a major role in neurodevelopment, also an outcome relevant to many toxic exposures of childhood. Individuals of lower socioeconomic status are at increased risk of exposure to several environmental toxicants (see Chapter 55). More than simply acting as confounders, however, social determinants of health may also modify the relationship between environmental exposures and outcomes. In other words, the concurrent presence of social stressors and chemical toxicants may act synergistically to produce toxicity.

Low income or poverty is itself not toxic but is a marker of factors that coincide with poverty (eg, chemical exposure, social stress, exposure to violence, social isolation). Low income is a proxy for social stressors and it is these factors, usually unmeasured, that cause the health effects of poverty. Traditionally, poverty has been believed to be a potential confounder of exposure to chemical toxicants, such as lead, with measures of poverty included in evaluations to account for its independent effects on developmental outcomes. A new paradigm has arisen in the last several years, and investigators are now studying whether poverty is not a confounder but is, instead, a modifier of lead toxicity and other environmental exposures. In this paradigm, there is synergism between environmental toxicants and factors that coincide with poverty. The concept of toxic stress—the unmitigated continuous stress often experienced by children living in poverty—has gained traction among pediatricians and others concerned about the effects of early exposures on one's life trajectory.[26] Pediatricians now are encouraged to screen families for toxic stress using Adverse Childhood Events (ACEs) screening tools.[27]

Figure 4-1 outlines the many factors to consider when unraveling the effects of lead exposure on cognitive function.

For example, Rauh et al[28] demonstrated an interaction between exposure to secondhand smoke (SHS) and maternal hardship on cognitive development among minority 24-month-old children in New York City. In their study, children with prenatal SHS exposure were twice as likely to be significantly delayed, and among children of mothers who reported significant unmet basic needs, the effect of exposure to SHS on cognitive function was significantly exacerbated. The reason for this interaction is uncertain, but several theories emerge. Mothers with fewer unmet needs may be better able to compensate for the toxic effect of exposure to SHS by providing positive developmental support for their children in the form of increased social interaction, an enhanced developmental environment, improved prenatal and postnatal nutrition, or reduced exposure to other developmental neurotoxicants also associated with poverty. Stress in pregnancy has been shown to modify the relationship between exposure to air pollution and childhood asthma, increasing the risk of disease when high stress is combined with higher exposure to air pollution.[29]

The cognitive effect of childhood exposure to lead, the most thoroughly studied developmental neurotoxicant, is also modified by social factors. In a cohort of children in Mexico City, increased maternal self-esteem attenuated the negative effect of lead exposure on cognitive development of 24-month-old children.[30] In addition, lead poisoning has been shown to alter the programming of cortisol rhythms in children. Cortisol rhythms are highly influenced by chronic stress, suggesting a further link between lead poisoning and social environment.[31] In a striking animal model, environmental enhancement was demonstrated to reverse the neurological effects of lead exposure. Guilarte et al[32] exposed rats to neurotoxic levels of lead and then randomized them to standard cages or enriched environments with shared cages, greater space allowance per rat, and interactive objects. Rats in enriched environments showed better spatial learning and recovery of gene expression in the hippocampus, specifically associated with lead-related neurotoxicity. In effect, the social environment served as an effective "treatment" for lead poisoning.

The effects of lead poisoning on neurodevelopment have been considered by many experts to be irreversible. Adults with a history of childhood lead exposure tend to have smaller brain volume, and higher childhood lead concentrations are associated with increased criminal arrests in early

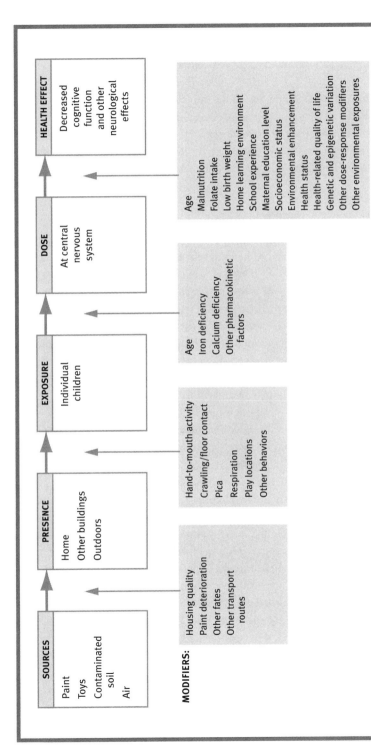

**SOURCES**

Paint
Toys
Contaminated
soil
Air

**PRESENCE**

Home
Other buildings
Outdoors

**EXPOSURE**

Individual
children

**DOSE**

At central
nervous
system

**HEALTH EFFECT**

Decreased
cognitive
function
and other
neurological
effects

**MODIFIERS:**

Housing quality
Paint deterioration
Other fates
Other transport
routes

Hand-to-mouth activity
Crawling/floor contact
Pica
Respiration
Play locations
Other behaviors

Age
Iron deficiency
Calcium deficiency
Other pharmacokinetic
factors

Age
Malnutrition
Folate intake
Low birth weight
Home learning environment
School experience
Maternal education level
Socioeconomic status
Environmental enhancement
Health status
Health-related quality of life
Genetic and epigenetic variation
Other dose-response modifiers
Other environmental exposures

For the prototypical example of lead poisoning, this diagram illustrates the many factors that may modify an individual's susceptibility.

**Figure 4-1. Biologic Impact Pathway of Lead on Cognitive Function**

adulthood.[33,34] Chelation therapy, the mainstay of treatment for acute child-hood lead poisoning, was shown in a multicenter study to have no significant effect in reversing lead-induced cognitive deficits caused by chronic lead exposure.[35] Chelation therapy clearly remains the treatment of choice for acute severe systemic lead poisoning. However, the findings of Guilarte et al,[32] which need to be validated in human populations, open the door to the possibility that some of the developmental effects associated with chronic "low level" lead exposure could be remediated, in part, through social interventions. This is a promising finding for a disease process with otherwise dim treatment prospects.

## NUTRITIONAL SUSCEPTIBILITY

Nutritional factors may affect both the absorption and the in vivo effects of environmental toxicants. This has been demonstrated particularly with heavy metals. Iron-deficiency anemia, which is independently known to negatively affect early development, is also associated with subsequent lead poisoning.[36,37] Iron-deficient individuals absorb a greater proportion of ingested lead, thought to occur because a common iron receptor in the gastrointestinal epithelium is up-regulated in the setting of iron deficiency.[38] Similarly, increased calcium intake has been associated with lower blood lead concentration.[39,40] Low dietary calcium, likewise, will increase lead absorption and also perhaps mobilize lead for deposit in bone cortex.[41]

A study of children in the rural Philippines showed an interaction between lead and folate concentrations on cognitive function.[42] Among these generally poor and undernourished children, higher folate concentrations appeared to have a protective effect against lead's neurotoxic effects. The pathophysiology of this relationship is unclear, but folate is known to play a major role in neuro-development and also influences DNA expression because of its indispensable role in DNA methylation. DNA methylation is known to regulate gene expression, and the study's findings might be explained by lead-induced changes in gene expression modified, in turn, by folate metabolism.

Together, these findings suggest multiple potential roles for nutritional supplementation in mitigating the effects of lead exposure. In one trial of this hypothesis in India, supplementing the diets of school children with iron-fortified rice decreased blood lead concentration, but the cognitive effects of such interventions have not been established.[43] A randomized trial in the United States of calcium supplementation among lead-exposed children failed to find a benefit in reducing the risk of lead poisoning.[44]

Nutrition plays a very important independent role in child health, particularly in neurodevelopment. These findings suggest that improved nutrition, in the form of specific micronutrients, may provide additional benefits to protect from environmental toxicants. Other elements of nutrition may also help protect against the effects of toxic exposures. For example, in multiple studies of fetal polychlorinated biphenyl (PCB) exposure, breastfeeding has been shown to protect against adverse neurodevelopmental outcomes.[45–48] It is unclear whether this effect is attributable to the nutritional benefits of breast-feeding compared with cow milk-based infant formula or to the enhanced social interaction between the mother and infant that may be inherent to breastfeeding.

## AGE

The concept of critical windows of susceptibility underlies all the susceptibility factors mentioned previously. The age at time of exposure is itself a suscep-tibility factor. Although there is some controversy regarding the effect of age of exposure on lead poisoning, data suggest that 2 years of age is the time of highest susceptibility.[49] This age also corresponds to the peak of synaptic pruning and network formation in the developing brain.[50] A separate study found older ages to be the most susceptible.[51] The widespread application in recent years of research into the developmental origins of health and disease further demonstrates the role of exposure timing in health. With the develop-ment of sophisticated exposure measures and models and more highly devel-oped statistical approaches, new methods to identify the time boundaries of critical windows have been introduced.[52]

## CONCLUSION

Genetic predisposition, social determinants of health, and nutritional quality are likely contributors to an individual's susceptibility to environmental toxicants. The relationship between environmental exposure and outcome is not linear; rather, it is a complex web of interconnecting and interdependent factors likely to be unique for each exposed individual.

These determinants of susceptibility are of tremendous clinical importance to clinicians caring for children exposed to environmental toxicants. The most effective way to address environmental health threats is primary prevention through prevention of exposure. Accordingly, primary prevention should be particularly emphasized among susceptible individuals, whether attributable to genetic, social, or nutritional risk factors.

When primary prevention is not possible and exposure has already occurred, treatment becomes the next best option. Although genetic predispo-sition may not (yet) be modifiable, nutritional status and social environment may well be. The data mentioned previously suggest that social and nutritional interventions may have real effects on environmental health outcomes. In the lead poisoning example, chelation therapy, the treatment of choice for acute high-dose lead poisoning, has not been associated with improved developmental outcomes after lead exposure. Social interventions, such as early intervention programs, and nutritional supplementation may be effective in improving these outcomes.

Social and nutritional interventions need not necessarily be complex to be effective. Every day, pediatricians see concerned parents who are worried about the myriad toxicants in the modern environment. What a powerful message it could be to say that one might ameliorate some effects of these exposures by providing a rich social environment and a complete and nutritious diet. Such a message does not mean that lead or other environmental poisons are not worrisome, nor is it meant to shift the blame for toxicity away from the chemical (or polluters causing the exposure) to parents. Instead, this message conveys that, while it may require significant effort, children may be able to overcome some or many of the toxic effects of chemical exposures and lead long and fruitful lives. Given that exposures to environmental toxicants frequently occur in disadvantaged communities, many of these issues, particularly regarding the nutritional components and social environments, can be seen as environmental justice issues. Addressing environmental contaminants should always include addressing the social and nutritional problems commonly experienced by children.

## References

1. Hall SD, Zaiqui W, Huang SM, et al. The interaction between St John's wort and an oral contraceptive. *Clin Pharamacol Ther.* 2003;74(6):525–535
2. Erlandsen H, Stevens RC. The structural basis of phenylketonuria. *Mol Genet Metab.* 1999;68(2):103–125
3. Koch R, Azen C, Friedman EG, Williamson ML. Paired comparisons between early treated PKU children and their matched sibling controls on intelligence and school achievement test results at eight years of age. *J Inherit Metab Dis.* 1984;7(2):86–90
4. Terrell TR, Abramson R, Barth JT, et al. Genetic polymorphisms associated with the risk of concussion in 1056 college athletes: a multicentre prospective cohort study. *Br J Sports Med.* 2018;52(3):192–198.
5. Myers RH, Schaefer EJ, Wilson PW, et al. Apolipoprotein E epsilon4 association with dementia in a population-based study: the Framingham study. *Neurology.* 1996;46(3):673–677
6. Ober C. Asthma genetics in the post-GWAS era. *Ann Am Thorac Soc.* 2016;13(Suppl 1):S85–S90
7. Martinez FD. CD14, endotoxins, and asthma risk: actions and interactions. *Proc Am Thorac Soc.* 2007;4(3):221–225
8. Baldini M, Lohman IC, Halonen M, Erickson RP, Holt PG, Martinez FD. A polymorphism in the 5' flanking region of the CD14 gene is associated with circulating soluble CD14 levels and with total serum immunoglobulin E. *Am J Respir Cell Mil Biol.* 1999;20(5):976–983
9. Eder W, Klimecki W, Yu L, et al. Opposite effects of CD14/-260 on serum IgE levels in children raised in different environments. *J Allergy Clin Immunol.* 2005;116(3):601–607
10. Martinez FD. Gene-environment interactions in asthma and allergies: a new paradigm to understand disease causation. *Immunol Allergy Clin North Am.* 2005;25(4):709–721

11. Simpson A, John SL, Jury F, et al. Endotoxin exposure, CD14, and allergic disease: an interaction between genes and the environment. *Am J Respir Crit Care Med*. 2006;174(4):386–392

12. Liu AH, Leung DY. Renaissance of the hygiene hypothesis. *J Allergy Clin Immunol*. 2006;117(5):1063–1066

13. Schaub B, Lauener R, van Mutius E. The many faces of the hygiene hypothesis. *J Allergy Clin Immunol*. 2006;117(5):969–977

14. Bollati V, Baccarelli A. Environmental epigenetics. *Heredity*. 2010; 105(1):105–112

15. Wright R, Saul RA. Epigenetics and primary care. *Pediatrics*. 2013;132(Suppl 3):S216–S223

16. Shahbazain MD, Zoghbi HY. Rett syndrome and MeCP2: linking epigenetics and neuronal function. *Am J Hum Genet*. 2002;71(6):1259–1272

17. McVeigh GE, Allen PB, Morgan DR, Hanratty CG, Silke B. Nitric oxide modulation of blood vessel tone identified by waveform analysis. *Clin Sci*. 2001;100(4):387–393

18. Dolinoy DC, Weidman JR, Jirtle RL. Epigenetic gene regulation: linking early developmental environment to adult disease. *Reprod Toxicol*. 2007;23(3):297–307

19. Bleich S, Lenz B, Ziegenbein M, et al. Epigenetic DNA hypermethylation of the HERP gene promoter induces down-regulation of its MRNA expression in patients with alcohol dependence. *Alcohol Clin Exp Res*. 2006;30(4):587–591

20. Wright RO, Baccarelli A. Metals and neurotoxicology. *J Nutr*. 2007;137(12):2809–2813

21. Jacob RA, Gretz DM, Taylor PC, et al. Moderate folate depletion increases plasma homocysteine and decreases lymphocyte DNA methylation in postmenopausal women. *J Nutr*. 1998;128(7):1204–1212

22. Hou L, Wang D, Baccarelli A. Environmental chemicals and microRNAs. *Mutat Res*. 2011; 714(1-2):105–112

23. Beck R, Styblo M, Sethupathy P. Arsenic exposure and type 2 diabetes: microRNAs as mechanistic links? *Curr Diab Rep*. 2017;17(3):18

24. Chou WC, Lee PH, Tan YY, et al. An integrative transcriptomic analysis reveals bisphenol A exposure-induced dysregulation of microRNA expression in human endometrial cells. *Toxicol In Vitro*. 2017;41:133–142

25. Su MW, Yu SL, Lin WC, Tsai CH, Chen PH, Lee YL. Smoking-related microRNAs and mRNAs in human peripheral blood mononuclear cells. *Toxicol Appl Pharmacol*. 2016;305:169–175

26. Block RW. Recognizing the importance of the social determinates of health. *Pediatrics*. 2015;135(2):e526–e527

27. American Academy of Pediatrics. Healthychildren.org. ACEs and Toxic Stress. https://www.aap.org/en-us/advocacy-and-policy/aap-health-initiatives/resilience/Pages/ACEs-and-Toxic-Stress.aspx. Accessed February 9, 2018

28. Rauh VA, Whyatt RM, Garfinkel R, et al. Developmental effects of exposure to environmental tobacco smoke and maternal hardship among inner-city children. *Neurotoxicol Teratol*. 2004;26(3):373–385

29. Rosa MJ, Just AC, Kloog I, et al. Prenatal particulate matter exposure and wheeze in Mexican children: effect modification by prenatal psychosocial stress. *Ann Allergy Asthma Immunol*. 2017;119(3):232–237

30. Surkan PJ, Schnaas L, Wright RJ, et al. Maternal self-esteem, exposure to lead, and child neurodevelopment. *Neurotoxicology*. 2008;29(2):278–285

31. Tamayo Y Ortiz M, Téllez-Rojo MM, Wright RJ, Coull BA, Wright RO. Longitudinal associations of age and prenatal lead exposure on cortisol secretion of 12-24 month-old infants from Mexico City. *Environ Health*. 2016;15:41

32. Guilarte TR, Toscano CD, McGlothan JL, Weaver SA. Environmental enrichment reverses cognitive and molecular deficits induced by developmental lead exposure. *Ann Neurol*. 2003;53(1):50–56

33. Cecil KM, Brubaker CJ, Adler CM, et al. Decreased brain volume in adults with childhood lead exposure. *PLoS Med.* 2008;5(5):e112

34. Wright JP, Dietrich KN, Ris MD, et al. Association of prenatal and childhood blood lead concentrations with criminal arrests in early adulthood. *PLoS Med.* 2008;5(5):e101

35. Rogan WJ, Dietrich KN, Ware JH, et al. The effect on chelation therapy with succimer on neuropsychological development in children exposed to lead. *New Engl J Med.* 2001;344(19):1421–1426

36. Lozoff B, Jimenez E, Wolf AW. Long-term developmental outcome of infants with iron deficiency. *N Engl J Med.* 1991;325(10):687–694

37. Wright RO, Tsaih SW, Schwartz J, Wright RJ, Hu H. Association between iron deficiency and blood lead level in a longitudinal analysis of children followed in an urban primary care clinic. *J Pediatr.* 2003;142(1):9–14

38. Barton JC, Conrad ME, Nuby S, Harrison L. Effects of iron in the absorption and retention of lead. *J Lab Clin Med.* 1978;92(4):536–547

39. Mahaffey KR, Gartside PS, Gluek CJ. Blood lead levels and dietary calcium intake in 1 to 11 year old children: the Second National Health and Nutrition Examination Survey, 1976 to 1980. *Pediatrics.* 1986;78(2):257–262

40. Lacasaña M, Romieu I, Sanin LH, Palazuelos E, Hernandez-Avila M. Blood lead levels and calcium intake in Mexico City children under five years of age. *Int J Environ Health Res.* 2000;10(4):331–340

41. Morris C, McCarron DA, Bennett WM. Low-level lead exposure, blood pressure, and calcium metabolism. *Am J Kidney Dis.* 1990;15(6):568–574

42. Solon O, Riddell TJ, Quimbo SA, et al. Associations between cognitive function, blood lead concentration, and nutrition among children in the central Philippines. *J Pediatr.* 2008;152(2): 237–243

43. Zimmerman MB, Muthayya S, Moretti D, Kurpad A, Hurrell RF. Iron fortification reduces blood lead levels in children in Bangalore, India. *Pediatrics.* 2006;117(6):2014–2021

44. Sargent JD, Dalton MA, O'Connor GT, Olmstead EM, Klein RZ. Randomized trial of calcium glycerophosphate-supplemented infant formula to prevent lead absorption. *Am J Clin Nutr.* 1999;69(6):1224–1230

45. Jacobson JL, Jacobson SW. Intellectual impairment in children exposed to polychlorinated biphenyls in utero. *N Engl J Med.* 1996;335(11):783–789

46. Patantin S, Lanting C, Mulder PG, Boersma ER, Sauer PJ, Weisglas-Kuperus N. Effects of environmental exposure to PCBs and dioxins on cognitive abilities in Dutch children at 42 months of age. *J Pediatr.* 1999;134(1):33–41

47. Walkowiak J, Wiener JA, Fastabend A, et al. Environmental exposure to polychlorinated biphenyls and quality of the home environment: effects on psychodevelopment in early childhood. *Lancet.* 2001;358(9293):1602–1607

48. Jacobson JL, Jacobson SW. Prenatal exposure to polychlorinated biphenyls and attention at school age. *J Pediatr.* 2003;143(6):780–788

49. Braun JM, Hoffman E, Schwartz J, et al. Assessing windows of susceptibility to lead-induced cognitive deficits in Mexican children. *Neurotoxicology.* 2012;33(5):1040–1047

50. Bressler J, Kim KA, Chakraborti T, Goldstein G. Molecular mechanisms of lead neurotoxicity. *Neurochem Res.* 1999;24(4):595–600

51. Hornung RW, Lanphear BP, Dietrich KN. Age of greatest susceptibility to childhood lead exposure: a new statistical approach. *Environ Health Perspect.* 2009;117(8):1309–1312

52. Hsu HH, Chiu YH, Coull BA, et al. Prenatal particulate air pollution and asthma onset in urban children. Identifying sensitive windows and sex differences. *Am J Respir Crit Care Med.* 2015;192(9):1052–1059

Chapter 5

# Taking an Environmental History and Giving Anticipatory Guidance

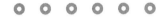

## KEY POINTS

- An environmental history is a basic component of a complete pediatric history.
- Basic areas of inquiry are age and condition of the home; secondhand smoke exposure; dietary exposure to mercury in fish and to arsenic in rice products and juice; exposure to ultraviolet radiation; exposure to noise; and parental/teen occupations and hobbies.
- Questions can be incorporated into health supervision visits, as well as visits for illnesses with known or potential environmental causes.
- Questions about the environment also are appropriate when symptoms are unusual, persistent, or when multiple people in the home (or child care setting, school, etc.) have similar symptoms.
- Information gathered from an environmental history may help prevent some potentially hazardous exposures and mitigate others.

## INTRODUCTION

During much of the 20th century, when house calls were routine, doctors could observe home environments. Making house calls is no longer part of standard practice. Today's pediatricians, therefore, must ask questions to find out about the home and other places where the child or adolescent lives or spends time, learns, plays, or works. Questions about these environments are basic to a comprehensive health history. The answers can help pediatricians understand a child's physical surroundings and offer guidance to prevent some exposures and mitigate other possibly hazardous exposures.

Questions can be incorporated into health supervision (well child and adolescent) visits, as well as visits for illnesses with known or potential environmental causes. Questions about the environment also are appropriate when symptoms are unusual, persistent, or when multiple people in the home (or child care setting, school, etc.) have similar symptoms.

Parents may face challenges in modifying their home environments. For example, renters may not know the age of the home or may not be able to undertake remedial work recommended as a result of mold investigations. Recommendations may be difficult or impossible to implement because of factors such as cost or lack of influence on a landlord. There may be discomfort with "raising a fuss" as in situations when a parent is advised to ask another parent or other family member to stop smoking inside the home. Recommendations may not be followed when families' cultural beliefs and practices differ from those of the pediatrician.

Keeping these caveats in mind, this chapter reviews key areas of a pediatric environmental history and reviews advice that may prevent or mitigate exposures. It is unlikely that busy practitioners will have the time to ask about everything. At minimum, it seems prudent to suggest that pediatricians inquire about the age and condition of the home, secondhand smoke (SHS) exposure, dietary exposure to mercury in fish and arsenic in rice products and juice, exposure to ultraviolet radiation, exposure to noise, and parental and teen occupation and hobbies. Asking additional questions depends on the situation of individual patients, taking into account factors such as the child's age, socioeconomic status, geographic location, and known hazards in the community.

Certain children are likely to be at higher risk of exposures and adverse health effects. These include children living in poverty or in ethnic minority communities, children whose parents are migrant or farm workers, and children living with parents who use tobacco or illicit substances or have mental health condition(s). Disparities often exist for members of minority groups even across socioeconomic lines.[1] Children adopted from or who have lived in or visited low- or middle-income countries (see Chapter 14) often are at higher risk for certain environmental exposures (such as exposure to lead) compared with children who have not been in these areas. Children who are adopted, or are in foster or kinship care, may have unknown or incomplete past histories; therefore, toxic exposures may need to be considered.

Laboratory testing of biological samples (such as blood or urine [see Chapter 6]) and/or of environmental samples (including air, water, soil, or dust [see Chapter 7]) may help clinicians evaluate children with potential environmental exposures or environmentally related disorders.

Health supervision visits are key elements of pediatric care in the United States.[2] Many areas must be reviewed during well visits, however, and time constraints are a common challenge. Environmental health history screening forms were developed to facilitate the history-taking process for practices in which information is collected using paper.[3] Pediatric practices using electronic health records (EHRs) may choose to customize their EHR to include questions about children's and adolescents' environments.

The following are basic areas of questioning about the child's and adolescent's environment:[3]

1. Physical surroundings;
2. Tobacco smoke exposure, tobacco use, and use of alternative nicotine products (such as electronic cigarettes) by household members;
3. Water sources;
4. Exposures from food;
5. Sun exposure and artificial exposure to ultraviolet radiation (UVR);
6. Noise exposure;
7. Exposures resulting from household member occupations and hobby activities.

Developmental stage is an important consideration. Table 5-1 suggests when to introduce environmental questions. Table 5-2 gives a summary of questions and where in the book to find additional information.

| Table 5-1. When to Introduce Environmental Questions[a] | |
|---|---|
| TOPIC | SUGGESTED TIME |
| Home environment including carbon monoxide, renovation, mold, secondhand smoke (SHS), water source, consumption of fish, noise, occupational exposures | Prenatal visit; newborn visit; new patient |
| SHS, sun exposure, mold, arsenic in rice products, juice | When the child is 2 months old |
| Risk of poisoning from chemicals and pesticides, lead poisoning | When the child is 6 months old |
| Wooden playsets and picnic tables, arts and crafts exposures | Preschool period |
| Occupational exposures, exposures from hobbies, deliberate sun tanning and tanning salons, noise | When the patient is a teenager |
| Lawn and garden products, lawn services, scheduled chemical applications, sun exposure | Spring and summer |
| Wood stoves and fireplaces, gas stoves | Fall and winter |

[a] Table is adapted from Balk SJ et al.[4]

| Table 5-2. Summary of Environmental Health Questions for Health Supervision Visits[a] | | |
|---|---|---|
| **AREA** | **QUESTIONS** | **FOR MORE INFORMATION, SEE CHAPTER ON** |
| **Surroundings** — At home | What type of home does your child live in or spend time in? | Child Care Settings, Indoor Air Pollutants, Lead |
| | What are the age and condition of your home? Is there lead, mold, asbestos, or formaldehyde? | Asbestos, Indoor Air Pollutants, Lead |
| | Is there ongoing or planned renovation? | Asbestos, Lead |
| | Do you have carbon monoxide (CO) detectors? | Carbon Monoxide |
| | What type of heating/air system does your home have? | Indoor Air Pollutants |
| | Where and how do you store chemicals and pesticides? | Pesticides |
| | Do you use chemicals in the garden or spray the lawn with pesticides? | Pesticides |
| | Have you tested your home for radon? | Radon |
| | Do you think there is lead in your soil? | Lead |
| | Do you have a playset or picnic table made of treated wood? | Arsenic |
| | Is there exposure to excessive noise? | Noise |
| — At school | Are there concerns about your child's school environment? | Schools |
| — In the community | Is there a source of pollution in your community? | Environmental Equity, Indoor Air Pollutants, Outdoor Air Pollutants, Waste Sites |
| **Tobacco smoke and nicotine exposure** | Does anyone living in or visiting your home use tobacco in any way? Who does? Where does this person smoke? Is that in the house? Does anyone smoke in the car?[5] Does anyone in the family use an alternative nicotine product (including electronic cigarettes)?[6] | Asthma, Tobacco Use and Tobacco Smoke Exposure, Electronic Cigarettes and other Alternative Nicotine Products |

| | | FOR MORE INFORMATION, |
|---|---|---|
| **AREA** | **QUESTIONS** | **SEE CHAPTER ON** |
| **Water sources** | Do you use tap water? Well water? | Lead, Nitrates, Water, Arsenic |
| **Dietary exposures** | What kind of cereal does your baby eat? Does your family eat rice? Does your child drink juice? Do you eat fish? Does your child eat fish? What kinds and how often? | Arsenic, Mercury, Persistent Organic Pollutants |
| **Sun and other exposure to ultraviolet radiation (UVR)** | Is your child protected from excessive sun exposure? Do you visit tanning salons or other indoor tanning facilities? | Ultraviolet Radiation |

**Table 5-2. Summary of Environmental Health Questions for Health Supervision Visits[a] (*continued*)**

[a]Table is adapted from Balk SJ et al.[4]

## 1. Physical Surroundings

### At Home

Young children spend 80% to 90% of their time indoors—in their own home or in a relative's home or child care setting.

Important questions related to the home include:

- What type of building environments does your child live in or spend time in?
- What are the age and condition of your home? Is there lead, mold, or asbestos?
- Is there ongoing or planned renovation?
- Do you have carbon monoxide (CO) detectors?
- What type of heating/air system does your home have?
- Where and how do you store chemicals and pesticides?
- Do you use chemicals in the garden or spray the lawn with pesticides?
- Have you tested your home for radon?
- Do you live in an area where elevated levels of lead in the soil could be a concern?
- Do your children play on a wooden playset or use a wooden picnic table?

### What type of building environments does your child live in or spend time in?

Is it a single-family home, apartment, mobile home, or temporary shelter? Single-family homes or apartments may have high levels of radon in basements or lower floors, or friable asbestos. Mobile homes may be constructed using materials such as particle board and pressed-wood products containing formaldehyde, a respiratory and dermal irritant.

## What are the age and condition of your home? Is there lead, mold, or asbestos?

*Lead:* Lead paint could be used in home construction until the late 1970s. Buildings constructed before 1950 are most likely to have leaded paint that may peel, chip, or chalk. Leaded paint is the most common and most concentrated source of lead for children living in older housing. Lead dust can be released from poorly maintained surfaces, and by friction, such as occurs at doors or windows.

*Recommendations:* Federal law requires testing of Medicaid-eligible children at 1 and 2 years of age. Other children should be tested according to state or local guidelines, or other risk factors. Immigrant, refugee, and internationally adopted children are at increased risk for lead poisoning; it is recommended that their blood lead concentrations be tested when they arrive in the United States.[7]

*Mold and Dampness:* Homes that have flooded or have leaky plumbing or roofs may have mold growth; exposure may be associated with respiratory symptoms. A damp or musty smell indicates the presence of mold. Ineffective and unused ventilation contributes to mold or dampness. Mold also may be associated with allergies; it can trigger exacerbations of asthma. Exposure to the mold *Stachybotrys atra* (also known as *Stachybotrys chartarum*) has been associated with the development of acute pulmonary hemorrhage in young infants. Exposure to secondhand smoke in the presence of mold increases the infant's risk of developing acute pulmonary hemorrhage.[8]

*Recommendations:* It is reasonable for pediatricians to advise that infants should not be exposed to *Stachybotrys atra*. Water leaks and other sources of water intrusion should be repaired, and all reservoirs of mold should be removed. Areas of visible mold measuring 3 feet by 3 feet or less can be removed using a household detergent and water or a dilute solution of chlorine bleach (1 part chlorine to 10 parts water).[9] It is important to use an adequately ventilated space if bleach is used. Infants, young children, and anyone with respiratory tract disease should avoid the area until it has been cleaned. Removal by a professional trained in mold remediation is recommended for moldy areas greater than 3 feet by 3 feet or if removal of building materials is required.[9] Mold present on hard surfaces can be wiped clean. Dry cleaning may be attempted for visible mold growth on clothing. Permeable and semipermeable materials, such as upholstered furniture and carpeting, should be discarded if there is mold growth. Surfaces in the cleaned area should then be vacuumed with a high-efficiency particulate air (HEPA) vacuum before resuming use of the area. Mold is ubiquitous, and the expectation of creating an entirely "mold-free" environment is unrealistic. A healthy environment, however, is dry and free of visible mold growth beyond that which normally occurs (eg, bathroom mold). Children (especially infants) and others should not be exposed to moldy environments.

Information about cleaning homes that have been flooded is available from the US Environmental Protection Agency (EPA).[10]

*Asbestos:* Asbestos was commonly used decades ago as insulation around boilers and pipes, in ceiling and floor tiles, and other areas. Asbestos coverings can deteriorate, or if disturbed, asbestos can be released into the air during renovation or other work. Airborne asbestos may be inhaled into the lungs, possibly resulting in mesothelioma or lung cancer years after exposure.

*Recommendations:* Asbestos can be identified visually by a certified inspector or by contacting the manufacturer of the product. Undamaged asbestos is best left alone. Asbestos in poor condition (more than a very small amount) must be removed by a certified asbestos contractor.[11]

## Is there ongoing or planned renovation?

Renovation of a bedroom is common to prepare for the birth of a baby or to update the room decor as the child grows. Improper renovation procedures may expose a pregnant woman, her fetus, or child to lead or other dusts, asbestos, and mold. Newly installed carpets may release irritating or toxic vapors.

*Recommendations:* Pregnant women and young children should vacate their premises during renovation if there is the possibility of exposure to lead, mold, or other contaminants. Only certified contractors should conduct renovation activities that involve removal of lead or asbestos. The premises should be ventilated to limit exposure to irritating or toxic vapors. Residents may return only after the areas are certified as free of lead or asbestos.

## Do you have CO detectors?

Unintentional CO poisoning causes hundreds of deaths in the United States each year.

*Recommendations:* Chimneys should be inspected and cleaned each year. Combustion appliances must be properly installed, maintained, and vented according to manufacturers' instructions. The Consumer Product Safety Commission recommends that parents install CO detectors meeting the most recent standards of the Underwriters Laboratories (UL) in every sleeping area.[12] Parents should never ignore an alarming CO detector. Note: children may already be symptomatic from excess CO when a CO monitor alarm sounds.

## What type of heating/air system does your home have?

Wood stoves and fireplaces emit respiratory irritants (nitrogen dioxide [$NO_2$], respirable particulates, and polycyclic aromatic hydrocarbons), especially when they are not properly vented and maintained. Gas stoves, which may produce $NO_2$, are used in more than half of US homes. Respiratory symptoms may occur when gas stoves are used as supplemental heat. Wood stoves, fireplaces, and other fuel-burning appliances may be sources of CO.

*Recommendations:* Parents should be advised to regularly maintain and clean heating systems. Use of wood-burning appliances should be discouraged, if possible, when children have asthma or other chronic respiratory conditions. Information about wood stoves, including health effects of exposure, and installing cleaner and more efficient stoves, is available from the US EPA.[13]

### Where and how do you store chemicals and pesticides?

Pesticides and other chemicals can cause acute poisoning and death as well as subacute and chronic poisoning.

*Recommendations:* Parents can be encouraged to use the least toxic options for pest control. Integrated pest management (IPM) is an approach that uses chemical and nonchemical methods to provide the least toxic alternative for pest control. IPM uses regular monitoring (rather than predetermined chemical applications) to determine whether and when treatments are needed. If toxic chemicals are used, they should be placed out of children's reach. Chemicals should be stored in original containers and never in containers such as soda or juice bottles.

### Do you use chemicals in the garden or spray the lawn with pesticides?

Children may inhale and absorb pesticide residues as they crawl or play on freshly sprayed outdoor surfaces, such as lawns and gardens, or on indoor surfaces, such as upholstery or rugs. Pesticide residues may adhere to plush toys.

*Recommendations:* Spraying or "bombing" with pesticides is hazardous, especially while children are young or when a woman is pregnant. Pediatricians should discourage using pesticides in the home or garden for ornamental purposes. There is no clearly established length of time that parents must prohibit children from playing in freshly sprayed lawns and gardens. If a parent has applied an herbicide, it is reasonable to wait at least 24 to 48 hours before a child has contact with the lawn. Insecticides are generally more toxic to animals than are compounds designed to kill plants. It is, therefore, reasonable to avoid contact for a longer time period, such as 48 to 72 hours, after insecticide application.[4]

### Have you tested your home for radon?

Approximately 10% of lung cancer in the United States is attributable to radon, a preventable exposure.

*Recommendations:* The US EPA and the US Surgeon General recommend testing homes below the third floor for radon.[14] The US EPA recommends that radon testing be performed before buying or selling a home.[14]

## Do you live in an area where elevated levels of lead in the soil could be a concern?

Lead contaminates soil when paint chips or dust from old buildings mixes with the soil. Lead was present in gasoline in the United States until the 1970s. Because lead moves little once deposited, lead that originated from auto emissions or deteriorating paint can be present in soil. In urban areas, soil lead levels are highest around building foundations. A garden located near heavily trafficked roads may have a high lead content and plants grown in these gardens can absorb lead.

*Recommendations:* The US EPA recommends placing doormats outside and inside all entryways and removing shoes before entering to avoid tracking contaminated soil into the home. The US EPA also recommends planting bushes close to the house to keep children from playing in soil next to the home.[15] If high levels of lead in soil are suspected and there are young children who play there, parents are encouraged to have the soil tested.

## Do your children play on a wooden playset or use a wooden picnic table?

Outdoor wooden playsets and picnic tables may have been treated with the preservative chromated copper arsenate (CCA) to protect wood from decay. Children's hand-mouth behavior may result in exposure to arsenic leaching from the CCA. Manufacturers reached a voluntary agreement with the US EPA to end the manufacture of CCA-treated wood for most consumer applications by December 31, 2003. Some stocks of wood treated before then were expected to be found on shelves until mid-2004. Hundreds of thousands of play structures, decks, and tables were built before the ban and some may still be in use.

*Recommendations:* If there is a wooden playset, deck, or picnic table manufactured before 2003, parents can call the manufacturer to determine whether it contains CCA. CCA in decks, play structures, or picnic tables should be treated with a clear sealant every 6 months to 1 year to decrease the amount of arsenic leaching from the wood. Alternatively, parents can choose to have the set or table safely dismantled. CCA-treated wood should not be burned or sawed because this will increase the amount of arsenic released. If parents keep a playset, they should wash children's hands with soap and water immediately after outdoor play, and especially before eating. Children should not eat while playing on CCA-treated playground equipment. It is prudent to cover a treated picnic table with a cloth before eating.

### At School

### Are there concerns about your child's school environment?

Many hazards found in home environments may also be encountered in school environments but schools also may have additional hazards (see Chapter 11).

Children engaging in arts and crafts activities may encounter potential hazards, such as felt-tip markers (containing aromatic hydrocarbons) and oil-based paints. Children with certain disabilities may be at more risk of toxic exposures. Visually impaired children working close to a project, or children with asthma, may be affected by fumes. Children unable to follow safety precautions may contaminate their skin or place art materials in their mouths. Emotionally disturbed children may abuse art materials, endangering themselves and others.

*Recommendations:* Parents concerned about possible exposures in the school should be encouraged to act as advocates for their child. Pediatricians may sometimes be helpful in the advocacy process.

### In the Community

**Is there a source of pollution in your community? Do you live near a major roadway, highway, or airport?**

Toxic hazards may exist in the community. Sources of exposure include polluted lakes and streams, industrial plants, and dump sites. Children can be exposed to lead if they live downwind from a lead smelter or to pesticides or other chemicals if they live on farms or at the urban-rural interface. Because small aircraft still use leaded fuel, children living very near small airports also can be exposed to lead. Air quality is often poorer around homes and buildings located within 300 meters of a major highway. Low-income communities and racial/ethnic minority communities are more likely to face toxic hazards, termed "environmental disparities" or "environmental injustice" (see Chapter 55).

A child or teenager may have experienced a disaster such as Superstorm Sandy, Hurricanes Katrina, Harvey or Maria, or the World Trade Center disaster. Exposure to catastrophic environmental occurrences may have long-term effects on physical and mental health.

Other aspects of "community" may affect health—for example, health is often influenced by the presence or absence of safe places to walk and exercise.

*Recommendations:* Parents concerned about possible exposures in their community should be encouraged to act as advocates for their family. Pediatricians can help with this process. If the family is planning a move, it may be relevant to consider the proximity of the new home to traffic pollution because air quality is affected near major highways. This is especially relevant if the child has a respiratory condition.

## 2. Tobacco Smoke Exposure

- Does your child live with anyone who uses tobacco?
- Does anyone who provides care for your child smoke?
- Does your child visit places where people smoke?
- Does anyone ever smoke in your home?

- Does anyone ever smoke in your car?
- Do you ever smell smoke from your neighbors in or near your home or apartment?[4]

Exposure to secondhand tobacco smoke (SHS) places exposed individuals at risk of significant morbidity and mortality. "Third-hand smoke" describes the mixture of gases and particles clinging to smokers' hair and clothing and to furniture and carpeting in a room. Third-hand smoke pollutants may linger after SHS has cleared from a room, accumulate on the hands of children who live in environments where tobacco is used, and may contribute to children's overall tobacco smoke exposure.[16]

*Recommendations:* If parents or other caregivers smoke or use other tobacco or nicotine products (such as electronic cigarettes or hookahs [see Chapter 28]), pediatricians should advise them to quit and offer help in doing so. Educating parents about the associations between SHS and their child's illness may help them quit. Parents can also be informed that their children are more likely to begin smoking if parents smoke. The US Preventive Services Task Force (USPSTF), an independent organization of experts who evaluate the effectiveness of clinical preventive health services, recommends that clinicians ask all adults about smoking at every clinical encounter and offer smokers at least a brief (1 to 3 minutes) intervention at each visit.[17] This recommendation received an "A" rating, meaning that "there is high certainty that the net benefit is substantial."[18]

Quit-smoking telephone counseling, available throughout the nation, is effective in helping smokers to quit. SmokefreeTXT (https://smokefree.gov/smokefreetxt) is a mobile text messaging service for US adults and young adults that offers encouragement, advice, and tips for smokers who want to quit. Whether or not parents choose to quit, they should introduce and enforce strict no-smoking bans in the home and car. If they have been smoking, parents and others should wash their hands and change clothes before interacting with their child. Parents should strive to avoid exposing children to any environment that contains tobacco smoke. Pediatricians should discuss the hazards of cigarette smoking with school-aged children and teenagers.

Teenagers who smoke should be advised to quit. Even if they are not smokers, teenagers should be asked about exposure to SHS because they may be exposed by family or friends who do smoke. Electronic cigarettes provide a new pathway to nicotine addiction in young people. Therefore, pediatricians should strongly discourage teens from using these and other alternative nicotine delivery products (see Chapter 28).

## 3. Water Sources

- Do you use tap water? Well water?

Water contaminants of particular concern for US infants and children are lead and nitrates.

*Lead:* Most large municipal water supplies maintain lead levels of less than the US EPA standard of 15 parts per billion (ppb). Most systems have acceptable lead levels. Until the late 1980s, lead solder was widely used to connect copper pipes; plumbing fixtures also may contain lead. It is possible for lead to leach from lead-containing components of water systems[7] and tap water used to reconstitute infant formula may be contaminated with lead.[19] Although water in a home may be free of lead, water in a child care setting, school, or playground may contain unacceptable lead levels.

Changes in water additives may increase lead leaching.[20] In Flint, MI in 2014, the city changed its water supply, prompted by a desire to save money. The switch to the more caustic Flint River water without proper corrosion control caused corrosion in the leaded pipes, resulting in leaching of lead and a public health crisis.[21]

*Recommendations:* Parents can be informed that in general, it is safe to assume that water from large municipal supplies is monitored to maintain recommended levels of lead. To decrease the possibility of contamination from leaded pipes and solder, water that has been standing in pipes overnight should be run until it becomes as cold as it can get, before it is used. Parents should use only water from the cold-water tap for drinking, cooking, and especially for making baby formula. Hot water is likely to contain higher levels of lead.[22] Parents can also choose to test their water for lead. They also can ask child care providers and school officials about testing all drinking water outlets in the building and playground, especially those supplying water used to drink, cook, and prepare infant formula.[23] Bottled water may be an acceptable, although expensive, alternative. Certain countertop filters and certain filters applied to the tap can remove lead.[22] Depending on the child's age, housing situation, and other risk factors, children should be tested according to the US Centers for Disease Control and Prevention (CDC) guidelines with a blood lead test.

*Nitrates and Coliforms:* Infants exposed to high levels of nitrates in well water may develop methemoglobinemia, which may result in death. Well water may also contain coliform bacteria. High levels of nitrates or coliforms in the water may indicate the presence of pesticides.

*Recommendations:* When buying or purchasing a home, parents should have their private wells tested for nitrates, coliforms, and inorganic compounds (total dissolved solids, iron, magnesium, calcium, chloride, and lead). Testing for nitrates and coliforms should be performed annually. Repeat testing for other contaminants should be considered if a new source of contamination becomes known (for example, if a neighbor discovers a new contaminant in his or her well).[24] Federal guidelines are available; local health or environmental departments can advise about testing.[25]

Well water should be tested for nitrates and coliforms before being offered to an infant. Water high in nitrates or coliforms should not be given to infants.

Boiling water for infant formula is rarely necessary. Overboiling water for infant formula preparation concentrates lead and nitrates. Water brought to a rolling boil for 1 minute kills microorganisms such as *Cryptosporidium* species without concentrating lead or nitrates; at altitudes greater than 6,562 feet (>2,000 m), water should be boiled for 3 minutes.[26]

## 4. Exposures from Food

- What kind of infant cereal do you plan to introduce to your baby? Does your family eat much rice? Does your child drink fruit juice?

### Arsenic in Rice Cereal, Juice, and Rice Products

Rice cereal traditionally is the first solid food given to babies. Rice cereal is easy to digest, is unlikely to cause allergies, and is fortified with iron needed as the infant outgrows iron stores. In 2012, the nonprofit Consumers Union called attention to research showing elevated levels of arsenic in rice products, including infant rice cereal. After Consumers Union called for regulation of arsenic in these products, in 2016 the US Food and Drug Administration (FDA) proposed draft guidance to industry to limit inorganic arsenic to 100 ppb in infant rice cereal.[27,28] Until FDA guidance is finalized, it is reasonable for pediatricians to recommend iron-fortified oatmeal, barley, or multigrain cereal as an infant's first food. Rice milk is not recommended for infants.

Rice is a staple food for many families. Because rice plants readily take up any arsenic from soil they are grown in, it is reasonable to advise families to include a variety of grains in their diet.[29]

Elevated arsenic levels were found in some apple and grape juice samples. As of 2013, the FDA proposed an action level of 10 ppb for inorganic arsenic in juice, identical to the US EPA's 2001 limit for drinking water.[30] Until these limits are finalized, it makes sense to vary the source of children's juice. Juice is not a necessary part of a child's diet. If parents decide to introduce juice, they should wait until their child reaches at least age 1.

### Fish

Do you eat fish?
- Does your child eat fish?
- What kinds and how often?

Although fish is an excellent source of protein and some fish contain high amounts of omega-3 fatty acids, certain fish may be contaminated with excessive amounts of mercury or polychlorinated biphenyls (PCBs). Exposure to these contaminants may have adverse effects, especially on fetuses and young children.

***Recommendations:*** Families eating commercially caught fish should choose fish low in mercury and other pollutants. The FDA issued guidance about fish low in mercury.[31] Children most often eat shrimp (low in mercury and PCBs but high in cholesterol and most often sourced from overseas using highly unsustainable practices), salmon (high in omega-3 fatty acids; historically, farm-raised salmon had higher PCB levels but this is less of a concern recently), and canned tuna (light or skipjack tuna has the lowest mercury content whereas yellowfin, albacore/white, and especially bluefin have higher mercury content). Families catching their own fish should follow fish advisories issued by state and local health departments to determine which fish are safe to eat.

### 5. Sun and Other Exposure to Ultraviolet Radiation (UVR)

- Is your child protected from excessive sun exposure?
- Do you visit tanning parlors?

About one quarter of a person's exposure to the sun occurs before age 18. Early exposure to UVR increases skin cancer risk. Teenagers, especially teen girls, often visit tanning salons, thereby also raising their skin cancer risk. This includes risk of melanoma, a common cancer in teenagers and young adults and the skin cancer most likely to result in fatality.

The USPSTF recommends that clinicians counsel fair-skinned individuals aged 6 months to 24 years to avoid excessive ultraviolet radiation exposure to decrease their skin cancer risk, giving this recommendation a "B" rating.[32] The B rating indicates "that there is high certainty that the net benefit is moderate or there is moderate certainty that the net benefit is moderate to substantial."[18]

*Recommendations:* Advice about sun protection includes covering up with clothing and hats, timing children's activities to avoid peak sun exposure, consulting the Ultraviolet Index, using sunscreen and reapplying frequently as needed, and wearing sunglasses. Teenagers and others should not visit tanning salons.

### 6. Noise Exposure

Noise, defined as unwanted or disturbing sound, often goes unrecognized as an individual and public health problem. Although noise generally is not appreciated as a serious public health issue, noise pollution affects millions of people in the United States.[33] Noise can affect hearing, learning, result in a physiologic stress response, and cause psychological harm. Because damage to hearing accumulates, noise exposures starting in earlier life are potentially more harmful as people age.

*Recommendations:* Pediatricians should discuss noise exposures with families. Advice includes avoiding toys, such as cap pistols, that make loud noises; and reducing the volume on televisions, computers, radios, and personal music devices. In particular, older children and teens should be cautioned to use their headphones and earbuds judiciously. Earplugs, noise-cancelling headphones, or noise-cancelling earbuds should be used if parents or children are attending loud events, such as rock concerts or dances. If the level of noise is perceived as uncomfortable or painful, it is prudent to leave the event.

## 7. Exposures Resulting From Occupations and Hobbies

- What are parents' and teenagers' jobs?
- What are parents' and teenagers' hobbies?

Parental occupations may produce hazards for a child. Workplace contaminants may be transported to the home on clothes, shoes, and skin surfaces.[34] Lead poisoning has been described in children of lead storage battery workers[35] and through take-home exposure from a father working in an electronic scrap recycling facility;[36] asbestos-related lung diseases have been found in families of shipyard workers, miners, insulators, and others;[37] and elevated mercury concentrations have been reported in children whose parents worked in a mercury thermometer plant.[38] Parents who work with art materials at home may expose children to toxicants, such as lead used in solder, pottery glazes, or stained glass.

Employment may help teenagers develop skills and responsibility and earn money, but work activities may carry the risk of toxic exposure or injury. Environmental exposures include UVR with outdoor work, SHS encountered in restaurants and bars, pesticides from lawn-care and farm work, and noise from operating equipment. Work may also interfere with an adolescent's education, sleep, and social behavior. Federal and state child labor laws regulate employment of children younger than age 18. These laws address the minimum ages for general and specific types of employment, maximum daily and weekly number of hours of work permitted, prohibition of work during night hours, prohibition of certain types of employment, and the registration of minors for employment.[39]

Hobby activity may pose a risk to school-aged children and adolescents. Shooting at an indoor firing range may result in lead exposure.[40] Toluene and other solvents may be encountered in glues used in model-building. Adolescents may be especially at risk of huffing (inhaling) if glue is present in their environments, resulting in easy access.

*Recommendations:* An occupational history may be obtained when information about family composition and the family history is obtained. Workers exposed to toxic substances are legally entitled to be notified of these exposures under federal "right-to-know" and "hazard communication" laws. Parents who work with toxic substances should shower, if possible, and change clothes and shoes before leaving work. At home, children should not be allowed in rooms where parents work with toxic substances.

## VISITS FOR ILLNESS: CONSIDERING ENVIRONMENTAL ETIOLOGIES IN THE DIFFERENTIAL DIAGNOSIS

Secondhand tobacco smoke is the most common toxicant associated with respiratory diseases, such as asthma; recurrent lower and upper airway disease; and persistent middle ear effusion. Lead poisoning may present with recurrent abdominal pain, constipation, irritability, developmental delay, seizures, or unexplained coma. Foods and medications brought from other countries may be sources of lead and other heavy metals. Headaches may be caused by acute and chronic exposure to CO from improperly vented heating sources, formaldehyde, and chemicals used on the job or in the home. Pediatricians should ask about mold and water damage in the home when they treat infants with acute pulmonary hemorrhage.

Environmental causes of illness may not always be apparent.[41] Because most environmental or occupational illnesses present as common medical problems or have nonspecific symptoms, the diagnosis may be missed unless an exposure history is obtained. This is especially important if the illness is atypical or unresponsive to treatment. The following questions may provide information about whether an illness is related to the environment.

1. Do symptoms subside or worsen in a particular location (eg, home, child care, school, a certain room)?
2. Do symptoms subside or worsen during a particular time? At a particular time of day? On weekdays or weekends? During a particular week or season?
3. Do symptoms worsen during a particular activity? While the child is playing outside, or engaging in hobby activities, such as working with arts and crafts?
4. Are siblings or other children experiencing similar symptoms?
5. What are parents' thoughts about why symptoms are occurring?

Three case examples illustrate integrating environmental health etiologies into the differential diagnosis:

## Case 1: Asthma

*A 5-year-old boy comes to your office for follow-up from a hospitalization for an asthma exacerbation. He was diagnosed with mild persistent asthma 2 years ago and has been on an inhaled corticosteroid to help control symptoms. Before increasing his dose of controller medications, or adding another controller, what else do you need to know?*

Environmental triggers that may precipitate asthma exacerbations include:

- Secondhand smoke
- Other air pollutants (eg, particulate matter or oxides of nitrogen [$NO_x$]) from wood burning stoves, fireplaces
- Molds, pollen
- Dust mites
- Cockroaches
- Animal allergens
- Odors
- Volatile organic compounds (such as formaldehyde) from air fresheners, paints, insecticides, cosmetics, cleaning products

Most of these triggers are amenable to environmental interventions. Asking about environmental exposures and suggesting ways to decrease exposures may result in improved symptoms (See Chapter 47).

## Case 2: Fever and Rash

*A 3-year-old boy comes in with a 1-week history of fever, rash, and difficulty walking. His medical history is unremarkable. Physical examination reveals an irritable child with temperature of 104°F (40°C), conjunctival injection, pharyngeal erythema, swelling of the hands and feet, and a macular rash. What is in your differential diagnosis?*

The differential diagnosis includes:

- Kawasaki disease
- Measles
- Scarlet fever
- Juvenile rheumatoid arthritis
- Acrodynia

Although the child described in this case is later diagnosed with Kawasaki disease, the differential diagnosis includes acrodynia ("pink disease"), a rare hypersensitivity reaction to mercury that occurs mainly in children. In the past, acrodynia was described after exposure to mercury-containing teething powders, and in more recent times after exposure to mercury-containing latex paint (voluntarily ceased in 1990) and mercury-containing diaper rinses. Prominent symptoms are neurologic, including irritability, photophobia, weakness, and paresthesias. Physical examination reveals an acral rash with edematous, painful, pink and red desquamating fingers and toes. Hypertension is a cardinal finding. Acrodynia now is a relatively rare condition. It is important to consider this diagnosis when there is a child with neurologic symptoms and signs, hypertension, and red, edematous, desquamating hands and feet.[42]

## Case 3: Seizure (adapted from Khine et al[43])

*A 3-year-old Hispanic girl with a history of seizures presents to the emergency department (ED) after a generalized tonic-clonic seizure. She received rectal diazepam at home before her arrival in the ED. She is awake but tired. She is afebrile and her physical examination is normal. The child's medical history is significant for a seizure disorder of unknown etiology diagnosed at age 3 months. An MRA/MRI of the brain and electroencephalogram (EEG) done 2 years previously were normal. What is in the differential diagnosis?*

The differential diagnosis includes:

- Seizure disorder of unknown etiology
- Infection
- Brain tumor
- Toxic ingestion
- Other toxic exposure

Alcohol, acetaminophen, aspirin, and iron are not detected on serum toxicology screening. The results of urine toxicology screening for drugs of abuse are negative.

A recent report has called attention to seizures occurring in children exposed to camphor, a known cause of seizures and reported after camphor ingestion, inhalation, and dermal absorption.[28] Camphor (alcanfor in Spanish) is commonly used as a natural remedy in certain populations. When questioned specifically about camphor, the mother reveals that she was rubbing a properly labeled camphor ointment over the child's upper chest, forehead, and back hourly for several hours before the onset of the seizure, to relieve her cold symptoms. The mother used camphor-containing products in various other ways, such as putting it in the vaporizer, placing it in a bowl with water under the crib, hanging camphor tablets in a meshed cloth on the posts of the crib, and spreading crushed tablets around the house to control roaches. Two of the mother's other children had seizure disorders; all had evaluations and normal imaging studies. The other siblings did not suffer seizures when they previously lived in the grandmother's apartment for 1 year. The grandmother did not allow the use of camphor during that time. Use of camphor products in the home was discontinued, and anticonvulsant medications were discontinued for the children. On follow-up 10 weeks after this seizure, no further episodes of seizures were reported in any of the children.

The US FDA restricts the camphor content to less than 11% in some products intended for medicinal use. Camphor products intended for use as pesticides must be registered with the US EPA. Nevertheless, many imported camphor-containing products fail to meet the requirements of the US FDA and the US EPA for labeling and content. This case illustrates the importance of asking about camphor use when a child has a seizure and of educating families about the risks of using camphor.

## Resources

### Agency for Toxic Substances and Disease Registry (ATSDR) Case Studies in Environmental Medicine

Elements of a pediatric environmental history are reviewed in "Principles of Pediatric Environmental Health," one of several monographs in the Case Studies in Environmental Medicine series available from the ATSDR. Web site: https://www.atsdr.cdc.gov/csem/csem.asp?csem=27&po=0

### ATSDR–PSR Environmental Health Toolkit

The ATSDR, the Greater Boston Physicians for Social Responsibility (PSR), and the University of California-San Francisco Pediatric Environmental Health Specialty Unit collaborated to develop an environmental health anticipatory guidance online training module with downloadable tools for use in clinical practice. The Toolkit includes materials to help provide guidance to clinicians and parents focused on preventing exposures to toxic substances and other substances affecting children's health.

Web sites: Toolkit materials

https://www.atsdr.cdc.gov/emes/health_professionals/pediatrics.html

www.psr.org/resources/pediatric-environmental-health-toolkit.html

## Bright Futures

Bright Futures, a national health promotion and prevention initiative, is led by the American Academy of Pediatrics (AAP) with support from the US Department of Health and Human Services, Health Resources and Services Administration (HRSA), and Maternal and Child Health Bureau (MCHB). The *Bright Futures Guidelines* provide theory-based and evidence-driven guidance for all preventive care screenings and well-child visits including guidance about several environmental exposures.

Web site: https://brightfutures.aap.org/Pages/default

## National Environmental Education Foundation (NEEF)

NEEF is a national nonprofit organization with several educational initiatives related to pediatric environmental health, including a Pediatric Environmental History Initiative. Resources include history forms for taking a general environmental history and for a child with asthma.

Web site: www.neefusa.org/health

## Pediatric Environmental Health Specialty Units

Pediatric Environmental Health Specialty Units (PEHSU) are composed of environmental health specialists located in several centers in North America. PEHSU staff respond to questions from clinicians, public health professionals, policy makers, and the public about the impacts of environmental factors on children's health and the health of reproductive-age adults. PEHSU staff offer webinars and courses, fact sheets, and experts who can answer questions about environmental health issues relevant to children.

Web site: www.pehsu.net

## References

1. Galvez MP, Balk SJ. Environmental risks to children: prioritizing health messages in pediatric practice. *Pediatr Rev.* 2017;38(6):263–277

2. Hagan JF, Duncan PM. Maximizing children's health: Screening, anticipatory guidance and counseling. In: *Nelson's Textbook of Pediatrics.* 20th edition. Kliegman RM, Behrman RE, St Geme JW, Schor NF, Behrman RE, eds. Philadelphia, PA: Saunders Elsevier; 2016

3. National Environmental Education Foundation. Pediatric Environmental History Forms. https://www.neefusa.org/resource/pediatric-environmental-history. Accessed April 20, 2018

4. Balk SJ, Forman JA, Johnson CL, Roberts JR. Safeguarding kids from environmental hazards. *Contemp Pediatr.* 2007;24(3):64–78

5. American Academy of Pediatrics Section on Tobacco Control. Clinical practice policy to protect children from tobacco, nicotine, and tobacco smoke. *Pediatrics.* 2015;136(5): 1008–1017

6. Walley SC, Jenssen BP, Section on Tobacco Control. Electronic nicotine delivery systems. *Pediatrics*. 2015;136(5):1018–1026

7. American Academy of Pediatrics Council on Environmental Health. Policy statement. Prevention of childhood lead toxicity. *Pediatrics*. 2016;38(1):e20161493

8. American Academy of Pediatrics, Committee on Environmental Health. Spectrum of noninfectious health effects from molds. *Pediatrics*. 2006;118(6):2582–2586

9. National Environmental Education Foundation. Mold/mildew and asthma. In: Environmental Intervention Guidelines and Patient Handouts. National Environmental Education Foundation; Washington DC, 2017. https://www.neefusa.org/sites/default/files/assets/health/guidelines/english/2016/Asthma_mold_mildew.pdf. Accessed April 20, 2018

10. US Environmental Protection Agency. Resources for Flood Cleanup and Mold. https://www.epa.gov/mold/resources-flood-cleanup-and-mold. Accessed April 20, 2018

11. US Environmental Protection Agency. Asbestos. Protect Your Family. https://www.epa.gov/asbestos/protect-your-family. Accessed April 20, 2018

12. Underwriters Laboratories. Exposing an invisible killer: The dangers of carbon monoxide. https://www.ul.com/newsroom/pressreleases/exposing-an-invisible-killer-the-dangers-of-carbon-monoxide. Accessed April 20, 2018

13. US Environmental Protection Agency. Burn Wise. https://www.epa.gov/burnwise. Accessed April 20, 2018

14. US Environmental Protection Agency. Radon. https://www.epa.gov/radon. Accessed April 20, 2018

15. US Environmental Protection Agency. Protect Your Family from Exposures to Lead. https://www.epa.gov/lead/protect-your-family-exposures-lead#soil. Accessed April 20, 2018

16. Mahabee-Gittens EM, Merianos AL, Matt GE. Preliminary evidence that high levels of nicotine on children's hands may contribute to overall tobacco smoke exposure. *Tob Control*. 2018;27(2):217–219

17. Agency for Healthcare Research and Quality. Treating Tobacco Use and Dependence: 2008 Update. https://www.ahrq.gov/professionals/clinicians-providers/guidelines-recommendations/tobacco/index.html. Accessed April 20, 2018

18. United States Preventive Services Task Force. Grade Definitions. https://www.uspreventiveservicestaskforce.org/Page/Name/grade-definitions#brec2. Accessed April 20, 2018

19. Baum CR, Shannon MW. The lead concentration of reconstituted infant formula. *J Toxicol Clin Toxicol*. 1997;35(4):371–375

20. Edwards M, Triantafyllidou S, Best D. Elevated blood lead in young children due to lead-contaminated drinking water: Washington, DC: 2001-2004. *Environ Sci Technol*. 2009;43(5):1618–1623

21. National Public Radio. Lead-Laced Water In Flint: A Step-By-Step Look At The Makings Of A Crisis. http://www.npr.org/sections/thetwo-way/2016/04/20/465545378/lead-laced-water-in-flint-a-step-by-step-look-at-the-makings-of-a-crisis. Accessed April 20, 2018

22. US Environmental Protection Agency. Basic Information about Lead in Drinking Water. https://www.epa.gov/ground-water-and-drinking-water/basic-information-about-lead-drinking-water#reducehome. Accessed April 20, 2018

23. US Environmental Protection Agency. Protect Your Family from Exposures to Lead. https://www.epa.gov/lead/protect-your-family-exposures-lead#protect. Accessed April 20, 2018

24. American Academy of Pediatrics, Committee on Environmental Health and Committee on Infectious Diseases. Drinking water from private wells and risks to children. *Pediatrics*. 2009;123(6):1599–1605

25. Centers for Disease Control and Prevention. Well Testing. http://www.cdc.gov/healthywater/drinking/private/wells/testing.html. Accessed April 20, 2018

26. Centers for Disease Control and Prevention. Parasites – Cryptosporidium (also known as "Crypto"). http://www.cdc.gov/parasites/crypto/health_professionals/bwa/public.html. Accessed April 20, 2018

27. Food and Drug Administration. Arsenic in Rice and Rice Products. https://www.fda.gov/food/foodborneillnesscontaminants/metals/ucm319870.htm. Accessed April 20, 2018

28. American Academy of Pediatrics. AAP Welcomes FDA Announcement on Limiting Arsenic in Infant Rice Cereal. https://www.aap.org/en-us/about-the-aap/aap-press-room/pages/AAP-Welcomes-FDA-Announcement-on-Limiting-Arsenic-in-Infant-Rice-Cereal.aspx. Accessed April 20, 2018

29. Consumer Reports. Arsenic in rice and rice products. http://www.consumerreports.org/video/view/healthy-living/food-nutrition/1895177516001/arsenic-in-rice-and-rice-products. Accessed April 20, 2018

30. Food and Drug Administration. Questions & Answers: Apple Juice and Arsenic. https://www.fda.gov/food/resourcesforyou/consumers/ucm271595.htm. Accessed April 20, 2018

31. Food and Drug Administration. Advice About Eating Fish. What Pregnant Women & Parents Should Know. January 2017. https://www.fda.gov/downloads/Food/ResourcesForYou/Consumers/UCM536321.pdf. Accessed April 20, 2018

32. United States Preventive Services Task Force Final Recommendation Statement: Skin Cancer Prevention: Behavioral Counseling. https://www.uspreventiveservicestaskforce.org/Page/Document/UpdateSummaryFinal/skin-cancer-counseling2?ds=1&s=skin%20cancer%20prevention. Accessed August 26, 2018.

33. US Environmental Protection Agency. Clean Air Act Title IV - Noise Pollution. https://www.epa.gov/clean-air-act-overview/clean-air-act-title-iv-noise-pollution. Accessed April 20, 2018

34. Chisolm JJ. Fouling one's own nest. *Pediatrics.* 1978;62(4):614–617

35. Whelan EA, Piacitelli GM, Gerwel B, et al. Elevated blood lead levels in children of construction workers. *Am J Public Health.* 1997;87(8):1352–1355

36. Newman N, Jones C, Page E, Ceballos D, Oza A. Investigation of childhood lead poisoning from parental take-home exposure from an electronic scrap recycling facility — Ohio, 2012. *MMWR Morb Mortal Wkly Rep.* 2015;64(27):743–745

37. Donovan EP, Donovan BL, McKinley MA, Cowan DM, Paustenbach DJ. Evaluation of take home (para-occupational) exposure to asbestos and disease: a review of the literature. *Crit Rev Toxicol.* 2012;42(9):703–731

38. Hudson PJ, Vogt RL, Brondum J, Witherell L, Myers G, Pascal DC. Elemental mercury exposure among children of thermometer plant workers. *Pediatrics.* 1987;79(6):935–938

39. Pollack SH. Adolescent occupational exposures and pediatric take-home exposures. *Pediatr Clin North Am.* 2001;48(5):1267–1289

40. Laidlaw MA, Filippelli G, Mielke H, Gulson B, Ball AS. Lead exposure at firing ranges-a review. *Environ Health.* 2017;16(1):34

41. Goldman LR. The clinical presentation of environmental health problems and the role of the pediatric provider. What do I do when I see children who might have an environmentally related illness? *Pediatr Clin North Am.* 2001;48(5):1085–1098

42. Mercer JJ, Bercovitch L, Muglia JL. Acrodynia and hypertension in a young girl secondary to elemental mercury toxicity acquired in the home. *Pediatr Dermatol.* 2012;29:199–201

43. Khine H, Weiss D, Graber N, Hoffman RS, Esteban-Cruciani N, Avner JR. A cluster of children with seizures caused by camphor poisoning. *Pediatrics.* 2009;123(5):1269–1272

Chapter 6

# Laboratory Testing of Body Fluids and Tissues

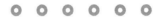

## KEY POINTS

- Most environmental chemical exposures occur at very low concentrations and measuring human exposure requires specialized laboratory technology not available in clinical laboratories.
- An exposure history is needed to decide which, if any, laboratory tests are appropriate.
- Except for tests to measure blood and urine metals, tests to measure exposure to environmental chemicals are usually not available from commercial clinical laboratories.
- Clinical interpretation or relevance of most environmental chemical tests are uncertain. Most test results are not predictive of current or future health effects. Before ordering tests, clinicians should consider whether test results will aid in diagnosis, management, or treatment.
- Clinicians who decide to order specialized tests for environmental chemical exposures are advised to consult with experts in these measurements, such as a medical toxicologist or their regional Pediatric Environmental Health Specialty Unit (PEHSU) for questions about testing.
- Because children excrete less creatinine in their urine compared with adults, a creatinine-corrected result may be unusually high. This occurs because the concentration is divided by (a small amount of) creatinine. Therefore, an "uncorrected" concentration may be a more accurate indicator of exposure.

## INTRODUCTION

Clinical laboratory testing is an important diagnostic, evaluation, and monitoring tool for many childhood disorders and diseases. For example, clinical chemistry results are indispensable in the diagnosis and management of diabetes mellitus and for determining the need for fluid therapy when gastroenteritis is severe. A few environmental chemical exposures, particularly several metals, may cause serious health consequences, and these can be diagnosed using clinical laboratory tests. However, clinical tests are of limited help for evaluating complex conditions that might be related to the typically low levels of environmental exposure. Because many laboratory tests for environmental exposures are not routinely available or used in clinical pediatrics, the challenge for the pediatrician is to understand the distinction between test results that mainly provide evidence of exposure and test results that aid in diagnosis, management, and treatment. The distinction is important because there are developmental or chronic conditions where an environmental exposure has been shown to be a risk factor; however, this does not mean that the exposure caused the condition. In fact, many such conditions are likely to be multifactorial. Although laboratory tests may document that exposure has occurred and actions should be taken to reduce the exposure, some results may be difficult to interpret or may not alter prognosis or therapy. Measurements of levels of metals in blood or urine may be done by many clinical laboratories, but other measurements may not be available outside of research or specialized laboratory settings.

## CONSIDERATIONS BEFORE ORDERING A CLINICAL LABORATORY TEST FOR CHILDREN

A detailed exposure history (see Chapter 5) should be taken for any child with a potential environmental chemical exposure or if symptoms could be related to an environmental exposure. Exposures to environmental chemicals or pollutants present special challenges. Few of these exposures can be accurately identified or quantified, and they may be intermittent or involve relatively low chemical concentrations. Children may present for assessment long after the exposure occurred, and it is usually not possible to identify the relative contributions from one or more chemical contaminants. If the chemical is rapidly eliminated from the body, it may be undetectable by the time a specimen can be collected. For chemicals that bioaccumulate or persist in the body, it may be impossible to determine when the exposure occurred. The utility and validity of laboratory testing to evaluate health effects of environmental chemicals is extremely limited, and a "shotgun" approach to test for multiple chemicals is not recommended or useful. Laboratory tests should be performed if the history suggests an exposure and if the results will influence patient management.

The effects of an environmental chemical exposure will depend on many factors, including the dose and duration, the child's age, genetics (eg, genetic polymorphisms for metabolizing or detoxifying enzymes, predisposition to chronic diseases or cancer, predisposition to asthma), and other environmental factors, including psychosocial, socioeconomic, cultural or ethnic, dietary, and other factors (see Chapter 4). Environmental chemicals also may act through epigenetic mechanisms that alter gene regulation and disease risk (eg, DNA methylation).[1,2]

## ASSESSMENT OF THE CHILD

Information gained from evaluating the child's symptoms and taking an exposure history, along with considering parental concerns, will help determine the need for laboratory testing. Some health complaints, such as asthma, allergies, or recurrent or recent onset of abdominal pain or headaches, may guide the exposure history questions. It is important to determine whether the exposure occurred before the onset of the problem or symptoms. If a chemical environmental exposure is suspected, it is essential to determine whether a laboratory test is available that will document the exposure or provide a result that indicates toxic effects. Finally, most chronic conditions or symptom complexes have multiple causal or contributing factors, and identifying one or a few environmental exposures that have contributed to the condition may not change the management or treatment. Reducing an environmental chemical exposure may be possible and desirable, even in the absence of laboratory testing. For example, if paint and glue fumes are generated during craft activities, improving ventilation or relocating the craft area may reduce exposure to offending volatile organic compounds and alleviate the headaches, respiratory irritation, or other symptoms related to the exposure.

## HELPFULNESS OF LABORATORY TESTING WHEN EVALUATING A POTENTIAL EXPOSURE

If the clinical picture suggests an environmental exposure, and a valid and relevant laboratory test is available to help to guide appropriate therapy, laboratory testing can be warranted. Evaluating a child with headaches may include carbon monoxide (CO) exposure in the differential diagnosis. For example, if the headaches occur in the morning and the child sleeps in a basement bedroom near the furnace, a blood carboxyhemoglobin (COHb) level should be measured if carbon monoxide exposure is possible (see Chapter 25). Because lead is a neurotoxicant, a child being evaluated for neurodevelopmental disorders should have a blood lead level measured, especially if excessive mouthing behaviors are noted or the child is younger than 3 years (see Chapter 32).[3] Some states require annual blood lead testing in younger children, even if the child is asymptomatic. Children who are enrolled in Medicaid are required to have blood lead tests at 12 and 24 months of age. In addition, any child between the ages of 24 and 72 months who is enrolled in Medicaid but does not have a blood lead test in his or her record is required to have one.

## ADDITIONAL RESOURCES FOR EVALUATING ENVIRONMENTAL CHEMICAL EXPOSURES

Finding specific information about suspected environmental chemical exposures may be difficult. Commercial and consumer products, such as glues, paints, household cleaners, and consumer products, have limited ingredient labeling. Safety Data Sheets (SDSs) often are available for consumer products and are designed to provide information needed by workers and emergency personnel to handle ingredient chemicals safely. The SDS includes physical information and chemical properties (eg, liquid, vapor), hazards (eg, flammability), toxicity and health effects including carcinogenicity, as well as occupational exposure limits, handling precautions, emergency measures, and contact information for a responsible party. Poison control centers often have access to detailed ingredient information and may be helpful in evaluating the relationship between symptoms and the exposure. If the source of a suspected environmental chemical exposure is outside the home, such as a playground or in soil or dust where the child plays, environmental sampling may be desirable. However, this is not within the usual scope of pediatric practice. Instead, local public health or environmental departments can be notified, especially when children may be exposed in group settings, such as child care or school, or from a shared exposure source, such as drinking water or a playground. Other helpful information resources for evaluating environmental exposures are the PEHSUs, which provide consultation and advice and are geographically distributed (www.pehsu.net).

## CONSIDERATIONS WHEN ORDERING LABORATORY TESTS

Once it is determined that a laboratory test is indicated and would be a diagnostic or therapeutic aid, additional considerations include involving what type of specimen to collect, proper specimen collection, and interpreting results. If the laboratory test is unfamiliar, it is advisable to contact a clinical laboratory consultant before ordering the test and to obtain information about the test, specimen and collection, and interpretation. A medical toxicologist available through a regional poison control center or regional PEHSU may also be of assistance. Cost of the testing may be another consideration if an insurer or payer limits coverage of laboratory services. Table 6-1 shows the laboratory tests and specimens used to evaluate some common environmental exposures.

### Specimen Selection

Validated laboratory tests use either blood (serum, plasma, or whole blood) or urine (a single or spot sample, or a 24-hour collection). Choice of either blood or urine depends on the chemical being measured and is usually specified by the laboratory. Some tests can be performed on both blood and urine, but the interpretation of the results may be different because of the toxicokinetics of

## Table 6-1. Laboratory Tests Used to Evaluate Specific Exposures

| EXPOSURE | SPECIMEN/TEST | COMMENT |
|---|---|---|
| Lead | Whole blood/lead | Current reference level is 5 mcg/dL. |
| Elemental or inorganic mercury | Urine/mercury | Urine total mercury is measured; preservative may be required. |
| Organic mercury (methyl mercury) | Whole blood/total mercury | Whole blood mercury is largely organic mercury, unless there is recent high-dose mercury vapor exposure. |
| Arsenic | Urine/speciated arsenic, if available; total arsenic will be elevated for 24–48 hours after seafood consumption. | Urine total arsenic consists of inorganic + organic arsenic. Organic arsenic (mainly from seafood) is nontoxic compared with inorganic arsenic. Subtracting organic arsenic from total arsenic gives a better estimate of the more toxic inorganic arsenic. |
| Cadmium | Urine/cadmium | Urine cadmium is an indicator of cadmium body burden or chronic exposure. |
| Cadmium | Whole blood/cadmium | Blood cadmium can be elevated with recent exposure. |
| Carbon monoxide | Blood carboxyhemoglobin | Smokers have higher carboxyhemoglobin levels compared with nonsmokers (usually <2%); ≥10% indicates significant and toxic carbon monoxide exposure. |

the chemical. Urine mercury is an indicator of inorganic mercury resulting from mercury vapor exposure, whereas whole blood mercury measures organic mercury, mainly methylmercury.[4] Although elevated blood lead concentrations may be associated with specific adverse health effects, urine lead measurements reflect only recent exposure, do not correlate with toxicity, and are not useful to evaluate childhood lead exposure.

## Collecting the Specimen

From a practical standpoint, specimen collection may not always be feasible before emergency treatment or intervention is begun. For example, measuring a COHb level could be diagnostic in a symptomatic child, but therapy will likely be initiated by emergency responders at the scene. If symptoms suggest exposure to mercury vapor, immediate actions to stop ongoing exposure and identify the source(s) are appropriate before specimen collection is begun.

The collection facility and staff need to be aware of any specific requirements or procedures to ensure the right specimen is obtained and collected properly, and whether timing of the collection is critical. To assess CO exposure, the blood COHb specimen needs to be collected and analyzed immediately following exposure because CO concentrations drop rapidly once a patient is removed from the exposure and/or receives supplemental oxygen. Urine for measurement of mercury, whether a spot sample or 24-hour specimen, may require refrigeration or a preservative added to the collection container to prevent the mercury from converting to elemental mercury, and subsequently off-gassing as mercury vapor. A preservative also may be required to prevent bacterial growth that can alter or metabolize the chemical during storage or transport of the specimen to an outside laboratory. Urine and blood specimens for metals and metalloids (eg, lead, mercury, cadmium, arsenic) must be collected with special precautions to avoid external contamination. Collection containers for metals should be certified as being "metal-free," or at least free of contamination by the metal to be measured. Because the concentrations of metals being measured are low (typically, parts per billion or mcg/L), trace amounts of contamination can considerably inflate the results. For several metals and metalloids (eg, cadmium, mercury, arsenic), a 24-hour urine collection may be preferred to a single "spot" urine; however, the likelihood of a complete collection over 24 hours, the ability to avoid contamination, and the urine storage conditions available during the collection time are important considerations. If urine arsenic is the chemical being measured, recent seafood consumption (within 3 days) should be documented because the total arsenic will be affected (increased because of seafood-derived arsenic). In this case, speciated urinary arsenic should be ordered to aid in the interpretation of the results (see Chapter 22).

## Interpreting Results

Blood and urine measurements of environmental chemicals require a basis for comparison, or a reference value or range. Unlike endogenous clinical chemistries, such as creatinine, electrolytes, glucose, cholesterol, and others, there is no "normal" physiologic value or range for exogenous chemical pollutants. Instead, results may be compared with age-adjusted population reference values, such as the median, 95th, or other percentile; with laboratory-based reference ranges; or, if they exist, with health-based thresholds. The 2005 childhood blood lead level of concern (10 mcg/dL) is an example of a health-based reference value.[5] However, no safe blood level has been identified, and the recent reference value of 5 mcg/dL is based on the measurements from an ongoing national survey, the National Health and Nutrition Examination Survey (NHANES). The reference value is defined as the 97.5th percentile, which means that 2.5% of American children ages 1 to 5 years had blood lead levels at or above 5 mcg/dL.[3] The blood methylmercury reference value of 5.8 mcg/L is also health-based, but it is derived from an estimated daily (lifetime) methylmercury intake at which the most sensitive person should not experience an adverse health effect.[6] The Centers for Disease Control and Prevention (CDC) has determined US population reference ranges for a number of environmental chemicals. Results are presented in tables that show selected percentiles (eg, median or 50th, 95th) categorized by age group, sex, and race/ethnicity.[7] These ranges consist of the values or concentrations that have been measured periodically in representative samples of the US population with "background" exposures or exposures encountered in activities of daily living. Reference ranges in children younger than 6 years are limited, but the CDC provides blood and urine measurements for more than 250 chemicals.[8]

## Urinary Creatinine-corrected Results

Results of metals and other exogenous chemicals measured in a single "spot" urine may be reported as creatinine "corrected" (eg, mcg/g of creatinine), in addition to the concentration per volume of urine (eg, mcg/L). Creatinine correction is done to adjust for urine dilution. The concentration of the chemical (usually in mcg/L) is divided by the concentration of creatinine in the specimen, with the result typically expressed as mcg/g of creatinine. Endogenous creatinine is produced in proportion to muscle mass; thus, males typically have higher creatinine excretion compared with females. Older age, greater body mass index, and non-Hispanic black race/ethnicity are associated with higher urinary creatinine.[7] In healthy persons, creatinine is largely eliminated by glomerular filtration, although 15% to 20% is actively secreted by the renal tubules.[9] Younger children typically excrete smaller amounts of urinary creatinine, so the creatinine-corrected results may be higher compared with the measured concentration of a chemical. Using 2011 and 2012 US population results for spot urine mercury as an example, the median or 50th percentile value in children aged 6 to 11 years was 0.24 mcg/L, and the creatinine-corrected value was 0.35 mcg/g creatinine. If the urine specimen is very dilute and the creatinine very low, the creatinine-adjusted value will be much higher than the measured concentration, leading to questions about the collection procedures and difficulty interpreting the results. In children, therefore, an "uncorrected" concentration may be a more accurate indicator of exposure.

## THE CLINICAL LABORATORY

Laboratories that conduct tests used for clinical purposes require ongoing quality control and formal accreditation. Because test results are used for diagnosis, evaluation, and treatment of humans, all US clinical laboratories must demonstrate reliable specimen processing and quality control, certification, and efficient reporting of results. The laboratories must be certified under the Clinical Laboratory Improvement Amendments (CLIA) program administered by the Centers for Medicaid & Medicare Services. The CLIA regulations include requirements for proficiency testing, quality control, test calibration, patient test management, personnel training and documentation of competency, and periodic inspections. Many laboratories seek additional accreditation from laboratory professional accrediting organizations, such as the College of American Pathologists.[10] Conversely, most research laboratories are not accredited to perform clinical tests or to interpret them because most research studies that measure environmental chemicals in human samples do not report the results to the study participants.

## WHEN PARENTS REQUEST INTERPRETATION OF UNUSUAL RESULTS

Parents may obtain laboratory testing results and then ask the pediatrician to interpret the results. This may be difficult for the pediatrician, but assistance may be available from a regional PEHSU or poison control center, or consultation with a medical toxicologist. The tests may be highly specialized or unfamiliar, the laboratory may or may not be accredited so results may be suspect, specifics about the analytical method may not be provided, and reference ranges (normal ranges) may not be available. Although the testing laboratory may provide a reference or "normal" range, it may not provide information about how it was determined, such as the analytical limit of detection and the sample of patients in whom the chemical was measured. A laboratory reference range is usually the range of values that were measured in 95% or 97.5% of the healthy patients in the sample group. Thus, a laboratory reference range can vary among laboratories. Alternatively, a laboratory may use a "no-effect" level as a toxic threshold for reporting results. The no-effect level for many chemicals is extrapolated from animal studies, includes uncertainty factors, is used mainly in regulatory activities, and is difficult to use in the interpretation of individual chemical results. The reference ranges used by the CDC are derived from the US population and presented by age categories; thus, these ranges may be helpful for comparison purposes, depending on the age of the child.[7] Unfortunately, the CDC measures few chemicals—mainly blood metals and serum cotinine—in children younger than 6 years. Prior to 2015, urine chemicals were measured only in children aged 6 and older; after 2015, urine collections were obtained from children as young as 3 years.

Physicians should understand that interpretations of these tests can be difficult because limited information is available on assessing and interpreting the burden of chemical contaminants in the bodies of children.

## TESTING OF UNCONVENTIONAL OR NONSTANDARD SPECIMENS

In research studies, a few chemicals have been tested in hair, fingernail clippings, or teeth, but these specimens are used exclusively for research and are usually a qualitative (presence or absence), rather than quantitative (concentration) indicator of exposure. Clinical interpretation of measurements using nonstandard specimens is uncertain because validated analytical or specimen preparation methods do not exist, and results cannot be correlated with conventional specimen results.[11] Hair products can either contaminate or remove chemicals in the hair, and hair-washing procedures to remove external contamination are not validated or standardized.[12] Even drug-of-abuse testing using hair measurement of cocaine metabolites, which can only come from internal metabolism, is plagued by uncertainties about thresholds and reliability of results.[13]

## FREQUENTLY ASKED QUESTIONS

Q   *Chemical X was measured in my child's blood, and I have been given a result. I am told that chemical X is a carcinogen. Does this mean my child will get cancer?*

A   Many chemicals have been classified as carcinogens based on studies in which animals were given high doses, often over long periods, or workers were exposed to large amounts of the chemical, usually over many years. Just because a person is exposed to a low level of a chemical, which is the usual situation with environmental exposures, *does not mean* that an adverse health effect or cancer will occur. Cancer is a complex process that develops over many years, and the likelihood of developing cancer is affected by a person's genetics; lifestyle habits, including smoking and alcohol; and even diet. Healthy eating that includes foods high in vitamins, antioxidants, and fiber, along with avoiding known carcinogens, especially tobacco and ultraviolet light, will help reduce the likelihood of cancer.

Q   *The laboratory reported my child's blood level of chemical X as being above the reference range. What does this mean?*

A   The laboratory reference range is usually the range of values that were measured by that laboratory in either 95% or 97.5% of patient samples. Depending on the chemical, there may be general population reference ranges available for comparison (www.cdc.gov/exposurereport). If the child's blood level is lower than the 95th percentile for that chemical, the interpretation is that the child's exposure is similar to the general population exposure. A result higher than the 95th percentile means that only 5% of the general population has higher values and greater exposure to the chemical.

Q *I paid a lot of money to have blood tests done on my child to identify the presence of harmful chemicals. The results showed that my child has harmful chemicals in his body and I want them removed. How do I get these harmful chemicals out of his body?*

A Unless your pediatrician or other health care provider ordered the test and was involved in the decision-making process, these tests may have been unnecessary. Your pediatrician may not be able to interpret or make recommendations based on these results for several reasons. Many of these tests are not performed in an accredited laboratory and reference ranges are not available; therefore, the results are not interpretable. In addition, finding of a measurable amount of a chemical in the body does not mean that the chemical causes a health problem.

Many of the chemicals may already have been deactivated (metabolized) and eliminated from the body. Some chemicals are very slowly eliminated from the body. Identifying and eliminating sources of the child's exposure to hazardous chemicals is the best course of action. Many therapies promoted to speed elimination of chemicals from the body are unproven or even dangerous. Consult with your pediatrician and, if needed, a pediatric environmental health specialist, to determine if your child has any health problems that may be related to the chemicals identified by laboratory testing. If such metals as lead, mercury, and cadmium were among the measurements, chelation therapy to remove any of these substances is not recommended and may be harmful. The only US Food and Drug Administration–approved indication for oral chelation therapy (succimer) is for blood lead levels greater than 45 mcg/dL. Other uses of chelation are unproven, experimental, and potentially hazardous. Consider consulting a poison control center or a physician with medical toxicology expertise if signs of metal toxicity are suspected.

Q *I have heard that laboratories can measure many harmful chemicals in my child's blood. Can you order all the possible tests for her?*

A Your pediatrician will use evidence-based practices when ordering, interpreting, and making recommendations based on laboratory tests to assess for exposures. It is not good clinical practice to order such tests because it is not yet known what the results mean. Interpreting the results is not possible because information on reference values and levels that may be linked to harmful effects is not available. Very few chemicals can be measured and interpreted accurately. In addition, the finding of a measurable amount of a chemical in the body does not mean that the chemical causes a health problem.

Q *What is the blood lead reference value?*

A In 2012, the blood lead "level of concern" was replaced by a reference value because no safe blood lead level has been identified. The reference value is based on the blood lead distribution during a specific period and is the 97.5th percentile of blood lead levels in American children aged 1 to 5 years, measured as part of the NHANES. The current reference value, 5 mcg/dL, comes from blood lead levels measured from 2007 through 2010. The reference value can be recalculated every 4 years as new blood lead data become available (eg, 2011 to 2014 data). The reference value is used to identify children with elevated blood lead levels; that is, the top 2.5% of blood lead levels. Children with elevated blood lead levels should be monitored but do not need chelation therapy unless the blood lead level is higher than 45 mcg/dL. Parents should be counseled about lead exposure sources, particularly lead paint hazards in housing and healthy nutrition to reduce lead absorption.

Q   *Can toxic chemicals or metals be measured reliably in hair?*

A   Hair samples have been used to measure environmental chemicals and metals, but the results cannot distinguish metals in the hair from those deposited from external contaminants. Hair methylmercury has been measured in research studies, according to strict protocols. Validated specimen preparation and analytical methods are not available. The wide range of hair treatments, shampoos, and conditioners that are used by Americans may contain metals or chemicals that leave deposits on the hair or may remove chemicals or metals from the hair. Thus, hair measurement is an unreliable indicator of what is inside a person's body. In addition, the results cannot be correlated with conventional results, such as blood or urine concentrations. Pediatricians may not be able to interpret results or make recommendations because of the unreliability of the result. In addition, there is no evidence to show that testing of hair for environmental chemicals or metals has any utility in the diagnosis or management of autism spectrum disorder (ASD).

Q   *Should I stop breastfeeding because I have been exposed to Chemical X, which can get into breast milk?*

A   Breastfeeding provides well-documented advantages for infants and mothers, as well as to families and society. Benefits of breastfeeding include immunologic advantages, lower obesity rates, greater cognitive development in the infant, and health advantages for the lactating mother. A number of environmental pollutants can cross from the mother into her breast milk, but breastfeeding need not be avoided or discontinued unless exceptional exposure has occurred (eg, an unintentional spill).[14,15] There is evidence that breastfeeding may even counter the subtle adverse effects associated with in utero exposure to some neurotoxic or endocrine disruptor substances at background levels.[16]

# References

1. Bakulski KM, Lee H, Feinberg JI, et al. Prenatal mercury concentration is associated with changes in DNA methylation at TCEANC2 in newborns. *Int J Epidemiol.* 2015;44(4):1249–1262

2. Ladd-Acosta C, Shu C, Lee BK, et al. Presence of an epigenetic signature of prenatal cigarette smoke exposure in childhood. *Environ Res.* 2016;144(Pt A):139–148

3. Advisory Committee on Childhood Lead Poisoning Prevention of the Centers for Disease Control and Prevention. Low level lead exposure harms children: a renewed call for primary prevention. http://www.cdc.gov/nceh/lead/acclpp/final_document_030712.pdf. Published January 4, 2012. Accessed January 7, 2018

4. Mortensen ME, Caudill SP, Caldwell KL, Ward CD, Jones RL. Total and methyl mercury in whole blood measured for the first time in the U.S. population: NHANES 2011-2012. *Environ Res.* 2014;134:257–264

5. Centers for Disease Control and Prevention. *National Report on Human Exposure to Environmental Chemicals, Updated Tables, March 2018.* http://www.cdc.gov/exposurereport. Updated March 2018. Accessed September 1, 2018

6. Centers for Disease Control and Prevention. *Preventing Lead Poisoning in Young Children.* Atlanta, GA: Centers for Disease Control and Prevention; 2005. https://www.cdc.gov/nceh/lead/publications/prevleadpoisoning.pdf. Accessed January 2, 2018

7. Barr DB, Wilder LC, Caudill SP, Gonzalez AJ, Needham LL, Pirkle JL. Urinary creatinine concentrations in the U.S. population: implications for urinary biologic monitoring measurements. *Environ Health Perspect.* 2005;113(2):192–200

8. US Environmental Protection Agency. Integrated Risk Information System (IRIS) Chemical Assessment Summary: Methylmercury (MeHg); CASRN 22967-92-6. http://cfpub.epa.gov/ncea/iris/iris_documents/documents/subst/0073_summary.pdf. Revised July 27, 2001. Accessed January 7, 2018

9. Boeniger MF, Lowry LK, Rosenberg J. Interpretation of urine results used to assess chemical exposure with emphasis on creatinine adjustments: a review. *Am Ind Hyg Assoc J.* 1993;54(10):615–627

10. College of American Pathologists. Accreditation. http://www.cap.org/web/home/lab/accreditation?_afrLoop=76503146869365#%40%3F_afrLoop%3D76503146869365%26_adf.ctrl-state%3D102jt0a53c_4. Accessed January 7, 2018

11. Pellizzari ED, Clayton CA. Assessing the measurement precision of various arsenic forms and arsenic exposure in the National Human Exposure Assessment Survey (NHEXAS). *Environ Health Perspect.* 2006;114(2):220–227

12. Rollins DE, Wilkins DG, Krueger GG, et al. The effect of hair color on the incorporation of codeine into human hair. *J Anal Toxicol.* 2003;27(8):545–551

13. Bortolotti F, Gottardo R, Pascali J, Tagliaro F. Toxicokinetics of cocaine and metabolites: the forensic toxicological approach. *Curr Med Chem.* 2012;19(33):5658–5663

14. American Academy of Pediatrics Section on Breastfeeding. Breastfeeding and the use of human milk. *Pediatrics.* 2012;129(3):e827–e841

15. Dórea JG. Policy statements on breastfeeding and human milk: additional comments. *Pediatrics.* 2012;130(2):e462–e464; author reply e465–e466

16. Marques RC, Dórea JG, Bernardi JV, Bastos WR, Malm O. Prenatal and postnatal mercury exposure, breastfeeding and neurodevelopment during the first 5 years. *Cogn Behav Neurol.* 2009;22(2):131–141

Chapter 7

# Environmental Measurements

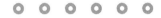

## KEY POINTS

- Environmental measurements are used to link a patient's diagnosis to an environmental exposure, assess short- and long-term health risks, develop health risk messages, and clarify when remediation is warranted.
- Soil, dust, water, and air sample results are compared with established reference values to understand environmental exposures.
- Widely varying sample collection methods are employed, and some samples are collected using methods that can be performed by the public.

## INTRODUCTION

This chapter provides an overview of evaluation tools used to measure environmental exposures—including contaminants in air, water, soil, and dust—to better equip pediatricians to address environmental exposure questions, request exposure characterization surveys, and evaluate exposure monitoring results. A basic understanding of environmental measurements helps clinicians to understand when and how exposure monitoring is important to case management, including prevention of future exposure. Examples include measuring formaldehyde that volatilizes (off-gasses) in a mobile home, heating oil that contaminates rural drinking well water, and lead dust that results from home renovation.

Although a clinician may suspect that a patient's diagnosis is attributable to an environmental exposure, acting on this assumption may be hampered by insufficient exposure information. In some cases, an exposure of concern may be identified through the environmental exposure history (see Chapter 5). In other cases, the exposure information is vague because of lack of understanding of the complex array of potential environmental exposures, such as chemicals with no odor or other warning properties. In addition, a patient or parent may be influenced by his or her belief system, media reports, or anxiety. The absence of exposure monitoring data limits a pediatrician's ability to attribute an illness to an environmental exposure, assess risk, or develop risk communication messages. Testing of the home, child care setting, school, or other sites can identify important exposures and provide objective data for comparison with established reference levels, such as the US Environmental Protection Agency (EPA) inhalation reference concentrations or other agency reference levels, and/or published values.

Biological monitoring tests, such as measurements in urine or blood, which characterize absorbed dose, may confirm a suspicion of exposure (see Chapter 6). Biological tests are useful because they integrate all routes of exposure (ingestion, inhalation, dermal absorption, transplacental). Unfortunately, biological monitoring tests are available for only a limited number of environmental toxicants, reference values frequently do not exist for children, and adult reference values are difficult to extrapolate to children. In addition, a biological test result does not provide insight into the relative importance of different sources of exposure when multiple sources are present. For example, an elevated blood lead level could result from exposure to sources including household paint dust, drinking water, or take-home exposure resulting from a parent's occupation. Identifying the significant sources of exposure is important for intervention and prevention efforts.

A clinician may be asked to comment on exposure monitoring results. Parents may expect their pediatrician to understand environmental exposure-assessment reports, interpret results, assess the child health risks associated with measured exposures, and communicate health risks. A clinician also may be asked to comment on the need for costly exposure mitigation interventions or post-remediation clearance sampling. Parents may seek guidance about when it is safe for a child to return to a remediated environment. In some instances, however, insufficient exposure information may limit the development of an exposure reduction plan to prevent future exposures. Assistance from environmental medicine pediatricians and other experts is available from the network of Pediatric Environmental Health Specialty Units funded by the Centers for Disease Control and Prevention and the US EPA at https://www.pehsu.net.

## ENVIRONMENTAL EXPOSURE EVALUATION

Several methods are available to measure chemical exposures in the environment.

### Environmental Monitoring and Reference Values

Collecting, analyzing, and interpreting environmental measurements in the absence of standardized exposure evaluation methods and health-based reference values are frequently problematic and are not recommended in the clinical setting. Published research protocols may describe sample collection and analysis methods. Without standardization, however, results from one laboratory may not be comparable to results from another. Further, the accuracy of the results may vary from batch to batch even at the same laboratory. Once exposure data exist, there may be significant momentum to interpret the data and provide a health risk message. In the absence of established reference values, interpretation of sample results is fraught with difficulty. The interpretation may vary from expert to expert, and the published literature may provide a limited framework for developing an interpretation. Even when health reference values exist, emerging research may modify the exposure interpretation framework.

The toxicological profiles produced by the Agency for Toxic Substances and Disease Registry (ATSDR) include a comprehensive list of regulations and advisories in each substance-specific profile (www.atsdr.cdc.gov/toxprofiles/index.asp). Profiles exist for approximately 175 common environmental contaminants. The regulations section includes a listing of regulations and guidelines for contaminants in air, water, soil, and food from organizations including the World Health Organization, the International Agency for Research on Cancer, the Occupational Safety and Health Administration (OSHA), the US EPA, the US Food and Drug Administration, individual states, and the American Conference of Governmental Industrial Hygienists. Reference values and exposure results may be reported in mass or parts per million units. Table 7-1 provides information about units used to measure liquid, solid, and air concentrations.

| Table 7-1. Units Used for Environmental Samples | | |
|---|---|---|
| **MATRIX** | **PARTS PER MILLION (PPM)** | **PARTS PER BILLION (PPB)** |
| Soil, house dust, or other solid | ppm = mg of contaminant/kg of solid matrix<br>1 ppm = 1 mg/kg = 1 mcg/g<br>1,000 ppm = 1 mg/g<br>1% = 10,000 ppm<br>1 ppm = 1,000 ppb | ppb = mcg/kg of solid matrix<br>1 ppb = 1 mcg/kg = 1 ng/g<br>1,000 ppb = 1 mcg/g<br>1 ppb = 1,000 parts per trillion (ppt) |
| Water or liquid | ppm = mg of contaminant/L of liquid matrix<br>1 ppm = 1 mg/L = 1 mcg/mL<br>1% = 10,000 ppm<br>1 ppm = 1,000 ppb | ppb = mcg/L of matrix<br>1 ppb = 1 mcg/L<br>1 ppb = 1,000 ppt |
| Air | ppm = one part of the chemical in one million parts of air<br>ppm to mg/m$^3$ conversion:<br>Y mg/m$^3$ = (X ppm) (molecular weight of substance) ÷ 24.45<br>mg/m$^3$ to ppm conversion:<br>X ppm = (Y mg/m$^3$) (24.45) ÷ (molecular weight)<br>1% = 10,000 ppm<br>0.001 ppm = 1 ppb = 1,000 ppt | ppb = one part of the chemical in one billion parts of air<br>ppb to mcg/m$^3$ conversion:<br>Y mcg/m$^3$ = (X ppb) (molecular weight) ÷ 24.45 mcg/m$^3$ to ppb conversion:<br>X ppb = (Y mcg/m$^3$) (24.45) ÷ (molecular weight)<br>1% = 10,000 ppm<br>0.001 ppm = 1 ppb = 1,000 ppt |

## Safety Data Sheets

For products used in work settings, chemical manufacturers are required by OSHA to create Safety Data Sheets (SDSs; formerly called Material Safety Data Sheets). Safety Data Sheets are health and safety information sheets that identify the chemical ingredients present at 1% of the formulation (except carcinogens that must be identified if present at 0.1%). Safety Data Sheets also describe health hazard information, including signs and symptoms of exposure and health problems associated with exposure, routes of exposure, regulatory limits, and other information. Asthma triggers, such as fragrance chemicals, however, may not be listed on the SDSs if they are present in concentrations of less than 1%. In addition, manufacturers may classify some ingredients as proprietary; disclosure of these ingredients is only possible through a regulatory mechanism of OSHA.

Safety Data Sheets are frequently available for household products, including cleaning agents, paints, stains, adhesives, and pesticides. The National Library of Medicine Household Products Database (see Resources at the end of the chapter) provides SDS information for hundreds of household products. Safety Data Sheets are also frequently available online at the product manufacturer's Web page or by directly contacting the product manufacturer or a local supplier.

## Environmental Consultants

The collection and interpretation of environmental samples may require a knowledgeable and experienced professional who can help to correctly identify the exposure, select the correct monitoring method and sampling plan, ensure correct timing of the sampling, and interpret results. Industrial hygienists, also called exposure scientists, are trained in the anticipation, identification, evaluation, and control of chemical, physical, and biological hazards in work, residential, or other settings. Industrial hygienists incorporate all potential routes of exposure in an exposure evaluation. They have expertise in sample collection and analytical methods, interpretation of results, and exposure control, reduction, and remediation strategies. During environmental health investigations, hygienists use visual, olfactory, and other sensory clues as well as occupants' symptoms. Although the field of industrial hygiene historically has focused on occupational settings, the exposure evaluation framework also applies to environmental exposures relevant to children. Other environmental science professionals may also have the qualifications necessary to effectively evaluate pediatric environmental exposures.

## OUTDOOR POLLUTANTS

Outdoor (ambient) air pollution is regulated by the US EPA in partnership with state governments. As described in Chapter 21, air pollutants that are monitored include ozone, particulate matter, lead, sulfur oxide compounds, nitrogen oxide compounds, carbon monoxide (CO), and approximately 185 other toxic chemicals associated with small and large industrial facilities, vehicle emissions, and other sources. Using these data in the context of individual patient care can be difficult because the patient may live some distance from the nearest monitoring station, and because local factors, such as prevailing winds and geography, may limit the applicability of the data to an individual. When industrial site emissions are of interest, it may be useful to contact the state agency responsible for air quality to learn whether monitoring data are available.

Although the federal Emergency Planning and Community Right-to-Know Act requires the EPA Toxics Release Inventory (TRI) Program to disclose toxic chemicals that are stored and/or released to the air, water, and land, the law is primarily designed to aid response planning in the event of a chemical spill or release. Disclosure is based on quantities stored or released and not on ambient air concentrations; therefore, the utility and specificity of the data for health care are limited. It is difficult to use the TRI to address concerns regarding chronic, low-dose exposures associated with industrial emissions. Although a chemical release report can be generated by zip code (www.epa.gov/triexplorer), the information is not specific enough for use in patient care, except under extreme release circumstances. The US EPA National Air Toxics Assessment program used the TRI, state and local pollution inventories, and other databases to model median outdoor concentrations of approximately 180 toxic air pollutants in 2014. (https://www.epa.gov/national-air-toxics-assessment/2014-national-air-toxics-assessment/2014-nata-map).

It is possible to characterize chemicals associated with industrial or other pollution sources when the chemicals have established analytical methods and reference standards for occupational exposures. Methods used to measure industrial chemical pollutants may not be applicable to measure community exposures that are typically orders of magnitude lower than occupational exposures. In addition, there are only a limited number of community exposure standards. Occupational standards are set to protect typical adults working 8 hours a day and 40 hours a week for 30 years, whereas community exposure standards are set to protect the most sensitive members of society and assume a 24-hour-a-day, 7-day-a-week, lifetime exposure pattern. In the absence of rigorous sample collection or analytical methods for contaminants found in the community at low concentrations, or in the absence of regulatory reference values, community exposure characterization is not recommended because it is extremely difficult to interpret results in the context of individual patient care.

## INDOOR POLLUTANTS

Unlike outdoor air pollution, indoor air pollutants are not routinely measured or regulated. The US EPA recommends, but does not require, radon testing in all homes located below the third floor (see Chapter 42). Air quality data can be used to identify important environmental exposures, explain a patient's symptoms, assess risk, develop risk communication messages, and clarify when exposure reduction strategies are warranted. Example situations when data on indoor air pollutants may be helpful are described as follows:

- To learn if a patient's headaches are the result of CO emitted from a malfunctioning furnace or other combustion device (see Chapter 25)
- To link a patient's irritant symptoms to formaldehyde off-gassing from new construction materials (see Chapter 20)
- To determine whether remediation is warranted to protect the developing fetus or newborn from mercury contamination (see Chapter 33)
- To prevent disease that is the result of infiltration of toxicants that affect indoor air quality, such as air pollution or contaminated plumes or groundwater located below structures in which children spend time

Commonly used methods to characterize airborne chemical exposures include meters with digital displays (direct-read instruments), colorimetric chemical detector tubes, passive samplers, or sampling pumps with specialized sample media. Some exposure measurement methods are relatively straightforward and can be performed by a layperson. Other methods require specialized equipment and/or the services of a trained professional. Table 7-2 summarizes the approach to measuring airborne contaminants and the approximate costs.

Direct-read instruments are available for a variety of contaminants and provide immediate information about contaminant concentration. For example, CO meters are commonly used by fire departments to evaluate furnaces and other combustion sources. Some instruments "datalog" or can measure and record contaminant concentrations for selected averaging windows (seconds, minutes, or hours) over an extended period (days to weeks). Datalogging provides average, maximum, and minimum exposure data and provides an opportunity to correlate events (eg, window cleaning) in time with contaminant spikes (eg, ammonia, Butyl Cellosolve [a chemical used in cleaning agents]) in the recorded data, which may be useful in identifying contaminant sources. Although these instruments are typically rented by trained professionals, they are available to the public and generally include instruction manuals. Rental costs vary depending on the type of equipment and duration of the rental.

Color diffusion or dosimeter tubes are available for some chemicals (gases and vapors) and can be successfully used by the public. Passive color tubes, the size of a small pen, rely on air diffusion to move the contaminant of interest through the medium. As the contaminant reacts with the material inside the tube, a color change occurs and the length of the colored stain is read using the scale printed on the outside of the glass tube. The user must carefully follow directions because the calibrated scale is based on the duration of sampling. With an error margin of ±25%, passive colorimetric tubes are useful screening tools for contaminants. Care must be taken when selecting a specific tube because many colorimetric tubes are designed for industrial settings with higher contaminant concentrations. To select a tube, the contaminant concentration should first be estimated by reviewing community air standards or results in published papers and then carefully checking the tube concentration ranges available to determine whether the detection range is appropriate for the situation. Carbon monoxide is an example of a chemical for which concentrations may be measured using colorimetric tubes.

Passive samplers can be used to characterize formaldehyde, radon, and other gases and vapors in indoor air. Samples are passively collected and then submitted to a laboratory for analysis. Passive sampler costs are generally higher and may or may not include laboratory costs.

## Table 7-2. Airborne Contaminants Measurement Approach and Cost

| AIRBORNE CONTAMINANT | RECOMMENDED METHODS AND COMMENTS | APPROXIMATE COST[a] |
|---|---|---|
| Carbon monoxide (furnace, emergency power generators, and other combustion sources) | If carbon monoxide exposure is suspected, vacate the premises immediately and contact the local fire department. To identify low-dose exposures, use passive colorimetric tube with level of detection <5 ppm.[b] | $ |
| Formaldehyde[b] | Passive tube for residential use with level of detection at 5 ppb | $ to $$ |
| Fungal mycotoxins | Sampling not recommended Sample collection and analysis methods not standardized Consensus reference levels not established Research method—not readily available commercially | NA |
| Gasoline or heating oil fingerprint | Hire a professional. Contact state department of ecology or public health for assistance. | $$$$ |
| Indoor mold and mold-related concerns | Sampling generally not needed. Stop water infiltration and remediate visible mold growth following recommended guidelines. Spore-trap sample results are occasionally used to identify other indoor air problems, such as fiberglass. | NA |
| Lead or asbestos clearance samples (post-remediation) | Hire a professional. | $$ |

| | | |
|---|---|---|
| Mercury (elemental) | Direct read instrument needed<br>Contact local fire department, health department, or hire a professional.<br>A single CFL or mercury thermometer break usually does not require testing provided that proper cleanup guidelines are followed. | Local government resources, if available; likely no cost<br>Professional $$$ |
| Radon[b] | Use a radon air test kit.<br>Work with state or local health department or private laboratory. | $ |
| Secondhand tobacco smoke | Research method—not readily available commercially | NA |
| Other contaminants | Work with state or local health department or private laboratory.<br>Hire a professional as needed. | $$ to $$$$ |

Abbreviations: CFL, compact fluorescent light; NA, not applicable; ppb, parts per billion; ppm, parts per million.
[a] Approximate cost ranges: $, <$100; $$, $100–$299; $$$, $300–$999; $$$$, >$1,000.
[b] Indicates that a layperson can generally successfully collect the sample.

Colorimetric tubes, passive samplers, or direct-read instruments are not available for many environmental contaminants. In these cases, an industrial hygienist or another environmental specialist is needed to measure contaminant levels. Sample collection involves using a small air pump that pulls air at a defined rate through filters or sorbent tubes in which the contaminant of interest is concentrated for analysis. When validated methods exist, this approach provides very accurate measurements in the lower concentration ranges expected in residential, school, or other environments in which children spend time. An evaluation by a professional typically includes the consultant's time, sampling equipment, laboratory costs for sample analysis, and a written report with an interpretation of the results.

## Radon

The US EPA recommends that all homes be tested below the third floor for radon using an air test kit. These kits are available through many state departments of health in which experts are available to assist with interpretation of the results and remediation resources. More information about radon can be found in Chapter 42.

## Mold

Environmental evaluation for molds is common and typically includes a careful indoor and outdoor inspection for visible mold growth, water damage, conditions conducive to water intrusion, and the presence of musty odors. Although visual inspection is often sufficient to identify problematic mold growth contributing to poor indoor air quality, air, wipe, tape-lift, and/or bulk samples are frequently collected and analyzed for molds and related indoor pollutants. If an inspection reveals extensive visible mold growth and/or damp indoor spaces, the water infiltration and/or moisture problems require correction and mold remediation is recommended. Extensive sampling to identify specific mold species or count spores is usually not required, except in the context of a research investigation.

Characterization of mold exposure and interpretation of results generally require the assistance of a trained professional, such as a certified industrial hygienist. Home test kits, such as "settle plates," are not recommended because the sample results are highly variable, difficult to interpret, and often inaccurate. Sampling in extremely contaminated areas may require use of respiratory protection and adherence to other safety precautions and may present a hazard to building occupants if not performed appropriately.

### Air Sample Collection

Two common air sample collection methods are the culturable or "viable" method and the spore-trap method that counts both viable and nonviable spores. With viable samples, a known volume of air is directed toward a nutrient medium that is then incubated for a specified period. Mold colonies are identified and enumerated by a skilled microscopist. Results are reported in colony-forming units per cubic meter of air sampled ($CFU/m^3$). The main advantage of viable sampling is the enhanced ability to identify some mold colonies. However, viable sampling underrepresents the airborne mold population because it does not detect nonviable spores, which may have toxic or allergenic properties.

With nonviable or spore-trap methodology, spores and other particulates are collected by directing a known volume of air onto a sticky surface, which is then analyzed. The spores, fibers, pollen, dander, skin cells, and other particulates are identified and enumerated by a skilled microscopist. Results are reported as the number of spores, fibers, or other particulates per $m^3$ of air sampled. Important spore-trap advantages are: (1) both fresh viable and old, nonviable spores are counted, providing a more accurate representation of total exposure; (2) nonfungal particles (eg, skin cells, fiberglass, pollens) that can contribute to poor indoor air quality can be identified and counted; and (3) spore chains, which indicate an active growth site nearby, can be identified. Nonviable sampling identifies mold spores by their morphology; because some molds have similar appearances, identification is less precise than with the viable method. For example, *Penicillium* and *Aspergillus* molds cannot be differentiated by this method.

Air samples are collected in problem indoor locations and, as a comparison location, outdoors. Sometimes samples are also collected in nonproblem indoor locations to provide additional comparison information. Comparison samples should be collected within hours of the samples collected in problem locations. Use of an accredited environmental microbiology laboratory is recommended to analyze all mold samples. Environmental Microbiology Laboratory Accreditation Program laboratories have met rigorous performance standards as defined by the American Industrial Hygiene Association.

### Bulk, Swab, and Tape-lift Samples

Bulk, swab, and tape-lift samples provide surface mold information. Bulk samples are collected from areas with visible mold growth. A sample the size of a dime or smaller of moldy drywall or other material, or a chunk of the mold, is submitted and identified via microscopy. Swab samples are collected by wiping a surface with a moistened, sterile swab. The material is then cultured and identified. In tape-lift sample collection, clear adhesive tape is gently pushed against the surface of interest. The tape is then placed on a standard glass microscope slide for direct microscopic examination. Nonfungal particles that can affect indoor air quality, such as fiberglass, can also be identified in tape-lift samples.

## Mold Results Interpretation

Interpreting mold monitoring data is challenging. No state or federal regulatory levels or consensus guidelines define mold counts indicative of indoor mold growth (or amplification) or mold exposure problems. Thus, experienced professionals may arrive at different conclusions regarding the likelihood of an indoor mold source when interpreting the same data. The most common approach to air sample interpretation is to compare specific mold colony or spore counts in problem indoor locations with the mold colony or spore counts outdoors and/or to the counts in nonproblem indoor locations. Outdoor counts generally are higher than indoor counts and typically reflect the same mix of molds. Generally, as the indoor count exceeds and dwarfs the outdoor count for a specific mold, the likelihood of a mold amplification problem increases. However, mold growth is also possible if the problem area count is higher than expected for that type of mold, or if a specific mold dominates the indoor sample count but does not dominate the comparison location(s) count. Because of the complexities of mold monitoring, exceptions to the rule are common. Interpretation is aided by knowledge of the unique characteristics of each mold identified, such as how frequently it is identified and typical concentrations outdoors and in damp environments, moisture requirements for growth, common growth substrates, and ease of spore generation.

Mold spore release is highly variable. Repeated fungal bioaerosol measurements can vary by orders of magnitude over the course of one day. This is compounded by the fact that sample collection duration is 15 minutes or less. This is in sharp contrast to the 8- or 24-hour (or longer) sampling approach used to characterize chemical concentrations in the environment. In addition, 1 or, at most, 2 samples are collected at each location during a typical survey, which is insufficient to capture within- and between-day mold spore variability. Seasonal spore release variability is also important. In addition, certain genera of mold spores or bacteria may be present in the air but do not compete well on the nutrient media selected for the survey, which is why they may be found infrequently despite their presence.

## Bulk Sample Interpretation

The utility of bulk, swab, and tape-lift samples is limited because there are no regulatory reference values or comparison sample locations (eg, an outdoor air sample). Swab and tape-lift samples may be collected on surfaces cleaned frequently, reflecting recent spore deposition, and are useful for clearance sampling. Swabs and tape lifts from rarely cleaned reservoirs, such as the tops of doorjambs, reflect deposition over an unknown period (months, years), which limits the utility of the information. Samples collected in ducted heating, air-conditioning, and ventilation systems can be very useful because these systems can be effective collectors as well as disseminators of bioaerosols associated with indoor environment contamination.

## Lead in Paint, Dust, and Soil

Potential residential lead hazards, described in Chapter 32, include interior and exterior paint, household dust, outdoor soil, lead-glazed pottery, toys and other household items, drinking water (addressed later in the chapter), spices, and herbal remedies. Soil, water, paint chips, household dust, and other materials can be tested for lead by a lead-accredited analytical laboratory. Some states offer lead programs to aid sample collection and analysis for homeowners.

Paint samples are relatively easy to collect if the paint is chipping, peeling, or damaged. Samples must contain all paint layers down to the wood because lead is often found in the older layers and not in the top layers. As an alternative, a direct-reading x-ray fluorescence (XRF) analyzer can be used. Portable XRF scanners use nondestructive methods to detect lead in paint independent of the thickness or composition of the various layers of paint. They also can be used to test toys and other surfaces; accuracy of XRF use for these purposes is under examination. X-ray fluorescence scanners require users to be trained and experienced technicians because these instruments contain a radioactive source.

Surface wipe samples are used to characterize the lead content in settled household dust and to verify that lead containment or lead dust cleanup efforts were effective. Wipe samples should be collected and analyzed by parties independent of the renovation or remediation contractors who did the work. Sample collection involves donning gloves, wiping a 4-inch$^2$ (10-cm$^2$) area (using tape or a template to delineate the area) with a wipe moistened with distilled water, and placing the wipe in the sealed container provided by an analytical laboratory (see National Institute of Occupational Safety and Health, lead in surface wipe sampling method at https://www.cdc.gov/niosh/docs/2003-154/pdfs/9100.pdf). Settled dust samples may be collected from floors, window sills, and troughs because reference values exist for those locations (Table 7-3). Lead surface test kits, which include wipes, sealed containers, distilled water, and gloves, are available from some lead-accredited laboratories.

Soil testing methods are described in detail (http://player-care.com/lead_handbk-2a.pdf). To reduce costs, individual samples can be combined into a composite sample. Comparison values are included in Table 7-3.

## Table 7-3. Lead Standards and Recommendations

| LEADED MATERIAL | STANDARD/RECOMMENDATION | REFERENCE |
|---|---|---|
| Lead-based paint definition | 1.0 mg lead/cm$^2$ (XRF) or 0.5% lead by weight (lab analysis of paint chip) | EPA TSCA 403[a] |
| Dust-lead hazard definition | 40 mcg/ft$^2$ of floor (wipe samples) 250 mcg/ft$^2$ interior window sills (wipe samples) | EPA TSCA 403<br><br>40 CFR §745[a] HUD 35.1320 |
| Lead abatement clearance requirements | 40 mcg/ft$^2$ of floor (wipe samples) 250 mcg/ft$^2$ interior window sills 400 mcg/ft$^2$ window wells | EPA TSCA 403<br><br>40 CFR §745[a] |
| Outside soil | 400 ppm lead in bare soil in a child's play area 1,200 ppm lead in bare soil in the rest of the yard | EPA TSCA 403<br><br>40 CFR §745[a] |
| Residential drinking water | Standing and running water sample (no more than 10% of samples can exceed the action level) Action level: 0.015 mg/L = 15 ppb | Safe Drinking Water Act Lead and Copper Rule, 56 FR 26460[b] |
| Voluntary school drinking water (Local recommendations may be lower.) | Standing and running water sample from any ONE outlet Action level: 0.020 mg/L = 20 ppb | 3Ts for Reducing Lead in Drinking Water in Schools (https://www.epa.gov/dwreginfo/3ts-reducing-lead-drinking-water-schools-and-child-care-facilities) |

Abbreviations: CFR, Code of Federal Regulations; EPA, US Environmental Protection Agency; FR, *Federal Register;* HUD, US Department of Housing and Urban Development; ppb, parts per billion; ppm, parts per million; TSCA, Toxic Substances Control Act; XRF, x-ray fluorescence.
[a] www.epa.gov/lead/pubs/leadhaz.htm.
[b] https://www.epa.gov/dwstandardsregulations.

To better ensure that laboratory test results are accurate, it is essential to use a lead-accredited laboratory. The US EPA maintains a list by state of currently accredited laboratories (https://www.epa.gov/lead/national-lead-laboratory-accreditation-program-nllap), which includes those participating in the National Lead Laboratory Accreditation Program. Accredited laboratories participate in periodic performance evaluations, including proficiency testing. Because some states also operate parallel lead and other laboratory accreditation programs, additional accredited laboratories may be available in a particular region. Some states operate an environmental laboratory that accepts samples from the public. Sample collection kits are available from many laboratories and include sample collection directions, sample containers, and sample handling procedures.

Home lead test kits to detect lead in paint, dust, soil, jewelry, vinyl, and other surfaces are not recommended for use by laypeople. Although readily available in hardware stores, research has shown these test kit results are inaccurate because interfering substances can cause false-negative and false-positive results.[1,2] The US EPA has recognized 3 lead paint test kits that are reliable when used by professionals. The US EPA maintains a list of these recognized kits and describes test kit limitations (https://www.epa.gov/lead/lead-test-kits).

## DRINKING WATER

Drinking water contaminants include organic and inorganic chemicals, such as radon, lead, bacteria, nitrate, gasoline, pesticides, and others. Public utilities must test sources of drinking water for a wide variety of contaminants. Well and source water contaminants also can be characterized by working with state or private laboratories.

Some contaminants, such as radon and lead, are relatively easy to measure by using inexpensive test kits available from state or private laboratories. If local plumbing-related contaminants, such as lead, are the concern, standing and running water samples are collected at a high-use location, such as the kitchen sink. Other contaminants (ie, gasoline, heating oil) require more complicated assessment procedures, which are identified by analyzing samples for a combination of compounds ("fingerprinting"). Chemicals linked to oil and gas fracking vary by region because of the geology of the oil shale. For example, the Pennsylvania Department of Environmental Protection has developed water testing parameters that include indicator chemicals for the shale in that region (see Resources at the end of the chapter). For detection of some drinking water contaminants, it is best to hire a professional.

Drinking water testing requires collection of a water sample for submission to an accredited laboratory for analysis. The US EPA Web portal (http://water.epa.gov/scitech/drinkingwater/labcert/index.cfm) lists accredited laboratories in specific areas. In some states, this search tool can be used to identify all laboratories accredited to analyze environmental samples. Accredited laboratories must meet performance standards, including proficiency testing, which help to ensure that test results are accurate. People interested in testing water are advised to choose an analytical laboratory that provides sample collection kits, which include sample collection directions, containers (including pretreated containers and/or sample preservatives), sample storage and transport guidelines, and other information to ensure the accuracy of analytical results. For example, lead testing requires acid-washed containers, and nitrate testing requires a preservative. Except for postage, sample collection kits are

## Table 7-4. Approaches to Measuring Drinking Water Contaminants and Approximate Costs

| CONTAMINANT | APPROXIMATE COST[a] |
|---|---|
| Lead, cadmium, copper, iron, other heavy metals[b] Arsenic and nitrate (well water)[b] | $$ |
| Radon[b] | $ |
| Microbiological (*E. coli*)[b] | $ |
| Organic chemicals:[b] PFOA and PFOS (perfluoroalkyl substances) Gasoline or heating oil fingerprint compounds Trihalomethanes Chloramines | $ to $$ depending on compound |
| Oil/gas fracking chemicals[b] | $$$ to $$$$ |
| Pesticides[b] | $$ to $$$ for common pesticides |

Abbreviations: PFOA, perfluorooctanoic acid; PFOS, perfluorooctanesulfonic acid.
[a] Approximate cost ranges: $, <$100; $$, $100–$299; $$$, $300–$999; $$$$, >$1,000.
[b] Work with county, state, or private lab to obtain sampling kit to include sample collection instructions, container, and storage/shipping information

typically included in the analysis cost. Table 7-4 summarizes the approach to measuring drinking water contaminants as well as the approximate costs.

Drinking water test results are compared with drinking water contaminant reference values available at www.epa.gov/safewater/contaminants/index.html. The US EPA has issued health advisories for some unregulated chemicals, such as perfluoroalkyl and polyfluoroalkyl substances (PFAS) (see Resources at the end of the chapter). For assistance with other chemicals, such as those associated with oil and gas fracking, contact local public health or ecology departments for assistance.

## TESTING OF DIETARY SUPPLEMENTS, SPICES, COSMETICS, AND FOOD PESTICIDES

Herbal remedies, dietary supplements, spices, candy, other food items, and cosmetics can be tested for metals such as lead or mercury, pesticides, and other contaminants. A local accredited laboratory will be able to provide guidance regarding pricing, sample collection, and submission. Table 7-5 summarizes the approach to measure contaminants in dietary supplements and spices and other miscellaneous contaminants.

**Table 7-5. Miscellaneous Contaminants Measurement Approach and Cost**

| CONTAMINANT | RECOMMENDED ACTION | APPROXIMATE COST[a] |
|---|---|---|
| Lead in paint, soil/dust<br>Lead and other heavy metals in spices, alternative medicines, teas, or herbal remedies | Work with county, state, or private lab to obtain sampling kit to include sample collection instructions, container, and storage/shipping information. | $ to $$ |
| Mercury in spices, alternative medicines, teas, or herbal remedies | Work with county, state, or private lab to obtain sampling kit to include sample collection instructions, container, and storage/shipping information. | $$ |
| Suspected asbestos-containing material | Hire a professional. | $$ to $$$ |
| Pesticide residues on food, grass, play equipment, toys | Work with county, state, or private lab to obtain sampling kit to include sample collection instructions, container, and storage/shipping information. | $$ |
| Contaminants in fish: mercury, PCBs, DDT | Sampling not recommended<br>Check for local fish advisories.<br>For patients frequently consuming fish meals, check US EPA and other fish testing databases for contaminant levels in relevant waterways. | NA |
| PCBs, dioxin, PBDEs in human milk | Sampling generally not recommended except for exceptional exposures<br>Laboratory methods not standardized<br>Consensus reference levels not established<br>Research method—not readily available commercially | NA |
| Fungal mycotoxins in dust | Sampling not recommended<br>Sample collection and analysis methods not standardized<br>Consensus reference levels not established<br>Research method—not readily available commercially | NA |
| Allergens (dust mites, cat, dog, bird, insects, rodent) in dust | Sampling not recommended<br>Consensus reference levels not established<br>Research method—not readily available commercially | NA |
| Endocrine disruptors:<br>bisphenol A, phthalates in food or water from plastic storage containers | Sampling not recommended<br>Sample collection and analysis methods not standardized<br>Consensus reference levels not established<br>Research method—not readily available commercially | NA |

Abbreviations: DDT, dichlorodiphenyltrichloroethane; NA, not applicable; PBDE, polybrominated diphenyl ether; PCB, polychlorinated biphenyl; US EPA, US Environmental Protection Agency.
[a] Approximate cost ranges: $, <$100; $$, $100–$299; $$$, $300–$999; $$$$, >$1,000.

## FREQUENTLY ASKED QUESTIONS

Q *Our home is being remodeled and the contractor is in the final steps of finishing the project. We recently learned that homes like ours, built before 1978, are likely to contain lead-based paint. What should we do before we move our children back into our home?*

A Discuss your lead dust exposure concern with your renovation contractor. The US EPA requires certification of contractors in lead-safe work practices to prevent lead dust contamination during renovation, repair, or painting activities in homes, schools, and child care facilities built before 1978. The rule requires the contractor to apply methods to limit the dispersal of dust during work and leave a work site that has passed a visually clean verification procedure by comparing a wipe sample visually to a cleaning verification reference card. Individual states may apply more stringent standards that require surface dust wipe samples to be collected and analyzed in a laboratory. If wipe samples results exceed the US EPA 40 mcg/ft$^2$ floor or 250 mcg/ft$^2$ interior window sill standards, further cleaning is necessary using a high-efficiency particulate air filter vacuum and by damp wiping all surfaces. When clean, additional sampling should be performed by a qualified and experienced independent contractor to verify effectiveness of the remediation and cleanup. If the home has a forced-air heating system, it may be necessary to damp wipe the furnace interior and ducts. Carpet, soft furnishings, and ducts with internal duct liners can be difficult to evaluate and decontaminate and may require disposal.

Homeowners with limited financial resources could collect samples for analysis in lieu of hiring a certified professional but should be warned that lead contamination may be unevenly distributed, so finding low concentrations in one area does not ensure low concentrations in others. The EPA Lead Renovation, Repair and Painting Web page describes the program in detail (https://www.epa.gov/lead/renovation-repair-and-painting-program).

Asbestos may also be present in homes built before 1986 in ceiling tiles, roll vinyl or tile floor coverings, insulation, and other materials. If asbestos-containing materials are disturbed, exposure control procedures are required to prevent asbestos contamination of the home. Contact a local US EPA office for more information.

Q *A compact fluorescent light (CFL) broke on a carpeted floor in our daughter's nursery and we followed the recommended cleanup procedures. Should we have the air tested to determine whether there is a mercury air problem in the nursery?*

A    Air testing following breakage of CFLs is not currently recommended when spill cleanup procedures are followed.[3] Seek additional advice from your local or state health or environmental agency as needed. Following breakage, open windows immediately and carefully follow cleanup procedures (https://www.atsdr.cdc.gov/mercury/docs/Residential_Hg_Spill_Cleanup.pdf).

## Resources

**ATSDR mercury small spill cleanup**
Web site: https://www.atsdr.cdc.gov/mercury/docs/Residential_Hg_Spill_Cleanup.pdf

**ATSDR toxicological profiles**
Web site: www.atsdr.cdc.gov/toxprofiles/index.asp

**Maine Department of Environmental Protection CFL Revised Cleanup Guidance**
Web site: www.maine.gov/dep/homeowner/cflreport/appendixe.pdf

**Maine Department of Environmental Protection Compact Fluorescent Lamp Study Report**
Web site: www.maine.gov/dep/homeowner/cflreport.html

**National Library of Medicine Household Products Database**
Web site: http://householdproducts.nlm.nih.gov

**Pennsylvania Department of Environmental Protection Recommended Basic Oil and Gas Pre-Drill Parameters**
Web site: https://www.dep.pa.gov/DataandTools/Reports/Oil%20and%20Gas%20Reports/Pages/default.aspx

**SKC catalogues**
Web site: www.skcltd.com/index.php/products

**US EPA accredited laboratories**
Web site: https://www.epa.gov/lead/national-lead-laboratory-accreditation-program-nllap

**US EPA AirNow ambient particulate matter and ozone Web portal**
Web site: http://airnow.gov

**US EPA Emergency Planning and Community Right-to-Know Act Web portal**
Web site: https://www.epa.gov/epcra

**US EPA fish advisories Web page**
Web site: www.epa.gov/waterscience/fish/states.htm

**US EPA Hazardous Air Pollutants Web portal**
Web site: https://www.epa.gov/haps

**US EPA lead paint test kits for use by professionals**
Web site: https://www.epa.gov/lead/lead-test-kits

**US EPA lead in paint, dust, and soil Web portal**
Web site: https://www.epa.gov/lead/
national-lead-laboratory-accreditation-program-nllap

**US EPA Mold Web site**
Web site: www.epa.gov/mold

**US EPA Mold Remediation in Schools and Commercial Buildings Guide (also applies to residences)**
Web site: https://www.epa.gov/mold/
mold-remediation-schools-and-commercial-buildings-guide

**US EPA National Air Toxics Assessment program**
Web site: https://www.epa.gov/national-air-toxics-assessment

**US EPA PFOA & PFOS Drinking Water Health Advisories**
Web site: https://www.epa.gov/sites/production/files/2016-06/documents/
drinkingwaterhealthadvisories_pfoa_pfos_updated_5.31.16.pdf

**US EPA TRI program Release Chemical Report queries**
Web site: www.epa.gov/triexplorer

## References

1. Cobb D, Hatlelid K, Jain B, Recht J, Saltzman LE. CPSC staff report: evaluation of lead test kits. https://www.cpsc.gov/s3fs-public/lead.pdf. Published October 2007. Accessed January 9, 2018
2. Rossiter WJ Jr, Vangel MG, McKnight ME, Dewalt G. Spot test kits for detecting lead in household paint: a laboratory evaluation. http://www.fire.nist.gov/bfrlpubs/build00/PDF/b00034.pdf. National Institute of Standards and Technology Publication No. 6398. Published May 2000. Accessed January 5, 2018
3. Salthammer T, Uhde E, Omelan A, Lüdecke A, Moriske HJ. Estimating human indoor exposure to elemental mercury from broken compact fluorescent lamps (CFLs). *Indoor Air.* 2012;22(4):289–298

# Chapter 8

# Toxic or Environmental Preconceptional and Prenatal Exposures

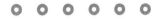

## KEY POINTS

- Maternal and paternal exposures before conception may affect fertility or fetal outcomes that may persist across generations.
- The effects of prenatal exposures to the fetus may be smaller, larger, or different depending on the stage of development.
- Strategies exist to decrease certain exposures at work and home.

## INTRODUCTION

Harmful environmental exposures associated with poor health outcomes may occur to genetic material across generations (genetic and epigenetic), ova and sperm before fertilization (preconceptional exposures), and in utero (potentially teratogenic). Further vulnerability to these environmental exposures may differ depending on concurrent stressors, such as poverty.[1] Occupational and environmental risks to the fetus are becoming increasingly important. Each parent may have different exposures.

Preconceptional exposures of ova or sperm to environmental contaminants may lead to the development of an abnormal fetus. In addition, a woman's exposure to contaminants may result in a delayed exposure to the developing fetus by the ongoing elimination of the chemical from the mother's body (secondary fetal exposure). Because the initial exposure is before conception, these exposures are nonconcurrent with the pregnancy. For some chemicals, such as organohalogens (eg, polychlorinated biphenyls [PCBs], which accumulate and persist in the body for many years), the fetus can be affected by nonconcurrent and concurrent maternal exposures.

Concern with prenatal exposures is based on the knowledge that there are certain periods during development—"critical windows"—when the fetus is much more vulnerable to the effects of exposures than at other times.[1–4] One detailed timeline highlights such windows of vulnerability by synthesizing research in animals and potential developmental effects of endocrine disruption across multiple organ systems.[5] A well-known example is the teratogen thalidomide; exposure to thalidomide in utero results in devastating limb-reduction defects. In a retrospective observational study, thalidomide exposure was also associated with a slightly higher incidence of autism spectrum disorders than expected for the general population.[4,6] A period of extreme vulnerability to ionizing radiation exists from gestational age 8 to 15 weeks; exposure during this period may result in microcephaly, poor somatic growth, and cognitive issues.[7,8] The importance of critical windows and ionizing radiation was emphasized by a primate model that demonstrated that the same ionizing radiation dose had differing neurodevelopmental effects depending on the timing of exposure.[9] Nevertheless, critical windows have not been clearly defined for most exposures. Effects (ie, neurodevelopmental effects, cancer) arising from preconceptional and prenatal exposures may be latent until later in childhood, adolescence, or adulthood.

This chapter describes overarching concepts regarding preconceptional and prenatal exposures and the spectrum of adverse outcomes known to be associated with select parental occupational and environmental exposures. For more detail on specific agents, refer to the corresponding chapter.

## TIMING OF EXPOSURES

### Exposures to the Ovum

The ovum from which the fetus is derived develops during the early fetal life of the mother and arrests in the prophase of the cell cycle until ovulation, which may occur up to 50 years later. Environmental contaminants that may affect the oocyte have been measured in samples of human follicular fluid (and in seminal plasma).[10]

One important reproductive outcome to measure is fertility. In general, few outcome studies on environmental exposures resulting in fertility loss or other adverse effects have been reported because such transgenerational studies require a lengthy period of observation between exposure and outcome.

Although it is beyond the scope of the chapter to detail every exposure related to infertility, several illustrative instances exist. An example of an exposure linked to infertility is exposure to tobacco smoke. Scientific evidence is sufficient to causally link maternal active smoking with infertility and earlier menopause, with mounting evidence to suggest exposure to secondhand smoke may have similar effects.[11] Infertility also has been associated with pesticide exposure.[1]

Another important class of chemicals associated with infertility are the endocrine disrupting chemicals (EDCs) which, depending on structure, may inhibit or have similar effects as endogenous hormones.[12] One well-known example of exposure to EDCs is the population of children whose mothers took diethylstilbestrol (DES), an estrogen analogue, to prevent pregnancy loss.[12] Compared with unexposed fetuses, girls exposed to DES in utero were more likely to develop clear cell adenocarcinoma of the vagina and other adverse genital and reproductive effects. Boys were more likely to develop nonmalignant cysts. Transgenerational effects from DES exposure (preconceptional effects in persons whose grandmothers took DES during pregnancy [ie, DES grandchildren]) also have been documented. These include an increased incidence of hypospadias in DES grandsons and ovarian cancer in granddaughters and decreased fertility in the second generation.[12,13] In general, there is mounting evidence both in animal and human studies that EDCs can affect ovarian development and ovulation and thus fertility.[14]

Infertility in adulthood also is clearly increased in survivors of childhood cancer. However, this setting has multiple potential exposures contributing to later reproductive outcomes. These multifactorial influences derive from surgery, chemotherapy, and radiation therapy to the areas proximal to the gonads or alternatively, to the head/brain affecting the hypothalamic/pituitary axis. A higher risk of infertility exists in female childhood cancer survivors, especially if they were treated with alkylating agents or exposed to radiation therapy (gonadal radiation at greater than 5 Gray (Gy) or hypothalamic/ pituitary radiation at greater than 22 to 30 Gy).[15] Further outcomes of female survivors may include spontaneous abortion, preterm labor, and low birth weight if the pelvic region was significantly exposed to radiation therapy.[16]

## Exposures to the Sperm

Similar to females, male infertility is also linked with risk factors, including higher doses of alkylating chemotherapeutic agents and testicular radiation above 4-7.5 Gy.[15] In contrast to effects on ova, however, effects on sperm can be measured relatively easily in the next generation. There is, therefore, more scientific evidence to suggest that paternal occupational exposures before conception may constitute a risk to the fetus. Medical conditions such as obesity, exposures to ionizing radiation, and exposures to tobacco, alcohol, or EDCs have been related to decreased sperm counts, sperm quality, or male infertility.[14,17-19] The sperm itself is vulnerable to the effects of mutagens; in its final form, the sperm has no DNA repair mechanisms. It has therefore been suggested that the sperm may be a vulnerable target for carcinogenesis. The association of paternal occupation with cancer risk in offspring has been extensively researched with studies reaching varying conclusions. Studies of paternal exposures and childhood cancers have inconsistencies from study to study attributed, in part, to imprecision in exposure assessment or null results, making it difficult to directly link paternal exposures with childhood cancers.[20-23] However, one recent study suggested positive associations with paternal periconceptional exposures to pesticides and childhood leukemias.[24]

Studies on the association of birth defects with paternal occupation were also reviewed and found to have many of the same limitations as studies of paternal occupation and cancer.[18,19] The National Birth Defects Prevention Study examined paternal occupational exposures and anomalies.[25] Interestingly, there were select paternal occupations associated with a constellation of anomalies, such as photographers and photo processing workers producing offspring with various eye deformities and the offspring of landscapers having a variety of gastrointestinal deformities.[25] In addition, artists had a higher risk of having offspring with different types of anomalies (of the eye, ear, palate, and gastrointestinal tract).[25]

## Secondary Fetal Exposure: Maternal Body Burden

Fetal exposure may result from ongoing excretion or mobilization of chemicals stored in the mother's body. This mobilization is sometimes termed "nonconcurrent" fetal exposure. Adipose tissue and skeletal tissue are known storage sites for various chemicals. For example, polychlorinated biphenyls (PCBs) are persistent pollutants stored in adipose tissue. Following a Taiwanese poisoning episode with PCBs, children born up to 6 years after maternal exposure had similar developmental abnormalities (developmental delays, mildly disordered behavior, and increased activity levels) as those found in children born within 1 year of maternal exposure.[26,27] The developmental delays persisted in these children at all times measured. Thus, these children had significant effects from maternal exposure to PCBs that occurred up to 6 years before their birth.

The major repository for lead is bone, where the half-life of lead is years to decades.[28] Chronic lead exposure may result in significant accumulation of lead in the skeleton. During pregnancy, calcium turnover is greatly increased, which increases mobilization of lead stores from bone.[28,29] Congenital lead poisoning because of an elevated maternal body burden was illustrated in 2 case reports of children born to women who were inadequately treated for childhood plumbism.[30,31] Maternal skeletal mobilization of lead is a major source of fetal exposure[29] and negatively affects a child's neurologic development.[32]

## Concurrent Maternal Prenatal Exposures

Prenatal exposures to the mother arise from sources including maternal occupation, paraoccupational exposure through a third party (such as a spouse or family member), air, water, and diet. Internet resources for estimating the risk of exposures to pregnant women are found in the Toxicology Data Network (TOXNET, http://toxnet.nlm.nih.gov), which includes the Developmental and Reproductive Toxicology Database (DART, www.healthdata.gov/dataset/developmental-and-reproductive-toxicology-database-dart).

## ROUTES OF EXPOSURES

### Maternal Occupational Exposures

Only a small fraction of chemicals found in the workplace has been assessed for reproductive toxicity, although more than 2,000 new chemicals are added each year.[33] Several maternal occupations increase the risk of a poor pregnancy outcome. Associations between workplace exposures and poor reproductive outcome (eg, spontaneous abortion, miscarriage, birth defects) have been found for lead, mercury, organic solvents, ethylene oxide, and ionizing radiation.[34] Recent data show a decreased risk of having an infant that is small for gestational age for women working in nursing, and higher risk of having a preterm delivery for women working in the food industry.[35] The National Birth Defects Prevention Study found that several maternal occupations were associated with anomalies. For example, janitors and cleaners had a higher risk of giving birth to infants with eye and gastrointestinal anomalies and oral clefts.[36] The study also determined that some occupations were protective or lowered the risk of certain birth defects; for example, teachers had fewer offspring with neural tube defects, gastroschisis, and septal defects.[36] Maternal occupational exposure to paint was found to be associated with a higher risk of offspring with acute myeloid leukemia.[37] More information is found in Chapter 48. The US Department of Labor Occupational Safety and Health Administration Web site on reproductive hazards provides many relevant resources, as does the European Agency for Safety and Health at Work Web site: (www.osha.gov/SLTC/reproductivehazards/index.html and https://oshwiki.eu/wiki/Reproductive_effects_caused_by_chemical_and_biological_agents). Cosmetologists, predominantly women who are nail technicians or hairdressers, have exposures to several potentially hazardous chemicals.[38] Nail products contain toluene, phthalates, acetone, ethyl methacrylate, and formaldehyde.[38] Hair products contain nitrosamines and formaldehyde.[38] It is difficult to determine reproductive effects of exposure to combinations of chemicals, especially because hair and nail services and their associated products may be located in the same salons.[38]

Occupational exposure to radiation is common in aviation and medical technology. The occupational limit is 0.005 Gy (0.5 rad) and dose monitoring should occur during pregnancy to ensure that a pregnant woman is not exposed to higher levels of ionizing radiation.[39] Non-cancer risks from radiation exposure during pregnancy may include pregnancy loss, congenital malformations, cognitive deficits, and fetal growth restriction. These risks increase with the dose of radiation received. There appears to be a threshold dose below which no effects occur.[8,39] The risk of childhood cancer seems to have no threshold.[8,39]

Aviation work results in a natural occupational exposure to ionizing radiation, mainly from high levels of galactic cosmic radiation found at altitudes maintained by commercial flights.[40] A flight crew's exposure varies depending on the length of time in flight, altitude, and latitude (one half exposure at the equator compared with polar regions).[40] Guidelines limit exposure to pregnant crewmembers.[40] Further considerations should include the risk of thromboembolic events with stasis, and dehydration that is the result of low cabin humidity.[41] Further recommendations are available about acceptable exposures to galactic radiation for pregnant air crewmembers.[40–42]

## Paraoccupational Exposure

A paraoccupational exposure occurs when the mother, father, or another household member brings or tracks home occupational chemicals, when the home itself is in an occupational setting, or when industrial chemicals are purposely brought home for home use. Chemicals may be brought into the house by others on skin, hair, clothing, and shoes.[33] These chemical exposures may be reduced by using proper personal protective equipment, leaving work clothes and showering at the location of occupation, and laundering work clothes separately from the clothing of other household members.[33] Key examples of household member "take-home" substances with health effects include beryllium, asbestos, and lead.[43,44]

## Air Pollution

Air pollution is an important source of exposure to a pregnant woman and her fetus, exposing them to many contaminants. For example, exposure of the mother to secondhand tobacco smoke is linked to preterm birth, decreased birth weight, increased risk of sudden infant death syndrome,[10,45,46] and obesity in the offspring.[47] Other examples of exposure through air include benzene and volatile compounds (see Chapter 20). The US Environmental Protection Agency (EPA) reviews 6 criteria pollutants (carbon monoxide, lead, nitrogen dioxide, particulate matter ($<$10 mcm and $<$2.5 mcm), sulfur dioxide, and ozone) and regulates them with the National Ambient Air Quality Standards (NAAQS) (https://www.epa.gov/naaqs). Ambient air pollution is a mixture of these components; therefore, it is challenging to isolate effects of a single pollutant. Nevertheless, there is increasing evidence that maternal exposure to ambient air pollution is associated with preterm delivery, delivery of an infant small for gestational age, and low birth weight at term.[48-53] In addition, there is emerging epidemiologic evidence linking air pollution to poorer neurodevelopmental outcomes such as attention-deficit/hyperactivity disorder, autism, and adverse cognitive effects.[54-56]

## Water

Because the fetus develops through multiple short critical periods, the quality of water consumed by a pregnant woman is a daily concern; methods that provide guidance by using a yearly average of contaminants will not be sufficient to protect the developing fetus. Public and well water supplies can vary greatly over the course of a year. A review of prenatal chemical exposures and reproductive and pregnancy outcomes examined the relationship of drinking water contaminants to adverse pregnancy outcomes.[34] It concluded that limited evidence exists to support an association between exposure to byproducts of chlorinated water disinfectants (such as trihalomethane) and increased risk of spontaneous abortions, stillbirths, or having an infant who is small for gestational age or who has a neural tube defect.[34] Arsenic in groundwater has been associated with stillbirth, spontaneous abortions, and neonatal and infant mortality.[57]

## Diet

Contaminants in the diet may result in important exposures. Methylmercury from an acetaldehyde-producing plant in Minamata, Japan contaminated the food chain in the 1950s.[58] Pregnant women living in fishing villages on Minamata Bay gave birth to severely neurologically damaged infants, whereas the women had only mild transient paresthesias or no symptoms at all. Pregnant women should avoid consumption of fish with high mercury content including shark, swordfish, king mackerel, and tile fish and limit their intake of other fish, such as white (albacore) tuna, that may have high mercury content (see Chapter 33).

## PATHWAYS OF FETAL EXPOSURE

### Placenta-dependent Pathways

For a placenta-dependent chemical to reach the fetus, it must first enter the mother's bloodstream and then cross the placenta in significant amounts. Not all environmental toxicants meet these criteria. Three properties that enable chemicals to cross the placenta are low molecular weight, fat solubility, and resemblance to nutrients that are specifically transported. Information about an individual chemical's ability to cross the placenta may be found by using the Toxicology Data Network (TOXNET http://toxnet.nlm.nih.gov), which includes the Developmental and Reproductive Toxicology Database,[59] or by reviewing the chemical's Safety Data Sheet.

An example of a low molecular weight compound is carbon monoxide (CO). Carbon monoxide is an asphyxiant because it displaces oxygen from hemoglobin, forming carboxyhemoglobin (COHb). If enough COHb accumulates in the circulation, cellular metabolism is impaired by the inhibition of oxygen transport, delivery, and use. Fetal COHb accumulates more slowly than maternal COHb but increases to a steady state approximately 10% greater than in the maternal circulation. Thus, nonfatal CO poisoning of the mother may prove fatal to the fetus.

Examples of fat-soluble chemicals that readily cross the placenta are ethanol and polycyclic aromatic hydrocarbons (PAHs), including benzo(a)pyrene, a carcinogen present in secondhand tobacco smoke. Alcohol causes fetal alcohol spectrum disorders; the most severe end of the spectrum is fetal alcohol syndrome. Alcohol use during pregnancy is considered the main preventable cause of intellectual disability.[60,61] In pregnant ewes, intravenous infusion of ethanol results in identical maternal and fetal blood alcohol concentrations.[62] PCBs have been measured in equal concentrations in fetal and maternal blood.[63]

Calcium is a nutrient that is actively transported across the placenta to provide the fetus with 100 to 140 mg/kg of calcium per day during the third trimester. It is thought that lead is transported by the calcium transporter. The average contribution of maternal skeletal lead mobilized to the infant's cord blood lead has been calculated to be 79%.[29] Calcium supplementation decreases maternal bone resorption, thereby lowering the amount of lead mobilized from maternal bone that would then become available to the fetus.[29] A randomized controlled trial conducted in Mexico City showed that women who received 1,200 mg daily of calcium carbonate had moderately lower lead concentrations during pregnancy.[64] This effect was greater in compliant mothers, in mothers with higher baseline lead concentrations, and during the second trimester.

## Placenta-independent Pathways

Placenta-independent hazards to the fetus include ionizing radiation, heat, noise, and possibly electromagnetic fields. Ionizing radiation is a well-characterized teratogen (see Chapter 31). Much of our knowledge about the effects of radiation comes from studies of survivors of the atomic bombings in Hiroshima and Nagasaki[65] and the Chernobyl nuclear disaster.[66,67]

Ionizing radiation is associated with birth defects such as microcephaly.[68] Exposure to low-dose cobalt-60 ionizing radiation was associated with increased time to pregnancy.[69] In an occupational setting, laboratory technicians working with radioactive materials had a higher risk of preterm delivery.[70] Not all forms of radiation are hazardous to the fetus; radon and ultraviolet radiation do not reach the fetus.

Heat may directly penetrate to the fetus; exposure to heat in the first trimester has been associated with neural tube defects.[71] Noise has a waveform, which may be transmitted to the fetus. Noise has been associated with certain birth defects, preterm birth, and low birth weight.[72]

Increasing attention has been given to intrauterine programming and epigenetic phenomena. These occur when environmental factors change gene expression through DNA methylation and chromatin remodeling; such alterations may continue to affect future generations.[2] One example is the association between maternal smoking during pregnancy and the increased risk of childhood obesity.[73] Another is concern about early exposure to endocrine disrupting chemicals such as bisphenol A and the development of adult chronic disease such as obesity.[2,73,74] Emerging evidence demonstrates that these epigenetic changes are heritable across generations.[75]

## SPECTRUM OF OUTCOMES

Developmental processes—from the fertilization of an egg to the birth of baby through the completion of adult development—are highly intricate. The sites of action of chemicals and radiation are numerous. An intrauterine exposure to radiation or chemicals may result in a broad array of phenotypic effects that often are not thought of as teratogenic effects. Table 8-1 lists some phenotypes that may be seen.

The environment has been strongly linked to birth defects. A study of 371,933 women investigated the relative risk of a child being born with a birth

| Table 8-1. Spectrum of Phenotypic Effects | |
|---|---|
| ■ Behavioral dysfunction | ■ Intrauterine growth retardation |
| ■ Cancer | ■ Major and minor malformations |
| ■ Cognitive dysfunction | ■ Metabolic dysfunction |
| ■ Deformations | ■ Microcephaly |
| ■ Effects on vision | ■ Preterm birth |
| ■ Endocrine dysfunction | ■ Pulmonary dysfunction |
| ■ Hearing loss | ■ Spontaneous abortion/ |
| ■ Infertility | miscarriage |

defect similar to the birth defect affecting the preceding sibling;[76] the relative risk of a similar birth defect was 11.6 (95% confidence interval, 9.3–14.0) and decreased by more than 50% when the mother changed her living environment between the 2 pregnancies.

Developmental neurotoxicity deserves special mention. The development of the central nervous system requires expression of unique proteins in specific cell populations during specific critical windows. There is concern that injury to these populations may result in neurodevelopmental disorders, such as intellectual disabilities, autism spectrum disorder, dyslexia, and attention-deficit/hyperactivity disorder. Parents report that nearly 8% of US children have a learning disability and that 13% have either a mental disorder (such as autism spectrum disorder or conduct disorder) or attention-deficit/hyperactivity disorder.[77] These developmental disabilities are increasing over time.[78] Some are caused by genetic aberrations (eg, Down syndrome, fragile X syndrome), some by perinatal anoxia or meningitis, and some by exposure to drugs (eg, alcohol, cocaine). For most neurodevelopmental disorders, however, the cause is unknown. Environmental chemicals such as lead, tobacco, PCBs, and mercury are known developmental neurotoxicants. Despite nearly ubiquitous exposures to multiple chemicals, such as endocrine disrupting compounds and pesticides, most have not been tested for developmental neurotoxicity; combinations of chemicals have generally not been evaluated.[77] It is possible that neurodevelopmental disabilities that become evident after birth are linked to in utero exposure to one or multiple chemicals.

## PREVENTION OF EXPOSURE

For women who are planning pregnancies, an occupational and environmental exposure history may be obtained during preconception or interconception health visits. Because approximately one half of all pregnancies are unplanned (https://www.cdc.gov/reproductivehealth/unintendedpregnancy/), it is important to obtain an exposure history for every woman of reproductive age. It is not enough to know the woman's occupation. The clinician must ask about the nature of her work, the nature of her partner's work, their hobbies and home activities, secondhand smoke exposure at home and elsewhere, and the characteristics of their residence and neighborhood. Additional areas of inquiry include the composition of the diet and use of tobacco, alcohol, or street drugs. The clinician should inquire about medicines (prescribed, over-the-counter, or natural/alternative/herbal) used during the pregnancy.[79] The Select Panel for Preconception Health and Health Care of the Centers for Disease Control and Prevention (CDC) created "Before, Between & Beyond Pregnancy," a Web site that includes a preconception curriculum for health care providers.[80]

Women who work have a right to know about the chemicals with which they work, and they have a right to be protected from harmful exposures. Safety data sheets are available to any employee who requests them. These sheets supply information about potential reproductive hazards. Personal protective gear should be available, and increased monitoring of potential exposures should be instituted. In certain instances, temporary job shifting may prevent exposure.

## Frequently Asked Questions

Q   *What can I do to improve the likelihood of having a healthy, full-term baby?*

A   The first step in having a healthy baby is ensuring that the mother is healthy. The mother's health begins before conception. If you are a woman of childbearing age, take a folic acid supplement every day. Ingesting 0.4 mg (400 mcg) of folic acid per day will prevent certain kinds of birth defects, particularly defects of the nervous system. Pregnant women should increase their folic acid intake to 0.6 mg (600 mcg) per day. Because many pregnancies are not planned and women may not know they are pregnant until the first trimester is well under way, folic acid should be taken by all women of childbearing age. Folic acid is available as part of many multivitamin supplements. Furthermore, iodine supplementation is important because iodine deficiency in the United States is occurring at least marginally in about one third of pregnant women.[81] This deficiency may be compounded by environmental exposures that are ubiquitous: for example, perchlorate (in food and water) may take the place of iodide and thus make iodide less available for the thyroid and for breast milk.[82,83] Adequate amounts of iodine range from 290 mcg to 1,100 mcg per day; this could include a supplement of 150 mcg of iodine as is included in most standard prenatal vitamin supplements.[84] Women should also use iodized salt to help maintain an adequate iodine intake. Make sure that any medications you take are safe to use during pregnancy. Do not drink alcohol, do not smoke tobacco or use electronic cigarettes, and try to avoid others who smoke. Avoid eating the 4 large, predatory fish that contain high amounts of mercury (swordfish, shark, tilefish, and king mackerel) and limit your intake of white (albacore) tuna. It is important to continue to consume regularly (at least two 3-oz [85 g] servings a week) other seafood before and during pregnancy, especially seafood rich in fatty acids and low in mercury (eg, salmon, pollock, scallops), to ensure that sufficient amounts of the essential fatty acids docosahexaenoic acid (DHA) and eicosapentaenoic acid (EPA) are available for the development of the fetal brain.[85] If you work with chemicals, become informed about the possible risks those chemicals could pose to your fetus and take necessary precautions. Remember that environmental hazards can exist not only at work but also at home or even as a result of other household members' exposures. Be aware of potential environmental exposures that might occur during preparation for the baby's arrival such as renovating the nursery—renovation could possibly result in lead exposure from removing lead-based paint.

Q *Is there any information about chemical exposures and risks to women who work in hair or nail salons?*

A Exposures at nail and hair salons involve multiple substances. Hair salons may use chemicals such as aromatic amines (hair dye) or formaldehyde-based disinfectants. Nail salons use solvents, such as acetone or toluene, and acrylates. Because of the presence of these multiple substances as well as differences in ventilation and time of exposure, true reproductive health risks are difficult to determine. Furthermore, very few human studies examine multiple substance exposures and associated health risks. Hairdressers should have a work environment that includes wearing gloves, avoiding standing for long periods of time, ensuring good ventilation, covering products and garbage when not in use, and maintaining separate areas to eat.[86] Nail salons have similar issues. Recommendations for nail salon workers include ensuring good ventilation, keeping products and garbage closed if not in use, removing garbage frequently, using appropriate dust masks for grinding nails, using gloves, and having separate places to eat. It is also recommended that products containing liquid methyl methacrylate (MMA) be avoided, mainly because studies in animals exposed to MMA show adverse respiratory and liver effects. Information about protecting nail salon workers may be found at the Nail Salons Project of the US EPA (https://www.epa.gov/saferchoice/protecting-health-nail-salon-workers-0).

## Resources

### Agency for Toxic Substances and Disease Registry (ATSDR)
Principles of Pediatric Environmental Health. How Can Parents' Preconception Exposures and In Utero Exposures Affect a Developing Child? https://www.atsdr.cdc.gov/csem/csem.asp?csem=27&po=8

### National Institute for Occupational Safety and Health (NIOSH), Reproductive Health and the Workplace
www.cdc.gov/niosh/topics/repro

### Occupational Safety and Health Administration (OSHA) Reproductive Hazards
www.osha.gov/SLTC/reproductivehazards
Information relevant to reproductive hazards in the workplace.

**Organization of Teratology Information Specialists (OTIS) Information Service MotherToBaby**

http://mothertobaby.org/
Provides fact sheets on different hazards and links to medical providers in the United States and Canada.

**Pediatric Environmental Health Specialty Units**

www.pehsu.net

**The March of Dimes**

www.marchofdimes.org/professionals/professional-education.aspx
Offers education for professionals about preconception issues.

**Toxicology Data Network (TOXNET)**

http://toxnet.nlm.nih.gov
A cluster of databases covering toxicology, hazardous chemicals, environmental health, and related areas. It is managed by the Toxicology and Environmental Health Information Program (TEHIP) in the Division of Specialized Information Services (SIS) of the National Library of Medicine (NLM). One such database on TOXNET is Developmental and Reproductive Toxicology Database (DART)—References to developmental and reproductive toxicology literature — http://www.healthdata.gov/dataset/developmental-and-reproductive-toxicology-database-dart.

**University of California San Francisco**
**Program on Reproductive Health and the Environment**

http://prhe.ucsf.edu/prhe/clinical_resources.html
Information for clinicians including link to a prenatal environmental history form.

## References

1. Di Renzo GC, Conry JA, Blake J, et al. International Federation of Gynecology and Obstetrics opinion on reproductive health impacts of exposure to toxic environmental chemicals. *Int J Gynaecol Obstet.* 2015;131(3):219–225

2. Grandjean P, Bellinger D, Bergman A, et al. The Faroes statement: human health effects of developmental exposure to chemicals in our environment. *Basic Clin Pharmacol Toxicol.* 2008;102(2):73–75

3. Etzel RA, Landrigan PJ. Children's exquisite vulnerability to environmental exposures. In: Landrigan PJ, Etzel RA, eds. *Textbook of Children's Environmental Health.* New York, NY: Oxford; 2014:18–27

4. Landrigan PJ. Children's environmental health: a brief history. *Acad Pediatr.* 2016;16(1):1–9

5. The Endocrine Disruption Exchange. Critical Windows of Development Timeline. http://endocrinedisruption.org/prenatal-origins-of-endocrine-disruption/critical-windows-of-development/timeline-test/. Accessed March 27, 2018

6.  Miller MT, Strömland K, Ventura L, Johansson M, Bandim JM, Gillberg C. Autism associated with conditions characterized by developmental errors in early embryogenesis: a mini review. *Int J Dev Neurosci.* 2005;23(2-3):201–219

7.  Yamazaki JN, Schull WJ. Perinatal loss and neurological abnormalities among children of the atomic bomb. Nagasaki and Hiroshima revisited, 1949 to 1989. *JAMA.* 1990;264(5):605–609

8.  Brent RL. Saving lives and changing family histories: appropriate counseling of pregnant women and men and women of reproductive age, concerning the risk of diagnostic radiation exposures during and before pregnancy. *Am J Obstet Gynecol.* 2009;200(1):4–24

9.  Selemon LD, Ceritoglu C, Ratanather JT, et al. Distinct abnormalities of the primate prefrontal cortex caused by ionizing radiation in early or midgestation. *J Comp Neurol.* 2013;521(5):1040–1053

10.  Younglai EV, Foster WG, Hughes EG, Trim K, Jarrell JF. Levels of environmental contaminants in human follicular fluid, serum, and seminal plasma of couples undergoing in vitro fertilization. *Arch Environ Contam Toxicol.* 2002;43(1):121–126

11.  Hyland A, Piazza K, Hovey KM, et al. Associations between lifetime tobacco exposure with infertility and age at natural menopause: The Women's Health Initiative Observational Study. *Tob Control.* 2016;25(6):706–714

12.  Sathyanarayana S, Focareta J, Dailey T, Buchanan S. Environmental exposures: how to counsel preconception and prenatal patients in the clinical setting. *Am J Obstet Gynecol.* 2012;207(6):463–470

13.  Newbold RR. Prenatal exposure to diethylstilbestrol (DES). *Fertil Steril.* 2008;89(2 Suppl):e55–e56

14.  Gore AC, Chappell VA, Fenton SE, et al. Executive summary to EDC-2: The Endocrine Society's second scientific statement on endocrine-disrupting chemicals. *Endocr Rev.* 2015;36(6):593–602

15.  Antal Z, Sklar CA. Gonadal function and fertility among survivors of childhood cancer. *Endocrinol Metab Clin North Am.* 2015;44(4):739–749

16.  Hudson MM. Reproductive outcomes for survivors of childhood cancer. *Obstet Gynecol.* 2010;116(5):1171–1183

17.  Sharma R, Harlev A, Agarwal A, Esteves SC. Cigarette smoking and semen quality: a new meta-analysis examining the effect of the 2010 World Health Organization laboratory methods for the examination of human studies. *Eur Urol.* 2016;70(4):635–645

18.  Frey KA, Navarro SM, Kotelchuck M, Lu MC. The clinical content of preconception care: preconception care for men. *Am J Obstet Gynecol.* 2008;199(6 Suppl 2):S389–S395

19.  Cordier S. Evidence for a role of paternal exposures in developmental toxicity. *Basic Clin Pharmacol Toxicol.* 2008;102(2):176–181

20.  Yang Q, Wen SW, Leader A, Chen XK, Lipson J, Walker M. Paternal age and birth defects: how strong is the association? *Hum Reprod.* 2007;22(3):696–701

21.  Bailey HD, Fritschi L, Metayer C, et al. Parental occupational paint exposure and risk of childhood leukemia in the offspring: findings from the Childhood Leukemia International Consortium. *Cancer Causes Control.* 2014;25(10):1351–1367

22.  Carlos-Wallace FM, Zhang L, Smith MT, Rader G, Steinmaus C. Parental, in utero, and early-life exposure to benzene and the risk of childhood leukemia: a meta-analysis. *Am J Epidemiol.* 2016;183(1):1–14

23.  Keegan TJ, Bunch KJ, Vincent TJ, et al. Case-control study of paternal occupation and social class with risk of childhood central nervous system tumors in Great Britain, 1962-2006. *Br J Cancer.* 2013;108(9):1907–1914

24.  Bailey HD, Fritchi L, Infante-Rivard C, et al. Parental occupational pesticide exposure and the risk of childhood leukemia in the offspring: findings from the Childhood Leukemia International Consortium. *Int J Cancer.* 2014;135(9):2157–2172

25. Desrosiers TA, Herring AH, Shapira SK, et al. Paternal occupation and birth defects: findings from the National Birth Defects Prevention Study. *Occu Environ Med.* 2012;69(8):534–542

26. Chen YC, Guo YL, Hsu CC, Rogan WJ. Cognitive development of Yu-Cheng ("oil disease") children prenatally exposed to heat-degraded PCBs. *JAMA.* 1992;268(22):3213–3218

27. Chen YC, Yu ML, Rogan WJ, Gladen BC, Hsu CC. A 6-year follow-up of behavior and activity disorders in the Taiwan Yu-Cheng children. *Am J Public Health.* 1994;84(3):415–421

28. Hu H, Shih R, Rothenberg S, Schwartz BS. The epidemiology of lead toxicity in adults: measuring dose and consideration of other methodologic issues. *Environ Health Perspect.* 2007;115(3):455–462

29. Gulson BL, Mizon KJ, Korsch MJ, Palmer JM, Donnelly JB. Mobilization of lead from human bone tissue during pregnancy and lactation—a summary of long-term research. *Sci Total Environ.* 2003;303(1-2):79–104

30. Shannon MW, Graef JW. Lead intoxication in infancy. *Pediatrics.* 1992;89(1):87–90

31. Thompson GN, Robertson EF, Fitzgerald S. Lead mobilization during pregnancy. *Med J Aust.* 1985;143(3):131

32. Hu H, Téllez-Rojo MM, Bellinger D, et al. Fetal lead exposure at each stage of pregnancy as a predictor of infant mental development. *Environ Health Perspect.* 2006;114(11):1730–1735

33. Grajewski B, Rocheleau CM, Lawson CC, Johnson CY. "Will my work affect my pregnancy?" Resources for anticipating and answering patients' questions. *Am J Obstet Gynecol.* 2016;214(5):597–602

34. Wigle DT, Arbuckle TE, Turner MC, et al. Epidemiologic evidence of relationships between reproductive and child health outcomes and environmental chemical contaminants. *J Toxicol Environ Health B Crit Rev.* 2008;11(5-6):373–517

35. Casas M, Cordier S, Martinez D, et al. Maternal occupation during pregnancy, birth weight, and length of gestation: combined analysis of 13 European birth cohorts. *Scand J Work Environ Health.* 2015;41(4):384–396

36. Herdt-Losavio ML, Lin S, Chapman BR, et al. Maternal occupation and the risk of birth defects: an overview from the National Birth Defects Prevention Study. *Occup Environ Med.* 2010;67(1):58–66

37. Bailey HD, Fritschi L, Metayer C, et al. Parental occupational paint exposure and risk of childhood leukemia in the offspring: findings from the Childhood Leukemia International Consortium. *Cancer Causes Control.* 2014;25(10):1351–1367

38. Pak VM, Powers M, Liu J. Occupational chemical exposures among cosmetologists. *Workplace Health Saf.* 2013;61(12):522–528

39. Williams PM, Fletcher S. Health effects of prenatal radiation exposure. *Am Fam Physician.* 2010;82(5):488–493

40. U.S. Department of Transportation Federal Aviation Administration. In-Flight Radiation Exposure. http://www.faa.gov/documentlibrary/media/advisory_circular/ac_120-61b.pdf. Accessed March 27, 2018

41. ACOG Committee on Obstetric Practice. ACOG Committee Opinion No. 443: air travel during pregnancy. *Obstet Gynecol.* 2009;114(4):954–955

42. US Federal Aviation Administration. Galactic Cosmic Radiation Exposure of Pregnant Aircrew Members. https://www.faa.gov/data_research/research/med_humanfacs/oamtechreports/2000s/media/00_33.pdf. Accessed March 27, 2018

43. NIOSH Protect your family: Reduce contamination at home. NIOSH 1997: DHHS (NIOSH) Publication No. 97-125;1-16. https://www.cdc.gov/niosh/docs/97-125/pdfs/wkhmcn.pdf. Accessed March 27, 2018

44. Protecting workers' families: A research agenda. NIOSH 2002: DHHS (NIOSH) Publication No. 2002-113;1-11. https://www.cdc.gov/niosh/docs/2002-113/pdfs/2002-113.pdf. Accessed March 27, 2018

45. Farber HJ, Walley SC, Groner JA, Nelson KE, American Academy of Pediatrics, Section on Tobacco Control. Clinical practice policy to protect children from tobacco, nicotine, and tobacco smoke. *Pediatrics*. 2015;136(5):1008–1017

46. Farber HJ, Groner J, Walley S, Nelson K, American Academy of Pediatrics, Section on Tobacco Control. Technical report protecting children from tobacco, nicotine, and tobacco smoke. *Pediatrics*. 2015;136(5):e1439–e1467

47. Oken E, Levitan EB, Gillman MW. Maternal smoking during pregnancy and child overweight: systematic review and meta-analysis. *Int J Obes (Lond)*. 2008;32(2):201–210

48. Pereira G, Evans KA, Rich DQ, Bracken MB, Bell ML. Fine particulates, preterm birth, and membrane rupture in Rochester, NY. *Epidemiology*. 2016;27(1):66–73

49. Sapkota A, Chelikowsky AP, Nachman KE, Cohen AJ, Ritz B. Exposure to particulate matter and adverse birth outcomes: a comprehensive review and meta-analysis. *Air Qual Health*. 2012;5:369–381

50. Lamichhane D, Leem JH, Lee JY, Kim HC. A meta-analysis of exposure to particulate matter and adverse birth outcomes. *Environ Health Toxicol*. 2015;30:e2015011

51. Salihu H, Ghaji N, Mbah AK, Alio AP, August EM, Boubakari I. Particulate pollutants and racial/ethnic disparity in feto-infant morbidity outcomes. *Matern Child Health J*. 2012;16(8):1679–1687

52. Brauer M, Lencar C, Tamburic L, Koehoorn M, Demers P, Karr C. A cohort study of traffic-related air pollution impacts on birth outcomes. *Environ Health Perspect*. 2008;116(5):680–686

53. Dadvand P, Parker J, Bell ML, et al. Maternal exposure to particulate air pollution and term birth weight: a multi-country evaluation of effect and heterogeneity. *Environ Health Perspect*. 2013;121(3):267–373

54. Raz R, Roberts AL, Lyall K, et al. Autism spectrum disorder and particulate matter air pollution before, during, and after pregnancy: a nested case–control analysis within the Nurses' Health Study II Cohort. *Environ Health Perspect*. 2015;123(3):264–270

55. Newman NC, Ryan P, LeMasters G, et al. Traffic-related air pollution exposure in the first year of life and behavioral scores at 7 years of age. *Environ Health Perspect*. 2013;121(6):731–736

56. Guxens M, Garcia-Esteban R, Giorgis-Allemand L, et al. Air pollution during pregnancy and childhood cognitive and psychomotor development: six European birth cohorts. *Epidemiology*. 2014;25(5):636–647

57. Quansah R, Armah FA, Essumang DK, et al. Association of arsenic with adverse pregnancy outcomes/infant mortality: a systematic review and meta-analysis. *Environ Health Perspect*. 2015:123(5):412–421

58. Harada M. Methyl mercury poisoning due to environmental contamination ("Minamata disease"). In: Oehme FW, ed. *Toxicity of Heavy Metals in the Environment*. New York, NY: Marcel Dekker; 1978:261

59. HealthData.gov. Developmental and Reproductive Toxicology Database (DART). http://www.healthdata.gov/dataset/developmental-and-reproductive-toxicology-database-dart. Accessed March 27, 2018

60. Centers for Disease Control and Prevention. Advisory on Alcohol Use in Pregnancy. http://www.cdc.gov/ncbddd/fasd/documents/SurgeonGenbookmark.pdf. Accessed March 27, 2018

61. Centers for Disease Control and Prevention. Fetal Alcohol Syndrome. Guidelines for Referral and Diagnosis. http://www.cdc.gov/ncbddd/fasd/documents/FAS_guidelines_accessible.pdf. Accessed March 27, 2018

62. Clarke DW, Smith GN, Patrick J, Richardson B, Brien JF. Activity of alcohol dehydrogenase and aldehyde dehydrogenase in maternal liver, fetal liver and placenta of the near-term pregnant ewe. *Dev Pharmacol Ther*. 1989;12(1):35–41

63. Bush B, Snow J, Koblintz R. Polychlorobyphenyl (PCB) congeners, p,p'-DDE, and hexachlorobenzene in maternal and fetal cord blood from mothers in upstate New York. *Arch Environ Contam Toxicol.* 1984;13(5):517–527

64. Ettinger AS, Lamadrid-Figueroa H, Téllez-Rojo MM, et al. Effect of calcium supplementation on blood lead levels in pregnancy: a randomized placebo-controlled trial. *Environ Health Perspect.* 2009;117(1):26–31

65. Blot WJ. Growth and development following prenatal and childhood exposure to atom radiation. *J Radiat Res.* 1975;16(Suppl):82–88

66. Harjulehto T, Aro T, Rita H, Rytömaa T, Saxén L. The accident at Chernobyl and outcomes of pregnancy in Finland. *BMJ.* 1989;298(6679):995–997

67. Hoffman W. Fallout from the Chernobyl nuclear disaster and congenital malformations in Europe. *Arch Environ Health.* 2001;56(6):478–484

68. Brent RL. Saving lives and changing family histories: appropriate counseling of pregnant women and men and women of reproductive age, concerning the risk of diagnostic radiation exposures during and before pregnancy. *Am J Obstet Gynecol.* 2009;200(1):4–24

69. Lin CM, Chang WP, Doyle P, et al. Prolonged time to pregnancy in residents exposed to ionising radiation in cobalt-60 contaminated buildings. *Occup Environ Med.* 2010;67(3):187–195

70. Zhu JL, Knudsen LE, Andrersen AM, Hjollund NH, Olsen J. Laboratory work and pregnancy outcomes: a study within the national birth cohort in Denmark. *Occup Environ Med.* 2006;63(1):53–58

71. Milunsky A, Ulcickas M, Rothman KJ, Willett W, Jick SS, Jick H. Maternal heat exposure and neural tube defects. *JAMA.* 1992;268(7):882–885

72. American Academy of Pediatrics, Committee on Environmental Health. Noise: a hazard for the fetus and newborn. *Pediatrics.* 1997;100(4):724–727

73. Trasande L, Cronk C, Durkin M, et al. Environment and obesity in the National Children's Study. *Environ Health Perspect.* 2009;117(2):159–166

74. Boekelheide K, Blumberg B, Chapin RE, et al. Predicting later-life outcomes of early-life exposures. *Environ Health Perspect.* 2012;120(10):1353–1361

75. Manikkam M, Guerrero-Bosagna C, Tracey R, Haque MM, Skinner MK. Transgenerational actions of environmental compounds on reproductive disease and identification of epigenetic biomarkers of ancestral exposures. *PLoS One.* 2012;7(2):e31901

76. Lie RT, Wilcox AJ, Skjaerven R. A population-based study of the risk of recurrence of birth defects. *N Engl J Med.* 1994;331(1):1–4

77. Lanphear BP. The impact of toxins on the developing brain. *Ann Rev Public Health.* 2015;36;211–230

78. Centers for Disease Control and Prevention. https://www.cdc.gov/reproductivehealth/unintendedpregnancy. Accessed March 27, 2018

79. Stephenson J, Heslehurst N, Hall J, et al. Before the beginning: nutrition and lifestyle in the preconception period and its importance for future health. *Lancet.* 2018;391(10132):1830–1841

80. Before, Between & Beyond Pregnancy. http://beforeandbeyond.org. Accessed March 27, 2018

81. Caldwell KL, Makhmudov A, Ely E, Jones RL, Wang RY. Iodine status of the U.S. population, National Health and Nutrition Examination Survey, 2005-2006 and 2007-2008. *Thyroid.* 2011;21(4):419–427

82. Blount BC, Valentin-Blasini L, Osterloh JD, Maulden JP, Pirkle JL. Perchlorate exposure of the US population, 2001-2002. *J Expo Sci Environ Epidemiol.* 2007;17(4):400–407

83. Murray CW, Egan SK, Kim H, Beru N, Bolger PM. US Food and Drug Administration's total diet study: dietary intake of perchlorate and iodine. *J Expo Sci Environ Epidemiol.* 2008;18(6):571–580

84. American Academy of Pediatrics Council on Environmental Health, Rogan WJ, Paulson JA, et al. Iodine deficiency, pollutant chemicals, and the thyroid: new information on an old problem. *Pediatrics*. 2014;133(6):1163–1166

85. Institute of Medicine. *Seafood Choices: Balancing Benefits and Risks*. 2006. http://nationalacademies.org/hmd/reports/2006/seafood-choices-balancing-benefits-and-risks.aspx. Accessed March 27, 2018

86. US Department of Labor. Occupational Safety and Health Administration. Hair Salons: Facts about Formaldehyde in Hair Products. https://www.osha.gov/SLTC/hairsalons/protecting_worker_health.html. Accessed March 27, 2018

# Chapter 9

# Community Design

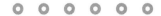

## KEY POINTS

- The design of communities and neighborhoods (including buildings, parks, transportation systems, and infrastructure such as roads and sewer systems) affects children's physical and mental health.
- Community design contributes to factors that influence health, including air quality, physical activity, safety, community connectedness, and access to healthy food and other resources.
- Pediatricians can be powerful advocates for urban planning practices that promote children's health.

## INTRODUCTION

Buildings, parks, infrastructure (ie, roads, sewer systems), and other elements of urban design influence children's physical and mental health. For example, physical activity can be encouraged and supported by community design elements that provide safe, accessible spaces for children to walk and play. The design of cities and communities also may contribute to risks of injury, respiratory disease, infections, and mood disorders. Vulnerable populations, including low-income and minority communities, are disproportionately affected by these risks.

The 20th century shift of many families from cities to suburbs and the modern dependence on cars for transportation fundamentally changed how many American children live.[1] Zoning laws were originally designed to separate people from the noxious fumes of industry. There has been commercial and governmental promotion of home and automobile ownership. Extra land was needed to fulfill this urban design strategy. Residential communities, therefore, were and often continue to be far from commercial areas, schools, and other regular destinations. This shift in lifestyle and community design occurred in parallel with extraordinary increases in obesity, asthma, mental health disorders, and other chronic conditions.

Activity levels, diet, and outdoor play are factors that modify the risk of these chronic illnesses in children, adolescents, and adults. Community design features, such as walkways, bikeways, and parks, provide opportunities for physical activity. These features also mitigate air pollution, traffic-related risks, and other safety risks to children and others. Access to trees and green spaces influences mental health, cognitive development, and school performance. Access to healthy food, infrastructure conferring resilience in relation to natural disasters, and neighborhood features that increase the perceptions of safety and community connectedness are other examples of health-promoting attributes of community design. Pediatricians are in a unique position to collaborate with urban planners and policy makers in designing communities that promote children's health.[2]

## RISK OF INJURIES

Many features of community design contribute to child safety. For example, high traffic speeds,[3] wide road lanes, and lack of safe pedestrian walkways[4] contribute to pedestrian injuries. Bicycle paths and traffic calming measures help to prevent injuries to bicyclists.[5]

Siting decisions can influence the risk of injury. For example, proximity of residences to high-speed, high traffic roads can increase the risk of traffic-related injury and increase exposure to traffic-related air pollution. Proximity to hazards, such as toxic waste sites, can impair air and water quality (see Chapter 13).

Neighborhood infrastructure components, such as parks, painted and marked crosswalks, and maintained vacant lots, also promote safety. Features such as these are associated with a reduction in adolescent homicide rates, likely the result of a complex interplay of factors including increasing opportunities for physical activity and social interaction, as well as decreasing the appearance of dilapidation and neglect.[6]

## OBESITY

Although evidence about the effects of community design on obesity is inconclusive,[7] it is clear that community design features can influence families' food choices and level of physical activity. Physical activity includes free play, sports, walking or cycling with friends, or walking or cycling to school. Community design features, such as planning of neighborhoods, location of schools, and access to recreation centers and green spaces, affect opportunities for physical activity.

## Access to Healthy Foods

Community design can affect nutrition through the availability, or lack thereof, of fresh fruits and vegetables, as well as the availability of unhealthy food outlets. Community gardens, farmers' markets, promoting the presence of chain supermarkets, and urban farms are efforts to increase proximity to healthy food outlets.[8] Especially in communities with low rates of car ownership, the relative proximity to large grocery stores increases fruit and vegetable intake, whereas the relative proximity to convenience stores decreases intake. Low-income, minority, and rural neighborhoods have less access (in proximity and transportation) to supermarkets and healthful food but have increased access to convenience stores and the nutrient-poor, high-calorie foods often found in these food outlets.[9] In a study of neighborhoods in Detroit, increased access to supermarkets increased fruit and vegetable consumption among adults by 0.69 servings per day. White, black, and Hispanic adults all consumed more servings of fruits and vegetables when a large grocery store was present in their neighborhood, with the highest increase for Hispanic adults; convenience stores significantly decreased fruit and vegetable intake among Hispanic adults.[10] In addition, a higher density of fast food outlets has been associated with increased weight gain and increased diagnosis of obesity among children.[11,12] Greater accessibility to fast food outlets has also been associated with increased insulin resistance (independent of obesity measures) among Hispanic children.[13] Adolescents with fast food outlets in close proximity to their schools, compared with their peers for whom this is not the case, consume fewer servings of fruit and vegetables and more soda, and are more likely to be overweight.[14] Disparities exist in the relative proximity of unhealthy food outlets to schools, with Hispanic and low-income students most likely to attend schools located near convenience stores and fast food outlets.[15-18] The long-term effects of city and state land use policies and public transportation routes that increase access to grocery stores on children's health remain to be seen.

Focus group data suggest that residents of low-income communities place the highest value on efforts to improve economic access to food; geographic access is an important secondary factor.[19] Although improving economic access to food is outside the scope of this chapter, it is important to remember that these efforts work hand in hand. Geographic access to healthy food alone is not sufficient to increase healthful food purchasing and intake. Food quality and store quality (ie, cleanliness, good upkeep, limiting traffic or panhandling in parking lots) are also important to community members.[19] As pediatricians and policy makers work to address the problem of healthy food access, it is important to include community stakeholders in designing and implementing solutions.

## Active Commuting to School

Active commuting to school, defined as walking or biking, can be an important source of regular physical activity in children. This form of activity has declined in the last half century. Between 1969 and 2001, national rates of elementary school students' active transportation to school declined from 41% to 13%.[20] School policies, community safety programs, and school siting have had important and sometimes unintended adverse effects on health promotion.

The significant decline in active commuting to school is partly explained by proximity to schools. The closer children live to their school, the more likely they are to actively commute. In 1969, 66% of students lived within 3 miles of school; in 2001, the number of students dropped to 49%. Proximity does not, however, fully explain the decline in walking. Over the past several decades, proximity between home and school seems to be playing a declining role in whether children actively commute. In 1977, if a child lived 1.9 miles (3 km) from school versus 1 mile (1.6 km), the odds of active commuting were decreased by a factor of 50. In 2001, the odds only decreased by a factor of 21.[20] Therefore, there are other factors in addition to distance from home to school that influence how frequently children actively commute to school.

Historically, small neighborhood schools served as "anchors" within the community and places for after-school programs, for social and recreational gathering, and as disaster shelters.[21] In 1953, the Council of Education Facilities Planners International recommended a minimum acreage of 10 acres (4.05 hectares) for elementary schools and an extra acre (0.40 hectares) for every 100 students over 600.[22] In the 1950s, many states established policies on the size and location of school buildings that met these standards. According to those guidelines, to receive state funding, schools required a minimum acreage; having more students meant that a larger amount of space was required.[20] Because untapped acreage sufficient to meet these standards is most often at the edge of an urban area, neighborhood schools (typically only 2 to 8 acres [0.81 to 3.24 hectares] in size) were frequently demolished or closed in favor of larger schools at the outskirts of communities. In 2004, the Council of Education Facilities Planners International (CEFPI) revised its guidelines, no longer recommending minimum acreage.[23] Since that time, many states' policy makers recognized the health benefits of walking to school, and there is increasing interest in supporting smaller schools. Change occurs slowly, however, with other factors influencing the maintenance of large acreage. District-level pressure to maintain large athletic facilities encourages larger acreage. There also is demand from policy makers and communities for larger parking lots because of the large number of children who are driven or drive to school. Evidence from 4 states shows that thus far, the on-the-ground impact of changes to acreage requirements has been slow, largely because of a lag in district-level school planning.[24] More research is needed to understand why district-level school planning has not led to siting more schools closer to homes, and to understand influences on individual behavior regarding active transportation.[24]

Parents' perceptions of crime and traffic safety may influence whether children actively commute to school. In a study of Australian children, 81% of parents of children aged 10 to 12 years reported a strong concern about strangers, and 78% expressed a strong concern about road safety. Forty-seven percent reported no lights or crossings, and 42% reported that their children had to cross several roads to get to school.[25] Road safety concern was the factor most strongly associated with the likelihood that children aged 10 to 12 years walked or biked to school. Lack of a road barrier on a busy road, no lights or crossings, a steep road without a barrier, and a school distance of more than 800 meters from home were associated with less active transport. Active commuting also was decreased if other children did not live in the area. When parents of American children were asked which possible barriers existed for children walking to school, long distance was identified by 50% of respondents; traffic danger by 40%; adverse weather conditions by 24%; crime danger by 18%; and opposing school policy by 7%. Sixteen percent of parents reported no barriers. Their children were 6 times more likely to walk or bike to school.[26]

The relationship between safety and physical activity is complex. Although road safety plays a role in active transportation to school, the relationship of fear of crime to physical activity is less well understood. Perceptions and the presence of neighborhood crime may affect physical activity. Crime prevention strategies themselves may unintentionally decrease physical activity, whether because of a physical barrier such as a fence that limits access to a recreation area or playground after hours, or because of increased validation of parental fears of crime.[27]

Many localities are making efforts to promote walking and biking to school because of the childhood obesity crisis. Measures include walk to school days, bike to school days, safety measures such as crossing guards at busy intersections, and collaboration between local police and schools to improve pedestrian safety near schools. There is hope for success for policies designed to promote safe walking to school. "Walking school bus" programs, in which groups of children walk to school with adult supervision, have been associated with increased prevalence of students walking to school, as well as an increase in general level of physical activity among students.[28] An observational study of 118 Toronto elementary schools found that pedestrian crosswalks, traffic lights, intersection density, and school crossing guards correlated positively with walking to school. The presence of a crossing guard could reduce the influence of other features of the environment on active transportation to school.[29]

## Walkability

The principle of walkability describes how community design relates to walking behavior. Just as walking to school is influenced by community design, walking for other utilitarian reasons, and for recreation, is also affected. Residential density, proximity, and ease of access to nonresidential land uses, street connectivity, walking or cycling facilities, aesthetics, pedestrian traffic safety, and crime safety play a role in walkability.[30] Hills, sidewalks, and proximity to destinations affect walkability.[31] Increased neighborhood walkability increases how much children walk to school.[32]

When looking at how a neighborhood is designed, one salient feature is the proximity of one residence to another. For example, some suburban neighborhoods are built with large lots with a single-family home on each lot. Homes may each be on as much as a third of an acre (0.14 hectare). In more urban neighborhoods, there are often multifamily dwellings built close together with smaller lot sizes. When homes are located more closely together, children walk more.[33] For adolescents, walkability can be affected by social features of their neighborhood. When adolescents are more likely to talk or wave to neighbors, they are also more likely to walk as a means of transportation.[34]

Geographic features of a neighborhood can have positive or negative influences on walking, depending on whether the individual is walking for utilitarian or recreational reasons. For example, although the presence of hills decreases walking for transportation to a destination, hills (and sidewalks) seem to increase rates of walking for recreation. Having destinations, such as a grocery store or park, nearby also can increase walking.

Although distance is the most important factor that influences the likelihood that children walk to school, other factors that increase daily walking have been demonstrated among adults; these may have a similar effect among children. Factors include mixed use zoning (blending residential, commercial, cultural, and other development in a physically and functionally integrated manner), vacant commercial center redevelopment, maintaining a historic district, and implementing traffic-calming methods (to slow motor vehicle speeds in urban and residential areas).[35]

## Public Transportation

The availability and use of public transportation increases physical activity among adults. In one study from the United Kingdom, adults who commuted using public transportation had a lower body mass index than those who commuted via car. Switching from commuting by car to public transportation was associated with an average weight loss of about 10 pounds (4.5 kg) in the first year.[36] Another study showed that new transit riders lost weight while former transit riders who switched to commuting by car gained weight.[37] Public transit commuters are more likely to get at least 30 minutes of physical activity daily.[38]

## Centers of Recreation

Parks, gyms, playgrounds, and sports fields offer important recreational opportunities for physical activity. For normal weight children aged 4 to 7 years and 8 to 12 years, an increase in per capita park area was associated with increased physical activity.[39] Access to parks predicts physical activity, especially for minority populations.[40] Significantly fewer centers of physical activity are available, however, in low-income neighborhoods and in neighborhoods with more ethnic minorities. In a study of 20,000 children in grades 7 to 12, those from neighborhoods characterized by low education levels and high proportions of ethnic minorities were half as likely to have access to a physical activity center (school, public park, gym, YMCA).[41] When more physical activity centers were located in a neighborhood, fewer children were overweight.

## AIR POLLUTION

Exposure to air pollution, of which vehicular pollution is a major source, is associated with health effects in children, including increasing the risk of low birth weight and prematurity, contributing to asthma severity, and impairing neurocognitive development.[42] Air pollution contributes to obesity[43] and the development of type 2 diabetes mellitus.[44] Many urban design features can reduce air pollution by (1) limiting urban sprawl; (2) zoning for "mixed use" so that residential areas are near to needed resources and amenities such as food outlets, retail, and recreational spaces; (3) providing infrastructure for multi-modal transportation, including walking, biking, and public transportation; and (4) increasing trees and green spaces. When residences and schools are located near high-traffic roadways, there is more exposure to vehicular air pollution, and proximity to these roadways is associated with increased asthma risk.[45]

## TREES AND GREEN SPACE

Urban trees improve air quality[46,47] and mitigate the urban heat island effect (the phenomenon of metropolitan areas having higher air temperatures than surrounding areas, caused both by urban land use and waste heat resulting from energy use). Urban trees reduce energy used for cooling and heating,[48] and make urban environments aesthetically more preferable.[49] Exposure to green spaces can be psychologically and physiologically restorative by promoting mental health,[50,51] reducing nonaccidental mortality,[52] reducing physician-assessed morbidity,[53] reducing income-related health inequality's effect on morbidity,[54] reducing blood pressure and stress levels,[55,56] reducing sedentary leisure time,[57] and promoting physical activity.[58,59]

## Mental Health, Cognitive Development, and Learning

Access to neighborhood green spaces is associated with lower levels of depression and anxiety.[60] Exposure to green spaces is associated with improved cognitive development among primary schoolchildren and the "greenness" of landscape surrounding schools is linked with improved academic performance.[61,62] The overall mental well-being of children, including their response to stress, attention, and behavior, in addition to their cognitive development and academic performance, is improved with increased access to green spaces.[63]

One pathway by which access to trees and green space may influence mental health is through restoration, the ability to recover from stress and regain attention and focus. Exposure to acute and chronic stress has effects on physical health, such as reduced immune function and fatigue. Once fatigue sets in, it is increasingly difficult for an individual to pay attention and inhibit impulses. In people with no underlying disorders of inattention, symptoms of inattention and impulsivity are reduced after exposure to natural settings and views.[64,65]

In a regional study[66] and a national study,[67] parents of children with attention-deficit/hyperactivity disorder (ADHD) reported that their children's attention and behavioral symptoms improved more after activities in green outdoor settings. This suggests a potential therapeutic benefit of exposure to natural settings for children with ADHD.

Being exposed to nature in neighborhoods is hypothesized to decrease loneliness by encouraging social interaction, and helping to create crucial social relationships that buffer stress.[68] Local parks are associated with increased play among children and social support between parents and non-family members.[69,70] Exposure to nature in neighborhoods is associated with an increase in moderate physical activity[71] and increased "nature affinity."[72] Nature affinity, in turn, reinforces ongoing park visits and is associated with decreased stress.[73] New clinic-based interventions are exploring pediatricians' roles in promoting nature exposure among low-income children living in urban settings.[74] Future research will illuminate the effects of such interventions on children's health and development.

## STORMWATER MANAGEMENT

In urban settings with a high concentration of impervious surfaces such as roofs and pavement, these surfaces can collect pollutants that are then washed into waterways during storm events. Water can pool on these surfaces, creating potential breeding areas for mosquitoes that may carry disease. Many cities have combined sewer systems that collect sewage and stormwater in the same pipes. During storm events, these systems can overflow and discharge a mix of untreated sewage and surface runoff into streams, rivers, and other bodies of water. These events can harm drinking water quality, render recreational waters unsafe, and contribute to the spread of waterborne and vectorborne illnesses.[75]

Stormwater management strategies include incorporating building and landscape features such as permeable pavement, green roofs, tree planting, and bioretention systems (landscaping features designed to slow stormwater runoff, remove pollutants, and then allow infiltration of treated water into native soil or direction to nearby drains). These strategies can help to mitigate stormwater runoff risks and protect communities from storm damage.

## COMMUNITY RESILIENCE

In light of events such as Hurricane Katrina in New Orleans, Hurricane Harvey in Houston, and Hurricane Maria in Puerto Rico, strategies to increase the physical resilience of communities and neighborhoods in the face of extreme weather events must be considered in urban planning policies and practices. These strategies include building siting practices, stormwater management infrastructure, and distributed power generation. In wildfire-prone areas, buildings and communities can be protected by brush clearing, barrier zones, and fire-resistant landscaping. Designing communities for resilience to climate change-related risks, including extreme weather events and rising sea levels, is critical to protect children's health.[76]

## VULNERABLE POPULATIONS

Hazardous neighborhood features such as unsafe housing, proximity to environmental health hazards such as air pollution, and lack of safe spaces for outdoor walking and play are more likely to be found in minority and low-income communities (see Chapter 56). Children with chronic illness and physical limitations also are particularly vulnerable to these hazards. The availability of neighborhood recreation centers, parks, and playgrounds is associated with increased physical activity in children with special health care needs.[77]

### Advocacy Efforts by Pediatricians

Pediatricians can be powerful advocates for urban planning practices that promote children's health. They can offer testimony to policy makers or during public comment periods when new community design features or regulations are considered. Pediatricians are uniquely positioned to discuss the child health impacts of interventions, such as road construction, public transportation infrastructure, streetscapes that are pedestrian- and bike-friendly, zoning laws, and parks and public spaces. Pediatricians can work with community organizations dedicated to improving access to healthy food and limiting access to unhealthy food, improving public transportation and roadways that support multiple modes of transportation, and developing trust and connectedness among community members. They can join community-wide coalitions working on safe and accessible "complete streets"—a policy and design approach requiring that streets are planned, operated, and maintained for all users regardless of what kind of transportation is used. Pediatricians can work with schools to promote walking and biking to school, and to promote students' access to green spaces. Pediatricians can be a strong voice for children from underrepresented and vulnerable communities that have historically borne the brunt of environmental health hazards. These include children from low-income and minority communities, and those with chronic illness and disabilities.[78]

## CONCLUSION

Policies and programs that promote active transportation, improve access to park space and green space, improve access to nutritious foods, improve social connectedness, and improve community resilience can be designed with children's health in mind. Great potential exists for innovative design and programming through collaboration among pediatricians, policy makers, developers, and designers.

## FREQUENTLY ASKED QUESTIONS

Q *How can I advocate for health-promoting design features in my neighborhood or city?*

A Specific examples will vary locally and regionally. In general, to advocate for measures supporting active transportation, relevant community organizations may include local bicycle coalitions, public transportation organizations, and regional transportation coordination agencies. Local school districts are important partners in advocating for active transportation to school, new school siting, access to green space, and schools' proximity to healthy and unhealthy food outlets. Citizens can also advocate with their city planning departments to make zoning decisions that promote active transportation and access to amenities such as healthy food outlets, trees and green spaces, and recreational areas. Additional resources are listed later in this chapter.

Q *We are thinking of moving to a new neighborhood. What can you recommend about what to look for when selecting a neighborhood?*

A Being able to walk or bike to school and other places is good for everyone's health. Consider whether your children will be able to walk or bike to school. Look for the nearest source of fresh fruits and vegetables. Look at the distance to shops and activities and consider whether these locations are sufficiently close for walking or biking. Ask potential neighbors how friendly and connected the neighbors are to each other. Ask whether they see children walking or biking to school. Find the nearest park or playground and consider whether it is within walking distance. Pay attention to the number of trees in the neighborhood.

## ADDITIONAL RESOURCES

**National Complete Streets Coalition**
Web site: https://smartgrowthamerica.org/program/national-complete-streets-coalition

**Safe Routes to School and the Transportation Alternatives Program**
Web site: www.saferoutespartnership.org/resources/fact-sheet/federal-funding-infographics

**The Children and Nature Initiative of the National Environmental Education Foundation (NEEF)**
Phone: (202) 833-2933
Web site: www.neefusa.org/health/children_nature.htm
NEEF's Children and Nature Initiative addresses preventing serious health conditions, including obesity and diabetes mellitus, and reconnecting children to nature. The Initiative educates pediatric health care providers about prescribing outdoor activities to children. The program also connects health care providers with local nature sites so that they can refer families to safe and easily accessible outdoor areas.

## REFERENCES

1. Brownson RC, Boehmer TK, Luke DA. Declining rates of physical activity in the United States: what are the contributors? *Annu Rev Public Health.* 2005;26:421–443
2. Allender S, Cavill N, Parker M, Foster C. 'Tell us something we don't already know or do!'— The response of planning and transport professionals to public health guidance on the built environment and physical activity. *J Public Health Policy.* 2009;30(1):102–116
3. Rosen E, Sander U. Pedestrian fatality risk as a function of car impact speed. *Accid Anal Prev.* 2009;41(3):536–542
4. National Highway Traffic Safety Administration. Traffic Safety Facts 2015 Data—Pedestrians. Washington, DC: US Department of Transportation; 20175. Publication no. DOT-HS-812-375. https://crashstats.nhtsa.dot.gov/Api/Public/ViewPublication/812375. Accessed July 14, 2018
5. Harris MA, Reynolds CC, Winters M, et al. Comparing the effects of infrastructure on bicycling injury at intersections and non-intersections using a case-crossover design. *Inj Prev.* 2013;19(5):303–310
6. Culyba AJ, Jacoby SF, Richmond TS, Fein JA, Hohl BC, Branas CC. Modifiable neighborhood features associated with adolescent homicide. *JAMA Pediatr.* 2016;170(5):473–480

7. Gascon M, Vrijheid M, Nieuwenhuijsen MJ. The built environment and child health: an overview of current evidence. *Curr Environ Health Reports*. 2016;3(3):250–257

8. Grimm K, Moore LV, Scanlon KS, Centers for Disease Control and Prevention. Access to healthier food retailers: United States, 2011. *MMWR*. 2013;62(Suppl 3):20–26

9. Larson N, Story M, Nelson MC. Neighborhood environments: disparities in access to healthy foods in the U.S. *Am J Prev Med*. 2009;36(1):74–81

10. Zenk SN, Lachance LL, Schulz AJ, Mentz G, Kannan S, Ridella W. Neighborhood retail food environment and fruit and vegetable intake in a multiethnic urban population. *Am J Health Promot*. 2009;23(4):255–264

11. Pearce M, Bray I, Horswell M. Weight gain in mid-childhood and its relationship with the fast food environment. *J Public Health (Oxf)*. 2018;40(2):237–244

12. Hamano T, Li X, Sundquist J, Sundquist K. Association between childhood obesity and neighbourhood accessibility to fast-food outlets: a nationwide 6-year follow-up study of 944,487 children. *Obes Facts*. 2017;10(6):559–568

13. Hsieh S, Klassen AC, Curriero FC, et al. Fast-food restaurants, park access, and insulin resistance among Hispanic youth. *Am J Prev Med*. 2014;46(4):378–387

14. Davis B, Carpenter C. Proximity of fast-food restaurants to schools and adolescent obesity. *Am J Public Health*. 2009;99(3):505–510

15. D'Angelo H, Ammerman A, Gordon-Larsen P, Linnan L, Lytle L, Ribisl KM. Sociodemographic disparities in proximity of schools to tobacco outlets and fast-food restaurants. *Am J Public Health*. 2016;106(9):1556–1562

16. Strum R. Disparities in the food environment surrounding US middle and high schools. *Public Health*. 2008;122(7):681–690

17. Neckerman KM, Bader MD, Richards CA, et al. Disparities in the food environments of New York City public schools. *Am J Prev Med*. 2010;39(3):195–202

18. Kestens Y, Daniel M. Social inequalities in food exposure around schools in an urban area. *Am J Prev Med*. 2010;39(1):33–40

19. Evans G, Banks K, Jennings R, et al. Increasing access to healthful foods: a qualitative study with residents of low-income communities. *Int J Behav Nutr Phys Act*. 2015;12(Suppl 1):S5

20. McDonald N. Active transportation to school: trends among U.S. schoolchildren, 1969 - 2001. *Am J Prev Med*. 2007;32(6):509–516

21. Passmore S. *Education and Smart Growth: Reversing School Sprawl for Better Schools and Communities: Translation Paper*. Coral Gables, Florida: Funder's Network for Smart Growth and Livable Communities.

22. Beaumont CE, Pianca EG. *Why Johnny Can't Walk to School*. Washington, DC: National Trust for Historic Preservation; 2002. https://www.americantrails.org/files/pdf/whyjohnnywalkschool.pdf. Accessed July 17, 2018

23. *Creating Connections: The CEFPI Guide for Educational Facility Planning*. Scottsdale, AZ: Council of Educational Facility Planners International (CEFPI); 2004

24. McDonald N, Salvesen DA, Kuhlman HR, Combs TS. The impact of changes in state minimum acreage policies on school siting practices. *Journal of Planning Education and Research*. 2014;34(2):169–179

25. Timperio A, Crawford D, Telford A, Salmon J. Perceptions about the local neighborhood and walking and cycling among children. *Prev Med*. 2004;38(1):39–47

26. Centers for Disease Control and Prevention. Barriers to children walking to or from school-United States, 2004. *MMWR Morb Mortal Wkly Rep*. 2005;54(38):949–952

27. Foster S, Giles-Corti B. The built environment, neighborhood crime and constrained physical activity: an exploration of inconsistent findings. *Prev Med*. 2008;47(3):241–251

28. Smith L, Norgate S, Cherrett T, Davies N, Winstanley C, Harding M. Walking school buses as a form of active transportation for children—a review of the evidence. *J Sch Health.* 2015;85(3): 197–210

29. Rothman L, To T, Buliung R, Macarthur C, Howard A. Influence of social and built environment features on children walking to school: an observational study. *Prev Med.* 2014;60:10–15

30. Moudon AV, Lee C, Cheadle AD, et al. Operational definitions of walkable neighborhood: theoretical and empirical insights. *J Phys Act Health.* 2006;3(Suppl 1):S99–S117

31. Lee C, Moudon AV. Correlates of walking for transportation or recreation purposes. *J Phys Act Health.* 2006;3(Suppl 1):S77–S98

32. Kerr J, Rosenberg D, Sallis JF, Saelens BE, Frank LD, Conway TL. Active commuting to school: associations with environment and parental concerns. *Med Sci Sports Exerc.* 2006;38(4):787–793

33. Roemmich JN, Epstein LH, Raja S, Yin L. The neighborhood and home environments: disparate effects on physical activity and sedentary behaviors in youth. *Ann Behav Med.* 2007;33(1):29–38

34. Carver A, Timperio AF, Crawford DA. Neighborhood road environments and physical activity among youth: the CLAN study. *J Urban Health.* 2008;85(4):532–544

35. Saelens BE, Handy SL. Built environment correlates of walking: a review. *Med Sci Sports Exerc.* 2008;40(7 Suppl):S550–S566

36. Flint E, Cummins S. Active commuting and obesity in mid-life: cross-sectional, observational evidence from UK Biobank. *Lancet Diabetes Endocrinol.* 2016;4(5):420–435

37. Brown BB, Werner CM, Tribby CP, Miller HJ, Smith KR. Transit use, physical activity, and body mass index changes: objective measures associated with complete street light-rail construction. *Am J Public Health.* 2015;105(7):1468–1474

38. Saelens BE, Moudon AV, Kang B, Hurvitz P, Zhou C. Relation between higher physical activity and public transit use. *Am J Public Health.* 2014;104(5):854–859

39. Roemmich JN, Epstein LH, Raja S, Yin L, Robinson J, Winiewicz D. Association of access to parks and recreational facilities with the physical activity of young children. *Prev Med.* 2006;43(6):437–441

40. Cohen D, McKenzie TL, Sehgal A, Williamson S, Golinelli D, Lurie N. Contribution of public parks to physical activity. *Am J Public Health.* 2007;97(3):509–514

41. Gordon-Larsen P, Nelson MC, Page P, Popkin BM. Inequality in the built environment underlies key health disparities in physical activity and obesity. *Pediatrics.* 2006;117(2):417–424

42. American Academy of Pediatrics Committee on Environmental Health. Ambient air pollution: health hazards to children. *Pediatrics.* 2004;114(6):1699–1707

43. McConnell R, Shen E, Gilliland FD, et al. A longitudinal cohort study of body mass index and childhood exposure to secondhand tobacco smoke and air pollution: the Southern California Children's Health Study. *Environ Health Perspect.* 2015;123(4):360–366

44. Alderete TL, Habre R, Toledo-Corral CM, et al. Longitudinal associations between ambient air pollution with insulin sensitivity, β-cell function, and adiposity in Los Angeles Latino children. *Diabetes.* 2017;66(7):1789–1796

45. McConnell R, Islam T, Shankardass K, et al. Childhood incident asthma and traffic-related air pollution at home and school. *Environ Health Perspect.* 2010;118(7):1021–1026

46. Nowak DJ, Crane DE, Stevens JC. Air pollution removal by urban trees and shrubs in the United States. *Urban Forestry & Urban Greening.* 2006;4:115–123

47. Nowak DC, Hirabayashi S, Bodine A, Greenfield E. Tree and forest effects on air quality and human health in the United States. *Environ Pollut.* 2014;193:119–129

48. Akbari H, Pomeranz M, Taha H. Cool surfaces and shade trees to reduce energy use and improve air quality in urban areas. *Solar Energy.* 2001;70(3):295–310

49. Smardon RC. Perception and aesthetics of the urban environment: review of the role of vegetation. *Landscape & Urban Planning.* 1988;15(1-2):85–106

50. Richardson EA, Pearce J, Mitchell R, Kingham S. Role of physical activity in the relationship between urban green space and health. *Public Health.* 2013;127(4):318–324

51. Hyun Q, Craig W, Janssen I, Pickett W. Exposure to public natural space as a protective factor for emotional well-being among young people in Canada. *BMC Public Health.* 2013;13:407

52. Villeneuve PJ, Jerrett M, Su JG, et al. A cohort study relating urban green space with mortality in Ontario, Canada. *Environ Res.* 2012;115:51–58

53. Maas J, Verheij RA, de Vries S, Spreeuwenberg P, Schellevis FG, Groenewegen PP. Morbidity is related to a green living environment. *J Epidemiol Community Health.* 2009;63(12):967–973

54. Mitchell R, Popham F. Effect of exposure to natural environment on health inequalities: an observational population study. *Lancet.* 2008;372(9650):1655–1660

55. Grahn P, Stigsdotter UA. Landscape planning and stress. *Urban Forestry & Urban Greening.* 2003;2:1–18

56. Pretty J, Peacock J, Sellens M, Griffin M. The mental and physical health outcomes of green exercise. *Int J Environ Health Res.* 2005;15(5):319–337

57. Storgaard, RL, Hansen HS, Aadahl M, Glumer C. Association between neighbourhood green space and sedentary leisure time in a Danish population. *Scand J Public Health.* 2013;41(8): 846–852

58. Kaczynski AT, Henderson KA. Environmental correlates of physical activity: a review of evidence about parks and recreation. *Leisure Sciences.* 2007;29:315–354

59. Humpel N, Owen N, Leslie E. Environmental factors associated with adults' participation in physical activity: a review. *Am J Prev Med.* 2002;22(3):188–199

60. Beyer KM, Kaltenbach A, Szabo A, Bogar S, Nieto JF, Malecki KM. Exposure to neighborhood green space and mental health: evidence from the survey of the health of Wisconsin. *Int J Environ Res Public Health.* 2014;11(3):3453–3472

61. Dadvand P, Nieuwenhuijsen MJ, Esnaola M, et al. Green spaces and cognitive development in primary schoolchildren. *Proc Natl Acad Sci U S A.* 2015;112(26):7937–7942

62. Wu CD, McNeely E, Cedeño-Laurent JG, et al. Linking student performance in Massachusetts elementary schools with the "greenness" of school surroundings using remote sensing. *PLoS One.* 2014;9(10):e108548

63. McCormick R. Does access to green space impact the mental well-being of children: a systematic review. *J Pediatr Nurs.* 2017;37:3–7

64. Kaplan S. The restorative benefits of nature: toward an integrative framework. *J Environ Psychol.* 1995;15:169–182

65. Kaplan R, Kaplan S. *The Experience of Nature.* New York, NY: Cambridge University Press; 1989

66. Taylor AF, Kuo F, Sullivan W. Coping with ADD: the surprising connection to green play settings. *Environ Behav.* 2001;33(1):54–77

67. Kuo FE, Taylor AF. A potential natural treatment for attention-deficit/hyperactivity disorder: evidence from a national study. *Am J Public Health.* 2004;94(9):1580–1586

68. de Vries S, van Dillen S, Groenewegen P, Spreeuwenberg P. Streetscape and greenery nd health: stress, social cohesion and physical activity as mediators. *Soc Sci Med.* 2013;94:26–33

69. Bedimo-Rung AL, Mowen AJ, Cohen DA. The significance of parks to physical activity and public health: a conceptual model. *Am J Prev Med.* 2005;28(2 Suppl 2):159–168

70. American Public Health Association Policy Statement. 2013. *Improving Health and Wellness through Access to Nature.* https://www.apha.org/policies-and-advocacy/public-health-policy-statements/policy-database/2014/07/08/09/18/improving-health-and-wellness-through-access-to-nature. Accessed July 17, 2018

71. Kaczynski AT, Henderson KA. Parks and recreation settings and active living: a review of associations with physical activity function and intensity. *J Phys Act Health.* 2008;5(4):619–632

72. Perkins H. Measuring love and care for nature. *J Environ Psychol.* 2010;30(4):455–463

73. Feda D, Seelbinder A, Baek S, Raja S, Yin L, Roemmich JN. Neighbourhood parks and reduction in stress among adolescents: results from Buffalo, New York. *Indoor and Built Environment.* 2015;24:631–639. http://journals.sagepub.com/doi/abs/10.1177/1420326X14535791. Accessed July 17, 2018

74. Razani N, Kohn MA, Wells NM, Thompson D, Hamilton Flores H, Rutherford GW. Design and evaluation of a park prescription program for stress reduction and health promotion in low-income families: The Stay Healthy in Nature Everyday (SHINE) study protocol. *Contemp Clin Trials.* 2016;51:8–14

75. Gaffield SJ, Goo RL, Richards LA, Jackson RJ. Public health effects of inadequately managed stormwater runoff. *Am J Public Health.* 2003;93(9):1527–1533

76. American Academy of Pediatrics Council on Environmental Health. Global climate change and children's health. *Pediatrics.* 2015;136(5):992–997

77. An R, Yang Y, Li K. Residential neighborhood amenities and physical activity among U.S. children with special health care needs. *Matern Child Health J.* 2017;21(5):1026–1036

78. Perdue WC, Stone LA, Gostin LO. The built environment and its relationship to the public's health: the legal framework. *Am J Public Health.* 2003;93(9):1390–1394

# Chapter 10

# Child Care Settings

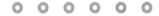

## KEY POINTS

- Environmental hazards in child care settings may include poor indoor air quality, secondhand and thirdhand smoke, lead, mold, pesticides, and phthalates among others.
- Key environmental health questions should be included in the routine health and safety inspection of a child care facility.
- Although disinfectants and sanitizers are essential to control communicable diseases in child care settings, they are potentially hazardous to children, particularly if the products are in concentrated form.

## INTRODUCTION

Every day, 12 million preschoolers—including 6 million infants and toddlers, regardless of their parents' work status—are in some form of nonparental care.[1] This accounts for approximately half of children younger than 6 years. Typical child care arrangements for young children when parents work outside the home are child care facilities (22%), family child care homes (17%), parents (22%), relatives (29%), and in-home caregivers other than a parent or relative (3%).[1] Children enter care as early as 6 weeks of age and can be in care for 40 or more hours per week until they reach school age.[1] Millions of school-aged children are in after-school and summer activities, and more than 6 million children are home alone on a regular basis.[1]

Child care settings are located in single-family homes or buildings specifically designed for child care or within office buildings, schools, churches, malls, health clubs, and other sites. The American Public Health Association and American

Academy of Pediatrics (AAP) recommend that these national child care settings be designed or modified to meet current standards published in *Caring for Our Children: National Health and Safety Performance Standards—Guidelines for Out-of-Home Child Care Programs, Third Edition.*[2] These standards, which apply to all aspects of child care settings, including environmental health aspects, should be met regardless of the setting or whether the care provided is full time or part time.

States establish and enforce child care licensing regulations that include health and safety requirements. The scope and intensity of state enforcement activities differ among the provider types within states as well as among states overall. For example, most states do not regulate some types of providers, such as relatives or in-home nannies and au pairs.[3] Child care centers typically have more health and safety regulations and oversight compared with family child care homes, hourly drop-off care, and parochial and preschool programs (particularly if they operate on a part–time basis). Compliance with regulations often depends on the degree to which child care providers agree with the rationale for the regulations as well as the quality and frequency of inspections. The licensing and enforcement activities most commonly considered to be critical are background checks, monitoring visits, sanctions, training for licensing staff, and caseload of licensing staff.[3]

The occurrence of environmental hazards in child care varies widely and is influenced by the following:

- Type of setting;
- Licensing requirements;
- Location, age, and condition of the structure;
- Past use of the land or structure;
- Current use of other parts of the structure;
- Behaviors and practices of adults in the setting; and
- Prevalence of hazards in the community.

Hazards in child care settings include those related to food and food sharing, with risks of food contamination and allergic reactions. These are covered in Chapter 18. Hazards related to using toxic arts and crafts materials are covered in Chapter 46. Information about the importance of handwashing, safety in the use of toys, selection and maintenance of equipment, and playground design to avoid choking, falling, and strangulation hazards is presented in *Caring for our Children: National Health and Safety Performance Standards—Guidelines for Out-of-Home Child Care Programs.*[2]

Hazards in a child care setting can adversely affect a group of children. On the other hand, children may benefit when hazards are reduced or controlled. For example, children exposed to secondhand tobacco smoke (SHS), radon, or lead paint at home may reduce their total daily exposure by spending time in child care if the child care setting is free of these hazards.

Environmental hazards in child care settings (see Table 10-1) may include poor indoor air quality and mold, SHS, lead, pesticides, and phthalates among others (see Chapters 20, 43, 32, 40, and 41, respectively).

## Table 10-1. Possible Environmental Hazards in Child Care Settings

| ENVIRONMENTAL HAZARD | INDOOR SOURCES | OUTDOOR SOURCES |
|---|---|---|
| Carbon monoxide (CO) | ▪ Malfunctioning or improperly vented fuel-burning appliances such as stoves, furnaces, fireplaces, clothes dryers, water heaters, and space heaters<br>▪ Poorly maintained home heating systems such as dirty furnace filters or blocked flues | ▪ Playground located near high-traffic area or near the exhaust outlet of a building<br>▪ Auto, truck, or bus exhaust from attached garages, nearby roads, or parking areas |
| Secondhand and thirdhand tobacco smoke | ▪ Smoking or vaping in the child care area<br>▪ Smoking or vaping allowed when children are not present<br>  — A multiple-use building with a smoking area that is not properly ventilated and exhausted to the outside<br>  — Smoke incursions travelling through walls and vents if the building allows smoking in some units | ▪ Fresh air intake (eg, doorway) located near an outside smoking area or an exhaust outlet that emits tobacco smoke in an area where children play |
| Molds and other biological pollutants | ▪ Plumbing leaks, roof leaks, and flooding provide moisture for molds and other biological pollutants | ▪ Water from river or sewer overflows<br>  — Humid climate |
| Volatile organic compounds (VOCs) | ▪ Building materials and furnishings (eg, formaldehyde), paints, cleaning supplies, and coverings on floors | |
| Lead and other heavy metals | ▪ Leaded dust or paint chips, particularly on floors, windowsills, and window wells, and during renovation of pre-1978 structures<br>  — Leaded water piping and soldered lead connections<br>▪ Leaded paint on furniture or toys, leaded ceramic dishware, remedies, and other sources<br>▪ Certain toys, arts and crafts supplies, paints, dishware, and lead plumbing | ▪ Leaded soil or leaded paint on the building's exterior, fences, sheds, or playground equipment<br>▪ Leaded water piping and soldered lead connections<br>  — Improperly contained materials from renovations in the vicinity of the setting<br>▪ Soil contamination at the site from prior industrial use or geological mineral deposits<br>▪ Toxic clays and play structures or contents of storage areas accessible to children |

**Table 10-1. Possible Environmental Hazards in Child Care Settings (*continued*)**

| ENVIRONMENTAL HAZARD | INDOOR SOURCES | OUTDOOR SOURCES |
|---|---|---|
| Pesticide sprays including lawn and garden chemicals, herbicides, insecticides, rodenticides | ▪ Improper storage, labeling, handling, or use of pesticides in any child care area, particularly in the following high-risk areas: diaper changing areas, food preparation and storage, carpeted areas, laundry, maintenance and custodial supply rooms, rooms where children eat and play, other areas prone to pest infestation<br>▪ Pest-infested food and storage areas, bedding, laundry rooms, spaces under sinks due to preventable problems such as poor sanitation, water leaks, and unprotected openings to the outside<br>— Old cardboard boxes<br>— Clutter | ▪ Improper storage, labeling, handling, or use of chemical products in any area accessible to children, particularly unsecured storage sheds<br>▪ Infested playgrounds and storage sheds, space under sheds, debris, and clutter or dense foliage near the foundation<br>▪ Location next to agricultural fields or contaminated sites<br>▪ Use of pesticide sprays |
| Sanitizers and disinfectants | ▪ Industrial strength and general cleaning products and room deodorizers used indoors<br>(See Table 10-3) | |
| Polybrominated diphenyl ether (PBDE) flame retardants | ▪ Electronic products such as cables, circuit boards and structural components<br>▪ Building products such as wood, insulation and other materials<br>▪ Foam products such as polyethylene and styrene foam<br>▪ Textiles used for upholstery, carpeting, bedding and draperies<br>▪ Clothing, furniture<br>▪ Heat-resistant coatings to protect structural steel elements from warping or buckling during a fire | ▪ Cars |
| Formaldehyde | ▪ Composite and pressed-wood furniture<br>▪ Carpets, carpet pads<br>▪ Paints, coatings<br>▪ Furniture fabrics, draperies<br>▪ Personal care products | ▪ Construction materials<br>▪ Permanent press clothing<br>▪ Personal care products |

**Other hazards**

| | | |
|---|---|---|
| Medications | Improper storage, labeling, handling, or use of medications. | |
| Cleaners, other chemicals | Improper storage, labeling, handling or using chemical products in any area accessible to children, particularly unsecured storage sheds | |
| Asbestos | Friable, nonintact asbestos in exposed insulation, ceilings, floors, or duct work; Renovation without appropriate asbestos containment | Disasters (eg, collapse of the World Trade Center towers) |
| Bisphenol A (BPA) | Consumer products such as baby bottles, sippy cups, toys with #3, 6, or 7; Protective coating on food cans, personal care products; Receipt paper | |
| Mercury | Ingestion of certain fish; broken fluorescent light bulbs, thermostats | Release from industrial processes such as mining and coal burning |
| Radon | Cracks and openings in foundations resulting in radon leakage from the ground into buildings | Naturally occurring in some areas |
| Phthalates | Vinyl flooring, plastic clothing (eg, rain coats), detergents, adhesives, personal care products (eg, fragrances, nail polish, soap), vinyl (eg, poly-vinyl chloride [PVC]) and plastic products (eg, toys, plastic bags) | |
| Fragrances/Perfumes | Household cleaning products, personal care products, air fresheners, scented detergents, hand lotions | |
| Ultraviolet radiation | | Excessive sun exposure because of inadequate shade in the playground, and inadequate use of sun-protective clothing, hats, and sunscreen |
| Noise | Room design or materials that amplify sounds | Adjacent roadways, airports, wind turbines or industrial sources of sound |

## INDOOR AIR QUALITY

Children spend 80% to 90% of their time indoors (home, child care, school, after-school care, etc), and indoor air quality is an important health concern (see Chapter 20) stimulating federal initiatives such as *Indoor Air Quality: Tools for Schools, Home\*A\*Syst/Farm\*A\*Syst,* and *HealthySEAT*.[4-6] Pollutants that contribute to poor indoor air quality include secondhand and thirdhand smoke, molds and other biological products, lead and heavy metals, pesticides, sanitizers, disinfectants, combustion byproducts, and volatile organic compounds (VOCs). One study of indoor air quality investigated carbon dioxide ($CO_2$) levels in 91 child care centers in Quebec, Canada. Ninety percent had $CO_2$ levels that exceeded the office building standard.[7] Increased $CO_2$ levels were associated with the number of children in a given area. A high $CO_2$ level (>1,000 parts per million [ppm]) can be used as a rough indicator of the effectiveness of ventilation and can serve as a marker for other indoor air pollutants.[7] Airflow in child care settings should be between 15 and 20 cubic feet/minute per person (0.42 to 0.57 cubic meter/minute per person) and result in more than 4 air changes per hour. Carbon dioxide levels, which are useful in determining the adequacy of ventilation, should be less than 1,000 ppm when a room has been occupied for 4 to 6 hours (see Chapter 11 and Ventilation for Acceptable Indoor Air Quality [www.ashrae.org]). A study in 2 North Carolina counties looked for 7 indoor air allergens in 89 child care facilities and found each allergen in most facilities.[8] The report indicates that children and child care professionals may be exposed to indoor allergens through their facilities. Another study in Singapore assessed indoor air quality measurements among 346 classrooms in 104 randomly selected child care centers. The types of ventilation systems were identified. When compared with air-conditioned buildings, naturally ventilated buildings had lower concentrations of indoor pollutants and $CO_2$ levels and were associated with the lowest occurrence of respiratory problems among children.[9] The negative effects that indoor air pollution has on children have been well documented.[10-12] In rural counties of New York State, an indoor air quality study of child care facilities observed high levels of pollutants such as lead, radon, carbon monoxide, asbestos, and mold.[11] As a result, recommendations were made to lower exposure levels in child care facilities.[13]

## SECONDHAND AND THIRDHAND TOBACCO SMOKE

The AAP recommends smoke-free child care environments. Some states have enacted laws to protect children from SHS exposure in commercial and home-based child care centers. As of December 2017, 44 states and US territories had smoking bans that applied to day care centers (up from 36 in 2007); of these 44 states, 39 banned smoking in both commercial and home day care centers,

4 states (AK, IN, NH, WI) banned smoking in commercial day care centers only, and 1 state (OK) banned smoking in home day care centers only. Certain states specify that smoking bans are only in effect when children are on the premises (11 commercial day care laws and 26 home day care laws). Toxicants in SHS, however, remain on surfaces and then revolatilize and resuspend, resulting in exposure from "thirdhand smoke." Children may, therefore, be exposed if employees are allowed to smoke when children are not present. Data suggest that state laws are more lenient toward home-based child care centers than commercial child care centers in allowing smoking when children are no longer present.[14] Children may incur additional exposure when there is smoking in another part of the building that shares a common ventilation system with the center. They can be exposed when a person who smokes transports children to or from the child care setting in a car, school bus, or van.[15] Day care vehicles should be kept smoke free at all times; as of December 2017, however, only 17 states had enacted laws to ban smoking in these vehicles, and 9 of these laws are were only in effect when the child is in the vehicle. Day care smoking bans should also apply to staff: custodial staff or drivers must never smoke. Child care workers who smoke outside the child care setting or on breaks should be asked to change clothes or wear a cover-up before working with children. Eliminating smoking at all times and implementing a total ban on smoking in child care centers is the only way to ensure that children avoid SHS exposure.

## LEAD

Few studies address lead hazards in child care. The prevalence of lead in family child care homes is most likely similar to the prevalence among homes in the community. A survey of schools, preschools, and child care centers conducted in Washington state found that 62% of 75 facilities built before 1979 contained leaded paint, and 31% contained elevated levels of lead in soil or dust.[16] The First National Environmental Health Survey of Child Care Centers, published in 2005, surveyed 168 licensed randomly selected child care facilities to measure lead in soil and dust samples.[17] Twenty-eight percent of the surveyed facilities contained lead-based paint, and 14% contained one or more significant lead-based hazards.[17] Significant lead-based paint hazards were 4 times as likely to be found in facilities in which the majority of children were black, compared with those in which the majority of children were white.[17]

Exposure to lead in child care settings may be underestimated by routine surveillance systems. When a child has an elevated blood lead concentration, sources in the home, such as lead-based paint, are tested for and identified. Sources of lead away from the home (such as child care settings) are more likely to be overlooked. Two studies of children attending child care centers with high environmental lead levels (in paint, dust, or soil) found only 1 child who had a confirmed blood lead concentration exceeding 10 mcg/dL (12 mcg/dL).[16,18] These results, however, cannot be generalized to all child care settings. In both studies, the average age of the participants was approximately 5 years, and in 1 study, the rate of participation was low.[16] Children in these 2 studies may have been protected from lead exposure by continual supervision, a high frequency of hand washing (averaging once per hour), and standard cleaning practices, including daily wet mopping of floors. The risk of exposure is higher for younger children, when children have poor hygiene, when maintenance practices are inadequate, or when housing renovations occur without appropriate testing and containment measures.

Another potential source of lead exposure is drinking water. Child care facilities (as well as schools) that have and/or operate their own public water systems must comply with the federal Safe Drinking Water Act (SDWA) that requires testing water for lead to comply with the US EPA action level of 15 parts per billion (ppb). According to US EPA estimates, approximately 8,000 child care facilities and schools are in this category. About 500,000 child care facilities and 98,000 public schools are not regulated under the SDWA. These facilities may or may not conduct voluntary drinking water testing. The US EPA's "3T's Toolkit"—"Training, Testing and Telling"—was developed to assist school officials in their efforts to reduce lead in drinking water.[19] Currently, only 7 states (Connecticut, Illinois, New Hampshire, New Jersey, Oregon, Rhode Island, and Washington) and 1 city (New York City) require licensed child care facilities served by community water systems to test their drinking water for lead.[20]

Federal regulations begin to address the problem of lead only in the child's home. Limited federal funding for remediation of lead hazards can be applied to homes, but not to child care settings.

## PESTICIDES AND OTHER POTENTIALLY TOXIC PRODUCTS

### Pesticides

Children are highly vulnerable to the adverse effects of pesticides (see Chapter 40). The first national survey of pesticide exposures in child care facilities demonstrated that among 63% of surveyed centers, the number of pesticides used in each ranged from 1 to 10.[21] Frequency of pesticide use ranged from 1 to 107 times annually.[21] The most commonly used pesticides were pyrethroids, followed by organophosphates.[21] In another survey of 89 child care providers in North Carolina, the majority responded that they use high-risk pesticide application methods.[22] A quarter of the respondents indicated using Integrated Pest Management (IPM) (see Chapter 40); those using pest-control contractors were less likely to use IPM for pest control.[22]

Communities in which children are at increased risk of exposure include agricultural areas as well as urban settings where pesticides are used extensively in schools, homes, and child care centers for control of cockroaches, rats, and other pests. Pesticide use in child care settings is common because young children spill food that attracts pests, and many of the buildings used for child care are old and poorly maintained for control of pests by other means. In some cases, facilities use regular pesticide application for prevention even when there is not an obvious problem, rather than increasing best practices, such as IPM, and reducing the opportunity to attract pests. Children may be exposed through sources such as:

- Residues from indoor or outdoor pesticide use (from the indoor air, surfaces, household dust, and soil/drift);
- Treatment for head lice;
- Pets treated with flea dips;
- Residues on food;
- Playground structures made of wood treated with wood-preserving pesticides, such as chromated copper arsenate;
- Lawn and garden products; and/or
- Insect repellents.

The incidence of poisoning by pesticides and other products (such as medications, arts and crafts materials, toxic plants, and petroleum products) was higher when children were in their own homes.[23] Children in child care centers may be protected somewhat because they usually are supervised by an adult, the facility and equipment are designed for children, and licensing procedures and public health inspections help to eliminate hazards. However, the potential for poisonings is real. In Colorado, health inspectors visiting child care settings 2 weeks after licensing inspections found that toxic chemicals were accessible to children in 68% of settings.[24] Products, such as pesticides, may be used as directed but still are not safe to use in child care settings.[25] Pediatricians should encourage parents to inquire about the type of pesticides and other chemicals used and any known or potential health implications for children. IPM should be recommended. IPM involves the careful consideration of all available pest control techniques that discourages the development of pest populations and keeps pesticide use and other interventions to levels that are economically justified while minimizing risks to human health and the environment.[26] IPM improves knowledge and pest control practices in child care facilities.[27,28]

## Cleaning Products

Sanitizing and disinfecting are important processes that help to promote clean and healthy child care settings. The terms cleaning, sanitizing, and disinfecting are sometimes used interchangeably, possibly resulting in confusion and using cleaning procedures that are not effective.[2]

The purpose of *cleaning* is to physically remove all visible dirt and contamination with a household soap or mild detergent.[2] *Sanitizing* is the process used after visible dirt is removed from a surface. Sanitizing is designed to greatly reduce the number of pathogens that are likely to cause disease. Sanitizing refers to applying heat or a chemical, such as household bleach, to clean surfaces so as to yield a 99.9% reduction in representative (but not all) disease-causing microorganisms of public health importance. An example of cumulative heat treatment is found in the operation of some household dishwashers. Household dishwashers that effectively sanitize dishes and utensils using hot water may be used to clean and sanitize the outer surfaces of plastic toys. However, dishwashers that use a heating element to dry dishes should be used with caution to avoid melting soft plastic toys. Some dishwashers may permit the heating element used for drying to be deactivated while retaining the sanitizing process. Child care staff can consult the manufacturer's user guide for instructions. Surfaces that have contact with children's mouths and with food (eg, crib railings, mouthing toys, dishes, high chair trays) should be sanitized. *Disinfecting* is more rigorous than sanitizing. Disinfecting refers to applying cumulative heat or a chemical to result in the elimination of almost all microorganisms from inanimate surfaces. Pathogens of public health importance and nearly all other microorganisms are eliminated, but not to the degree achieved by sterilization. Surfaces such as changing tables and counter tops should be disinfected. *Caring for Our Children: National Health and Safety Performance Standards—Guidelines for Out-of-Home Child Care Programs* contains more details.[2] See Appendix K at http://cfoc.nrckids.org/WebFiles/AppendicesUpload/AppendixK.pdf. Although it is common for child care facilities to perform all 3 of these tasks, it is important to avoid using harsh and irritating products whenever possible. There are alternatives for facilities to consider, such as dilute vinegar solution and mild soap and water for sanitation needs. Third-party certifications, such as GreenSeal and EcoLogo, are recommended to assist with identification of cleaning products with reduced or no harsh chemicals. If a bleach solution is used to sanitize or disinfect a surface, providers must be sure to adhere to the suggested water-to-bleach formula. A funnel should be used when mixing bleach and water to minimize creating droplets in the air and irritating the lungs.

## Plastics

In 2008, the National Toxicology Program of the National Institutes of Health raised concerns about exposure to bisphenol A (BPA) during pregnancy and childhood because of a potential effect on human growth and development.[29] In January 2010, the US Food and Drug Administration expressed concern about the possible effects of bisphenol A on the brain and prostate gland of the fetus, infant, and child and also raised concerns about effects on behavior.[30]

More research was recommended. Existing research has suggested connections between low-dose bisphenol A exposure and conditions such as cancer, obesity, early puberty, hyperactivity, and diabetes mellitus.[29] Bisphenol A is used in products including some baby bottles, sippy cups, reusable water bottles, and microwaveable plastic containers.[29] Parents and child care providers should be encouraged to purchase and use bisphenol A-free bottles, sippy cups, and other containers.[29] Bisphenol A can leak from scratches, so scratched or worn bisphenol A-containing bottles and cups should be discarded. Very hot liquids should not be placed into containers made with bisphenol A, and labels should be checked to ensure microwave safety before microwaving foods and liquids. In response to consumer preferences, the 6 largest manufacturers of baby bottles are already producing baby bottles without bisphenol A. Canada has banned bisphenol A from children's products.[30]

## Formaldehyde

In 2012, the California Air Resources Board released a report that highlighted research conducted at the UC Berkeley Center for Environmental Research and Children's Health.[31] Using a variety of sampling and analytical methods to test the indoor air and floor dust of 40 US child care facilities in California's Alameda and Monterey counties, this study measured and analyzed a variety of pollutants in center- and home-based facilities. Although the levels of most pollutants measured resembled similar findings in California schools and residences, 35 of the 40 facilities displayed levels of formaldehyde that exceeded California's 8-hour chronic reference exposures levels.[32] Formaldehyde is a known carcinogen associated with acute irritation of the eyes, skin, and respiratory tract.[31]

## Medications

Adhering to the "five rights of medication administration"—right child, right time, right medication, right dose, and right route—may help to prevent accidental poisoning through a medication error. Child care providers should have clear guidelines to govern administration of medication in the child care setting. Guidelines include having clear instructions, ensuring that medications are placed in child-resistant containers, and obtaining permission from the parent or guardian to administer the medication. Storage procedures include keeping medications out of the reach of children, assessing the need for refrigeration of medication, and ensuring that an emergency medication will be readily accessible. Unused medications should be returned to parents for safe disposal. The AAP developed an online medication administration training for child care providers as part of *Healthy Futures* that is available at: https://www.aap.org/en-us/advocacy-and-policy/aap-health-initiatives/healthy-child-care/Pages/Healthy-Futures.aspx.

## CHARACTERISTICS OF CHILD CARE SETTINGS THAT MAY EXACERBATE HAZARDS

Characteristics of child care facilities may affect environmental quality. First, low salaries (the average salary of a child care worker ranges from $14,100 to $22,780 per year, depending on the state) and lack of benefits result in a high turnover rate among child care providers.[33] Because approximately one third of child care providers leave their centers each year, child care service operators need to continually educate new employees.[33] Keeping staff training current is a significant challenge for child care centers. Approximately 2.3 million individuals provide child care and education for children younger than 5 years. Of those, an estimated 1.2 million are working within a formal child care setting, and the remaining 1.1 million providers are paid relatives, friends, or neighbors.[34] In addition, 36 states require no training in early childhood care and education, intensifying the need for voluntary continuing education.[35] Provider education, retention, and compensation are key indicators for child care quality.[36] Second, child care businesses usually operate with a low profit margin. The largest portion of a family child care home or center budget is dedicated to staff salaries. Tuition funded by public assistance often is at low, fixed dollar amounts. These conditions result in limited funds for preventive measures, such as ventilation maintenance, lead hazard abatement, remodeling, or renovation. It is difficult for centers to close temporarily to implement measures to reduce or eliminate environmental hazards. Finally, when a center is located within a larger facility, such as a church or office building, hazards may arise as a result of practices that occur in other parts of the facility.

## MEASURES TO PREVENT OR CONTROL ENVIRONMENTAL HAZARDS IN CHILD CARE SETTINGS

*Caring for Our Children: The National Health and Safety Performance Standards—Guidelines for Out-of-Home Child Care Programs* identifies measures for prevention and control of environmental hazards.[2] Some of these are discussed here. The standards should be consulted for details on the features of the facility and the operational activities that reduce environmental risks. An important aspect of prevention is frequent handwashing; children should be encouraged to wash their hands or use hand sanitizer throughout the day, especially after toileting and outdoor play and before eating meals or snacks.

### Primary Prevention

#### Site Selection

An environmental audit, conducted from both a child's and adult's perspective, should be performed before selecting a child care site and before new construction begins or an existing building is renovated. The audit should at least include assessments of (1) historical land use to determine the potential for soil contamination with toxic or hazardous waste, such as old gasoline storage; (2) mold, lead, and asbestos in older buildings; (3) potential sources of infestation, noise, air pollution, and toxic exposures; (4) location of the playground in relation to stagnant water, roadways, industrial emissions, and building exhaust outlets; and (5) access to a safe drinking water supply (public or private), a public sewer or approved septic tank system, and other utilities such as electricity. Although geologic factors may suggest potential radon exposure, there are no reliable methods of testing for radon prior to construction.

### Architectural Design and Building Materials

Modern homes and buildings are more tightly sealed, and mechanical cooling and heating systems are common in all climate zones. Thousands of new materials used as goods, finishes, and furnishings have resulted in increased indoor pollution.[37] From the perspective of architectural design and building materials, indoor air quality depends on (1) the absence of pollutants (source management—includes removal, substitution, and encapsulation); (2) the power of ventilation systems to supply fresh indoor air; (3) the ability of local exhaust systems and air filters to remove pollutants; and (4) controlling exposure to pollutants, such as cleaning products, through the principles of time of use and location of use.[38] Prevention and control measures include ensuring frequent air exchanges and sufficient ventilation of air to the outside; having some windows that open, preferably offering cross-ventilation, especially in bathrooms, diapering areas, and kitchens; and properly placing fresh-air intakes, which prevent exhaust from automobiles and building systems from reaching hazardous levels indoors. Pesticide use can be reduced by sealing openings and using screens on doors and windows. Less toxic building materials, paints, cleaners, and other products can be selected to minimize levels of toxic substances.[37] Less toxic building materials include renewable and environmentally responsible products that reduce negative health outcomes with contact. Selection criteria for material selections include resource efficiency, indoor air quality implications, energy efficiency, and water conservation opportunities.

### Child Care Regulation and Monitoring

To prevent environmental hazards, it is essential to consult an environmental health specialist (such as one located in a local health department) before construction or remodeling begin to review construction or remodeling plans. Child care settings should be monitored by trained licensers who visit during construction or remodeling, inspect them before the center opens and routinely during operation, and investigate complaints. All parts of the child care setting, not only the food service area, must be inspected to identify potential environmental hazards so preventive actions can be implemented. Table 10-2 provides key environmental health questions to include in a routine health and safety inspection of a child care facility. Providers may refer to *Caring for Our Children: National Health and Safety Performance Standards—Guidelines for Out-of-Home Child Care Programs* for a comprehensive listing of standards and rationale.[2]

State or local health departments may need to develop additional environmental health regulations that specifically address child care facilities.

---

### Table 10-2. Some Key Questions to Assess Potential Environmental Hazards in a Child Care Setting

- Is the setting smoke-free? Is there a smoke-free policy? Is smoking allowed when children are not present? Is smoking allowed in other parts of the building?
- Does the facility appear clean, in good repair, and without water-marked areas or areas of peeling and chipping paint?
- Is there evidence of water damage or mold? Have flooding or plumbing problems occurred? Are there musty odors?
- Are the rooms adequately ventilated?
- Has the child care center or home been tested for radon?
- Are fuel-burning furnaces, stoves, or other equipment in use?
- Are medications and chemical products properly labeled and stored in areas inaccessible to children and in a manner so as not to contaminate food? Are staff members trained in the safe use of chemical products and administration of medications?
- Are arts and crafts supplies free of hazardous substances and labeled in compliance with the American Society for Testing and Materials?
- Are the kitchen and bathroom areas operated in compliance with health department regulations?
- Are scented and unscented candles or air fresheners allowed?
- Are hand-washing policies followed and monitored? Are soap and clean towels always available? Paper towels, rather than cloth towels, generally are preferred in child care settings. Individual cloth towels may be used for each child but must be changed frequently.
- Are indoor and outdoor storage closets and sheds locked so their contents are inaccessible to children? All maintenance, lawn care and other hazardous equipment, and chemical products (such as gasoline, paints, pesticides, and cleaning products) must be inaccessible to children.
- When sanitizing and disinfecting, are the least toxic options used? When agents are used, are they used only for their intended purpose and according to label instructions?
- Is chlorine bleach used only when required by state and local authorities? If used, is chlorine bleach limited to only when needed for disinfection?

## Table 10-2. Some Key Questions to Assess Potential Environmental Hazards in a Child Care Setting (*continued*)

- Is a carbon monoxide detector present and in working order?
- If the building was constructed before 1978, has the building been assessed for lead paint, dust, and soil hazards? Homes and other buildings built before 1978 may contain lead, and those built before 1950 have the most lead. If remodeling or renovation work is under way, have lead and asbestos hazards been assessed, and have children been protected from the release of these potentially hazardous toxicants?
- Is the tap water tested at least annually for contaminants of concern? Old lead piping is a source for lead poisoning.
- Are the least toxic cleaning products used?
- Are furniture and carpet in good condition, without foam or inside stuffing exposed? Is furniture made of solid wood or low VOC products? Is there wall to wall carpeting?
- Are plastics and plastic toys made of PVC (such as chew toys, rubber duckies, soft vinyl dolls, and beach balls) avoided?
- Is there standing water inside or outside of the facility?
- Is integrated pest management (IPM) used?
- Are fruits and vegetables thoroughly washed to avoid possible exposure to pesticides?
- Are there adequate shady areas for play outside?
- Is there a playground or deck made with chromated copper arsenate-treated wood (pre-2004)? If so, are at least 2 coats of waterproof stain or sealant used once a year?
- Are vehicles prevented from idling outside during drop off and pick up?

### Education

In Sweden, continuing education of child care providers was shown to be a strong predictor of having few safety hazards in child care centers.[38] Providers with specialized training are more likely to be nurturing, reinforce early literacy skills, and enhance early learning.[39] Many states have established a health consultation system that responds to the needs of child care providers for health and safety education.[40] Often, this system includes personnel from local health departments who have expertise in environmental hazards, communicable diseases, injury control, nutrition, sanitation, and/or safety. Health professionals who provide child care consultation can assist child care providers to identify environmental hazards, understand health risks, and implement preventive actions. Many times, child care providers seek consultation directly from their community's pediatricians and other health professionals. More information for health professionals, including strategies for advocacy, training, consultation, and policy making, may be obtained in *The Pediatrician's Role in Promoting Health and Safety in Child Care* (www.healthychildcare.org/PedsRole.html). Another useful resource is the National

Eco-Healthy Child Care (EHCC) program. This program has been working to train child care professionals about environmental health and promoting safer and healthier child care facilities for over a decade (www.cehn.org/our-work/eco-healthy-child-care/).

To prevent environmental health hazards, all employees, including maintenance personnel, should be included in continuing education. Janitorial and custodial staff should be regularly monitored to ensure the safest practices. The Occupational Safety and Health Administration requires that Safety Data Sheets be kept on file to explain health hazards from chemicals that are used, proper use and storage procedures, and emergency procedures in case of toxic chemical exposure. Staff also may use Safety Data Sheets to choose nontoxic chemicals. Parents have a right to ask for the Safety Data Sheets for chemicals used at child care facilities.

Child care providers may not have knowledge about, or experience or supervisory support in, administering medications. To avoid having child care providers administer medications to children, pediatricians may consider prescribing formulations that require fewer dosages or altering the time of administration. When medications must be given while a child is in child care, specific written instructions should be on the bottle and on a separate piece of paper. Instructions are especially important for medications that are used on an as-needed basis. Instructions are needed for prescription and nonprescription medications and topical preparations, including sunscreen.

### Child Care Program Policies and Procedures

Child care providers are well positioned to respond quickly and appropriately to environmental hazards. By developing child care policies, safer practices can become part of the everyday routine. For example, (1) smoking should be prohibited (even among noncaregivers in a family child care home) while children are present and at all other times; (2) plumbing leaks, roof leaks, and flooding should be cleaned up within 24 hours and wet areas should be cleansed with detergent and water to prevent growth of molds and other biological pollutants; (3) emergency preparedness plans should include procedures for responding to hazardous material incidents and chemical/biological/radiologic threats; and (4) staff should receive education in administration of medications and use of chemicals. Some states have specific regulations and training that conform to those regulations.

## Secondary Prevention

It is possible to avoid some hazardous situations by educating providers and others working in child care settings about how to recognize and appropriately control hazards (eg, by properly storing or using chemicals). Other hazards may require more costly and complex measures. For example, when extensive mold is found, interim control measures may be needed before full remediation is possible. Remediation procedures should meet applicable standards and regulations. If conditions are potentially hazardous, the center may need to be shut down. When the facility has limited financial resources, environmental health regulators play an important role in ensuring that children's health is not jeopardized. This may require community collaboration to offset the burden of cost.

## ILLNESS OR DEATH OCCURRING IN A CHILD WHO ATTENDS OUT-OF-HOME CHILD CARE

When a child's illness or symptoms may have an environmental etiology, parents, health care personnel, and public health investigators should evaluate potential exposures in the child's home environment and out-of-home settings. An increased risk of Sudden Infant Death Syndrome (SIDS) has been documented in out-of-home child care settings, but the reason is not understood.[41] Environmental exposures in the child care setting should be considered as part of the death scene investigation.

---

### Available Resources to Help Protect Children in Child Care Facilities

■ **American Academy of Pediatrics and American Public Health Association.**
*Caring for Our Children: National Health and Safety Performance Standards—Guidelines for Out-of-Home Child Care Programs*, 3rd ed. This resource is available in electronic format at the National Resource Center for Health and Safety in Child Care's Web site at http://nrckids.org and in hard copy through the American Academy of Pediatrics and the American Public Health Association. Child care regulations for every state are available through the federally funded National Resource Center for Health and Safety in Child Care's Web site at http://nrckids.org. This site also has a search engine for accessing specific child care topics by state.

## Available Resources to Help Protect Children in Child Care Facilities (*continued*)

■ **The National Eco-Healthy Child Care® (EHCC) Program**
www.cehn.org/ehcc
This national program for child care providers throughout the United States works with child care professionals to eliminate or reduce environmental health hazards found in and around child care facilities. This work is accomplished by education/training work and 2-year endorsements of child care facilities that meet the expected protective health actions. The Eco-Healthy Child Care® Program was created in 2010 through a merger of the Oregon Environmental Council's eco-healthy child care program, which began as an Oregon-based initiative in 2005, and the Healthy Environments for Child Care Facilities and Pre-schools program, created by the Washington, DC-based Children's Environmental Health Network. The EHCC program offers a variety of resources and best practices on the program site.

■ **Agency for Toxic Substances and Disease Registry**
Choose Safe Places for Early Child Care and Education Guidance Manual. This manual is a resource to help keep children in the community safe and healthy in places where they receive early care and education.
https://www.atsdr.cdc.gov/safeplacesforECE/cspece_guidance/foreword.html

## Frequently Asked Questions

Q   *How can I make my child care facility safer for children with asthma?*

A   The 2 most important steps that a child care facility can take to prevent asthma attacks in children are to prohibit smoking and to keep the facility free of molds and other biological pollutants. Of the 13 million children 5 years and younger enrolled in child care in the United States, an estimated 1.4 million have asthma (approximately 1 child in 11).[42] Child care programs need specific information on file (provided by the parent or guardian and the child's physician) for every child with asthma. The information should explain known triggers for the child's asthma (eg, fragrances, perfumes, pet dander, pests), medications and how to use them, symptoms indicating when the asthma is worsening, and what to do in an emergency.

The Asthma and Allergy Foundation of America, New England Chapter, has an "Asthma-Friendly Child Care Checklist" available in English, Spanish, Haitian Creole, and Portuguese, with information for making child care environments safe for children with asthma and allergies. It can be ordered through: www.asthmaandallergies.org/Articles/Asthma%20Friendly%20 Child%20Care.pdf or by calling 877-2-ASTHMA. The National Heart, Lung, and Blood Institute has a similar but shorter checklist—"How Asthma-Friendly Is Your Child Care Setting?"—available in English and Spanish, which includes an extensive list of resources for child care providers, available at: www.nhlbi.nih.gov/health/public/lung/asthma/child_ca.htm.

Q   *Are sandboxes, sand, and chemically treated wood play areas safe for children?*

A   Sandboxes are safe if constructed and filled with appropriate materials and properly maintained. Sandbox frames are sometimes made with inexpensive railroad ties, which may cause splinters and may be saturated with creosote, a carcinogen. Nontoxic landscaping timbers or nonwood containers are preferred.

In 1986, concern was first expressed that some types of commercially available play sand contained tremolite, a fibrous substance found in some crushed limestone and crushed marble (see Chapter 23). It was hypothesized that the long-term effects of exposure to tremolite would be identical to those of asbestos. Despite these concerns, the US Consumer Product Safety Commission denied a petition prohibiting marketing of play sand containing significant levels of tremolite. The Consumer Product Safety Commission currently has no standards or labeling requirements regarding the source or content of sand.

Parents and directors of facilities may have difficulty determining which sand is safe. They should attempt to buy only natural river sand or beach sand. They should avoid products that are made from crushed limestone, crushed marble, crushed crystalline silica (quartz) or those that are obviously dusty. When there is doubt, parents may send a sample to a laboratory to determine whether the sand contains tremolite or crystalline silica. Information about reliable laboratories can be obtained from the US EPA Regional Asbestos Coordinators (see Resources, Chapter 23).

Once installed, the sandbox should be covered to prevent contamination with animal feces and parasites. Sand should be raked regularly to remove debris and dry it out. A sand rake does a better job than a garden rake.

Chromated copper arsenate (CCA) is a chemical wood preservative containing chromium, copper, and arsenic, used to protect pressure-treated wood from insect and microbial-induced rot. Prior to 2004, many residential outdoor structures, such as playground sets, picnic tables, benches, and decks, were manufactured using CCA-treated wood. However, because of health concerns related to arsenic, a known carcinogen, the manufacture of CCA-treated products was phased-out for residential and consumer uses. Structures currently in use, built with CCA-treated wood prior to 2004, could potentially be a source of arsenic exposure to children. To reduce exposure, children should immediately wash their hands with mild soap and water after playing on CCA-treated wood.[43]

Q   *Which disinfectants and sanitizers are recommended in child care settings?*

A   Although disinfectants and sanitizers are essential to control communicable diseases in child care settings, they are potentially hazardous to children, particularly if the products are in concentrated form. Child care standards require disinfection solutions to be used on set schedules for use on items such as diaper changing tables, crib railings, hand washing sinks, and bathrooms (including toilet bowls, toilet seats, training rings, soap dispensers, potty chairs, door and cabinet handles).[44]

Products must be stored in their original labeled containers and in places inaccessible to children. Diluted disinfectants and sanitizers in spray bottles must be labeled and stored out of the reach of children. Solutions should not be sprayed when children are nearby to avoid inhalation and exposing skin and eyes.

Before using any cleaning products, child care providers should read the product label and manufacturer's Safety Data Sheet. They should consult public health personnel with questions. It is important to follow label instructions. Questions to consider when selecting a disinfectant are: Is it inactivated by organic matter? Is it affected by hard water? Does it leave a residue? Is it corrosive? Is it a skin, eye, or respiratory irritant? Is it toxic (by skin absorption, ingestion, or inhalation)? What is its effective shelf life after dilution? Household bleach (chlorine as sodium hypochlorite) is active against most microorganisms, including bacterial spores and can be used as a disinfectant or sanitizer, depending on its concentration. Bleach is available at various strengths. Household or laundry bleach is a solution of 5.25%, or 52,500 ppm, of sodium hypochlorite. The "ultra" form is only slightly more concentrated and should be diluted and used in the same fashion as ordinary strength household bleach. Higher-strength industrial bleach solutions are not appropriate to use in child care settings. See Table 10-3 for instructions on diluting bleach with water.

Household bleach is effective, economical, convenient, and available at grocery stores. It can be corrosive to some metal, rubber, and plastic materials. Each state has a water-to-bleach ratio that is recommended for

## Table 10-3. Diluting Bleach

For use on diaper changing tables, hand washing sinks, bathrooms (including toilet bowls, toilet seats, training rings, soap dispensers, potty chairs), door and cabinet handles, etc.

**DISINFECTING SOLUTIONS**

| WATER | BLEACH STRENGTH* 2.75% | BLEACH STRENGTH* 5.25%–6.25% | BLEACH STRENGTH* 8.25% |
|---|---|---|---|
| 1 Gallon | 1/3 Cup, plus 1 Tablespoon | 3 Tablespoons | 2 Tablespoons |
| 1 Quart | 1½ Tablespoons | 2¼ Teaspoons | 1½ Teaspoons |

**SANITIZING SOLUTIONS**

For use on eating utensils, food use contact surfaces, mixed use tables, high chair trays, crib frames and mattresses, toys, pacifiers, floors, sleep mats, etc.

| 1 Gallon | 1 Tablespoon | 2 Teaspoons | 1 Teaspoon |
|---|---|---|---|
| 1 Quart | 1 Teaspoon | ½ Teaspoon | ¼ Teaspoon |

Disinfection of nonporous non-food contact surfaces can be achieved with 600 parts per million (ppm) of chlorine bleach. To make measuring easier, the strengths listed in this table represent approximately 600 to 800 ppm of bleach for disinfecting, and approximately 100 ppm for sanitizing. Chlorine test strips with a measuring range of 0 to 800 ppm or higher can also be used to determine the strength of the solution. Use a funnel to pour the bleach into the water to avoid aerial contamination and possible asthma attacks.

**Contact your local health jurisdiction** for further instructions on cleaning and disinfecting if specific disease or organisms are identified as causing illness in your program.

*****Use only plain unscented bleach** that lists the percent (%) strength on the manufacturer's label. Read the label on the bleach bottle to determine the bleach strength. For example, Sodium Hypochlorite–6.25% or 8.25%.

use in child care facilities. Bleach solutions gradually lose their strength, so fresh solutions must be prepared daily, and stock solutions must be replaced every few months. In child care settings, a bleach solution is typically applied using spray bottles. Spray bottles should be labeled with the name of the solution and the dilution. Contact time is important. What is typically observed in a child care setting is "spray and wipe." Bleach solution should be left on for at least 2 minutes before being wiped off. It can be allowed to dry because it leaves no residue.

Household bleach can be used to sanitize dishes and eating utensils. The concentration of chlorine used in the process is much less than that used for disinfecting other objects. One rationale for sanitizing (as opposed to disinfecting) dishes and eating utensils is that these objects are typically contaminated by only one person and are washed and rinsed thoroughly before being treated with the sanitizing agent. Other objects typically are contaminated by more than one person and less thoroughly washed, resulting in a potentially greater microbial load and diversity of microorganisms.

Q   *Is it beneficial to use cleaners that contain disinfectants?*

A   By separating out the cleaning and disinfecting processes, you will reduce the amount of disinfectant chemicals used. Soiled objects or surfaces will block the effects of a disinfectant or sanitizer. Therefore, proper disinfection or sanitizing of a surface requires that the surface be cleaned (using mild soap or detergent and a water rinse) before disinfecting or sanitizing.[2] Bleach (the sanitizer/disinfectant) and ammonia (the cleaner) should never be mixed because the mixture produces a poisonous gas. Not all items and surfaces require sanitizing or disinfecting. Guidelines for cleaning, sanitizing, and disinfecting can be found in *Caring for Our Children: National Health and Safety Performance Standards—Guidelines for Out-of-Home Child Care Programs.*[2]

Q   *What are alternative or less toxic homemade cleaning products? Are they safe?*

A   Alternative or less toxic cleaners are made from ingredients such as baking soda, liquid soap, and vinegar. For example, an all-purpose floor cleaner might consist of 2 tablespoons of liquid soap or detergent and 1 gallon of hot water (29 mL in 3.8 liters of water). Many of the ingredients are inexpensive, so you may save money over time. They also may require more exertion; you may have to scrub harder. Although the ingredients in homemade cleaners (eg, baking soda for scrubbing, vinegar for cutting grease) are safer, not all are nontoxic. Treat them as you would any other cleaner, with caution.

Q   *Should I place my child in child care if there isn't a "no smoking" and "no vaping" policy in place?*

A   No. The American Academy of Pediatrics states that in schools, child care programs, and other venues for children, there should be no tobacco use in or around the premises, regardless of whether children are present.[45] Children should not be exposed to vaping or secondhand or thirdhand smoke, and smoke-free policies should be written or stated, enforced, and monitored by the director of the center and parents.

Q  *I know that there are health concerns related to carpeting. What precautions should I take?*

A  The ideal floor is warm to the touch, skid-proof, easily cleanable, moisture resistant, nontoxic, and does not generate static electricity. This can best be achieved by using hard flooring materials. Carpets are an easy gathering place for biological pollutants, such as molds and dust mites, as well as lead dust and pesticide residues. Instead of wall-to-wall carpeting, consider using area rugs (that are secured to avoid slipping) on hard surfaces; these tend to be easier to clean than installed carpeting. Carpets, pads, and adhesives emit ("off-gas") volatile organic compounds. For children, the elderly, and people with lung conditions, allergies, and allergic-type sensitivities, exposure to fairly low amounts of volatile organic compounds may result in problems such as headaches; nausea; irritation to eyes, nose, and throat; and difficulty breathing. If installing new carpet, look for low–volatile organic compound-emitting carpets and nontoxic adhesives and pads. Ask the carpet store or installer to air out the carpet for at least 24 to 48 hours in the store or warehouse. During installation, make sure the room is well ventilated. After the carpet is installed, continue to ventilate and wait at least 72 hours before using the room. Other preventive measures include: vacuum daily using a good HEPA filtering vacuum cleaner; leave shoes worn outdoors at the entry way; choose carpet that cleans easily; do not saturate the carpet when wet-cleaning, and ensure the carpet is dry within 24 hours; and use low- or no-solvent cleaning products. Thoroughly clean and dry water-damaged carpets within 24 hours or remove and replace them. Be aware that some carpet comes already treated with antimicrobial products. When possible, avoid the use of pesticides on carpeting.[46]

Q  *Are air cleaners that generate ozone safe and effective to use in my child care program?*

A  No. Ozone generators that are sold as air cleaners intentionally produce the gas ozone. Manufacturers and vendors of ozone devices often use terms such as "energized oxygen" or "pure air" to suggest that ozone is a healthy kind of oxygen.[47] Ozone is a toxic gas. For more information, see the US EPA indoor air quality publications at www.epa.gov/iaq/pubs/ozonegen.html.

Q  *Should pets be allowed in child care settings?*

A  Many child care providers who care for children in their homes have pets, and many centers include pets as part of their educational program. Other than service dogs, animals should be avoided or limited in schools and child care settings.[48]

If a pet is in the child care setting, guidelines to protect health and safety and to avoid risks should be followed. Health and safety concerns for children include allergies, injuries (eg, dog and cat bites), and infections (eg, salmonellosis caused by common bacteria carried by animals such as chickens, iguanas, and turtles). Healthy Child Care Washington has developed a concise handout, "Animals and Domestic Pets" (2007), available at: www.healthychildcare-wa.org/Health Risks from Animals.pdf.

Q  *I just got a call from my neighbor, who would like to donate her home playground equipment to my child care program. I have a copy of the Consumer Product Safety Commission Handbook for Public Playground Safety (www.cpsc.gov/cpscpub/pubs/playpubs.html), and her playground equipment does not seem to meet their guidelines, but I'm not sure. What should I do?*

A  Playground equipment is a leading source of childhood injury. Many deaths and injuries have occurred on home playgrounds.[49] Since 1981, the Consumer Product Safety Commission has worked to strengthen playground safety guidelines and standards. If you are uncertain whether the playground equipment meets Consumer Product Safety Commission guidelines, get professional advice. Contact your local parks and recreation office or the National Recreation and Park Association (www.nrpa.org), and they will connect you with a certified playground inspector in the area. This person can determine the safety of the equipment, provide advice about the types of equipment to best suit the ages of the children in your care and your physical space, and the type and amount of shock-absorbing surfacing needed around play equipment.

## References

1. Children's Defense Fund. *Child Care Basics. Children's Defense Fund Issue Basics: April 2005.* http://www.childrensdefense.org/child-research-data-publications/data/child-care-basics.pdf. Accessed February 9, 2018

2. American Public Health Association, American Academy of Pediatrics, National Resource Center for Health and Safety in Child and Early Education. *Caring for Our Children: National Health and Safety Performance Standards. Guidelines for Out-of-Home Child Care Programs.* 3rd ed. Washington, DC: American Public Health Association; and Elk Grove Village, IL: American Academy of Pediatrics; 2011

3. General Accounting Office. *Child Care: State Efforts to Enforce Safety and Health Requirements.* http://www.gao.gov/new.items/he00028.pdf. Accessed February 9, 2018

4. US Environmental Protection Agency, Indoor Environments Division. *IAQ Tools for Schools Action Kit.* IAQ Coordinator's Guide. https://www.epa.gov/iaq-schools/indoor-air-quality-tools-schools-action-kit. Accessed February 9, 2018

5. *Help Yourself to a Healthy Home: Protect Your Children's Health.* https://www.epa.gov/sites/production/files/2016-08/documents/2016-08-r9-rtoc-presentation-help-yourself-to-healthy-home.pdf. Accessed February 9, 2018

6.  US Environmental Protection Agency, Healthy School Environments. *Healthy School Environments Assessment Tool (HealthySEAT)*. https://nepis.epa.gov/Exe/ZyPURL. cgi?Dockey=2000D006.txt. Accessed February 9, 2018

7.  Daneault S, Beausoleil M, Messing K. Air quality during the winter in Quebec day-care centers. *Am J Public Health*. 1992;82(3):432–434

8.  Arbes Jr S, Sever M, Mehta J, Collette N, Thomas B, Zeldin D. Exposure to indoor allergens in day-care facilities: results from 2 North Carolina counties. *J Allergy Clin Immunol*. 2005;116(1): 133–139

9.  Zauraimi MS, Tham KW, Chew FT, Ooi PL. The effect of ventilation strategies of child care centers on indoor air quality and respiratory health of children in Singapore. *Indoor Air*. 2007;17(4):317–327

10. Roberts JW, Dickey P. Exposure of children to pollutants in house dust and indoor air. *Rev Environ Contam Toxicol*. 1995;143:59–78

11. Subedi B, Sullivan KD, Dhungana B. Phthalate and non-phthalate plasticizers in indoor dust from childcare facilities, salons, and homes across the USA. *Environ Pollut*. 2017;230:701–708

12. Hoang T, Castorina R, Gaspar F, et al. VOC exposures in California early childhood education environments. *Indoor Air*. 2017;27(3):609–621

13. Laquatra J, Maxwell LE, Pierce M. Indoor air pollutants: limited-resource households and child care facilities. *J Environ Health*. 2005;67(7):39–43

14. Centers for Disease Control and Prevention. National Center for Chronic Disease Prevention and Health Promotion. CDC STATE Tobacco Legislation Database. https://chronicdata.cdc. gov/Legislation/CDC-STATE-System-Tobacco-Legislation-Smokefree-Ind/32fd-hyzc. Accessed February 9, 2018

15. Centers for Disease Control and Prevention. National Center for Chronic Disease Prevention and Health Promotion. State System Vehicles Fact Sheet. State Smoking Restrictions in Vehicles (Private Employer, Government-Owned, Day Care Centers, and Personal Vehicles) https://data.cdc.gov/download/dh22-5kgj/application/pdf. Accessed February 9, 2018

16. Washington State Department of Health. *Environmental Lead Survey in Public and Private School Preschools and Day Care Centers*. Olympia, WA: Washington State Department of Health; 1995:1–20

17. Fraser A, Marker D, Rogers J, Viet SM. First National Environmental Health Survey of Child Care Centers, Final Report, July 15, 2003. Volume I: Analysis of Lead Hazards. Washington, DC: U.S. Department of Housing and Urban Development, Office of Healthy Homes and Lead Hazard Control; 2003

18. Weismann DN, Dusdieker LB, Cherryholmes KL, Hausler W Jr, Dungy CI. Elevated environmental lead levels in a day care setting. *Arch Pediatr Adolesc Med*. 1995;149(8):878–881

19. US Environmental Protection Agency. *3 Ts for Lead in Drinking Waters in Schools and Child Care Facilities*. https://www.epa.gov/dwreginfo/3ts-reducing-lead-drinking-water-schools-and-child-care-facilities. Accessed August 26, 2018.

20. McCormick LA, Lovell SC. *Putting children first: Tackling lead in water at child care facilities*. Washington, DC: Environmental Defense Fund, 2018. https://www.edf.org/sites/default/files/documents/edf_child_care_report-062518.pdf. Accessed August 26, 2018.

21. Tulve NS, Jones PA, Nishioka MG, et al. Pesticide measurements from the first national environmental health survey of child care centers using a multi-residue GC/MS analysis method. *Environ Sci Technol*. 2006;40(20):6269–6274

22. Toxic Free North Carolina. *Toxic Free Kids*. http://www.toxicfreenc.org/programs/toxic-free-kids/. Accessed February 11, 2018

23. Gunn WJ, Pinsky PF, Sacks JJ, Schonberger LB. Injuries and poisoning in out-of-home child care and home care. *Am J Dis Child*. 1991;145(7):779–781

24. Aronson SS. Role of the pediatrician in setting and using standards for child care. *Pediatrics.* 1993;91(1 Pt 2):239–243

25. Fenske RA, Black KG, Elkner KP, Lee CL, Methner MM, Soto R. Potential exposure and health risks of infants following indoor residential pesticide applications. *Am J Public Health.* 1990;80(6):689–693

26. Kass D, McKelvey W, Carlton E, et al. Effectiveness of an integrated pest management intervention in controlling cockroaches, mice, and allergens in New York City public housing. *Environ Health Perspect.* 2009;117(8):1219–1225

27. Alkon, A, Nouredini, S, Swartz, A, et al. Integrated pest management intervention in child care centers improves knowledge, pest control, and practices. *J Pediatr Health Care.* 2016;30(6): e27–e41

28. Stephens M, Hazard K, Moser D, Cox D, Rose R, Alkon A. An integrated pest management intervention improves knowledge, pest control, and practices in family child care homes. *Int J Environ Res Public Health.* 2017;14(11):1299

29. California Childcare Health Program. Risks Associated with Bisphenol A in baby bottles. https://cchp.ucsf.edu/sites/cchp.ucsf.edu/files/BisphenolEn0908.pdf. Accessed August 24, 2018

30. US Food and Drug Administration. Bisphenol A (BPA). Update on Bisphenol A (BPA) for Use in Food: January 2010. http://www.fda.gov/newsevents/publichealthfocus/ucm064437.htm. Accessed August 24, 2018

31. Bradman A, Gaspar F, Castorina R, et al. Formaldehyde and acetaldehyde exposures in California early childhood education environments. *Indoor Air.* 2017;27(1):104–113

32. US EPA Environmental Protection Agency. Technology Transfer Network Air Toxics Web Site: Formaldehyde. https://www.epa.gov/sites/production/files/2016-09/documents/formaldehyde.pdf. Accessed August 24, 2018

33. National Association of Child Care Resource and Referral Agencies. What Child Care Providers Earn. 2006 Annual Mean Wage. http://www.naccrra.org/randd/child-care-workforce/provider_income.php. Accessed February 11, 2018

34. Bank H, Behr A, Schulman K. *State Developments in Child Care, Early Education, and School-Age Care.* Washington, DC: Children's Defense Fund; 2000:57. http://www.childrensdefense.org/pdf/2000_state_dev.pdf. Accessed February 11, 2018

35. Center for the Child Care Workforce. Estimating the Size and Components of the U.S. Child Care Workforce and Caregiving Population. http://www.naccrra.org/randd/child-care-workforce/cc_workforce.php. Accessed February 11, 2018

36. Early Childhood Education and Care: key lessons from research for policy makers European Commission: 2009. Available at: http://www.nesse.fr/nesse/activities/reports/activities/reports/ecec-report-pdf. Accessed March 4, 2018

37. Olds AR. *Child Care Design Guide.* New York, NY: McGraw-Hill; 2001

38. US Environmental Protection Agency. *IAQ Design Tools for Schools.* https://www.epa.gov/iaq-schools/indoor-air-quality-design-tools-schools. Accessed February 11, 2018

39. Sellstrom E, Bremberg S. Education of staff—a key factor for a safe environment in day care. *Acta Paediatr.* 2000;89(5):601–607

40. National Association of Child Care Resource and Referral Agencies. *Building a National Community-Based Training System for Child Care Resource and Referral.* Arlington, VA: National Association of Child Care Resource and Referral Agencies; 2005:7

41. Kiechl-Kohlendorfer U, Moon RY. Sudden infant death syndrome (SIDS) and child care centres (CCC). *Acta Paediatr.* 2008;97(7):844–845

42. Asthma and Allergy Foundation of America, New England Chapter. *For Child Care Providers.* http://asthmaandallergies.org/programs-services/childcare-training/. Accessed February 11, 2018

43. Agency for Toxic Substances and Disease Registry. Public Health Statement: Arsenic. August 2007. https://www.atsdr.cdc.gov/PHS/PHS.asp?id=18&tid=3. Accessed February 11, 2018

44. Washington State Department of Health. Disinfecting and Sanitizing with Bleach: Guidelines for Mixing Bleach Solutions for Child Care and Similar Environments. http://here.doh.wa.gov/materials/guidelines-for-bleach-solutions/13_Disinfect_E15L.pdf. Accessed February 11, 2018

45. Farber HJ, Groner J, Walley S, Nelson K, Section on Tobacco Control. Protecting children from tobacco, nicotine, and tobacco smoke. *Pediatrics.* 2015;136(5):e1439–e1467

46. Vermont Department of Health. Burlington, VT: Vermont Department of Health. http://www.healthvermont.gov/health-environment/healthy-schools/best-practices. Accessed February 11, 2018

47. US Environmental Protection Agency. *Ozone Generators that are Sold as Air Cleaners: An Assessment of Effectiveness and Health Consequences.* https://www.epa.gov/indoor-air-quality-iaq/ozone-generators-are-sold-air-cleaners. Accessed February 11, 2018

48. American Academy of Pediatrics Committee on School Health, National Association of School Nurses. *Health, Mental Health, and Safety Guidelines for Schools.* Taras H, Duncan P, Luckenbill D, et al, eds. Elk Grove Village, IL: American Academy of Pediatrics; 2004

49. US Consumer Product Safety Commission. *Home Playground Equipment-Related Deaths and Injuries.* https://www.cpsc.gov/PageFiles/122137/270.pdf. Accessed February 11, 2018

Chapter 11

# Schools

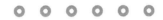

**KEY POINTS**

- The average school-aged child spends much of his or her waking time at school. The school environment therefore plays a large role in the child's attainment of social skills and cognitive knowledge.
- Schools are complex environments with multiple roles including classroom education, sports and physical activity, and food service. The details of how a specific school addresses each of these functions can affect the health and well-being of each child. Many schools are in excellent condition, but many others unfortunately need major repairs or renovation.
- Parents should remain in frequent communication with teachers and school administrators to anticipate potential issues impacting their children. Topics of concern should be discussed with school leaders. A child's pediatrician can serve as a valuable resource in addressing school health concerns.

**INTRODUCTION**

The typical school-aged child spends approximately 1,170 hours per year at school—which translates into more than 2,300 days during the 13 years between kindergarten and 12th grade.[1] That figure can increase by thousands of hours if children also participate in after-school programs or extracurricular activities. This chapter describes how physical, nutritional, and psychosocial aspects of the school environment can affect a child's health and well-being. This chapter also discusses the importance of the environmental health history in identifying school-related adverse health factors, and steps to promote improved safety, health, and wellness in schools. Additional specific guidance is available in the *Health, Mental Health and Safety Guidelines for Schools* (available at www.nationalguidelines.org).

## PHYSICAL DIMENSIONS OF THE SCHOOL ENVIRONMENT

### School Buildings

Most schools in the United States were built before 1984 and have not undergone major renovation since that time.[2] Because of this, they are likely to contain materials such as asbestos (see Chapter 23), lead (see Chapter 32), and polychlorinated biphenyls (see Chapter 38). The risk of exposure to such substances is greatest when buildings are being renovated or fall into disrepair—a common situation in some cities and poorly resourced rural areas. Routine inspection of school buildings and construction sites to identify hazards is critical.

Renovations are often undertaken to address shortcomings of the school building. Such projects should optimally occur during periods when the school, or at least that portion of the school building, is not in use, such as during summer breaks or during weekends or holidays. Following this timeline minimizes exposure of staff and students to the noise and emissions occurring during construction, and also minimizes staff noncompliance with optimal construction practices (such as failure to wear safety equipment while in the construction area).

#### *High-performance Schools*

High-performance school buildings are efficient in their use of energy, water, and materials and are also safe, secure, stimulating, and healthy. They require careful attention to site selection and design. They also require commissioning, a systematic process of ensuring that the buildings perform interactively and in a way consistent with design intent and operational needs. The Collaborative for High-Performance Schools (www.chps.net) and the National Clearinghouse for Educational Facilities (www.edfacilities.org) provide information about designing and commissioning high-performance schools. The US Environmental Protection Agency (US EPA) Healthy Buildings Tool Kit (www.epa.gov/schools-healthy-buildings) is a series of free downloadable programs that can be used to systematically track and manage information about school environmental conditions, recommend possible improvements, and address school compliance with government regulations and voluntary school program requirements.

### Utilization of Space

Understanding the school environment requires an assessment of how space is used. Schools are primarily established to provide children with an education, and they also may serve other community functions. They often serve as sites for before- and after-school child care and enrichment programs, recreation, adult education, artistic performances, and public meetings. School-based health centers and social service providers may co-locate in schools. During disasters and other emergencies, schools often serve as shelters or command posts. These uses raise concerns about safety and security as well as the possibility that utilizing makeshift and converted spaces exposes users to existing environmental hazards.

Information about the benefits and challenges of schools serving as focal points for academic, health, social service, community development, and community engagement efforts is available (www.communityschools.org).

## Crowding

Objectively, crowding occurs when people inhabit a space beyond its capacity or when people in a space have very little room per person. Subjectively, crowding occurs when an individual feels that his or her ability to control interaction with other people is impaired or that other people interfere with an individual's activities. Crowding is linked to increased transmission of infectious diseases. Crowding is stressful. It can cause overstimulation, interfere with concentration, create social friction, and increase aggression. This, in turn, can interfere with learning and precipitate problematic behavior—especially for children with autism spectrum disorder (ASD), attention-deficit/hyperactivity disorder (ADHD) or other attention disorders, sensory integration dysfunction, or learning disabilities (also known as learning differences). Teachers are likely to feel stressed in crowded environments, where they often spend more time on discipline and classroom management.

## Acoustics and Noise

Poor classroom acoustics can interfere with children's ability to learn and communicate.[3] Noise—unwanted sound—can interfere with student concentration, motivation, and memory. It can be stressful, especially if loud or persistent, and can result in elevated blood pressure.[4] Students with sensory impairment, auditory processing disorders, ADHD, and ASD may be particularly sensitive to noise.[5,6] In many cases, improved acoustics and noise reduction can be achieved by simple interventions such as furniture reconfiguration, designation of quiet areas, replacement of noisy lighting fixtures and equipment, and changes in scheduling (eg, staggering lunchtimes to reduce hallway traffic during instructional periods). In other cases, soundproofing and other building modifications may be necessary. Information on classroom acoustics and noise reduction is available from the Acoustical Society of America (http://asa.aip.org/classroom.html) and Quiet Classrooms (www.quietclassrooms.org). See Chapter 35 on Noise.

## POTENTIAL TOXIC HAZARDS IN THE SCHOOL ENVIRONMENT

### Learning Environments and Activities

Certain learning activities may pose health risks because of the nature of the learning space or the materials and equipment used.

- Industrial arts projects often involve potentially toxic chemicals. Students should be taught about the potential toxicity and how to avoid exposure. Workshops typically contain tools and equipment that may cause cuts, abrasions, burns, lifting injuries, or more serious injuries, such as amputations. Students may be exposed to noise, flying objects, chemical fumes, intense heat, and sharp edges; protective gear (eg, goggles, ear plugs, gloves, masks) must be used in potentially hazardous situations. In wood shops, dust and shavings in the air can trigger asthma exacerbations and use of a protective mask should be considered.

- Certain materials used for art and craft projects are potentially toxic (see Chapter 46). Nontoxic materials certified by the Art & Creative Materials Institute (www.acminet.org) should be used whenever possible. Kilns can emit chemicals that may cause respiratory problems. Adequate ventilation is crucial.

- Chemistry and biology classrooms and labs may contain potentially toxic materials that require proper storage and handling. The US EPA provides information and tools for managing these risks.[7] Other potential injuries include burns and cuts. Handling live animals may lead to bites, scratches, allergic reactions, or zoonotic diseases.[8] Animals should only be maintained as necessary for curricula and should be carefully confined in suitable, sanitary, self-contained enclosures appropriate for their size.[9]

- Traumatic injuries may occur in gym classes and with recreational activities involving movement. Risks can be reduced by ensuring adequate supervision and space. Floors and equipment should be in good repair and cleaned regularly. Indoor pools should be properly maintained and well ventilated.

When schools utilize modular buildings (trailers) for educational space, care should be taken to ensure that the modular building meets all requirements for functioning as an effective and healthy place in which to learn. Because of the often extensive use of manufactured wood products within these structures, off-gassing of formaldehyde and other volatile organic compounds (VOCs) occurs at high levels. Temperature control within the structure may be uneven or unsatisfactory because of the nature of the construction and limited insulation used in the walls, floor, and ceiling of the modular unit. When these structures are designed for short-term, temporary use, but are left in service far longer than originally intended, their physical condition may deteriorate.

## Bathrooms and Locker Rooms

Bathrooms and locker rooms are locations where students may be exposed to microorganisms, such as molds and bacteria carried on the skin and in the digestive tract, especially when there are plumbing leaks or when toilets overflow. Students may come into contact with infectious agents by interacting with other students and through fomites. Waste containers, soap, and paper towels should be readily available. Students should wash hands or use hand sanitizer throughout the day, especially after toileting, outdoor play, and before eating. School personnel should aim to prevent young children from ingesting hand sanitizer because of possible ethanol toxicity. Bathroom areas should be well ventilated because sewer gases, cigarette smoke, air fresheners, hair sprays, and perfumes may contribute to poor air quality. Each of these exposures is a potential asthma trigger. Good lighting and anti-slip measures should be used to reduce the risk of injuries in showers and areas where water tends to be tracked. The water temperature should be set low enough to prevent scalding; best practice calls for water temperature to be maintained below 120°F (49°C).

## Food Preparation, Storage, and Service Areas

Pest management is particularly important in food-related areas. Other important considerations in selecting, purchasing, and preparing food in the school setting include choosing foods of high quality and reducing foods that are common food allergens to the extent feasible. Food quality can be enhanced by providing fresh fruits and vegetables whenever possible rather than canned products. Providing organic fruits and vegetables when feasible reduces the amount of pesticides ingested by students and others who eat at school.

Food service staff and students involved in food preparation or service should be trained in proper food storage and handling techniques to reduce the risk of spread of infectious disease, food contamination, and spoilage. Equipment should be cleaned and maintained properly to reduce the risk of biological contaminants or nonfood objects affecting food. It is important to clean equipment properly to avoid cross-contamination that can trigger food allergy. The National Coalition for Food-Safe Schools (www.foodsafe-schools.org) and the US EPA (https://www.epa.gov/managing-pests-schools/introduction-integrated-pest-management) are excellent sources of information on this topic.

## Lighting

Lighting quality affects students' ability to see and process visual information. Students may have difficulty attending and learning if available light is insufficient, unbalanced (contrasting bright spots and shadows), or gloomy. Glare may cause fatigue, eye strain, and headaches. Modern school designs tend to better integrate natural light into lighting design. Students tend to perform better when natural light contributes to classroom lighting and may experience a subtle, positive effect on their mood and behavior.[10]

Children with visual impairment, learning disabilities, sensory processing/integration disorder, ADHD, and ASD are often very sensitive to lighting environments. They may disengage from the learning process or engage in problematic behavior if distracted, annoyed, or stressed by glare or malfunctioning (flickering, humming) light fixtures. Interventions include repairing or replacing lighting fixtures, strategic use of window coverings, repositioning classroom furniture, and assigning students to optimally lighted classroom areas.

In schools with fluorescent light fixtures manufactured before 1978, leakage of polychlorinated biphenyls (PCBs) can occur. The best way to reduce PCB contamination in schools is for schools to systematically replace old ballasts with PCB-free ballasts manufactured since 1978.[11]

## Ergonomics

Ergonomics is the science of taking human characteristics into account when designing and using objects or equipment. Providing child-friendly seating, workstations, equipment, and furniture can be especially challenging given the wide variation in children's sizes, body proportions, and growth rates. Children who use adaptive equipment or who have specific areas of difficulty or disability may present additional challenges. Information about backpacks is available from the American Academy of Pediatrics (AAP) (https://www.healthychildren.org/English/safety-prevention/at-play/Pages/Backpack-Safety.aspx); information about ergonomic aspects of backpacks, computers, and other items associated with school is available through Healthy Computing (www.healthycomputing.com/kids), the Cornell University Ergonomics Web site (http://ergo.human.cornell.edu/MBergo/schoolguide.html), and Ergonomics 4 Schools (http://ergonomics4schools.com). Information on inspecting and retrofitting bleachers to reduce the risk of injury is available from the US Consumer Product Safety Commission (https://www.cpsc.gov/PageFiles/122347/330.pdf).

## Thermal Conditions

Temperature, relative humidity, and air velocity are important parts of the physical environment (see Chapter 26). Thermal conditions influence mold growth and the release of chemical and microbiological agents into the air. Relatively small changes in thermal conditions can influence student comfort. Students are less able to learn if they are uncomfortable. Factors such as student clothing and activity level; radiant heat transfer from heat-producing equipment (eg, computers); season; air flow; heating, ventilating, and air conditioning (HVAC) unit performance; sunlight penetration; and building construction should be considered when managing the thermal environment.

The national consensus standard for outside air ventilation is ASHRAE (American Society of Heating, Refrigerating and Air-Conditioning Engineers) Standard 62.1-200, Ventilation for Acceptable Indoor Air Quality (available online via www.ashrae.org) and its published Addenda. This standard is often incorporated into state and local building codes and specifies the amounts of outside air that must be provided by natural or mechanical ventilation systems to various areas of schools, including classrooms, gymnasiums, kitchens, and other special-use areas. Airflow in schools should be between 15 and 20 cubic feet/minute per person (0.42 to 0.57 cubic meters/minute per person) and result in more than 4 air changes per hour.[12,13] Carbon dioxide levels, which are useful in determining the adequacy of ventilation, should be less than 1,000 parts per million (ppm) when a room has been occupied in its typical use for 4 to 6 hours.[14] The optimal temperature for most classrooms is 69.8°F to 73.4°F (21°C to 23°C).[15]

The relative humidity should be between 30% and 60%. High temperature, especially in combination with low relative humidity, can increase eye, skin, and mucosal irritation and may also result in fatigue, lethargy, poor concentration, and headache. High relative humidity, often manifested as surfaces that feel damp, is problematic because it stimulates dust mite multiplication as well as growth of bacteria and mold. This is a particular problem in portable classroom structures. Mold can be a potent trigger for asthma exacerbations. High humidity may be caused by flooding, wet carpet, inadequate bathroom ventilation, and kitchen-generated moisture. Other sources of moisture include humidifiers, dehumidifiers, air conditioners, and drip pans under refrigerator cooling coils. Means of reducing moisture include proper maintenance of HVAC systems, using exhaust fans in high-moisture environments (eg, kitchens, pool areas), repairing leaks, and promptly drying or removing wet carpeting. Regular walk-throughs and inspections can help to identify these hazards before they cause harm.

## Air Quality

Poor air quality in schools places children at risk of short- and long-term health problems and can have a negative effect on learning and performance. An analysis of school-level data from the 2006 School Health Policies and Programs Study showed that 51.4% of schools had a formal indoor air quality management program and that those schools were significantly more likely to have policies and use strategies to promote indoor air quality than were schools without a program.[16]

## Outdoor Air Pollution

Air quality around schools depends on factors such as traffic patterns, nearby industrial activities, proximity to waste sites, local herbicide and pesticide use, atmospheric conditions, and geography. Outdoor air pollution is linked to respiratory problems in children, including decreased lung function, coughing, wheezing, more frequent respiratory illness, and asthma exacerbations (see Chapter 21). Children are primarily exposed to outdoor air pollutants while traveling to or from school and when playing outside. Pollutants also may enter through doors, windows, vents, and drains. Carbon monoxide (see Chapter 25), nitrogen dioxide, and particles found in vehicle exhaust may be present at high levels in schools located close to busy roadways or where busses, delivery trucks, or passenger vehicles idle nearby for long periods of time. Carbon monoxide detectors in schools are required by law in only a few states.[17] School officials can reduce traffic-related emissions by discouraging vehicle idling and improving school-related traffic flow and by using the free toolkit available from the US EPA's Clean School Bus USA program (https://www.epa.gov/cleandiesel/clean-school-bus). They should also consider outdoor air quality when scheduling recess, sports, and other outdoor activities. Information about ozone levels and smog alerts is available through local media and the US EPA's Air Now Web site (http://airnow.gov).

## Indoor Air Quality

Many factors contribute to indoor air quality (see Chapter 20). The concentration of indoor air pollutants can vary from room to room and even within a single classroom. Levels also may vary according to the activity occurring in the space (eg, higher levels during craft activities) and variations in airflow (eg, caused by opening windows). Secondhand smoke exposure and exposure to smoke carried on clothing, occurring more intensively in certain areas, may contribute to worse air quality in those areas.

Pollen, soot, fiberglass fibers, chalk dust, lead, and other airborne particulates can cause respiratory and other health problems. Smoking should not be allowed within the school or any part of the school property, including sporting fields and bleachers. Secondhand smoke exposure (see Chapter 43) can occur if schools restrict smoking to designated areas.

Schools built between the 1950s and the late 1970s may have fluorescent light ballasts that contain PCBs. Congress banned their use in 1976. These old fluorescent ballasts can leak PCBs into the indoor air of the classroom. They should be replaced with energy-efficient lighting (see Chapter 38).

Toxic gases can affect air quality. Although some can be detected by odor, others are odorless and require specific equipment for detection. An estimated 19.3% of US schools have at least 1 room with radon levels at or above 4 picocuries per liter (pCi/L).[18] Formaldehyde may cause irritation of the mouth, throat, nose, and eyes; worsen asthma symptoms; and cause headache and nausea. Exposure may be especially likely in portable classrooms containing composite wood products (eg, plywood, particleboard).[19] Paints, adhesives, carpets, cleaning products, and building materials may contain VOCs which are associated with respiratory and other health problems. Unhealthy concentrations of VOCs may be especially common in portable classrooms in which thermal conditions tend to facilitate off-gassing, especially in the first few years of use.[19]

Poor indoor air quality may give rise to a building-related illness or "sick building syndrome." Building-related illnesses are disorders that can be directly attributed to chemical or physical agents in a particular building.[20] Sick building syndrome is a phenomenon whereby several occupants in the same building experience similar acute or lingering symptoms with no obvious etiology. Symptoms appear to be linked to a particular building or area within a building. Sick building syndrome has been linked to inadequate fresh air intake, poor air flow caused by poorly designed and maintained HVAC systems, biological and chemical contaminants, overly warm temperatures, and high relative humidity.[21,22] Very low levels of specific pollutants and other physical factors may act synergistically or in combination to cause sick building syndrome.[23] Often, symptoms of sick building syndrome and building-related illnesses disappear when the people are not in the building. Some of the symptoms of sick building syndrome may overlap with symptoms of idiopathic environmental intolerance (see Chapter 60).[24,25]

Free materials related to indoor air quality in schools are available on the US EPA's Tools for Schools Web site (www.epa.gov/iaq/schools).

Biological air pollutants are found to some degree in every school. They may generate toxic or allergic reactions, particularly with excessive exposure. Sources include outdoor air, animals, human occupants, insects, and water reservoirs (eg, humidifiers).

- Molds characteristically thrive in warm, moist climates and release spores into the air that are associated with allergic reactions in susceptible individuals, asthma exacerbations, coughing, wheezing, and upper respiratory symptoms in otherwise healthy people.[26]
- Hair and dander of cats, dogs, and other animals may be shed by classroom pets, laboratory animals, service animals, visiting pets, and vermin. They may be carried to school on children's clothes. Classroom allergen levels may become high enough to cause sensitization or induce asthma in children who do not have pets at home or come into direct contact with animals. Other than service dogs, animals should be avoided or limited in schools and in child care settings.[9]

- Dust mite allergens may become airborne and cause asthma, rhinitis, or atopic dermatitis in predisposed individuals. Reservoirs in schools include upholstered furniture, pillows, carpets, and books.
- Rodent and cockroach allergens can be significant factors in the development and exacerbation of asthma in children.[27] When such pests are present in the school setting, appropriate steps should be taken to eradicate them.

Among children with clinical complaints related to the environment, appropriate allergic and psychological consultation should be considered. Viral respiratory tract infections peak in prevalence at the onset of school, and children with asthma often have increased respiratory symptoms from those viral respiratory tract infections. Mold spores and animal dander in the school can cause inhalant allergy symptoms in susceptible allergic children; these problems can be identified by appropriate clinical assessment and often are readily treatable. For the individual child in whom treatment is not successful, special arrangements may be needed.

Although it is important to eliminate undesirable insects and other pests, routine spraying of pesticides inside and outside the building can adversely affect indoor air quality and can leave toxic residues that can be ingested or absorbed through the skin (see Chapter 40). To control pests in a more environmentally sensitive and cost-effective way, schools should generally adopt integrated pest management (IPM) programs. IPM involves the judicious use of pesticides in conjunction with other strategies informed by knowledge about specific pests and their interactions with the environment. When chemicals are used, the treatments are timed according to the pest's life cycle (eg, breeding, egg laying) to maximize effect. Materials related to IPM in schools are available from the US EPA (https://www.epa.gov/managing-pests-schools/introduction-integrated-pest-management), the National School IPM Information Source (http://schoolipm.ifas.ufl.edu), and the National Pest Management Association (www.pestworld.org).

### Cleaning Materials and Practices

Children's health and well-being may be enhanced or compromised by products and practices used to clean and maintain schools.[28] Cleaning, sanitizing, and disinfecting are useful methods for protecting people against viruses and bacteria. Cleaning refers to using soaps or detergents and water to physically remove visible dirt and contamination from surfaces or objects. Sanitizing is used after visible dirt is removed from a surface. Sanitizing greatly reduces the number of pathogens to levels unlikely to cause disease. Disinfecting, a process that is more rigorous than sanitizing, involves applying cumulative heat or a chemical to result in the elimination of almost all microorganisms from inanimate surfaces.

Routine procedures differ from place to place and may include use of disinfectants on frequently touched surfaces and objects. Although it is important to maintain surfaces to ensure a low risk of infection, excessive use of disinfectants often contributes to respiratory irritation and worse indoor air quality when these compounds become airborne. More information on cleaning, sanitizing, and disinfecting can be found in Chapter 10.

Many chemicals used to clean floors, desks, and tables are potentially toxic. String mops used to clean bathroom floors may promote the spread of infectious agents to uncontaminated areas. Although cleaning is important to remove particulate matter from floors, carpets, and other surfaces, many cleaning activities, such as rag dusting and use of a vacuum cleaner with a cloth bag, resuspend particulate matter rather than remove it. School staff should vacuum regularly using well-constructed cleaners with high-efficiency particulate air (HEPA) filters or near-HEPA filters. Dusters should be made of materials that trap, rather than simply push, dust particles.

Many schools have adopted "green" cleaning programs that minimize the effects of cleaning materials on health and protect the environment. Such programs emphasize the thoughtful use and proper storage of cleaning materials. They incorporate healthier, environmentally conscious policies, procedures, and training. Information can be obtained from the Healthy Schools Campaign (www.healthyschoolscampaign.org), the National Clearinghouse for Educational Facilities (www.ncef.org), and The Cleaning for Healthy Schools Toolkit (www.cleaningforhealthyschools.org).

## Water Quality

Lead contamination may be a significant water-related concern in schools. The public health crisis that occurred in Flint, Michigan in 2014 as a result of high lead levels in the water supply extended to schools (see Chapter 32). The American Civil Liberties Union of Michigan then sued Michigan's state education department and the Flint schools, contending that students' exposure to high lead levels violated federal education laws.[29] More than 57% of Philadelphia's public schools had water lead levels exceeding the US EPA action level at the time of 20 parts per billion (ppb).[30] More than 28% had water with mean lead levels in excess of 50 ppb. Lead most frequently enters drinking water by leaching from plumbing materials and fixtures as water moves through plumbing.[31] High concentrations of lead can accumulate in water overnight, on weekends, and over school holidays because of the increased time that the water remains in the water distribution system. Lead concentration in water is often highest within the first 90 seconds after the faucet is turned on.

Schools and child care facilities that have and/or operate their own public water system are required to comply with the federal Safe Drinking Water Act

(SDWA) and must therefore test their water for lead to comply with the US EPA action level. According to the US EPA, an estimated 8,000 schools and child care facilities fall into this category. Approximately 98,000 other public schools and 500,000 child care facilities are not regulated under the SDWA and may or may not conduct voluntary testing of drinking water. The US EPA developed the "3T's Toolkit"—"Training, Testing and Telling"—to assist school officials with reducing lead in drinking water.[32]

The current US EPA action level for lead in water is 15 ppb. The amount of lead in water should be below this level. Schools should meet or exceed federal and state laws for lead and other water quality measures. Those with private wells should have water tested periodically for bacterial and chemical contamination. Information about water quality is available from the US EPA Safewater program (https://www.epa.gov/ground-water-and-drinking-water).

Water may also contain other unhealthful compounds, including hydrocarbons, flame-retardant chemicals, and bacteria, depending on the source of the water. Optimally, schools should periodically check on the quality of their water intended for drinking. Obtaining drinking water from water sources within the school other than water fountains, drinking water dispensers, and similar sources intended for supplying potable water, should be discouraged to avoid potential hazards from use of nonpotable water for drinking.

## Other Toxicants

Children may be exposed to a wide variety of other toxicants in schools. For a summary of selected toxicants, see the table at the beginning of the chapter on Child Care Settings (Chapter 10).

## Playgrounds and Outdoor Athletic Spaces

Playgrounds, athletic fields, and green areas provide spaces for play, physical activity, socializing, and relaxation (see Chapter 9). They allow contact with the natural world and can facilitate learning about local wildlife. With these benefits come potential risks related to air pollution, ultraviolet (UV) radiation, contaminated soil, contaminated groundwater, play surfaces, and equipment, as well as contact with birds, animals, and people from the larger community.

Many schools utilize artificial turf for outdoor play areas, with the goal of reducing maintenance, maintaining year-round availability, and eliminating the need for grass cultivation, fertilization, and herbicide use. Concerns about potential health impacts of older styles of artificial turf have generally been addressed in recent designs. Before installing or reinstalling artificial turf, it is prudent to carefully investigate the properties of the specific product(s) being considered. Injury risks to students playing on artificial turf are difficult to compare with risks of playing on natural grass because of many potentially confounding factors.

Excessive exposure to UV radiation (see Chapter 44) places children at higher risk of skin cancers and other serious health problems later in their lives.[33] Schools can schedule children's outdoor activities before or after the hours when UV rays are strongest (ie, avoiding outdoor activities from 10 am to 4 pm). They can implement policies that encourage students to wear protective clothing, hats, and sunglasses and to apply sunscreen during outdoor activities. They can implement educational programs, such as the National Environmental Education Foundation's SunWise Program (https://www.neefusa.org/sunwise), to encourage and reinforce preventive behaviors. Information on increasing outdoor shading using strategies is suggested by Shade Planning for America's Schools (www.cdc.gov/cancer/skin/pdf/shade_planning.pdf). Several states have enacted legislation to allow students to use sunscreen in schools and similar legislation is pending in other states.[34]

Toxicants may be present in the soil and groundwater near schools, especially those built in areas of high air pollution or on land contaminated by industrial waste. Lead (see Chapter 32) may be found in high concentrations near school walls, where paint has flaked off and accumulated, or throughout the grounds if the school is located near a point source, such as a smelter or battery manufacturing plant. High levels of PCBs may be found in and near buildings with PCB-containing caulk.[35] Sufficient exposure to herbicides and pesticides used on school grounds can cause skin and eye irritation as well as abdominal pain and vomiting.

Play areas should be designed and maintained to meet the needs of all students, including students with disabilities. An informative reference, *Accessible Play Areas: A Summary of Accessibility Guidelines for Play Areas*, is available at https://www.access-board.gov/guidelines-and-standards/recreation-facilities/guides/play-areas/.

Playgrounds are common sites of serious injury at school. Emergency departments in the United States treat more than 200,000 children aged 14 and younger for playground-related injuries every year. Approximately 75% of playground-related injuries occur on public playgrounds, with most occurring at a place of recreation or at school.[36] More than one half of these injuries are fractures and contusions or abrasions.[36] Such injuries can often be reduced by modifying playground equipment and layout, as well as installing shock-absorbing safety surfaces. Information is available from the National Program for Playground Safety (www.playgroundsafety.org) and in the Public Playground Safety Handbook developed by the Consumer Product Safety Commission (CPSC) (www.cpsc.gov//PageFiles/122149/325.pdf).

The risk of athletic injuries increases if students have insufficient space, are exposed to physical hazards (eg, rocks, holes, sharp objects, animal droppings) on playing fields, or engage in sports on hard, loose, or uneven terrain.

Artificial turf containing recycled tire crumb may be used on playing fields and playgrounds.[37] Playing spaces should be clearly marked. Where appropriate, nets and other barriers should be used to protect spectators from stray balls or other play-related hazards.

## Travel Routes to and From School

Hazards around school driveways, parking lots, and other paths of travel increase the risk of injury. These areas should be clearly marked, well-lighted, and well-maintained, especially when weather conditions cause them to be slippery or difficult to traverse. Areas where students are picked up and dropped off should offer adequate protection from the elements as well as from traffic and vehicle exhaust. During peak traffic times, additional safety measures, such as having crossing guards and making alterations in traffic light timing, can help reduce the risk of accidents. The Pedestrian and Bicycle Information Center (www.pedbikeinfo.org) provides information to enhance biking and walking safety. The Centers for Disease Control and Prevention (CDC)'s KidsWalk-to-School program (https://stacks.cdc.gov/view/cdc/11316/) and the National Center for Safe Routes to School (www.saferoutesinfo.org) provide information to encourage children to walk and bicycle to and from school.

Children who walk, bicycle, or take public transportation may be vulnerable to street crime. Students may be more inclined to engage in truant, delinquent, or risky behavior if nearby parks, stores, abandoned buildings, or wooded areas prove to be tempting hangouts. It is prudent for school officials to investigate any potential dangers in nearby areas such as construction sites, industrial sites, and water bodies.

## THE SCHOOL NUTRITIONAL ENVIRONMENT

Most children eat meals or snacks at school. Although some food and beverages are brought from home or purchased off-site, much is obtained from the cafeteria or purchased from on-site vending machines. Schools may play an important role in influencing children's food intake, eating habits, and knowledge of nutrition. Food often plays a significant part in school events (eg, fund-raising, class parties). Information about food and nutrition is often incorporated into health, science, home economics, and vocational curricula. Status among peers may be affected by a child's eating habits, such as whether a child eats a school lunch or brings lunch from home, contents of lunches and lunch containers brought from home or provided by a family member during the lunch period, whether one shares food, where and with whom (if anyone) one sits at lunch, and whether the environment provides opportunity for activities that might make a child rush or skip lunch.[38] School breakfast and lunch programs are often subsidized for students meeting certain criteria, such as low family incomes. Optimal practice calls for avoiding any potential stigma from participation in such programs, perhaps by separating the payment for school breakfast and lunch from the actual distribution of the food. Food should not be used as a reward for good performance.

Many students, both boys and girls, may feel pressured to engage in unhealthy eating practices or use potentially dangerous diet supplements or performance-enhancing compounds. Other students may be inclined to overeat if they find the school environment stressful or are on restrictive diets at home.

Although significant effort has been undertaken to improve the nutritional value of foods offered and eaten at school, some foods consumed at school can be high in calories and have limited nutritional value, thereby increasing the risk of obesity and diabetes mellitus. This risk may be especially relevant for children from low-income families, whose diets may be especially lacking in nutrients. Ideally, food and drinks available at schools should conform to the federal nutrition guidelines established for schools participating in the National School Lunch and Breakfast programs. Foods served at schools have been occasionally linked to widespread illness among children.[39]

Meal planning can be challenging given budgetary constraints, bulk food purchasing policies, concerns about food allergies, and children's food preferences. The US Department of Agriculture's Food and Nutrition Services Web site (www.fns.usda.gov) and the School Nutrition Association (www.school nutrition.org) offer information on school nutrition assistance programs, school meal planning, and nutrition. Information on improving the school nutritional environment and encouraging physical activity is available from the Action for Healthy Kids (www.actionforhealthykids.org) and the Healthy Schools campaign (www.healthyschoolscampaign.org).

## PSYCHOSOCIAL DIMENSIONS OF THE SCHOOL ENVIRONMENT

Historically, environmental health research and practice has focused on toxicants and physical hazards. A more holistic perspective recognizes the significant influence of psychosocial factors. School affords children the opportunity to develop social skills, form friendships, learn teamwork, achieve a sense of belonging, and develop a positive self-image. School can also be a site where animosities foment and children feel physically or emotionally vulnerable to other students, teachers, cliques, or gangs.

### School Violence and Intimidation

Violent crime on school grounds represents a real threat to student health and well-being. Some 841,100 violent crimes on school property—including 26 homicides—were reported during the 2013–2014 school year alone.[40] Many students' school experiences are affected by concerns about violence; 3% of students reported being afraid of attack or harm at school in 2015. Those attending schools in urban or suburban areas were more likely to feel unsafe. Approximately 15% of students attending urban schools reported the presence of gangs in their school, while those attending suburban or rural schools reported lower rates (10.2% and 3.9%, respectively). Among students in grades 9 through 12, 7% of males and 4.6% of females reported having been threatened or injured with a weapon on school property in the past year. Some 5% reported having skipped classes or extracurricular activities, avoided certain places on school grounds, or stayed home from school in the previous 6 months because of fear of attack or harm. All of these rates are lower than in previous surveys over the past decade.

Bullying was defined, in 2014, by CDC and the US Department of Education to include "direct bullying" and "indirect bullying."[41] Direct bullying comprises events that occur in the presence of the targeted individual, while indirect bullying encompasses events that are not directly expressed to the target (such as spreading rumors about the bullied individual). This definition also categorizes four types of bullying to include physical acts, verbal acts, relational bullying (by attempting to harm the reputation or relationships of the target), and acts intended to damage property. Bullying can also utilize electronic media and computer technology or social media to perform verbal and relational acts (cyberbullying). Cyberbullying can extend into property damage if the target's stored electronic information is altered or destroyed.

The Indicators of School Crime and Safety 2016 report also found that 7% of students 12 to 18 years of age reported that someone at school had used hate-related words against them, having to do with their race, ethnicity, religion, disability, gender, or sexual orientation. Twenty-seven percent reported seeing hate-related graffiti at school. The reported incidence of these hate-related acts has decreased since 2000. Twenty percent of students aged 12 to 18 years had been bullied at school during the previous 6 months.[40] The bullying involved pushing, shoving, tripping, or being spit upon in approximately 5% of students. The prevalence of cyberbullying (through e-mail, text messages, or Web sites) in 2015–2016 was reported by 8% of students. Resources are available from the Stop Bullying Now campaign at www.stopbullying.gov.[42]

## Substance Use

Substance use and abuse occurs on school property. Thirty-two percent of students in grades 9 to 12 reported having consumed at least 1 alcoholic drink on school property during the previous 30 days.[35] One in 5 (20.1%) students smoked cigarettes, cigars, cigarillos, or little cigars or used chewing tobacco, snuff, or dip (a form of smokeless tobacco) at least 1 day during the past 30 days.[43] Information about youth tobacco use is available from the CDC Youth Risk Behavior Surveillance System (www.cdc.gov/HealthyYouth/yrbs/) and the

Youth Tobacco Survey (www.cdc.gov/tobacco/data_statistics/surveys/yts/index.htm).[43]

More than 1 in 5 students (21.6% of respondents) reported using marijuana anywhere during the past 30 days in 2015. Data about marijuana use at school were not collected in 2013 or 2015; in 2011, about 25% of students reporting marijuana use anywhere reported having used marijuana on school property during that period.[43] The use of inhalants (huffing) is a concern at school because the school is where students may access glues, markers, paints, solvents, and other substances with mind-altering effects. Information about youth substance abuse is available from the National Institute on Drug Abuse (www.drugabuse.gov) and the National Inhalant Prevention Coalition (www.inhalants.com).

## Positive Influences and Effects

School is a place where children are taught facts and develop academic skills. It is also a place where children can learn how to ask questions, problem-solve, relate, communicate, act responsibly, and lead. For many children, school is a place where their learning disabilities, emotional and behavioral problems, social difficulties, or maltreatment are first noticed and addressed. School may serve as a temporary haven for those with chaotic home lives.

Many children encounter teachers and other positive role models who inspire, encourage, and support them. They are afforded opportunities to feed their curiosity and expand their interests, as well as develop and be recognized for their artistic, athletic, and intellectual talents. School is often a place where good memories are formed and important friendships take root. These positive aspects can enhance mental health, bolster resiliency, and pave the way for healthy adult relationships and personal success.

## STUDENTS AS ACTIVE PARTICIPANTS IN SCHOOL ENVIRONMENTAL HEALTH EFFORTS

Students can play active roles in promoting healthy school environments. For example, they can participate in school walk-throughs to identify potential health hazards; initiate and promote recycling programs, help cultivate school-yard wildlife habitats (see the US Fish and Wildlife Service's School Habitat Program at https://www.fws.gov/cno/conservation/schoolyard.html), and help implement anti-bullying campaigns. Student interest in school environmental health can be sparked through materials and lessons such as those offered by the National Environmental Education Foundation (www.neefusa.org), the National Institute of Environmental Health Sciences (www.niehs.nih.gov/health/scied/teachers/index.cfm), and the US EPA Teaching Center (https://www.epa.gov/students/lesson-plans-teacher-guides-and-online-resources-educators ).

## THE PEDIATRICIAN'S ROLE IN SCHOOL ENVIRONMENTAL HEALTH

### The Pediatrician as School District Consultant

AAP School Health policy recommends that each school district work closely with one or more pediatricians who serve in a formal consulting manner, advising about school health and school health policies.[44] Pediatricians often closely collaborate with school nurses and other school leaders in activities promoting student and staff wellness, frequently through the activities of a "School Wellness Advisory Committee."

### Taking a School Environmental Health History

Taking a school environmental health history can be important when a child presents with respiratory problems; unexplained illness and nonspecific symptoms suggestive of toxicant exposure; or behavioral and social problems associated with sensory integration difficulties, ADHD, or autism spectrum disorders. It can be valuable when addressing chronic conditions with implications across multiple domains, such as obesity, asthma, diabetes mellitus, hypertension, and mood disorders. The history-taking process provides opportunities to educate children, families, and educators about how school environmental factors can enhance or compromise children's health and well-being.

It can be helpful to ask the student to recount his or her activities and interactions over the course of a typical week. Younger children may have difficulty providing detailed information, but their input is nonetheless valuable because it may yield information about the physical environment and provide insight into their experience of school. Older students are likely to have more complicated schedules that vary from one day or marking period to the next.

In addition to focusing on the health of individual children, pediatricians are uniquely poised to promote the health, development, and wellness of children in the community. Pediatricians' expertise, interests, and concerns afford the opportunity to contribute to or lead efforts to improve the school environment by participating in on-site inspections of school buildings, grounds, and play equipment; encouraging schools to promote good nutrition; supporting efforts to increase physical activity; educating parents, students, and school personnel about using protective clothing and equipment; encouraging exploration of and integrating concern for nature and the environment into curricula (see Appendix C) and into students' daily experiences; serving on school committees addressing health, wellness, and emergency preparedness; and supporting school nurse efforts to make the school a positive focus for child health in the community.

## Frequently Asked Questions

*Q*  *Asbestos was recently discovered in ceilings at my child's school. What should the school do? Should my child have a chest x-ray? Will she develop cancer?*

*A*  Asbestos was extensively used as insulation in school construction until the 1970s. Because asbestos release is typically episodic (eg, when materials are fractured during renovation) and usually missed by air sampling, visual inspection is required to establish the nature of the asbestos risk. All schools must maintain an asbestos management plan and undergo systematic inspection every 3 years. Normally, asbestos removal is not necessary unless children are likely to come into direct contact with it or building renovation is about to occur. More often, the fibers are simply contained by installing drywall, drop ceilings, or other enclosures. Under Federal law, you have the right to request a copy of your school's asbestos management plan, which provides information about building inspections, as well as asbestos removal and containment activities. The risk of lung cancer or mesothelioma from a brief exposure is very low. A chest x-ray will not be helpful because asbestos does not produce acute changes in the lungs.

*Q*  *How do I know if there is a problem with lead in our school?*

*A*  Schools built before the 1970s are likely to contain leaded materials on walls, woodwork, stairwells, and window casings and sills. Other sources include deteriorating paint, lead pipes, lead-lined water coolers, water fixtures, and lead-containing art supplies. Many schools also have potential exposure to lead from drinking water supplied through leaded distribution pipes, present in many cities with long-established municipal water systems. Periodic testing of water at points of intended use can ascertain the concentration of lead in water. It is prudent to obtain water for drinking or cooking only from fixtures intended for providing drinking water, and to avoid using bathroom sinks or utility sinks for obtaining potable water.

You can contact school officials to ask for copies of any inspections or test results. You can also contact health department officials to learn about regulations related to lead hazards.

*Q*  *What is an artificial turf field?*

*A*  Today's artificial turf fields are made of three basic layers:
  1. The top layer is a long-pile "carpet" of plastic artificial grass fibers.
  2. A second layer of infill material lies within the carpet, to support the "grass" and provide cushioning. It can be made of sand, recycled rubber crumbs ("crumb rubber") or an alternate material.
  3. Underneath is a perforated woven backing holding the carpet in place.

Underlying drainage systems prevent these fields from becoming waterlogged.

Q  *What are the benefits of artificial turf over natural grass?*

A  Artificial turf has become a popular alternative to natural grass because of a variety of features:

1. *Waste reduction:* Scrap tires are a major waste disposal challenge. According to the Rubber Manufacturers Association, in 2007, crumb rubber infill for artificial fields kept 300 million pounds of tires out of landfills. However, infill must be replaced every 5 to 10 years so disposal concerns are deferred but not eliminated.

2. *Increased hours of playability:* Artificial turf fields offer more playable hours than natural grass.[45] Newer fields with underlying drainage systems, however, may increase their playable hours.

3. *No need to mow, water, or fertilize:* According to a University of California Berkeley study in 2010, a 1,000 square foot natural field requires 70,000 gallons of water each week and 15 to 20 pounds of fertilizer each year, plus herbicides and pesticides.[45] New natural fields, however, can require less input.

4. *Increased access to sports:* Artificial fields can be placed on historically contaminated soils, increasing access to field spaces.[46]

Q  *What are the health concerns for artificial turf?*

A  1. *They are hot.* Artificial fields are composed of several heat-retaining materials that become much hotter than natural grass. This increases risk of heat-related injuries, such as heat blisters, or illnesses such as heat exhaustion and heat stroke.

2. *They contain chemicals.* Artificial turf made from recycled tires contains numerous concerning chemicals.[47] These chemicals include but are not limited to known and suspected carcinogens (eg, benzene, arsenic, cadmium, polycylic aromatic hydrocarbons), respiratory irritants, neurotoxicants (eg, volatile organic compounds, crystalline silica, chromium, particulate matter, lead, zinc), allergens (latex), and reproductive toxicants (phthalates). Children can be exposed through inhalation, ingestion, and dermal contact. Exposure is influenced by the age of the field and environmental conditions, such as temperature, field ventilation, and the individual's activity. Chemical composition of fields is highly variable and manufacturers are not required by law to disclose a turf field's chemical content.[48]

To date, limited research shows that these fields do not present dangerous exposure levels. These studies have been small, have not assessed exposure under realistic playing conditions, have not assessed all routes of exposure, and involve no long-term follow-up of exposed children. Exposures vary according to composition and age of the field and environmental conditions including temperature and ventilation.

Therefore, uncertainty remains about what quantities of these chemicals enter the bodies of active children. Risk may also depend on environmental conditions and field age.

3. *Injuries.* New fields appear to have similar rates of injury as natural grass, although the types of injury may vary.[49]

4. *Infections.* Artificial turf may have lower concentrations of bacteria but cause more skin abrasions that could lead to infection. The sum of these effects is not certain.[50]

Q  *What are the environmental concerns for artificial turf?*

A  1. *Contamination of waterways.* Turf fields can leach toxic zinc into waterways, harming aquatic life.[51,52]

2. *Heat island effect.* Turf fields may retain even more heat than paved surfaces, worsening the "heat island" effect of cities and communities.[46]

3. *Displacement of natural environments.* Natural environments offer many physical and psychological benefits. Artificial fields can reduce these natural settings.

Q  *What can be done to reduce health risks with today's artificial turf fields?*

A  Families and communities can research the safest turf options available. They may consult with a Pediatric Environmental Specialty Unit to discuss the newest natural field options. It is prudent to be aware that terms such as "green" and "organic" are not regulated for turf products and have no defined meaning.

To reduce children's exposures, consider this Tips for Safer Play from the Children's Environmental Health Center's Artificial Turf Health Based Consumer Guide.[48]

Q  *I understand that the caulk used in some older schools may contain PCBs. What can I do to protect my child?*

A  Until it can be safely removed, limit exposure to caulk containing PCBs by keeping children from touching caulk or surfaces near it, washing children's toys often, washing their hands with soap and water before eating, and using wet cloths to clean surfaces and cleaning frequently to reduce dust.[53,54]

Q  *Where else can I find information about school health issues?*

A  School health information on a variety of topics is available from the American Academy of Pediatrics (AAP) School Health Web site maintained by the AAP Council on School Health (www.aap.org/sections/schoolhealth),

the American School Health Association, (www.ashaweb.org), the
CDC Division of Adolescent and School Health (DASH) (www.cdc.gov/
HealthyYouth/index.htm), Center for Health and Health Care in Schools
(www.healthinschools.org), and the National Association of School Nurses
(www.nasn.org).

---

## Tips for Safer Play on Artificial Turf Surfaces

- If you select a turf field that does contain chemicals of concern, post a safety warning on your field to keep players and spectators safe
- Avoid use on very hot days
- Avoid use for passive activities (ie, sitting, lounging, picnicking)
- Ensure good ventilation of indoor fields by opening doors and windows and utilizing fans
- Monitor young children to prevent accidental ingestion
- Always wear shoes on artificial turf
- Wash hands before eating, drinking, or adjusting mouth guards
- Clean cuts and abrasions immediately
- Brush hair thoroughly after play
- Remove and clean shoes and gear outside before getting in car
- At home, take off shoes and shake out your children's equipment and clothes outside or over the garbage
- Shower immediately after playing on artificial turf and vacuum any infill that comes into your home[48]

---

## Resources

**Healthy Schools Network, Inc.**

Advocates for the protection of children's environmental health in schools.
Web site: www.healthyschools.org

# References

1. Silva E. *On the Clock: Rethinking the Way Schools Use Time.* Washington, DC: Education Sector; 2007

2. National Center for Education Statistics. *How Old Are America's Public Schools?* Washington, DC: National Center for Education Statistics; 1999

3. Shield BM, Dockrell JE. The effects of noise on children at school: a review. *Building Acoustics.* 2003;10(2):97–106

4. Evans GW, Lercher P, Meis M, Ising H, Kofler WW. Community noise exposure and stress in children. *J Acoust Soc Am.* 2001;109(3):1023–1027

5. Alcántara, JI, Weisblatt EJ, Moore BC, Bolton PF. Speech-in-noise perception in high-functioning individuals with autism or Asperger's syndrome. *J Child Psychol Psychiatry.* 2004;45(6):1107–1114

6. Dobbins M, Sunder T, Soltys S. Nonverbal learning disabilities and sensory processing disorders. *Psychiatric Times.* 2007;24(9). http://www.psychiatrictimes.com/articles/nonverbal-learning-disabilities-and-sensory-processing-disorders. Accessed February 15, 2018

7. US Environmental Protection Agency. Sensible steps to healthier school environments. https://www.epa.gov/schools/sensible-steps-healthier-school-environments. Accessed February 15, 2018

8. Pickering LK, Marano N, Bocchini JA, Angulo FJ, American Academy of Pediatrics Committee on Infectious Diseases. Exposure to nontraditional pets at home and to animals in public settings: risks to children. *Pediatrics.* 2008;122(4):876–886

9. American Academy of Pediatrics, Committee on School Health; National Association of School Nurses. *Health, Mental Health and Safety Guidelines for Schools.* Taras H, Duncan P, Luckenbill D, et al, eds. Elk Grove Village, IL: American Academy of Pediatrics; 2004

10. Heschong Mahone Group. *Daylighting in Schools: An Investigation into the Relationship Between Daylighting and Human Performance.* HMG Project No. 9803. San Francisco, CA: Pacific Gas and Electric Company; 1999

11. US Environmental Protection Agency. Practical actions for reducing exposure to PCBs in schools and other buildings. https://www.epa.gov/sites/production/files/2016-03/documents/practical_actions_for_reducing_exposure_to_pcbs_in_schools_and_other_buildings.pdf. Accessed February 15, 2018

12. Etzel RA. Indoor air pollutants in homes and schools. *Pediatr Clin North Am.* 2001;48(5):1153–1165

13. US Environmental Protection Agency. Heating, Ventilation, and Air-Conditioning (HVAC) Systems. Codes and Standards. http://www.epa.gov/iaq/schooldesign/hvac.html#Codes and Standards. Accessed February 15, 2018

14. American Society of Heating, Refrigerating and Air-Conditioning Engineers Inc. Standard 62-2007, Ventilation for Acceptable Indoor Air Quality. Atlanta, GA: American Society of Heating, Refrigerating and Air-Conditioning Engineers Inc; 2007

15. Jaakkola JJK. Temperature and humidity. In: Frumkin H, Geller R, Rubin IL, Nodvin J, eds. *Safe and Healthy School Environments.* New York, NY: Oxford University Press; 2006:46–57

16. Everett Jones S, Smith AM, Wheeler LS, McManus T. School policies and practices that improve indoor air quality. *J Sch Health.* 2010;80(6):280–286

17. National Conference of State Legislatures. Carbon Monoxide Detector Requirements, Laws and Regulations. http://www.ncsl.org/research/environment-and-natural-resources/carbon-monoxide-detectors-state-statutes.aspx. Accessed February 15, 2018

18. US Environmental Protection Agency. Radon Measurement in Schools (Rev Ed). EPA Publication 402-R-92-014. https://www.epa.gov/radon/radon-schools. Accessed February 15, 2018

19. Jenkins PL, Phillips TJ, Waldman J. *California Portable Classrooms Study Project: Executive Summary. Final Report, Vol. III.* Sacramento, CA: California Department of Health Services; 2004. http://www.arb.ca.gov/research/indoor/pcs/leg_rpt/pcs_r2l.pdf. Accessed February 15, 2018

20. Menzies D, Bourbeau J. Building-related illnesses. *N Engl J Med.* 1997;337(21):1524–1531

21. Gammage RB, Kaye SV. *Indoor Air and Human Health.* Chelsea, MI: Lewis Publishers; 1985

22. Reinikainen LM, Jaakkola JJK. Effect of temperature and humidification in the office environment. *Arch Environ Health.* 2001;56(4):365–368

23. US Environmental Protection Agency. *Indoor Air Facts No. 4: Sick Building Syndrome (Rev).* https://www.epa.gov/sites/production/files/2014-08/documents/sick_building_factsheet.pdf. Accessed February 15, 2018

24. Salvaggio JE. Psychological aspects of "environmental illness," "multiple chemical sensitivity," and building-related illness. *J Allergy Clin Immunol.* 1994;94(2 Pt 2):366–370

25. Ryan CM, Morrow LA. Dysfunctional buildings or dysfunctional people: an examination of the sick building syndrome and allied disorders. *J Consult Clin Psychol.* 1992;60(2):220–224

26. Institute of Medicine. *Damp Indoor Spaces and Health.* Washington, DC: National Academy of Sciences; 2004

27. Gruchalla RS, Pongracic J, Plaut M, et al. Inner city asthma study: relationships among sensitivity, allergen exposure, and asthma morbidity. *J Allergy Clin Immunol.* 2005;115(3):478–485

28. American Academy of Pediatrics. *Red Book: 2018 Report of the Committee on Infectious Diseases.* Kimberlin DW, Brady MT, Jackson MA, Long SS, eds. 31st ed. Itasca, IL: American Academy of Pediatrics; 2018

29. Reuters. Lawsuit filed over student exposure to lead in Flint, Michigan, schools. https://www.reuters.com/article/us-michigan-water/lawsuit-filed-over-student-exposure-to-lead-in-flint-michigan-schools-idUSKCN12I2J8. Accessed February 15, 2018

30. Bryant D. Lead-contaminated drinking waters in the public schools of Philadelphia. *J Toxicol Clin Toxicol.* 2004;42(3):287–294

31. US Environmental Protection Agency. *3Ts for Reducing Lead in Drinking Water in Schools: Revised Technical Guidance.* http://nepis.epa.gov/Exe/ZyPURL.cgi?Dockey=P100H93Z.txt. Accessed February 15, 2018

32. US Environmental Protection Agency. *Drinking Water Requirements for States and Public Water Systems: Lead in Drinking Water in Schools and Childcare Facilities.* https://www.epa.gov/dwreginfo/lead-drinking-water-schools-and-childcare-facilities. Accessed June 8, 2018

33. Balk SJ. American Academy of Pediatrics Council on Environmental Health and Section on Dermatology. Technical Report—ultraviolet radiation: a hazard to children and adolescents. *Pediatrics.* 2011;127(3):e791–e817

34. National Conference of State Legislatures. Relaxing School Sunscreen Regulations. http://www.ncsl.org/documents/legisbriefs/2017/lb_2528.pdf. Accessed February 15, 2018

35. Herrick RF, Lefkowitz DJ, Weymouth GA. Soil contamination from PCB-containing buildings. *Environ Health Perspect.* 2007;115(2):173–175

36. Centers for Disease Control and Prevention. Playground Safety. https://www.cdc.gov/safechild/playground/index.html. Accessed February 15, 2018

37. US Environmental Protection Agency. Federal Research on Recycled Tire Crumb Used on Playing Fields. https://www.epa.gov/chemical-research/federal-research-recycled-tire-crumb-used-playing-fields. Accessed September 1, 2018

38. Thorne B. Unpacking school lunch: structure, practice, and the negotiation of differences. In: Cooper CR, ed. *Developmental Pathways Through Middle Childhood: Rethinking Contexts and Diversity as Resources.* Philadelphia, PA: Lawrence Erlbaum; 2005:63–87

39. Centers for Disease Control and Prevention. Outbreaks of gastrointestinal illness of unknown etiology associated with eating burritos—United States, October 1997-October 1998. *MMWR Morb Mortal Wkly Rep.* 1999;48(10):210–213

40. Musu-Gillette L, Zhang A, Wang K, Zhang J, Oudekerk BA. *Indicators of School Crime and Safety: 2016.* Washington, DC: US Departments of Education and Justice; 2017. NCES Publication 2017-064/NCJ 250650

41. Gladden RM, Vivolo-Kantor AM, Hamburger ME, Lumpkin CD. Bullying surveillance among youths: uniform definitions for public health and recommended data elements. Atlanta, GA: US Centers for Disease Control and Prevention; 2014

42. Stopbullying.gov. Washington, DC: US Department of Health and Human Services. http://stopbullying.gov. Accessed February 15, 2018

43. Teplitskaya A, Gerzoff RB. Surveillance Summary: Youth Tobacco Use—Selected U.S. States, 2012-2013. Atlanta, GA: US Centers for Disease Control and Prevention. https://www.cdc.gov/tobacco/data_statistics/surveys/yts/pdfs/yts_ss_2012-2013-508tagged.pdf. Accessed August 27, 2018

44. Devore CD, Wheeler LS, American Academy of Pediatrics Council on School Health. Role of the school physician. *Pediatrics.* 2013;131(1):178–182

45. Simon R. University of California, Berkeley Laboratory for Manufacturing and Sustainability. Review of the impacts of crumb rubber in artificial turf applications. *Green Manufacturing and Sustainable Manufacturing Partnership.* 2010

46. Toronto Public Health. Health impact assessment of the use of artificial turf in Toronto. April, 2015

47. Cheng H, Hu Y, Reinhard M. Environmental and health impacts of artificial turf: a review. *Environ Sci Technol.* 2014;48(4):2114–2129

48. Mount Sinai Children's Environmental Health Center. Artificial Turf: A Health Based Consumer Guide. http://icahn.mssm.edu/files/ISMMS/Assets/Departments/Environmental%20Medicine%20and%20Public%20Health/CEHC%20Consumer%20Guide%20to%20Artificial%20Turf%20May%202017.pdf. Accessed February 15, 2018

49. Dragoo JL, Braun HJ. The effect of playing surface on injury rate: a review of the current literature. *Sports Med.* 2010;40(11):981–990

50. California Department of Resources Recycling and Recovery. Safety study of artificial turf containing crumb rubber infill made from recycled tires: measurements of chemicals and particulates in the air, bacteria in the turf, and skin abrasions caused by contact with the surface. October, 2010

51. Connecticut Academy of Science and Engineering. Committee report: Peer review of an evaluation of the health and environmental impacts associated with synthetic turf playing fields. June 15, 2010

52. Lim l, Walker R. An assessment of chemical leaching, releases to air and temperature at crumb-rubber in filled synthetic turf fields. 2009. http://www.dec.ny.gov/docs/materials_minerals_pdf/crumbrubfr.pdf. Accessed February 15, 2018

53. US Environmental Protection Agency. Renovations and Polychlorinated Biphenyls (PCBs) for a Healthy School Environment. https://www.epa.gov/schools-healthy-buildings/renovations-and-polychlorinated-biphenyls-pcbs-healthy-school-environment. Accessed June 14, 2018

54. Western States Pediatric Environmental Health Specialty Units. Polychlorinated Biphenyls (PCBs) in Schools: How children are exposed, health risks, and tips to reduce exposure. https://wspehsu.ucsf.edu/wp-content/uploads/2017/10/final_pcbs_facts_2017.pdf. Accessed June 14, 2018

# Chapter 12

# Workplaces

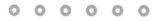

## KEY POINTS

- Many adolescents work, sometimes in jobs that have significant hazards and for which they are not adequately trained or supervised. This includes hazards associated with heights, burn risks, use of dangerous equipment or chemicals, or contact with large animals.
- Parents may assume incorrectly that employers are ensuring a safe environment or that the government adequately regulates work environments for youth.
- Clinicians need to be aware of child labor laws and include attention to employment in routine health histories and anticipatory guidance with adolescents and their parents.

## INTRODUCTION

Although adolescents spend much of their time in school, many will also have jobs sometime before high school graduation. Some have multiple part-time jobs and many work longer hours during the summer months. Although work has many developmental and financial benefits for youth, including an association with reduction in mortality during the teenage years, there are avoidable risks in the work environment.[1] By addressing work as an element of primary care with adolescents, clinicians can help assess potential risks associated with work and provide valuable guidance to teens and their parents. This chapter describes the major types of work done by adolescents and the risks and outcomes they encounter in these environments. The chapter also provides resources to help the clinician access additional information to guide their discussions with patients and families.

## NATURE OF ADOLESCENT WORK

Because of varying laws across the states relating to youth work and whether permits are required, there is no authoritative estimate of the number of adolescents working for someone else's business. Even less information is available about youth who are self-employed (eg, doing lawn care, babysitting, housework). However, national surveys conducted by the US Department of Labor indicate that 60% of youth aged 16 to 24 years were working in spring 2015.[2] About 70% were working in either leisure and hospitality or retail trade jobs, while 11% worked in education and health services jobs and 8% in professional and business settings. Four percent were working in construction and 2% in agriculture. These industry proportions vary by region of the country and by demographics. Typically, labor force participation is greater for white youth than for minorities; for example, in 2016 the US Bureau of Labor Statistics reported that 32.2% of white youth aged 16 to 19 years were employed compared with 21.3% of African American youth and 18.8% of Asian youth of the same age.[3] Some evidence exists showing that minority youth may be more likely to experience an injury at work[4] and that higher parental socioeconomic status may be protective against youth workplace injury.[5] Another study did not find racial differences in reporting occupational injuries but found differences in the duration of absence from work.[6]

Unlike many adult workers who assume specific occupational roles with defined tasks, adolescents frequently work in environments in which they are doing a wide variety of jobs. For example, a fast food worker may be expected to unload deliveries, use fryers, clean equipment or the premises, mow the grass, take orders, operate payment equipment, and handle cash. Similarly, in some settings such as construction or agriculture, the young worker may be exposed to environments with widely varying weather conditions, presence of heavy equipment or large animals that impose risks even if the youth are not, themselves, operating the equipment or handling the animals directly.

Despite being inexperienced in work in general and in specific jobs, many young workers receive little job training and often what training they do receive does not include training on safety.[7,8] Few report being provided or using protective equipment even though safety standards recommend protective equipment for the particular job task.[9,10] Furthermore, supervision is often inconsistent. For example, in one national study, adolescents younger than age 18 years working in retail and service sector jobs indicated they had worked completely alone during daylight hours, while others work alone at night when robberies and workplace assaults are most common.[7,11] Nationally, among these 14- to 17-year-old teenagers working in retail and service jobs, 26% reported having worked without adult supervision for at least 1 day, and 40% reported having their work checked less often than once a day, creating multiple opportunities for unsafe practices and inadequate protection.[7]

Although many parents express confidence that employers are ensuring a safe work environment for their children, it should not be assumed that they are actually aware of the risks in the environments where their children work or that they are knowledgeable about the laws governing young worker safety.[12,13] Even when teen workers themselves detect risks, they are often reluctant to speak up, wanting to appear more competent than they are or fearing loss of their jobs.[14]

Work is regulated by both the federal and state government. The Fair Labor Standards Act is a federal law that limits the hours and types of work that adolescents of different ages can do.[15] States have differing laws that restrict work environments and hours for youth and whether youth are required to obtain work permits before taking a job. The details for each state are available on the US Department of Labor Web site.[16] Federal laws prevail unless state laws are more stringent. States also vary on whether youth are required to obtain any sort of work permit to take a job and what information is required as part of the permitting process. Although it is the employer's responsibility to adhere to the child labor laws, it is wise for clinicians to be aware of these laws in their own states so they can properly counsel parents and youth about the restrictions and their rights as workers.

## DEATH AND INJURY AMONG YOUNG WORKERS

In 2013, 67 US workers younger than age 20 years and 268 between 20 and 24 years died as a result of work-related injuries.[17] Among all those younger than 25 years, 139 were killed in transportation events and 71 were victims of homicide. The industries with the highest rates of young worker deaths are mining, agriculture, and construction.[18]

National data systems do not allow full capture of nonfatal injuries, but data captured by the Bureau of Labor Statistics at the US Department of Labor indicate that for every death of an adolescent worker younger than age 20 there are 325 injuries severe enough to limit normal activities, with a total of nearly 23,000 nonfatal injuries in 2014.[19] The median days away from work because of work injuries or illnesses are 4 for those aged 16 to 19 years and 5 for persons aged 20 to 24 years.[20]

The patterns of nonfatal injuries by industry are different than for fatalities, with most injuries occurring in retail and service trades, where youth most commonly experience burns, falls, and cuts. In agriculture, they are exposed to encounters with equipment as well as to a variety of chemicals, depending on the type of work they do. Adolescents working with heavy equipment also experience more severe nonfatal injuries such as amputation.

## HAZARDS IN DIFFERENT TYPES OF ADOLESCENT WORK SETTINGS

### Injury

Hazards include physical risks that result in injuries, such as falls, cuts, burns, or broken bones. Chemical exposures can result in burns, respiratory effects, and neurobehavioral effects. Although fatalities are relatively rare in the leisure, hospitality, retail, and service sectors, young workers experience several major categories of injury in these sectors. Restaurant workers are particularly vulnerable to falls, cuts, burns, and assault. Falls are often associated with slippery flooring from grease or water spills. Burns often occur in the process of cooking, particularly with grease, or working with steam tables. Workers in grocery settings are exposed to cutting hazards (eg, box cutters), as well as working with sharp or powered equipment (eg, box crushers, food slicers, forklifts).

In any establishment in which there is exchange of cash, workers are at risk for robbery, assaults, and threats from customers and coworkers.[21-23] Homicide is the largest cause of worker mortality in this setting, accounting for over half of retail-related fatalities among all ages.[24]

### Toxic Exposures

Several common chemical exposure hazards exist in industries in which adolescents are commonly employed, such as restaurants, janitorial work, landscaping, and nail salons, although there is relatively little research specific to adolescents. Work in these and related jobs may involve contact with chemical hazards such as cleaning products, packaging materials, solvents, lubricants, and pesticides. Studies indicate that exposure to bisphenol A (BPA) and phthalates, which are widely present in plastics, food packaging materials, and cosmetics, may result in cardiovascular, developmental, and other health effects in adolescents and young adults.[25,26] Working as a cashier, a common job for youth, may result in exposure to BPA, which is present in thermal paper used for electronic transaction receipts.[27,28] Youth who work in hair or nail salons may be exposed to skin and airborne hazards, such as irritants and volatile organic compounds, at levels high enough to affect health.[29-31] Culturally appropriate interventions have been shown to be effective in reducing worker exposure in immigrant adults in nail salons, but the peer-reviewed literature has little information on the overall effectiveness of exposure reduction interventions for youth in the industries in which they are commonly employed.[32]

## Biological and Physical Hazards

Working adolescents may be exposed to biological, physical, or ergonomic hazards, such as allergens, noise, heat and cold, or repetitive motion that may lead to injury. All these hazards may require personal protective equipment (PPE) or worksite redesign to prevent injury or death. Young workers often are not provided with, properly trained, or required by the employer to use appropriate PPE for the job. Depending on the task, proper PPE may include gloves, slip-resistant shoes, hearing protection, and eye protection.[9] Furthermore, proper work practices and health promotion may include regular hydration, rest breaks, and use of sunscreen where needed.[33] Legal requirements for worksite safety for adults are often assumed to protect children and adolescents, but beyond child labor laws there are few additional requirements for preventing exposure to these hazards in younger workers. Moreover, if adolescents are employed in a setting or role that is not in compliance with current law or regulation, it is possible their risk and exposure to these hazards may even be greater.

Agricultural work on family farms is exempt from many legal or regulatory requirements. Children and adolescents who live and work on farms owned by their families are exposed to numerous risks and there are virtually no restrictions on what a child can do (eg, a 5-year-old child is not prohibited from driving a tractor). In the United States, children start work in agriculture at an earlier age than in other sectors, with more than half of children who live on farms working on the farm.[34] Some also work on farms operated by others, including as migrant or seasonal workers, in which some protections apply. For example, migrant workers on non-family farms must be 18 years old to handle chemicals. Youth older than age 16 may legally work in any farm job, even though many of these jobs are highly dangerous (eg, operating tractors and power-takeoff devices attached to tractors that operate other trailing equipment), working with large animals; working in grain bins in which workers may be sucked in and die of suffocation; and being exposed to toxic chemicals (eg, pesticides, herbicides). In these settings they are also exposed to the elements (eg, sun, lightning, cold) and using assorted farm vehicles (eg, trucks, all-terrain vehicles) as well as to labor involved in lifting or bending and using sharp tools (eg, machetes) for harvesting or to exposure to the crops themselves (eg, tobacco sickness). The North American Guidelines for Agricultural Tasks provide guidelines to families or supervisors as to what may be reasonable to expect of youth at different stages of development (see: www.nagcat.org). The introduction of these guidelines has been associated with a decreased risk of serious and fatal illness and injury.

Deaths of young workers most often occur in the context of vehicle or machinery-related events, with tractors (eg, rollovers, run overs) accounting for over half.[34] Nonfatal injuries are more likely associated with animals and vehicles, especially, all terrain vehicles.[34] Higher numbers of both fatal and nonfatal injuries occur among males compared with females, most likely as a function of being assigned work in more dangerous circumstances, sometimes working in settings or conditions in violation of safety laws.[35,36] As many as 40% of youth who sustain nonfatal injuries experience long-term disabilities, ranging from traumatic brain and spinal cord injury to amputations and sequelae of crushing injuries or ingestions.[34]

Even children not working on the farm may be exposed to the hazards of the farm by virtue of living and playing there. Depending on the accessibility of childcare facilities in the community, farm children may be exposed to limited supervision or may be joining their parents in the farm work environment at a very young age.

Although young agricultural workers are likely exposed to solvents, petroleum, and cleaning and disinfection products, there is little available research on young worker exposures. The chemical hazards that have been most extensively investigated among adolescents are pesticides used on crops and in animal husbandry.[37] The limited research in this area suggests that adolescents using pesticides have deficits in neurobehavioral performance compared with controls, and that the risk of these effects increases with years of exposure.[37] Although many adolescent farm workers report being exposed to pesticides, relatively few recall receiving pesticide safety training and those who do score lower on assessments of pesticide safety knowledge compared with older adults.[38] This is of potential concern because adolescents' bodies and nervous systems are still developing, and they have more future years of life to develop adverse health outcomes compared with adult workers.

Nonfatal injuries in construction are most commonly strains, sprains, contusions, and lacerations, although young workers also experience more severe outcomes, such as amputations or severe injuries resulting from falls or in vehicle crashes.[39] A national analysis published in 2003 described fatal injuries among young construction workers as most often associated with electrocution, being struck by falling objects, falls from heights, and drowning. In half of the incidents the employer was violating child labor laws that prohibit certain types of work. This included working at heights (eg, roofing), operating power-driven equipment, being an electrician's helper, or working in trenches.[40] In one state study of all adolescents getting work permits to work in construction over the summer, the teens reported performing a wide variety of tasks, with more than half reporting tasks of cleaning the work area, using sharp instruments, using adhesives, or working as a spotter. More than 80% of these same workers reported performing tasks that were in violation of child labor restrictions, most reporting multiple illegal tasks including working at heights, doing electrical work, working in trenches, operating heavy equipment, and using powered saws or nail guns. One-fifth of these workers reported having worked alone, without anyone in hearing range.[41] The youth reported varying levels of use of protective equipment, such as earplugs, dust masks, fall protection, hard hats, and safety vests, further indicating that employers may be lax in following worker safety laws.

## BALANCING WORKPLACE SAFETY WITH ADOLESCENT DEVELOPMENT

Employment, when not overly intensive such that it detracts from school or other activities, can have benefits for adolescent development. Employment can provide youth with a sense of satisfaction and empowerment in their ability to develop new skills and manage increasing responsibility, including financial responsibility.[42] The quality of the job (perceived quality of job tasks and pay) is associated with a greater sense of satisfaction.[43]

### Work and School

A few studies have shown a relationship between employment and worse school performance.[44] Some have hypothesized that the relationship reflects a selection effect whereby adolescents who seek out employment, and more hours of employment, do so because of a lack of interest in school or that there may be correlations between other family characteristics associated with both employment and poorer school performance. Longitudinal studies and those attempting to control for confounding variables have found mixed support for this idea.[43-45]

### Work and Sleep

Sleep deprivation has been associated with increased risk of workplace injuries in adults, but fewer studies have examined how adolescent employment affects the amount of sleep adolescents get and thereby increases the risk of injury on the job.[46,47] One study using a daily diary method found that employed students got less sleep than those who did not work, an average of half an hour on school days.[48] Adolescents have greater sleep requirements than adults, and given the competing demands of school work while employed, may have difficulty sleeping sufficient hours.[48-50]

### Work and Substance Use

Substance use (eg, tobacco, alcohol, illicit drug use) is more prevalent among adolescents who are employed, with a pattern of more hours worked more strongly associated with substance use.[51-55] However, several studies have found these effects are reduced or disappear once other demographic factors, such as age, gender, and race/ethnicity, are taken into account.[52,53,56] Other personal and social variables, such as parental involvement, school performance, and peer relationships, are likely related.[57]

## ROLE OF THE CLINICIAN IN ADDRESSING ADOLESCENT WORK ISSUES

The clinical encounter with adolescent patients provides an opportunity to ask about their work involvement as part of routine history-taking. This enables the clinician to understand the amount of work the adolescent is doing and in what types of work environments. A simple mnemonic device may be helpful for this: WORKS, asking about Work hours (eg, number of hours, late hours on school nights), Organization (eg, working alone versus with adequate supervision); Risks related to work (eg, exposure to equipment, chemicals), Kinds of training received to perform the job safely, and Safety precautions (eg, use of protective clothing or devices).[58]

Having information about the adolescent's work also provides the clinician the opportunity to detect illnesses that may be work-related (eg, chronic fatigue in an adolescent who makes silk screens can be caused by chronic solvent intoxication if the teenager works or sleeps in an area with inadequate ventilation) or work situations that may exacerbate chronic problems such as asthma.

Although clinicians may not always have the advanced training necessary to make the work-illness link, they can seek guidance from industrial hygienists, union or corporate health and safety employees, and local Committee on Occupational Safety and Health groups. State-based Occupational Safety and Health Administration training sections may be helpful. These units are usually located in either state health or labor departments. The Migrant Clinicians Network is also a resource.[59]

### Anticipatory Guidance to Adolescents and Parents

Clinicians also can provide guidance to teens and their parents about potential benefits and risks of their work, much as they might discuss teen driving, sexuality, and experimentation with smoking or drinking. By discussing these issues with parents, clinicians can provide encouragement to parents to help the adolescent explore safety issues within the context of their particular work environment and become familiar with their rights as workers (eg, to know what chemicals they are using and to be provided proper training and protective devices). Clinicians should be prepared to explore the potential for risks. They should be able to help parents understand and access information about the types of work that are prohibited for teens of certain ages, and the restrictions on work hours based on age and whether it is a school year or not. They should also urge parents to familiarize themselves with their child's specific work environment and raise concerns with supervisors if warranted.

## Policy Engagement

Finally, clinicians working with adolescents are in a good position to influence policies that affect safety for young workers. By becoming familiar with state and federal worker safety provisions, clinicians can identify problem areas and bring this to the attention of regulatory authorities within state government. Informed clinicians can also be advocates for policy improvements to enhance the safety of working youth; for example, addressing challenges in protecting children working on family farms for which regulatory authority is practically nonexistent.

## Frequently Asked Questions

Q  *My teenager has asthma, for which she takes daily medication. She wants to get a part-time job. Can I help direct her to work that won't cause her asthma to flare up?*

A  Teenagers need to ask potential employers about the tasks they will be doing and whether they may be exposed to any chemical respiratory irritants, cold, or allergens. Although increasingly infrequent because of indoor smoking bans in many states, a restaurant with a smoking section is not a wise choice for a teenager with asthma. A customer service or cashier job should provide a better respiratory environment, or the teenager with asthma may seek work in an ice cream store that does not allow smoking, as long as he or she is not also required to use cleaning materials that are respiratory irritants. In any job, parents should be concerned about adult supervision, job training, and safety training. It is important for parents to visit the workplace. A job that requires personal protective equipment suggests a possible risk that should be explored and discussed with the adolescent. Potential chemical exposures in vocational education, shop or art classes, work-study, and volunteer work or hobbies should be considered.

Q  *Are teenagers less vulnerable to workplace exposures because they are young and healthy? When we were young, we worked without all these protections.*

A  Risks of exposures can be small or life-threatening, depending on the chemical. Teenagers and children are just as vulnerable to enclosed space exposures as older workers. Like adults, they will die in an oxygen-deprived environment, such as in a tank they are cleaning that was previously full of chemicals. Theoretically, if a chemical becomes less toxic when metabolized, and teenagers metabolize better or faster than adults, then its effects could be less toxic for a young worker. If the metabolite itself is poisonous, however, teenagers could be at increased risk. Because one is unlikely to know in advance which situation pertains for any given chemical, testing the situation may involve risking illness or death. Thus, protection from exposure is always the best approach.

*Q* *Are teenagers more vulnerable to work exposure than adults because their
systems (especially immune systems) are not yet fully developed?*

A  Adolescents may be more vulnerable in some respects but not because of
their immune systems. Although there are no definitive data to answer this
question at present, by adolescence, the immune system is essentially fully
developed, so it is not likely to be more vulnerable. When advocating for
adolescent occupational health and safety, it is important not to exaggerate
the risks that exist; this may lessen our credibility about the real risks.
If we know, however, that an exposure is hazardous for adults, we should
assume that it is likely to be at least as hazardous for adolescents and protect
them from that exposure. Exposure to potentially cancer-causing (carcinogenic) substances and to substances that may produce birth defects (teratogens) may create increased risk for adolescents because they have more
future years. There may be higher risks of early life exposure to substances
(especially carcinogenic ones) associated with diseases that occur only
after long latency periods. If a substance accumulates in the body over
time and the effects are dose-related, teen workers may be at risk because
their exposure started earlier in life. It is possible that exposure to a potential carcinogen during the rapid growth period of adolescence may increase
cancer risk. Given that adolescence is a time of endocrine changes, there may
be increased vulnerability to chemicals (including certain pesticides) that are
endocrine disrupters. Because adolescents are of childbearing age, acute and
latent reproductive effects of chemicals are potentially of concern.

*Q* *Is it safe for a teenager who is still growing to do manual labor with heavy
equipment?*

A  Current knowledge about occupational back injury and about overuse
injuries among young gymnasts and baseball players suggests that periods
of rapid growth may put an individual at increased risk of severe and
chronic musculoskeletal injuries, especially if there are too many repeti-
tions of a movement.[55] This has implications for farm work, cashier work,
and any work with repetitive motion.

## Resources

### Child Labor Coalition

Web site: www.stopchildlabor.org/index.html
This is a coalition of diverse organizations and individuals (including the
American Academy of Pediatrics, consumer groups, medical professionals,
universities, unions, and religious organizations) interested in international
and US child labor. They organize conferences, meet monthly, and maintain
one of the most up-to-date watches in the nation on federal and state child
labor law changes.

**Committees on Occupational Safety and Health (COSH)**

Most community-based COSH groups maintain staff capable of answering questions about occupational exposures. COSH groups coordinate national advocacy efforts, share educational and training resources, and develop and disseminate strategies for improving worker safety. See: www.coshnetwork.org/about-us

**Labor Departments**

Each state Department of Labor has information on child labor laws; wages; hours of work; safety regulations, including Hazard Orders that prohibit specific types of hazardous exposures; and problems with any of those areas. A poster summarizing child labor law often is available. In some states, a caller will be told to call the local office of the US Department of Labor. The US Department of Labor Web site provides information about the laws in each state at: www.dol.gov/whd/childlabor.htm

**Migrant Clinicians Network**

Phone: 512-327-2017

Web site: www.migrantclinician.org

Migrant Clinicians Network creates practical solutions at the intersection of poverty, migration, and health.

**National Child Labor Committee**

Phone: 212-840-1801

Web site: www.nationalchildlabor.org

This committee, founded in 1904, has historical and legal information related to child labor and advocates for the safe employment of adolescents.

**National Institute for Occupational Safety and Health (NIOSH)**

Phone: 800-356-4674

Web site: www.cdc.gov/niosh/, with special section related to young workers: www.cdc.gov/niosh/topics/youth/

The Web site of this federal agency contains information on hours and safety regulations, hazards, and how to protect against them, including a sheet for teenagers. The Division of Safety Research in the Morgantown, WV, NIOSH office (phone: 304-285-5894) has expertise in the scientific, research, and educational aspects. The NIOSH office in Cincinnati, OH, works on exposures in vocational/technical education settings. In May 1995, NIOSH published *Alert-Request for Assistance in Preventing Deaths and Injuries of Adolescent Workers*. This booklet (Department of Health and Human Services Publication No. 95-125, available from NIOSH) has background information and a tear-out page to post in the office or to copy for adolescent patients and their parents or for community work. NIOSH funds educational resource centers and academic departments of occupational medicine.

### North American Guidelines for Children's Agricultural Tasks

Web site: www.nagcat.org/nagcat

The North American Guidelines for Children's Agricultural Tasks, published by the Marshfield Clinic Research Foundation, were developed to assist parents in assigning farm jobs to their children 7 to 16 years of age, living or working on farms. The guidelines can help answer questions from parents and professionals about the role of their child in agricultural work.

### Occupational Safety and Health Administration (OSHA)

Phone: 800-321-OSHA (6742)

Web site: www.osha.gov

This federal agency deals with regulatory and enforcement issues. If a teenager has a question about a specific hazard, the teenager or parent (with permission) can call OSHA for assistance. This can be done anonymously, but sometimes an employee may be identifiable. Pediatricians should consider this agency especially when there is concern about imminent danger to other adolescents in that workplace. OSHA offices can be found in local phone directories.

### Poison Control Centers

Poison control centers can provide information on toxicity of specific chemicals, clinical guidance, expertise, and treatment advice by phone. All poison control centers can be reached by calling the same telephone number: 1-800-222-1222.

## References

1. Davila EP, Christ SL, Caban-Martinez AJ, et al. Young adults, mortality, and employment. *J Occup Environ Med.* 2010;52(5):501–504
2. US Bureau of Labor Statistics. Summer Youth Labor Force News Release. 2015. http://www.bls.gov/news.release/youth.htm. Accessed February 3, 2018
3. US Bureau of Labor Statistics. Employment Status of the Civilian Noninstitutional Population by Age, Sex, and Race. 2016. https://www.bls.gov/cps/cpsaat03.pdf. Accessed February 3, 2018
4. Zierold KM, Anderson HA. Racial and ethnic disparities in work-related injuries among teenagers. *J Adolesc Health.* 2006;39(3):422–426
5. Rauscher KJ, Myers DJ. Socioeconomic disparities in the prevalence of work-related injuries among adolescents in the United States. *J Adolesc Health.* 2008;42 (1):50–57
6. Strong LL, Zimmerman FJ. Occupational injury and absence from work among African American, Hispanic, and non-Hispanic white workers in the national longitudinal survey of youth. *Am J Public Health.* 2005;95(7):1226–1232

7. Runyan CW, Schulman M, Dal Santo J, Bowling JM, Agans R, Ta M. Work-related hazards and workplace safety of US adolescents employed in the retail and service sectors. *Pediatrics.* 2007;119(3):526–534

8. Zierold KM, Garman S, Anderson H. Summer work and injury among middle school students, aged 10–14 years. *Occup Environ Med.* 2004;61(6):518–522

9. Runyan CW, Vladutiu CJ, Rauscher KJ, Schulman M. Teen workers' exposures to occupational hazards and use of personal protective equipment. *Am J Ind Med.* 2008;51(10):735–740

10. Woolf A, Alpert HR, Garg A, Lesko S. Adolescent occupational toxic exposures: a national study. *Arch Pediatr Adolesc Med.* 2001;155(6):704–710

11. Schaffer KB, Casteel C, Kraus JF. A case-site/control-site study of workplace violent injury. *J Occup Environ Med.* 2002;44(11):1018–1026

12. Runyan CW, Schulman M, Dal Santo J, Bowling JM, Agans R. Attitudes and beliefs about adolescent work and workplace safety among parents of working adolescents. *J Adolesc Health.* 2009;44(4):349–355

13. Rauscher K, Runyan CW, Schulman MD. Awareness and knowledge of the U.S. child labor laws among a national sample of working adolescents and their parents. *J Adolesc Health.* 2010;47(4):414–417

14. Vladutiu CJ, Rauscher KJ, Runyan CW, Schulman M, Villaveces A. Hazardous task recognition among U.S. adolescents working in the retail or service industry. *Am J Ind Med.* 2010;53(7): 686–692

15. Fair Labor Standards Act. Vol 29 USC 201, CFR 570–5801938

16. U.S. Department of Labor. Youth Rules! Preparing the 21st Century Workforce. http://youthrules.dol.gov/law-library/state-laws/index.htm. Accessed February 3, 2018

17. U.S. Bureau of Labor Statistics. *Revisions to the 2013 Census of Fatal Occupational Injuries (CFOI) counts.* Office of Occupational Safety and Health Statistics. 2015

18. Centers for Disease Control and Prevention. Occupational injuries and deaths among younger workers—United States, 1998–2007. *MMWR Morb Mortal Wkly Rep.* 2010;59(15): 449–455

19. Bureau of Labor Statistics. Nonfatal Occupational Injuries and Illnesses Requiring Days Away from Work. Press release November 19, 2015. https://www.bls.gov/news.release/archives/osh2_11192015.htm. Accessed February 3, 2018

20. U.S. Bureau of Labor Statistics. *Median days away from work and incidence rate of injuries and illnesses, by age of worker, 2008.* https://www.bls.gov/iif/oshwc/osh/os/oshs2008_37.pdf. Accessed June 26, 2018

21. Runyon C, Schulman M, Hoffman C. Understanding and preventing violence against adolescent workers: what is known and what is missing? *Clin Occup Environ Med.* 2003;3(4):711–720

22. Loomis D, Marshall SW, Wolf SH, Runyan CW, Butts JD. Effectiveness of safety measures recommended for prevention of workplace homicide. *JAMA.* 2002;287(8):1011–1017

23. Rauscher KJ. Workplace violence against adolescents in the US. *Am J Ind Med.* 2008;51(7):539–544

24. Injuries, Illnesses & Fatalities in Wholesale and Retail Trade in 2005: A Chartbook. [WRT Chartbook]. Cincinnati, OH: U.S. Department of Health and Human Services, Public Health Service, Centers for Disease Control and Prevention, National Institute for Occupational Safety and Health. https://www.cdc.gov/niosh/docs/2012-106/. Accessed February 3, 2018. DHHS (NIOSH) Publication No. 2012–106 December 2011

25. Lin CY, Shen FY, Lian GW, et al. Association between levels of serum bisphenol A, a potentially harmful chemical in plastic containers, and carotid artery intima-media thickness in adolescents and young adults. *Atherosclerosis.* 2015;241(2):657–663

26. Meeker JD, Ferguson KK. Relationship between urinary phthalate and bisphenol A concentrations and serum thyroid measures in U.S. adults and adolescents from the National Health and Nutrition Examination Survey (NHANES) 2007-2008. *Environ Health Perspect.* 2011;119(10):1396–1402

27. Ndaw S, Remy A, Jargot D, Robert A. Occupational exposure of cashiers to bisphenol A via thermal paper: urinary biomonitoring study. *Int Arch Occup Environ Health.* 2016;89(6): 935–946

28. Biedermann S, Tschudin P, Grob K. Transfer of bisphenol A from thermal printer paper to the skin. *Anal Bioanal Chem.* 2010;398(1):571–576

29. Mounier-Geyssant E, Oury V, Mouchot L, Paris C, Zmirou-Navier D. Exposure of hairdressing apprentices to airborne hazardous substances. *Environ Health.* 2006;5:23

30. Alaves VM, Sleeth DK, Thiese MS, Larson RR. Characterization of indoor air contaminants in a randomly selected set of commercial nail salons in Salt Lake County, Utah, USA. *Int J Environ Health Res.* 2013;23(5):419–433

31. Quach T, Gunier R, Tran A, et al. Characterizing workplace exposures in Vietnamese women working in California nail salons. *Am J Public Health.* 2011;101(Suppl 1):S271–S276

32. Quach T, Varshavsky J, Von Behren J, et al. Reducing chemical exposures in nail salons through owner and worker trainings: an exploratory intervention study. *Am J Ind Med.* 2013;56(7): 806–817

33. American Academy of Pediatrics Council on Sports Medicine and Fitness and Council on School Health. Policy Statement—Climatic heat stress and exercising children and adolescents. *Pediatrics.* 2011;128(3):1–7

34. Wright S, Marlenga B, Lee B. Childhood agricultural injuries: an update for clinicians. *Curr Probl Pediatr Adolesc Health Care.* 2013;43(2):20–44

35. U.S. Bureau of Labor Statistics. Women Experience Fewer Job-related Injuries and Deaths than Men. 1998; https://www.bls.gov/opub/btn/archive/women-experience-fewer-job-related-injuries-and-deaths-than-men.pdf. Accessed February 3, 2018

36. McCall BP, Horwitz IB, Carr BS. Adolescent occupational injuries and workplace risks: an analysis of Oregon workers' compensation data 1990-1997. *J Adolesc Health.* 2007;41(3): 248–255

37. Rohlman DS, Nuwayhid I, Ismail A, Saddik B. Using epidemiology and neurotoxicology to reduce risks to young workers. *Neurotoxicology.* 2012;33(4):817–822

38. John E. Survey of residents of Northwest Orchard Community shows high levels of perceived pesticide risk and lack of pesticide training. *MCN Streamline.* 2010;16(4):4–5

39. Schoenfisch AL, Lipscomb HJ, Shishlov K, Myers DJ. Nonfatal construction industry-related injuries treated in hospital emergency departments in the United States, 1998-2005. *Am J Ind Med.* 2010;53(6):570–580

40. Suruda A, Philips P, Lillguist D, Sesek R. Fatal injuries to teenage construction workers in the US. *Am J Ind Med.* 2003;44(5):510–514

41. Runyan CW, Dal Santo J, Schulman M, Lipscomb H, Harris T. Work hazards and workplace safety violations experienced by adolescent construction workers. *Arch Pediatr Adolesc Med.* 2006;160(7):721–727

42. Staff J, Messersmith EE, Schulenberg JE. Adolescents and the World of Work. In: Lerner R, Steinberg L, eds. *Handbook of Adolescent Psychology.* Vol 3. New York, NY: John Wiley and Sons; 2009:270–313

43. Mortimer JT. The benefits and risks of adolescent employment. *Prev Res.* 2010;17(2):8–11

44. Marsh HW, Kleitman S. Consequences of employment during high school: character building, subversion of academic goals, or a threshold? *Am Educ Res J.* 2005;42(2):331–369

45. Staff J, Schulenberg JE, Bachman JG. Adolescent work intensity, school performance, and academic engagement. *Sociol Educ*. 2010;83(3):183–200

46. Sparks K, Cooper C, Fried Y, Shirom A. The effects of hours of work on health: a meta-analytic review. *J Occupational and Organizational Psychology*. 1997;70(4):391

47. Lombardi DA, Folkard S, Willetts JL, Smith GS. Daily sleep, weekly working hours, and risk of work-related injury: US National Health Interview Survey (2004–2008). *Chronobiol Int*. 2010;27(5):1013–1030

48. Kalenkoski CM, Pabilonia SW. Time to work or time to play: the effect of student employment on homework, sleep, and screen time. *Labour Economics*. 2012;19(2):211–221

49. Laberge L, Ledoux É, Auclair J, Gaudreault M. Determinants of sleep duration among high school students in part-time employment. *Mind, Brain, and Education*. 2014;8(4):220–226

50. Institute of Medicine. *Protecting Youth at Work: Health, Safety, and Development of Working Children and Adolescents in the United States*. Washington, DC: 1998

51. Valois RF, Dunham AC, Jackson KL, Waller J. Association between employment and substance abuse behaviors among public high school adolescents. *J Adolesc Health*. 1999;25(4):256–263

52. Wu LT, Schlenger WE, Galvin DM. The relationship between employment and substance use among students aged 12 to 17. *J Adolesc Health*. 2003;32(1):5–15

53. Bachman JG, Schulenberg J. How part-time work intensity relates to drug use, problem behavior, time use, and satisfaction among high school seniors: are these consequences or merely correlates? *Developmental Psychology*. 1993;29(2):220–235

54. Kingston S, Rose A. Do the effects of adolescent employment differ by employment intensity and neighborhood context? *Am J Community Psychol*. 2015;55(1-2):37–47

55. Morris BJ, Uggen C. Alcohol and employment in the transition to adulthood. *J Health Soc Behav*. 2000;41(3):276–294

56. Osilla KC, Miles JN, Hunter SB, D'Amico EJ. The longitudinal relationship between employment and substance use among at-risk adolescents. *J Child Adolesc Behav*. 2015;3(3):202

57. Paschall MJ, Flewelling RL, Russell T. Why is work intensity associated with heavy alcohol use among adolescents? *J Adolesc Health*. 2004;34(1):79–87

58. Runyan CW. Advocating the inclusion of adolescent work experience as part of routine preventive care. *J Adolesc Health*. 2007;41(3):221–223

59. Migrant Clinicians Network. (2014, September 23). http://www.migrantclinician.org/. Accessed February 3, 2018

Chapter 13

# Waste Sites

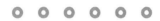

## KEY POINTS

- Millions of children are potentially at risk of exposure to waste site hazards.
- A child may be exposed by waste migrating into groundwater, surface water, drinking water, air, surface soil, sediment, dust, or plant and/or animal food sources.
- The overall impact of hazardous waste sites on local and national health is difficult to assess because of conflicting information from epidemiologic studies and limitations of the methodologies used.

## INTRODUCTION

According to the US Environmental Protection Agency (EPA), "hazardous waste is a waste with properties that make it dangerous or capable of having a harmful effect on human health or the environment."[1] "An uncontrolled hazardous waste site is an area where an accumulation of hazardous substances creates a threat to the health and safety of individuals or the environment or both."[2] Those sites where risk of harm is highest are placed on a National Priorities List (NPL) of sites. The US EPA determines which sites are eligible for placement on this list through a formal assessment process. The NPL is a list of hazardous waste sites with high levels of contamination requiring long-term remediation under the Superfund Program. This federal program locates, investigates, and cleans up the worst uncontrolled and abandoned toxic waste sites.[3] The NPL is intended primarily to guide the US EPA in determining which sites warrant further investigation. On the basis of the NPL hazard ranking system, there were 1,341 NPL sites in the United States at the end of 2017.[3]

Locations of sites containing hazardous waste may be a source of concern to families and health professionals. With the exception of North Dakota (which has none), all states have at least 1 NPL site; 5 states (California, Michigan, New Jersey, New York, Pennsylvania) contain 34% of all the sites and 28% of all the children and youth ( from birth through age 17) in the United States.[4,5] An estimate of the proximity of children by age group is presented in Table 13-1. These data highlight that millions of children are potentially at risk of exposure to waste site hazards.

In addition, 1,555,950 women of childbearing age (aged 15 to 44 years) live within 1 mile (1.6 kilometers) of an NPL site. Of those women of childbearing age, it is estimated that 52,327 and 316,303 pregnant women live within 1 mile (1.6 kilometers) of NPL sites and Comprehensive Environmental Response, Compensation, and Liability Act (CERCLA) sites, respectively.[7]

Most uncontrolled hazardous waste sites (65% to 70%) in the United States are waste storage/treatment facilities (including landfills) or former industrial properties.[8] Many of these properties have been abandoned, and most have more than one chemical contaminant that poses serious risk to human health. Less common uncontrolled hazardous waste sites are waste recycling facilities and mining sites, which may be active, inactive, or abandoned.

Some of the substances found in uncontrolled hazardous waste sites are heavy metals, such as lead, chromium, and arsenic; and organic solvents, such as trichloroethylene and benzene.[9] Arsenic and lead have been found in more than 1,100 and 1,200 current and former NPL sites, respectively, and ranked No. 1 and 2 on the Agency for Toxic Substances and Disease Registry (ATSDR)/US EPA priority list of hazardous chemicals in 2017.[9] Children living in urban areas may have greater risks of exposure to hazardous waste because of nearby industrial

| Table 13-1. US Population of Children Within 1 and 3 Miles of Superfund Remedial Sites[6] | | | | | |
|---|---|---|---|---|---|
| DEMOGRAPHICS | (APPROXIMATE) POPULATION WITHIN 1 MILE (1.6 km) OF SITES | | (APPROXIMATE) POPULATION WITHIN 3 MILES (4.8 km) OF SITES | | (APPROXIMATE) US POPULATION |
| Under 5 years of age | 7.0% | 842,716 | 6.7% | 3,520,737 | 6.4% | 20,052,112 |
| Under 18 years of age | 23.7% | 2,839,619 | 23.3% | 12,262,899 | 23.7% | 73,877,478 |

From: https://www.epa.gov/sites/production/files/2015-09/documents/webpopulationrsuperfundsites9.28.15.pdf

sites designated as "brownfields." A brownfield site is a piece of land that has been developed and used for industrial purposes and polluted, abandoned, and later designated by municipalities for commercial and/or residential redevelopment. The US EPA estimates that there are more than 450,000 brownfields in the United States (https://www.epa.gov/brownfields/brownfield-overview-and-definition). The ATSDR is working with communities to address concerns about brownfields in the United States. More information on this initiative can be found at: www.atsdr.cdc.gov/sites/brownfields/overview.html.

An additional group of hazardous waste sites is associated with federal government facilities, in particular, military facilities and nuclear energy complexes that include some NPL sites. The US Government Accountability Office (GAO) reported finding:

> The US Departments of Agriculture (USDA), the Interior (DOI), Defense (DOD), and Energy (DOE) have identified thousands of contaminated and potentially contaminated sites on land they manage but do not have a complete inventory of sites, in particular, for abandoned mines. The GAO reported in January 2015 that the USDA had identified 1,491 contaminated sites and many potentially contaminated sites. However, the USDA did not have a reliable, centralized site inventory or plans and procedures for completing one, in particular, for abandoned mines. For example, officials at the USDA's Forest Service estimated that there were from 27,000 to 39,000 abandoned mines on its lands—approximately 20% of which may pose some level of risk to human health or the environment. The GAO also reported that the DOI had an inventory of 4,722 sites with confirmed or likely contamination. However, the DOI's Bureau of Land Management had identified over 30,000 abandoned mines that were not yet assessed for contamination, and this inventory was not complete. The DOD reported to Congress in June 2014 that it had 38,804 sites in its inventory of sites with contamination. The DOE reported that it had 16 sites in 11 states with contamination.[10]

Certain types of waste sites and chemical contaminants are in preponderance in distinct regions of the country. For example, the New England states have many sites related to old economy industries, such as mills, radium clock factories, and metal plating and tanning facilities; common contaminants at these sites are lead, arsenic, chromium, radium, and mercury. In contrast, several southwestern states have waste sites related to oil refining and petrochemicals, wood treatment, and mining and smelting; common contaminants at these sites are volatile organic compounds (VOCs), pentachlorophenol, lead, arsenic, and creosote.[11]

Although not explicitly a waste site, the Great Lakes areas of concern present their own unique exposures to women of childbearing age and children. Each lake has a unique set of contaminants, but chemicals of interest include: polychlorinated biphenyls (PCBs), polycyclic aromatic hydrocarbons (PAHs), heavy metals, various pesticides, and other persistent organic pollutants. This contamination was created by decades of industrial and municipal discharges, combined sewer overflows, and urban and agricultural non-point source runoff. There are an estimated 1,411,722 women of childbearing age (aged 15 to 44 years) living within 1 mile (1.6 km) of these areas of concern.[12]

Responsibility for regulating and addressing cleanup was assigned to the US EPA under a number of legislative acts. In addition, the US Department of Health and Human Services' ATSDR was assigned roles in conducting health assessments and other nonregulatory functions to protect human health. Table 13-2 provides a short overview of the federal legislation covering ATSDR and US EPA roles related to waste sites and unintentional releases of hazardous substances.

| Table 13-2. US Legislation Covering Waste Sites and Unintentional Releases |
|---|
| **1980** The Comprehensive Environmental Response, Compensation, and Liability Act (CERCLA), also referred to as the Superfund Act, of 1980 provides a Federal "Superfund" to clean up uncontrolled or abandoned hazardous waste sites as well as accidents, spills, and other emergency releases of pollutants and contaminants into the environment. Through CERCLA, the US EPA was given power to seek out those parties responsible for any release and ensure their cooperation in the cleanup. |
| The US EPA cleans up orphan sites when potentially responsible parties cannot be identified or located, or when they fail to act. Through various enforcement tools, the US EPA obtains private party cleanup through orders, consent decrees, and other small party settlements. The US EPA also recovers costs from financially viable individuals and companies once a response action has been completed. |
| The US EPA is authorized to implement the Act in all 50 states and US territories. Superfund site identification, monitoring, and response activities in states are coordinated through the state environmental protection or waste management agencies. |
| ATSDR as an agency of the Public Health Service was given mandates to (1) establish a National Exposure and Disease Registry; (2) create an inventory of health information on hazardous substances; (3) create a list of closed and restricted-access sites; (4) provide medical assistance during hazardous substance emergencies; and (5) determine the relationship between hazardous substance exposures and illness. |
| https://www.epa.gov/laws-regulations/summary-comprehensive-environmental-response-compensation-and-liability-act |

| Table 13-2. US Legislation Covering Waste Sites and Unintentional Releases (*continued*) | |
|---|---|
| **1984** | The Resource Conservation and Recovery Act (RCRA) is the US's primary law governing the disposal of solid and hazardous waste. RCRA was amended and strengthened by Congress in November 1984 with the passing of the Federal Hazardous and Solid Waste Amendments (HSWA). These amendments to RCRA required phasing out land disposal of hazardous waste. <br><br> RCRA, as amended in 1984, mandated that ATSDR work with the US EPA to (1) identify new hazardous waste sites to be regulated; (2) conduct health assessments at RCRA sites at the US EPA's request; and (3) consider petitions for health assessments by the public or states. <br><br> RCRA has been amended on two occasions since: <br><br> 1. Federal Facility Compliance Act of 1992 – strengthened enforcement of RCRA at federal facilities. <br><br> 2. Land Disposal Program Flexibility Act of 1996 – provided regulatory flexibility for land disposal of certain wastes. <br><br> RCRA focuses only on active and future facilities and does not address abandoned or historical sites, which are managed under CERCLA—commonly known as Superfund. <br><br> https://www.epa.gov/rcra/resource-conservation-and-recovery-act-rcra-overview |
| **1986** | The Superfund Amendments and Reauthorization Act (SARA) of 1986 reauthorized CERCLA to continue cleanup activities around the country. Several site-specific amendments, definitions, clarifications, and technical requirements were added to the legislation, including additional enforcement authorities. Also, Title III of SARA authorized the Emergency Planning and Community Right-to-Know Act (EPCRA). <br><br> SARA broadens ATSDR's responsibilities in the areas of public health assessments, establishment and maintenance of toxicological databases, information dissemination, and medical education. <br><br> https://www.epa.gov/laws-regulations/summary-comprehensive-environmental-response-compensation-and-liability-act |

## ROUTES AND SOURCES OF EXPOSURE

For a hazardous substance to result in a health impact, the substance must have a pathway into the body. This pathway is achieved through 3 routes of exposure. These routes are ingestion, inhalation, and dermal absorption. A child or adult may be exposed by waste migrating into groundwater, surface water, drinking water, air, surface soil, sediment, dust, or plant and/or animal food sources.

The exposures a pregnant woman experiences are often shared with the developing fetus. Many harmful substances cross the placenta and expose the fetus. Growing evidence shows that early life exposures in fetal development and early childhood have the potential to result in disease outcomes and disease susceptibilities later in life. Exposures during fetal development can produce epigenetic modifications that operate as "on/off switches" to regulate, either increasing or decreasing, gene expression. "Epigenetic modifications that function as a rheostat are often driven by environmental conditions, particularly those that are extreme, and are thought to function as a cellular memory of previous environmental conditions . . . so that future environments can be physiologically anticipated."[13]

Children are at higher risk of environmental exposures than adults. Child physiology, diet, and behavior contribute to unique exposure risks to hazardous environmental substances. From birth, children breathe more air, drink more water, and eat more food per unit of body weight than adults do. Young children typically have limited food sources that may lead to greater exposures to contaminants, such as pesticide residues, unique to certain foods, such as apple or rice products, common in a child's diet. In addition, children have a higher surface area to body mass ratio that increases their exposure to substances absorbed through the skin. Young children also are developmentally less able to process and eliminate toxic substances from their bodies.[14]

Age-specific behaviors also put children at increased risks of exposure. For infants and toddlers, normal play includes crawling on floors and hand-to-mouth behavior. These behaviors increase exposure to dust, dirt, and other particles that may contain toxic substances found on floors, carpets, lawns, and toys that children explore during play. Older children may find waste sites interesting. They may ignore or fail to notice warning signs, find or create openings in fences, or otherwise gain access to restricted places on or near a site. These factors change as a child ages.

## CLINICAL EFFECTS

Absent an exposure pathway, no health impact should result from a hazardous waste site. If completed exposure pathways exist, potential health effects on infants, children, and adolescents from exposure to hazardous substances are related to the chemical properties of the pollutant, the total and peak dose received, the toxicity of the substance, and the child's individual susceptibility.

The overall impact of hazardous waste sites on human health is difficult to assess because of conflicting information from epidemiologic studies and limitations of the methodologies used.[15] Many study results have been interpreted as "insignificant," meaning that no statistically significant increase in adverse health effects was found. These observations may reflect the true absence of adverse effects or the inability to detect such effects because of inadequacies in study design or sample size. For example, many studies that found little, if any, excess risks of adverse effects defined their target populations crudely, based on linear distance from a site, instead of examining documented environmental pathways and routes of exposure. Likewise, study results interpreted as "significant" may reflect a true effect or other types of study design flaws, such as misclassification of exposure, insufficient time for health effects to manifest, or inappropriate choice of comparison groups.[15]

Advances in analytical chemistry and molecular biology are identifying new classes of biomarkers. These "biomarkers are capable of detecting early manifestations of chemical-induced cell injury and cell death."[16] Applied in computational modeling, these evolving analytical tools are providing "new insights into initial mechanisms of chemical-induced toxicity."[17] Concepts and study methods are also emerging that have the capacity to examine mixtures of substances over time.[15] One concept is the exposome, defined as "the measure of all the exposures of an individual in a lifetime and how those exposures relate to health."[16] The exposome provides a framework to apply new analytical tools and investigate specific biological responses and mechanistic connections between exposures and adverse health outcomes across the lifespan.[18] These and other advances hold greater promise for demonstrating that exposure to certain waste site contaminants may have adverse health effects later in life.

Adverse health effects have been reported in some, but not all, investigations of communities around hazardous waste sites.[15] These effects have ranged from nonspecific symptoms (eg, headache, fatigue, skin rashes)[19] to congenital heart defects,[20] low/reduced birth weight,[20–23] and other birth outcomes.[21–23] In communities surrounding waste facilities that utilize incineration techniques, effects found include cancer of the lung and larynx, non-Hodgkin's lymphoma, and congenital malformations.[24,25]

Most investigations have included some children in the study population, but only a few have focused primarily on health effects among infants and children. In these studies, it is difficult to know whether proximity to the waste site or some other factor(s) is responsible for the health outcome. Some of the studies that support concerns were conducted by governmental agencies and findings of those studies have not always been reported in peer-reviewed literature, making access to such documents difficult. Table 13-3 offers findings of health impacts during pregnancy and childhood associated with close proximity to hazardous waste sites in the United States.

An array of information resources is available on hazardous waste sites in the United States and on the health hazards of more than 200 individual toxic substances. This information is provided by the ATSDR in a variety of formats intended for different audiences. The ATSDR Toxicological Profiles critically review the literature on toxicology, pharmacokinetics, epidemiology, exposure, environmental fate, and transport of the substances found at waste sites.

## Table 13-3. Health Impacts During Pregnancy and Childhood Associated With Hazardous Waste Sites

| POPULATION AND LOCATION | SUBSTANCE | HEALTH IMPACT OBSERVED |
|---|---|---|
| Children living in a zip code containing a hazardous waste site | Persistent organic pollutants (POPs) | Zip code containing a POPs waste site significantly increased the frequency of hospitalization for asthma and infectious respiratory disease.[26] |
| Women residing 1 mile or less (1.6 km) from pesticide-containing waste sites in Washington State | Pesticides | Fetal death risk increased among women residing ≤1 mile (1.6 km) from pesticide-containing sites.[27] |
| Maternal residence during pregnancy of 1 mile (1.6 km) or less from urban waste sites in Washington State | | Living <5 miles (8 km) from a hazardous waste site was associated with increased risk of any malformations in offspring.[28] |
| Mothers who lived in the Emergency Declaration Area of Love Canal New York and were of reproductive age sometime during that time period | More than 200 distinct organic chemical compounds found, including dioxin[29] | ■ Significantly elevated risk of preterm birth[22]<br>■ Ratio of male to female births was lower[22]<br>■ Frequency of congenital malformations was greater than expected among Love Canal boys born from 1983 to 1996[22] |
| Women living within a New York State zip code close to a PCB waste site or contaminated body of water | Polychlorinated biphenyls (PCBs) | A 6% increased risk of giving birth to a male infant of low birth weight and 3% for female infant of low birth weight[30] |
| Pregnant women working in a former Navy facility in Massachusetts | Trichloroethylene (TCE) in the air above a level of health concern | May be at risk for having an unborn child with damage of the heart[31] |
| Children exercising in a former Navy facility in Massachusetts | Tetrachloroethylene (perchloroethylene or PCE) in the air above a level of health concern | May be at an increased risk of damage to the immune system[31] |
| Autism spectrum disorder (ASD) cohort in New Jersey | | A statistically significant correlation with the rate of ASD and the number of identified Superfund sites per 1,000 residents in 49 of 50 states[32] |
| Prevalence of students with autism spectrum disorder (ASD) in Minnesota school districts | | A significantly higher ASD prevalence among school districts having one or more NPL sites within both a 10- and 20-mile (16 and 32 km) radius[33] |

Additional information specific to children's health and developmental issues is provided in profiles covering the most commonly encountered substances on the US EPA's National Priority List of sites. Individual profiles are available for health professionals through the ATSDR Toxic Substances Portal at www.atsdr.cdc.gov/substances/index.asp.

## DIAGNOSTIC METHODS

An exposed infant or child can remain asymptomatic, acquire nonspecific symptoms, or acquire signs and symptoms frequently associated with common medical conditions. Because of this range of outcomes, a history of environmental exposure should be obtained when evaluating the etiology of unexplained symptoms. Standardized approaches to taking an exposure history are available.[34,35]

### Individual Evaluation

As in other aspects of medicine, the patient history guides laboratory testing. Blood or urine tests may be indicated when a child is symptomatic and there is a recent history of a specific exposure (eg, when a child has climbed over a fence and played in a site known to be contaminated with a specific toxicant). Generally, laboratory tests to document exposure are not recommended in the absence of signs or symptoms. However, diagnostic blood testing of children potentially exposed to lead may be indicated, and other diagnostic tests may be indicated for specific children on the basis of known effects of the particular contaminant.

### Community Studies

In formal epidemiologic studies, laboratory biological tests may be useful to determine whether there is an association between exposure and any adverse health effects.

A biomarker of exposure provides a reasonable measure of the internal body level of a substance over a period that depends on the pharmacokinetics of that substance. Testing may be performed on blood ( for lead), urine ( for metallic mercury, arsenic), or tissue specimens. Analytical methods and human reference ranges are available for many of the substances found most commonly at hazardous waste sites. In some cases, age-specific reference ranges are available through the National Health and Nutritional Examination Survey (NHANES) to facilitate interpretation of levels found in infants and children.[36] It may be difficult to interpret the results, however, when reference ranges for children are not available.

Highly sensitive standardized medical test batteries are available for use in epidemiologic studies to evaluate subclinical and clinical organ damage or dysfunction.[16] Because of their low specificity, these test batteries are not useful to assess effects of community exposures outside the context of a formal research study.

## TREATMENT

Treatment of acute exposure to one or more substances from a hazardous waste site depends on the substance; the route, dose, and duration of exposure; and the presence of any symptoms or ill effects. Treatment should generally be undertaken in consultation with a medical toxicologist or an expert in pediatric environmental health. Local Poison Control Centers and the Pediatric Environmental Health Specialty Units (PEHSUs) are sources for acute and chronic exposure concerns. The ATSDR offers information on Managing Hazardous Materials Incidents (MHMIs). It is a 3-volume set (with a video) comprised of recommendations for on-scene (prehospital) and hospital medical management of patients exposed during a hazardous materials incident.[37]

## CONSULTATION

Consultation is available on potentially toxic exposures and possible ill effects from such exposures. A national network of PEHSUs can provide information, receive referrals, and offer training in the diagnosis and treatment of illnesses associated with exposure to toxic substances and other environmental health risks (see Resources).

## PREVENTION OF EXPOSURE

In the United States, the US EPA is responsible for cleaning up waste sites under the Superfund Act. Experience at hundreds of communities near waste sites has demonstrated the value and importance of early and extensive community engagement. Community-involved engagement not a simple process. Government agencies have made considerable progress in these areas by forming community assistance panels; awarding assistance grants; and developing valid methods of needs assessment, providing health risk communication, and community outreach. These methods have enhanced the agencies' abilities to recognize the value of community input, address community needs, and focus attention on those needed areas. Table 13-4 lists ways to prevent or limit exposure to waste site contaminants.

## Table 13-4. Preventing or Limiting Exposure

**Personal Preventive Actions**

Comply with advisories (eg, warnings about eating fish or swimming in certain waters)

Connect to a safer water supply

Establish play areas through fencing and landscape methods to reduce potential for exposures to contaminated soil

**Engineering Controls**

Destroy contaminants by incineration or by chemical or biological reactions

Remove the contaminants to a safer location

Disrupt the exposure pathway (eg, an alternate water supply or perimeter fence)

Use dust control and other measures to protect workers and neighbors during the cleanup process

Develop engineering solutions to eliminate relatively small, acute problems (removal actions)

Develop "remedial actions," engineering solutions that involve complex planning to permanently solve a complicated waste site problem

**Administrative Controls**

Temporarily or permanently relocate residents

Restrict deeds (eg, to prevent future use of the land for residential or child care purposes)

Enact ordinances to control future land use

Communicate health advisories

## Frequently Asked Questions

Q   *I am confused by the conflicting information I hear about the risks to my children from waste sites. Can you clarify this?*

A   The risks depend on the amount, type, and duration of exposure and the types of chemicals involved; therefore, each case is different and the risks cannot be generalized. It is difficult to know the exact details of a child's exposure, so it is difficult to know the risk precisely. For any health effects to be seen, there must be a complete exposure pathway via ingestion, inhalational, or dermal. An example of each are: dermal contact with contaminated soil, inhalation of methane gas, and ingestion of contaminated water. In addition, for many chemicals, the effects of exposure in childhood are not well known and only can be estimated from the toxic effects found in experiments with animals.

Q   *Did exposure from a waste site cause my child's illness?* or *One of my children has an illness that is linked to the waste site. Will my other children also become ill?*

A   It is difficult to establish that one child's illness was caused by exposure to one particular waste site. Most of the illnesses that can be caused by exposure to toxic chemicals have more than one possible cause. Also, not every child who is exposed becomes ill. A linkage is more likely if several children (or adults) become ill at about the same time, at the same place, and/or following the same exposure.

Q   *Will my child get cancer from exposure to a waste site?*

A   Although a number of chemicals found at waste sites are carcinogens (known or predicted to cause cancer), the chance of getting cancer from exposure to a waste site is thought to be small. If the child was exposed to one or more carcinogens, the risk to the child depends on the amount and duration of the exposure and type of carcinogen, among other considerations. Most experts believe that development of cancer is unlikely unless there has been exposure for many years (see Chapter 49).

Q   *Is my child's learning disability (or attention-deficit/hyperactivity disorder) caused by exposure to a waste site?*

A   A number of chemicals found at waste sites may affect the nervous system, including a child's developing nervous system. These chemicals include heavy metals (eg, lead, mercury), organic solvents (eg, toluene), and certain types of pesticides (eg, carbamates, organophosphates). The risk to the child depends on how long the child was exposed, the child's age at exposure, the degree of exposure, and the child's genetic susceptibility.

Q   *How can I protect my child from future exposure to hazardous waste sites?*

A   It is best to avoid areas where soil is contaminated by hazardous waste. Explain to children the meaning and importance of posted warning signs, and strongly advise children to stay out of restricted areas. Do not let children swim in streams or other bodies of water that are known to be contaminated. Such conditions usually are posted, but if there is doubt, contact the local health department. Know the source of your household drinking water, and if uncertain about contaminants, have it tested. Children, pregnant women, and others should not eat certain fish caught from contaminated waters. Fishing license brochures available locally list advisories about which fish are safe to eat. If a parent or other caregiver works at a hazardous waste site, soiled work clothes should not be brought into the home. Dust can be a source of exposure for children. Stay engaged and vigilant during the development of remediation plans and the actual remediation process to ensure that proper dust control and other safety procedures are in place and followed.

Q   *My home is near a landfill. Is my child at risk?*

A   The risk depends on the types of chemicals at the site and the quantity, route, and duration of exposure. Because it is extremely difficult to determine the precise nature of any exposure, it is not easy to measure the real risk for your child. In addition, more scientific information is needed about the ways that many chemicals, such as those found in landfills, affect children's health. It is best to keep your child away from the site, monitor activities that could cause exposure to chemicals, and regularly test drinking water from nearby wells. Investigate whether your local community holds household hazardous waste collection days, which help prevent toxic chemicals from entering municipal waste streams and landfills. Substitute less toxic alternatives in your home, minimize your family's use of hazardous chemicals, and advocate for these healthier practices within your local community.

## Resources

### Agency for Toxic Substances and Disease Registry (ATSDR)

Educational materials, medical management guidelines for acute toxicity, toxicity information for individual chemicals, Toxicological Profiles, publications and information: https://www.atsdr.cdc.gov/substances/index.asp

Phone: Contact CDC/ATSDR: 800-232-4636 / TTY: 888-232-6348

Chemical emergencies and accidental releases: 1-770-488-7100 (information available 24 hours a day).

The CDC/ATSDR provides 24-hour technical and scientific support (emergency operation center: 770-488-7100) for chemical emergencies (including terrorist threats) such as spills, explosions, and transportation accidents throughout the United States. The ATSDR also provides health consultations for people exposed to individual substances or mixtures. The 3-volume reference text, Managing Hazardous Materials Incidents: Medical Management Guidelines for Acute Chemical Exposures[37] is available at: https://www.atsdr.cdc.gov/substances/ToxEmergency.asp

Other resources provided by ATSDR include:
—Cases Studies in Environmental Medicine
—Grand Rounds in Environmental Medicine (information for clinicians on specific exposures):
    https://www.atsdr.cdc.gov/substances/ToxMedical.asp
—ToxFAQs (frequently asked questions about contaminants found at hazardous waste sites):
    www.atsdr.cdc.gov/toxfaqs/index.asp
—Public Health Statements (a series of summaries about hazardous substances):
    https://www.atsdr.cdc.gov/substances/ToxCommunity.asp

### CDC/National Center for Environmental Health (NCEH)

Located within the Centers for Disease Control and Prevention, NCEH addresses diverse environmental health issues.
Web site: www.cdc.gov/nceh

**Chemical poisoning emergencies**
Web site: www.poison.org
Phone: 1-800-222-1222

**Dartmouth Toxic Metals Research Program**
Web site: www.dartmouth.edu/,toxmetal

**EPA EJSCREEN (Environmental Justice Screening and Mapping Tool) Tool**
Web site: https://www.epa.gov/ejscreen

**EPA Response to Chemical spills, oil spills, threats**
Phone: 800-424-8802
Web site: www.epa.gov/oilspill/oilhow.htm

**EPA Superfund Program (general description)**
Web site: www.epa.gov/superfund

**National Institute of Environmental Health Sciences (NIEHS)/EPA Children's Environmental Health and Disease Prevention Research Centers**
Web site: https://www.niehs.nih.gov/research/supported/centers/prevention/index.cfm

**National Library of Medicine TOXNET: Toxicology Data Network**
Web site: http://toxnet.nlm.nih.gov/cgi-bin/sis/htmlgen?TOXLINE

**Pediatric Environmental Health Specialty Units**
Provide consultation and professional education free of charge
Web site: www.www.pehsu.net

## References

1. U.S. Environmental Protection Agency. Hazardous Waste. Learn the Basics of Hazardous Waste. https://www.epa.gov/hw/learn-basics-hazardous-waste. Accessed March 30, 2018

2. HAZWOPER Definitions and Key Terms. Occupational Safety and Health Administration. https://www.hazmatstudent.com/hazwoper-training/hazwoper-definitions/. Accessed March 30, 2018

3. U.S. Environmental Protection Agency. Superfund: National Priorities List. https://www.epa.gov/superfund/superfund-national-priorities-list-npl. Accessed March 30, 2018

4. U.S. Environmental Protection Agency. National Priorities List (NPL) Sites – by State. https://www.epa.gov/superfund/national-priorities-list-npl-sites-state. Accessed March 30, 2018

5. U.S. Census Bureau. Annual Estimates of the Resident Population: April 1, 2010 to July 1, 2014 https://www.census.gov. Accessed April 28, 2018

6. U.S. Environmental Protection Agency. Population surrounding 1,388 Superfund remedial sites. OSWER/Office of Communications, Partnerships, and Analysis. September 2015. https://www.epa.gov/sites/production/files/2015-09/documents/webpopulationrsuperfundsites9.28.15.pdf. Accessed March 30, 2018

7. Agency for Toxic Substances and Disease Registry. 2016. Geospatial analysis performed by GRASP. Dec, 2016

8. Agency for Toxic Substances and Disease Registry. *Report to Congress,* 1993, 1994, 1995. US Department of Health and Human Services, Public Health Service. 1999

9. Agency for Toxic Substances and Disease Registry. *Priority List of Hazardous Substances.* Updated Feb 2016. https://www.atsdr.cdc.gov/spl/. Accessed March 30, 2018

10. U.S. Government Accountability Office. Hazardous Waste Cleanup: Numbers of Contaminated Federal Sites, Estimated Costs, and EPA's Oversight Role. Testimony before the Subcommittee on Environment and the Economy, Committee on Energy and Commerce, House of Representatives. Statement of J. Alfredo Gómez, Director, Natural Resources and Environment. September 2015. https://www.gao.gov/assets/680/672464.pdf. Accessed March 30, 2018

11. Amler RW, Falk HF. Opportunities and challenges in community environmental health evaluations. *Environ Epidemiol Toxicol.* 2000;2:51–55

12. U.S. Environmental Protection Agency. Contaminated Sediment in the Great Lakes. Updated Sept 2016. https://www.epa.gov/greatlakes/contaminated-sediment-great-lakes. Accessed March 30, 2018

13. Boekelheide K, Blumberg B, Chapin RE, et al. Predicting later-life outcomes of early-life exposures. *Environ Health Perspect.* 2012;120(10):1353–1361. https://www.ncbi.nlm.nih.gov/pmc/articles/PMC3491941/. Accessed March 30, 2018

14. Western States Pediatric Environmental Health Specialty Units. Pediatric Environment Health Toolkit: Key Concepts. http://peht.ucsf.edu/index.php. Accessed March 30, 2018

15. Elliott P, Briggs D, Morris S, et al. Risk of adverse birth outcomes in populations living near landfill sites. BMJ. 2001;323(7309):363–368. https://www.ncbi.nlm.nih.gov/pmc/articles/PMC37394/. Accessed March 30, 2018

16. National Institute for Occupational Safety and Health. Exposome and Exposomics. Centers for Disease Control and Prevention. https://www.cdc.gov/niosh/topics/exposome/default.html. Accessed March 30, 2018

17. Fowler BA. *Molecular Biological Markers for Toxicology and Risk Assessment.* Elsevier; 2016. http://www.sciencedirect.com/science/article/pii/B9780128095898000019. Accessed March 30, 2018

18. Dennis KK, Auerbach SS, Balshaw DM, et al. The importance of the biological impact of exposure to the concept of the exposome. *Environ Health Perspect.* 2016;124(10):1504–1510. https://www.ncbi.nlm.nih.gov/pmc/articles/PMC5047763/. Accessed March 30, 2018

19. Brender JD, Pichette JL, Suarez L, Hendricks KA, Holt M. Health risks of residential exposure to polycyclic aromatic hydrocarbons. *Arch Environ Health.* 2003;58(2):111–118

20. Brender JD, Maantay JA, Chakraborty J. Residential proximity to environmental hazards and adverse health outcomes. *Am J Public Health.* 2011;101(Suppl 1):S37–S52

21. Baibergenova A, Kudyakov R, Zdeb, Carperter DO. Low birth weight and residential proximity to PCB-contaminated waste sites. *Environ Health Perspect.* 2003;111(10):1352–1357. https://www.ncbi.nlm.nih.gov/pmc/articles/PMC1241618/pdf/ehp0111-001352.pdf. Accessed March 30, 2018

22. Austin AA, Fitzgerald EF, Pantea CI, et al. Reproductive outcomes among former Love Canal residents, Niagara Falls, New York. *Environ Res.* 2011;111(5):693–701. http://www.sciencedirect.com/science/article/pii/S0013935111000995?via%3Dihub. Accessed March 30, 2018

23. Gilbreath S, Kass PH. Adverse birth outcomes associated with open dumpsites in Alaska native villages. *Am J Epidemiol.* 2006;164(6):518–528. http://citeseerx.ist.psu.edu/viewdoc/download?doi=10.1.1.333.3220&rep=rep1&type=pdf. Accessed March 30, 2018

24. Franchini M, Rial M, Buiatti E, Bianchi F. Health effects of exposure to waste incinerator emissions: a review of epidemiological studies. *Ann Ist Super Sanita*. 2004;40(1):101–115. http://www.iss.it/publ/anna/2004/1/401101.pdf. Accessed March 30, 2018

25. Porta D, Milani S, Lazzarino AI, Perucci CA, Forastiere F. Systematic review of epidemiological studies on health effects associated with management of solid waste. *Environ Health*. 2009;8:60. https://www.ncbi.nlm.nih.gov/pmc/articles/PMC2805622/. Accessed March 30, 2018

26. Ma J, Kouznetsova M, Lessner L, Carpenter DO. Asthma and infectious respiratory disease in children—correlation to residence near hazardous waste sites. *Paediatr Respir Rev*. 2007;8(4):292–298. http://www.prrjournal.com/article/S1526-0542(07)00072-3/fulltext. Accessed March 30, 2018

27. Mueller BA, Kuehn CM, Shapiro-Mendoza CK, Tomashek KM. Fetal deaths and proximity to hazardous waste sites in Washington State. *Environ Health Perspect*. 2007;115(5):776–780. https://www.ncbi.nlm.nih.gov/pmc/articles/PMC1867977/. Accessed March 30, 2018

28. Kuehn CM, Mueller BA, Checkoway H, Williams M. Risk of malformations associated with residential proximity to hazardous waste sites in Washington State. *Environ Res*. 2007;103(3):405–412

29. Love Canal: A Special Report to the Governor and Legislature: April 1981. New York State Department of Health. https://www.health.ny.gov/environmental/investigations/love_canal/lcreport.htm#toxicological. Accessed March 30, 2018

30. Baibergenova A, Kudyakov R, Zdeb M, Carpenter DO. Low birth weight and residential proximity to PCB-contaminated waste sites. *Environ Health Perspect*. 2003;111(10):1352–1357. https://www.ncbi.nlm.nih.gov/pmc/articles/PMC1241618/pdf/ehp0111-001352.pdf. Accessed March 30, 2018

31. Agency for Toxic Substances and Disease Registry. Health Consultation: The Navy Yard Mills Site, Dracut MA. April 10, 2014. Department of Health and Human Services. https://www.atsdr.cdc.gov/HAC/pha/NavyYardMillsSite/NavyYardMills%20_HC_04-10-2014_508.pdf. Accessed March 30, 2018

32. Ming X, Brimacombe M, Malek JH, Jani N, Wagner GC. Autism spectrum disorders and identified toxic land fills: co-occurrence across States. *Environ Health Insights*. 2008;2:55–59. https://www.ncbi.nlm.nih.gov/pmc/articles/PMC3091342/. Accessed March 30, 2018

33. DeSoto MC. Ockham's Razor and autism: the case for developmental neurotoxins contributing to a disease of neurodevelopment. *Neurotoxicology*. 2009;30(3):331–337. http://cdn.harmonyapp.com/assets/4c6ff4d3dabe9d392d000021/autism_and_superfund_sites.pdf. Accessed March 30, 2018

34. Agency for Toxic Substances and Disease Registry. Case Studies in Environmental Medicine: Taking a Pediatric Exposure History. U.S. Department of Health and Human Services. 2013. https://www.atsdr.cdc.gov/csem/csem.html. Accessed March 30, 2018

35. Agency for Toxic Substances and Disease Registry. Case Studies in Environmental Medicine: Principles of Pediatric Environmental Health. U.S. Department of Health and Human Services. 2014. https://www.atsdr.cdc.gov/csem/csem.html. Accessed March 30, 2018

36. Centers for Disease Control and Prevention. National Report on Human Exposure to Environmental Chemicals: Updated Tables, March 2018. U.S. Department of Health and Human Services. https://www.cdc.gov/exposurereport/index.html. Accessed March 30, 2018

37. Agency for Toxic Substances and Disease Registry. Managing Hazardous Materials Incidents: Medical Management Guidelines for Acute Chemical Exposures. U.S. Department of Health and Human Services, Public Health Service. 2001

# Chapter 14

# Considerations for Children from Low- and Middle-income Countries

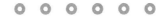

## KEY POINTS

- Children living in low- and middle-income countries are at increased risk for health compromise from environmental hazards including toxic metal exposures, tobacco smoke, pesticides, indoor and outdoor air contaminants, persistent organic pollutants, vector-borne disease, and climate change.
- Household air pollution from biomass burning for cooking and heating is a leading cause of global death and disability.
- Pediatricians should consider these exposures when caring for children living inside the United States as immigrants, refugees, and adoptees, and when caring for children residing in low- and middle-income countries.

## INTRODUCTION

Most of the world's children live in low- and middle-income countries (LMICs), settings with environmental conditions that may be detrimental to health. Awareness of the environmental health conditions in other parts of the world provides a perspective on the roles of the United States and other governments, nonprofit institutions, and international organizations in improving global child health.

Pediatricians in the United States, particularly in urban areas and areas with large immigrant populations, may examine and care for children—including adoptees and refugees—who previously resided outside of the United States. Most immigrant children are not adoptees or refugees. The major countries of origin of most immigrants to the United States in 2015 were India, Mexico, China, and Canada.[1]

In 2015, there were 5,648 children adoptees to the United States. In that year, the highest numbers arrived from China, Ethiopia, the Republic of Korea, and Ukraine.[2] Each year, thousands of persons who face persecution in their country of nationality seek asylum or refugee status in the United States. In 2016, the leading countries of origin for refugees included Myanmar (formerly known as Burma), Democratic Republic of Congo (also known as Zaire), Somalia, Iraq, Bhutan, Syria, and Iran.[3] Children and families from Mexico and Central America, Cuba, and Haiti also immigrate to and seek asylum in the United States. Refugees frequently have encountered displacement from their homes, family disruption, violence, and other traumatic events. Children from low-income families generally face greater risks than children from more affluent families. The lifestyle, cultural, and environmental factors associated with country of origin also often greatly influence health status for children who come to the United States from LMICs.

This chapter will provide an overview of global pediatric environmental health issues and discuss the key exposures to consider in the care of international immigrants, adoptees, and refugees from LMICs.

## GLOBAL PEDIATRIC ENVIRONMENTAL HEALTH: DEFINING THE POPULATION, KEY PROBLEMS, AND ORGANIZATIONS

Children aged 0 to 14 years comprise 17%, 26%, and 43% of the population of high-, middle-, and low-income countries, respectively.[4] The total global population is projected to increase from the current 7.6 billion to 9.8 billion by the year 2050, with essentially all growth in LMICs, concentrated among the poorest populations in urban areas.[5]

One out of every 4 deaths worldwide in 2012 were a result of living or working in an unhealthy environment.[6] The World Health Organization (WHO) estimates that the impacts of environment are greatest on young children (younger than age 5). Figure 14-1 demonstrates that the most significant fraction of disease and disability in LMICs could be improved through addressing environmental components. This unequal disease burden on the poorer nations may be further aggravated by differences in access to health care.

Urbanization, unregulated industrialization, outsourcing by high-income countries to less regulated regions, extraction industries, population growth and displacement, and increased pressure on limited natural resources

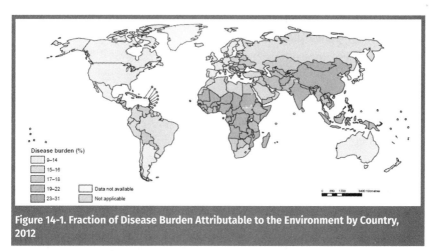

**Figure 14-1. Fraction of Disease Burden Attributable to the Environment by Country, 2012**

Reproduced with permission from Prüss-Üstün A, Wolf J, Corvalan C, Bos R, Neira M. Preventing disease through healthy environments: a global assessment of the burden of disease from environmental risks. World Health Organization. ISBN 978 92 4 156519 6 http://apps.who.int/iris/bitstream/10665/204585/1/9789241565196_eng.pdf.

underlie the environmental hazards in poorer nations. Mitigation measures are often unaddressed in the quest for economic development. Obstacles to protecting pediatric environmental health in LMICS include inadequate medical and public health infrastructure and financial resources, shortage of laboratory equipment and trained technical personnel, and distrust between the public and governmental agencies.

Core agencies in the United Nations (UN) monitor trends, identify priorities, and promote programs and activities designed to improve pediatric environmental health in LMICs. The WHO, the UN's public health arm, provides national profiles and tracks health indicators in the lower resourced regions of the world, and estimates burden of disease and disability attributable to environmental factors. Capacity-building activities and resource development relevant to LMIC countries are ongoing. The International Pediatric Association, an organization of national pediatric societies, has a program focusing on environmental health. The International Network for Children's Health, Environment and Safety also focuses on this topic (see Resources section at end of chapter).

The following primary areas of concern in global child health and environment are well recognized and briefly described in this chapter.

- Unsafe water, poor sanitation, and hygiene
- Vector-borne diseases
- Household air pollution

- Tobacco and secondhand tobacco smoke
- Traffic-related pollution and traffic injury
- Industrialization and hazardous materials
- Pesticides
- Climate change and severe weather events

## Unsafe Water, Poor Sanitation, and Hygiene

Access to improved drinking water sources are available for 66%, 92%, and 100% of low-, middle-, and high-income countries, respectively.[7] In 2015, the WHO estimated that 2.4 billion people had no access to sanitary means of excreta disposal. Of them, 946 million defecate in the open.[8] Access to safe drinking water and sanitation is particularly low in the poor, rural areas of low-income countries.

With proper sanitation, proper hygiene, and safe drinking water, diarrhea can be decreased by one third.[9] However, rapid growth of cities in LMICs represents a serious challenge to efforts to provide proper housing, drinking water, and sanitation. Given that diarrhea accounts for 8% of deaths of children younger than age 5, improvements in water and sanitation are critical to child health.[10] In addition, improved sanitation and safe drinking water will help to eradicate guinea worm disease, hookworm, schistosomiasis, and other waterborne diseases that influence the health and development of children in low-income countries, especially in sub-Saharan Africa.

High levels of chemical contaminants, such as nitrates, arsenic, and fluoride, are common in drinking water supplies in many rural areas. High levels of naturally occurring arsenic have been found in many LMICs, particularly in South Asia and South America, exposing approximately 200 million individuals.[11] Accumulating epidemiologic evidence from these areas links early life exposure to arsenic to an increased risk of adverse neurodevelopmental outcomes including cognitive deficits and immunotoxicity.[12,13] These findings raise concern, although methodological limitations and differences across studies limit firm conclusions. Ingestion of naturally occurring arsenic from drinking water also is linked to a higher risk for the development of lung, bladder, and skin cancer (see Chapter 22). Fluorosis is a potentially crippling disease caused by the ingestion of too much fluoride in drinking water.[14] High concentrations of fluoride occur naturally in groundwater and coal in many LMICs. Fluorosis is endemic in many countries including India, Mexico, China, Bangladesh, and some African countries.[15] Pesticide contamination is also common because approximately two thirds of rural people in poor countries are engaged in agricultural work.[16] Persistent organic pollutants have been documented in water supplies throughout LMICs (see Chapter 38).[17]

## Vector-borne Diseases

Environmental degradation can lead to increased vector-borne disease. Poorly designed irrigation and water systems and poor waste disposal and water storage can contribute to malaria, dengue fever, leishmaniasis, and Zika virus. According to the most recent WHO estimates, there were 216 million cases of malaria in 2016 and 445,000 deaths.[18] African children younger than age 5 are the highest risk group. Dengue fever, with associated dengue hemorrhagic fever, is the world's fastest growing vector-borne disease.[19]

Progress in malaria eradication occurred from 2010 to about 2015; there was an increase in the number of malaria cases in 2016.[20] The United Nations Environment Programme (UNEP) has identified links between increased malaria and worsening environmental conditions.[21] The expansion of extractive industries has been associated with an increased incidence of malaria. For example, in Sri Lankan gem-mining areas, shallow pits left behind by gem miners become ideal mosquito breeding areas. Studies from Brazil suggest that mercury used in small-scale gold mining may increase susceptibility to malaria by depressing immune systems in humans. Deforestation and road building disrupt forest and river systems that may increase the habitats for malaria-carrying mosquitoes. Migration of workers into previously inaccessible areas increases the population at risk. In addition, the WHO recently estimated that 6% of malaria cases in parts of the world during the last 25 years are the result of climate change.

## Household Air Pollution

In LMICs, household air pollution from solid fuel burning for cooking and heating is an important risk factor that contributes to disease and death overall.[22] Solid fuel use is most prevalent in Africa, and South and Southeast Asia where more than 60% of households cook with solid fuels.[23] These fuels include wood, dung, coal, charcoal, and crop waste, which are burned indoors on open fires or in poorly ventilated stoves. This creates levels of gas and particulate pollutant mixtures many times greater indoors than permitted under typical regulatory limits.[24] Community ambient air can also be significantly impacted. The WHO global burden of disease study reported that household air pollution was responsible for 4.3 million deaths, and 7.7% of the global mortality in 2012.[25] Women of childbearing age are traditionally responsible for cooking, and consequently, exposures are highest for them and for their infants and young children, who are often carried on their mothers' backs. Child exposures also occur at school, where biomass fuel is commonly used. Indoor air pollution is estimated to cause 1 million deaths in infants and young children by causing acute lower respiratory infections.[26]

In some countries, kerosene is used as a substitute because it seems to burn "cleaner." As with biomass fuel, indoor kerosene burning leads to the accumulation of multiple toxic constituents including volatile organic compounds and polycyclic aromatic hydrocarbons. Intervention studies using improved stoves or trials to provide liquid petroleum gas are ongoing in poor, rural communities where access to alternative fuels is very limited. These studies demonstrate that pollution levels can be lowered significantly but sustained implementation and adoption have been problematic.[27] In recent years, initiatives have expanded to develop access and adoption of use of clean fuels, such as liquid petroleum gas to reduce household air pollution[28] (see Chapter 20).

## Tobacco and Secondhand Tobacco Smoke (SHS)

Tobacco use is the world's leading killer, causing 1 in 10 (or 5.4 million) deaths annually among adults worldwide. Unless urgent action is taken, there will be more than 8 million tobacco deaths annually by 2030, with more than 80% occurring in LMICs. Smokers are not the only ones affected. One in 100 people around the world dies from exposure to secondhand tobacco smoke (SHS) each year and nearly two thirds of these deaths occur in children.[29]

Nearly two thirds of the world's smokers live in 10 countries, with tobacco use growing fastest in low-income countries as populations grow, and as tobacco companies turn their attention away from the increasingly regulated US and European markets. With approximately 350 million smokers, China has the biggest smoking population in the world. Smokers in China consume an estimated 1.7 trillion cigarettes per year and roughly 540 million Chinese people are exposed to SHS. Of Chinese smokers, 61% are men, and fathers who smoke account for 60% of children's exposure to SHS; 98% of smokers smoke at home, and an estimated 43% of Chinese people are exposed to SHS outside the home.[30]

India is the third largest tobacco-producing country in the world after China and Brazil, and a large part of that production is consumed within the country. With a population of 1.15 billion, India represents 17% of the Earth's population. A high prevalence of tobacco use is found in the Indian population, with 57% of males and 3% of females using tobacco; 26.6% of Indian children are exposed to SHS indoors and more than 40% are exposed outside their homes.[30]

Although there are strong cultural differences in smoking behaviors in different countries and regions, the WHO Framework Convention on Tobacco Control, a multilateral treaty ratified by 173 parties, developed a blueprint for countries to halt the tobacco epidemic and move toward a tobacco-free world. Although the United States signed the Framework Convention on Tobacco Control, it has never been ratified by the Senate; thus, the United States is not among the parties to the treaty. To help countries fulfill the promise of the Convention, the WHO established the MPOWER package, which includes the 6 most important and effective tobacco-control policies proven to reduce tobacco use and SHS exposure: raising taxes and prices; banning advertising and promotion of tobacco products and sponsorship of sporting events by tobacco companies; protecting people from SHS; warning people about the dangers of tobacco; offering help to people who want to quit; and carefully monitoring the epidemic and prevention policies.[31]

## Traffic-related Pollution and Traffic Injury

Urban air pollution is largely and increasingly derived from vehicular combustion and power generation, leading to significant contamination from hazardous air pollutants including diesel particulates, nitrogen oxides, and sulfur dioxide (see Chapter 21). In the rapidly growing megacities of Asia, Africa, and Latin America, concentrations of pollutants rival and exceed those experienced in the industrialized countries in the early 20th century.[32] Outdoor air pollution is made worse in many LMICs because of the types of vehicles driven. In Southeast Asia and several other LMICs, most vehicles are 2- and 3-wheelers, including mopeds, motorcycles, scooters, and auto rickshaws. These types of vehicles use the more polluting 2-stroke engine technology, which contributes greatly to air pollution in urban areas.

Lead contamination from leaded gasoline has been a significant problem in rapidly industrializing countries. Currently, all but 3 countries have phased out the use of lead in non-aviation fuels.[33] Recycling of lead from vehicle batteries is also a significant contributor to community contamination and lead poisoning among children in LMICs.[34]

A WHO review of published childhood blood lead surveillance data found that 40% of children worldwide had blood lead concentrations greater than 5 mcg/dL, and 20% had blood lead concentrations greater than 10 mcg/dL.[35] Ninety percent of these high blood lead concentrations were observed in children who lived in LMICs. Fewer than 10% of the children had blood lead concentrations greater than 20 mcg/dL, but 99% of those children lived in these LMIC regions (see Chapter 32).

Road traffic injuries are a major public health problem. The 2009 WHO Global Status Report on Road Safety notes that death rates are twice as high in LMICs compared with high-income countries.[36] By 2020, road traffic deaths are expected to increase 92% in China and 147% in India, with an average increase of 80% in many other LMICS. Unlike high-income countries, where traffic injuries predominantly affect drivers, a far higher proportion of road deaths in LMICs occur among "vulnerable road users" including pedestrians, bicyclists, other non-motorized traffic, motorcyclists and moped riders, and passengers of buses and trucks.

## Industrialization and Hazardous Materials

Fossil fuel power plants, steel factories, and extraction operations with relatively little regulatory oversight or environmental impact reduction procedures have created severe air, water, and soil contamination in much of Central and Eastern Europe and other parts of the world. Many of the world's smelters are located in LMICs. Pollutants from these operations include mercury vapor, sulfur dioxide, nitrogen oxides, particulate matter, lead, chromium, arsenic, cadmium, zinc, copper, and heavy metals in mine tailings.

Metal contamination with mercury from gold mining and other heavy metals from uranium mines is a serious problem because these waste products are often disposed of in open dumps. Scavenging in these open dumps, particularly by children, has become a cottage industry and a means of support for many young people. Children and pregnant women also are exposed through participation in electronic waste recycling.[37] Small-scale industries, such as mining and battery recycling, are present in many LMICs.[38] Artisanal gold mining at the household level led to a fatal outbreak of lead poisoning in Nigeria.[39] Mercury contamination associated with small-scale gold mining and processing presents a major hazard in multiple countries in Latin America, Asia, and Africa.[40]

## Pesticides

Pesticides, including some banned in more developed countries, are widely used in LMICs. Lack of regulatory oversight, protective measures, and education increases the risk of significant exposure. Children experience exposure through pathways that may include exposures from household members who work with pesticides (so-called "take-home" exposures), drift from nearby spraying, residue on food crops, contact with treated foliage, contaminated water, or their own occupational or residential use of pesticides.

Although the sale of pesticides is higher in high-income countries, pesticide-related poisoning is more frequent in lesser resourced countries.[41] Pesticides marketed in LMICs may not meet internationally accepted quality standards and represent more toxic and environmentally persistent chemicals.[42] Data about poisoning among the general population in low-resourced countries are lacking, although up to one third of agricultural workers in low-income countries report a poisoning episode in the last year.[43] Data on worldwide prevalence of poisoning are difficult to obtain given the limited efforts at surveillance, even in high-income countries. Few worldwide data specific to children's exposures and poisonings are available. Most regional estimates are derived from hospitalizations and represent the most severe cases. Available studies suggest an incidence rate in the general population (non-occupational) of approximately 35 cases of acute pesticide poisoning per 100,000 people[44] (see Chapter 40).

## Climate Change

Some of the primary public health impacts of climate change include increased heat stress, worsened air quality, changes in vector-borne disease, extreme weather events, droughts, floods, and water scarcity (see Chapter 58). LMICs are the most vulnerable by virtue of having fewer resources to adapt socially, technologically, and financially. The rapid economic development and concurrent urbanization of poorer countries may lead to their increasing contribution to the problem, although at present, their contribution is lowest in terms of greenhouse gas emissions. In a comprehensive, peer-reviewed analysis of climate change effects on health, the WHO estimated that the changes that have occurred since the mid-1970s are causing more than 250,000 deaths per year.[45] These effects result from increases in diarrheal diseases, heat stress, malaria, and malnutrition that occur mainly in low-income countries.[45] Regions at highest risk include coastlines along the Pacific and Indian Oceans and sub-Saharan Africa. Large sprawling cities, with their urban "heat island" effect, are also prone to temperature-related health problems. The African region is gravely at risk of warming-related effects on infectious disease incidence and consequences.[46] An estimated 22 million climate refugees are present worldwide, and these populations are not officially protected under the 1951 Refugee Convention. As such, they are at high risk of lacking basic needs including access to food, clean water, and health care, including mental health care.[47]

## IMPLICATIONS FOR IMMIGRANT CHILDREN, INCLUDING FOREIGN ADOPTEES

A child's previous environmental setting or cultural identity and practices will guide a pediatrician's specific environmental health evaluation beyond routine screening and preventive health guidelines for adoptees and immigrant children.[48] Table 14-1 summarizes the key environmental exposures to consider for children who are immigrants. An environmental history can reveal potential hazardous exposures, such as residence near waste dumps or gold mining operations; living in home-based cottage industries involving lead exposure; consumption of potentially contaminated fish; or family use of ethnic remedies that may result in heavy metal exposure. Pediatricians who are not well acquainted with how to assess and manage a child's potential hazardous exposure can consult with a pediatric environmental health specialist (www.pehsuclassroom.net/lms).

Because elevated blood lead concentrations have been commonly observed among immigrant, refugee, and foreign adoptees from LMICs, it is appropriate to perform a blood lead test for these high-risk children. The Centers for Disease Control and Prevention issued specific guidance for testing of all immigrant and refugee children (www.cdc.gov/nceh/lead/Publications/RefugeeToolKit/Refugee_Tool_Kit.htm).

**Table 14-1. Identified Sources of Toxic Environmental Exposures Among Immigrant Populations**

| POTENTIAL TOXICANT | POSSIBLE EXPOSURE | ASSOCIATED CHAPTER FOR ADDITIONAL INFORMATION |
|---|---|---|
| Lead | Imported spices<br>Herbal, traditional, or imported medicinals<br>Imported, traditional cosmetics<br>Proximity to or work in lead battery recycling<br>Lead glaze in dishware or crystal | Chapter 32, Lead |
| Mercury | Contaminated fish<br>Proximity to or work in gold mining operations<br>Rituals (eg, Santeria) | Chapter 33, Mercury |
| Pesticides | Proximity to treated croplands, parent occupational exposures | Chapter 40, Pesticides |
| Arsenic | Imported spices<br>Herbal, traditional, or imported medicinal products<br>Groundwater contamination | Chapter 22, Arsenic<br>Chapter 19 Herbs, Dietary Supplements, and Other Remedies |
| Alcohol | Prenatal exposure | Chapter 8, Preconceptional and Prenatal Exposures<br>Chapter 48, Birth Defects and Other Adverse Developmental Outcomes |
| Radioactivity | Residential proximity to waste sites, spills | Chapter 31, Ionizing Radiation |
| Hazardous waste materials | Residential proximity to waste sites, spills | Chapter 13, Waste Sites |
| Tobacco, secondhand tobacco smoke | Prenatal and/or postnatal exposure<br>Work in tobacco fields | Chapter 43, Tobacco Use and Tobacco Smoke Exposure |

Alcohol consumption patterns vary widely among countries. Data on fetal alcohol exposure and related morbidity by country are limited, although available data find the highest rates in Croatia and South Africa.[49] Established protocols for assessment of fetal alcohol syndrome and effects should be used if there is suspicion based on phenotype or other features noted on physical examination or exposure assessment.

Biological assessment of mercury exposure may be considered for children who have lived in settings with presumed environmental contamination (eg, gold mining operations), participated in waste recycling, or where consumption of contaminated fish, medicinals, or spices is suspected.

People from several ethnic groups may use remedies that could contain toxic substances. Such remedies include azarcon, a lead-containing orange powder, and greta, a lead-containing yellow powder used by Mexican and Mexican-American people; pay-loo-ah, a lead- and arsenic-containing orange powder used by Hmong people; and ghasard, bala goli, and kandu, lead-containing brown, black, or red powders used by some American Indian people. Some Ayurvedic (pertaining to a traditional system of medicine native to India) medicines may contain lead or arsenic. Ritual practices may result in exposure to environmental contaminants. For example, some Hispanic people who practice Santeria may sprinkle elemental mercury in the house, possibly resulting in elevated levels of mercury in indoor air.

Because of increased monitoring, it is known that the population affected by arsenic contamination of groundwater is expanding. A careful physical examination can identify stigmata of arsenic exposure (eg, hyperkeratotic lesions of the palms and/or soles), although skin changes are unlikely until years after chronic exposure and generally occur only in settings of very high exposure. Biomarker assessment of arsenic exposure is limited by its rapid excretion. Urinary arsenic concentrations are useful for exposure assessment only if conducted within days of exposure; therefore, measurement will not be useful in most situations. In most cases of suspected exposure, it is prudent to consult with a pediatric environmental health specialist to best assess risk and improve communication with families (see Chapter 22).

## FUTURE DIRECTIONS AND NEEDS IN GLOBAL CHILDREN'S ENVIRONMENTAL HEALTH

Data on sources of specific contaminants, disease incidence, and biological monitoring in many LMICs are sparse. Efforts to measure children's environmental health risks, develop policies and programs to mitigate exposures worldwide, and strengthen efforts to address these problems are needed. This includes enhancing the education of pediatricians and others who care for children to recognize, treat, and promote prevention of pediatric environmental health hazards. International health tracks in pediatric residencies should also foster this education.

## Frequently Asked Questions

Q   *My partner and I are planning to adopt a child from outside of the United States. How can I find information about environmental exposures he or she may have been exposed to?*

A  Because exposure to lead and lead poisoning are more common in other nations, you may want to obtain a sample of the child's blood to determine the lead level. Other exposures depend on the country of origin. Consultation with an expert from the Pediatric Environmental Health Specialty Unit, or an expert in adoption, can help to determine any next steps.

## Resources

### AAP Red Book

https://redbook.solutions.aap.org/
Provides information about treating children with parasitic diseases or other infectious diseases associated with environmental hazards.

### Foreign adoption medicine resources

Web site: http://pediatrics.aappublications.org/content/pediatrics/early/2011/12/21/peds.2011-2381.full.pdf.
Many universities and hospitals have specialty international adoption medicine clinics that can provide specialty expertise for caring for foreign adoptees. The American Academy of Pediatrics Section on Adoption and Foster Care can help locate the closest resource.

### International Network for Children's Health, Environment and Safety

Web site: www.inchesnetwork.net

### International Pediatric Association

Web site: www.ipa-world.org

### World Health Organization (WHO) Children's Environmental Health

Web site: www.who.int/ceh/en
Links to publications and resources regarding national profiles, fact sheets, workshops, and statistics.

## References

1. Lopez G, Bialik K. Key findings about U.S. immigrants. Pew Research Center. May 3, 2017. http://www.pewresearch.org/fact-tank/2017/05/03/key-findings-about-u-s-immigrants. Accessed March 31, 2018

2. Bureau of Consular Affairs, U.S. Department of State. FY 2015 Annual Report on Intercountry Adoption. https://travel.state.gov/content/dam/aa/pdfs/2015Annual_Intercountry_Adoption_Report.pdf. Accessed March 31, 2018

3. Igielnik R, Krogstad JM. Key Facts. Where Refugees to the U.S. come from. Pew Research Center. February 3, 2017. http://www.pewresearch.org/fact-tank/2017/02/03/where-refugees-to-the-u-s-come-from/. Accessed March 31, 2018

4. World Bank. Population Ages 0-14 (% of total). https://data.worldbank.org/indicator/SP.POP.0014.TO.ZS. Accessed March 31, 2018

5. United Nations Department of Economics and Social Affairs. World Population Prospects: The 2017 Revision. June 21, 2017. https://www.un.org/development/desa/publications/world-population-prospects-the-2017-revision.html. Accessed March 31, 2018

6. Prüss-Ustün A, Wolf J, Corvalán C, Bos R, Neira M. Preventing Disease Through Healthy Environments 2016. WHO. http://apps.who.int/iris/bitstream/10665/204585/1/9789241565196_eng.pdf?ua=1. Accessed March 31, 2018

7. World Bank. Improved Water Source (% of population with access). http://data.worldbank.org/indicator/SH.H2O.SAFE.ZS. Accessed March 31, 2018

8. WHO/UNICEF. Progress on sanitation and drinking water 2015 update and MDG assessment. http://www.who.int/water_sanitation_health/publications/jmp-2015-update/en/. Accessed March 31, 2018

9. Mara D, Lane J, Scott B, Trouba D. Sanitation and health. *PloS Med*. 2010;7(11):e1000363

10. UNICEF Data: Monitoring the Situation of Children and Women. December 2017. Diarrheal Disease: Current Status and Progress. Updated December 2017. http://data.unicef.org/topic/child-health/diarrhoeal-disease/. Accessed March 31, 2018

11. George CM, Sima L, Arias MH, et al. Arsenic exposure in drinking water: an unrecognized health threat in Peru. *Bull World Health Organ*. 2014;92(8):565–572

12. Naujokas MF, Anderson B, Ahsan H, et al. The broad scope of health effects from chronic arsenic exposure: update on a worldwide public health problem. *Environ Health Perspect*. 2013;121(3):295–302

13. Bellinger D. Inorganic arsenic exposure and children's neurodevelopment: a review of the evidence. *Toxics*. 2013;1(1):2–17

14. World Health Organization. Water Sanitation Hygiene. Water related Diseases. Fluorosis. http://www.who.int/water_sanitation_health/diseases-risks/diseases/fluorosis/en/. Accessed March 31, 2018

15. Sun L, Gao Y, Liu H, et al. An assessment of the relationship between excess fluoride intake from drinking water and essential hypertension in adults residing in fluoride endemic areas. *Sci Total Environ*. 2013;443:864–869

16. Roser M. Employment in Agriculture. Our World in Data. 2017. https://ourworldindata.org/employment-in-agriculture. Accessed March 31, 2018.

17. European Environment Agency. *Children's Health and Environment: A Review of Evidence. A Joint Report from the European Environment Agency and the WHO Regional Office for Europe*. Environmental Issue Report No. 29. Copenhagen, Denmark: European Environment Agency; 2002. http://www.eea.europa.eu/publications/environmental_issue_report_2002_29. Accessed March 31, 2018

18. World Health Organization. Malaria Fact Sheet 2016. http://www.who.int/mediacentre/factsheets/fs094/en/. Accessed March 31, 2018

19. World Health Organization. Health and Environment Linkages Initiative. Vector-borne Disease. 2017. http://www.who.int/heli/risks/vectors/vector/en/. Accessed March 31, 2018

20. World Health Organization. World Malaria Report 2017. http://www.who.int/malaria/publications/world-malaria-report-2017/report/en/. Accessed March 31, 2018

21. United Nations Environment Programme. *Geo YearBook 2004/5: An Overview of Our Changing Environment*. Nairobi, Kenya: United Nations Environment Programme; 2005. https://wedocs.unep.org/rest/bitstreams/14963/retrieve. Accessed March 31, 2018

22. Martin WJ II, Glass RI, Araj H, et al. Household air pollution in low- and middle-income countries: health risks and research priorities. *PLoS Med*. 2013;10(6):e1001455

23. Bonjour S, Adair-Rohani H, Wolf J, et al. Solid fuel use for household cooking: country and regional estimates for 1980–2010. *Environ Health Perspect*. 2013;121(7):784–790

24. World Health Organization Guidelines for Indoor Air Quality: Household Fuel Combustion. 2014. http://apps.who.int/iris/bitstream/10665/141496/1/9789241548885_eng.pdf?ua=1. Accessed March 31, 2018

25. WHO Global Health Observatory Data. Mortality from Household Air Pollution. Situation and Trends. http://www.who.int/gho/phe/indoor_air_pollution/burden/en/. Accessed March 31, 2018

26. Rinne ST, Rodas EJ, Rinne ML, Simpson JM, Glickman LT. Use of biomass fuel is associated with infant mortality and child health in trend analysis. *Am J Trop Med Hyg.* 2007;76(3): 585–591

27. Lewis JJ, Pattanavak SK. Who adopts improved fuels and cookstoves? A systematic review. *Environ Health Perspect.* 2012;120(5):637–645

28. National Institutes of Health Office of Strategic Coordination. Household Air Pollution Investigation Network. https://commonfund.nih.gov/globalhealth/hapinresources. Accessed March 31, 2018

29. World Health Organization Tobacco Fact Sheet May 2017. http://www.who.int/mediacentre/factsheets/fs339/en/. Accessed March 31, 2018

30. Wipfli H, Avila-Tang E, Navas-Acien A, et al. Secondhand smoke exposure among women and children: evidence from 31 countries. *Am J Public Health.* 2008;98(4):672–679

31. World Health Organization. WHO Report on the Global Tobacco Epidemic, 2008. The MPOWER Package. Geneva, Switzerland: World Health Organization; 2008. http://www.who.int/tobacco/mpower/mpower_report_full_2008.pdf. Accessed March 31, 2018

32. Krzyzanowski M, Apte JS, Bonjour SP, Brauer M, Cohen AJ, Pruss-Ustun AM. Air pollution in the mega-cities. *Curr Environ Health Rpt.* 2014;1(3):185–191

33. UNEP. Leaded Petrol Phase-out: Global Status as of March 2017. https://wedocs.unep.org/bitstream/handle/20.500.11822/17542/MapWorldLead_March2017.pdf?sequence=1&isAllowed=y. Accessed March 31, 2018

34. Daniell WE, Van Tung L, Wallace RM, et al. Childhood lead exposure from battery recycling in Vietnam. *BioMed Res Int.* 2015;2015:193715

35. World Health Organization. *Quantifying Environmental Health Impacts. Annex 4. Estimating the Global Disease Burden of Environmental Lead Exposure.* http://www.who.int/quantifying_ehimpacts/publications/en/9241546107ann4-5.pdf. Accessed March 31, 2018

36. World Health Organization Global Status Report on Road Safety. Time for Action. https://books.google.com/books?hl=en&lr=&id=Ndrf6DuCQHMC&oi=fnd&pg=PP2&ots=tedFErhXXD&sig=EjsKq3BzRhxG8rS81mT7X2ig_SY#v=onepage&q&f=false. Accessed March 31, 2018

37. Grant K, Goldizen FC, Sly P, et al. Health consequences of exposure to e-waste: a systematic review. *Lancet Glob Health.* 2013;1(6):e350–e361

38. Dowling R, Caravanos J, Grigbsby P, et al. Estimating the prevalence of toxic waste sites in low- and middle-income countries. *Ann Glob Health.* 2016;82(5):700–710

39. Dooyema CA, Neri A, Lo Y-C, et al. Outbreak of fatal childhood lead poisoning related to artisanal gold mining in northwestern Nigeria, 2010. *Environ Health Perspect.* 2012;120(4):601–607

40. Gibb H, O'Leary KG. Mercury exposure and health impacts among individuals in the artisanal and small-scale gold mining community: a comprehensive review. *Environ Health Perspect.* 2014;122(7):667–672

41. Kesavachandran CN, Fareed M, Pathak MK, Bihari V, Mathur N, Srivastava AK. Adverse health effects of pesticides in agrarian populations of developing countries. *Rev Environ Contam Toxicol.* 2009;200:33–52

42. Ecobichon DJ. Pesticide use in developing countries. *Toxicology*. 2001;160(1-3):27–33

43. Corriols M, Marin J, Berroteran J, Lozano LM, Lundberg I. Incidence of acute pesticide poisonings in Nicaragua: a public health concern. *Occup Environ Med*. 2009;66(3):205–210

44. Thundiyil JG, Stover J, Besbelli N, Pronczuk J. Acute pesticide poisoning: a proposed classification tool. *Bull World Health Organ*. 2008;86(3):205–209

45. World Health Organization Climate Change and Health Fact Sheet. July 2017. http://www.who.int/mediacentre/factsheets/fs266/en/. Accessed March 31, 2018

46. Patz JA, Campbell-Lendrum D, Holloway T, Foley JA. Impact of regional climate change on human health. *Nature*. 2005;438(7066):310–317

47. UNHCR The UN Refugee Agency. Climate Change and Disasters. http://www.unhcr.org/en-us/climate-change-and-disasters.html. Accessed March 31, 2018

48. Seery T, Boswell H, Lara A. Caring for refugee children. *Pediatr Rev*. 2015;36:323–338

49. Lange S, Probst C, Gmel G, Rehm J, Burd L, Popova S. Global prevalence of fetal alcohol spectrum disorder among children and youth: a systematic review and meta-analysis. *JAMA Pediatr*. 2017;171(10):948–956

Chapter 15

# Human Milk

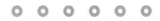

## KEY POINTS

- The benefits of breastfeeding greatly outweigh the potential risks in nearly every circumstance of possible contamination.
- The relatively high concentration of fat in human milk means that fat-soluble contaminants will, in effect, concentrate there. The quantities transferred can leave breastfed children with detectably higher body burdens of pollutants for years.
- Despite literature spanning over 50 years, there are very few instances in which morbidity has been described in an infant from a pollutant chemical in human milk and there is good evidence that little, if any, morbidity occurs from the more common and well-studied chemical agents.
- It is important to eliminate exposure to persistent bioaccumulating toxic chemicals to decrease the bioburden in children. The manufacture and use of dichlorodiphenyltrichloroethane (DDT), cyclodienes, and most polychlorinated biphenyls (PCBs) has been discontinued in the United States, but not in many other parts of the world.

## INTRODUCTION

Breastfeeding provides ideal nutrition for the healthy growth and development of infants. The World Health Organization (WHO),[1,2] the US Surgeon General,[3] and the American Academy of Pediatrics (AAP), both in previous editions of this book and in a policy statement,[4,5] have considered the problem of environmental contaminants in human milk and continue to recommend breastfeeding. Extensive research has documented the broad and compelling advantages for infants, mothers, families, and society related to breastfeeding. Some of the many benefits include immunological advantages, lower obesity rates, and greater cognitive development for the infant, as well as many health advantages for the lactating mother.[4] Although a number of environmental pollutants readily pass to the infant through human milk, the advantages of breastfeeding continue to greatly outweigh the potential risks in nearly every circumstance. Thus, the AAP recommends avoidance of breastfeeding only under exceptional circumstances (such as after incidents that are associated with release of chemicals into the environment) when the levels of environmental chemicals in breast milk may be significantly elevated.[5] So far, despite literature spanning over 50 years, there are very few instances in which morbidity has been described in an infant from a pollutant chemical in milk. There is good evidence that little, if any, morbidity occurs from the more common and well-studied chemical agents. This chapter will discuss chemicals that are known to appear in human milk.

In 1951, Laug et al[6] reported the presence of the persistent pesticide dichlorodiphenyltrichloroethane (DDT) in human milk. DDT or one of its derivatives, usually the very stable metabolite dichlorodiphenyldichloroethylene (DDE), has since been found in the lipid of essentially all human milk tested worldwide. Hexachlorobenzene; the cyclodiene pesticides, such as dieldrin, heptachlor, and chlordane (all organochlorines); and industrial chemicals, such as polychlorinated biphenyls (PCBs) and similar compounds, have been, and in some cases continue to be, common contaminants. These residues are present in the milk of women without occupational or other special exposures (see Table 15-1).[7] Following regulations aimed at reducing exposure to these compounds, levels of PCBs and persistent pesticides have declined. Levels of

## Table 15-1. Chemicals That May Be Found in Human Milk

| | |
|---|---|
| Chlordane | PCBs (polychlorinated biphenyls) |
| DDT (dichlorodiphenyltrichloroethane), DDE (dichlorodiphenyldichloroethylene) | PCDDs (polychlorinated dibenzodioxins) |
| Heptachlor | PCDFs (polychlorinated dibenzofurans) |
| Hexachlorobenzene | Perchlorate |
| Metals | PFOA (perfluorooctanoic acid) |
| Mycotoxins (ochratoxin A, aflatoxin M1, zearalenone) | PFOS (perfluorooctane sulfonate) |
| Nicotine and other components of tobacco smoke | Phthalates |
| | Sunscreens (ultraviolet [UV] filters) |
| PBDEs (polybrominated diphenyl ethers) | Volatile organic compounds |

the flame retardants polybrominated diphenyl ethers (PBDEs) have, however, increased.[8] Infant formula is free of these residues because the lipid comes from coconuts or other sources low on the food chain. Dairy cows do not have much exposure; in addition, a cow makes tons of milk during her lifetime, keeping the concentrations of pollutants low in any given volume of cow milk.

Human milk is the major dietary source of these stable pollutants for young children. The persistent lipophilic chemicals found in human milk are preferentially stored in the mother's adipose tissue. To create milk for her infant, a woman's body mobilizes lifetime fat stores and, therefore, transmits a portion of her stores of environmental contaminants to her newborn during breast-feeding. The relatively high concentration of fat in human milk means that fat-soluble substances will, in effect, concentrate there. Because hindmilk has a higher fat concentration (approximately 4% or more) than foremilk (approximately 2.5%), it is likely that fat-soluble contaminants would have higher concentrations in hindmilk. The quantities transferred can leave breastfed children with detectably higher body burdens of pollutants for years.[9]

The persistent fat-soluble chemicals that are discussed here are the most-studied human milk contaminants because they are lipophilic (and therefore, persistent) and there is a relatively large database about these chemicals in human milk. These data can be used to determine trends in chemicals over time and to examine associations between levels of chemicals and characteristics of the mother/infant.[10] Volatile organic hydrocarbons, phthalates, metals, and organometals also can contaminate human milk, although almost always at levels that are of much less toxicological concern than the persistent fat-soluble agents. Asbestos fibers or fine particulate air pollutants are not found in human milk. Much of this material was reviewed in a "mini-monograph" of the journal *Environmental Health Perspectives* in June 2002.[11]

## SPECIFIC AGENTS

Persistent organic pollutants (POPs) are a chemical class manufactured either for a specific purpose (eg, pesticides or flame retardants) or produced as a by-product of incinerated waste. POPs are released into the air, soil, and water, and find their way into the food chain. They are stable compounds that are not readily degraded in the environment, nor are they completely metabolized or excreted by organisms. POPs are ubiquitous and are usually low-level contaminants in humans worldwide.[12]

### DDT and DDE

DDT, an organochlorine pesticide once used widely in the United States, was banned from manufacture in 1972 after 4 decades of extensive global use. This decision was based on, among other things, its widespread appearance in human tissue and its effects on wildlife, especially reproduction in pelagic birds (those living in open oceans or seas rather than in waters near land). The metabolites *o,p'*-DDT and DDE are weak estrogens. The possibility that DDE may interfere with lactation performance or have other toxicities (an association with preterm birth has been reported)[13] became relevant with the resurgence of interest in DDT for malaria control.[14] An estrogen-like effect of DDE (ie, shortened duration of lactation) was seen in 2 studies, one in North Carolina and the other in Mexico.[15] Although a similar-sized effect was seen among Michigan women,[16] studies in upstate New York[17] and Mexico[18] saw no association between DDE and weaning. Similarly, high levels of DDT in human milk from South African mothers did not affect duration of lactation.[19] An inverse relationship between head circumference and DDT exposure was reported in a Turkish cohort.[20] Results from a Catalonian[21] birth cohort showed that prenatal exposure to *p,p'*-DDE was associated with a delay in mental and psychomotor development at age 13 months; a study in mostly migrant women in California showed similar developmental delays, but in association with DDT, the parent compound.[22] Long-term breastfeeding was found to be beneficial to neurodevelopment in both studies, despite exposure to these chemicals through human milk. In contrast, in a cohort of mother-infant pairs in North Carolina, lactational exposure to DDT and DDE was not associated with adverse infant neurodevelopment at age 12 months.[23] Control of malaria vectors with affordable, effective methods in developing countries will present public health dilemmas if DDT is deemed the most suitable agent and yet increases the risk of preterm birth and early weaning.[24] It is important to note that DDT concentrations in human milk have declined in most areas of the world, consistent with restrictions on its use.[25]

## PCBs, PCDFs, and PCDDs

PCBs, PCDFs, and PCDDs are widespread environmental contaminants. Numerous animal studies have indicated that PCBs, PCDFs, and PCDDs are neurotoxic.[26–29] Perinatal exposure to these compounds has been shown to affect brain dopamine concentrations and alter steroidal and thyroid hormone status in rats.[30]

PCBs are used as heat-exchange fluids in electrical transformers and capacitors, and as additives in paint, carbonless copy paper, and plastics. Persistence of PCBs varies with the degree of halogenation, with an estimated half-life of 10 years. Exposure to commonly encountered levels of PCBs can disrupt neuropsychological development[31] and is associated with lower developmental/IQ test scores. These include lower psychomotor scores from the newborn period through age 2 years, defects in short-term memory in children aged 7 months and 4 years, lowered IQs in children aged 42 months and 11 years, and other effects. Prenatal exposure to PCBs from the mother's body burden, rather than exposure through human milk, seems to account for most of the findings.[32] In a large cohort of Spanish children, increasing prenatal PCB-153 concentrations were associated with worse mental and psychomotor scores, although statistical significance was reached only for psychomotor development. Of note, the association between exposure and effects weakened during the postnatal period, suggesting that although breastfeeding increases children's blood POP levels during postnatal life, the deleterious effects of PCB-153 on neurodevelopment were primarily attributable to prenatal exposures.[33] More recently, total serum burden of organochlorine compounds was determined from birth until adolescence in 2 birth cohorts established in 1997 in Ribera d'Ebre and the island of Menorca, Spain. Although the overall concentrations of all organochlorine compounds decreased from birth until adolescence, the total serum burden of PCBs was higher in adolescents than at birth. Furthermore, increases in total serum burden of organochlorines occurred both in breastfed and non-breastfed children, but was significantly higher in children who were breastfed compared with those who were not breastfed.[34] A review of 41 studies found limited evidence of an association between prenatal exposure to these compounds (DDE, PCBs, and dioxins) and risk of respiratory infections.[35]

PCDFs are partially oxidized PCBs and are by-products of high-temperature processes, such as incomplete combustion (after waste incineration or automobile operation) and production of pesticides and PCBs. PCDFs were responsible for some of the toxicity seen in workers cleaning up office building transformer fires[36] and also in 2 Asian outbreaks of PCB poisoning from contaminated cooking oil[37] (see Chapter 38). In the Asian poisonings, infants seem to have been affected by exposure through human milk.[38,39] Background exposure to PCDFs likely comes mostly from diet, especially contaminated fish.[40]

PCDDs are similar to PCBs and PCDFs in that they have 2 linked phenyl rings with varying numbers of chlorines. The dioxins have 2 oxygen molecules between the phenyl rings. These compounds were formed during the manufacture of hexachlorophene, pentachlorophenol, and the phenoxy acid herbicides 2,4,5 trichlorophenoxyacetic acid (a component of Agent Orange, used as a defoliant during the Vietnam War) and silvex, under what would now be considered poorly controlled conditions. Significant pollution with dioxins also occurred during the Industrial Revolution in the mid-19th century. Dioxins also are formed, albeit at very low yield, during paper bleaching and waste incineration. One dioxin congener, 2,3,7,8-tetrachlorodibenzo-*p*-dioxin, may be the most toxic synthetic chemical known.[41] In a large study of Danish infants, dioxin levels in human milk samples, used as a proxy for maternal/prenatal exposure, were associated with lower weight and percent fat at birth, accelerated height and weight gain in infancy, and increased insulin-like growth factor-1 (IGF-1) concentrations at age 3 months.[42]

## Chlordane

In 1970, inadvertent injection of chlordane, an organochlorine insecticide, into the heating ducts of military homes resulted in air contamination when the heat was turned on. The US Air Force performed studies in almost 500 dwellings and found that although most homes had very little chlordane in the air, values were as high as 260 mcg/m$^3$. The symptoms abated and the air cleared when appropriate repairs were made.[25] Among women who lived in homes treated with chlordane, human milk levels of chlordane increased during the following 5 years.[43] In Japan, concentration of persistent organochlorines, including chlordane, in human milk from primiparous mothers was found to be significantly higher than from multiparous mothers, implying elimination of organochlorines via lactation. In addition, there was a significant positive correlation between organochlorine levels in human milk and the age of primiparous mothers.[44] In lactating Korean women, leptin levels in human milk were negatively associated with maternal serum chlordane levels, suggesting that exposure to POPs, such as chlordane, may be associated with alteration of lipid metabolism in lactating women.[45] However, there are no reports of infant morbidity attributable to this exposure. Furthermore, in countries with restrictions on chlordane use, levels in human milk have declined substantially over time.[8]

## Heptachlor

The agricultural use of heptachlor, an organochlorine cyclodiene pesticide, led to 2 major incidents in Hawaii and Arkansas. In January 1982, routine analysis of cow milk by the Hawaii State Health Department turned up an unexpected amount of heptachlor epoxide, the stable metabolite. The contamination was traced to the practice of feeding dairy cows "green chop," which is the leafy portion of the pineapple plant. In this case, the pineapple plants had been treated with heptachlor to control aphids and were harvested too soon. Retrospective testing of green chop samples showed that heptachlor was present as far back as June 1981. Human milk in Hawaii had previously been quite low in heptachlor epoxide; during this incident, the levels increased threefold but into the range of values reported from the US mainland.[46] In 1986, cow milk in Arkansas was found to be contaminated. This time, the cows had been fed mash left over from the fermentation of grain to produce ethanol for addition to gasoline. Analysis was conducted on 942 samples collected contemporaneously with the exposure, and human milk concentrations of heptachlor epoxide did not seem to be higher in Arkansas than in the adjoining southeastern states.[47] Thus far, no morbidity has been attributable to these exposures, but research continues in Hawaii.[48] The use of heptachlor in the United States is now limited to fire ant control.

## Hexachlorobenzene

Hexachlorobenzene was first introduced in the 1940s as a fungicide to treat seeds on food crops. This fungicide in human milk has caused disease in breastfed infants. After an epidemic of hexachlorobenzene poisoning in Turkey (1957–1959), porphyria did not develop in breastfed children as seen in adults but rather *pembe yara* (pink sore), characterized by weakness, convulsions, and an annular papular rash, was seen. The case-fatality rate was approximately 95%, and cohorts of children died in some of the villages. The chemical was present in human milk but not quantitated at the time; 20 years later, 20 samples that were analyzed had an average of 0.23 parts per million (ppm) of hexachlorobenzene.[49] If it is assumed that analysis was per g of milk fat, then levels remained approximately 15 times background levels, 20 years after the original poisoning.

Limited data are available on the levels of hexachlorobenzene in human milk in the United States. Other countries, however, have reported significant decreases in hexachlorobenzene levels in human milk since its discontinuation as a fungicide.[7] In Norwegian women, hexachlorobenzene levels in human milk were associated with lower birth weight and increased odds of being small for gestational age; however, after stratification, this association was present only amongst smokers.[50] In contrast, prenatal exposure to hexachlorobenzene in a Spanish cohort was shown to be positively associated with rapid weight gain and overweight in infancy.[51]

## Nicotine and Other Components of Tobacco Smoke

Nicotine, cotinine,[52] thiocyanate (a compound present in tobacco smoke derived from hydrogen cyanide), and other components of cigarette smoke[53] appear in the milk of smokers. A case report showed neonatal nicotine withdrawal in an infant exposed to heavy cigarette smoke both pre- and postnatally.[54] Smokers tend to wean their infants early, but whether this is a result of smoking is not known.[55] Limited evidence exists about a smoking effect on the child from components of smoke in human milk. Smoking immediately prior to breastfeeding may alter infants' sleep/wake patterning.[56] Although nursing mothers who smoke should be counseled about smoking cessation, the benefits of breastfeeding outweigh the deleterious effects of nicotine exposure. Some evidence has shown the protective effects of breastfeeding against lower respiratory tract illnesses in the offspring of smoking mothers.[57] Furthermore, breastfeeding may mitigate the adverse effects of maternal smoking during pregnancy on fetal neurodevelopment.[58]

The Internet has facilitated the process of sharing and selling human milk among women with abundance and families in need of extra human milk. Health authorities, however, do not support this informal sharing of unpasteurized human milk outside the purview of a recognized milk bank. A recent study of human milk samples purchased via the Internet showed that approximately half of the samples had detectable levels of nicotine or cotinine, indicative of active smoking or secondhand smoke exposure.[59] Buyers of human milk from the Internet should be aware that advertisements do not always include accurate information regarding the health status of the milk donors. Chapter 43 contains more information about tobacco and Chapter 28 contains information about electronic nicotine delivery systems.

## Perchlorate

Perchlorate is a powerful oxidant that is primarily used in rocket fuel, munitions, blasting operations, and fireworks, but is also present as a trace contaminant in some fertilizers. Perchlorate is a common contaminant of human milk because it is commonly found in water and food. In lactating mothers from Central New Jersey, average perchlorate levels in breast milk were $6.8 \pm 8.76$ ng/mL, suggesting widespread perchlorate exposure, and that human milk may be a source of perchlorate exposure in infants.[60] Perchlorate competes with iodide for uptake into the thyroid, thus interfering with thyroid hormone production.[61] One study found that 9 of 13 breastfeeding infants were ingesting perchlorate at a level exceeding the reference dose (an estimate of a daily oral exposure that is likely to be without an appreciable risk of adverse health effects over a lifetime) suggested by the National Academy of Sciences, and 12 of 13 infants did not have an adequate intake of iodine as defined by the Institute of Medicine.[62] To obtain sufficient iodine, lactating women should be encouraged to use iodized salt.

## Polybrominated Diphenyl Ethers and Persistent Perfluorinated Chemicals

Polybrominated diphenyl ethers (PBDEs) (see Chapter 37) are flame-retardant compounds used in a wide variety of consumer products throughout the world. They have been detected in human milk for the last 2 decades, and concentrations in North America are among the highest. Some of these compounds have neurological or developmental toxicity in laboratory animals, but it is unclear whether exposure is sufficient to produce detectable toxicity.[63] In Spanish mothers, increasing PBDE concentration in colostrum, particularly BDE-209, was associated with worse infant mental development, but not psychomotor development; after adjustment for other POPs, this association became slightly weaker.[64] In animal models, some of the PBDEs have been shown to interfere with thyroid hormone homeostasis; however, in a Norwegian cohort of lactating mothers, there was no association between PBDEs in human milk and TSH levels in the newborn. Of note, the PBDE levels in this cohort were comparable with those reported from some other European countries and Asia, but not from the United States or Canada, where reported levels are approximately one order of magnitude higher.[65] Furthermore, concentrations of PBDEs in human milk samples from lactating mothers in the United Kingdom did not decrease during 12 months of lactation.[66] Because of their potential toxicity and persistence, the industrial production of some of the PBDEs is restricted under the Stockholm Convention, a treaty to control and phase out major POPs.

Perfluoroalkyl and polyfluoroalkyl substances, such as perfluorooctane sulfonate (PFOS) and perfluorooctanoic acid (PFOA), can be found in human milk. These manmade organic chemicals have developmental toxicity in laboratory animals. Although PFOS and PFOA were detected in human milk from French women, no effect was observed between these levels and birth weight.[67] Exposure to PFOA prenatally and via human milk was positively associated with higher T4 levels in Dutch girls but not boys, suggesting that PFOA may be associated with T4 in a sex-specific manner.[68] Serum concentrations of polyfluoroalkyl substances were determined in girls aged 6 to 8 years living in Greater Cincinnati and the San Francisco Bay area; the duration of breastfeeding was associated with higher polyfluoroalkyl substance levels at both sites.[69] The effects of these substances on human infants have yet to be determined.[70,71]

## Phthalates

Phthalates are plasticizers found in flooring, personal care products, medical devices, and some food packaging. Some phthalates have been demonstrated to be antiandrogens in laboratory studies, resulting in altered Leydig cell differentiation and function, and decreased fetal testosterone production.[72–75] A Danish study of boys with cryptorchidism measured phthalates in human milk and endogenous sex hormones in the participants at age 3 months.[76] Although the authors found no difference in phthalate exposure between the boys with cryptorchidism and controls, boys whose mothers had higher levels of certain phthalates in their milk had lower concentrations of serum testosterone and higher concentrations of luteinizing hormone.[76] Analysis of human milk samples collected from lactating mothers in the Republic of Korea indicates that the median daily intake estimates of phthalates, including both monoester and diester forms, through human milk consumption range between 0.91 to 6.52 mcg/kg body weight for di-ethyl-hexyl phthalate (DEHP) and between 0.38 to 1.43 mcg/kg body weight for di-n-butyl phthalate (DnBP). Based on the estimated daily intake, 8% of infants exceeded the reference dose of antiandrogenicity for DEHP and 6% of infants exceeded the daily tolerable intake for DnBP.[77] The clinical significance of these findings is unknown. Phthalates are discussed further in Chapter 41, and endocrine disruptors are discussed in Chapter 29.

## Volatile Organic Compounds

Because halothane has been detected in the milk of a lactating anesthesiologist,[78] it may be presumed to be present in lactating women who undergo anesthesia using halothane. Volatile agents similar to anesthetic gases may be excreted through expired air, and their concentration in human milk should decline rapidly once exposure ceases. Many other commonly encountered volatile organic compounds, such as benzene, Freon, and methylene chloride, have been found in human milk but are of no known clinical significance.[79]

## Metals

Lead concentrations in human milk are low, and there are no modern reports of lead toxicity in a child who was breastfed by an asymptomatic mother. Lead was known historically to be toxic to breastfed infants of women who worked with it. Decades ago, there was much more lead in canned formula and evaporated milk than in human milk because of the soldered seams in the cans. The levels in formula are now quite low; formula must be prepared with lead-free water to remain that way (see Chapters 16 and 17). Lead in human milk can be a problem among women with unusually high exposures; this may include women born overseas, or those with pica or occupational and environmental exposures. In Turkey, lead levels in human milk samples were reported to be $391.45 \pm 269.01$ mcg/L in a small cohort; however, the authors did not report on lead levels in the infants.[80] A significant and strong correlation between lead levels in the mother and her child has been reported. Environmental maternal exposure to lead resulting in lead levels of less than 5 mcg/dL in pregnant mothers had no effect on infant birth weight or the fatty acid profile of human milk.[81] Among healthy pregnant women in Japan, lead levels in cord red blood cells (RBCs) were found to be approximately 60% of maternal levels, and remained constant in infant RBCs after 3 months of breastfeeding.[82] The Centers for Disease Control and Prevention's Advisory Committee on Childhood Lead Poisoning Prevention has published guidance on this topic and encourages mothers with lead levels of less than 40 mcg/dL to breastfeed.[83]

Levels of cadmium, arsenic, and metallic mercury are low in human milk. Methyl mercury, although relatively nonpolar, associates with protein and appears in human milk at concentrations lower than those in serum. In Iraq in 1972, methyl mercury-treated seed wheat inadvertently used to make bread produced mercury concentrations in human milk of approximately 200 parts per billion (ppb), which is 50 to 100 times the background exposure. There were thousands of cases of illness (see Chapter 33), including some that may have resulted from exposure to human milk alone.[84] The upper end of background exposure to methyl mercury has been studied among children in the Seychelle Islands[85] and the Faroe Islands,[86] where there is a relatively high dietary exposure from ocean fish or mammals; these studies show inconsistent results, with some effects seen from transplacental exposure in the Faroe Islands but not in the Seychelles. In neither case were effects seen that could be attributed to human milk exposure. In Japan, the mercury level in cord RBCs was 1.5 times higher than in the mothers, and it declined by approximately 60% in RBCs from infants after 3 months of breastfeeding, suggesting that breastfeeding did not pose a great risk to this population. In the same study, selenium levels in cord RBCs were comparable to maternal levels, and declined by 75% after 3 months of breastfeeding.[82]

## Sunscreens (UV filters)

Potential adverse effects induced by UV filters in experimental animals include reproductive/developmental toxicity and disturbance of the hypothalamic-pituitary-thyroid axis.[87,88] Researchers in Europe asked nursing mothers about their use of sunscreens and cosmetics that contained the sunscreen ingredients benzophenone 2, benzophenone 3, 3-benzylidene camphor, 4-methylbenzylidene camphor (4-MBC), octyl methoxycinnamate (OMC), homosalate, octocrylene, and octyl-dimethyl para amino benzoic acid (PABA). Responding to questionnaires, 78.8% of the women reported using products that contained sunscreens; 76.5% of human milk samples contained these chemicals. A high correlation was reported between mothers' use of these chemicals and their concentrations in human milk. Except for lipsticks (the ingestion of which is probably important), the authors stated that their results agree with studies in animals and humans showing dermal sunscreen absorption.[89] Other studies have reported that approximately 85% of human milk samples contained UV filters.[90,91] Given that some of these chemicals have endocrine activity in animals, exposures can be lessened if mothers abstain from using these products during their children's sensitive life stages.

## Mycotoxins

Mycotoxins are lipid-soluble toxins produced by molds. A number of mycotoxins, including ochratoxin A, aflatoxin M1, and zearalenone, may be found in the milk of exposed women.[92,93]

### Ochratoxin A

Ochratoxin A, a nephrotoxic and carcinogenic mycotoxin, is a worldwide contaminant of both human and animal food and is found frequently in human biological fluids. Ochratoxin A ingested by nursing mothers can appear in breast milk and be passed on to the infant during breastfeeding. In a longitudinal study of Chilean infants exposed to ochratoxin A, parallel collection of maternal blood, milk, and of infant urine samples was performed over a 6-month period. Ochratoxin A was detected in almost all maternal blood plasma, at concentrations ranging between 72 and 639 ng/L. The ochratoxin A concentrations in breast milk were, on average, one quarter of those measured in plasma, but a higher fraction of circulating ochratoxin A was excreted in colostrum than with mature milk. It was estimated that Chilean infants had an average intake of 12.7 ± 9.1 ng/kg body weight during the first 6 days after delivery, whereas intake with mature milk averaged close to 5.0 ng/kg body weight/day.[94] Similarly, ochratoxin A was found in 66% of human milk samples from a Brazilian cohort[95] and 96% of human milk samples from an Iranian cohort.[96] Infant morbidity related to exposure to ochratoxin A via breastfeeding has not been reported.

### Aflatoxin M1 and Zearalenone

Aflatoxin B1 is detoxified to aflatoxin M1, which is found in human milk[97,98] and has been determined by the International Agency for Research on Cancer as a possible human carcinogen.[99] Zearalenone is an endocrine disruptor that has been monitored in human milk in Italy.[100]

## DIAGNOSTIC METHODS

Many laboratories have equipment needed to measure some or all of the contaminant residues in human milk. However, any such analysis must be regarded as research because there are no standard quality assurance methods, no established normal values, and some evidence that, at least for PCBs, the variability of test results between laboratories is too great to allow a single sample to be interpretable. Analysis of human milk for these chemicals is not clinically useful.

## REGULATIONS

No regulations exist for chemical contaminants in human milk. Although it is tempting to apply the numbers used for infant formula, the risk-benefit analysis is not comparable. It is likely that all human milk is contaminated. The most difficult situation is encountered with the persistent fat-soluble agents, such as PCBs, because their levels in human milk have been at or near the upper regulatory allowances for formula or infant foods. For the other environmental contaminants, amounts in human milk are relatively low.

The most important action is to eliminate exposure to persistent bioaccumulating toxic chemicals. The manufacture and use of DDT, all of the cyclodienes, and most PCBs have been stopped in the United States, but not in many other parts of the world. Because 25% of the US food supply is imported, global action is necessary.

### Frequently Asked Questions

Q   *Should I get my breast milk tested for chemical pollutants?*

A   No. Residue levels of many chemicals can be found in milk; quantitating them is difficult, and there are no programs to promote quality assurance. Even if a very good laboratory generates results, there are no accepted normal or safe values against which to evaluate them. In most instances, the benefits of breastfeeding far outweigh any risks posed by most chemical contaminants.

Q   *Could my child's illness be caused by a contaminant in my breast milk?*

A   Nursing infants have been poisoned by contaminant chemicals in human milk, although in most cases, the mother herself also was ill. This phenomenon is extraordinarily rare. Investigating such a case would be regarded as research.

Q   *If I diet while I am breastfeeding, will that increase the levels of contaminants in my body because the same amount of contaminants will be dissolved in a smaller amount of fat? If I lose weight, will that lead to the contaminants coming out of fat and allow them to increase in my breast milk?*

A   No one has measured the levels of these chemicals in human milk during weight loss. The greatest reported average weight loss among women who breastfeed long-term is 4.4 kg[101] at 1 year, compared with a 2.4-kg loss in non-breastfeeding women. Other studies find little or no weight loss among breastfeeding women.[102] Overweight breastfeeding women who exercise and restrict calories can achieve that weight loss faster, and lose it mostly as fat.[103] Theoretically, because the same amount of chemical would be stored in 4.4 kg less tissue, mostly fat, weight loss might increase the concentration of the fat-soluble contaminants by up to 25%.

Breastfeeding does decrease the amount of these contaminants in a mother's body. The concentration per unit of milk would be higher if the mother had lost body fat, but there should be no "mobilization" beyond that. Little evidence exists that shows background exposure to contaminated human milk produces any ill consequences in children. Conversely, there is reasonable evidence that obesity in the mother does have consequences. Therefore, it is reasonable for a woman to follow a sensible diet and to exercise while she is breastfeeding her baby.

Q   *If I smoke, should I breastfeed?*

A   Human milk is ideal for infants, regardless of whether a mother smokes. Breastfeeding mothers should not smoke, however, because nicotine, thiocyanate, and other toxicants are transferred through the human milk to the infant. Another reason not to smoke and breastfeed is that infants of women who smoke are weaned at an earlier age. If a mother does continue to smoke, she should never breastfeed while smoking because a high concentration of smoke will be in close proximity to the infant. It is also advised not to smoke immediately before breastfeeding.[55]

Q   *What advice can be given to women affected by ⌐ radiation disaster, such as a reactor meltdown?*

A   Radioiodine and potassium iodide (KI) are secreted into human milk. A mother can continue to breastfeed her infant when the risk of exposure to radioactive iodine is temporary and if appropriate KI doses are given to the mother and infant within 4 hours of the radiation contamination. If this is not the situation, the mother and infant should receive priority for protective measures, such as evacuation. "Breastfeeding mothers should consider temporarily stopping breastfeeding and switching either to expressed milk (that was pumped and stored before the exposure) or ready-to-feed infant formula until the mother can be seen by a doctor for appropriate treatment with KI. If no other source of food is available for the infant, the mother should continue to breastfeed, after washing the nipple and breast thoroughly with soap and warm water and gently wiping around and away from the infant's mouth."[104]

## References

1. World Health Organization. Safe food: Crucial for child development. http://www.who.int/ceh/publications/en/poster15new.pdf. Accessed May 17, 2018

2. Consultation on assessment of the health risk of dioxins; re-evaluation of the tolerable daily intake (TDI): executive summary. *Food Addit Contam.* 2000;17(4):223–240

3. The Surgeon General's Call to Action to Support Breastfeeding. Washington, DC: US Dept of Health and Human Services, Office of the Surgeon General. 2011

4. Johnston M, Landers S, Noble L, Szucs K, Viehmann L. American Academy of Pediatrics, Section on Breastfeeding: Policy statement. Breastfeeding and the use of human milk. *Pediatrics.* 2012;129(3):e827–e841

5. Dorea JG. Policy statements on breastfeeding and human milk: additional comments. *Pediatrics.* 2012;130(2):e462–e464

6. Laug EP, Kunze FM, Prickett CS. Occurence of DDT in human fat and milk. *AMA Arch Ind Hyg Occup Med.* 1951;3(3):245–246

7. Solomon GM, Weiss PM. Chemical contaminants in breast milk: time trends and regional variability. *Environ Health Perspect.* 2002;110(6):A339–A347

8. Noren K, Meironyte D. Certain organochlorine and organobromine contaminants in Swedish human milk in perspective of past 20-30 years. *Chemosphere.* 2000;40(9-11):1111–1123

9. Longnecker MP, Rogan WJ. Persistent organic pollutants in children. *Pediatr Res.* 2001;50(3):322–323

10. LaKind JS, Amina Wilkins A, Berlin CM, Jr. Environmental chemicals in human milk: a review of levels, infant exposures and health, and guidance for future research. *Toxicol Appl Pharmacol.* 2004;198(2):184–208

11. Landrigan PJ, Sonawane B, Mattison D, McCally M, Garg A. Chemical contaminants in breast milk and their impacts on children's health: an overview. *Environ Health Perspect.* 2002;110(6):A313–A315

12. Nickerson K. Environmental contaminants in breast milk. *J Midwifery Womens Health.* 2006;51(1):26–34

13. Longnecker MP, Klebanoff MA, Zhou H, Brock JW. Association between maternal serum concentration of the DDT metabolite DDE and preterm and small-for-gestational-age babies at birth. *Lancet.* 2001;358(9276):110–114

14. Roberts DR, Manguin S, Mouchet J. DDT house spraying and re-emerging malaria. *Lancet.* 2000;356(9226):330–332

15. Gladen BC, Rogan WJ. DDE and shortened duration of lactation in a northern Mexican town. *Am J Public Health.* 1995;85(4):504–508

16. Karmaus W, Davis S, Fussman C, Brooks K. Maternal concentration of dichlorodiphenyl dichloroethylene (DDE) and initiation and duration of breast feeding. *Paediatr Perinat Epidemiol.* 2005;19(5):388–398

17. McGuiness B, Vena JE, Buck GM. The effects of DDE on the duration of lactation among women in New York State Angler Cohort. *Epidemiology.* 1999;10:359

18. Cupul-Uicab LA, Gladen BC, Hernandez-Avila M, Weber JP, Longnecker MP. DDE, a degradation product of DDT, and duration of lactation in a highly exposed area of Mexico. *Environ Health Perspect.* 2008;116(2):179–183

19. Bouwman H, Kylin H, Sereda B, Bornman R. High levels of DDT in breast milk: intake, risk, lactation duration, and involvement of gender. *Environ Pollut.* 2012;170:63–70

20. Yalcin SS, Orun E, Yalcin S, Aykut O. Organochlorine pesticide residues in breast milk and maternal psychopathologies and infant growth from suburban area of Ankara, Turkey. *Int J Environ Health Res.* 2015;25(4):364–372

21. Ribas-Fito N, Julvez J, Torrent M, Grimalt JO, Sunyer J. Beneficial effects of breastfeeding on cognition regardless of DDT concentrations at birth. *Am J Epidemiol.* 2007;166(10):1198–1202

22. Eskenazi B, Marks AR, Bradman A, et al. In utero exposure to dichlorodiphenyltrichloroethane (DDT) and dichlorodiphenyldichloroethylene (DDE) and neurodevelopment among young Mexican American children. *Pediatrics.* 2006;118(1):233–241

23. Pan IJ, Daniels JL, Goldman BD, Herring AH, Siega-Riz AM, Rogan WJ. Lactational exposure to polychlorinated biphenyls, dichlorodiphenyltrichloroethane, and dichlorodiphenyldichloroethylene and infant neurodevelopment: an analysis of the pregnancy, infection, and nutrition babies study. *Environ Health Perspect.* 2009;117(3):488–494

24. Longnecker MP. Invited commentary: why DDT matters now. *Am J Epidemiol.* 2005;162(8):726–728

25. Smith D. Worldwide trends in DDT levels in human breast milk. *Int J Epidemiol.* 1999;28(2):179–188

26. Bowman RE, Heironimus MP, Barsotti DA. Locomotor hyperactivity in PCB-exposed rhesus monkeys. *Neurotoxicology.* 1981;2(2):251–268

27. Schantz SL, Bowman RE. Learning in monkeys exposed perinatally to 2,3,7,8-tetrachlorodibenzo-p-dioxin (TCDD). *Neurotoxicol Teratol.* 1989;11(1):13–19

28. Schantz SL, Levin ED, Bowman RE, Heironimus MP, Laughlin NK. Effects of perinatal PCB exposure on discrimination-reversal learning in monkeys. *Neurotoxicol Teratol.* 1989;11(3):243–250

29. Tilson HA, Davis GJ, McLachlan JA, Lucier GW. The effects of polychlorinated biphenyls given prenatally on the neurobehavioral development of mice. *Environ Res.* 1979;18(2):466–474

30. Morse DC, Groen D, Veerman M, et al. Interference of polychlorinated biphenyls in hepatic and brain thyroid hormone metabolism in fetal and neonatal rats. *Toxicol Appl Pharmacol.* 1993;122(1):27–33

31. Ribas-Fito N, Sala M, Kogevinas M, Sunyer J. Polychlorinated biphenyls (PCBs) and neurological development in children: a systematic review. *J Epidemiol Community Health.* 2001;55(8):537–546

32. Schantz SL, Widholm JJ, Rice DC. Effects of PCB exposure on neuropsychological function in children. *Environ Health Perspect.* 2003;111(3):357–576

33. Gascon M, Verner MA, Guxens M, et al. Evaluating the neurotoxic effects of lactational exposure to persistent organic pollutants (POPs) in Spanish children. *Neurotoxicology.* 2013;34:9–15

34. Gascon M, Vrijheid M, Gari M, et al. Temporal trends in concentrations and total serum burdens of organochlorine compounds from birth until adolescence and the role of breastfeeding. *Environ Int.* 2015;74:144–151

35. Gascon M, Morales E, Sunyer J, Vrijheid M. Effects of persistent organic pollutants on the developing respiratory and immune systems: a systematic review. *Environ Int.* 2013;52:51–65

36. Schecter A, Tiernan T. Occupational exposure to polychlorinated dioxins, polychlorinated furans, polychlorinated biphenyls, and biphenylenes after an electrical panel and transformer accident in an office building in Binghamton, NY. *Environ Health Perspect.* 1985;60:305–313

37. Rogan WJ, Gladen BC, Hung KL, et al. Congenital poisoning by polychlorinated biphenyls and their contaminants in Taiwan. *Science.* 1988;241(4863):334–336

38. Harada M. Intrauterine poisoning: clinical and epidemiological studies and significance of the problem. *Bull Inst Const Med.* 1976;25(Suppl):1–66

39. Yu ML, Hsu CC, Gladen BC, Rogan WJ. In utero PCB/PCDF exposure: relation of developmental delay to dysmorphology and dose. *Neurotoxicol Teratol.* 1991;13(2):195–202

40. Wang RY, Needham LL. Environmental chemicals: from the environment to food, to breast milk, to the infant. *J Toxicol Environ Health B Crit Rev.* 2007;10(8):597–609

41. Baarschers W. Eco-facts and Eco-fiction: Understanding the Environmental Debate. New York, NY: Routledge; 1996:221

42. Wohlfahrt-Veje C, Audouze K, Brunak S, et al. Polychlorinated dibenzo-p-dioxins, furans, and biphenyls (PCDDs/PCDFs and PCBs) in breast milk and early childhood growth and IGF1. *Reproduction.* 2014;147(4):391–399

43. Lillie TH. Chlordane in Air Force Family Housing: A study of houses treated after construction. Brooks Air Force Base, Tc: USAF Occupational and Environmental Health Laboratory, Brooks Air Force Base. Report No: OEHL 81-45 1981

44. Kunisue T, Muraoka M, Ohtake M, et al. Contamination status of persistent organochlorines in human breast milk from Japan: recent levels and temporal trend. *Chemosphere.* 2006;64(9):1601–1608

45. Kim S, Park J, Kim HJ, et al. Association between several persistent organic pollutants in serum and adipokine levels in breast milk among lactating women of Korea. *Environ Sci Technol.* 2015;49(13):8033–8040

46. Pesticide HAP: Heptachlor epoxide in mother's milk, Oahu, August 1981-November 1982. Manoa, HI: University of Hawaii at Manoa; 1983

47. Mattison DR, Wohlleb J, To T, et al. Pesticide concentrations in Arkansas breast milk. *J Ark Med Soc.* 1992;88(11):553–557

48. Luderer U, Kesner JS, Fuller JM, et al. Effects of gestational and lactational exposure to heptachlor epoxide on age at puberty and reproductive function in men and women. *Environ Res.* 2013;121:84–94

49. Cripps DJ, Peters HA, Gocmen A, Dogramici I. Porphyria turcica due to hexachlorobenzene: a 20 to 30 year follow-up study on 204 patients. *Br J Dermatol.* 1984;111(4):413–422

50. Eggesbo M, Stigum H, Longnecker MP, et al. Levels of hexachlorobenzene (HCB) in breast milk in relation to birth weight in a Norwegian cohort. *Environ Res.* 2009;109(5):559–566

51. Valvi D, Mendez MA, Garcia-Esteban R, et al. Prenatal exposure to persistent organic pollutants and rapid weight gain and overweight in infancy. *Obesity* (Silver Spring). 2014;22(2): 488–496

52. Dahlstrom A, Ebersjo C, Lundell B. Nicotine exposure in breastfed infants. *Acta Paediatr.* 2004;93(6):810–816

53. Zanieri L, Galvan P, Checchini L, et al. Polycyclic aromatic hydrocarbons (PAHs) in human milk from Italian women: influence of cigarette smoking and residential area. *Chemosphere.* 2007;67(7):1265–1274

54. Vagnarelli F, Amarri S, Scaravelli G, Pellegrini M, Garcia-Algar O, Pichini S. TDM grand rounds: neonatal nicotine withdrawal syndrome in an infant prenatally and postnatally exposed to heavy cigarette smoke. *Ther Drug Monit.* 2006;28(5):585–588

55. Counsilman JJ, Mackay EV. Cigarette smoking by pregnant women with particular reference to their past and subsequent breast feeding behaviour. *Aust N Z J Obstet Gynaecol.* 1985;25(2): 101–107

56. Mennella JA, Yourshaw LM, Morgan LK. Breastfeeding and smoking: short-term effects on infant feeding and sleep. *Pediatrics.* 2007;120(3):497–502

57. Nafstad P, Jaakkola JJ, Hagen JA, Botten G, Kongerud J. Breastfeeding, maternal smoking and lower respiratory tract infections. *Eur Respir J.* 1996;9(12):2623–2629

58. Batstra L, Neeleman J, Hadders-Algra M. Can breast feeding modify the adverse effects of smoking during pregnancy on the child's cognitive development? *J Epidemiol Community Health.* 2003;57(6):403–404

59. Geraghty SR, McNamara K, Kwiek JJ, et al. Tobacco metabolites and caffeine in human milk purchased via the Internet. *Breastfeed Med.* 2015;10(9):419–424

60. Borjan M, Marcella S, Blount B, et al. Perchlorate exposure in lactating women in an urban community in New Jersey. *Sci Total Environ.* 2011;409(3):460–464

61. Ginsberg GL, Hattis DB, Zoeller RT, Rice DC. Evaluation of the U.S. EPA/OSWER preliminary remediation goal for perchlorate in groundwater: focus on exposure to nursing infants. *Environ Health Perspect.* 2007;115(3):361–369

62. Dasgupta PK, Kirk AB, Dyke JV, Ohira S. Intake of iodine and perchlorate and excretion in human milk. *Environ Sci Technol.* 2008;42(21):8115–8121

63. Costa LG, Giordano G. Developmental neurotoxicity of polybrominated diphenyl ether (PBDE) flame retardants. *Neurotoxicology.* 2007;28(6):1047–1067

64. Gascon M, Fort M, Martinez D, et al. Polybrominated diphenyl ethers (PBDEs) in breast milk and neuropsychological development in infants. *Environ Health Perspect.* 2012;120(12): 1760–1765

65. Eggesbo M, Thomsen C, Jorgensen JV, Becher G, Odland JO, Longnecker MP. Associations between brominated flame retardants in human milk and thyroid-stimulating hormone (TSH) in neonates. *Environ Res.* 2011;111(6):737–743

66. Harrad S, Abdallah MA. Concentrations of polybrominated diphenyl ethers, hexabromocyclododecanes and tetrabromobisphenol-A in breast milk from United Kingdom women do not decrease over twelve months of lactation. *Environ Sci Technol.* 2015;49(23):13899–13903

67. Antignac JP, Veyrand B, Kadar H, et al. Occurrence of perfluorinated alkylated substances in breast milk of French women and relation with socio-demographic and clinical parameters: results of the ELFE pilot study. *Chemosphere.* 2013;91(6):802–808

68. de Cock M, de Boer MR, Lamoree M, Legler J, van de Bor M. Prenatal exposure to endocrine disrupting chemicals in relation to thyroid hormone levels in infants - a Dutch prospective cohort study. *Environ Health.* 2014;13:106

69. Pinney SM, Biro FM, Windham GC, et al. Serum biomarkers of polyfluoroalkyl compound exposure in young girls in Greater Cincinnati and the San Francisco Bay Area, USA. *Environ Pollut.* 2014;184:327–334

70. von Ehrenstein OS, Fenton SE, Kato K, Kuklenyik Z, Calafat AM, Hines EP. Polyfluoroalkyl chemicals in the serum and milk of breastfeeding women. *Reprod Toxicol.* 2009;27(3-4): 239–245

71. Karrman A, Ericson I, van Bavel B, et al. Exposure of perfluorinated chemicals through lactation: levels of matched human milk and serum and a temporal trend, 1996-2004, in Sweden. *Environ Health Perspect.* 2007;115(2):226–230

72. Borch J, Dalgaard M, Ladefoged O. Early testicular effects in rats perinatally exposed to DEHP in combination with DEHA—apoptosis assessment and immunohistochemical studies. *Reprod Toxicol.* 2005;19(4):517–525

73. Borch J, Ladefoged O, Hass U, Vinggaard AM: Steroidogenesis in fetal male rats is reduced by DEHP and DINP, but endocrine effects of DEHP are not modulated by DEHA in fetal, prepubertal and adult male rats. *Reprod Toxicol.* 2004;18(1):53–61

74. Foster PM, Mylchreest E, Gaido KW, Sar M: Effects of phthalate esters on the developing reproductive tract of male rats. *Hum Reprod Update.* 2001;7(3):231–235

75. Gray LE Jr, Ostby J, Furr J, Price M, Veeramachaneni DN, Parks L. Perinatal exposure to the phthalates DEHP, BBP, and DINP, but not DEP, DMP, or DOTP, alters sexual differentiation of the male rat. *Toxicol Sci.* 2000;58(2):350–365

76. Main KM, Mortensen GK, Kaleva MM, et al. Human breast milk contamination with phthalates and alterations of endogenous reproductive hormones in infants three months of age. *Environ Health Perspect.* 2006;114(2):270–276

77. Kim S, Lee J, Park J, et al. Concentrations of phthalate metabolites in breast milk in Korea: estimating exposure to phthalates and potential risks among breast-fed infants. *Sci Total Environ.* 2015;508:13–19

78. Cote CJ, Kenepp NB, Reed SB, Strobel GE. Trace concentrations of halothane in human breast milk. *Br J Anaesth.* 1976;48(6):541–543

79. Pellizzari ED, Hartwell TD, Harris BS, Waddell RD, Whitaker DA, Erickson MD. Purgeable organic compounds in mother's milk. *Bull Environ Contam Toxicol.* 1982;28(3):322–328

80. Gurbay A, Charehsaz M, Eken A, et al. Toxic metals in breast milk samples from Ankara, Turkey: assessment of lead, cadmium, nickel, and arsenic levels. *Biol Trace Elem Res.* 2012;149(1):117–122

81. Baranowska-Bosiacka I, Kosinska I, Jamiol D, et al. Environmental lead (Pb) exposure versus fatty acid content in blood and milk of the mother and in the blood of newborn children. *Biol Trace Elem Res.* 2016;170(2):279–287

82. Sakamoto M, Chan HM, Domingo JL, Kubota M, Murata K. Changes in body burden of mercury, lead, arsenic, cadmium and selenium in infants during early lactation in comparison with placental transfer. *Ecotoxicol Environ Saf.* 2012;84:179–184

83. Centers for Disease Control and Prevention. Guidelines on the Identification and Management of Lead Exposure in Pregnant and Lactating Women. Atlanta, Georgia. http://www.cdc.gov/nceh/lead/publications/LeadandPregnancy2010.pdf. Accessed May 17, 2018

84. Bakir F, Damluji SF, Amin-Zaki L, et al. Methylmercury poisoning in Iraq. *Science.* 1973;181(4096):230–241

85. Clarkson TW, Magos L, Myers GJ. The toxicology of mercury—current exposures and clinical manifestations. *N Engl J Med.* 2003;349(18):1731–1737

86. Grandjean P, Weihe P, White RF, et al. Cognitive deficit in 7-year-old children with prenatal exposure to methylmercury. *Neurotoxicol Teratol.* 1997;19(6):417–428

87. Faass O, Schlumpf M, Reolon S, et al. Female sexual behavior, estrous cycle and gene expression in sexually dimorphic brain regions after pre- and postnatal exposure to endocrine active UV filters. *Neurotoxicology.* 2009;30(2):249–260

88. Schreurs R, Lanser P, Seinen W, van der Burg B. Estrogenic activity of UV filters determined by an in vitro reporter gene assay and an in vivo transgenic zebrafish assay. *Arch Toxicol.* 2002;76(5-6):257–261

89. Schlumpf M, Durrer S, Faass O, et al. Developmental toxicity of UV filters and environmental exposure: a review. *Int J Androl.* 2008;31(2):144–151

90. Krause M, Klit A, Blomberg Jensen M, et al. Sunscreens: are they beneficial for health? An overview of endocrine disrupting properties of UV-filters. *Int J Androl.* 2012;35(3):424–436

91. Schlumpf M, Kypke K, Wittassek M, et al. Exposure patterns of UV filters, fragrances, parabens, phthalates, organochlor pesticides, PBDEs, and PCBs in human milk: correlation of UV filters with use of cosmetics. *Chemosphere.* 2010;81(10):1171–1183

92. Marroquín-Cardona AG, Johnson NM, Phillips TD, Hayes AW. Mycotoxins in a changing global environment—A review. *Food Chem Toxicol.* 2014;69:220–230

93. Warth B, Braun D, Ezekiel CN, Turner PC, Degen GH, Marko D. Biomonitoring of mycotoxins in human breast milk: current state and future perspectives. *Chem Res Toxicol.* 2016;29(7): 1087–1097

94. Munoz K, Blaszkewicz M, Campos V, Vega M, Degen GH. Exposure of infants to ochratoxin A with breast milk. *Arch Toxicol.* 2014;88(3):837–846

95. Iha MH, Barbosa CB, Heck AR, Trucksess MW. Aflatoxin M1 and ochratoxin A in human milk in Ribeirão Preto-SP, Brazil. *Food Control.* 2013;40:310–313

96. Dehghan P, Pakshir K, Rafiei H, Chadeganipour M, Akbari M. Prevalence of ochratoxin A in human milk in the Khorrambid Town, Fars Province, South of Iran. *Jundishapur J Microbiol.* 2014;7(7):e11220

97. Ishikawa AT, Takabayashi-Yamashita CR, Ono EYS, et al. Exposure assessment of infants to aflatoxin M1 through consumption of breast milk and infant powdered milk in Brazil. *Toxins (Basel).* 2016;8(9):E246

98. Atasever M, Yildirim Y, Atasever M, Tastekin A. Assessment of aflatoxin M1 in maternal breast milk in Eastern Turkey. *Food Chem Toxicol.* 2014;66:147–149

99. International Agency for Research on Cancer. Aflatoxins. Lyon, France. 2018. https://monographs.iarc.fr/wp-content/uploads/2018/06/mono100F-23.pdf. Accessed September 17, 2018

100. Massart F, Micillo F, Rivezzi G, et al. Zearalenone screening of human breast milk from the Naples area. *Toxicol Environ Chem.* 2016;98:128–136

101. Dewey KG, Heinig MJ, Nommsen LA. Maternal weight-loss patterns during prolonged lactation. *Am J Clin Nutr.* 1993;58(2):162–166

102. Schauberger CW, Rooney BL, Brimer LM. Factors that influence weight loss in the puerperium. *Obstet Gynecol.* 1992;79(3):424–429

103. Lovelady CA, Garner KE, Moreno KL, Williams JP. The effect of weight loss in overweight, lactating women on the growth of their infants. *N Engl J Med.* 2000;342(7):449–453

104. Paulson JA, American Academy of Pediatrics Council on Environmental Health. Pediatric considerations before, during, and after radiological/nuclear emergencies. *Pediatrics.* (in press)

Chapter 16

# Infant Formula

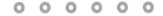

## KEY POINTS

- Although breastfeeding is recommended by the American Academy of Pediatrics and the World Health Organization, formula is widely used for infant feeding.
- Soy-based formulas contain isoflavones, a class of phytoestrogens.
- Genistein, an isoflavone found in soy-based formula, can bind to estrogen receptors. Although there is strong evidence of genistein's toxicity in animal models, data are insufficient to determine conclusively if ingestion of soy formula by infants results in adverse effects.
- Soy formulas are only indicated for infants with galactosemia, primary lactase deficiency, some infants with secondary lactase deficiency, and in situations where a vegan diet is preferred.
- The use of contaminated well water or other contaminated water to reconstitute infant formulas may result in exposure to chemicals such as lead, nitrates, arsenic, pesticides, and fluoride, and to bacteria, viruses and protozoa.

## INTRODUCTION

Although breastfeeding is recommended by the American Academy of Pediatrics (AAP) and the World Health Organization (WHO), formula is widely used for infant feeding. In the United States in 2011, approximately 20% of newborn infants and 50% of infants aged 6 months were fed formula. Although other formulas are available for special indications, nearly all formulas sold in the United States are based either on protein from cow milk or soybeans. The scope of this chapter is limited to people living in the rich countries of the world. For low-income countries, contamination of infant formula with infectious agents is a major issue.

This chapter focuses mainly on isoflavones in soy infant formula and briefly describes contaminants in or from the use of soy formula or cow milk-based formula (ie, aluminum and manganese, bacteria, melamine, contaminated water sources, and plasticizers in baby bottles). Some of these contaminants are described in more detail in Chapters 18 and 38.

## SOY FORMULA

Indications are few for the use of soy formulas (also known as soy-based formula or soy protein-based formula).[1] Soy formulas are lactose free and, thus, are indicated for infants with galactosemia, primary lactase deficiency (an extremely rare condition), some infants with secondary lactase deficiency, and in situations in which a vegan diet is preferred.[1] Sensitization to soy has been reported in infants with IgE-mediated cow milk allergy[2,3] and cow milk protein-induced enteropathy or enterocolitis; therefore, the AAP recommends using extensively hydrolyzed protein formula in these infants.[1] Soy formulas are not recommended for preterm infants.

Among infants in the United States who received formula, National Health and Nutrition Examination Survey (NHANES) data suggest that 69% consumed cow's milk formula, 12% consumed soy formula, and 11% consumed special formulas.[4] Based on 2009 market data, sales of soy formula in the United States represent about 12% of the total dollar sales for infant formula—almost a 50% decrease from 1999. The sale of soy formula varies geographically, ranging from 2% to 7% of infant formula sales in the United Kingdom, Italy, and France, to 13% in New Zealand, and to 31.5% in Israel.[5]

### Isoflavones in Soy Protein-based Formulas

Soy formulas contain isoflavones, a class of phytoestrogens. Phytoestrogens are plant-based compounds found in many foods, including tofu and soy milk,[6] that are able to produce some or all of the effects of estrogen. It is the presence of these compounds that led to the promotion of soy products to alleviate menopausal and other symptoms in adults. Genistein and daidzein, the primary isoflavones in soy formula, have structures similar to 17-β estradiol, can bind to estrogen receptors, and have weak estrogenic effects.[7] An infant fed soy formula has a daily exposure to total isoflavones that may be 6 to 11 times higher on a body weight basis than the dose that may affect menstrual cycle function in women ingesting soy proteins.[7] Whole blood genistein levels in infants fed soy formula are almost 50 times higher than in infants fed cow milk formula, 70 times higher than in breastfed infants, and 20 times higher than in vegetarians and vegans in Oxford, England.[8] The United Kingdom, Australia, New Zealand, and Israel have issued position statements suggesting restricted use of soy infant formulas.[9] The concern is based largely on studies in laboratory animals and *in vitro* experiments. The 2008 policy statement from the AAP Committee on Nutrition regarding soy formula provides relatively limited indications for its use in US infants.[1]

## Soybean Protease Inhibitor and Phytates in Soy Formulas

Soybean-based products contain heat-labile factors, such as soybean protease inhibitor, which have properties of an antitrypsin, antichymotrypsin, and antielastin;[10] 80% to 90% of this inhibitor is inactivated by heating soybean protein isolate, and thus is nutritionally irrelevant in soy formulas. Soy formulas also contain 1.5% phytates that bind minerals (20% more calcium and phosphorus compared with cow milk-based formulas; iron and zinc); therefore, soy protein-based formulas are fortified with iron, zinc, phosphorus, and calcium.

## Aluminum and Manganese in Soy Formulas

Aluminum, one of the most common metals on earth, has no known biological function. It is widely used in manufacturing and packaging and thus is a common contaminant of water, food, and medication. The main route of exposure is ingestion, but aluminum is poorly absorbed from the gastrointestinal tract. Aluminum that is absorbed is cleared by the kidneys; therefore, there is concern about aluminum toxicity for people with renal disease. Aluminum is present in cow milk-based formula and soy formulas; aluminum concentrations in both types of formula are higher than what is found in human milk. Although there is no evidence thus far of aluminum toxicity related to formula ingestion, there have been calls for reducing the aluminum concentration in infant formulas. More studies are needed to better describe effects, if any, from aluminum in formula, especially among children who are preterm or have renal or gastrointestinal diseases.

Infants fed soy infant formula consume greater amounts of manganese than do breastfed infants. The high concentration of manganese in soy-based formula (367 mcg/L, not fortified) is likely the result of high concentrations in soy.[12] Excessive manganese exposure is neurotoxic, especially in the presence of hepatic dysfunction. In cynomolgus macaque monkeys, chronic exposure to manganese was associated with subtle deficits in spatial working memory, modest decreases in spontaneous activity and manual dexterity, and an increase in stereotypic or compulsive-like behaviors such as compulsive grooming.[13] However, under normal circumstances, reduced gastrointestinal absorption, enhanced liver metabolism, and increased biliary excretion regulate manganese homeostasis and protect the infant from the effects of excessive dietary intake of manganese.

## ROUTES OF EXPOSURE

The levels of isoflavones in cord blood, amniotic fluid, human milk, and infant plasma and urine have been measured, providing evidence that isoflavones pass from the mother to the infant and that they are absorbed from infant formulas.[7,14–16] Infants ingesting human milk or cow milk-based formulas consume less than 1/200th as much isoflavones daily as do infants ingesting soy formula. Infants and adults who consume soy products also absorb isoflavones.

## HEALTH EFFECTS OF SOY PROTEIN-BASED INFANT FORMULAS

Few studies have been conducted in experimental animals of the effects of soy infant formula on reproduction and development; thus, direct observation of soy formula's adverse effect has been limited. More often, ingestion or injection of genistein is used in these animal studies. Although the effects of genistein ingestion or injection may not be directly extrapolated to human infants fed soy formula, the endpoints in animal studies have been relevant in suggesting possible effects of soy formula in humans, given the scarcity of human studies.

### Reproductive Effects

Experimental animal models or *in vitro* studies indicate that exposure to genistein may adversely affect growth and possibly survival, and may result in lower neonatal testosterone concentrations[17] but normal testosterone levels in adult marmoset monkeys.[18] Puberty onset, progression, and adulthood fertility were not affected in the soy formula-fed marmosets.[18] Shorter anogenital distance and hypospadias were reported in male mice exposed prenatally to genistein.[19,20] In contrast to male reproduction, the effects of genistein exposure on female reproductive function have received more attention. Studies in rodents given subcutaneous injections of genistein revealed a dose-dependent increase in the numbers of multi-oocyte follicles in the ovary, similar to observations following use of other endogenous and synthetic estrogens (ie, 17-B estradiol, diethylstilbestrol [DES], bisphenol A [BPA]).[21] Although the reproductive consequences of multi-oocyte follicles are not clear, this may signal permanently altered ovarian differentiation and decreased fertility later in life. Genistein also may affect hypothalamic-pituitary-gonadal function, disrupt estrous cyclicity, and reduce fertility. Chronic genistein exposure during fetal and immediate postnatal life has led to ductal/alveolar hyperplasia of the mammary gland in pups.[22] Neonatal exposure to genistein induced uterine adenocarcinoma in experimental animal models.[23] Studies from the National Toxicology Program (NTP) suggest a higher risk of mammary and pituitary gland adenomas and adenocarcinomas in female rats fed genistein for up to 2 years.[24] Other reproductive effects of genistein exposure include accelerated vaginal opening, decreased anogenital distance, and alterations in uterine and ovarian histopathology.[25]

Despite convincing evidence of relatively high exposures, the biologic activity of isoflavones in infants fed soy formulas remains unclear. Nearly all phytoestrogens in soy formula are bound to sugar molecules and these phytoestrogen-sugar complexes ("glucosides") are not generally considered hormonally active.[6,14] Once absorbed, as much as 97% to 99% of circulating phytoestrogens in human blood are in a conjugated form.[7]

A report from Puerto Rico found that soy formula use was associated with premature thelarche in girls before age 2 years.[26] Other factors, including maternal history of ovarian cysts, consumption of fresh chicken, and exposure to phthalate have been considered but the cause of premature thelarche in Puerto Rican girls remains unknown.[26] These findings have not been observed in other populations, and thus the association between soy formula use and premature thelarche remains speculative. Phthalate exposure was also considered by other investigators. Another study compared children fed soy formula with those fed other formulas for signs of precocious puberty, but the sample size was very small.[27] An Israeli study found that girls fed soy formula had a higher prevalence of palpable breast buds in the second year of life, suggesting prolonged presence of infantile breast tissue.[28] In a very small pilot study, 6-month-old girls fed soy formula had a tendency toward a more "estrogenized" profile of their vaginal epithelial cells (shed cells collected with a cotton-tipped swab of the introitus); the authors emphasized the potential utility of this method for assessing estrogen exposure rather than any effect of formula.[29]

The only epidemiologic study among adults who were fed soy formula during infancy indicated longer duration of menstrual bleeding and more discomfort with menstrual periods in women but did not find associations with age at menarche or with menstrual cycle length or regularity.[30] This study was not large enough to demonstrate the safety of soy formula use on reproduction, and there have been no similar studies with a larger sample size on adult fertility and pregnancy outcomes.

## Thyroid Function

In a rodent model, genistein exposure was shown to inhibit thyroid peroxidase but had no effect on serum triiodothyronine, thyroxine, and thyroid-stimulating hormone (TSH) concentrations.[31]

Limited information is available on the effects of soy formula on thyroid function in newborns. Before 1959, development of goiter after soy formula consumption was reported,[32] but its incidence was eliminated after adding iodine to the formulas. There are case reports of insensitivity to thyroxine treatment in infants with congenital hypothyroidism at the time of soy formula use, and switching to cow milk-based formula improved the treatment effect.[33,34] Furthermore, prolonged increase in TSH levels has been reported in soy formula-fed infants with congenital hypothyroidism compared with infants with congenital hypothyroidism who were fed non-soy formula.[35] It may be that the phytates in soy protein isolate interfere with iodine metabolism and thyroid hormone.[36] A case-control study of children with autoimmune thyroid diseases (Hashimoto thyroiditis or Graves disease) indicated a higher percentage of soy formula use in these cases than in healthy siblings or unrelated control children.[37] It is not clear whether this can be explained by a greater likelihood of soy formula consumption in atopic infants who have such antibodies. Currently, limited information is available on the use of soy formula and its effects on TSH or thyroid hormone.

## Immune Function

Results of animal studies on genistein's immunotoxicity are not consistent.[25] Early studies in rodents found decreased thymic weight and a reduced number of thymocytes. The feeding study in twin marmosets did not find a difference in thymic weight between soy formula-fed and cow milk-fed monkeys.[18] Genistein was found to inhibit both humoral and cell-mediated immune responses in some studies, but other studies did not find such effects.[38] It is possible that the effect of isoflavones on immune function vary by age, sex, species, and dosing regimens.

Soy formula use does not prevent allergic diseases[39] and does not affect the immune response. Although some older soy formulations may have interfered with immune response,[6] more recent studies found that soy formula-fed babies have a normal immune response to vaccinations.[40,41] However, soy formula-fed babies had higher levels of antibody to *Haemophilus influenza* type b at ages 7 and 12 months compared with the group fed cow milk formula or human milk, and their polio viral neutralization antibody at age 12 months was lower.[40] Soy formula-fed babies had immune cell counts similar to those babies fed cow milk formula or human milk, except that the percentage of CD57$^+$ natural killer T-cells was lower at age 12 months in infants fed soy formula.[41] A meta-analysis showed that the number of episodes of respiratory infections or acute diarrhea was similar between infants fed soy formula compared with infants fed human milk or cow milk-based formula.[42]

## Other Effects

One study compared cholesterol fractional synthesis rate (FSR), an indicator of endogenous cholesterol synthesis, in infants fed human milk, cow milk-based formula, and soy formula at age 4 months.[43] Soy formula-fed babies had the highest FSR, probably because of the absence of cholesterol contents in soy formula. Human milk-fed infants had the lowest FSR, and supplementing soy formula with cholesterol only slightly lowered the FSR, compared with no supplementation. Other studies examined the effect of soy infant formula on type 1 diabetes mellitus and cognitive function in children, but these studies were relatively small or designed for other purposes.[44,45] High levels of maternal soy consumption have been linked to the development of infant leukemia (acute lymphoblastic leukemia [ALL] and acute myeloid leukemia [AML]).[46]

## Growth and Development

Studies have documented normal growth trajectories in full-term babies fed soy infant formulas.[1,42] Soy formulas are not recommended for preterm babies however, because studies of mostly very low birth weight (less than 1,500 g) infants fed soy formula showed decreased growth rates, albumin concentrations, and bone mineralization in the first several months of life.[1,11]

The short- and long-term effects of soy formula use in childhood and adult life remain to be determined by well-designed, large-scale epidemiologic studies.

Studies in humans of soy formula use are summarized in Table 16-1.

## CONTROVERSIES REGARDING EFFECTS OF ISOFLAVONES IN SOY INFANT FORMULA

Although soy infant formulas have been used for approximately 50 years, relatively few studies have described the potential health risks in human infants or children. Many effects of environmental exposures, however, can only be revealed by well-designed epidemiologic studies, as in the cases of secondhand smoke and lead exposure. High levels of isoflavone intake and strong evidence of genistein's toxicity in animal models lead to legitimate concerns, but clear advice on soy formula use in infants needs relevant studies in humans. Studies in laboratory animals have found that high doses of genistein can disrupt reproduction and development. There are documented differences, however, in physiology between humans and laboratory animals, exposures (soy formula versus genistein), route of exposure (ingestion versus injection), and dosage (ad lib feeding versus repeated high dose). Integration of data from human studies with the results of laboratory experiments is not yet possible. A better estimate of the estrogenicity of isoflavones is still needed because this is relevant to the strength of an estrogenic effect in humans. Genistein has a higher affinity for estrogen receptor $\beta$ than for estrogen receptor $\alpha$. However, the 2 estrogen receptors are not equally distributed in tissues; thus, the estrogenic effects vary by tissue. The lack of large-scale epidemiologic studies and clinical observations in children fed soy formula as infants complicates the situation. Recognizing the controversy, several advisory committees in Australia, New Zealand, and Europe suggested limiting soy formula use in infants if other alternatives are available.[9] In 2006, the National Toxicology Program Center for Evaluation of Risk to Human Reproduction (NTP-CERHR) evaluated reproductive and developmental toxicity of genistein

## Table 16-1. Human Studies of Soy Infant Formula Use

| OUTCOME | AUTHOR, YEAR OF PUBLICATION | METHODS AND SUBJECTS | FINDINGS |
|---|---|---|---|
| Premature thelarche | Freni-Titulaer et al,[26] 1986 | Case-control study of 120 girls with premature thelarche and 120 matched controls | Soy formula use increased risk |
| Reproductive development | Giampietro et al,[27] 2004 | 48 soy formula-fed children and 18 controls | No signs of precocious puberty in girls or of gynecomastia in boys |
| Breast bud persistence | Zung et al,[28] 2008 | Cross-sectional study of 92 soy formula-fed and 602 human milk- or cow milk formula-fed female infants | Soy group had higher prevalence of breast buds (1.5 cm) than milk group in the second year of life but not in the first year |
| Adult reproduction | Strom et al,[30] 2001 | Controlled but not randomized feeding study in infancy, follow-up at early adulthood, 120 males and 128 females fed soy formula, 295 males and 268 females fed cow milk formula | Soy formula use increased duration of menstrual bleeding and discomfort with menstrual periods but did not affect puberty or menstrual cycle length or regularity |
| Breast cancer development | Boucher et al,[47] 2008 | Population-based case-control study of women aged 25-74 years diagnosed with breast cancer, 372 women with cancer, and 356 women without cancer, who were fed soy formula, cow milk formula, or human milk | A reduced, but not significant, association was found between soy formula intake and breast cancer |

## Table 16-1. Human Studies of Soy Infant Formula Use (*continued*)

| OUTCOME | AUTHOR, YEAR OF PUBLICATION | METHODS AND SUBJECTS | FINDINGS |
|---|---|---|---|
| Autoimmune thyroid disease | Fort et al,[37] 1990 | Case-control study of 59 children with autoimmune thyroid disease, 76 healthy siblings, and 54 healthy unrelated control children | Patients with autoimmune thyroid disease had higher percentages of soy formula feeding (31%) than did healthy siblings (12%) or healthy controls (13%) |
| Immune function | Ostrom et al,[40] 2002 Cordle et al,[41] 2002 | Randomized feeding study of 94 infants fed soy formula with added nucleotides and 92 infants fed soy formula without added nucleotides, plus nonrandomized groups of 81 infants fed human milk or cow milk formula | Total IgG concentrations similar. Soy-fed infants had higher *H influenzae* type b antibody and lower polio neutralizing antibody concentrations. Soy-fed infants had more physician-reported diarrhea. Immune cell (B, T, natural killer cells) status similar; soy-fed infants had lower CD57$^+$ natural killer T-cells |

and soy formula; they concluded that purified genistein can produce reproductive and developmental toxicity in rodents,[25] but the effects of soy formula in humans could not be determined because of insufficient data.[6] In 2008, the AAP Committee on Nutrition reviewed the existing studies on isoflavones in soy formula and child health but found no conclusive evidence that dietary soy isoflavones can adversely affect human development, reproduction, or endocrine function.[1] Similarly, in 2009, the NTP-CERHR reevaluated reproductive and developmental toxicity related to soy formula and concluded that there was "minimal concern" for adverse developmental effects in infants fed soy formula.[48] A more recent meta-analysis assessing the safety of soy-based formula concluded that there were no differences in growth patterns; bone health; neurocognitive functioning; and metabolic, reproductive, endocrine, and immune functions between infants fed soy formula versus either cow milk formula or human milk.[42] Currently, there are insufficient human data to determine conclusively if there are adverse effects of soy infant formula on reproduction, development, thyroid hormones, or immune function.[1,6,49]

## DIAGNOSTIC METHODS

Soy formula use can be identified through infant feeding history. Isoflavone concentrations in plasma samples have previously been quantified.[50] Urine samples in diapers and saliva samples also can be used to analyze isoflavone excretion in infants.[8,51] These assays, however, are only available in research settings.

## TREATMENT OF CLINICAL SYMPTOMS

Currently, data are insufficient to define clinical symptoms from isoflavones in soy infant formula. However, if isoflavones cause any symptoms, switching to cow milk-based formula may alleviate the symptoms.

## PREVENTION OF EXPOSURE

Consumption of soy infant formula usually is voluntary (ie, at the discretion of parents). To prevent isoflavone intake, parents can simply decide to use human milk or cow milk-based formula. Infants who have cow milk protein-induced enteropathy or enterocolitis can be provided formula with hydrolyzed protein or synthetic amino acid.[1]

Infant formula is regulated as food by the Food and Drug Administration (FDA). The FDA has requirements for nutrients in infant formulas; however, it does not regulate isoflavone levels in soy formula. Isoflavone levels in soybeans can vary by geographic location, climate, and other environmental conditions. Depending on isoflavone levels in soy formula and daily formula consumption, infants consuming soy formula have an estimated intake of total isoflavones (in unconjugated isoflavone equivalents) of 2 to 12 mg/kg of body weight per day.[6] The intake of genistein, expressed in aglycone equivalents, is estimated to range between 1 to 6 mg/kg of body weight.[49] Efforts can be directed toward reducing isoflavone concentrations in soy protein isolates in the future (ie, using ion exchange technology) if isoflavones in soy formula remain a continuing source of concern.

## POSSIBLE CONTAMINANTS IN INFANT FORMULA

The use of well water or other contaminated water sources to reconstitute formulas may lead to infant exposure to lead, nitrates, arsenic, pesticides, and fluoride, and to bacteria, viruses and protozoa.

## Lead

Lead is a well-documented neurotoxic metal. Although the intake of lead from infant formulas is relatively low, lead contamination of water used to reconstitute formula can result in increased exposure. Effects of lead exposure in childhood are described in Chapter 32.

## Organochlorine Compounds

Organochlorine compounds, such as polychlorinated dibenzo-*p*-dioxins (PCDDs), polychlorinated dibenzofurans (PCDFs), and polychlorinated biphenyls (PCBs), represent a class of widely distributed environmental contaminants. Ingestion is generally recognized as the main source of exposure to these compounds. Limited information is available regarding infant exposure to these compounds via formula feeding. Evaluation of PCB intake by formula-fed Spanish children showed that the ingestion of PCBs via formulas did not exceed the tolerable daily intake of 2 pg WHO-TEQ (toxic equivalents)/kg body weight/day recommended by the Scientific Committee on Food nor the threshold value of 10 ng/kg body weight/day proposed by the Institute of Public Health and the Environment, Bilthoven, Netherlands.[52] A subsequent study evaluating PCDD, PCDF, and PCB intake in non-breastfed European infants showed dietary exposure of greater than 2 pg WHO-TEQ/kg body weight in infants aged 0 to 4 months who were consuming 'starting' hypoallergenic formula.[53] (See Chapter 38)

## Nitrates

Infants who consume formula that is prepared using well water remain a high-risk group for excessive nitrate consumption. Nitrates are natural constituents of plant material, and the effect of commercial nitrate-containing fertilizers on the nitrate content of vegetables is inconsistent.[54] For infants, a desirable target concentration of nitrate nitrogen for food is less than 100 parts per million (ppm). The potential hazard of nitrates lies in its conversion to methemoglobin-producing nitrites before and/or after ingestion. The nitrite ion oxidizes ferrous ion in hemoglobin to the ferric state. The resulting compound, methemoglobin, is incapable of binding molecular oxygen, thus causing a leftward shift in the oxygen-dissociation curve, and subsequent hypoxemia. Absorbed nitrate that has not been converted to nitrite can be readily excreted in the urine without adverse effects. Breastfed infants are not at risk of nitrate poisoning from mothers who ingest water with high nitrate content (up to 100 ppm nitrate nitrogen) because nitrate concentration does not increase significantly in human milk.[55] (See Chapter 34)

## Arsenic

Arsenic occurs naturally in bedrock and is a common contaminant of well water. Formula powder can contain low concentrations of arsenic.[56-58] Thus, both components of reconstituted formula (the powder and the water with which it is mixed) can be sources of arsenic for formula-fed infants. If infants receive formula with added rice cereal, they may receive additional arsenic from the rice cereal.[59,60]

Conversely, breast milk has relatively low concentrations of arsenic,[61] even in women with high exposure via drinking water.[62] Early life exposure to high concentrations of arsenic from drinking water has been associated with increased fetal mortality, decreased birth weight, and diminished cognitive function and IQ in childhood.[63,64] Furthermore, the effects of chronic high-dose early life exposure can continue into adult life, as indicated by an increased occurrence and/or severity of lung and cardiovascular disease, as well as cancers later in life.[65,66]

## Fluoride

The optimal fluoride concentration in drinking water, as established by the US Public Health Service, is 0.7 to 1.2 ppm, a range that has shown to be beneficial in reducing caries.[67] In some areas, naturally occurring fluoride levels may be above or below these concentrations. Most bottled waters contain a concentration of fluoride that is less than optimal, and the fluoride content varies among brands.[68,69]

Both milk- and soy-based infant formulas also contain fluoride, with ready-to-feed formulas containing a lower fluoride concentration compared with formula powder or concentrate.[70] Because powdered and liquid concentrates contain fluoride, the final concentration of fluoride in these formulas depends largely on the fluoride content of the water used to reconstitute them.[70,71] Ingestion of excessive amounts of fluoride during critical periods of tooth development may result in fluorosis, a type of hypomineralization of the enamel. The severity and distribution of fluorosis depend on the amount and duration of fluoride intake; the stage of tooth development at exposure; and the child's susceptibility to the condition.[72]

After reviewing the available data, the American Dental Association Council on Scientific Affairs concluded that clinicians should be aware that children are exposed to multiple sources of fluoride during the period of tooth development, and that reducing fluoride intake from reconstituted infant formula alone would not eliminate the risk of fluorosis. Breastfed infants are not at risk for the development of fluorosis because human milk has consistently low levels (0.005 to 0.01 ppm) of fluoride.[73,74]

## Bacteria

Liquid infant formula is sterile. Powdered infant formula is not sterile; there-fore, bacterial contamination may occur. Powdered infant formula consump-tion has been associated with reported cases of *Cronobacter* (previously known as *Enterobacter sakazakii*) infection, which can kill 40% to 80% of infected infants.[75] *Cronobacter* was found in 2.4% of powdered infant formula samples in 2003, but a recent review found that invasive *Cronobacter* disease was rare (only 46 cases reported from 1958 to 2005).[75] More details on infant infec-tion with *Cronobacter* can be found on the Centers for Disease Control and Prevention Web site: www.cdc.gov/cronobacter/technical.html. Other bacteria have been found in powdered infant formula. Formula also may be contami-nated during preparation if it is mixed with contaminated water, or if dirty bottles or utensils are used.

## Bisphenol A

Previously, baby bottles often contained bisphenol A (BPA), a weak estrogenic compound, which can migrate from the bottle to its liquid contents, especially when the liquid is hot. Increased migration of BPA from the bottle is also noted after repeated dishwashing, boiling, and brushing.[76] A report from the National Toxicology Program estimated that formula-fed infants had a range of exposure to BPA of 1 to 11 mcg/kg per day.[77] In a recent study evaluating 22 liquid and 28 powder formulas, BPA concentrations were found to range between 0.003 and 0.375 mcg/g (median 0.015 mcg/g). Importantly, there were no differences in the concentrations of BPA between liquid and powder formu-las even though the samples were packaged in different types of containers.[78]

The National Toxicology Program considers current exposure levels to cause some concern for possible adverse effects on the brain, behavior, and prostate gland in infants and children.[77] In 2012, the FDA granted 2 petitions requesting that it amend its food additive regulations to no longer provide for the use of certain BPA-based materials in baby bottles, sippy cups, and infant formula packaging. Subsequently, in a memorandum drafted in 2014, the FDA noted that exposure to BPA was expected to decrease based on recent amend-ments to the food additive regulations that no longer authorized the use of polycarbonate resins in infant feeding bottles and spill-proof cups, or the use of BPA-based epoxy resins as coatings in packaging for infant formulas.[79] See Chapter 41 for more detailed information.

## Melamine

In 2008, an outbreak of kidney stones and renal failure in infants consuming melamine-contaminated powdered milk formula occurred in China, result-ing in at least 3 deaths and 13,000 hospitalizations.[80] Melamine, an industrial material that is not permitted for use as a food additive, and its derivative cyanuric acid, were associated with renal failure in US pets in 2007.[81] Melamine was deliberately added to raw milk in China to increase protein readings, but its renal toxicity in human infants led to the large-scale international market withdrawal of contaminated formulas and other dairy products. No such infant formulas, however, were imported to the US market. In experimental studies, melamine and cyanuric acid produced significant renal damage and crystals in nephrons.[81] Reports of adverse effects among human infants consuming melamine-contaminated formulas have been published.[82–85]

## Frequently Asked Questions

Q   Can my daughter switch to soy formula because she has lactose intolerance? Will isoflavones in soy formula cause harmful effects in her?

A   When thinking about what formula to give to an infant, it is important to remember that it is very unusual for an infant to be born with lactose intolerance. Lactose intolerance, if it develops, usually occurs later in childhood. Nevertheless, many infants are given soy infant formula because soy protein-based formula is lactose free. Lactose-free and reduced-lactose cow milk-based formulas are also available. Soy formula contains much higher levels of isoflavones than does human milk or cow milk-based formula. Experimental studies in animals have found that high-level genistein (one compound in the isoflavone category) can cause adverse effects in reproduction and development. However, studies using soy infant formula in experimental animals were not conclusive. Currently, there are some data on the effects of isoflavone exposure in human infants who were fed soy formula. More research is needed in this area.[86]

Q   Are the phytoestrogens in soy formula related to precocious puberty?

A   Soy infant formula contains phytoestrogens that are weak estrogenic compounds. However, isoflavones in soy formula have estrogenic effects that are probably orders of magnitude lower than estradiol, the natural human estrogen. There is one report of soy infant formula use and premature breast development in girls aged younger than 2 years, but that study was small and inconclusive.[26] Precocious puberty in girls aged younger than 8 years or boys younger than 9 years may be caused by exogenous hormone exposure, but the role of soy infant formula has not been clearly demonstrated.

Q   Is it possible to reduce isoflavone levels in soy infant formula?

A   Isoflavone levels vary in soybeans depending on geographic location and meteorologic conditions. This variation can probably be exploited to produce soy protein isolates with lower concentrations of isoflavones. In the future, manufacturers may be able to consider processes that modify isoflavone levels from soy protein isolates. Isoflavone levels are not currently labeled on soy infant formula packages.

Q    *Is BPA in baby bottles harmful to my formula-fed baby?*

A    Experimental studies in animals have found adverse effects of bisphenol A (BPA) on reproduction and development from relatively low-level exposures that may be experienced by infants. Although some studies suggest that BPA exposure can adversely affect brain development and increase the risk for the development of obesity later in life, more research is needed in this area. Recent amendments to food additive regulations no longer authorize the use of BPA in infant feeding bottles and spill-proof cups, or the use of BPA-based epoxy resins as coatings in packaging for infant formulas.

Q    *Can melamine contamination happen again, and does internationally produced formula come into the United States?*

A    In the Chinese incident of adulterated infant formula, melamine was added to falsely increase the apparent protein content because melamine contains nitrogen. This practice has been banned in China. Melamine is not approved in the United States for addition to foods. When the FDA tested milk (Yili Pure Milk and Yili Sour Milk produced by Nationwide HUA XIA Food Trade, USA, Flushing, NY), they found melamine contamination.[87] Currently, there are no Chinese-made infant formulas for sale in the United States.

Q    *What is the recommended way to prepare infant formula?*

A    Water used for mixing infant formula must be from a safe water source as defined by the state or local health department. If you are concerned or uncertain about the safety of tap water, you may use bottled water or bring cold tap water to a rolling boil for 1 minute (no longer), then cool the water to room temperature for no more than 30 minutes before it is used. Warmed water should be tested in advance to make sure it is not too hot for the infant. The easiest way to test the temperature is to shake a few drops on the inside of your wrist. Otherwise, a bottle can be prepared by adding powdered formula and room temperature water from the tap just before feeding. Bottles made in this way from powdered formula can be ready for feeding because no additional refrigeration or warming is required. Prepared formula must be discarded within 1 hour after serving to an infant. Prepared formula that has not been given to an infant may be stored in the refrigerator for 24 hours to prevent bacterial contamination. An open container of ready-to-feed, concentrated formula, or formula prepared from concentrated formula should be covered, refrigerated, and discarded after 48 hours if not used.[88,89]

## Resources

### National Institute of Environmental Health Sciences

Web site: www.niehs.nih.gov

Available publications include NTP-CERHR Monograph on Soy Infant Formula (https://ntp.niehs.nih.gov/ntp/ohat/genistein-soy/soyformula/soymonograph2010_508.pdf) and

NTP-CERHR Expert Panel Report on the Reproductive and Developmental Toxicity of Genistein (www.ncbi.nlm.nih.gov/pmc/articles/PMC2020434)

### US Food and Drug Administration

Web site: www.fda.gov

Frequently Asked Questions about FDA's Regulation of Infant Formula: www.fda.gov/food/guidanceregulation/guidancedocumentsregulatory information/ucm056524.htm

## References

1. Bhatia J, Greer F, American Academy of Pediatrics Committee on Nutrition. Use of soy protein-based formulas in infant feeding. *Pediatrics*. 2008;121(5):1062–1068

2. Zeiger RS, Sampson HA, Bock SA, et al. Soy allergy in infants and children with IgE-associated cow's milk allergy. *J Pediatr*. 1999;134(5):614–622

3. Klemola T, Vanto T, Juntunen-Backman K, Kalimo K, Korpela R, Varjonen E. Allergy to soy formula and to extensively hydrolyzed whey formula in infants with cow's milk allergy: a prospective, randomized study with a follow-up to the age of 2 years. *J Pediatr*. 2002;140(2):219–224

4. Rossen LM, Simon AE, Herrick KA. Types of infant formulas consumed in the United States. *Clin Pediatr (Phila)*. 2016;55(3):278–285

5. National Institute of Environmental Health Sciences. Soy Infant Formula. https://www.niehs.nih.gov/health/topics/agents/sya-soy-formula/index.cfm. Accessed May 20, 2018

6. Rozman KK, Bhatia J, Calafat AM, et al. NTP-CERHR expert panel report on the reproductive and developmental toxicity of soy formula. *Birth Defects Res B Dev Reprod Toxicol*. 2006;77(4):280–397

7. Chen A, Rogan WJ. Isoflavones in soy infant formula: a review of evidence for endocrine and other activity in infants. *Annu Rev Nutr*. 2004;24:33–54

8. Cao Y, Calafat AM, Doerge DR, et al. Isoflavones in urine, saliva, and blood of infants: data from a pilot study on the estrogenic activity of soy formula. *J Expo Sci Environ Epidemiol*. 2009;19(2):223–234

9. Agostoni C, Axelsson I, Goulet O, et al. Soy protein infant formulae and follow-on formulae: a commentary by the ESPGHAN Committee on Nutrition. *J Pediatr Gastroenterol Nutr*. 2006;42(4):352–361

10. Liener IE. Implications of antinutritional components in soybean foods. *Crit Rev Food Sci Nutr*. 1994;34(1):31–67

11. Corkins MR, American Academy of Pediatrics Committee on Nutrition. Technical Report. Aluminum toxicity in infants and children. *Pediatrics* (in press)

12. Cockell KA, Bonacci G, Belonje B. Manganese content of soy or rice beverages is high in comparison to infant formulas. *J Am Coll Nutr*. 2004;23(2):124–130

13. Schneider JS, Decamp E, Koser AJ, et al. Effects of chronic manganese exposure on cognitive and motor functioning in non-human primates. *Brain Res*. 2006;1118(1):222–231

14. Setchell KD, Zimmer-Nechemias L, Cai J, Heubi JE. Isoflavone content of infant formulas and the metabolic fate of these phytoestrogens in early life. *Am J Clin Nutr.* 1998;68(6 Suppl): 1453S–1461S

15. Tuohy PG. Soy infant formula and phytoestrogens. *J Paediatr Child Health.* 2003;39(6):401–405

16. Essex C. Phytoestrogens and soy based infant formula. *BMJ.* 1996;313(7056):507–508

17. Sharpe RM, Martin B, Morris K, et al. Infant feeding with soy formula milk: effects on the testis and on blood testosterone levels in marmoset monkeys during the period of neonatal testicular activity. *Hum Reprod.* 2002;17(7):1692–1703

18. Tan KA, Walker M, Morris K, Greig I, Mason JI, Sharpe RM. Infant feeding with soy formula milk: effects on puberty progression, reproductive function and testicular cell numbers in marmoset monkeys in adulthood. *Hum Reprod.* 2006;21(4):896–904

19. Fielden MR, Samy SM, Chou KC, Zacharewski TR. Effect of human dietary exposure levels of genistein during gestation and lactation on long-term reproductive development and sperm quality in mice. *Food Chem Toxicol.* 2003;41(4):447–454

20. Vilela ML, Willingham E, Buckley J, et al. Endocrine disruptors and hypospadias: role of genistein and the fungicide vinclozolin. *Urology.* 2007;70(3):618–621

21. Jefferson WN, Couse JF, Padilla-Banks E, Korach KS, Newbold RR. Neonatal exposure to genistein induces estrogen receptor (ER)alpha expression and multioocyte follicles in the maturing mouse ovary: evidence for ERbeta-mediated and nonestrogenic actions. *Biol Reprod.* 2002;67(4):1285–1296

22. Delclos KB, Bucci TJ, Lomax LG, et al. Effects of dietary genistein exposure during development on male and female CD (Sprague-Dawley) rats. *Reprod Toxicol.* 2001;15(6): 647–663

23. Newbold RR, Banks EP, Bullock B, Jefferson WN. Uterine adenocarcinoma in mice treated neonatally with genistein. *Cancer Res.* 2001;61(11):4325–4328

24. Program NT. Toxicology and carcinogenesis studies of genistein (Cas No. 446-72-0) in Sprague-Dawley rats ( feed study). *Natl Toxicol Program Tech Rep Ser.* 2008;(545):1–240

25. Rozman KK, Bhatia J, Calafat AM, et al. NTP-CERHR expert panel report on the reproductive and developmental toxicity of genistein. *Birth Defects Res B Dev Reprod Toxicol.* 2006;77(6):485–638

26. Freni-Titulaer LW, Cordero JF, Haddock L, Lebron G, Martinez R, Mills JL. Premature thelarche in Puerto Rico. A search for environmental factors. *Am J Dis Child.* 1986;140(12):1263–1267

27. Giampietro PG, Bruno G, Furcolo G, et al. Soy protein formulas in children: no hormonal effects in long-term feeding. *J Pediatr Endocrinol Metab.* 2004;17(2):191–196

28. Zung A, Glaser T, Kerem Z, Zadik Z. Breast development in the first 2 years of life: an association with soy-based infant formulas. *J Pediatr Gastroenterol Nutr.* 2008;46(2):191–195

29. Bernbaum JC, Umbach DM, Ragan NB, et al. Pilot studies of estrogen-related physical findings in infants. *Environ Health Perspect.* 2008;116(3):416–420

30. Strom BL, Schinnar R, Ziegler EE, et al. Exposure to soy-based formula in infancy and endocrinological and reproductive outcomes in young adulthood. *JAMA.* 2001;286(7):807–814

31. Chang HC, Doerge DR. Dietary genistein inactivates rat thyroid peroxidase in vivo without an apparent hypothyroid effect. *Toxicol Appl Pharmacol.* 2000;168(3):244–252

32. Shepard TH, Pyne GE, Kirschvink JF, Mclean M. Soy bean goiter: report of three cases. *N Engl J Med.* 1960;262:1099–1103

33. Chorazy PA, Himelhoch S, Hopwood NJ, Greger NG, Postellon DC. Persistent hypothyroidism in an infant receiving a soy formula: case report and review of the literature. *Pediatrics.* 1995;96(1 Pt 1):148–150

34. Jabbar MA, Larrea J, Shaw RA. Abnormal thyroid function tests in infants with congenital hypothyroidism: the influence of soy-based formula. *J Am Coll Nutr.* 1997;16(3):280–282

35. Conrad SC, Chiu H, Silverman BL. Soy formula complicates management of congenital hypothyroidism. *Arch Dis Child.* 2004;89(1):37–40

36. Simmen RC, Eason RR, Till SR, et al. Inhibition of NMU induced mammary tumorigenesis by dietary soy. *Cancer Lett.* 2005;224(1):45–52

37. Fort P, Moses N, Fasano M, Goldberg T, Lifshitz F. Breast and soy-formula feedings in early infancy and the prevalence of autoimmune thyroid disease in children. *J Am Coll Nutr.* 1990;9(2):164–167

38. Cooke PS, Selvaraj V, Yellayi S. Genistein, estrogen receptors, and the acquired immune response. *J Nutr.* 2006;136(3):704–708

39. Osborn DA, Sinn J. Soy formula for prevention of allergy and food intolerance in infants. *Cochrane Database Syst Rev.* 2006;(4):CD003741

40. Ostrom KM, Cordle CT, Schaller JP, et al. Immune status of infants fed soy-based formulas with or without added nucleotides for 1 year: part 1: vaccine responses, and morbidity. *J Pediatr Gastroenterol Nutr.* 2002;34(2):137–144

41. Cordle CT, Winship TR, Schaller JP, et al. Immune status of infants fed soy-based formulas with or without added nucleotides for 1 year: part 2: immune cell populations. *J Pediatr Gastroenterol Nutr.* 2002;34(2):145–153

42. Vandenplas Y, Castrellon PG, Rivas R, et al. Safety of soya-based infant formulas in children. *Br J Nutr.* 2014;111(8):1340–1360

43. Cruz ML, Wong WW, Mimouni F, et al. Effects of infant nutrition on cholesterol synthesis rates. *Pediatr Res.* 1994;35(2):135–140

44. Fort P, Lanes R, Dahlem S, et al. Breast feeding and insulin-dependent diabetes mellitus in children. *J Am Coll Nutr.* 1986;5(5):439–441

45. Malloy MH, Berendes H. Does breast-feeding influence intelligence quotients at 9 and 10 years of age? *Early Hum Dev.* 1998;50(2):209–217

46. Azarova AM, Lin RK, Tsai YC, Liu LF, Lin CP, Lyu YL. Genistein induces topoisomerase IIbeta- and proteasome-mediated DNA sequence rearrangements: implications in infant leukemia. *Biochem Biophys Res Commun.* 2010;399(1):66–71

47. Boucher BA, Cotterchio M, Kreiger N, Thompson LU. Soy formula and breast cancer risk. *Epidemiology.* 2008;19(1):165–166

48. National Toxicology Program. Center for Evaluation of of Risks to Human Reproduction. Final CERHR expert panel report on soy infant formula. Reseach Triangle Park, NC: 2010. https://ntp.niehs.nih.gov/ntp/ohat/genistein-soy/soyformula/soymonograph2010_508.pdf. Accessed May 21, 2018

49. McCarver G, Bhatia J, Chambers C, et al. NTP-CERHR expert panel report on the developmental toxicity of soy infant formula. *Birth Defects Res B Dev Reprod Toxicol.* 2011;92(5):421–468

50. Setchell KD, Zimmer-Nechemias L, Cai J, Heubi JE. Exposure of infants to phyto-oestrogens from soy-based infant formula. *Lancet.* 1997;350(9070):23–27

51. Irvine CH, Shand N, Fitzpatrick MG, Alexander SL. Daily intake and urinary excretion of genistein and daidzein by infants fed soy- or dairy-based infant formulas. *Am J Clin Nutr.* 1998;68(6 Suppl):1462S–1465S

52. Loran S, Conchello P, Bayarri S, Herrera A. Evaluation of daily intake of PCDD/Fs and indicator PCBs in formula-fed Spanish children. *Food Addit Contam Part A Chem Anal Control Expo Risk Assess.* 2009;26(10):1421–1431

53. Pandelova M, Piccinelli R, Lopez WL, et al. Assessment of PCDD/F, PCB, OCP and BPA dietary exposure of non-breast-fed European infants. *Food Addit Contam Part A Chem Anal Control Expo Risk Assess.* 2011;28(8):1110–1122

54. Phillips WE. Naturally occurring nitrate and nitrite in foods in relation to infant methaemoglobinaemia. *Food Cosmet Toxicol.* 1971;9(2):219–228

55. Greer FR, Shannon M, American Academy of Pediatrics Committee on Nutrition, American Academy of Pediatrics Committee on Environmental Health. Infant methemoglobinemia: the role of dietary nitrate in food and water. *Pediatrics.* 2005;116(3):784–786

56. U.S. Food and Drug Administration. Analytical Results from Inorganic Arsenic in Rice and Rice Products Sampling. 2014. https://www.fda.gov/downloads/food/ foodborneillnesscontaminants/metals/ucm352467.pdf. Accessed May 21, 2018

57. Jackson BP, Taylor VF, Punshon T, Cottingham KL. Arsenic concentration and speciation in infant formulas and first foods. *Pure Appl Chem.* 2012;84(2):215–223

58. Ljung K, Palm B, Grander M, Vahter M. High concentrations of essential and toxic elements in infant formula and infant foods: a matter of concern. *Food Chem.* 2011;127(3):943–951

59. Carignan CC, Punshon T, Karagas MR, Cottingham KL. Potential exposure to arsenic from infant rice cereal. *Ann Glob Health.* 2016;82(1):221–224

60. Shibata T, Meng C, Umoren J, West H. Risk assessment of arsenic in rice cereal and other dietary sources for infants and toddlers in the U.S. *Int J Environ Res Public Health.* 2016;13(4):361

61. Bjorklund KL, Vahter M, Palm B, Grander M, Lignell S, Berglund M. Metals and trace element concentrations in breast milk of first time healthy mothers: a biological monitoring study. *Environ Health.* 2012;11:92

62. Fangstrom B, Moore S, Nermell B, et al. Breast-feeding protects against arsenic exposure in Bangladeshi infants. *Environ Health Perspect.* 2008;116(7):963–969

63. National Research Council. Critical Aspects of EPA's IRIS Assessment of Inorganic Arsenic, Interim Report. Washington, DC: National Academies Press; 2014

64. Wasserman GA, Liu X, Loiacono NJ, et al. A cross-sectional study of well water arsenic and child IQ in Maine schoolchildren. *Environ Health.* 2014;13(1):23

65. Smith AH, Marshall G, Yuan Y, et al. Increased mortality from lung cancer and bronchiectasis in young adults after exposure to arsenic in utero and in early childhood. *Environ Health Perspect.* 2006;114(8):1293–1296

66. Naujokas MF, Anderson B, Ahsan H, et al. The broad scope of health effects from chronic arsenic exposure: update on a worldwide public health problem. *Environ Health Perspect.* 2013;121(3):295–302

67. Centers for Disease Control and Prevention. Engineering and administrative recommendations for water fluoridation. *MMWR Recomm Rep.* 1995;44(RR-13):1–40

68. Ayo-Yusuf OA, Kroon J, Ayo-Yusuf IJ. Fluoride concentration of bottled drinking waters. *SADJ.* 2001;56(6):273–276

69. Quock RL, Chan JT. Fluoride content of bottled water and its implications for the general dentist. *Gen Dent.* 2009;57(1):29–33

70. Siew C, Strock S, Ristic H, et al. Assessing a potential risk factor for enamel fluorosis: a preliminary evaluation of fluoride content in infant formulas. *J Am Dent Assoc.* 2009;140(10):1228–1236

71. Buzalaf MA, Damante CA, Trevizani LM, Granjeiro JM. Risk of fluorosis associated with infant formulas prepared with bottled water. *J Dent Child (Chic).* 2004;71(2):110–113

72. DenBesten PK, Thariani H. Biological mechanisms of fluorosis and level and timing of systemic exposure to fluoride with respect to fluorosis. *J Dent Res.* 1992;71(5):1238–1243

73. Ericsson Y. Fluoride excretion in human saliva and milk. *Caries Res.* 1969;3(2):159–166

74. Ekstrand J, Spak CJ, Falch J, Afseth J, Ulvestad H. Distribution of fluoride to human breast milk following intake of high doses of fluoride. *Caries Res.* 1984;18(1):93–95

75. Bowen AB, Braden CR. Invasive Enterobacter sakazakii disease in infants. *Emerg Infect Dis.* 2006;12(8):1185–1189

76. Brede C, Fjeldal P, Skjevrak I, Herikstad H. Increased migration levels of bisphenol A from polycarbonate baby bottles after dishwashing, boiling and brushing. *Food Addit Contam.* 2003;20(7):684–689

77. Shelby MD. NTP-CERHR monograph on the potential human reproductive and developmental effects of bisphenol A. *NTP CERHR MON.* 2008;(22):v, vii-ix, 1–64

78. Cirillo T, Latini G, Castaldi MA, et al. Exposure to di-2-ethylhexyl phthalate, di-n-butyl phthalate and bisphenol A through infant formulas. *J Agric Food Chem.* 2015;63(12):3303–3310

79. Food and Drug Administration. 2014. https://www.fda.gov/downloads/NewsEvents/Public HealthFocus/UCM424266.pdf. Accessed May 21, 2018

80. World Health Organization. Outbreak news. Melamine contamination, China. *Wkly Epidemiol Rec.* 2008;83(40):358

81. Dobson RL, Motlagh S, Quijano M, et al. Identification and characterization of toxicity of contaminants in pet food leading to an outbreak of renal toxicity in cats and dogs. *Toxicol Sci.* 2008;106(1):251–262

82. Guan N, Fan Q, Ding J, et al. Melamine-contaminated powdered formula and urolithiasis in young children. *N Engl J Med.* 2009;360(11):1067–1074

83. Ho SS, Chu WC, Wong KT, et al. Ultrasonographic evaluation of melamine-exposed children in Hong Kong. *N Engl J Med.* 2009;360(11):1156–1157

84. Wang IJ, Chen PC, Hwang KC. Melamine and nephrolithiasis in children in Taiwan. *N Engl J Med.* 2009;360(11):1157–1158

85. Langman CB. Melamine, powdered milk, and nephrolithiasis in Chinese infants. *N Engl J Med.* 2009;360(11):1139–1141

86. Nielsen IL, Williamson G. Review of the factors affecting bioavailability of soy isoflavones in humans. *Nutr Cancer.* 2007;57(1):1–10

87. Ingelfinger JR. Melamine and the global implications of food contamination. *N Engl J Med.* 2008;359(26):2745–2748

88. American Academy of Pediatrics. How to Safely Prepare Formula With Water. https://www.healthychildren.org/English/ages-stages/baby/feeding-nutrition/Pages/How-to-Safely-Prepare-Formula-with-Water.aspx. Accessed May 21, 2018

89. WHO, Food and Agriculture Organization of the United Nations. Guidelines for safe preparation, storage and handling of powdered infant formula. 2007. http://www.who.int/foodsafety/publications/micro/pif_guidelines.pdf?ua=1. Accessed June 29, 2018

Chapter 17

# Drinking Water

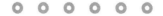

## KEY POINTS

- Safe drinking water is key to the health of the population.
- In the United States, federal and state standards apply to community drinking water supplies serving 25 or more customers. These regulations result in very safe water most of the time.
- Private wells are not regulated; it is therefore the responsibility of the individual homeowner to test water from private wells for certain chemicals and other possible contaminants.
- Bottled water is becoming more popular with consumers but is not recommended over tap water in most circumstances.

## INTRODUCTION

Safe drinking water is of primary importance to the health of children and all others. Drinking water is used for drinking, but also for cooking and preparing infant formulas for children who are not breastfed. The food supply may become contaminated when crops are irrigated with polluted water or when fish and shellfish from polluted waters are consumed. Although water is important for bathing and swimming, contaminated water can result in exposures to children who may swallow or have skin contact with pollutants. In developing countries, access to safe water is a major determinant of child health (see Chapter 14).

Although 70% of the earth is covered by water, only 3% of the earth's water is fresh. Of that 3%, two thirds is frozen in glaciers and ice caps, leaving only 1%

available for human use. Freshwater is classified as either groundwater, such as underground aquifers (0.7%), or surface water, such as lakes and rivers (0.3%), but less than half of the liquid freshwater in the world is readily accessible.[1] In the United States, approximately half of drinking water comes from groundwater, with the other half coming from either surface water or mixed surface water and groundwater sources. Preserving an adequate supply of quality freshwater is essential to public health and ecologic integrity but is threatened by increasing population pressure and industrial and agricultural production, which can result in pollution.

Water pollution results from sources of contamination termed either point or nonpoint. Point sources of pollution include municipal wastewater treatment plant discharges and industrial wastewater discharges into surface waters. Nonpoint sources are more difficult to identify and control and include agricultural runoff, urban runoff, soil contamination, and atmospheric deposition. Pollutants contaminate surface waters or soils directly and seep into underground aquifers to contaminate groundwater.

Contaminated drinking water has long been identified as a potential threat to public health, going back to prehistory with the construction in ancient Rome of systems to purify and purvey drinking water to urban communities. Water pollutants can be categorized as biological agents, chemicals, or radionuclides (see Table 17-1). Hundreds of biological agents and thousands of chemical agents may be found in water. For many water pollutants, little is known of their long-term health effects. In the United States, federal water regulations were not required until passage of the Safe Drinking Water Act of 1974; regulations exist for only a small percentage of the contaminants that have been identified in water. Federal standards apply to community water supplies serving 25 or more customers. Some states have standards for smaller suppliers, but private wells are not regulated. Internationally, similar systems are in place in many countries. The World Health Organization (WHO) has established guidelines for drinking water quality.[2] In addition, many states establish standards for drinking water that must be at least as protective, or more protective, than federal standards. Modern water treatment facilities have made drinking water safe in most of the world, eliminating most waterborne infectious illnesses as well as contamination by lead and other harmful substances. In many parts of the United States, however, drinking water supplies are threatened by contaminants. The true effects of drinking water contamination are difficult to determine, but it is estimated that in the United States, millions of illnesses each year are caused by microbial contaminants. Even where water treatment facilities are regulated, drinking water outbreaks can be caused by breaches in municipal water treatment and distribution processes, source water contamination, treatment plant inadequacies, and minor intrusions in the distribution system caused by water main breaks.[3]

## Table 17-1. Examples of Some Water Pollutants, Common Sources, and Systems Affected

| POLLUTANT CATEGORY (SPECIFIC EXAMPLES) | COMMON SOURCES | SYSTEMS AFFECTED/ HEALTH EFFECTS |
|---|---|---|
| **Biological Agents** | | |
| **Bacteria** | | |
| *Campylobacter* species | Feces: human, animal | Gastrointestinal tract |
| *Escherichia coli* | Feces: human, animal | Gastrointestinal tract |
| *Salmonella* species | Feces: human, animal | Gastrointestinal tract |
| *Shigella* species | Feces: human | Gastrointestinal tract |
| *Vibrio* species | Feces: human, animal | Gastrointestinal tract |
| *Legionella pneumophilia* | Found naturally in freshwater environments | Respiratory tract |
| **Viruses** | | |
| Calicivirus | Feces: human | Gastrointestinal tract |
| Enterovirus | Feces: human | Gastrointestinal tract, neurologic |
| Hepatitis A virus | Feces: human | Gastrointestinal tract (liver) |
| Rotavirus | Feces: human | Gastrointestinal tract |
| **Parasites** | | |
| *Balantidium coli* | Feces: human, animal | Gastrointestinal tract |
| *Cryptosporidium parvum* | Feces: human, animal | Gastrointestinal tract |
| *Entamoeba histolytica* | Feces: human | Gastrointestinal tract |
| *Giardia intestinalis* | Feces: human, animal | Gastrointestinal tract |
| **Natural Toxins** | | |
| Microcystins *Pfiesteria* toxins | Cyanobacteria *Pfiesteria piscicida* | Gastrointestinal tract, neurologic Neurologic, dermatologic |
| Phytoplankton (Dinoflagellate) toxins | *Alexandria catarella Pseudonitzchia pungens* | Neurologic |
| **Chemicals** | | |
| **Inorganic** | | |
| Arsenic | Ores, smelting, pesticides | Lung, kidney, and skin cancer; cardiovascular; neurodevelopmental |
| Chromium | Ores, steel and pulp mills | Cancer (chromium VI) |
| Lead | Pipes, solder, soil | Neurologic, cardiovascular |
| Mercury (inorganic) | Waste incineration, burning coal, mercury use, volcanoes | Kidney damage, neurologic |

## Table 17-1. Examples of Some Water Pollutants, Common Sources, and Systems Affected (*continued*)

| POLLUTANT CATEGORY (SPECIFIC EXAMPLES) | COMMON SOURCES | SYSTEMS AFFECTED/ HEALTH EFFECTS |
|---|---|---|
| Nitrates | Nitrogen fertilizer, leaching from septic tanks, sewage; erosion of natural deposits | Methemoglobinemia in infants |
| **Organic** | | |
| Benzene, other organic chemicals | Leaking gasoline storage tanks | Leukemia, aplastic anemia |
| Perfluoroalkyl and polyfluoroalkyl substances (PFAS) | Nonstick cookware, clothing, stain repellents, and aerospace | Developmental effects, cancer |
| Perchlorate | Storage, manufacture, and testing of solid rocket motors | Thyroid |
| Pesticides | Agricultural use, urban runoff | Multiple |
| Polychlorinated biphenyls | Transformers, industry | Multiple |
| Trichloroethylene | Degreasing, dry cleaning | Cancer |
| **Disinfectants and Disinfection Byproducts** | | |
| Chloramines | Water chlorination | Eye irritation, upper and lower airway irritation; stomach discomfort, anemia |
| Chlorine | Water chlorination | Eye/nose irritation; stomach discomfort |
| Chlorine dioxide | Water chlorination | Anemia; nervous system effects |
| Haloacetic acid | Byproduct of drinking water disinfection | Increased risk of cancer |
| Trihalomethanes | Byproduct of drinking water disinfection | Increased risk of cancer |
| **Radionuclides** | | |
| Radon | Natural uranium | Lung cancer |

In the United States, there is increasing concern about how aging drinking water infrastructures may adversely impact health. Older drinking water systems with corroded pipes and sluggish flow may harbor unconventional microbial contaminants. For example, in Flint, Michigan, corroded pipes associated with lead contamination were found also to be linked to outbreaks of *Legionella* infections.[4] Moreover, changes in source waters attributable to global climate change are expected to create management problems including conditions that favor growth and survival of certain pathogens and intrusion of sodium into groundwater in coastal areas.

The discussion in this chapter will be limited to representative examples of each of the categories of water pollutants. Although biological contamination of drinking water represents the largest threat to human health worldwide, it will not be extensively discussed in this chapter. See the American Academy of Pediatrics (AAP) *Red Book* for information about infectious diarrheal diseases.[5] Details about specific pollutants can be found in other chapters in this book.

## ROUTES AND SOURCES OF EXPOSURE

Children drink more water per kg of body weight than do adults. For example, infants aged 6 to 12 months consume 4 times the amount of water per unit of body weight compared with adults. Drinking water is consumed in several forms: as water; as an addition to infant formula powder or concentrate, juice, and other drinks; and in cooking. To the extent that children consume human milk or drinks from outside the home (eg, fresh milk and juice, premixed formulas, sodas), they have less consumption of household tap water.

Household water supplies can result in inhalation exposures. If volatile substances (eg, organic solvents) or gases (eg, radon gas) are present, these will enter the home during showering, bathing, and other activities. It has been estimated that 50% of the total exposure to volatile organic compounds in drinking water is via this inhalation route.

Water can cause exposure via other pathways. When contaminated water is used for irrigation of foods, the foods may become contaminated (see Chapter 18). Fish and shellfish harvested from polluted fresh and marine waters also are important sources of exposure to water pollutants; in many cases, pollutants are concentrated by shellfish and fish. Contaminated bathing water can result in exposures via ingestion or dermal contact. Young children particularly are at risk because they swallow more water when bathing than do older children and adults. Flood water may adversely affect human health by bringing children in contact with metals, such as lead and cadmium, in the soil of flood plains.[6]

The fetus may be exposed to pollutants when a pregnant woman ingests foods in the aquatic food chain in which water pollutants have bioaccumulated. Methylmercury and polychlorinated biphenyls (PCBs) in fish are particularly important in this regard because they accumulate in the body and are not readily excreted. These toxicants may be found in the body years after exposure.

# CONTAMINANTS IN WATER

## Biological Agents

### Microorganisms

Drinking and bathing water may contain numerous pathogens that can survive in the water for variable periods. Some of these agents are listed in Table 17-1. Some agents (eg, certain parasites) form small cysts that pass through standard filters and are quite resistant to water disinfectants. Waterborne illness usually results in mild gastroenteritis with diarrhea but can also result in nongastrointestinal tract disease. Even when water systems comply with federal and local regulations, sporadic and epidemic illnesses occur.[3] This is of particular concern for infants and immunocompromised persons exposed to pathogens, such as *Cryptosporidium* species, despite state-of-the-art water treatment. In the United States, it is rare to have serious dysentery or enteric fever attributable to *Vibrio cholerae* and *Salmonella typhi*, even in areas where water quality is compromised. Viral upper respiratory and gastrointestinal tract infections can be transmitted by contaminated bathing water. Syndromes associated with illnesses from various pathogens are described in the AAP *Red Book*.[5]

### Natural Toxins and Algal Blooms

Natural toxins may produce acute or chronic illnesses and a variety of clinical syndromes. Water from ponds and lakes as well as municipal and recreational waters, under certain conditions, may contain toxin-producing cyanobacteria (blue-green algae [eg, *Microcystis aeruginosa*]) or phytoplankton, which may result in toxic shellfish poisoning. Cyanotoxins, such as microcystins, are hepatotoxic and neurotoxic compounds. They have been linked to liver failure and death in rare outbreaks in communities in which uncontrolled algal growth occurred in the absence of appropriate water treatment.[7] Water from the rivers flowing into the Chesapeake Bay on the eastern shore of the United States or mussel-growing areas in the Pacific Northwest periodically may be contaminated with dinoflagellates (*Pfiesteria piscicida, pseudonitzchia pungens*) that can produce neurotoxins.[8] The rate of contamination by toxin-producing organisms is not well characterized but thought to be infrequent.

## Chemical Contaminants

Water and sediments in water are the ultimate sinks for many chemicals produced and used by humans. Each year in the United States, more than 15,000 chemicals are produced in amounts of more than 10,000 pounds each, and thousands of new chemicals are introduced into use. Few of these chemicals have been evaluated to assess their effects on human health. Even among the 2,800 chemicals used at more than a million pounds per year, more than half have not been tested for toxic effects on humans.[9] Thousands of synthetic organic chemicals are used in agricultural and industrial processes. For example, drinking water supplies near natural gas production sites can be contaminated by chemicals used in hydraulic fracturing ("hydrofracking" or "fracking"), a process to extract natural gas from shale (see Chapter 57).

According to the US Geological Survey, many industrial chemicals, antibiotics, other pharmaceuticals (including estrogens), and pesticides frequently are found in the waters of the United States, particularly downstream from factories and cities.[10]

## Inorganic Chemicals

### Arsenic

Arsenic, a ubiquitous metal, can be found in the environment in organic and inorganic forms and in valence states of 0, 3, and 5. Drinking water and food are the major sources of arsenic for humans. Clinical effects of arsenic are discussed in Chapter 22 and include developmental neurotoxicity; skin, bladder, and lung cancers; peripheral neuropathy (in adults); hyperkeratotic skin lesions; and chronic lung disease (in adults). Arsenic is a known human carcinogen; its natural occurrence in drinking water and the expense of removal, however, have led the US Environmental Protection Agency (EPA) to allow a drinking water standard that is less protective than is usual for carcinogens.[11] Increasingly, associations are being made between high levels of arsenic in drinking water and neurodevelopmental effects, including loss of IQ points.[12]

### Chromium

Chromium in drinking water is regulated to protect against exposure to one of the valence states of chromium—chromium VI (hexavalent chromium) (see Chapter 24). The US EPA is reviewing this contaminant in a process that was announced in 2010 and is not yet completed. In 2014, the State of California adopted a maximum contaminant level (MCL) of 10 parts per billion (ppb) for chromium VI, based on cancer risk.

### Fluoride

In 2011, the US Department of Health and Human Services and the US EPA set the recommended level of fluoride in drinking water at 0.7 mg/L, which is the lower limit of the prior standard (0.7 to 1.2 mg/L). This lower standard is expected to reduce the incidence of fluorosis in the United States.[13]

### Lead

Drinking water represents a potential source of exposure to lead. In the past 2 decades, expanded regulations and monitoring have made most large municipal water supplies safe from exposure to lead. Nevertheless, water in some homes and schools in the United States contains lead above acceptable levels.

Chicago, Boston, and other cities historically used 100% lead piping to connect water mains to homes. Millions of these lead connectors (also known as lead service lines) still exist. In addition, lead solder, used to connect copper pipes, was widely used until the late 1980s. Drinking water, particularly water that is "soft" (ie, low in calcium or magnesium), or below a neutral pH, causes lead to leach from lead service lines, soldered joints, or lead-containing fixtures.[14] Clinical effects of lead exposure are discussed in Chapter 32. Entire towns can be affected. The case of Flint, Michigan, illustrates how sources of drinking water, drinking water treatment systems, and old lead service lines can interact to cause unhealthy levels of lead exposure in children. For economic reasons, in 2014 Michigan decided to switch the source of Flint's drinking water from Lake Huron to the Flint River. Flint River water was dirtier and more corrosive than Lake Huron water but drinking water officials failed to treat the water's corrosiveness. Over a relatively short period of time, the Flint River water began to leach lead from the service pipes that had been used to construct the system. By 2015, physicians had detected higher lead levels in children in Flint.[15] Flint River water also was responsible for outbreaks of *Legionella* in Flint. Massive efforts have been required to provide the people of Flint with safe drinking water, to remove the old lead service lines, and to restore their drinking water system to safety.

The standard for lead in drinking water, called the Lead and Copper Rule, is acknowledged to be outdated, and has been in revision for several years. The standard is not health-based but instead is aimed at technologies that result in limiting the levels of lead in drinking water across systems. Lead in drinking water is controlled by limiting the corrosiveness of the water (ie, the ability of the water to leach lead from pipes, connectors, and fixtures) and eliminated by removing lead pipes or pipes with lead solder. Increased levels of lead in drinking water have been found in some older systems with lead service lines after the disinfectant chlorine was replaced with less explosive chloramines.[16]

### Methylmercury

Mercury in fish originates from natural sources (such as volcanoes) and from combustion sources that release mercury into the air, such as coal-fired power plants used for generating electrical energy and municipal waste incinerators that burn garbage.[17] Atmospheric mercury is ultimately deposited into lakes and rivers by dustfall, rain, and snow. In the aquatic environment, mercury is converted by sediment bacteria into methylmercury, which becomes concentrated in the muscle tissues of fish by direct absorption from the water and by biomagnification up through the aquatic food chain. Clinical effects of mercury exposure are discussed in Chapter 33. Although mercury is regulated as a drinking water contaminant, the most important source of methylmercury exposure for most children is through consumption of contaminated fish (typically long-lived species such as swordfish, shark, and tuna).

## Organic Chemicals

### Gasoline and its Additives

In underground tanks that store gasoline, leaks may develop over the years, causing toxic chemicals to rapidly move into groundwater and eventually into drinking water. The most toxic component of gasoline probably is benzene. Along with other gasoline constituents (some of which also are very toxic), it enters the water when gasoline is spilled or when gasoline tanks leak into the ground and from other industrial sources. Benzene is known to cause leukemia in humans, and at high doses results in aplastic anemia. Thousands of other compounds in gasoline have unknown toxicity. One toxic compound in gasoline found in drinking water sources is methyl tertiary butyl ether (MTBE).[18] The US EPA issued a drinking water advisory for MTBE, including recommendations for preventing unpleasant odor and taste (occurring at levels between 20 and 40 ppb). California regulates MTBE on the basis of taste and odor (5 ppb) and as a carcinogen (13 ppb) (see Chapter 30).

### Nitrates

Nitrates enter the water supply from urban and agricultural runoff of nitrogen fertilizers and also are produced by bacterial action on animal waste runoff. Nitrates themselves are not toxic to humans but can be converted by gut bacteria to more reactive and toxic nitrites. Nitrates in drinking water above the US EPA level of 10 mg/L may cause fatal methemoglobinemia in infants (see Chapter 34).

### Pesticides

Pesticides may not be removed by conventional drinking water treatment (see Chapter 40). As detection technologies have improved, increasingly low concentrations of common insecticides, herbicides, and fungicides have been documented in drinking water sources.[11] Some older pesticides (such as dichlorodiphenyltrichloroethane [DDT]) were designed to persist in the environment for years and can be found distributed worldwide in water and soil. Newer pesticides degrade more quickly but still contaminate water and may persist for long durations in groundwater. Concentrations in water often correlate with growing seasons in agricultural areas and rainy seasons in more urban settings. Private drinking water wells are particularly susceptible to contamination by agricultural chemicals, especially in higher risk agricultural areas with sandy soils and high water tables. The US EPA is required to consider contributions of exposures from drinking water when establishing standards for pesticides in foods.

## Polychlorinated Biphenyls and Dioxins

Polychlorinated biphenyls (PCBs) and dioxins have very low solubility in water and are not found in drinking water. They are a problem because they readily bioaccumulate in the fat of wildlife, are very resistant to biological degradation, and remain in the environment for decades. The sediments of many lakes and rivers are contaminated with PCBs and/or dioxins. Contaminated sediments, a nonpoint source, are still the major source of PCBs and dioxins found in fish and wildlife. Exposures to certain dioxins and PCBs are associated with risks of cancer and developmental toxicity (see Chapter 38).[19,20]

## Trichloroethylene

In 1986, an association was found between childhood leukemia and drinking water supplied from 2 municipal wells in Woburn, MA.[21] Childhood leukemia rates in Woburn reported between 1964 and 1983 were twice the national rates. Some chemical disposal pits, used for several decades, were suspected as the source of trichloroethylene, a chlorinated product, and other chlorinated chemicals. Although the 2 affected wells were shut down immediately on discovery of the contamination, exposure to these carcinogens is believed to have occurred for many years. At this time, trichloroethylene is classified as a known human carcinogen based on strong evidence in animals and human epidemiologic evidence.[19]

## Disinfectants and Disinfection Byproducts

In the 1970s, chlorination of waters with high natural organic content (eg, humic and tannic acids) was found to cause the formation of chloroform and other chlorinated compounds called trihalomethanes. Some residual levels of the disinfectants chlorine and chlorine dioxide are found in tap water. Epidemiologic studies show a correlation between drinking water that contains trihalomethanes and increased rates of rectal and bladder cancer.[22] In 1981, as a result of extensive testing of water supplies in the United States, cancer risk analysis of the chemicals found, and suggestive epidemiologic studies, the US EPA issued a maximum contaminant level (MCL) for trihalomethanes in water. Studies have found associations between trihalomethanes and spontaneous abortion and birth defects; it appears, however, that the evidence for these associations is not strong at currently allowable levels in the United States.[23,24] A consistent conclusion is that disinfecting drinking water reduces waterborne diseases, a benefit that far outweighs risks resulting from traces of disinfection byproducts in drinking water. Chlorination of swimming pool water is also a common practice. Some studies have indicated a possible relationship between chloramines found in pool water and childhood asthma among swimmers.[25]

## Emerging Chemical Risks

### Perchlorate

Perchlorate occurs naturally but is present in drinking water because of its use as an oxidizer in rocket propellants, munitions, fireworks, airbag initiators for vehicles, and other products. It is an endocrine disrupting chemical with thyroid hormone blocking actions (see Chapter 37), and is especially a health concern for the fetus, infant, and child.[26] Perchlorate contamination occurs around sites where it has been manufactured and used. Massachusetts and California established standards for perchlorate and several other states have issued guidance requiring monitoring and clean-up.[27]

### Perfluoroalkyl and Polyfluoroalkyl Substances (PFAS)

The family of fluorinated organic chemicals has entered drinking water via many uses in manufacture of nonstick cookware, clothing, stain repellents, and aerospace, automotive, and electronics equipment. PFAS are quite prevalent in drinking water in areas around facilities that have manufactured and used them.[10,28] Two PFAS, perfluorooctanoic acid (PFOA) and perfluorooctanesulfonate (PFOS), are associated with developmental effects as well as cancer (see Chapter 36). In 2016, the US EPA issued a health advisory recommending steps that drinking water systems and public health officials can take to reduce excessive levels of these chemicals and to inform the public about them. This advisory is not enforceable.

## Radionuclides

### Radon

Radon gas, a product of the radioactive decay of uranium, enters the water supply naturally and becomes aerosolized during use of tap water. Radon further breaks down into radon "daughters" or "progeny." Radon in water is important because radon may be inhaled during showering. Lung cancer in adults has been linked to inhalation of radon progeny (see Chapter 42).[29]

## PREVENTION OF EXPOSURE

The 20th century public health successes that eliminated epidemic cholera and typhoid fever are dramatic evidence of the importance of prevention in managing drinking and recreational water supplies. Historically, water and waste management were local responsibilities. During the environmental movement in the 1970s, Congress enacted laws that unified standards, resulting in the development of high-quality drinking and recreational waters.

## Public Water Supplies

The US EPA and state agencies require that municipal or commercial water suppliers serving more than 25 people meet all standards developed under the Safe Drinking Water Act of 1974 and its amendments (see Table 17-2). At this time, the US EPA has one new standard under development, for perchlorate, discussed previously. The US EPA also is reviewing hexavalent chromium for possible standard development. The Water Pollution Control Act (1972) and the Resource Conservation and Recovery Act (1976) require industrial, commercial, and municipal facilities to meet requirements to prevent contamination of surface and ground waters. The US EPA and state environmental agencies also require municipal water supplies to meet specific standards for pesticides found in groundwater and surface water. Restrictions have been placed on the use of certain pesticides that have a propensity to leach into waters.

| Table 17-2. Selected National Primary Drinking Water Regulations (http://www.epa.gov/safewater/contaminants/index.html)[a] | | |
|---|---|---|
| **CONTAMINANT** | **TYPE OF STANDARD[b]** | **STANDARD** |
| **Microbiologic Contaminants** | | |
| *Cryptosporidium* species | TT | 99% removal[c] |
| Fecal coliforms and *Escherichia coli* | MCL | ≤5.0% of samples/month allowed to contain fecal coliforms and *Escherichia coli* |
| *Giardia lamblia* | TT | 99.9% removal/inactivation |
| Heterotrophic plate count (HPC)[d] | TT | ≤500 bacterial colonies/mL |
| *Legionella* species | TT | No limit, but EPA believes that if *Giardia* and viruses are removed/inactivated, *Legionella* will also be controlled |
| Total coliforms | TT | ≤5.0% of samples/month allowed to contain coliforms and every sample with coliforms must be tested for either fecal coliforms or *Escherichia coli* |
| Turbidity[e] | TT | Can never exceed 1 turbidity unit; <0.3 unit in 95% of daily samples (per month) |
| Viruses (enteric) | TT | 99.99% removal/inactivation |

## Table 17-2. Selected National Primary Drinking Water Regulations (http://www.epa.gov/safewater/contaminants/index.html)[a] (*continued*)

| CONTAMINANT | TYPE OF STANDARD[b] | STANDARD |
|---|---|---|
| **Inorganic Chemicals** | | **Standard (mg/L = parts per million)** |
| Antimony | MCL | 0.006 |
| Arsenic | TT | 0.010 |
| Asbestos (fiber >10 mcm) | MCL | 7 million fibers/L |
| Barium | MCL | 2 |
| Beryllium | MCL | 0.004 |
| Cadmium | MCL | 0.005 |
| Chromium (total) | MCL | 0.1 |
| Copper | TT | 1.3 |
| Fluoride | MCL | 4.0 |
| Lead | TT | Action level = 0.015 |
| Mercury (inorganic) | MCL | 0.002 |
| Nitrate (measured as nitrogen) | MCL | 10 |
| Nitrite (measured as nitrogen) | MCL | 1 |
| Selenium | MCL | 0.05 |
| Thallium | TT | 0.002 |
| **Organic Chemicals** | | |
| Acrylamide | TT | If used, 0.05% dosed at 1 mg/L (or equivalent) |
| Alachlor | MCL | 0.002 |
| Atrazine | MCL | 0.003 |
| Benzene | MCL | 0.005 |
| Benzo(a)pyrene | MCL | 0.0002 |

(*continued*)

## Table 17-2. Selected National Primary Drinking Water Regulations (http://www.epa.gov/safewater/contaminants/index.html)[a] (*continued*)

| CONTAMINANT | TYPE OF STANDARD[b] | STANDARD |
|---|---|---|
| Carbofuran | MCL | 0.04 |
| Carbon tetrachloride | MCL | 0.005 |
| Chlordane | MCL | 0.002 |
| Chlorobenzene | MCL | 0.1 |
| Cyanide | MCL | 0.2 |
| 2,4-D | MCL | 0.07 |
| Dalopon | MCL | 0.2 |
| 1,2-Dibromo-3-chloropropane (DBCP) | MCL | 0.0002 |
| o-Dichlorobenzene | MCL | 0.6 |
| p-Dichlorobenzene | MCL | 0.075 |
| 1,2-Dichloroethane | MCL | 0.005 |
| 1,1-Dichloroethylene | MCL | 0.007 |
| Cis-1,2-Dichloroethylene | MCL | 0.07 |
| Trans-1,2-Dichloroethylene | MCL | 0.1 |
| Dichloromethane | MCL | 0.005 |
| 1,2-Dichloropropane | MCL | 0.005 |
| Di(2-ethylhexyl) adipate | MCL | 0.4 |
| Di (2-ethylhexyl) phthalate | MCL | 0.006 |
| Dinoseb | MCL | 0.007 |
| Dioxin (2,3,7,8-TCDD) | MCL | 0.00000003 |
| Diquat | MCL | 0.02 |
| Endothall | MCL | 0.1 |
| Endrin | MCL | 0.002 |

## Table 17-2. Selected National Primary Drinking Water Regulations (http://www.epa.gov/safewater/contaminants/index.html)[a] (*continued*)

| CONTAMINANT | TYPE OF STANDARD[b] | STANDARD |
|---|---|---|
| Epichlorohydrin | TT | If used, 0.01% dosed at 20 mg/L (or equivalent) |
| Ethylbenzene | MCL | 0.7 |
| Ethelyne dibromide | MCL | 0.00005 |
| Glyphosate | MCL | 0.7 |
| Heptachlor | MCL | 0.0004 |
| Heptachlor epoxide | MCL | 0.0002 |
| Hexachlorobenzene | MCL | 0.001 |
| Hexachlorocyclopentadiene | MCL | 0.05 |
| Lindane | MCL | 0.0002 |
| Methoxychlor | MCL | 0.04 |
| Oxamyl | MCL | 0.2 |
| Pentachlorophenol | MCL | 0.001 |
| Picloram | MCL | 0.5 |
| Polychlorinated biphenyls | MCL | 0.0005 |
| Simazine | MCL | 0.004 |
| Styrene | MCL | 0.1 |
| Tetrachloroethylene | MCL | 0.005 |
| Toluene | MCL | 1 |
| Toxaphene | MCL | 0.003 |
| 2,4,5-T, Silvex | MCL | 0.05 |
| 1,2,4-Trichlorobenzene | MCL | 0.07 |
| 1,1,1-Trichloroethane | MCL | 0.2 |
| 1,1,2-Trichloroethane | MCL | 0.005 |

(*continued*)

## Table 17-2. Selected National Primary Drinking Water Regulations (http://www.epa.gov/safewater/contaminants/index.html)[a] (*continued*)

| CONTAMINANT | TYPE OF STANDARD[b] | STANDARD |
|---|---|---|
| Trichloroethylene | MCL | 0.005 |
| Vinyl chloride | MCL | 0.002 |
| Xylenes (total) | MCL | 10 |
| **Disinfectants/Disinfectant Byproducts** | | |
| Bromate | MCL | 0.01 |
| Chloramines (as $Cl_2$) | MRDL | 4.0 |
| Chlorine (as $Cl_2$) | MRDL | 4.0 |
| Chlorine dioxide (as $ClO_2$) | MRDL | 0.8 |
| Chlorite | MCL | 1.0 |
| Haloacetic acid | MCL | 0.06 |
| Total trihalomethanes | MCL | 0.08 |
| **Radionuclides** | | |
| Alpha particles | MCL | 15 pCi/L |
| Beta particles and photon emitters | MCL | 4 mrem/y |
| Radium-226 & radium-228 (combined) | MCL | 5 pCi/L |
| Uranium | MCL | 30 mcg/L |

[a] From US Environmental Protection Agency[30]
[b] MCL, maximum contaminant level; MRDL, maximum residual disinfectant level; mrem, millirem; pCi, picocurie; TT, treatment technique.
[c] http://www.epa.gov/envirofw/html/icr/gloss_path.html
[d] Heterotrophic plate count (HPC): HPC has no health effects but is an analytic method used to measure the variety of bacteria common in water. The lower the concentration of bacteria in water, the better maintained is the water system.
[e] Turbidity: a measure of water cloudiness used to determine water quality and filtration effectiveness. Higher turbidity levels are often associated with higher levels of disease-producing organisms.

## Private Wells

Private wells are not federally regulated. However, the US EPA and/or state drinking water standards are used to interpret the results of tests on private wells. The US EPA estimates that 15% to 20% of the US population obtains drinking water from private wells. Infants and children may drink well water at home and if they are on vacation, traveling, or in child care or other locations. Contamination of well water can occur if the well is shallow, in porous soil, old, poorly maintained, near a leaky septic tank, or downhill from agricultural fields or intensive livestock operations. Flooding associated with extreme weather events can carry pollutants into private wells. Each state has different testing procedures, sometimes requiring testing only at transfer of land ownership. Testing of private wells is the responsibility of individual homeowners but in some states may be performed at no cost by the health department if testing is recommended by a health care provider. In rural areas, physicians can ask patients if their wells have been tested for coliforms and nitrates by local or county health departments within the last year. Guidance for testing and water treatment for owners of private wells is available from the American Academy of Pediatrics.[31]

In agricultural areas, higher-than-normal levels of nitrates (discussed previously) or coliform bacteria may indicate the presence of pesticides. If so, parents can contact state health and environmental agencies to determine whether their well water should be tested for specific pesticides. State agencies may conduct the testing without cost or may recommend private laboratories. Extensive pesticide testing should not be encouraged because of the cost and the rarity of pesticide contamination.

## Home Water-treatment Systems

Home water-filtration and treatment systems that remove lead, chlorine byproducts, traces of organic compounds, and bacteria are increasingly popular. These systems, which may attach to the end of a water faucet, generally provide limited health benefits. Most drinking water sources keep contaminants below US EPA standards and state criteria. In addition, small, end-of-the-faucet filtration systems or water pitcher-based filters are not always highly effective in removing trace substances.[32] If not properly maintained, filters using activated carbon can provide media for the growth of bacteria. Unless the carbon filter is frequently replaced, the first morning draw of tap water can have unacceptable levels of bacteria. It is therefore important to change the filter according to the manufacturer's instructions. Despite potential drawbacks, some home water-filtration systems can be effective in removing lead and other toxic substances. These systems, however, do not remove fluoride.

Home drinking treatment systems or filters are not encouraged unless a chemical problem has been identified. Even then, it is more effective, on a community-wide basis, to have the municipal or commercial water source personnel correct the problem as required by law than to have homeowners assume the responsibility. However, if families prefer to treat water, it is important to ensure that the treatment system removes the pollutants of concern and that the system is maintained so that it functions well and does not become contaminated. Moreover, in the case of lead, the source of the contaminant can be the home plumbing system itself so that the onus is on the property owner to correct the problem.

A basic pediatric environmental history should include questions about the source of the child's drinking water (private well or municipal water supply) and use of home water-filtration systems.

## Bottled Water

Bottled water is another drinking water option. Industry estimates indicate that in 2016, per capita consumption of bottled water was 39.3 gallons, compared with 38.5 gallons of carbonated soda beverages; 2016 was the first year that bottled water consumption was higher. Although bottled water is preferable to sweetened beverages, unless there are known contamination problems of drinking water, bottled water is not preferable to tap water. Bottled water is not required to meet higher standards than tap water and can cost 500 to 1,000 times as much. In addition, although it may contain adequate levels of fluoride as a natural constituent, bottled water is not required to have sufficient fluoride to prevent tooth decay and promote oral health. In general, bottled water products labeled as de-ionized, purified, demineralized, or distilled do not contain enough fluoride unless fluoride is specifically listed as an added ingredient. Unless fluoride is added to bottled water, the US Food and Drug Administration (FDA, the agency that regulates bottled water) does not require that fluoride amounts be listed. Families should not be encouraged to buy bottled water in most circumstances. For more information, see www.fda.gov/Food/ResourcesForYou/Consumers/ucm046894.htm.

## Contaminants in Fish

Physicians living in active fishing areas with advisories related to PCBs or mercury should ask patients if their consumption of fish is in accordance with federal- and state-issued fish advisories. Freshwater fish generally have higher levels of contaminants than do saltwater fish. Saltwater fish, generally low in contaminants, are the main fish purchased in the marketplace. However, a few saltwater fish may have higher levels of contaminants than freshwater fish. They include swordfish, shark, king mackerel, tuna, and tilefish, which are long-lived, predatory fish capable of bioaccumulating methylmercury. See Chapter 33 for more information about methylmercury in fish.

## To reduce hazards from fish consumption, inform parents to:

- Eat pan fish rather than large predator fish (shark, swordfish, tuna).

- Eat small game fish rather than large fish.

- Eat fewer fatty fish (mackerel, carp, catfish, lake trout), which accumulate higher levels of chemical toxicants.

- Trim skin and fatty areas where contaminants, such as PCBs and DDT, accumulate. (Note: Trimming fatty areas will have no effect on removing methylmercury, which accumulates in fish muscle).

- Follow fish advisories for women of childbearing age, pregnant women, nursing mothers, and young children.

- Be aware of federal and state fish advisories issued by health, environmental, and conservation departments.

### Frequently Asked Questions

Q  *Does my pitcher-based water filter remove lead?*

A  Water-filtration pitchers are commonly used because of their affordability. Most water pitchers use granular-activated carbon and resins to bond with and trap contaminants. These filters are effective at improving the taste of water, and many will also reduce levels of lead and other contaminants. Specific contaminants removed vary by model. Carbon filters have a specified shelf life and should be replaced regularly according to the manufacturer's instructions.[32]

Q  *Are the chemicals in swimming pools a health concern?*

A  Concern is emerging about the health effects of chemicals accumulating above a swimming pool, "off-gassed" from the water into the air breathed by swimmers or pool workers. Chemicals used in pools are irritating to eyes, skin, and upper and lower airways. Exposures may also be associated with development of asthma in predisposed atopic children.[33] Children who frequently swim or work in poorly ventilated indoor pools may be at higher risk.[34] Swimming is a popular and healthy form of exercise for children. Showering before swimming to remove organic matter (eg, sweat, dirt, lotions) which can react with pool chemicals to form chloramines helps to prevent their formation. Proper disinfection practices and ventilation will reduce exposure.

Q  *Should I boil my baby's water or use a home water-treatment system?*

A  If a family uses a public water supply that meets standards, parents should not boil their infant's drinking water or use a home water-treatment system unless the drinking water is contaminated. Drinking water should be boiled only when the water supplier or health or environmental agency issues such instructions. The Centers for Disease Control and Prevention and the US EPA state that people with special health needs (eg, those who are immunocompromised) may wish to boil or treat their drinking water. Boiling tap water for 1 minute inactivates or destroys biological agents, but boiling water longer than 1 minute may concentrate contaminants. Point-of-use filters also may be considered but only if they are clearly labeled to remove particles 1 mcm or less in diameter. Unless they are well maintained on schedule, home water-treatment systems often are ineffective and may even contribute to exposure to waterborne bacteria.

Q  *Is it true that federal and state regulations ensure the safety of drinking water?*

A  Federal and state regulations have oversight for water distributions systems that serve at least 25 homes. In most cases, regulations result in very safe water. Nonetheless, almost 10% of the population drinks water that does not meet regulations. Violations are higher where water supply systems serve fewer than 1,000 people. Some standards (eg, for *Cryptosporidium* species) only apply to systems that serve more than 10,000 people. Information on drinking water quality and violations can be obtained from the water supplier or state health and environmental agencies. Even water that complies with all standards may contain harmful contamination. Consumers are given annual written statements of any violations by their public water supply in consumer confidence reports. Many public water suppliers maintain Web sites with current surveillance information. Private wells are not regulated, so determining safety of water from those sources requires the attention of well owners.

Q  *Should I get my water tested?*

A  Under most circumstances, it is not necessary to have drinking water tested. If the local water supply fails to meet a standard, pressure should be exerted on politicians to correct the problem, rather than having people test their own water. As a precaution, people who use private wells less than 50 feet (15 meters) deep and who have septic systems should have wells tested yearly for coliforms (see Table 17-2). In the case of private wells, quarterly testing for 1 year is recommended, followed by yearly testing for nitrates if results of quarterly tests are normal.

Q  *How do I know that my water is safe for infant formula?*

A  Water used for mixing infant formula must be from a safe water source, as defined by the state or local health department. If there are concerns or uncertainty about the safety of tap water, bottled water or cold tap water that has been brought to a rolling boil for 1 minute (no longer), then cooled to room temperature for no more than 30 minutes, may be used.

Q  *How do I test my water for lead and what should I do about the results?*

A  Public water systems test for lead but homes may have internal plumbing materials containing lead. Because you cannot see, taste, or smell lead dissolved in water, testing is the only sure way to know whether there are harmful quantities of lead in your drinking water. State or local drinking water authorities maintain lists of laboratories certified for testing drinking water for lead. The US EPA maintains a Web site providing a list of all such laboratories: https://www.epa.gov/dwlabcert/contact-information-certification-programs-and-certified-laboratories-drinking-water. The cost of testing is between $20 and $100. You may also contact your water supplier because the supplier may have useful information, including whether the service connector used in your home or area is made of lead. A number of steps can be taken to reduce the amount of lead exposure from drinking water at home:

— Use only water from the cold tap for drinking, cooking, and making baby formula. The water from the hot water tap may have higher levels of lead.

— Regularly clean your faucet's screen (also known as an aerator).

— Consider using a water filter certified to remove lead and know when it is time to replace the filter. (See the guidance on home water filtration.)[32]

— Before drinking, flush your pipes by running your tap, taking a shower, or doing laundry or a load of dishes.

Q  *Is it okay to flush unused prescription drugs down the toilet?*

A  Residues of birth control pills, antidepressants, painkillers, shampoos, and many other pharmaceuticals and personal care products have been found in water, in trace amounts. These chemicals are flushed into rivers from sewage treatment plants or leach into groundwater from septic systems. The discovery of these substances in water probably reflects better sensing technology. The health effects, if any, from exposure to these substances in water is not yet known.

In many cases, these chemicals enter water when people excrete them or wash them away in the shower. Some chemicals, however, are flushed or washed down the drain when people discard outdated or unused drugs. Recent federal guidelines state that prescription or over-the-counter medications should not be flushed down the toilet or poured down a sink unless patient information material specifically states that it is safe to do so (https://www.fda.gov/drugs/resourcesforyou/consumers/buyingusingmedicinesafely/ensuringsafeuseofmedicine/safedisposalofmedicines/ucm186187.htm).

If no disposal instructions are given on the prescription drug labeling, then follow these FDA guidelines to dispose of these products properly and to prevent harm from accidental exposure or intentional misuse after they are no longer needed:

— "Follow any specific disposal instructions on the prescription drug labeling or patient information that accompanies the medicine. Do not flush medicines down the sink or toilet unless this information specifically instructs you to do so.

— Take advantage of programs that allow the public to take unused drugs to a central location for proper disposal. Call your local law enforcement agencies to see if they sponsor medicine take-back programs in your community. Contact your city's or county government's household trash and recycling service to learn about medication disposal options and guidelines for your area.

— Transfer unused medicines to collectors registered with the Drug Enforcement Administration (DEA). Authorized sites may be retail, hospital or clinic pharmacies, and law enforcement locations. Some offer mail-back programs or collection receptacles ("drop-boxes"). Visit the DEA's Web site (www.deadiversion.usdoj.gov/drug_disposal/index.html) or call 1-800-882-9539 for more information and to find an authorized collector (www.deadiversion.usdoj.gov/pubdispsearch/spring/main?execution=e1s1) in your community.

— If no disposal instructions are given on the prescription drug labeling and no take-back program is available in your area, throw the drugs in the household trash following these steps:

  • Remove them from their original containers and mix them with an undesirable substance, such as used coffee grounds, dirt, or kitty litter (this makes the drug less appealing to children and pets, and unrecognizable to people who may intentionally go through the trash seeking drugs).

  • Place the mixture in a sealable bag, empty can, or other container to prevent the drug from leaking or breaking out of a garbage bag."[35]

## Resources

### Agency for Toxic Substances and Disease Registry
Web site: www.atsdr.cdc.gov

### US Environmental Protection Agency
Web site: www.epa.gov/ost/fish
EPA Safe Drinking Water Hotline: 800/426-4791. Regional offices are listed in the local telephone book.

## US Environmental Protection Agency: Private Drinking Water Wells
Web site: www.epa.gov/privatewells/publications.html

## US Fish and Wildlife Service, Department of the Interior
Web site: www.fws.gov

## US Food and Drug Administration
FDA Regulates the Safety of Bottled Water Beverages Including Flavored Water and Nutrient-Added Water Beverages

Web site: www.fda.gov/Food/ResourcesForYou/Consumers/ucm046894.htm

## Wisconsin Department of Natural Resources
Information for Homeowners with Private Wells

Web site: www.dnr.state.wi.us/org/water/dwg/prih2o.htm

## References

1. Okum D. Water quality management. In: Last JM, Wallace RB, eds. *Maxcy-Rosenau-Last Public Health and Preventive Medicine.* 13th ed. East Norwalk, CT: Appleton & Lange; 1992;619–648

2. World Health Organization. *Guidelines for Drinking-Water Quality. Incorporating First Addendum. Vol 1, Recommendations.* 4th ed. Geneva, Switzerland: World Health Organization; 2011

3. Reynolds KA, Mena KD, Gerba CP. Risk of waterborne illness via drinking water in the United States. *Rev Environ Contam Toxicol.* 2008;192:117–158

4. Schwake DO, Garner E, Strom OR, Pruden A, Edwards MA. Legionella DNA markers in tap water coincident with a spike in Legionnaires' Disease in Flint, MI. *Environmental Science & Technology Letters.* 2016;3:311–315

5. American Academy of Pediatrics. *Red Book: 2015 Report of the Committee on Infectious Diseases.* Pickering LK, Baker CJ, Kimberlin DW, Long SS, eds. 30th ed. Elk Grove Village, IL: American Academy of Pediatrics; 2015

6. Albering HJ, van Leusen SM, Moonen EJC, et al. Human health risk assessment: a case study involving heavy metal soil contamination after the flooding of the river Meuse during the winter of 1993-1994. *Environ Health Perspect.* 1999;107(1):37–43

7. Otten TG, Paerl HW. Health effects of toxic cyanobacteria in U.S. drinking and recreational waters: our current understanding and proposed direction. *Curr Environ Health Rpt.* 2015;2:75–84

8. Friedman MA, Levin BE. Neurobehavioral effects of harmful algal bloom (HAB) toxins: a critical review. *J Int Neuropsychol Soc.* 2005;11(3):331–338

9. Goldman LR, Koduru S. Chemicals in the environment and developmental toxicity to children: a public health and policy perspective. *Environ Health Perspect.* 2000;108(Suppl 3):443–448

10. Glassmeyer ST, Furlong ET, Kolpin DW, et al. Nationwide reconnaissance of contaminants of emerging concern in source and treated drinking waters of the United States. *Sci Total Environ.* 2017;581–582:909–922

11. National Research Council, Committee on Toxicology. *Arsenic in Drinking Water: 2001 Update.* Washington, DC: National Research Council

12. Tolins M, Ruchirawat M, Landrigan P. The developmental neurotoxicity of arsenic: cognitive and behavioral consequences of early life exposure. *Ann Glob Health.* 2014;80(4):303–314

13. Centers for Disease Control and Prevention. Community Water Fluoridation: Questions and Answers. http://www.cdc.gov/fluoridation/fact_sheets/cwf_qa.htm. Accessed April 26, 2018

14. American Academy of Pediatrics Council on Environmental Health. Prevention of childhood lead toxicity. *Pediatrics*. 2016;138(1). Correction available at: http://pediatrics.aappublications.org/content/140/2/e20171490

15. Zahran S, McElmurry SP, Kilgore PE, et al. Assessment of the Legionnaires' disease outbreak in Flint, Michigan. *Proc Natl Acad Sci U S A*. 2018;115(8):E1730–E1739

16. Miranda ML, Kim D, Hull AP, Paul CJ, Galeano MA. Changes in blood lead levels associated with use of chloramines in water treatment systems. *Environ Health Perspect*. 2007;115(2):221–225

17. Goldman LR, Shannon MW. Technical report: mercury in the environment: implications for pediatricians. *Pediatrics*. 2001;108(1):197–205

18. Moran MJ, Zogorski JS, Squillace PJ. MTBE and gasoline hydrocarbons in ground water of the United States. *Ground Water*. 2005;43(4):615–627

19. US Department of Health and Human Services, National Toxicology Program. *Report on Carcinogens, 14th ed*. Research Triangle Park, NC: US Department of Health and Human Services, Public Health Service; 2016

20. Jacobson JL, Jacobson SW. Prenatal exposure to polychlorinated biphenyls and attention at school age. *J Pediatr*. 2003;143(6):780–788

21. National Research Council. *Environmental Epidemiology: Public Health and Hazardous Wastes*. Washington, DC: National Academies Press; 1991

22. Villanueva CM, Fernandez F, Malats N, Grimalt JO, Kogevinas M. Meta-analysis of studies on individual consumption of chlorinated drinking water and bladder cancer. *J Epidemiol Community Health*. 2003;57(3):166–173

23. Savitz DA, Singer PC, Herring AH, Hartmann KE, Weinberg HS, Makarushka C. Exposure to drinking water disinfection by-products and pregnancy loss. *Am J Epidemiol*. 2006;164(11):1043–1051

24. Nieuwenhuijsen MJ, Toledano MB, Eaton NE, Fawell J, Elliott P. Chlorination disinfection byproducts in water and their association with adverse reproductive outcomes: a review. *Occup Environ Med*. 2000;57(2):73–85

25. Goodman M, Hays S. Asthma and swimming: a meta-analysis. *J Asthma*. 2008;45(8):639–647

26. National Research Council. 2005. Health Implications of Perchlorate Ingestion. National Research Council of the National Academies. Washington, DC: National Academies Press

27. US Environmental Protection Agency. Perchlorate in Drinking Water Frequent Questions. https://www.epa.gov/dwstandardsregulations/perchlorate-drinking-water-frequent-questions. Accessed April 26, 2018

28. US Environmental Protection Agency. Fact Sheet. PFOA & PFOS Drinking Water Health Advisories. https://www.epa.gov/sites/production/files/2016-06/documents/drinkingwaterhealthadvisories_pfoa_pfos_updated_5.31.16.pdf. Accessed April 26, 2018

29. Bean JA, Isacson P, Hahne RM, Kohler J. Drinking water and cancer incidence in Iowa. II. Radioactivity in drinking water. *Am J Epidemiol*. 1982;116(6):924–932

30. US Environmental Protection Agency, Office of Ground Water and Drinking Water. *National Primary Drinking Water Regulations*. https://www.epa.gov/ground-water-and-drinking-water/national-primary-drinking-water-regulations. Accessed April 26, 2018

31. American Academy of Pediatrics Committee on Environmental Health, Committee on Infectious Diseases, Rogan WJ, Brady MT. Drinking water from private wells and risks to children. *Pediatrics*. 2009;123(6):1599–1605

32. NSF International. Home Water Treatment System Selection. http://www.nsf.org/consumer-resources/water-quality/water-filters-testing-treatment/home-water-treatment-system-selection. Accessed April 26, 2018

33. Bernard A, Carbonnelle S, de Burbure C, Michel O, Nickmilder M. Chlorinated pool attendance, atopy, and the risk of asthma during childhood. *Environ Health Perspect*. 2006;114(10):1567–1573

34. Centers for Disease Control and Prevention. Ocular and respiratory illness associated with an indoor swimming pool—Nebraska, 2006. *MMWR Morb Mortal Wkly Rep*. 2007;56(36):929–932

35. US Food and Drug Administration. Where and How to Dispose of Unused Medicines. Silver Spring, MD: US FDA; 2017. https://www.fda.gov/ForConsumers/ConsumerUpdates/ucm101653.htm. Accessed April 26, 2018

Chapter 18

# Food Safety

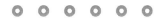

## KEY POINTS

- Although the US food supply is among the safest in the world, an estimated 47.8 million foodborne illnesses occur in the United States every year, with infants and young children among those most at risk for complications.
- Pediatricians have important roles to play in monitoring the safety of the food supply by reporting incidents of foodborne illnesses to local and state public health agencies.
- Current evidence does not support any meaningful nutritional benefits or deficits from eating organic foods compared with conventionally grown foods.
- The pesticide residue levels of organic foods are consistently lower than nonorganic foods; washing and peeling nonorganic foods prior to consuming can reduce pesticide exposure.

## INTRODUCTION

This chapter focuses on topics including foodborne illness and food contaminants, food irradiation, organic foods, food labeling, food additives, and pesticides. Contamination of food by lead and mercury is described in Chapters 32 and 33, respectively.

## FOODBORNE ILLNESSES

Although the US food supply is among the safest in the world, the Foodborne Diseases Active Surveillance Network, a collaborative program among the Centers for Disease Control and Prevention (CDC) and other federal and state agencies, documented 24,029 infections, 5,512 hospitalizations, and 98 deaths that were the result of infections that were confirmed in 2016, with the very young, elderly, and/or immunocompromised most at risk for complications.[1-3] The American Academy of Pediatrics (AAP) *Red Book* describes the diagnosis and treatment of illnesses caused by foodborne pathogens. Symptoms, timing, and food consumed are crucial in determining the cause, treatment, and prognosis. Contaminants in foods include:

- Viruses: hepatitis A, norovirus, and rotavirus;
- Parasites: *Toxoplasma gondii, Cryptosporidium parvum, Cyclospora species, Giardia lamblia, Taenia* species, *and Trichinella spiralis;*
- Bacteria: *Salmonella* species, *Shigella* species, *Campylobacter* species, *Escherichia coli, Vibrio cholerae, Vibrio vulnificus, Yersinia enterocolitica, Brucella species*, and *Listeria* species;
- Toxins produced by bacteria: *Staphylococcus aureus, Bacillus cereus, Clostridium perfringens, Clostridium botulinum,* and *E. coli* O157:H7;
- Toxins produced by molds: aflatoxins, vomitoxin, and other mycotoxins;
- Prions: can cause abnormal folding of protein (eg, Creutzfeldt-Jakob disease);
- Heavy metals: tin, copper, cadmium, iron, zinc;
- Products accumulated in the food chain of fish and shellfish: scombroid, saxitoxin, ciguatera toxin, tetrodotoxin, and domoic acid.

For a complete list including symptoms, timing, and cause, please refer to the AAP *Red Book* (https://redbook.solutions.aap.org/chapter.aspx?sectionId=88187334&bookId=1484&resultClick=1#91031943).

The American Medical Association, the Centers for Disease Control and Prevention (CDC), the Food Safety and Inspection Service (FSIS), and the US Food and Drug Administration (FDA) produced a primer for physicians that describes the diagnosis and management of foodborne illnesses.[3]

### Pathogenic Hazards

Infectious organisms are ubiquitous in the environment and can enter the food supply in many ways. Chickens infected with *Salmonella* species can excrete these organisms into their eggs before the shells are formed or excrete the organisms in feces that can contaminate egg shells. Shellfish and other seafood can become contaminated by pathogens, such as the hepatitis A virus and *Anisakis simplex* (a roundworm) in sushi. Animal feces can contaminate foods via polluted irrigation water, unsafe handling of manure, and unsanitary production and processing activities. Food can become contaminated in retail facilities, institutional settings, and homes because of inappropriate food handling.

The food production system is becoming more centralized and global, adding to the complexity of foodborne pathogen exposures. For example, in the United States large outbreaks of infection were caused by the presence of *Cyclospora* in fresh produce.[4] In a 2013 multistate outbreak, 631 cases occurred; cilantro was identified as the most common vehicle of infection.[4] In late 2017, up to 15 states and Canada reported severe outbreaks of hemolytic-uremic syndrome and death caused by leafy greens contaminated with *E. coli* O157:H7.[5] Twenty-five people became infected, including 9 who were hospitalized. One death was reported. The CDC reports several *E. coli* O157:H7 outbreaks annually. More recently, widespread outbreaks of *Salmonella* were traceable to contaminated ground peanut products (*S.* Typhimurium) and contaminated imported jalapeno peppers (*S.* Saintpaul). Increases in *Campylobacter* infections among children have been linked to extreme precipitation events.[6]

Since 1996, the CDC has used the FoodNet system to track the incidence and trends of foodborne infections. The general trend from 2011 to 2014 was a lower incidence of Shiga toxin-producing *E. coli* O157:H7 (STEC O157:H7) and a higher incidence of STEC non-O157:H7; otherwise, there were no changes in infections caused by *Cryptosporidium* species, *Cyclospora* species, *Listeria* species, *Salmonella* species, *Shigella* species, or *Yersinia* species.[1] With the exception of *Listeria, Vibrio,* and *Cyclospora,* the incidence of these infections was highest among children younger than age 5 years. Many pathogens are particularly virulent for children. *Salmonella, Listeria, Cyclospora, Cryptosporidium, E. coli* O157:H7, *Shigella,* and *Campylobacter* are among many foodborne pathogens that pose risks to young children.[1] Standards for pathogens are established for meat, poultry, and egg products by the FSIS and for all other foods by the FDA. State public health agencies, along with local public health officers, monitor the incidence of foodborne illness, and the US Environmental Protection Agency (US EPA) regulates the discharge of pollutants into waters that may later contaminate food.

Every year, *Listeria* has been associated with more than 1,600 illnesses in people in the United States. It is fatal in up to 20% of patients. In July 2012, a multistate and international outbreak was investigated and identified imported soft cheese as the source.[7] Rarely, fresh produce may be a vehicle for listeriosis which was the case in an outbreak that occurred in late 2015 to early 2016.[8] The earliest case in the cluster occurred in July 2015, but the source was not detected until November 2015 because the tool used for surveillance did not include leafy green vegetables. When included, all interviewed patients reported consuming leafy greens the month prior to illness onset. In the United States, 19 persons from 9 states met the case definition. All were hospitalized; one died. Meningitis developed in one otherwise healthy child.

The prion, the agent responsible for transmissible spongiform encephalopathies, is neither a virus nor a bacterium, but an abnormal form of a normal glycoprotein. Prion diseases include bovine spongiform encephalopathy (mad cow disease), scrapie in sheep, chronic wasting disease in deer and elk, and Creutzfeldt-Jakob disease and variant Creutzfeldt-Jakob disease in humans.[9] In the United Kingdom, an epidemic of variant Creutzfeldt-Jakob disease followed the epidemic of bovine spongiform encephalopathy.[10] Although 4 cases of variant Creutzfeldt-Jakob disease have been identified in the United States, these patients were born outside of the United States and presumed to have acquired the disease from that location during the risk period (1980 to 1996).[11] These cases are to be differentiated from the cases of Creutzfeldt-Jakob disease in the United States secondary to injection of pituitary growth hormone extracted from pituitaries of infected individuals. Those cases resulted in removal of pituitary-derived growth hormone from the market; now only recombinant growth hormone is available.

## Toxic Hazards

Toxic chemicals in food can be grouped into the following broad categories:

- Residues of pesticides deliberately applied to food crops or to stored or processed foods
- Colorings, flavorings, and other chemicals deliberately added during processing (direct food additives) and substances used in food-contact materials including adhesives, dyes, coatings, paper, paperboard, and polymers (plastics) that may come into contact with food as part of packaging or processing equipment but are not intended to be added directly to food (indirect food additives)
- Contaminants that inadvertently or purposefully enter the food supply, such as aflatoxins, nitrites, polychlorinated biphenyls (PCBs), perchlorate, bisphenol A (BPA), BPA analogs such as BPX, dioxins, metals including lead, mercury and arsenic, persistent pesticide residues such as dichlorodiphenyltrichloroethane (DDT), and vomitoxin.

### Pesticides and Organic Foods

Pesticides are applied extensively to food crops around the world. More than 400 different pesticidal active ingredients are formulated into thousands of products. Pesticides are used at all stages of food production to protect against pests in the field, in shipping, and in storage. In 2012, more than 1.1 billion pounds of pesticides were used in the United States.[12] The US EPA sets "tolerances," standards for allowable levels of pesticides on food. In the United States, pesticides must be registered with the US EPA and the state before distribution. The FDA and the FSIS monitor the food supply for pesticide residues.

The Food Quality Protection Act (FQPA) of 1996 required that the US EPA provide an additional margin of safety when the toxic risks for children are uncertain. This requirement aims to ensure that children are adequately protected from excessive pesticide exposure.[13] Acute and chronic exposure to pesticides can have adverse effects on health. Numerous pesticides have potential carcinogenicity but there also are impacts on cognitive functioning, behavior, birth outcomes, and asthma. Exposure is mainly through ingestion but also includes dermal absorption (eg, from clothes) and inhalation.[14] The FQPA also considers cumulative effects of all pesticides, endocrine disruption, age-appropriate estimates of dietary consumption, reassesses tolerances every 10 years, and reviews all pesticides every 15 years.

Several methods can be used to reduce potential exposure to pesticides. Because diet is the main exposure source, changing the diet may help to decrease exposure. Regulations exist for foods labeled "organic." The US Department of Agriculture (USDA) developed the National Organic Program after the Organic Foods Production Act.[15] Under the National Organic Program, food (animals and crops) must not be grown or raised using hormones, genetic engineering, chemicals, antibiotics, or irradiation. Specifically, organically grown food can be labeled as such if the food was grown and processed using no synthetic fertilizers or pesticides. Approved pesticides are present in organic foods in quantities less than that found in nonorganic foods. Yearly inspection is conducted to ensure continued compliance with regulations.[16]

Parents frequently ask about food labeling, including "organic," "humane," and "antibiotic free." Organic farming avoids synthetic chemicals, hormones, antibiotics, genetic engineering, and irradiation. To qualify as organic, crops must be produced on farms that have not used most synthetic pesticides, herbicides, and fertilizers for 3 years before harvest, and have a sufficient buffer zone to decrease contamination from adjacent lands. Organic livestock must be reared without the routine use of antibiotics or growth hormones and be provided with access to the outdoors.

Diet is the main source of childhood pesticide exposure;[17] other sources and routes are described in Chapter 40. Pesticide residue levels in organic foods are consistently lower than in nonorganic foods.[18] In one study, children who ate organic foods had lower urinary excretion of pesticides compared with those who ate a conventional diet.[19] Washing or peeling produce and removing fat and skin from meat and fish (higher concentrations of some pesticides can be found in fat) can also decrease exposure.

Although pesticide consumption is less with organic food, the long-term clinical significance of this is to be determined.[20] An important consideration is that organic foods are more costly (up to 10% to 40% more) than nonorganic foods. This economic reality may lead families to eat fewer fruits and vegetables overall.

A common misconception about organic food is that it provides more nutrients than conventional food.[17,21] Organic farming has less of an environmental impact compared with conventional agricultural approaches but the nutritional and health benefits of organic foods have not been demonstrated to be significant.[22] The reaffirmed policy from the AAP (Organic Foods: Health and Environmental Advantages and Disadvantages) found no direct evidence of relevant nutritional differences between organic and conventional produce.[17] Studies have shown improved health with organic food consumption, but this may be better correlated with healthy lifestyle indicators rather than the nutritional value of the food itself.[21] Families will have better nutritional outcomes if they are reassured that having a well-rounded diet is more important than eating only organically grown and raised foods.

Understanding organic food labeling can be daunting and confusing. Certain labels are held to strict standards by the USDA, whereas other labels are not. For example, terms such as "100% organic" hold the product responsible to be made from 100% organically produced ingredients and processing aids (excluding water and salt).[16] Other terms, such as "no drugs," "no growth hormones used," "free range," or "sustainably harvested," are held to less stringent standards or restrictions. Another common label is "all natural." This label, closely regulated by the USDA, implies that products contain no artificial flavoring, color ingredients, or chemical preservatives. The USDA provides clear guidance on their Web site to indicate the meaning and implications that each label implies.[16]

### Food Additives

The FDA provides oversight of more than 80% of the food in the US food supply and, within the FDA, the Center for Food Safety and Applied Nutrition Office of Food Additive Safety reviews the safety of food ingredients and packaging.[23] More than 10,000 chemicals are allowed to be added to food and food contact materials in the United States, either directly or indirectly, under the 1958 Food Additives Amendment to the 1938 Federal Food, Drug, and Cosmetic Act.[24] Each added substance is evaluated by the FDA and is determined to, directly or indirectly, become a component or effect a component of the food.

Chemical agents that exhibit antimicrobial activity may be used to achieve food preservation by inhibiting growth of undesirable microorganisms. Food preservatives can be added to food to reduce the risk of foodborne infections, decrease microbial spoilage, and preserve the nutritional quality of the food. Although there are physical techniques used for food preservation— dehydration, freezing, refrigeration, freeze-drying, canning, curing, and pickling—chemical preservatives are used more often commercially. These chemicals may be synthetic compounds intentionally added to foods or naturally occurring, biologically derived substances.

The Federal Food, Drug, and Cosmetic Act allows for the use of a chemical preservative in foods if (1) it is "generally recognized as safe" or GRAS, (2) not used in a way to conceal damage or make the food appear better than it is, and (3) is properly declared on the label.[25] The Food Additive Status List omits, however, certain categories including those that are GRAS, certain synthetic flavorings, indirect food additives such as a pesticide chemical, and color additives. A pesticide chemical as a residue in or on a food is not considered a food additive, but instead must comply with tolerances as set by the US EPA but regulated by the FDA.[26] Substances are determined to be safe under the conditions of their intended use by qualified experts external to the FDA. According to the 1958 Food Additives Amendment, manufacturers determine when an additive is GRAS. Thus, substances that are GRAS are not considered food additives and do not require premarket approval by the FDA. Manufacturers may submit a substance through a GRAS affirmation petition process, but this is not mandatory. The FDA has been criticized for this program based on conflicts of interest that arise from individuals who review petitions.[27] More than 70% of GRAS petitions to the FDA are affirmed with no questions to the manufacturer.[28]

Food additives include diet-enriching and potentially hazardous additives. Examples of diet-enriching additives include vitamins, iron, iodine, and folic acid. Regulations exist about the type and amount of additive(s) that can be added to food; the additives are listed on food labels.

Some food additives may cause adverse reactions in children and others. Tartrazine (also known as FD&C—food dye and coloring—yellow No. 5) is a dye used in some foods and beverages. Cake mixes, candies, canned vegetables, cheese, chewing gum, hot dogs, ice cream, orange drinks, salad dressings, seasoning salts, soft drinks, and catsup may contain tartrazine. An estimated 0.12% of the general population is intolerant to tartrazine. Tartrazine may cause urticaria and asthma exacerbations in people who are sensitive to it.

Monosodium glutamate (MSG) is associated with the so-called "Chinese restaurant syndrome" of headache, nausea, diarrhea, sweating, chest tightness, and a burning sensation along the back of the neck. It seems to be linked to consuming large amounts of MSG, not only in Chinese foods, but also in other foods in which a large concentration of MSG is used as a flavor enhancer.

Sulfites are used to preserve foods and sanitize containers for fermented beverages. They may be found in soup mixes, frozen and dehydrated potatoes, dried fruits, fruit juices, canned and dehydrated vegetables, processed seafood products, jams and jellies, relishes, and some bakery products. Some beverages, such as hard cider, wine, and beer, also contain sulfites. Because sulfites can cause asthma exacerbations in sulfite-sensitive patients, the FDA ruled that packaged foods must be labeled if they contain more than 10 parts per million (ppm) of sulfites.

## Food Contact Substances

Indirect food additives enter the food supply through contact with food in manufacturing, packing, packaging, transport, or holding, even though the substances are not intended to have effects on food. More than 3,000 such substances are recognized by the FDA. One category is called "food contact substances;" these include packaging materials (adhesives and compounds of coatings, paper and paperboard products, polymers, adjuvants [agents added to increase the effect of the product], and production aids) and an array of other materials.

Certain plastic substances have come under increased scrutiny as food contact items. One is bisphenol A (BPA, 2,2-bis[4-hydroxyphenyl]propane), which is made by combining acetone and phenol and is one of the highest-volume chemicals produced worldwide. BPA acts as a weak estrogen. It is used mainly as a material for the production of epoxy resins used to line metal cans and in hard plastics. In the recent past, BPA had been found in hard plastic baby bottles, water bottles, and many other food containers. In a US national sample comparing data on BPA exposure from 2003 to 2004 to data from 2011 to 2012, the geometric mean urinary BPA levels significantly decreased from 2.64 ng/mL to 1.5 ng/mL; the highest intakes were in persons aged 12 to 19 years.[29] In 2012 and 2013, the FDA granted petitions requesting an amendment to regulations to no longer provide for the use of certain BPA-based materials in baby bottles, sippy cups, and infant formula packaging because their use had been abandoned.[30] This voluntary change was a result of the public's push for BPA removal from products and likely led to the significant decrease in BPA exposure, even before actions by the FDA.

Numerous analogs of BPA are collectively referred to as BPX. BPXs are not well studied but these analogs bind estrogen receptors to varying degrees and have varying activity levels. Phthalates, a class of plasticizers used in soft plastics, also may come into contact with food.[31] Phthalates are weakly estrogenic and anti-androgenic (androgen blocking) chemicals. Some phthalates are suspected of causing cancer. Phthalates have numerous industrial uses (eg, in industrial plastics, inks, and dyes and adhesives in food packaging), consumer uses (eg, in cosmetics and vinyl clothing), and medical uses (as a softener in polyvinyl chloride intravenous tubing, blood bags, and dialysis equipment). Over the years, phthalate compounds were used in pacifiers, baby bottle nipples, and teething toys, and then removed from these uses by the US Consumer Product Safety Commission (CPSC).

The Consumer Product Safety Improvement Act mandated that as of 2009, it is unlawful for any person to manufacture for sale, offer for sale, distribute in commerce, or import into the United States any children's toy or child care article that contains concentrations of more than 0.1% of the most commonly used phthalates diethylhexyl phthalate (DEHP), dibutyl phthalate (DBP), or benzyl butyl phthalate (BBP), and that it is unlawful for any person to manufacture for sale, offer for sale, distribute in commerce, or import into the United States any children's toy that can be placed in a child's mouth or child care article that contains concentrations of more than 0.1% of diisononyl phthalate (DINP), diisodecyl phthalate (DIDP), or di-*n*-octylphthalate (DnOP).

The FDA allows the use of phthalates in food contact items and has found that exposures are very low. The CDC tracks trends of phthalates in the human population. Bisphenol A and phthalates are discussed in Chapter 41.

### Mycotoxins

Mycotoxins are toxins produced by certain molds. Mycotoxins are present in many agricultural products such as peanuts, corn, and wheat.[32] The best-known mycotoxin, aflatoxin, is produced by the *Aspergillus* fungus. Others include patulin, citrinin, zearalenone, vomitoxin, and the trichothecenes.

The principal human exposure to aflatoxins is from food. The International Agency for Research on Cancer concluded that aflatoxin is a carcinogen[33] based on studies conducted in areas with a high incidence of hepatocellular carcinoma, such as in Asia, where the incidence of chronic hepatitis B viral infections also is high. Aflatoxin $B_1$ is an important risk factor for hepatocellular carcinoma in humans.[34,35] Vomitoxin, also known as deoxynivalenol, is a frequent contaminant of corn and wheat products, and can lead to epidemics of vomiting within hours of consuming contaminated food. Symptoms usually are self-limited.[36]

### Dioxins and Polychlorinated Biphenyls

Dioxins and furans are inadvertently produced during the manufacture of certain chemicals and by incineration. Polychlorinated biphenyls (PCBs) were manufactured for use as fire retardants and in electrical transformers and capacitors. Dioxins and PCBs are persistent and bioaccumulative chemicals; the highest levels are found in fish in contaminated areas. They can enter the food supply via animal feed. In the United States in 1998 and in Belgium in 1999 there were episodes in which a large proportion of the food supply (chickens, eggs, and catfish in the United States and chicken and eggs in Belgium) became contaminated by dioxins because of adulteration of animal feeds.[37,38] In 2001, the European Commission established a tolerable weekly intake of dioxins and dioxin-like PCBs in the diet.[39] The FDA established temporary tolerance levels for residues of PCBs as "unavoidable environmental or industrial contaminants" for multiple foods including milk and dairy products; poultry and eggs; animal feed, fish, and shellfish; and food packaging materials.[40] In 2012, the US EPA established a chronic oral reference dose for non-cancer effects for

2,3,7,8-tetrachlorodibenzo-*p*-dioxin (TCDD, the chemical used as the reference dioxin).[41] A reference dose is a level that is not likely to have long-term health effects over a lifetime, including for high-risk populations.

### Melamine

Melamine is a monomeric chemical that when polymerized makes a hard material that can be molded into dishes or containers, or used as a laminate. The polymer also is called melamine. Each molecule of melamine contains 4 nitrogen atoms. Melamine was identified as an illegal additive found in certain foods from China including infant formula, various milk and milk-derived products, and dog and cat food. The melamine problem was first identified in China in 2007 when mysterious illnesses including urinary stones and renal failure, and death developed in several cats and small dogs. Illnesses were linked to melamine in a wide variety of pet foods, eventually traced to a single source of protein powder.[42] It had been a standard practice to test the protein content of foods by assessing the total number of nitrogen atoms. Melamine was used as a food additive to defraud purchasers by artificially inflating the protein content of foods, thereby falsely making them appear suitable for consumption. In urine, melamine and its breakdown products precipitate to form calculi. In 2007 and 2008, thousands of infants across China were reported to have urinary tract symptoms involving calculi; an unknown number of deaths were linked to melamine-contaminated infant formula.[43,44] One specific brand of infant formula was identified; it is not marketed in the United States. Melamine, however, has now been identified in other foods in the United States, at much lower levels. At this time, the FDA is not concerned about these lower levels of melamine. Melamine dishware has not been implicated as a source for melamine contamination of food.

### Arsenic

Rice and seafood are the most commonly ingested foods known to be contaminated with arsenic. Inorganic arsenic is more toxic than organic arsenic. Inorganic arsenic is found in rice because rice plants absorb arsenic from the soil in which they are grown, and the content of arsenic in soil varies in the United States and around the world. Organic arsenic is found in seafood and is much less toxic. Most testing does not differentiate between inorganic and organic arsenic. Using data from the National Health and Nutrition Examination Survey (NHANES) study, researchers found that total urinary arsenic concentration increased 14.2% with each 0.25 cup increase in cooked rice consumption.[45] In 2012, the FDA suggested that some rice products had higher levels of inorganic arsenic than others with higher concentrations found in infant/toddler foods and snacks.[46] The FDA suggested that industry adopt a voluntary approach to decrease arsenic levels to below 50 mcg/kg, a level higher than the level found in most adult food products. In a study that assessed arsenic content in common infant and toddler rice cereals in US supermarkets, however, the average total arsenic and inorganic arsenic concentrations in infant rice cereal were 174.4 and 101.4 mcg/kg, respectively.[47] In response to these findings, the AAP suggested that cereals from other grains, such as oatmeal and wheat, as well as other pureed foods (eg, finely chopped meats and vegetable purees) are equally acceptable as rice cereal to introduce to infants as first foods. Other thickeners, such as finely ground oats, could be considered in children with swallowing difficulty.[48] As of this printing, no further guidance on arsenic in foods has been suggested.

### Perchlorate

Perchlorate is a molecule found in drinking water and some foods.[49] Perchlorate is manmade and also occurs naturally. Most perchlorate probably enters foods through contact during production and/or processing with water treated previously with chlorinated biocidal products for disinfection purposes. If ingested in large enough quantities, perchlorate can cause thyroid dysfunction and therefore may result in abnormalities of growth and neurologic development. If the level of perchlorate in public drinking water is greater than 15 parts per billion (ppb), bottled water or water that has perchlorate filtered out should be used to reconstitute infant formula. The US EPA established a reference dose of 0.7 mcg/kg body weight/day. For infants and young children, the estimated intake from food is 0.17 to 0.29 mcg/kg body weight/day. (https://www.fda.gov/Food/FoodborneIllnessContaminants/ChemicalContaminants/ucm077572.htm)

## FOOD IRRADIATION

Food irradiation is a process by which food is exposed to a controlled source of ionizing radiation to prolong shelf life and reduce food losses, improve microbiological safety, and/or reduce the use of chemical fumigants and additives. It can be used to reduce insect infestation of grain, dried spices, and dried or fresh fruits and vegetables; inhibit sprouting in tubers and bulbs; retard post-harvest ripening of fruits; inactivate parasites in meats and fish; eliminate spoilage microbes from fresh fruits and vegetables; extend shelf life in poultry, meats, fish, and shellfish; decontaminate poultry and beef; and sterilize food and feed.[50] Food irradiation can be useful when washing or heating of consumed products is minimal or when proper cold storage of produce is overlooked during transport.

The dose of ionizing radiation determines the effects of the food irradiation process on foods. Low-dose irradiation (up to 1 kilogray [kGy]) is used primarily to delay ripening of produce or to kill or render sterile insects and other higher organisms that may infest fresh food. Medium-dose irradiation (1 to 10 kGy) reduces the number of pathogens and other microbes on food and prolongs shelf life. High-dose irradiation (greater than 10 kGy) sterilizes food and is subject to higher regulations.[51] Intense pulsed light has also been studied as a means of food disinfection and has been approved by the FDA.[52] Different studies have shown microorganism sensitivities to pulsed light disinfection, but they have not been directly compared in one study. Sensitive organisms include fungal spores; bacterial endospores; yeasts, parasites, and viruses; and vegetative bacteria (in order of individually observed sensitivity).[36]

Food irradiation is considered a "process" by many nations. The US Congress explicitly included sources of irradiation as "food additives" under the 1958 Food Additives Amendment to the Federal Food, Drug, and Cosmetic Act (FDCA) of 1938.[53] Thus, irradiated food is defined as adulterated and illegal to market unless irradiation conforms to specified federal rules. The technical effect on the food, dosimetry, and environmental controls must be defined and in compliance with the FDCA. Facilities also must pass an environmental impact study to comply with the National Environmental Policy Act of 1969. Nutritional adequacy as well as radiologic, toxicologic, and microbiologic safety must be ensured under FDA regulations.

All irradiated food sold in the United States must be labeled with the international sign of irradiation, the radura (Figure 18-1). Current labeling rules do not require that the dose of radiation or the purpose of the irradiation be specified.[51] Thus, it is not possible for consumers to know whether food has been treated to reduce pathogen loads or merely to prolong shelf life. Furthermore, current rules do not require food services to identify irradiated foods they serve or for multi-ingredient products to identify which ingredients have been irradiated.

In terms of radiologic safety, neither the food nor the packaging materials become radioactive as a result of irradiation.[54] The sources of radiation

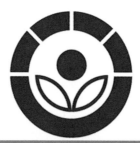

Figure 18-1. The Radura

approved for use in food irradiation are limited to those producing energy too low to induce formation of radioactive compounds or radioactive atomic species. Although in theory, radiation could cause undesired reactions of food chemicals and create toxic compounds, hundreds of studies have failed to identify any unique toxic compounds created during irradiation (versus canning, freezing, drying, etc) in amounts large enough to cause harm. Feeding studies and analytical chemical modeling studies have failed to identify any unusual toxicity associated with irradiation.[51] Recent studies found that food irradiation can result in medical adverse effects, such as leukoencephalopathy in cats; the doses (greater than 25 kGy) to which these cats were exposed, however, is much greater than most standard doses used in food irradiation.[54] In addition, heat-processed foods can contain 50 to 500 times the number of changed molecules than do irradiated foods.[55]

Microbes in food include those added intentionally to produce fermentation, those that cause spoilage rendering it unpalatable, and pathogens including invasive and toxigenic bacteria, toxigenic molds, viruses, and parasites.[51] Microbial safety of irradiated foods mainly has to do with pathogens that are relatively resistant to radiation. Irradiation kills microbes primarily by fragmenting DNA. Viruses, spores, cysts, toxins, and prions are quite resistant to the effects of irradiation because they contain little or no DNA and/or are in highly stable resting states. In general, irradiated food would most likely spoil long before becoming pathogenic. However, sporulating toxin-producing bacteria are approximately 10 times more resistant to radiation than are non-spore formers. For example, *Clostridium botulinum* type E, found in fish and seafood, can survive non-sterilizing doses of irradiation intended to extend shelf life. When refrigerated long enough at 50°F (10°C) or higher, toxin formation can occur. Thus, it may be possible for food to become toxic with botulinum toxin before it is obviously spoiled.[56] Conditions that allow for toxin formation before spoilage, such as inadequate refrigeration, are well understood, and regulations can be designed to mitigate against such occurrences. This concern also applies to other non-sterilizing food processing technologies, such as heat, to which spore-forming bacteria also are relatively resistant. Similar concerns exist about mycotoxins. Experimental data show conflicting results, but some studies show an increase in mycotoxin formation after irradiation.[57]

Irradiation can have a negative effect on some nutrients, similar to effects from cooking, canning, and other heat processing of foods. Slight loss of essential polyunsaturated fatty acids occurs with irradiation, but fats and oils that are major dietary sources of these nutrients tend to become rancid when irradiated and are not good candidates for this treatment.[58] The nutritional quality of protein is rarely altered because of irradiation.[51] Vitamin loss is the largest nutritional concern when foods are irradiated. Whole foods exert a protective effect on vitamins because most of the radiation dose is absorbed by macromolecules (proteins, carbohydrates, and fats). Losses can be minimized by irradiating at low temperatures, at low doses, and by excluding oxygen and light.[51] When studied in pure solution, the water-soluble vitamins most sensitive to irradiation are thiamine ($B_1$), pyridoxine ($B_6$), riboflavin ($B_2$), and vitamin C.[59] Of the fat-soluble vitamins, E and A are sensitive.[43] More than 50% of thiamine (found in meats, milk, whole grains, and legumes) can be lost after irradiation,[43] although other studies have shown that low- or medium-dose irradiation of food can effectively retain 100% of its individual items.[59] If all sources of thiamine come from irradiated products, a deficiency condition could develop, but this is unlikely in the United States. Vitamin E loss also can be significant after irradiation, especially in conjunction with cooking.[55] Many sources of vitamin E—cereal grains, seed oils, peanuts, soybeans, milk fat, and turnip greens—are unlikely to be treated with radiation and should provide for adequate alternative sources in a balanced and varied diet. In general, irradiated food is quite nutritious. As long as a diet is balanced and food choices are varied, deficiency states are unlikely to develop.

Palatability—taste, texture, color, and smell—can be affected by food irradiation, particularly in foods with high fat content. Modified conditions, such as excluding oxygen from the atmosphere, lowering the temperature, excluding light, reducing water content, or lowering the radiation dose, can minimize or eliminate these changes. These same modifications also can minimize vitamin loss.

Irradiated food is safe and nutritious and produces no unusual toxicity as long as best management practices are followed. Food irradiation, however, does not substitute for careful food handling from farm to fork.[57] Widespread use of food irradiation would require construction of irradiation facilities in the United States and other countries. The benefits of expanding this technology and the risks involved must be thoroughly debated. Pediatricians should participate in the dialogue. As with any technology, unforeseen consequences are possible. Therefore, careful monitoring and continuous evaluation of this and all food processing techniques are prudent precautions.

## PREVENTION OF FOOD CONTAMINATION

Care must be taken during food production and preparation to ensure that pathogens and other contaminants are not introduced into the food supply. When used in the manufacturing process, these methods are referred to as Hazard Analysis and Critical Control Point (HACCP) systems. HACCP systems require that food manufacturers identify points at which contamination is likely to occur and implement control processes to prevent it. Other important steps include preventing antibiotic resistance; controlling the use food additives; preventing environmental contamination of food; educating consumers about properly preparing and storing foods; pasteurization; irradiation; protecting the health of animals; and preventing the discharge of pathogens and nitrogen into water bodies. Integrated pest management (IPM), which uses information about pest biology to control pests, is a method employed to reduce the risks and use of pesticides (see Chapter 40).

Enforcing food safety laws is important at all levels and is supported by the federal Food Safety Modernization Act. Regulation and enforcement involve a complex network of federal, state, and local laws and regulations. Some enforcement efforts involve routine monitoring and surveillance of the food supply; other efforts occur in response to reports of problems and incidents. Pediatricians have important roles in reporting foodborne illnesses to local and state public health agencies. For example, physician reports of outbreaks of hemolytic-uremic syndrome caused by *E. coli* O157:H7 led to stronger enforcement efforts to ensure that foods, such as hamburger meat and apple juice, are safe to consume. Table 18-1 lists steps to reduce the likelihood of foodborne illness resulting from pathogens.

Four food safety rules can help families prevent foodborne illnesses: (1) hands, surfaces, and utensils should be cleaned frequently and thoroughly, (2) there should be no cross-contamination, keeping food groups separated during the cooking process, (3) refrigerate foods that are perishable, and

---

**Table 18-1. Steps to Reduce the Likelihood of Foodborne Illness Resulting From Pathogens in Food**

- Thoroughly wash fruits and vegetables with water to remove some pathogens and many pesticide residues. Wash before you peel. Do not peel anything you would not normally peel. It is unnecessary to use soap or chemicals when washing food.
- Do not consume raw eggs, fish, meat, or unpasteurized milk products.
- Thoroughly cook meat, poultry, and eggs to ensure that pathogens are killed. For hamburgers, a thermometer inserted into the center should read 160°F (71°C).
- After preparing raw poultry, make sure to wash hands, cutting boards, and implements used with soap and hot water. Cook stuffing for poultry separately rather than inside the birds.
- Store food appropriately. Refrigerating prepared food prevents the growth of many microorganisms responsible for food poisoning.
- Use soap and water to wash hands and surfaces to prevent transmission of pathogens from food. Incorporation of chemical agents into high-chair trays and cutting boards, and similar practices do not have a role in preventing foodborne infections. It also is unnecessary to use chemical disinfectants for washing hands in the home; soap and water are quite effective.

promptly after cooking, and (4) ensure that food is cooked to the appropriate temperature. (https://redbook.solutions.aap.org/chapter.aspx?sectionId=8818 7333&bookId=1484&resultClick=1#91031911)

## SEX STEROIDS AND BOVINE GROWTH HORMONE

Steroids and growth hormones are sometimes given to food animals and their use has been controversial. Cattle treated with sex steroids tend to have greater muscle mass which leads to better yield. Some concern exists that biologically active drugs or metabolites may be passed from the meat to the consumer and result in adverse health effects. Similarly, data have suggested that estrogens in cow's milk may be absorbed and result in gonadotropin secretion suppression that may affect sexual maturation of prepubertal children.[60] The potential for human exposure, however, is poorly understood.

Growth hormone is used to increase milk production in cows. No evidence has shown that the gross composition of milk is altered by treatment with bovine growth hormone, nor is there evidence that the vitamin and mineral contents of milk are changed by growth hormone treatment. Approximately 90% of bovine growth hormone in milk is destroyed during pasteurization. In addition, no evidence has shown that conventional milk contains significantly increased amounts of bovine growth hormone compared with organic milk. Growth hormone is destroyed in the gastrointestinal tract when ingested and must be injected to retain biologic activity. Furthermore, bovine growth hormone is species-specific and therefore is biologically inactive in humans. Because of this finding, any bovine growth hormone present in food products has no physiological effect on humans.[61,62]

## FOODS DEVELOPED USING BIOTECHNOLOGY

Food engineered through biotechnology is now common. Unique traits can be inserted into the genes of plants and animals through genetic engineering, causing the organism to predictably express the new trait. This technology has been controversial. Many clinicians argue that newly expressed traits are harmless and that selecting desirable traits has gone on for centuries using other methods. Others argue that there are too many uncertainties in the new technology, or that genetic engineering can lead to problems such as increased allergenicity, gene transfer, or outcrossing (mixing genes of genetically modified plants with conventional plants which could lead to difficulties with food safety and security).[63] Recommendations to perform post-marketing surveillance have been made but not initiated. Herbicide resistance has been introduced into many plants so that applying herbicides during the growing season does not affect the growth of treated crops. This invariably leads to greater use of herbicides; there generally is little to no effect on crops but there may be a potentially hazardous effect on consumers. Labeling of genetically engineered plants currently is voluntary.

Although debate continues, genetically engineered foods likely will be maintained in the United States as new products are developed and approved. Genetically modified foods now include corn, soybeans, rice, potatoes, milk, and about a dozen other products. The overall safety of genetically modified food continues to be thoroughly evaluated. Studies reveal that compared with conventional counterparts, genetically modified foods have considerably advanced increases in the micronutrient content in staple crops[63,64] but at the risk to the environment and ecosystems.[65] Before any genetically modified food products are commercialized, however, the FDA, US EPA, and USDA conduct scientific reviews to help ensure their safety. Specifically, the FDA conducts a premarket notification and safety review of bioengineered foods to ensure that they meet the safety standards of the FDCA that are expected in conventional foods. If products have been genetically modified to express a pesticide for insect or disease control, the US EPA is responsible for conducting a rigorous scientific review to ensure that the product will not cause unreasonably adverse effects on people or the environment. The USDA conducts premarket reviews to ensure that the new technology does not jeopardize existing plants or animals. As government regulatory processes and the science underlying biotechnology evolve and improve, questions about safety remain. Governmental, scientific, and medical communities must remain vigilant to ensure the safety of foods produced using biotechnology, and to monitor them for possible adverse effects, particularly as demand for food production increases.

## FREQUENTLY ASKED QUESTIONS

Q   *What do the different food labels mean? Are there some that have more meaning than others?*

A   Labels of foods have many different meanings and each meaning implies a certain standard of regulation. A good resource to further understand food labeling is "Food Labeling Fact Sheets" found on the US Department of Agriculture Web site: https://www.fsis.usda.gov/wps/portal/fsis/topics/food-safety-education/get-answers/food-safety-fact-sheets/food-labeling.

Q   *How should food be stored or heated?*

A   This depends on the type of food. The US Food and Drug Administration has information on Safe Food Handling: https://www.fda.gov/food/foodborneillnesscontaminants/buystoreservesafefood/ucm255180.htm.

Q   *How should human milk be stored and heated?*

A   Human milk can be stored at room temperature for 4 hours, in the refrigerator for 3 days, and in the freezer for 9 months. Human milk should be heated by placing the filled bottle in a warm container or pot. It is important not to submerge the bottle. Always test the milk on the inside of your wrist to make sure it is not too hot to give to your baby.

Q *Does artificial coloring cause attention-deficit/hyperactivity disorder (ADHD)?*

A Artificial colors and flavors have not been shown to cause hyperactivity. Research in the 1970s showed a possible correlation between artificial coloring and hyperactivity, but no definite link was made and more studies are needed. A subgroup of children were shown to have some hyperactivity; this finding has led to current studies to determine why some children are more sensitive.[66]

Q *Are there pesticides on fresh vegetables found in the store?*

A Pesticides commonly are found on fruits and vegetables in the store. Because no labeling is required, parents and other consumers cannot tell which fruits and vegetables contain pesticides. Even organically grown fruits and vegetables are not necessarily free of pesticides. It is a good idea to scrub all fruits and vegetables under running water to remove superficial particle residues. Fruits and vegetables are good for children because they provide vitamins, minerals, and roughage. Because of these health benefits, children should continue to consume a wide variety of fruits and vegetables, particularly those grown in season.

Q *Are there pesticides in store-bought baby food?*

A Processed foods generally contain lower residues of pesticides than fresh fruits and vegetables, in part because federal standards are stricter for processed foods. Some baby food manufacturers voluntarily make their products free of all pesticide residues, although they do not advertise this action. Arsenic, a natural metal-like element found in soil, was used as a pesticide in the past. Arsenic has been found in high concentrations in infant and toddler cereals and snacks. The FDA has recommended voluntary limits of arsenic in food. Despite this, it is important to provide infants and toddlers a variety of foods.

Q *Could cancer develop in my child because of exposure to pesticides?*

A Many factors contribute to cancer, including genetics, contact with viruses, and diet. More research is needed to determine how and why cancers develop during childhood. No causal relationship between exposure to pesticides in food and childhood cancer has been established. A number of pesticides can cause tumors in laboratory animals and are associated with cancer in some farm workers exposed to very high doses.

Q *Are pesticides in foods 10 times more hazardous for children than adults?*

A Many scientists recognize that children may be more susceptible to the effects of pesticides and other chemicals. To account for this difference, which often has not been quantified, standards for pesticides in foods generally include a 10-fold margin of safety.

Q   *I heard that hot dogs can cause brain cancer in children. Should my children avoid hot dogs?*

A   Sodium nitrite is used as a food preservative and prevents the growth of *Clostridium botulinum* in meat products. Published studies of exposure to nitrate and cancer risk are not all in agreement, but the International Agency for Research on Cancer has determined that ingesting nitrate under conditions that are likely to increase formation of endogenous *N*-nitroso compounds probably increases the risk for cancer. Although health benefits have been seen with diets that include nitrate-rich vegetables, high intake of preserved meats (ie, bacon, hot dogs, ham) can lead to higher nitrate levels and an increased risk for formation of nitrosamines. Children should eat a balanced diet, and an occasional hot dog may be a part of that diet. Young children, however, should not be given hot dogs because of the danger of choking.

Q   *What can I do to prevent my children from eating products contaminated with prions (the agents of mad cow disease)?*

A   Avoid consumption of brains or any food containing nerve tissue. Although there have been no cases of bovine spongiform encephalopathy (mad cow disease) reported in the United States, there have been confirmed cases of chronic wasting disease, a spongiform encephalopathy of deer and elk, in western and midwestern states. Avoid feeding children products made with deer or elk from areas known to have chronic wasting disease.

Q   *I am worried that the nonnutritive or artificial sweeteners will cause cancer, but I am also worried about my child's weight, so what should I do?*

A   There are 5 nonnutritive sweeteners that have FDA approval in the United States. These substances are hundreds of times sweeter than sugar, so only minute amounts are needed to sweeten foods. No studies have found a link between use of nonnutritive sweeteners and cancer in humans. A study in rats done in the 1970s found an association between bladder cancer and use of saccharine; however, the mechanism for cancer development in rats from saccharine exposure may not apply to humans. A wide range of nutritive and nonnutritive sweeteners are available in the food supply that can be blended to keep intakes of nonnutritive sweeteners in children well below acceptable daily intakes and reduce excessive calories or other negative effects of nutritive sweeteners. Drinking water is a good alternative to artificially sweetened drinks.

Q   *Are bioengineered food products required to be labeled?*

A   No. The FDA does not require labeling to indicate whether a food or food ingredient is a bioengineered product. Currently, the FDA has guidance available for companies that wish to voluntarily label their bioengineered food products.

Q   *Will irradiation eliminate foodborne illness?*

A   No. Most foodborne illness (approximately 67%) is caused by viruses, which are not killed by food irradiation. Among all illnesses attributable to foodborne transmission, only about 30% are caused by bacteria and about 3% are caused by parasites. Thus, an estimated 33% of foodborne illness (those attributable to bacteria and parasites) may potentially be prevented by food irradiation.[67]

Q   *Will irradiation kill prions?*

A   No. Irradiation does not kill prions, the agents of bovine spongiform encephalopathy.

## RESOURCES

**Gateway to Government Food Safety Information: Food Irradiation**
Web site: www.fsis.usda.gov

**International Atomic Energy Agency**
Web site: https://www.iaea.org/topics/food-safety-and-quality
Facts about food irradiation: www.iaea.org/icgfi/documents/foodirradiation.pdf

**Iowa State University**
Web site: www.extension.iastate.edu/foodsafety/rad/irradhome.html

**US Department of Agriculture**
Meat and Poultry Hotline: 800-535-4555
Web site: www.usda.gov

## REFERENCES

1.  Marder EP, Cieslak PR, Cronquist AB, et al. Incidence and trends of infections with pathogens transmitted commonly through food and the effect of increasing use of culture-independent diagnostic tests on surveillance-Foodborne Diseases Active Surveillance Network, 10 U.S. Sites, 2013-2016. *MMWR Morb Mortal Wkly Rep.* 2017;66(15):397–403

2.  American Academy of Pediatrics. *Red Book: 2018-2021 Report of the Committee on Infectious Diseases.* Kimberlin DW, Brady MT, Jackson MA, Long SS, eds. 31st ed. Itasca, IL: American Academy of Pediatrics; 2018

3.  American Medical Association, Centers for Disease Control and Prevention, Food and Drug Administration, Food Safety and Inspection Service. *Diagnosis and Management of Foodborne Illnesses: A Primer for Physicians.* Chicago, IL: American Medical Association; 2004

4.  Abanyie F, Harvey RR, Harris Jr, et al. 2013 multistate outbreaks of Cyclospora cayetanesis infections associated with fresh produce: focus on the Texas investigations. *Epidemiol Infect.* 2015;143(16):3451–3458

5.  Centers for Disease Control and Prevention. Multistate Outbreak of Shiga toxin-producing *Escherichia coli* O157:H7 infections linked to leafy greens. https://www.cdc.gov/ecoli/2017/o157h7-12-17/index.html. Accessed May 24, 2018

6. Soneja S, Jiang C, Romeo Upperman C, et al. Extreme precipitation events and increased risk of campylobacteriosis in Maryland, U.S.A. *Environ Res.* 2016;149:216–221

7. Heiman KE, Garalde VB, Gronostaj M, et al. Multistate outbreak of listeriosis caused by imported cheese and evidence of cross-contamination of other cheeses, USA, 2012. *Epidemiol Infect.* 2106;144(13):2678–2708

8. Self JL, Conrad A, Stroika S, et al. Notes from the Field: Outbreak of Listeriosis associated with consumption of packaged salad — United States and Canada, 2015–2016. *MMWR Morb Mortal Wkly Rep.* 2016;65(33):879–881

9. Whitley RJ, MacDonald N, Asher DM. American Academy of Pediatrics Committee on Infectious Diseases. Technical report: transmissible spongiform encephalopathies: a review for pediatricians. *Pediatrics.* 2000;106(5):1160–1165

10. Spencer MD, Knight RS, Will RG. First hundred cases of variant Creutzfeldt-Jakob disease: retrospective case note review of early psychiatric and neurological features. *BMJ.* 2002;324(7352):1479–1482

11. Centers for Disease Control and Prevention. Probable variant Creutzfeldt-Jakob disease in a U.S. resident—Florida, 2002. *MMWR Morb Mortal Wkly Rep.* 2002;51(41):927–929

12. Atwood D, Paisley-Jones C. *Pesticide Industry Sales and Usage: 2008-2012 Market Estimates.* Washington, DC: US Environmental Protection Agency, Office of Chemical Safety and Pollution Prevention; 2017

13. Goldman LR. Children—unique and vulnerable. Environmental risks facing children and recommendations for response. *Environ Health Perspect.* 1995;103(Suppl 6):13–18

14. American Academy of Pediatrics Council on Environmental Health. Policy Statement. Pesticide exposure in children. *Pediatrics.* 2012;130:e1757–e1763

15. Office of the Law Revision Counsel. United States Code. Title 7-Agriculture. Chapter 94. Organic Certification. Section 6503. National organic production program. http://uscode. house.gov/view.xhtml?req=granuleid:USC-prelim-title7-section6503&num=0&edition= prelim. Accessed May 24, 2018

16. U.S. Department of Agriculture. Agricultural Marketing Service. National Organic Program. Strategic Plan 2015–2018. https://www.ams.usda.gov/sites/default/files/media/ NOP-2015StrategicPlan.pdf. Accessed May 24, 2018

17. Forman JA, Silverman J, American Academy of Pediatrics Committee on Nutrition, Council on Environmental Health. Organic foods: health and environmental advantages and disadvantages. *Pediatrics.* 2012;130(5):e1406–e1415

18. National Research Council. *Pesticides in the Diets of Infants and Children.* Washington, DC: National Academies Press; 1993

19. Lu C, Toepel K, Irish R, Fenske R, Barr D, Bravo R. Organic diets significantly lower children's dietary exposure to organophosphorus pesticides. *Environ Health Perspect.* 2006;114(2): 260–263

20. Lu C, Barr DB, Pearson MA, Waller LA. Dietary intake and its contribution to longitudinal organophosphorus pesticide exposure in urban/suburban children. *Environ Health Perspect.* 2008;116(4):537–542

21. Brantsaeter AL, Ydersbond TA, Hoppin JA, Haugen M, Meltzer HM. Organic food in the diet: exposure and health implications. *Ann Rev Public Health.* 2017;38:295–313

22. Baker B, Benbrook C, Groth III E, Benbrook K. Pesticide residues in conventional, integrated pest management (IPM)-grown and organic foods: insights from three US data sets. *Food Addit Contam.* 2002;19(5):427–446

23. Food and Drug Administration. About the Center for Food Safety and Applied Nutrition. https://www.fda.gov/AboutFDA/CentersOffices/OfficeofFoods/CFSAN/. Accessed May 24, 2018.

24. Food and Drug Administration. Everything Added to Food in the United States (EAFUS). https://www.fda.gov/Food/IngredientsPackagingLabeling/FoodAdditivesIngredients/ucm115326.htm. Accessed May 24, 2018

25. Food and Drug Administration. Generally Recognized as Safe (GRAS). https://www.fda.gov/food/ingredientspackaginglabeling/gras/default.htm. Accessed May 24, 2018

26. Food and Drug Administration. Pesticide Residue Monitoring Program Questions and Answers. https://www.fda.gov/Food/FoodborneIllnessContaminants/Pesticides/ucm583711.htm. Accessed May 24, 2018

27. Neltner TG, Alger HM, O'Reilly JT, Krimsky S, Bero LA, Maffini MV. Conflicts of interest in approvals to food determined to be generally recognized as safe: out of balance. *JAMA Intern Med*. 2013;173(22):2032–2036

28. Food and Drug Administration. GRAS Notices. https://www.accessdata.fda.gov/scripts/fdcc/?set=grasnotices. Accessed May 24, 2018

29. Lakind JS, Naiman DQ. Temporal trends in bisphenol A exposure in the United States from 2003-2012 and factors associated with BPA exposure: spot samples and urine dilution complicate data interpretation. *Environ Res*. 2015;142:84–95

30. Food and Drug Administration. Question and Answers on Bisphenol A (BPA) Use in Food Contact Applications. https://www.fda.gov/Food/IngredientsPackagingLabeling/FoodAdditivesIngredients/ucm355155.htm. Accessed May 24, 2018

31. Carlos KS, de Jager LS, Begley TH. Investigation of the primary plasticisers present in polyvinyl chloride (PVC) products currently authorized as food contact materials. *Food Addit Contam Part A Chem Anal Control Expo Risk Assess*. 2018;35(6):1214–1222

32. Petrov V, Qureshi MK, Hille J, Gechev T. Occurrence, biochemistry and biological effects of host selective plant mycotoxins. *Food Chem Toxicol*. 2018;112:251–264

33. International Agency for Research on Cancer. Aflatoxins: naturally occurring aflatoxins (group 1). Aflatoxin M1 (group 2B). *IARC Monogr*. 2002;82:171

34. Moore MM, Schoeny RS, Becker RA, White K, Pottenger LH. Development of an adverse outcome pathway for chemically induced hepatocellular carcinoma: case study of AFB1, a human carcinogen with a mutagenic mode of action. *Crit Rev Toxicol*. 2018;48(4):312–337

35. Chu YJ, Yang HI, Wu CH, et al. Aflatoxin $B_1$ exposure increases the risk of hepatocellular carcinoma associated with hepatitis C virus infection or alcohol consumption. *Eur J Cancer*. 2018;94:37–46

36. Pinton P, Oswald IP. Effect of deoxynivalenol and other Type B trichothecenes on the intestine: a review. *Toxins*. 2014;6(5):1615–1643

37. Bernard A, Hermans C, Broeckaert F, De Poorter G, De Cock A, Houins G. Food contamination by PCBs and dioxins. *Nature*. 1999;401(6750):231–232

38. Hayward D, Nortrup D, Gardiner A, Clower M. Elevated TCDD in chicken eggs and farm-raised catfish fed a diet containing ball clay from a Southern United States mine. *Environ Res*. 1999;81(3):248–256

39. European Commission. Commission Press Release: Dioxin in food. Byrne welcomes adoption by Council of dioxin limits in food [press release]. Brussels, Belgium: European Commission; November 29, 2001. Report No. IP/01/1698

40. Food and Drug Administration. Code of Federal Regulations Title 21, Part 109, Subpart B-Tolerances for Unavoidable Poisonous or Deleterious Substances. https://www.accessdata.fda.gov/scripts/cdrh/cfdocs/cfcfr/CFRSearch.cfm?fr=109.30. Accessed May 24, 2018

41. Integrated Risk Information System (IRIS). National Center for Environmental Assessment. U.S. Environmental Protection Agency. 2,3,7,8-Tetrachlorodibenzo-*p*-dioxin (TCDD); CASRN 1746-01-6. https://cfpub.epa.gov/ncea/iris/iris_documents/documents/subst/1024_summary.pdf#nameddest=rfd. Accessed May 24, 2018

42. Melamine adulterates component of pellet feeds. *J Am Vet Med Assoc.* 2007;231(1):17

43. Zhang L, Wu LL, Wang YP, Liu AM, Zou CC, Zhao ZY. Melamine-contaminated milk products induced urinary tract calculi in children. *World J Pediatr.* 2009;5(1):31–35

44. Chen JS. A worldwide food safety concern in 2008—melamine-contaminated infant formula in China caused urinary tract stone in 290,000 children in China. *Chin Med J (Engl).* 2009;122(3):243–244

45. Davis MA, Mackenzie TA, Cottingham KL, Gilbert-Diamond D, Punshon T, Karagas MR. Rice consumption and urinary arsenic concentrations in U.S. children. *Environ Health Perspect.* 2012;120(10):1418–1424

46. Pediatric Environmental Health Specialty Units. Fact Sheets. Arsenic in Food Guidance for Parents and Families. October 2012. http://www.pehsu.net/_Library/facts/Arsenic_in_Food.pdf. Accessed May 24, 2018

47. Juskelis R, Li W, Nelson J, Cappozzo JC. Arsenic speciation in rice cereals for infants. *J Agric Food Chem.* 2013;61(45):10670–10676

48. American Academy of Pediatrics Arsenic in Rice Expert Work Group. AAP group offers advice to reduce infants' exposure to arsenic in rice. *AAP News.* 2014;35:13

49. Food and Drug Administration. Perchlorate Questions and Answers. https://www.fda.gov/Food/FoodborneIllnessContaminants/ChemicalContaminants/ucm077572.htm. Accessed May 24, 2018

50. Shea KM, American Academy of Pediatrics Committee on Environmental Health. Technical report: irradiation of food. *Pediatrics.* 2000;106(6):1505–1510

51. Food and Drug Administration. Subchapter B. Radiation and radiation sources. Irradiation in the production processing and handling of food. Code of Federal Register. 21CFR179. Revised as of April 1, 2017. Accessed May 24, 2018

52. Kramer B, Wunderlich J, Muranyi P. Recent findings in pulsed light disinfection. *J Appl Microbiol.* 2017;122(4):830–856

53. Derr D. International regulatory status and harmonization of food irradiation. *J Food Prot.* 1993;56:882–886, 892

54. Child G, Foster DJ, Fougerre BJ, Milan JM, Rozmanec M. Ataxia and paralysis in cats in Australia associated with exposure to an imported gama-irradiated commercial dry pet food. *Aust Vet J.* 2009;87(9):349–351

55. Diehl J. *Safety of Irradiated Food.* 3rd ed. New York: Marcel Dekker; 1999

56. Farkas J. Microbiological safety of irradiated foods. *Int J Food Microbiol.* 1989;9(1):1–15

57. Thayer D. Food irradiation: benefits and concerns. *J Food Qual.* 1990;13:147–169

58. World Health Organization. *Safety and Nutritional Adequacy of Irradiated Food.* Geneva, Switzerland: World Health Organization; 1994

59. Shahbaz HM, Akram K, Ahn JJ, Kwon JH. Worldwide status of fresh fruits irradiation and concerns about quality, safety and consumer acceptance. *Crit Rev Food Sci Nutr.* 2016;56(11):1790–1807

60. Maruyama K, Oshima T, Ohyama K. Exposure to exogenous estrogen through intake of commercial milk produced from pregnant cows. *Pediatr Int.* 2010;52(1):33–38

61. Food and Drug Administration. *Report on the Food and Drug Administration's Review of the Safety of Recombinant Bovine Somatotropin.* http://www.fda.gov/AnimalVeterinary/SafetyHealth/ProductSafetyInformation/ucm130321.htm. Accessed May 24, 2018

62. Collier RJ, Bauman DE. Update on human health concerns of recombinant bovine somatotropin use in dairy cows. *J Anim Sci.* 2014;92(4):1800–1807

63. Mogendi JB, De Steur H, Gellynck X, Makokha A. Consumer evaluation of food with nutritional benefits: as systemic review and narrative synthesis. *Int J Food Sci Nutri.* 2016;67(4):355–371

64. Qaim M. Benefits of genetically modified crops for the poor: household income, nutrition, and health. *New Biotech*. 2010;27(5):552–557

65. Tsatsakis AM, Nawaz MA, Tutelyn VA, et al. Impact on environment, ecosystem, diversity and health from culturing and using GMOs as feed and food. *Food Chem Toxicol*. 2017;107 (Pt A):108–121

66. Stevens LJ, Kuczek T, Burgess JR, Stochelski MA, Arnold LE, Galland L. Mechanisms of behavioral, atopic, and other reactions to artificial food colors in children. *Nutr Rev*. 2013;71(5):268–281

67. Etzel R. Epidemiology of foodborne illness—role of food irradiation. In: Loaharanu P, Thomas P, eds. *Irradiation for Food Safety and Quality*. Lancaster, PA: Technomic Publishing Co; 2001:50–54

Chapter 19

# Herbs, Dietary Supplements, and Other Remedies

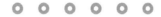

**KEY POINTS**

- Herbs and dietary supplements are commonly used by parents for their children and adolescents to maintain their good health and/or to treat chronic medical conditions.
- Herbs and dietary supplements are not subject to the same rigorous oversight by the US Food and Drug Administration as are pharmaceuticals; some may not be safe or effective when used to treat children's illnesses or to preserve their health.
- Pediatric health care providers should be key sources of authoritative information for parents on the safety and effectiveness of specific herbs and dietary supplements.
- Parents and guardians should be encouraged to disclose use of any special diets, herbal remedies, or other dietary supplements for their children during the interview portion of routine well child care.

**INTRODUCTION**

A dietary supplement can be defined as a product (other than tobacco) intended to supplement the diet that contains one or more of the following ingredients: a vitamin, a mineral, an herb or other botanical, or an amino acid; a dietary substance that supplements the normal diet; or a concentrate, metabolite, constituent, extract, or combination of the above ingredients (see Table 19-1).[1] This chapter will not address caffeine or a few botanicals not ordinarily considered as dietary supplements, such as marijuana, khat, or *Salvia divinorum*.

Unfortunately, herbal products and dietary supplements are virtually unregulated. Congress passed legislation, the Dietary Supplement Health and Education Act of 1994, which does not include all the consumer protections that are applied to medications.[1] Pharmacologically active substances, such as melatonin, yohimbine, and dehydroepiandrosterone, can be marketed as dietary supplements, provided that no therapeutic claims are made for them.

International conventions in naming plants do not exist, and many confusing synonyms do exist. The common names of plants and herbal remedies can be archaic and variable depending on the geographic region. For example, *cohosh* can refer to several different species of plants depending on where a person lives. Little regulation is mandated for the manufacture, quality, purity, concentration, or labeling claims of herbal remedies and dietary supplements. Errors in labeling may be inadvertent; however, intentional mislabeling also has been problematic. For example, one study revealed that products sold as ginseng actually contained substitutes such as scopolamine and reserpine.[2] Just over 50% of all Class I drug recalls by the US Food and Drug Administration (FDA) from 2004 to 2012 were classified as dietary supplements, as opposed to pharmaceuticals, with sexual enhancement products, bodybuilding supplements, and weight loss supplements being the most

### Table 19-1. Categories of Dietary Supplements[a]

**The term "dietary supplement" means**

1. A product (other than tobacco) intended to supplement the diet that bears or contains one or more of the following dietary ingredients:

   - Vitamin
   - Mineral
   - Herb or other botanical
   - Amino acid
   - Dietary substance that supplements the normal diet
   - Concentrate, metabolite, constituent, extract, or combination of any ingredients described in the previous entries

2. A product that is

   - Intended for ingestion
   - Not represented for use as a conventional food or as a sole item of a meal in the diet

[a]Dietary Supplement Health & Education Act, 1994

## Dietary Supplement Health and Education Act of 1994

■ Premarketing testing or oversight protections of the FDA licensing process for an herbal remedy or dietary supplement are not required.

■ The use of child-resistant containers or safe packaging for herbs or dietary supplements is not mandated.

■ Nutritional support claims made in the labeling or marketing of an herb or dietary supplement do not require FDA approval.

■ Pharmacologically active substances can be marketed as dietary substances, provided that no unsubstantiated claims concerning the cure of specific illnesses or conditions are made for them.

■ The Secretary of the US Department of Health and Human Services is empowered to act to remove a dietary supplement only when it "poses an imminent hazard to public health or safety."

■ There is no regulatory provision for mandatory reporting of adverse health effects associated with the use of herbs or dietary supplements.

common products recalled for containing unapproved drug ingredients.[3] A 2015 study found that mandatory government disclaimers warning of "unapproved use" on the labels of dietary supplements would not provide much influence on consumers' perceptions of their safety or effectiveness or their purchasing behaviors.[4]

### PREVALENCE AND TRENDS

The use of herbs and dietary supplements by Americans is growing. Sales of herbs and dietary supplements in the United States have continued to increase annually—by 2013, total sales exceeded $13 billion.[5] A review of data collected in the National Health and Nutrition Examination Survey (NHANES) from 2007 to 2010 indicated that 31% of US children aged birth through 19 years used dietary supplements, the most common of which were multivitamins/multiminerals (>90% of the childhood supplement users).[6] The 2007-2012 National Health Interview Survey (NHIS) found that 11.6% of children in the United States aged 4 to 17 years used some sort of complementary and alternative medicine, with use of non-mineral, non-vitamin dietary supplements being the most common complementary and alternative medicine practice pursued for children.[7] Such products are now being marketed to parents for the treatment of their children's illnesses as well as to maintain their overall health. In that same 2012 pediatric survey, fish oil, melatonin, probiotics, echinacea, garlic, ginseng, cranberry, glucosamine, chondroitin, and combination herbal pills were the most commonly used complementary and alternative medicine products; they were given for a variety of health complaints, including coughs and colds, musculoskeletal pain, depression, attention-deficit/hyperactivity disorder (ADHD), and insomnia.[7] One study (also using the 2012 NHIS database) of children aged 4 to 17 years suffering from chronic pain syndromes found that, of the 26.6% reporting various pain conditions, 21% used complementary and alternative medicine; of these, 47% used special diets and dietary supplements.[8] The rate of complementary and alternative medicine use by children in a Detroit, MI, survey of 1,013 families was 12%.[9] Of these, the most frequent therapies used included herbs (43%), high-dose vitamins and other nutritional supplements (34.5%), and folk/home remedies (28%). A 2005 to 2007 survey of mothers with infants found that a substantial number (9%) gave teas or dietary botanical supplements to their infants who were less than 1 year of age.[10] One New Zealand study found that most families do not report the use of complementary and alternative medicine to their primary care physician; parental use of complementary and alternative medicine was the strongest predictor of use of complementary and alternative medicine by the children.[11]

Good scientific evidence is available for the efficacy and safety of some herbs and dietary supplements when used in children with specific nutritional deficiencies or for some health issues. Some pediatric health care providers prescribe such supplements routinely in office practice. Examples include melatonin, ginger, probiotics, minerals, and/or vitamins (see Table 19-2). Families whose children have chronic conditions, such as autism or cystic fibrosis, may be particularly likely to use dietary supplements as part of their treatment regimen. The American Academy of Pediatrics has published guidelines for discussing such issues with parents.[12]

Use of herbal products increases in adolescence. Adolescents may use herbs and dietary supplements in addition to prescribed medications to treat their chronic illnesses (eg, allergies, seizures, cystic fibrosis, cancer, ADHD, autism, diabetes, lupus, or other autoimmune disease). Healthy adolescents commonly use herbs and supplements to boost energy, build strength and athletic performance, improve alertness, or for weight loss or to otherwise enhance their personal appearance. Student athletes may be influenced both by supplement claims of enhanced body-building and personal appearance as well as by claims of improved alertness, endurance, strength, and athletic performance. A national population-weighted online survey of 1,280 adolescents found that 46.2% had used dietary supplements in their lifetime—29.1%

## Table 19-2. Examples of Herbs Used for Children

| DIETARY SUPPLEMENT | SCIENTIFIC STUDIES | POTENTIAL ADVERSE EFFECTS AND CONTRAINDICATIONS |
|---|---|---|
| Echinacea | One trial of *Echinacea purpurea* in children who had upper respiratory tract infection found no significant difference in duration or symptoms.[13] | Allergic reactions |
| Melatonin | May promote sleep onset in children with attention-deficit/hyperactivity disorder or autistic spectrum disorder[14] | Possibly morning grogginess, increased bedwetting, headaches |
| German chamomile (*Matricaria recutita*) | Chamomile/pectin combinations have had positive effects on diarrhea.[15] Chamomile in combination with other herbs was found effective for treating infantile colic.[16–18] | Individuals allergic to the *Compositae* family (ragweed, chrysanthemum) may be allergic to chamomile. Chamomile can cause atopic and contact dermatitis and rare cases of anaphylaxis.[18,19] |
| Ginger (*Zingiber officinale*) | Clinical trials showed good results for ginger as a treatment for postoperative nausea and vomiting.[20] Ginger has proven helpful in treating hyperemesis gravidarum.[21] | Heartburn Contraindications: patients who have gallstones (ginger's cholagogue effect) |
| Lemon balm (*Melissa officinalis*) | Clinical trials of lemon balm/valerian combinations have shown modest enhanced sleep quality.[22–24] | Allergic reactions |
| Valerian (*Valeriana officinalis*) | See 'lemon balm' category above. | Allergic reactions, headaches, insomnia |

Table modified from Gardner and Riley.[25]

in the previous month.[26] One analysis of 1999 to 2002 NHANES data found that 27% of adolescents aged 11 to 19 years had used one or more supplements in the preceding month, with multivitamins and vitamin C being the most commonly cited.[27] Another study of youth in Monroe County, NY, found that more than 25% of high school students reported that they use herbs.[28] In that study, herbal use by adolescents was associated with substance abuse. A study of college students at 5 US universities found that 66% used some sort of dietary supplement weekly.[29] Among these, multivitamins with or without minerals, vitamin C, protein/amino acids, calcium, caffeine, and fish oil were most commonly reported. Students in this study reportedly most commonly used supplements to promote their general health (73%), provide more energy (29%), increase muscle strength (20%), and enhance endurance and athletic performance (19%).[29]

A "natural" product is advertised as such to imply that it is not synthetic in origin; "organic" implies growing methods that eschew the use of hormones, pesticides, and other chemicals. However, consumers frequently confuse terms such as "natural" or "organic" with "safe." "Natural" strychnine, extracted from the nut of the plant *Strychnos nux vomica,* still has the same potentially life-threatening toxicity. The definitions are ambiguous because the terms are used in different contexts by food and dietary supplement manufacturers, consumers, scientists, and policy makers. Chemical structures do not change, regardless of their origin. Synthesized ascorbic acid has the same structure as ascorbic acid found in orange juice or rose hips. Marketing of herbs in the form of pills or capsules using terms such as "safe" or "natural" may be misleading to consumers. A survey of dietary supplements advertised in popular health and bodybuilding magazines showed that no human toxicology data were available in the peer-reviewed scientific literature for approximately 60% of ingredients in the products advertised.[30] Student athletes may be influenced by the performance-enhancing claims of the purveyors of herbs and dietary supplements that contain ingredients such as caffeine, amino acids, proteins, or creatine. Adolescents and young adults are particularly easy targets for such promotional tactics.

## DEFINITIONS

Herbs used for medicinal purposes come in a variety of forms. Active parts of a plant may include leaves, flowers, stems, roots, seeds and/or berries, and essential oils.[31] They may be taken internally as liquids, capsules, tablets, or powders; dissolved into tinctures or syrups; or brewed in teas, infusions, and decoctions. Although few products are available as rectal suppositories, a wide variety of substances, in particular herbal products, are used in solutions for "therapeutic enemas." Table 19-3 lists some terms used in the context of herbal therapy.

## THERAPEUTIC EFFICACY

To give better advice to patients and their families, pediatricians should understand the pharmacologic activity of the active ingredients in products and whether animal or human studies demonstrate effectiveness.[32] For example, one study found that use of a supplement could increase micronutrients found

## Table 19-3. Definitions and Types of Preparations

| PREPARATION | DEFINITION |
|---|---|
| Abortifacient | Agent that induces an abortion. |
| Aromatherapy | Inhalation of volatile oils in the treatment of certain health conditions. |
| Carminative | Agent that aids in expelling gas from the gastrointestinal tract. |
| Carrier oil | A fixed oil (nonvolatile, long-chain fatty acid, such as safflower oil) into which a few drops of the potent, essential oils are added to dilute them for topical uses. |
| Decoction | A dilute aqueous extract prepared by boiling an herb in water and straining and filtering the liquid, similar to an infusion. |
| Discipline of signatures | Historical term suggesting that the appearance of a plant gives a clue as to its medical value (eg, the extract of St John's wort is red, thus it is believed to be restorative for conditions involving the blood). |
| Elixir | A clear sweetening hydroalcoholic solution for oral use. |
| Emmenagogue | Agent that influences menstruation. |
| Essential oil | Class of volatile oils composed of complex hydrocarbons (often terpenes, alkaloids, and other large molecular weight compounds) extracted from a plant. |
| Excipient | Another ingredient, such as a binder or filler, used to make a supplement product. |
| Extract | A concentrated form of a natural substance, which can be a powder, liquid, or tincture. The concentration varies from 1:1 in a fluid extract to 1:0.1 in a tincture. |
| "Natural" product | The term "natural" defies accurate definition because, strictly speaking, everything is derived from nature. In common usage it is intended to imply a substance that is not synthetic or is not grown using pesticides or other chemicals. |
| Poultice | Salve used in a preparation that is applied to skin, scalp, or mucous membrane. |
| Resin | Solid or semisolid organic substance found in plant secretions and applied topically in a cream or ointment. |
| Rubefacient | Agent that warms and reddens the skin by local cutaneous vasodilation. |

to be inadequate in the diets of children older than 8 years, such as magnesium, phosphorus, and vitamins A, C, and E.[33] In clinical studies, some herbs have shown promising results. For example, *Artemisia* species compared favorably with chloroquine in the treatment of some types of malaria, *Astragalus membranaceus* extracts enhanced the antibody response in immunosuppressed mice, and herbal teas containing chamomile seemed to have a salubrious effect on infantile colic.[34-36] The beneficial medicinal properties of some herbs are available in science-based published reviews.[25] Table 19-2 describes studies of some herbs commonly used for children.

## ETHNIC REMEDIES

Pediatricians should be culturally competent in their approach to the diagnosis and treatment of children in families from diverse ethnic backgrounds, whose health beliefs and practices may differ from those of Western medicine. For example, "*empacho,*" described as an illness in which food, saliva, or other matter becomes "stuck" to the intestines, is accepted among some Hispanic people as the etiology of gastrointestinal tract symptoms and treated with a variety of home-based remedies (such as greta or azarcon) as well as visits to a traditional healer.[37] More than half of patients of Southeast Asian descent using one Seattle, WA, primary care clinic used one or more traditional practices, such as moxibustion, cupping, coining, aromatic oils, or massage.[38] The formation of a therapeutic alliance among physician, parent, and child requires a sensitivity to the family's background and interests, with the goals of optimizing communications and facilitating a team approach in the clinical care of the child. For example, ethnomedical remedies practiced by the Puerto Rican community may hold some medical risks but also considerable benefits in decreasing the symptoms of asthma.[39] *Cao gio,* or coin rubbing of the skin to alleviate symptoms of illness, is an innocuous traditional Vietnamese practice that has unfortunately been confused by some Western physicians as traumatic abuse, leading to instances of distrust and avoidance of health care by people who practice it.[40] Certain Afro-Caribbean and Hispanic practices, such as the exposure to vapors of elemental mercury, have risks of toxicity.[41] Some treatments for *empacho,* such as greta or azarcon, are contaminated by significant amounts of lead. Table 19-4 lists some of the common folk remedies that can produce toxic effects. Authorities recommend an approach of education and community outreach to effect changes in potentially harmful practices. The pediatrician can be helpful in assessing the traditional practices families may be using to treat their children by listening carefully to their rationales, beliefs, and concerns. In the course of building a therapeutic alliance, the pediatrician can then counsel the family knowledgeably about possible benefits and/or adverse or harmful effects of such ethnic remedies, including interactions with other currently prescribed medications.

## Table 19-4. Examples of Toxicity of Some Ethnic Remedies and Dietary Supplements

| PRODUCT/ REMEDY | TOXIC AGENT | REGION WHERE COMMONLY USED | ADVERSE EFFECTS | REFERENCE |
|---|---|---|---|---|
| Ayurvedic remedies | Lead, arsenic | South Asia | Plumbism, arsenic poisoning (weight loss, myalgias, neuropathy, shock, death) | 42 |
| Azarcon, Alarcon | Lead | Latin America, Mexico, Dominican Republic | Plumbism | 43 |
| Ghasard, bala goli, kandu | Lead | South Asia | Plumbism | 44 |
| Glycerite asafoetida | Terpenes, undifferentiated | Caribbean | Methemoglobinemia | 45 |
| Greta | Lead | Latin America | Plumbism | 43 |
| Pay-loo-ah | Lead, arsenic | Asia | Plumbism, arsenic poisoning | 46 |
| Santeria, palo, voodoo, espiritismo | Mercury | Caribbean | Rash, neuropathy, seizures | 41, 47 |
| Tongue powders | Lead | Asia | Plumbism | 48 |

## ADVERSE EFFECTS

Products that are natural are frequently promoted to consumers as having no adverse effects; however, many potent drugs are derived from natural products (eg, ergot alkaloids, opiates, digitalis, estrogen), and other natural substances and plants are poisonous (eg, aconite, certain types of molds and mushrooms, snake venom, hemlock). On occasion, foragers who seek herbal remedies will mistakenly collect one plant, confusing it with another. This can be a lethal error if, for example, water hemlock is mistakenly harvested and eaten after being identified as wild ginseng.[49] Other mishaps related to misidentification of medicinal herbs are well documented.[50] Table 19-5 provides other examples of

## Table 19-5. Examples of Known Herbal Ingredients and Their Associated Toxic Effects

| HERBAL PRODUCT | TOXIC CHEMICALS | EFFECT OR TARGET ORGAN | REFERENCES |
|---|---|---|---|
| Chamomile *Matricaria chamomilla Anthemis nobilis* | Allergens: *Compositae* species | Anaphylaxis, contact dermatitis | 51 |
| Chaparral *Larrea divericata Larrea tridentate* | Nordihydroguaiaretic acid | Nausea, vomiting, lethargy Hepatitis | 52,53 |
| Cinnamon oil *Cinnamomum spp* | Cinnamaldehyde | Dermatitis, stomatitis, abuse syndrome | 54,55 |
| Coltsfoot *Tussilago farfara* | Pyrrolizidines | Hepatic veno-occlusive disease | 56–60 |
| Comfrey *(Symphytum officinale)* | Pyrrolizidines | Hepatic veno-occlusive disease | 56–60 |
| *Crotalaria* spp | Pyrrolizidines | Hepatic veno-occlusive disease | 56–60 |
| *Echinacea Echinacea augustifolia* (*Compositae* spp) | Polysaccharides | Asthma, atopy, anaphylaxis, urticaria, angioedema | 61 |
| Eucalyptus *Eucalyptus globules* | 1,8 cineole | Drowsiness, ataxia, seizures, coma Nausea, vomiting, respiratory failure | 62,63 |
| Garlic *Allium sativum* | Allicin | Dermatitis, chemical burns | 64 |
| Germander *Teucrium chamaedrys or Teucrium polium* | Teucrin A, teuchamaedryn A | Hepatotoxicity | 65 |
| Ginseng *Panax ginseng* | Ginsenoside | Ginseng abuse syndrome: diarrhea, insomnia, anxiety, hypertension, allergy | 66 |

## Table 19-5. Examples of Known Herbal Ingredients and Their Associated Toxic Effects (*continued*)

| HERBAL PRODUCT | TOXIC CHEMICALS | EFFECT OR TARGET ORGAN | REFERENCES |
|---|---|---|---|
| Glycerated asafetida | Oxidants | Methemoglobinemia | 45 |
| Groundsel *Senecio longilobus* | Pyrrolizidines | Hepatic veno-occlusive disease | 56–60 |
| Heliotrope, turnsole *Heliotropium* species *Crotalaria fulva* *Cynoglossum officinale* | Pyrrolizidines | Hepatic veno-occlusive disease | 56–60 |
| Jin bu huan *Stephania* species *Corydalis* species | L-Tetrahydro palmitine | Hepatitis, lethargy, coma | 67,68 |
| Kava kava *Piper methysticum* | Flavokavain B, pipermethysticin | Hepatotoxicity | 69,70 |
| Kratom *Mitragyna speciose* | Mitragynine, 7-hydroxymitragynine | Stimulant or opioid-like effects | 71 |
| Laetrile | Amygdalin; Cyanogenic glycosides | Coma, seizures, death | 72 |
| Licorice *Glycyrrhiza glabra* | Glycyrrhetic acid | Hypertension, hypokalemia, cardiac arrhythmias | 73 |
| Ma huang *Ephedra sinica* | Ephedrine | Cardiac arrhythmias, hypertension, seizures, stroke | 74–76 |
| Monkshood *Aconitum napellus* *Aconitum columbianum* | Aconite | Cardiac arrhythmias, shock, seizures, weakness, coma, paresthesias, vomiting | 77,78 |
| Nutmeg *Myristica fragrans* | Myristicin, eugenol | Hallucinations, emesis, tachycardia, dizziness, agitation, abdominal pain, nausea, headache | 79,80 |

(*continued*)

| HERBAL PRODUCT | TOXIC CHEMICALS | EFFECT OR TARGET ORGAN | REFERENCES |
|---|---|---|---|
| Strychnine *Nux vomica* | Strychnine | Seizures, abdominal pain, respiratory arrest | 81,82 |
| Pennyroyal *Mentha pulegium* or *Hedeoma* species | Pulegone | Centrilobular liver necrosis, shock Fetotoxicity, seizures, abortion | 83–85 |
| Ragwort (golden) *Senecio jacobaea* (*Senecio aureus* or *Echium*) | Pyrrolizidines | Hepatic veno-occlusive disease | 56–60 |
| Wormwood *Artemisia absinthium* | Thujone | Seizures, dementia, tremors, headache, renal failure | 86,87 |
| Yohimbe *Corynanthe Yohimbe* | Yohimbine | Tachycardia, hypertension, hypotension, anxiety, insomnia, tremors, disorientation, agitation, seizures | 88,89 |

**Table 19-5. Examples of Known Herbal Ingredients and Their Associated Toxic Effects (*continued*)**

some of the potent chemicals present in certain herbs and ethnic remedies and their potential uses, toxic effects, and/or drug-herb interactions.

The concentration of active ingredients as well as other chemicals in plants varies by the part of the plant harvested and sold as a remedy, the maturity of the plant at the time of harvest, and the time of year at harvest. Geography and soil conditions where the plant is grown; soil composition and its contaminants; and year-to-year variations in soil acidity, water, and weather conditions and other growth factors also can affect the concentration of the herb's active ingredients. Because of this variability in herbal product ingredients, the actual dose of active ingredients being consumed often is variable, unpredictable, or simply unknown. Children are particularly susceptible to such dosage considerations because of their smaller size and different capacity for detoxifying chemicals compared with adults. For some herbs, such as those containing pyrrolizidine alkaloids (eg, coltsfoot, comfrey, red tassel flower, golden ragwort), there may be no safe dose for children. The duration of use is another consideration, with longer courses of herbal therapy exposing the patient to a higher risk of acute and cumulative or chronic adverse effects.

Adverse effects resulting from consumption of dietary supplements may involve one or more organ systems. In some cases, a single ingredient can have multiple adverse effects. More than one dietary supplement product may be consumed concurrently, and many products may contain more than one physiologically active ingredient. Plants have complex mixtures of terpenes, sugars, alkaloids, saponins, and other chemicals. For example, more than 100 different chemicals have been identified in tea tree oil.[90] Certain herbs and dietary supplements can cause unexpected reactions when used with medications. Effects on a drug's pharmacokinetics may be pronounced and lead to either toxicity or therapeutic ineffectiveness. For example, St John's wort induces hepatic cytochromes and may decrease blood levels of medications such as indinavir, digoxin, and cyclosporin, causing loss of their effectiveness.[91–93] Pediatric patients who take oral anticoagulants, cardiovascular medications, psychiatric drugs, diabetes medications, immunosuppressive agents, or antiretroviral agents for HIV may experience a serious reduction in the efficacy of their medications with the concomitant use of certain herbs or dietary supplements.[94]

Contaminants and adulterants of herbal products and dietary supplements can be pharmacologically active and responsible for unexpected toxicity. For example, infants have sustained significant lead poisoning from spices brought into the United States from other countries.[95] Herbal plants may be harvested from contaminated soils or cleaned improperly such that they contain illness-producing microorganisms or soil contaminants. Contaminated Ayurvedic medications have been known to cause lead poisoning in children. (Ayurvedic medicine, or "ayurveda," is a system of health that has been practiced in India for more than 5,000 years.) Saper et al[96] tested a "market basket" of Ayurvedic remedies purchased in the United States and found that 20% were contaminated with metals such as lead, cadmium, arsenic, or mercury. Asian traditional medicines (also known as Asian patent remedies, Asian natural remedies, Chinese herbal medicines, Southeast Asian herbal remedies, Chinese traditional medicines) may contain undisclosed drugs such as phenylbutazone, barbiturates, benzodiazepines, or warfarin-like chemicals, as well as contaminants such as lead, cadmium, or arsenic. An analysis of raw Chinese herbs found metal and/or pesticide contaminants (in at least trace amounts) in all of them.[97]

Parents may be tempted to give herbs to children on the basis of product advertising, information from a magazine or Web site, or advice from friends or relatives, without any guidance from a knowledgeable source. Such experimentation can be expensive and risks exposure of the child to adverse effects. Herbal products are misused in excessive doses or in combinations without any known rationale. Some products are sold as mixtures of 10 or more different plants, vitamins, minerals, etc. The stacking of many different herbs increases the risk of toxicity from any of them or from their interactions.

The allergic potential of plants is well known. Infants and young children may be particularly sensitive to their first introduction to chemicals in herbs and dietary supplements. Manifestations may include dermatitis, wheezing, rhinitis, conjunctivitis, itchy throat, and other allergic manifestations. In infants, allergies also may cause nonspecific effects, such as irritability, colic, poor appetite, or gastrointestinal tract disturbances. Angelica and rue, which contain psoralen-type furocoumarins, and hypericin, the active ingredient in St John's wort, can cause photosensitization.[98]

Children differ from adults in their absorption and detoxification of some substances. However, they also have developing nervous and immune systems that may make them more sensitive to the adverse effects of herbs. For example, some herbs, such as buckthorn, senna, and aloe, are known cathartics, and some herbal teas and juniper oil contain powerful diuretic compounds.[98,99] Their actions may quickly cause clinically significant dehydration and electrolyte disturbances in an infant or young child. Children with underlying chronic illnesses may be especially vulnerable to the toxic effects of some herbs or supplements. For example, children with either liver or kidney disease may more slowly metabolize and/or excrete the parent chemical compounds or active metabolic products of supplements; therefore, additional caution should be employed in those children.

Although the chemicals in herbs may have carcinogenic effects, this concern has not been adequately investigated. Some chemicals found in plants are known carcinogens, for example, pyrrolizidines (comfrey, coltsfoot, *Senecio*), safrole (*Sassafras*), aristolochic acids (wild ginger), and catechin tannins (betel nuts).[99] Whether such chemicals pose a threat for children, who are particularly vulnerable because their developing organ systems and their longer life spans allow a long latency to tumor induction, is unknown.

Toxic effects of herbs on the male or female reproductive systems are of concern but have not been adequately investigated. Some essential oils, for example, have cytotoxic properties or cause cellular transformation in cell culture studies performed in vitro.[100] In many cases, the effects of herbs on the embryo and fetus are not known. It is possible that herbal chemicals may be transported through the placenta to cause toxic effects on the sensitive growing fetus. For example, Roulet et al[59] reported the case of a newborn infant whose mother drank senecionine-containing herbal tea daily for the duration of her pregnancy (senecionine is one of the pyrrolizidine alkaloids associated with hepatic venous injury). The infant was born with hepatic veno-occlusive disease and died. Animal studies have confirmed the teratogenicity of some herbs (eg, the popular Eastern European herb *Plectranthus fruticosus)*.[101] The excretion of chemicals from herbs and dietary supplements into human milk is a concern to pediatricians because some have lipophilic ingredients that might be expected to concentrate in human milk, although there are little data to confirm or refute this.

## ADVERSE EFFECT REPORTING

One recent study estimated that there were over 23,000 emergency department visits annually in the United States attributed to adverse events related to dietary supplements, with just over 3,000 of these involving children aged 19 years and younger.[102] In that report, the most common products involved included multivitamins, iron, weight loss supplements, and supplements for sleep, sedation, or anxiolysis. Clinicians may play a critical role in recognizing toxicity associated with herbal products and dietary supplements and identifying, reporting, and preventing adverse effects from dietary supplements. A special segment of the MedWatch program, administered by the FDA, has been dedicated to documenting adverse events involving such products. The reporting of adverse events likely underestimates the true rates because reporting of events to the FDA is voluntary.

## MedWatch & Poison Control Center Reporting

- To report adverse reactions or unexpected effects to the FDA, the MedWatch telephone number is:
  800-FDA-1088

- To fax a report of an adverse reaction or unexpected effects, the MedWatch fax telephone number is:
  800-FDA-0178

- Consumers can also report an adverse effect to the FDA Consumer Hotline at:
  888-INFO-FDA

- Poison Control Centers in the United States are a resource for both health professionals managing adverse effects of herbs and dietary supplements and members of the public who may be experiencing adverse effects:
  800-222-1222

## ADVICE TO PARENTS

The assessment of children whose parents may be seeking complementary and alternative medicine options requires strategies that promote the therapeutic interaction among physician, parent, and child. Physicians and other health professionals should ask questions about the use of dietary supplements, minerals, vitamins, or herbs as well as the reasons or health conditions for which these products are used. Guidelines have been suggested for physicians in the assessment of a patient whose parents may be seeking medical solutions involving complementary and alternative medicine.[103,104] These suggestions are modified here to make them more specific to the needs of pediatricians.

- Carry out a thorough medical evaluation.
- Communicate with parents and patients using straightforward, understandable language, provide clear advice and conclusions, and acknowledge when evidence is lacking.
- Obtain a complete medical history, including the presence of chronic diseases (in some of which the use of various supplements may be contraindicated).
- Obtain a complete medication profile to ensure that the current medications are compatible with the supplement.
- Explore conventional therapeutic options—establish a dialogue with the parents about what, in your opinion, is the best treatment for the condition as well as what may be untested alternatives. Keep an open mind and research what beliefs the parents may bring to the discussion.
- Ask the unasked question—find out about the current beliefs of the parents and any current alternative therapies, herbs, and/or other traditional or ethnic remedies in use by the family and given to children, using explicit terms such as 'alternative,' 'natural,' and 'herbal.'
- Document requests for complementary and alternative medicine or therapeutic refusals in the medical record. If you disagree with the plan, discuss why and document your disagreement in the record.
- Understand that the scope of the physician's duty to disclose and explain treatment alternatives as part of the process of obtaining informed consent may extend to complementary and alternative medicine therapies, where these have attained sufficient scientific evidence so as to be accorded prevailing medical acceptance of safety and efficacy.
- Obtain consultations as needed—for example, if the child has frequent unresolved ear infections, suggest that the parents follow up on your referral of the child to an otolaryngologist before trying herbs.
- Use the regional Poison Control Center (nationwide toll-free telephone number 1-800-222-1222) for help in identifying ingredients in specific herbal products and commercially sold supplements, as well as for clinically important, toxicological information about them.

The best interests of the child are always paramount. When the pediatrician disagrees with the family's intended actions, such disagreement should be voiced along with the reasons behind it. In other circumstances, the pediatrician can and should support the parents' decision to pursue herbal remedies or dietary supplements when the risk of harm is low, the possibility of benefit is backed by scientific evidence, and the parents can be engaged in an integrative approach to the child's care. All of this presumes that the pediatrician is sufficiently knowledgeable about the health aspects of the herbs and dietary supplements in question, using reliable sources of information.

## Frequently Asked Questions

Q  *Conventional medications have many side effects. Shouldn't I worry more about the known side effects?*

A  Conventional pharmaceutical products have been through extensive testing for safety and efficacy by manufacturers and through FDA review processes, and through this process, side effects and prevalence have been identified and are listed in package inserts or available sources. Less is known about side effects associated with children's use of certain herbs and dietary supplements because these products do not need to undergo this level of premarketing scrutiny.

Q  *Does my child need extra vitamins/food supplements? Won't they help my child grow, eat, and study better?*

A  A diet that provides enough calories and is balanced in all the major food groups generally provides adequate nutrition for an otherwise healthy growing child. Infants and young children may gain dental benefits from fluoride supplements if they drink only nonfluorinated bottled or well water or live in communities that do not fluoridate public water sources. Additional vitamin or dietary supplements may be necessary for children to reach recommended amounts of vitamin D. AAP guidelines recommend that breastfed infants, formula-fed infants, children, and teenagers who are consuming less than 1 quart per day of vitamin D-fortified formula or milk should receive a vitamin D supplement of 400 IU per day.[105] Guidelines from the Institute of Medicine and from the AAP recommend that children 1 year and older have a total of 600 IU of vitamin D daily from food and supplemental sources.[106,107] Guidelines for supplementation with iron, zinc, and other essential nutrients should be followed.[108]

Q  *Doesn't the FDA approve herbs and dietary supplements?*

A  No. Legislation enacted in 1994 made dietary ingredients exempt from FDA premarket approval that apply to drugs and food additives. Manufacturers no longer must prove that an ingredient is safe. The FDA needs to prove the ingredient is hazardous if it believes there is a risk.

*Q   Is it OK to give my child chamomile or spearmint tea?*

A   Weak teas made from the leaves and flowers of chamomile or spearmint probably pose a negligible threat of an adverse effect, although there is little evidence of clear therapeutic benefits on children's health from such teas. Keep in mind that children as well as adults might experience allergic reactions to any plant-derived products such as mint (*Mentha* species) and chamomile (*Compositae* species).

*Q   Is zinc of any value in the treatment of colds?*

A   Zinc is an essential metal for good health, and zinc deficiencies can weaken the immune system. Zinc supplementation was recently found to improve the survival of infants who were small for their gestational age. Its value in the treatment of childhood upper respiratory tract infections has yet to be shown in carefully controlled studies.

*Q   Are over-the-counter herbs of any value in treating my child's colds?*

A   Many laboratory or animal-based studies of certain herbs, such as *Echinacea* or *Astragalus,* have shown them to have remarkable effects on the immune system. However, such results may not necessarily be extrapolated to imply a benefit in the management of a sick child. Investigations of the use of *Echinacea* to treat colds in a randomized controlled trial in children showed no benefit. It is important to understand that some herbal remedies, such as camphor or eucalyptus oil, may be soothing if inhaled but also can have harmful effects, including seizures or coma, if ingested by children.

## Resources

### American Botanical Council

Web site: www.herbalgram.org

### Dr Duke's Phytochemical and Ethnobotanical Databases

Web site: www.ars-grin.gov/duke

### Food & Drug Administration, Center for Food Safety and Applied Nutrition

Web site: www.fda.gov/AboutFDA/CentersOffices/Officeoffoods/CFSAN/default

### Herb Research Foundation

Web site: www.herbs.org

### Memorial Sloan-Kettering Cancer Center

Web site: www.mskcc.org/aboutherbs

## National Center for Complementary and Alternative Medicine
Web site: www.nccam.nih.gov

## National Certification Commission for Acupuncture and Oriental Medicine
Web site: www.nccaom.org

## National Council Against Health Fraud
Web site: www.ncahf.org

## Quackwatch
Web site: www.quackwatch.org

## University of Florida, College of Pharmacy, Center for Drug Interaction Research & Education
Web site: www.druginteractioncenter.org

## US Department of Agriculture, National Agricultural Library, Food & Nutrition Information Center
Web site: www.nal.usda.gov/fnic

## References

1. Dietary Supplement Health and Education Act of 1994. https://health.gov/dietsupp/ch1.htm. Accessed March 5, 2018
2. Siegel R. Kola, ginseng, and mislabeled herbs. *JAMA*. 1978;237:25
3. Harel Z, Harel S, Wald R, Mamdani M, Bell CM. The frequency and characteristics of dietary supplement recalls in the United States. *JAMA Intern Med*. 2013;173(10):926–928
4. Kesselheim AS, Connolly J, Rogers J, Avorn J. Mandatory disclaimers on dietary supplements do not reliably communicate the intended issues. *Health Affairs (Milwood)*. 2015;34(3):438–446
5. Millman J. Americans are ignoring the science and spending billions on dietary supplements. Washington Post. February 5th 2015. https://www.washingtonpost.com/news/wonk/wp/2015/02/04/americans-are-ignoring-the-science-and-spending-billions-on-dietary-supplements/. Accessed March 6, 2018
6. Bailey RL, Gahche JJ, Thomas PR, Dwyer JT. Why U.S. children use dietary supplements. *Pediatr Res*. 2013;74(6):737–741
7. Black LI, Clarke TC, Barnes PC, Stussman BJ, Nahin RL. Use of complementary approaches among children aged 4-17 years in the United States: National Health Interview Survey 2007-2012. National Health Statistics Reports. February 10, 2015. Vol 78: 1–19. http://www.cdc.gov/nchs/data/nhsr/nhsr078.pdf. Accessed March 6, 2018
8. Groenewald CB, Beals-Erickson SE, Ralston-Wilson J, Rabbitts JA, Palermo TM. Complementary and alternative medicine use by children with pain in the United States. *Acad Pediatr*. 2017;17(7):785–793
9. Sawni-Sikand A, Schubiner H, Thomas RL. Use of complementary/alternative therapies among children in primary care pediatrics. *Ambulatory Pediatr*. 2002;2(2):99–103
10. Zhang Y, Fein EB, Fein SB. Feeding of dietary botanical supplements and teas to infants in the United States. *Pediatrics*. 2011;127(6):1060–1066

11. Wilson K, Dowson C, Mangin D. Prevalence of complementary and alternative medicine use in Christchurch, New Zealand: children attending general practice versus paediatric outpatients. *N Z Med J.* 2007;120(1251):U2464

12. American Academy of Pediatrics, Committee on Children with Disabilities. Counseling families who choose complementary and alternative medicine for their child with chronic illness or disability. *Pediatrics.* 2001;107(3):598–601

13. Taylor JA, Weber W, Standish L, et al. Efficacy and safety of echinacea in treating upper respiratory tract infections in children: a randomized controlled trial. *JAMA.* 2003;290(21):2824–2830

14. Wasdell MB, Jan JE, Bomben MM, et al. A randomized, placebo-controlled trial of controlled release melatonin treatment of delayed sleep phase syndrome and impaired sleep maintenance in children with neurodevelopmental disabilities. *J Pineal Res* 2008;44(1):57–64

15. Becker B, Kuhn U, Hardewig-Budny B. Double-blind, randomized evaluation of clinical efficacy and tolerability of an apple pectin-chamomile extract in children with unspecific diarrhea. *Arzneimittelforschung.* 2006;56(6):387–393

16. de la Motte S, Bose-O'Reilly S, Heinisch M, Harrison F. [Double-blind comparison of an apple pectin-chamomile extract preparation with placebo in children with diarrhea]. [Article in German.] *Arzneimittelforschung.* 1997;47(11):1247–1249

17. Savino F, Cresi F, Castagno E, Silvestro L, Oggero R. A randomized double-blind placebo-controlled trial of a standardized extract of Matricariae recutita, Foeniculum vulgare and Melissa officinalis (ColiMil) in the treatment of breastfed colicky infants. *Phytother Res.* 2005;19(4):335–340

18. Gardiner P. Complementary, holistic, and integrative medicine: chamomile. *Pediatr Rev.* 2007;28(4):e16–e18

19. Paulsen E. Contact sensitization from Compositae-containing herbal remedies and cosmetics. *Contact Dermatitis.* 2002;47(4):189–198

20. Chaiyakunapruk N, Kitikannakorn N, Nathisuwan S, Leeprakobboon K, Leelasettagool C. The efficacy of ginger for the prevention of postoperative nausea and vomiting: a meta-analysis. *Am J Obstet Gynecol.* 2006;194(1):95–99

21. Borrelli F, Capasso R, Aviello G, Pittler MH, Izzo AA. Effectiveness and safety of ginger in the treatment of pregnancy-induced nausea and vomiting. *Obstet Gynecol.* 2005;105(4):849–856

22. Bent S, Padula A, Moore D, Patterson M, Hehling W. Valerian for sleep: a systematic review and meta-analysis. *Am J Med.* 2006;119(12):1005–1012

23. Koetter U, Schrader E, Kaufeler R, Brattstrom A. A randomized, double blind, placebo-controlled, prospective clinical study to demonstrate clinical efficacy of a fixed valerian hops extract combination (Ze 91019) in patients suffering from non-organic sleep disorder. *Phytother Res.* 2007;21(9):847–851

24. Muller SF, Klement S. A combination of valerian and lemon balm is effective in the treatment of restlessness and dyssomnia in children. *Phytomedicine.* 2006;13(6):383–387

25. Gardiner P, Riley DS. Herbs to homeopathy—medicinal products for children. *Pediatr Clin North Am.* 2007;54(6):859–874

26. Wilson KM, Klein JD, Sesselberg TS, et al. Use of complementary medicine and dietary supplements among U.S. adolescents. *J Adolesc Health.* 2006;38(4):385–394

27. Gardiner P, Buettner C, Davis RB, Phillips RS, Kemper KJ. Factors and common conditions associated with adolescent dietary supplement use: an analysis of the National Health and Nutrition Examination Survey (NHANES). *BMC Complement Altern Med.* 2008;8:9

28. Yussman SM, Wilson KM, Klein JD. Herbal products and their association with substance use in adolescents. *J Adolesc Health.* 2006;38(4):395–400

29. Lieberman HR, Marriott BP, Williams C, et al. Patterns of dietary supplement use among college students. *Clin Nutr.* 2015;34(5):976–985

30. Philen RM, Ortiz DI, Auerbach SB, Falk H. Survey of advertising for nutritional supplements in health and bodybuilding magazines. *JAMA.* 1992;268(8):1008–1011

31. Woolf A. Essential oil poisoning. *J Toxicol Clin Toxicol.* 1999;37(6):721–727

32. Angell M, Kassirer JP. Alternative medicine—the risks of untested and unregulated remedies. *N Engl J Med.* 1998;339(12):839–841

33. Bailey RL, Fulgoni VL, Keast DR, Lentino CV, Dwyer JT. Do dietary supplements improve micronutrient sufficiency in children and adolescents? *J Pediatr.* 2012;161(5):837–842

34. White NJ, Waller D, Crawley J, et al. Comparison of artemether and chloroquine for severe malaria in Gambian children. *Lancet.* 1992;339(8789):317–321

35. Zhao KS, Mancini C, Doria G. Enhancement of the immune response in mice by *Astragalus membranaceus* extracts. *Immunopharmacology.* 1990;20(3):225–233

36. Weizman Z, Alkrinawi S, Goldfarb D, Bitran C. Efficacy of herbal tea preparation in infantile colic. *J Pediatr.* 1993;122(4):650–652

37. Pachter LM. Culture and clinical care. Folk illness beliefs and behaviors and their implications for health care delivery. *JAMA.* 1994;271(9):690–694

38. Buchwald D, Panwala S, Hooton TM. Use of traditional health practices by Southeast Asian refugees in a primary care clinic. *West J Med.* 1992;156(5):507–511

39. Pachter LM, Cloutier MM, Bernstein BA. Ethnomedical (folk) remedies for childhood asthma in a mainland Puerto Rican community. *Arch Pediatr Adolesc Med.* 1995;149(9):982–988

40. Yeatman GW, Dang VV. Cao gio (coin rubbing). Vietnamese attitudes toward health care. *JAMA.* 1980;244(24):2748–2749

41. Forman J, Moline J, Cernichiari E, et al. A cluster of pediatric metallic mercury exposure cases treated with meso-2,3 dimercaptosuccinic acid (DMSA). *Environ Health Perspect.* 2000;108(6):575–577

42. Moore C, Adler R. Herbal vitamins: lead toxicity and developmental delay. *Pediatrics.* 2000;106(3):600–602

43. Risser AL, Mazur LJ. Use of folk remedies in a Hispanic population. *Arch Pediatr Adolesc Med.* 1995;149(9):978–981

44. Centers for Disease Control and Prevention. Lead poisoning-associated death from Asian Indian folk remedies—Florida. *MMWR Morb Mortal Wkly Rep.* 1984;33(45):638, 643–645

45. Kelly KJ, Neu J, Camitta BM, Honig GR. Methemoglobinemia in an infant treated with the folk remedy glycerited asafoetida. *Pediatrics.* 1984;73(5):717–719

46. Centers for Disease Control and Prevention. Folk remedy-associated lead poisoning in Hmong children—Minnesota. *MMWR Morb Mortal Wkly Rep.* 1983;32(42):555–556

47. Riley DM, Newby CA, Leal-Almeraz TO, Thomas VM. Assessing elemental mercury exposure from cultural and religious practices. *Environ Health Perspect.* 2001;109(8):779–784

48. Woolf AD, Hussain J, McCullough L, Petranovic M, Chomchai C. Infantile lead poisoning from an Asian tongue powder: a case report and subsequent public health inquiry. *Clin Toxicol.* 2008;46(9):841–844

49. Centers for Disease Control and Prevention. Water hemlock poisoning—Maine, 1992. *MMWR Morb Mortal Wkly Rep.* 1994;43(13):229–231

50. Maeda K, Idehara R, Kusaka S. Mistaken identity: severe vomiting, bradycardia, and hypotension after eating a wild herb. *Clin Toxicol.* 2012;50(6):532–533

51. Benner MH, Lee HJ. Anaphylactic reaction to chamomile tea. *J Allergy Clin Immunol.* 1973;52(5):307–308

52. Grant KL, Pharm D, Boyer LV, Erdman BE. Chaparral-induced hepatotoxicity. *Integrative Med.* 1998;1:83–87

53. Centers for Disease Control and Prevention. Chaparral-induced toxic hepatitis—California and Texas. *MMWR Morb Mortal Wkly Rep.* 1992;41(43):812–814

54. Miller RL, Gould AR, Bernstein ML. Cinnamon-induced stomatitis venenata, clinical and characteristic histopathologic features. *Oral Surg Oral Med Oral Pathol.* 1992;73(6):708–716

55. Perry PA, Dean BS, Krenzelok EP. Cinnamon oil abuse by adolescents. *Vet Hum Toxicol.* 1990;32(2):162–164

56. Allgaier C, Franz S. Risk assessment on the use of herbal medicinal products containing pyrrolizidine alkaloids. *Regul Toxicol Pharmacol.* 2015;73(2):494–500

57. Ridker PM, Ohkuma S, McDermott WV, Trey C, Huxtable RJ. Hepatic venoocclusive disease associated with the consumption of pyrrolizidine-containing dietary supplements. *Gastroenterology.* 1985;88(4):1050–1054

58. Wiedenfeld H. Plants containing pyrrolizidine alkaloids: toxicity and problems. *Food Addit Contam Part A Chem Anal Control Expo Risk Assess.* 2011;28(3):282–292

59. Roulet M, Laurini R, Rivier L, Calame A. Hepatic veno-occlusive disease in the newborn infant of a woman drinking herbal tea. *J Pediatr.* 1988;112(3):433–436

60. Bunchorntavakul C, Reddy KR. Review article: herbal and dietary supplement hepatotoxicity. *Aliment Pharmacol Ther.* 2013;37(1):3–17

61. Mullins RJ, Heddle R. Adverse reactions associated with echinacea: the Australian experience. *Ann Allergy Asthma Immunol.* 2002;88(1):42–51

62. Tibballs J. Clinical effects and management of eucalyptus oil ingestion in infants and young children. *Med J Aust.* 1995;163(4):177–180

63. Webb NJ, Pitt WR. Eucalyptus oil poisoning in childhood: 41 cases in south-east Queensland. *J Paediatr Child Health.* 1993;29(5):368–371

64. Garty BZ. Garlic burns. *Pediatrics.* 1993;91(3):658–659

65. Sezer RG, Bozaykut A. Pediatric hepatotoxicity associated with polygermander (teucrium polium). *Clin Toxicol (Phila).* 2012;50(2):153

66. Paik DJ, Lee CH. Review of cases of patient risk associated with ginseng abuse. *J Ginseng Res.* 2015;39(2):89–93

67. Centers for Disease Control and Prevention. Jin bu huan toxicity in children—Colorado 1993. *MMWR Morb Mortal Wkly Rep.* 1993;42(33):633–635

68. Horowitz RS, Feldhaus K, Dart RC, Stermitz FR, Beck JJ. The clinical spectrum of Jin Bu Huan toxicity. *Arch Intern Med.* 1996;156(8):899–903

69. Teschke R, Schulze J. Risk of kava hepatotoxicity and the FDA consumer advisory. *JAMA.* 2010;304(19):2174–2175

70. Teschke R. Kava hepatotoxicity: pathogenetic aspects and prospective considerations. *Liver Int.* 2010;30(9):1270–1279

71. Warner ML, Kaufman NC, Grundmann O. The pharmacology and toxicology of kratom: from traditional herb to drug of abuse. *Int J Legal Med.* 2016;130(1):127–138

72. Hall AH, Linden CH, Kulig KW, Rumack BH. Cyanide poisoning from laetrile ingestion: role of nitrite therapy. *Pediatrics.* 1986;78(2):269–272

73. Walker BR, Edwards CR. Licorice-induced hypertension and syndromes of apparent mineralocorticoid excess. *Endocrinol Metab Clin North Am.* 1994;23(2):359–377

74. Samenuk D, Link MS, Homoud MK, et al. Adverse cardiovascular events temporally associated with ma huang, an herbal source of ephedrine. *Mayo Clin Proc.* 2002;77(1):12–16

75. Haller CA, Benowitz NL. Adverse cardiovascular and central nervous system events associated with dietary supplements containing ephedra alkaloids. *N Engl J Med.* 2000;343(25):1833–1838

76. Woolf AD, Litovitz T, Smolinske S, Watson WA. The severity of toxic reactions to ephedra: comparisons to other botanical products and national trends from 1993-2002. *Clin Toxicol (Phila).* 2005;43(5):347–355

77. Fatovich DM. Aconite: a lethal Chinese herb. *Ann Emerg Med.* 1992;21(3):309–311

78. Chan TY. Aconite poisoning. *Clin Toxicol (Phila).* 2009;47(4):279–285

79. Abernethy MK, Becker LB. Acute nutmeg intoxication. *Am J Emerg Med.* 1992;10(5):429–430

80. Carstairs SD, Cantrell FL. The spice of life: an analysis of nutmeg exposures in California. *Clin Toxicol (Phila).* 2011;49(3):177–180

81. Katz J, Prescott K, Woolf AD. Strychnine poisoning from a Cambodian traditional remedy. *Am J Emerg Med.* 1996;14(5):475–477

82. Jacob J, Tarabar AF. A rare case of combined strychnine and propoxur toxicity from a single preparation. *Clin Toxicol (Phila).* 2012;50(3):224

83. Gordon P, Khojasteh SC. A decades-long investigation of acute metabolism-based hepatotoxicity by herbal constituents: a case study of pennyroyal oil. *Drug Metab Rev.* 2015;47(1):12–20

84. Anderson IB, Mullen WH, Meeker JE, et al. Pennyroyal toxicity: measurement of toxic metabolite levels in two cases and review of the literature. *Ann Intern Med.* 1996;124(8): 726–734

85. Gordon WB, Forte AJ, McMurtry RJ, Gal J, Nelson SD. Hepatotoxicity and pulmonary toxicity of pennyroyal oil and its constituent terpenes in the mouse. *Toxicol Appl Pharmacol.* 1982;65(3):413–424

86. Arnold WN. Vincent van Gogh and the thujone connection. *JAMA.* 1988;260(20):3042–3044

87. Weisbord SD, Soule JB, Kimmel PL. Poison on line-acute renal failure caused by oil of wormwood purchased through the Internet. *N Engl J Med.* 1997;337(12):825–827

88. Cimolai N, Cimolai T. Yohimbine use for physical enhancement and its potential toxicity. *J Diet Suppl.* 2011;8(4):346–354

89. Giampreti A, Lonati D, Locatelli C, Rocchi L, Campailla MT. Acute neurotoxicity after yohimbine ingestion by a body builder. *Clin Toxicol (Phila).* 2009;47(8):827–829

90. Carson CF, Riley TV. Toxicity of the essential oil of *Melaleuca alternifolia* or tea tree oil. *J Toxicol Clin Toxicol.* 1995;33(2):193–194

91. Piscitelli SC, Burstein AH, Chaitt D, Alfaro RM, Falloon J. Indinavir concentrations and St John's wort. *Lancet.* 2000;355(9203):547–548

92. Johne A, Brockmoller J, Bauer S, Maurer A, Langheinrich M, Roots I. Pharmacokinetic interaction of digoxin with an herbal extract from St John's wort (*Hypericum perforatum*). *Clin Pharmacol Ther.* 1999;66(4):338–345

93. Ruschitzka F, Meier PJ, Turina M, Luscher TF, Noll G. Acute heart transplant rejection due to Saint John's wort. *Lancet.* 2000;355(9203):548–549

94. Gardiner P, Phillips R, Shaughnessy AF. Herbal and dietary supplement-drug interactions in patients with chronic illnesses. *Am Fam Physician.* 2008;77(1):73–78

95. Woolf AD, Woolf NT. Childhood lead poisoning in two families associated with spices used in food preparation. *Pediatrics.* 2005;116(2):e314–e318

96. Saper RB, Kales SN, Paquin J, et al. Heavy metal content of ayurvedic herbal medicine products. *JAMA.* 2004;292(23):2868–2873

97. Harris ES, Cao S, Littlefield BA, et al. Heavy metal and pesticide content in commonly prescribed individual raw Chinese herbal medicines. *Sci Total Environ.* 2011;409(20):4297–4305

98. Toxic reactions to plant products sold in health food stores. *Med Lett Drugs Ther.* 1979;21(7):29–32

99. Saxe TG. Toxicity of medicinal herbal preparations. *Am Fam Physician.* 1987;35(5):135–142

100. Pecevski J, Savkovic D, Radivojevic D, Vuksanovic L. Effect of oil of nutmeg on the fertility and induction of meiotic chromosome rearrangements in mice and their first generation. *Toxicol Lett.* 1981;7(3):239–243

101. Pages N, Salazar M, Chamorro G, et al. Teratological evaluation of *Plectranthus fruticosus* leaf essential oil. *Planta Med.* 1988;54(4):296–298

102. Geller AI, Shehab N, Weidle NJ, et al. Emergency department visits for adverse events related to dietary supplements. *N Engl J Med.* 2015;373(16):1531–1540

103. Gilmour J, Harrison C, Vohra S. Concluding comments: maximizing good patient care and minimizing potential liability when considering complementary and alternative medicine. *Pediatrics.* 2011;128(Suppl 4):S206–S212

104. Eisenberg DM. Advising patients who seek alternative medical therapies. *Ann Intern Med.* 1997;127(1):61–69

105. Wagner CL, Greer FR, American Academy of Pediatrics, Section on Breastfeeding and Committee on Nutrition. Prevention of rickets and vitamin D deficiency in infants, children, and adolescents. *Pediatrics.* 2008;122(5):1142–1152

106. Institute of Medicine. *Dietary Reference Intakes for Calcium and Vitamin D.* November 30, 2010. http://www.nationalacademies.org/hmd/Reports/2010/Dietary-Reference-Intakes-for-Calcium-and-Vitamin-D.aspx. Accessed May 12, 2018

107. Golden NH, Abrams SA, American Academy of Pediatrics Committee on Nutrition. Optimizing bone health in children and adolescents. *Pediatrics.* 2014;134(4):e1229–e1243

108. American Academy of Pediatrics Committee on Nutrition. *Pediatric Nutrition Handbook, 7th Edition.* Kleinman RE, ed. Elk Grove Village, IL: American Academy of Pediatrics; 2013

Chapter 20

# Air Pollutants, Indoor

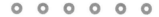

## KEY POINTS

- Children spend 80% to 90% of their time indoors and therefore are often exposed to pollutants in indoor air.
- Major sources of indoor air pollutants are tobacco smoke, gas stoves and wood stoves, pets and pests, molds and other biologicals, furnishings, and construction materials.
- The most important step to reduce the concentration of indoor pollutants in the home is to prohibit smoking indoors.
- Water damage should be cleaned up promptly; exposure to molds may result in infectious, allergic, or toxic health effects.
- Clinicians evaluating a child with a persistent or unusual respiratory symptom should consider exposure to an indoor air pollutant as a possible etiology.

## INTRODUCTION

Indoor air quality often affects children's health. There has been increasing concern in recent years as higher energy costs have led to building designs that reduce air exchanges. New synthetic materials have become more widely used in furnishings. Furthermore, children spend an estimated 80% to 90% of their time indoors at home, child care settings, or at school. Indoor environments have a range of airborne pollutants, including particulate matter, gases, vapors, biological materials, and fibers that may have adverse effects on health. In the home, smoking is a major cause of indoor air pollution.[1] Other common sources of air pollutants include gas stoves and wood stoves, and furnishings and construction materials that may release organic gases and vapors. Allergens and biological agents include animal dander, pest allergens from mice and cockroaches, fecal material from house dust mites and other insects, mold spores, and bacteria (see Chapter 47). Pollutants such as particulate matter may be brought into the indoor environment from the outdoor air by natural and mechanical ventilation. Pesticides may be sprayed in the home to reduce insect infestations. This chapter describes indoor air pollution from combustion products, ammonia, volatile organic compounds (VOCs), and molds. Other chapters in the book focus on outdoor air pollution (see Chapter 21), asbestos (see Chapter 23), carbon monoxide (see Chapter 25), radon (see Chapter 42), and secondhand and thirdhand smoke (see Chapter 43).

## COMBUSTION POLLUTANTS

### Route and Sources of Exposure

The route of exposure to combustion products is through inhalation. Combustion pollutants in the home arise primarily from gas ranges and gas heat, particularly when they malfunction or are used as space heaters, and from improperly vented wood stoves and fireplaces.

Combustion of natural gas results in the emission of nitrogen dioxide ($NO_2$) and carbon monoxide (CO). Levels of $NO_2$ in the home generally are increased during the winter, when ventilation is reduced to conserve energy and heat fueled by gas may be used. During the winter, average indoor concentrations of $NO_2$ in homes with gas cooking stoves are as much as twice as high as outdoor levels. Some of the highest indoor $NO_2$ levels have been measured in homes in which ovens were used as space heaters. Residential levels of CO generally are low unless appliances are inadequately ventilated.

Cooking or heating with wood results in the emission of liquids (suspended droplets), solids (suspended particles), and gases such as $NO_2$ and sulfur dioxide ($SO_2$). The aerosol mixture of very fine solid and liquid particles or "smoke" contains particles in the inhalable range, less than 10 μm in diameter. Measurements of wood smoke performed in indoor environments in the United States demonstrate that concentrations of inhalable particles are higher in homes with wood stoves, compared with homes without wood stoves. Depending on the frequency and duration of cooking or heating with wood and the adequacy of ventilation, the concentration of inhalable particles may exceed outdoor air standards. With adequate ventilation, however, operating a wood stove or fireplace may not adversely affect indoor air quality.

### Systems Affected

The nervous system, the cardiovascular system, the respiratory tract, and the mucous membranes of the eyes, nose, and throat are affected.

## Clinical Effects

Clinical symptoms attributable to exposure are usually acute and short lived and generally cease with elimination of exposure. Exposure to CO, which affects the nervous system and the cardiovascular system, is covered in Chapter 25. Exposure to high levels of $NO_2$ and $SO_2$ may result in acute mucocutaneous irritation and respiratory tract effects. The relatively low water solubility of $NO_2$ results in minimal mucous membrane irritation of the upper airway; the principal site of toxicity is the lower respiratory tract. If patients with asthma are exposed either simultaneously or sequentially to $NO_2$ and an aeroallergen, the risk of an exaggerated response to the allergen is increased.[2] The high water solubility of $SO_2$ makes it extremely irritating to the eyes and upper respiratory tract. Whether exposure to the relatively low levels of this gas attained in houses is associated with health effects remains to be determined.

Exposure to inhaled particles in wood smoke may result in irritation and inflammation of the upper and lower respiratory tract resulting in rhinitis, cough, wheezing, and worsening of asthma.[3]

## Diagnostic Methods

If CO poisoning is suspected, the family should vacate the premises immediately, and carboxyhemoglobin levels should be measured promptly (see Chapter 25).

For an indoor air pollution-related respiratory illness, a specific etiology may be difficult to establish because most respiratory signs and symptoms are nonspecific and may only occur in association with significant exposures. Effects of lower exposures may be milder and more vague. Furthermore, signs and symptoms in infants and children may be atypical. Multiple pollutants may be involved in each situation. Establishing the environmental cause of a respiratory illness is further complicated by the similarity of effects to those associated with allergies and respiratory infections. The clinician should ask whether anyone smokes in the home, whether anyone else in the family is ill, and whether the child's symptoms abate when away from the home and recur upon return. The clinician should also ask whether the family burns wood in a wood stove or fireplace. Use of space heaters, kerosene lamps or heaters, and gas ovens or ranges as home heating devices should raise concerns about exposure to combustion products, particularly if there is any indication that appliances may not be properly vented to the outside or that heating equipment may be in disrepair.

## Prevention of Exposure

Measures that may help to minimize exposure include periodic professional inspection and maintenance of furnaces, gas water heaters, and clothes dryers;

venting such equipment directly to the outdoors; and regular cleaning and inspection of fireplaces and wood stoves. Charcoal (in a hibachi or grill) should never be burned indoors or in a tent or camper.

## Guidelines

Levels of outdoor air pollution are regulated by the US Environmental Protection Agency (EPA), but there is no regulation of levels of pollution indoors. Although there are no standards for indoor air quality in the United States, the World Health Organization (WHO) published a global update on air quality guidelines in 2005. The air quality guidelines in Table 20-1 are recommended to be achieved everywhere (indoors and outdoors) to significantly reduce the adverse health effects of pollution.[4]

## AMMONIA

Ammonia is a major component of many common household cleaning products (eg, glass cleaners, toilet bowl cleaners, metal polishes, floor strippers, wax removers).

### Table 20-1. World Health Organization Air Quality Guidelines

| POLLUTANT | AIR QUALITY GUIDELINE VALUE | AVERAGING TIME |
|---|---|---|
| Carbon monoxide | 100 mg/m$^3$ | 15 min |
| | 60 mg/m$^3$ | 30 min |
| | 30 mg/m$^3$ | 1 h |
| | 10 mg/m$^3$ | 8 h |
| Nitrogen dioxide | 200 mcg/m$^3$ | 1 h |
| | 40 mcg/m$^3$ | Annual |
| Ozone | 100 mcg/m$^3$ | 8 h, daily maximum |
| Particulate matter | | |
| PM$_{2.5}$ | 10 mcg/m$^3$ | 1 y |
| | 25 mcg/m$^3$ | 24 h |
| PM$_{10}$ | 20 mcg/m$^3$ | 1 y |
| | 50 mcg/m$^3$ | 24 h |

Abbreviations: PM$_{2.5}$, particles <2.5 mcm in diameter; PM$_{10}$, particles <10 mcm in diameter.

## Route and Sources of Exposure

The route of exposure to ammonia is through inhalation. People are frequently exposed to ammonia while using household products. Household ammonia solutions usually contain 5% to 10% ammonia in water. Ammonia is found in smelling salts and in swine confinement buildings. It is liberated during combustion of nylon, silk, wood, and melamine, and used in the production of explosives, pharmaceuticals, pesticides, textiles, leather, flame retardants, plastics, pulp and paper, rubber, petroleum products, and cyanide. People who live near farms or cattle feedlots, poultry confinement buildings, or in the vicinity of other areas with high animal populations may be exposed to elevated ammonia levels. In enclosed animal confinement buildings, ammonia is adsorbed by dust particles that transport it more directly to small airways.

## Systems Affected

The respiratory tract and eyes are affected.

## Clinical Effects

Symptoms including rhinorrhea, scratchy throat, chest tightness, cough, dyspnea, and eye irritation usually subside within 24 to 48 hours. Symptoms have reportedly developed within minutes of entering animal confinement buildings. Typical environmental ammonia concentrations have not been reported to cause adverse health effects in the general population. However, low levels of ammonia may harm some people with asthma and other sensitive individuals.[5]

## Diagnostic Methods

If the causes of the child's respiratory symptoms are not apparent, questions about the use of household products containing ammonia and exposures to animal confinement buildings should be included in the environmental history.

## Prevention of Exposure

For household cleaning, a less toxic substitute for ammonia-containing household products is a vinegar and water solution or baking soda and water. If ammonia is used, it should never be mixed with bleach because toxic chloramines can be released, which cause lung injury.

## VOLATILE ORGANIC COMPOUNDS

Volatile organic compounds (VOCs) are chemicals that produce vapors readily at room temperature and normal atmospheric pressure.

## Routes and Sources of Exposure

The route of exposure to VOCs occurs through inhalation and dermal contact with surfaces on which they are deposited. Many household furnishings and products release ("off-gas") VOCs. These chemicals include aliphatic and aromatic hydrocarbons (including chlorinated hydrocarbons), alcohols, and ketones in products such as finishes, rug and oven cleaners, paints and lacquers, and paint strippers.

Because product labels may not always specify the presence of organic compounds, the specific chemicals to which a product user may be exposed may be difficult to discern. Over the normal range of room temperatures, VOCs are released as gases or vapors from furnishings or consumer products. Table 20-2 lists some common VOCs, their uses, and sources of indoor exposure.

Measurements in residential and nonresidential buildings show that exposure to VOCs is widespread and highly variable. In general, levels of VOCs are likely to be higher in recently constructed or renovated buildings compared with older buildings. Off-gassing of VOCs is greatest when materials containing VOCs are new and decreases over time. Once building-related emissions decrease, consumer products (including cigarettes) are likely to remain the predominant source of exposure to VOCs. Concentrations of VOCs (measured using a personal monitor) are greater indoors than outdoors; breath levels correlate better with air exposures in a person's breathing zone than with outdoor air levels, and inhalation accounts for more than 99% of exposure for many VOCs.

### Benzene

Benzene in indoor air comes primarily from cigarette smoking and consumer products, including off-gassing from particle board. Children's urine benzene levels are known to increase with the amount of smoking in the home.[6] In homes with attached garages, higher benzene levels have been measured than in homes with detached garages.

### Formaldehyde

Formaldehyde, one of the most ubiquitous indoor air contaminants, is found primarily in building materials and home furnishings. It is used in hundreds of products, such as urea-formaldehyde and phenol-formaldehyde resin (used to bond laminated wood products and to bind wood chips in particle board); as a carrier solvent in dyeing textiles and paper products; and as a stiffener and water repellent in floor coverings (eg, rugs, linoleum). Urea-formaldehyde foam insulation, one source of formaldehyde used in home construction until the early 1980s, is no longer used. The addition of new furniture to a home increases indoor formaldehyde concentrations. Mobile homes and classrooms, which have small enclosed spaces, low air exchange rates, and many particle board furnishings, may have much higher concentrations of formaldehyde than other types of homes and classrooms.[7] Formaldehyde can also be released from the formaldehyde-releasing resins used to make stain- and wrinkle-resistant

## Table 20-2. Common Volatile Organic Compounds (VOCs)

| VOC | USES | SOURCES OF INDOOR EXPOSURE |
|---|---|---|
| 1,1,1-Trichloroethane | As a dry-cleaning agent, a vapor degreasing agent, and a propellant | Wearing dry-cleaned clothes, using aerosol sprays and fabric protectors |
| 1,3-Butadiene | Used to produce synthetic rubber | Breathing cigarette smoke, motor vehicle exhaust, or wood fire smoke |
| 1,4-Dichlorobenzene | As an air deodorant and an insecticide | Using air fresheners, mothballs, and toilet-deodorizer blocks |
| 2-Butanone | As a solvent, and in the surface coating industry, in manufacturing synthetic resins | Smoking cigarettes, using paints and glues, breathing motor vehicle exhaust |
| Acetone | As a solvent in the production of lubricating oils and as an intermediate in pharmaceuticals and pesticides | Using household chemicals, nail polish, and paint, breathing cigarette smoke |
| Acetaldehyde | In adhesives, coatings, lubricants, inks, nail polish remover, room air deodorizers | Breathing cigarette smoke; wood smoke; using room air deodorizers, nail polish remover, adhesives, coatings, lubricants, inks |
| Benzene | Constituent in motor fuels, solvent for fats, inks, oils, paints, plastics, and rubber; also used in the manufacturing of detergents, pharmaceuticals, explosives, and dyestuffs | Breathing cigarette smoke, motor vehicle exhaust |
| Carbon tetrachloride | Used to make refrigeration fluid and propellants for aerosol cans | Using industrial-strength cleansers |
| Chlorobenzene | Used in the manufacture of dyestuffs and pesticides | Living near a waste site containing chlorobenzene |
| Chloroform | As a solvent; widely distributed in atmosphere and water | Showering |

(continued)

## Table 20-2. Common Volatile Organic Compounds (VOCs) (*continued*)

| VOC | USES | SOURCES OF INDOOR EXPOSURE |
|------|------|----------------------------|
| Ethylbenzene | As a solvent and in the manufacture of styrene-related products; emitted vapors at filling stations and from motor vehicles | Breathing motor vehicle exhaust |
| Formaldehyde | In particle board, insulation (UFFI), carpeting, mobile homes, temporary classrooms, and trailers | Breathing cigarette smoke, living in a mobile home or going to school in temporary classroom, using particle board furniture |
| *m*-Xylene, *p*-Xylene, and *o*-Xylene | As solvents, constituents of paint, lacquers, varnishes, inks, dyes, adhesives, cement, and aviation fluids; also used in the manufacture of perfumes, insect repellants, pharmaceuticals, and the leather industry | Using paints, adhesives; breathing motor vehicle exhaust |
| Naphthalene | In mothballs and deodorant cakes. Comes from burning wood, tobacco, or fossil fuels | Eating naphthalene mothballs or deodorant cakes or coming in close contact with clothing or blankets stored in naphthalene mothballs |
| Perchloroethylene | In dry cleaning | Wearing dry-cleaned clothes |
| Styrene | At high temperature, becomes a plastic; used in the manufacture of resins, polyesters, insulators, and drugs | Breathing motor vehicle exhaust, cigarette smoke; using photocopiers |
| Toluene | Used in the manufacture of benzene, as a solvent for paints and coatings, and as a component of car and aviation fuels | Using paints, breathing motor vehicle exhaust |
| Trichloroethylene | As a solvent in vapor degreasing, for extracting caffeine from coffee, as a dry-cleaning agent, and as an intermediate in production of pesticides, waxes, gums, resins, tars, and paints | Using wood stains, varnishes, finishes, lubricants, adhesives, typewriter correction fluid, paint removers, cleaners |

Abbreviations: UFFI, urea-formaldehyde foam insulation.

clothing. Cigarette smoke is an important source of formaldehyde and other VOCs including acrylonitrile, 1,3-butadiene, acrolein, and acetaldehyde.

### Naphthalene

Naphthalene in the indoor air comes from mothballs, unvented kerosene heaters, and tobacco smoke.

### Microbial Volatile Organic Compounds

Some molds can give off VOCs; these are known as microbial VOCs.

## Systems Affected

Exposure to VOCs leads mainly to respiratory, dermal, and mucocutaneous effects. Cancer may result from exposure to certain compounds.

## Clinical Effects

Depending on the dominant compounds and route and level of exposure, signs and symptoms may include upper respiratory tract and eye irritation, rhinitis, nasal congestion, wheeze, rash, pruritus, headache, nausea, and vomiting.[8] Symptoms are usually nonspecific and may be insufficient to permit identification of the offending compounds. One recent study documented that high exposure to total VOCs during mid- to late pregnancy was linked to decrements in birth weight among infants in Korea.[9] There also is evidence that early childhood exposure to VOCs resulting from renovation activities may increase the risk for wheeze among infants.[10] Some VOCs (including benzene and formaldehyde) cause cancer in humans, and others (1,3 butadiene, styrene, and naphthalene) cause cancer in animals and possibly cause cancer in humans.[11-14] An association between household paint and solvent exposure and leukemia has been described as well as an association between VOCs and pulmonary function deficits.[15-18] Clinical effects of some common VOCs are described in the following paragraphs. Microbial VOCs are further discussed under molds.

### Benzene

The effects of exposure to benzene are described in Chapter 30. Both the International Agency for Research on Cancer (IARC) and the US EPA assigned benzene their highest cancer classification, Group 1 ("is carcinogenic to humans") and Category A ("known human carcinogen"), respectively.[7,19] Epidemiologic studies provide conclusive evidence of a causal association between benzene exposure and leukemia, acute nonlymphocytic leukemia, and also possibly chronic nonlymphocytic and chronic lymphocytic leukemias.[19] Occasional reports have surfaced showing an increased risk in humans of other neoplastic changes in the blood or lymphatic system, including Hodgkin and non-Hodgkin lymphoma and myelodysplastic syndrome.[19]

### Formaldehyde

Formaldehyde, which smells like pickles, can cause health effects even when an odor cannot be detected. Exposure to airborne formaldehyde may result in conjunctival and upper respiratory tract irritation (ie, burning or tingling sensations in the eyes, nose, and throat); these symptoms are temporary and resolve with cessation of exposure.[20] Children may be more sensitive to formaldehyde-induced respiratory toxicity than adults. Formaldehyde may exacerbate asthma in some infants and children.[21,22] In 2004, the IARC determined that there was sufficient evidence to conclude that formaldehyde causes nasopharyngeal cancer in humans and reclassified it as a Group 1, known human carcinogen (previous classification: Group 2A–limited evidence of carcinogenicity in humans and sufficient evidence in animals).[12] The IARC also reported there was limited evidence to conclude that formaldehyde exposure causes nasal cavity and paranasal cavity cancer and "strong but not sufficient" evidence linking formaldehyde exposure to leukemia.[12,23]

### Naphthalene

Exposure to large amounts of naphthalene may result in hemolytic anemia, resulting in jaundice and hemoglobinuria in children with glucose-6-phosphate dehydrogenase (G6PD) deficiency. Nausea, vomiting, and diarrhea also may occur. Newborn infants appear to be susceptible to naphthalene-induced hemolysis, presumably because of a decreased ability to conjugate and excrete naphthalene metabolites. Naphthalene is possibly carcinogenic to humans (Group 2B–limited evidence of carcinogenicity in humans and less than sufficient evidence in animals).[24,25]

## Diagnostic Methods

Asking about environmental exposures is part of a complete evaluation when a child has a persistent or unusual respiratory symptom. Clinicians generally consider infection, allergy, asthma, and foreign bodies as possible causes. Several questions may help to identify an environmental etiology for a respiratory symptom. Does anyone smoke in the home? Is there an attached garage? Does the family live in a mobile home or a new home with large amounts of pressed wood products? Is there new pressed wood furniture? Are mothballs being used? Have household members recently worked with crafts or graphic materials? Are chemical cleaners used extensively? Has remodeling recently been done? Has anyone recently used paints, solvents, or sprays in the home? Do the parents store paints or other chemicals in the home? Are soaked materials and solvents being disposed of properly? Do the symptoms clear when the child is removed from the home and reappear when the child returns?

## Treatment

If VOCs are thought to be the cause of symptoms, the source should be identified and, if possible, removed. Measuring levels of VOCs in the air usually is not necessary or practical.

## Prevention of Exposure

The single most important step to reduce the concentrations of VOCs in the home is to prohibit smoking indoors. Another important prevention strategy is the modification of building codes to require detached garages. Attached garages should be isolated from living and working spaces by closing doorways, sealing the structures, and ensuring that there is a proper air pressure difference between the garage and other indoor spaces.

Many sources of VOCs exist around a typical home including leftover chemicals, such as paints, varnishes, solvents, adhesives and caulks. It is prudent to place these chemicals in a shed or a place that is not frequently visited. Some home furnishings, such as carpets and upholstered furniture, tend to off-gas more VOCs when they are new. Persons who wish to avoid VOC exposure should avoid doing their own painting and use no-VOC paint.

Homes or classrooms in which new materials have been installed or that have undergone renovation should receive increased outdoor air ventilation. In the initial months after building completion, the ventilation should operate 24 hours/day, 7 days/week. Installation of new products or renovation work should preferably occur when the space is unoccupied and will remain unoccupied until off-gassing of the strongest volatile organic compounds has occurred. Steps should be taken to reduce the relative humidity to 30% to 50% to reduce the growth of molds and microbial VOCs. Parents should avoid storing opened containers of unused paints and similar materials in the home and should dispose of soaked materials and solvents properly.

Items made of composite wood will off-gas more VOCs when they are new. If a home has large amounts of pressed wood products that cannot be removed, the exposure to formaldehyde can be reduced by coating cabinets, paneling, and other furnishings with polyurethane or other nontoxic sealants and by increasing the amount of ventilation in the building. Formaldehyde concentrations decrease rapidly over the first year after a product is manufactured. Textiles that have been coated with formaldehyde resins (draperies and some permanent-press clothes) should first be washed before using. Formaldehyde levels on treated fabrics greatly subside with each washing.

Infants should not be exposed to textiles (clothing/bedding) that have been stored for long periods with naphthalene-containing moth repellents. If families use naphthalene-containing moth repellents, the material should be enclosed in containers that prevent vapors from escaping and kept out of the reach of children. Blankets and clothing stored with naphthalene-containing moth repellents should be aired outdoors to remove naphthalene odors and washed before they are used.

## Guidelines

The total of all VOCs measured in an air sample is called total VOCs. The concentration of total VOCs is expressed as mcg/m$^3$ of air. The concentration of total VOCs in a building or home is a good indicator of whether there are elevated levels. Using data from German homes, researchers suggested that 300 mcg/m$^3$ of total VOCs (the average value of the study) should not be exceeded.[26,27]

At present, there are no US standards for total VOCs. The European Community prepared a target guideline value for total VOCs of 300 mcg/m$^3$ in which no individual VOC should exceed 10% of the total VOC concentration.[27] Levels higher than this may result in irritation to some occupants. However, lower levels can also be an issue if a particularly toxic substance or odorant is present.[28] The INDEX project in the European Union proposed that indoor air concentrations of benzene and formaldehyde should be kept as low as reasonably achievable because of their known carcinogenicity. A long-term guideline value of 10 mcg/m$^3$ for naphthalene was proposed.[29]

The WHO has guidelines to protect public health from risks caused by a number of chemicals commonly present in indoor air. The substances considered in the guidelines (ie, benzene, carbon monoxide, formaldehyde, naphthalene, nitrogen dioxide, polycyclic aromatic hydrocarbons [especially benzo(*a*) pyrene], radon, trichloroethylene, and tetrachloroethylene), have indoor sources, are known to be hazardous to health, and are often found indoors in concentrations of health concern.

For formaldehyde, a short-term (30-minute) guideline of 0.1 mg/m$^3$ is recommended as preventing sensory irritation in the general population.[30] For naphthalene, the WHO established a guideline value of 0.01 mg/m$^3$. This guideline value should be applied as an annual average.

## MOLD

Fungi are a kingdom of usually multicellular eukaryotic organisms that are heterotrophs (ie, they cannot make their own food and live by decomposing and absorbing the organic material in which they grow). There are more than 200,000 species of fungi, including molds, yeast, mushrooms, smuts, and rusts. More than 100,000 mold species have been identified. Mildew is lay term for a conspicuous mass of white threadlike hyphae and fruiting structures produced by various fungi.

## Routes and Sources of Exposure

Exposure to molds occurs via inhalation of contaminated air and dermal contact with surfaces on which they are deposited. Molds are ubiquitous in the outdoor environment and can enter the home through doorways, windows, air conditioning systems, and heating and ventilation systems. Molds are also common in the indoor environment. In healthy homes, there are fewer molds in the indoor air than in the air outside the home.

Molds proliferate in environments that contain excessive moisture, such as from leaks in plumbing, roofs, walls, and pet urine and plant pots. The most common molds found indoors are *Cladosporium, Penicillium, Aspergillus,* and *Alternaria* species.[31]

If a building is extremely wet for an extended period, other molds with higher water requirements, including *Stachybotrys* and *Trichoderma* species, can grow.[31]

## Systems Affected

The eyes, nose, throat, and respiratory tract are affected by exposure to molds. Exposure to molds can also affect the skin and nervous system.

## Clinical Effects

Exposure to molds may result in infectious, allergic, or toxic health effects. The American Academy of Pediatrics (AAP) *Red Book* provides guidance on fungal infections.[32] The Institute of Medicine and the AAP have published comprehensive reviews of the spectrum of health effects from dampness and molds.[33-35] Children's exposure to molds is associated with a higher risk of persistent upper respiratory tract symptoms such as rhinitis, sneezing, and eye irritation as well as lower respiratory tract symptoms, such as coughing and wheezing.[33-36] Some, but not all, studies show that atopic children may be more susceptible to the effects of moisture damage and mold.[37-39] The Institute of Medicine and the AAP have concluded that moisture in buildings is associated with the exacerbation of asthma in children. A guideline from the WHO also found that there was sufficient evidence to conclude that there is an association between exposure to molds and the development of asthma.[40]

The mechanism by which exposure to molds might result in the development of asthma is not fully understood. Studies in laboratory animals have suggested a non-IgE-mediated adjuvant-like effect of mold exposure that can increase the airway inflammatory response to other allergenic exposures.[41] Mice exposed to chitin, a structural element found in mold cell walls, have eosinophilic lung inflammation despite the lack of allergic sensitization.[42] In mice sensitized to ovalbumin and challenged, co-exposure with the mycotoxins gliotoxin and patulin resulted in an augmented eosinophilic airway response and greater airway hyperreactivity.[43]

Toxic effects of molds may be attributable to inhalation of mycotoxins, lipid-soluble toxins readily absorbed by the airways.[44] Species of mycotoxin-producing molds include *Fusarium, Trichoderma,* and *Stachybotrys.* A single mold species may produce several different toxins, and a given mycotoxin may be produced by more than one species of mold. Furthermore, toxin-producing molds do not necessarily produce mycotoxins under all growth conditions, with production being dependent on the substrate, temperature, water content, and humidity.[45] Exposure to an extremely moldy home has been associated with multifocal choroiditis in an adult.[46]

Exposure to *Stachybotrys chartarum (atra)* and other molds has been associated with acute pulmonary hemorrhage among young infants in Cleveland, OH, Kansas City, MO, Delaware, and New Zealand.[47–54] Exposure to *Trichoderma* species and other molds has been associated with acute pulmonary hemorrhage in an infant in North Carolina.[55] In California, a family of 6 became ill while living in a severely water-damaged home; their 16-month-old boy died from a pulmonary hemorrhage and mycotoxins were identified in the home and the lungs, liver, and brain of the deceased child.[56]

Studies of acute intratracheal exposure to the metabolites of *Stachybotrys* species in male rats demonstrate lung tissue injury. The studies concluded that lung cell damage was more likely attributable to toxins than fungal cell wall components.[57–60]

A variety of neurologic symptoms have been associated with living in moldy environments, including fatigue, difficulty concentrating, and headaches.[44] Although few studies of children have been performed, it is biologically plausible that these symptoms could be associated with mold exposures. Many mycotoxins that have been isolated from spores, mold fragments, and dust from moldy areas are significantly toxic. In vitro and in vivo studies have demonstrated adverse effects, including immunotoxic, neurologic, respiratory, and dermal responses, after exposure to specific toxins, bacteria, molds, or their products. Many pure microbial toxins, such as the products of *Fusarium* species ( fumonisin $B_1$, deoxynivalenol), *Stachybotrys* species (satratoxin G), *Aspergillus* species (ochratoxin A), and *Penicillium* species (ochratoxin A, verrucosidin), have been shown to be neurotoxic in vitro and in vivo.[61–66] In the indoor environment, various microbiological agents with diverse, fluctuating inflammatory and toxic potential are present simultaneously with other airborne compounds, inevitably resulting in interactions. Such interactions may lead to unexpected responses, even at low concentrations.[40]

Early postnatal exposure to mold was significantly associated with poorer cognitive function in 6-year-old children followed as part of a prospective birth cohort study in Poland.[67]

## Diagnostic Methods

Pediatricians must have a high index of suspicion because mold is considered to be a "great masquerader."[68] Several key questions about the child's home environment may help to identify potential exposure to molds. These questions include: Has the home been flooded? Is there any water-damaged wood or cardboard in the house? Has there been a roof or plumbing leak? Have occupants seen any mold or noticed a musty smell? Has anyone else in the home been ill? Do the child's symptoms resolve when away from the home and recur upon return to the home? Guidance for clinicians about recognizing and managing health effects related to mold exposure and moisture indoors has been published by the University of Connecticut Health Center.[69] Table 20-3 lists sentinel health conditions that may suggest mold or moisture in the absence of an alternative explanation. The concept of a "sentinel condition" has great utility in occupational and environmental health. The diagnosis of an individual with a sentinel illness associated with exposures in a particular environment may indicate that these exposures may also deleteriously affect others.[70,71] Intervention in the environment to limit such identified exposures is an opportunity for primary prevention.[69]

Testing the environment for specific molds usually is not necessary.[72,73] When testing is performed, indoor mold measures should be interpreted in the context of outdoor mold levels. Even then, the results may be difficult to interpret because there are no agreed-on standards. There are, however, some rules of thumb for assessing the number of mold spores found in the indoor air. Some investigators have categorized mean levels of culturable mold counts into 5 groups.[74]

| Table 20-3. Sentinel Conditions | |
|---|---|
| **SYMPTOMS AND SYNDROMES THAT MAY SUGGEST MOLD OR MOISTURE IN THE ABSENCE OF AN ALTERNATIVE EXPLANATION** | |
| **CONDITIONS OF CONCERN** | **PRECURSOR CONDITIONS** |
| New-onset asthma<br>Exacerbated asthma<br>Interstitial lung disease<br>Hypersensitivity pneumonitis<br>Sarcoidosis<br>Pulmonary hemorrhage in infants | Mucosal irritation<br>Recurrent rhinitis/sinusitis<br>Recurrent hoarseness |

Reprinted with permission from the University of Connecticut Health Center, Farmington, CT, from Guidance for Clinicians on the Recognition and Management of Health Effects Related to Mold Exposure and Moisture Indoors. https://health.uconn.edu/occupational-environmental/wp-content/uploads/sites/25/2015/12/mold_guide.pdf

Group 1:  Low ($<$100 colony forming units [CFUs]/$m^3$)
Group 2:  Medium (101–300 CFUs/$m^3$)
Group 3:  High (301–1,000 CFUs/$m^3$)
Group 4:  Very high (1,001–5,000 CFUs/$m^3$)
Group 5:  Extremely high ($>$5,000 CFUs/$m^3$)

Techniques for identifying specific molds at the genus level are elaborate and cost-intensive.[75] Tests to measure specific mycotoxins or mycotoxin adducts in urine have been developed for research purposes.[76,77] An adduct (from the Latin, adductus, "drawn toward") is a species formed by the union of 2 species (usually molecules) held together by a coordinate covalent bond.

Currently, there is no clinically available diagnostic test for mycotoxins in human tissue. Testing for antibodies to mold antigens may not be helpful because of cross-reacting antigens from related organisms. For these reasons, a questionnaire-based assessment of visible mold may serve as an adequate indicator of the indoor environment.[78,79]

Microbial VOCs produced by molds are responsible for the characteristic odors produced by molds, often described as musty, earthy, or moldy. Microbial VOCs include certain aldehydes, alcohols, and ketones that are not typically found to emit from building materials. Frequently found microbial VOCs include geosmin, hexanone, and octanols. Some of these microbial VOCs have been found to be irritants to humans and contribute to sick building syndrome (see Chapter 11). Microbial VOCs can be easily measured in the air at very low levels, and their presence is an indication of mold contamination. Because mold is frequently found inside walls and other inaccessible areas, measurements of microbial VOCs are sometimes used as a way of confirming and locating mold contamination.

## Prevention of Exposure

Prevention strategies include cleaning up water and removing all water-damaged items (including carpets) within 24 hours of a flood or leak. If these actions are taken, mold will not have the opportunity to grow. Interventions to reduce dampness and mold have been demonstrated to reduce asthma exacerbations among children.[80] Guidance on preventing mold exposure is available from the American Industrial Hygiene Association.[72]

## GUIDELINES

The WHO has produced Guidelines on Indoor Air Quality.[40]

## Frequently Asked Questions

Q *What are the most important things I can do to protect my child from indoor air pollution?*

A Do not smoke and do not allow anyone to smoke in your home. Preventing children from being exposed to secondhand and thirdhand smoke is important. Keep your home dry and fix all water leaks promptly. Wood stoves and fireplaces should be checked yearly by a professional to make sure they are clean and running efficiently. A carbon monoxide detector should be installed on each sleeping level in your home, but this should not be used as a replacement for annual furnace inspections. If you have an attached garage, make sure that you keep the door between the garage and the house tightly closed to reduce the amount of benzene that comes in to the house. Gas ovens should not be used to provide supplemental heat. Children should not come into contact with mothballs because they contain dangerous chemicals. Air fresheners do not improve air quality; they use artificial chemicals to provide scent.

Q *Are air fresheners hazardous?*

A Air fresheners release many different chemicals, including acetaldehyde, ethyl acetate, butylated hydroxytoluene (BHT), propylene glycol, and 1,3-dichloro-2-proponal. Some air fresheners contain phthalates. Limited information is available about the potential health effects of using air fresheners. One study linked blood levels of 1,4-dichlorobenzene, a volatile organic compound often used in air fresheners, to reduced pulmonary function in adults. The long-term effects have not been studied. Scented candles also off-gas volatile organic compounds. The list of ingredients may not indicate all the chemicals present in household air fresheners or scented candles. To avoid phthalates, do not purchase products with "fragrance" on the label because these products may contain phthalates.

Q *My child has had a persistent runny nose. Could this be caused by the new carpet we installed last month?*

A The symptom could be caused by viruses, bacteria, allergies, or perhaps a foreign body in the nose. It also is possible that the symptoms relate to something in the child's environment, such as secondhand smoke or the chemical compounds released from a new carpet. Sometimes an exact diagnosis is difficult to determine. Symptoms from colds are temporary, and symptoms from environmental irritants tend to improve once exposure to the irritant is eliminated. If possible, have your child play and sleep in another room to see if symptoms improve. It may take some time and a visit to your health care provider to determine the cause of the child's symptoms.

Q   *What are the effects of exposure to mothballs?*

A   Two products, *p*-dichlorobenzene and naphthalene, are used as moth
repellents. Reports of occupational exposure to the active ingredients of
mothballs are available. Studies documenting health effects from residential exposure are limited. The active ingredient in mothballs usually is
*p*-dichlorobenzene. Exposure to *p*-dichlorobenzene may cause irritation
of the eyes, nose, and throat; swelling around the eyes; headache; and a
runny nose, which usually subside 24 hours after exposure ends. Prolonged
occupational exposure to *p*-dichlorobenzene may result in loss of appetite,
nausea, vomiting, weight loss, and liver damage. Consider replacing
mothballs with cedar products.

Q   *What can be done to reduce the levels of particulates from wood stoves and
fireplaces?*

A   Measures to reduce the levels of particulate matter from a wood stove
include ensuring that the stove is placed in a room with adequate ventilation and properly vented directly to the outdoors. Newer stoves are
designed to emit less particulate matter into the air. Information on
improved wood stoves can be found at www.epa.gov/burnwise.

Q   *What are ionizers and other ozone-generating air cleaners? Should they be
used?*

A   Ion generators act by charging the particles in a room so that they are
attracted to walls, floors, tabletops, draperies, or occupants. Abrasion can
result in resuspension of these particles into the air. In some cases, these
devices contain a collector to attract the charged particles back to the unit.
Although ion generators may remove small particles (eg, those in secondhand smoke), they do not remove gases or odors and may be relatively
ineffective in removing large particles, such as pollen and house dust allergens. Ozone generators are specifically designed to release ozone to purify
the air.

Ozone is produced indirectly by ion generators and some electronic air
cleaners and produced directly by ozone generators. Although indirect
ozone production is of concern, there is even greater concern with the
direct and purposeful introduction of ozone into indoor air. No difference exists, despite the claims of some marketers, between ozone in smog
outdoors and ozone produced by ozone generators. Under certain conditions, these devices can produce levels of ozone high enough to be harmful
to a child. Ozone-generating air cleaners may also contribute to indoor
formaldehyde concentrations. They are not recommended for use in homes
or schools.

Q   *Can other air cleaners help?*

A   Other air cleaners include mechanical filters, electronic (eg, electrostatic precipitators), and hybrid air cleaners using 2 or more techniques. The value of any air cleaner depends on its efficiency, proper selection for the pollutant to be removed, proper installation, and appropriate maintenance. Drawbacks include inadequate pollutant removal, re-dispersal of pollutants, deceptive masking of the pollutant rather than its removal, generation of ozone, and unacceptable noise levels. The US EPA and Consumer Product Safety Commission have not taken a position either for or against the use of these devices.

Effective control at the source of a pollutant is key. Air cleaners are not a solution but are an adjunct to source control and adequate ventilation. The state of California regulates air cleaners. The California Air Resources Board lists the models of air cleaners that have been certified by the Air Resources Board as meeting the testing and certification requirements of the state's air cleaner regulation. The certified air cleaner models may be viewed at www.arb.ca.gov/research/indoor/aircleaners/certified.htm.

Q   *Should I consider buying a portable HEPA purifier?*

A   Some studies have documented that using portable HEPA (high efficiency particulate air) purifiers can reduce indoor concentrations of particulate matter by about 25% to 50% and reduce asthma symptoms and exacerbations.[81,82]

Q   *I am about to purchase a new vacuum cleaner for my home. Should I buy one with a HEPA filter?*

A   HEPA (high efficiency particulate air) filters reduce dust by trapping small particles and not rereleasing them into the air as you vacuum. Although widely advertised for use in homes in which children with asthma or allergies are living, it is not clear whether using a vacuum with a HEPA filter reduces symptoms or medication use in children with asthma. The use of HEPA filters should not substitute for other allergen-reduction methods.

Q   *When I bring clothes home from the dry cleaners, are the chemicals released from the clothes dangerous to my child?*

A   Perchloroethylene is the chemical most widely used in dry cleaning. In laboratory studies, it has been shown to cause cancer in animals. Recent studies indicate that people breathe low levels of this chemical both in homes where dry-cleaned goods are stored and as they wear dry-cleaned clothing. Dry cleaners recapture the perchloroethylene during the dry-cleaning process to save money by reusing it, and they remove more of the chemical during the pressing and finishing processes. Some dry cleaners, however, do not remove as much perchloroethylene as possible all the time. Taking steps to minimize your exposure to this chemical is prudent. If dry-cleaned goods have a strong chemical odor when you pick them up, do not accept them until they have been properly dried. If goods with a chemical odor are returned to you on subsequent visits, try a different dry cleaner.

Of more concern is whether the home is located directly above or adjacent to a dry-cleaning establishment. If so, the amount of daily exposure may be enough to cause adverse health effects.

Q   *Can exposure to chemicals from carpets make people sick?*

A   New carpet may emit volatile organic compounds, as do products such as adhesives and padding that accompany carpet installation. Some people report symptoms including eye, nose, and throat irritation; headaches; skin irritation; shortness of breath or cough; and fatigue, which may be associated with new carpet installation. Carpet also can act as a "sink" for chemical and biological pollutants including pesticides, dust mites, and molds.

Anyone seeking to purchase new carpet can ask retailers for information to help them select carpet, padding, and adhesives that emit lower amounts of volatile organic compounds. Before new carpet is installed, the retailer should unroll and air out the carpet in a clean, well-ventilated area. Opening doors and windows reduces the level of chemicals released. Ventilation systems should be in proper working order and operated during installation, and for 48 to 72 hours after the new carpet is installed.

Q   *What about using vapor rub when my baby has a cold?*

A   A few studies have shown that vapor rub use can irritate the airways and increase mucus production. Doctors treated an 18-month old child in whom severe respiratory distress occurred after vapor rub was applied directly under the nose. Studies of animals whose windpipes were exposed to vapor rub demonstrated that mucus secretion increased and clearance of mucus decreased.[83] Cold symptoms generally resolve on their own and using chemical products, such as vapor rub, will not help resolve symptoms. If you choose to use this product, it should be used according to the directions on the label: only on children older than 2 years and never directly under the nose. Saline nose drops are recommended to help with a baby's nasal congestion.

Q   *Can plants control indoor air pollution?*

A   Reports in the media and promotions by representatives of the decorative houseplant industry characterize plants as "nature's clean air machine," claiming that research by the National Aeronautics and Space

Administration shows that plants remove indoor air pollutants. Although it is true that plants remove carbon dioxide from the air, and the ability of plants to remove certain other pollutants from water is the basis for some pollution control methods, the ability of plants to control indoor air pollution is less well established. The only study of plants used to control indoor air pollutants in an actual building could not determine any benefit. As a practical means of pollution control, the plant removal mechanisms seem to be inconsequential when compared with common ventilation and air exchange rates. Overdamp planter soil conditions may promote growth of molds.

Q　*How do I keep my fireplace safe?*

A　There are several suggested measures to increase fireplace safety.

If possible, keep a window cracked open while the fire is burning.

Be certain the damper or flue is open before starting a fire. Keeping the damper or flue open until the fire is out will draw smoke out of the house. The damper can be checked by looking up into the chimney with a flashlight.

Use dry and well-aged wood. Wet or green wood causes more smoke and contributes to soot buildup in the chimney.

Smaller pieces of wood placed on a grate burn faster and produce less smoke.

Levels of ash at the base of the fireplace should be kept to 1 inch or less because a thicker layer restricts the air supply to logs, resulting in more smoke.

The chimney should be checked annually by a professional. Even if the chimney is not due for cleaning, it is important to check for animal nests or other blockages that could prevent smoke from escaping.

Q　*Are there potential problems with incense burning?*

A　Incense burning in homes can emit particulates, volatile organic compounds such as benzene, nitrogen dioxide, and carbon monoxide. Carbon monoxide levels from incense burning can reach a peak concentration of 9.6 mg/m$^3$, which could exceed the US EPA National Ambient Air Quality Standard of 10 mg/m$^3$ for an 8-hour average depending on the room volume, ventilation rate, and the amount of incense burned. Incense burning might be a significant contributor to indoor air pollution in cultures in which incense is burned frequently, for example when people use incense during religious rituals.

Q　*What is your advice about disposing of solvents?*

A　To avoid the problem of disposal, consider using safer alternatives, such as vinegar and water. If you purchase a hazardous material such as a solvent, buy a small amount so that it is more likely that you will use it up completely.

Read the label regarding the proper storage and disposal of the product. Always follow manufacturer's directions, not only for use but afterwards as well. There may be household hazardous product roundups in your community. Many local waste companies offer this service a few times a year. Consider contacting refuse companies found in the phone book or online for more options. Leave the product in its original packaging and seal the container tightly. This will keep the hazardous material from contaminating anything else and always leave labels intact, even when throwing an empty container away. Check with neighbors and friends to see whether they have any use for any extra product that you may have, instead of disposing of the unused portion. To prevent unintentional poisoning, keep the product out of the reach of small children.

## Resources

### American Lung Association
Phone: 800-LUNG-USA
Web site: www.lungusa.org

### Indoor Air Quality Scientific Findings Resource Bank
Web site: https://indoor.lbl.gov/

### National Center for Healthy Housing, Pediatric Environmental Home Assessment
Web site: www.healthyhomestraining.org/Nurse/PEHA.htm

### US Consumer Product Safety Commission
Phone: 800-638-CPSC
Web site: www.cpsc.gov
Provides information on particular product hazards.

### US Environmental Protection Agency
*Indoor Air Quality Information Clearinghouse*
Phone: 800-438-4318
Web site: www.epa.gov/iaq
Additional resources from the US EPA include EPA regional offices and state and local departments of health and environmental quality. For regulation of specific pollutants, contact the EPA Toxic Substances Control Act Assistance Information Service: 202-554-1404.

*Care for Your Air: A Guide to Indoor Air Quality*
Understand indoor air in homes, schools, and offices.
Web site: www.epa.gov/iaq/pubs/careforyourair.html

# References

1. Klepeis NE, Bellettiere J, Hughes SC, et al. Fine particles in homes of predominantly low-income families with children and smokers: key physical and behavioral determinants to inform indoor-air-quality interventions. *PLoS One.* 2017;12(5):e0177718

2. Hansel NN, Breysse PN, McCormack MC, et al. A longitudinal study of indoor nitrogen dioxide levels and respiratory symptoms in inner-city children with asthma. *Environ Health Perspect.* 2008;116(10):1428–1432

3. Robin LF, Less PS, Winget M, et al. Wood-burning stoves and lower respiratory illnesses in Navajo children. *Pediatr Infect Dis J.* 1996;15(10):859–865

4. World Health Organization. *Air Quality Guidelines: Global Update 2005.* 2006. http://www.euro.who.int/__data/assets/pdf_file/0005/78638/E90038.pdf. Accessed February 25, 2018

5. Agency for Toxic Substances and Disease Registry. *Toxicological Profile for Ammonia.* 2004. http://www.atsdr.cdc.gov/toxprofiles/tp.asp?id=11&tid=2. Accessed February 25, 2018

6. Protano C, Andreoli R, Manini P, Guidotti M, Vitali M. A tobacco-related carcinogen: assessing the impact of smoking behaviours of cohabitants on benzene exposure in children. *Tob Control.* 2012;21(3):325–329

7. Branco PT, Nunes RA, Alvim-Ferraz MC, Martins FG, Sousa SI. Children's exposure to indoor air in urban nurseries—Part II: gaseous pollutants' assessment. *Environ Res.* 2015;142:662–670

8. Mendell MJ. Indoor residential chemical emissions as risk factors for respiratory and allergic effects in children: a review. *Indoor Air.* 2007;17(4):259–277

9. Chang M, Park H, Ha M, et al. The effect of prenatal TVOC exposure on birth and infantile weight: the Mothers and Children's Environmental Health study. *Pediatr Res.* 2017;82(3):423–428

10. Franck U, Weller A, Röder SW, et al. Prenatal VOC exposure and redecoration are related to wheezing in early infancy. *Environ Int.* 2014;73:393–401

11. International Agency for Research on Cancer. *IARC Monographs Supplement 7. Benzene.* 1987. http://monographs.iarc.fr/ENG/Monographs/suppl7/Suppl7-24.pdf. Accessed February 25, 2018

12. International Agency for Research on Cancer. *IARC Monograph on the Evaluation of Carcinogenic Risks to Humans.* 2006. http://monographs.iarc.fr/ENG/Monographs/vol88/index.php. Accessed February 25, 2018

13. International Agency for Research on Cancer. *IARC Monograph on the Evaluation of Carcinogenic Risks to Humans. Vol 82. Some Traditional Herbal Medicines, Some Mycotoxins, Naphthalene and Styrene.* 2002. http://monographs.iarc.fr/ENG/Monographs/vol82/index.php. Accessed February 25, 2018

14. International Agency for Research on Cancer. *IARC Monograph on the Evaluation of Carcinogenic Risks to Humans. Vol 97. 1,3 Butadiene, Ethylene Oxide and Vinyl Halides.* 2008. http://monographs.iarc.fr/ENG/Monographs/vol97/index.php. Accessed February 25, 2018

15. Freedman DM, Stewart P, Kleinerman RA, et al. Household solvent exposures and childhood acute lymphoblastic leukemia. *Am J Public Health.* 2001;91(4):564–567

16. Lowengart RA, Peters JM, Cicioni C, et al. Childhood leukemia and parents' occupational and home exposures. *J Natl Cancer Inst.* 1987;79(1):39–46

17. Scélo G, Metayer C, Zhang L, et al. Household exposure to paint and petroleum solvents, chromosomal translocations, and the risk of childhood leukemia. *Environ Health Perspect.* 2009;117(1):133–139

18. Elliott L, Longnecker MP, Kissling GE, London SJ. Volatile organic compounds and pulmonary function in the Third National Health and Nutrition Examination Survey, 1988–1994. *Environ Health Perspect.* 2006;114(8):1210–1214

19. US Environmental Protection Agency. *Integrated Risk Information System (IRIS) on Benzene.* Center for Environmental Assessment, Office of Research and Development; 2002. https://cfpub.epa.gov/ncea/iris2/chemicalLanding.cfm?substance_nmbr=276. Accessed February 25, 2018

20. Wantke F, Demmer CM, Tappler P, Gotz M, Jarisch R. Exposure to gaseous formaldehyde induces IgE-mediated sensitization to formaldehyde in school-children. *Clin Exp Allergy.* 1996;26(3):276–280

21. McGwin G, Lienert J, Kennedy JI. Formaldehyde exposure and asthma in children: a systematic review. *Environ Health Perspect.* 2010;118(3):313–317

22. Smedje G, Norbäck D, Edling C. Asthma among secondary school children in relation to the school environment. *Clin Exp Allergy.* 1997;27(11):1270–1278

23. Zhang L, Steinmaus C, Eastmond DA, Xin XK, Smith MT. Formaldehyde exposure and leukemia: a new meta-analysis and potential mechanisms. *Mutat Res.* 2009;681(2-3):150–168

24. Dobson CP, Neuwirth M, Frye RE, Gorman M. Index of suspicion. *Pediatr Rev.* 2006;27(1):29–33

25. Athanasious M, Tsantali C, Trachana M, Hatziioannides C. Hemolytic anemia in a female newborn infant whose mother inhaled naphthalene before delivery. *J Pediatr.* 1997;130(4):680–681

26. Seifert B. Regulating indoor air. In: Walkinshaw DS, ed. *Indoor Air '90. Proceedings of the 5th International Conference on Indoor Air Quality and Climate.* Vol 5. Toronto, Canada, July 29-August 3, 1990:35–49

27. European Commission Joint Research Centre. *European Collaborative Action 'Indoor Air Quality and Its Impact on Man'. Total Volatile Organic Compounds (TVOC) in Indoor Air Quality Investigations.* Report No 19. EUR 17675 EN. Luxembourg: Office for Official Publications of the European Community; 1997

28. Health Canada. *Indoor Air Quality in Office Buildings: A Technical Guide.* http://publications.gc.ca/collections/Collection/H46-2-93-166Erev.pdf. Accessed February 27, 2018

29. Kotzias D, Koistinen K, Kephalopoulos S, et al. *The INDEX Project. Critical Appraisal of the Setting and Implementation of Indoor Exposure Limits in the EU.* Ispra, Italy: European Commission, Institute for Health and Consumer Protection, Physical and Chemical Exposure Unit; 2005:1–50. http://ec.europa.eu/health/ph_projects/2002/pollution/fp_pollution_2002_frep_02.pdf. Accessed February 27, 2018

30. World Health Organization Regional Office for Europe. WHO Guidelines for indoor air quality: selected pollutants. Copenhagen: WHO; 2010

31. Centers for Disease Control and Prevention and US Department of Housing and Urban Development. *Healthy Housing Reference Manual.* 2006. https://www.cdc.gov/nceh/publications/books/housing/housing_ref_manual_2012.pdf. Accessed February 27, 2018

32. American Academy of Pediatrics. *Red Book: 2018 Report of the Committee on Infectious Diseases.* Kimberlin DW, Brady MT, Jackson MA, Long SS, eds. 31st ed. Itasca, IL: American Academy of Pediatrics; 2018

33. Institute of Medicine. *Damp Indoor Spaces and Health.* Washington, DC: National Academy of Sciences; 2004

34. American Academy of Pediatrics, Committee on Environmental Health, Kim JJ, Mazur LJ. Policy statement: spectrum of noninfectious health effects from molds. *Pediatrics.* 2006;118(6):2582–2586

35. Mazur LJ, Kim JJ, American Academy of Pediatrics, Committee on Environmental Health. Technical report: spectrum of noninfectious health effects from molds. *Pediatrics.* 2006;118(6):e1909–e1926

36. Antova T, Pattenden S, Brunekreef B, et al. Exposure to indoor mould and children's respiratory health in the PATY study. *J Epidemiol Community Health.* 2008;62(8):708–714

37. Pekkanen J, Hyvarinen A, Haverinen-Shaughnessy U, Korppi M, Putus T, Nevalainen A. Moisture damage and childhood asthma: a population-based incident case-control study. *Eur Respir J*. 2007;29(3):509–515

38. Tisher CG, Hohmann C, Thiering E, et al. ENRIECO consortium. Meta-analysis of mould and dampness exposure on asthma and allergy in eight European birth cohorts: an ENRIECO initiative. *Allergy*. 2011;66(12):1570–1579

39. Karvonen AM, Hyvarinen A, Korppi M, et al. Moisture damage and asthma: a birth cohort study. *Pediatrics*. 2015;135(3):e598–e606

40. World Health Organization. *Guidelines for Indoor Air Quality: Dampness and Mold*. Copenhagen, Denmark: World Health Organization; 2009. http://www.euro.who.int/__data/assets/pdf_file/0017/43325/E92645.pdf. Accessed February 27, 2018

41. Rabinovitch N. Household mold as a predictor of asthma risk: recent progress, limitations, and future directions. *J Allergy Clin Immunol*. 2012;130(3):645–646

42. Van Dyken SJ, Garcia D, Porter P, et al. Fungal chitin from asthma-associated home environments induces eosinophilic lung infiltration. *J Immunol*. 2011;187(5):2261–2267

43. Schütze N, Lehmann I, Bönisch U, Simon JC, Polte T. Exposure to mycotoxins increases the allergic response in a murine asthma model. *Am J Respir Crit Care Med*. 2010;181(11):1188–1199

44. Croft WA, Jarvis BB, Yatawara CS. Airborne outbreak of trichothecene toxicosis. *Atmos Environ*. 1986;20(8):549–552

45. Burge HA, Ammann HA. Fungal toxins and B(1-3)-D-glucans. In: Macher J, ed. *Bioaerosols: Assessment and Control*. Cincinnati, OH: American Conference of Governmental and Industrial Hygienists; 1999:24-1–24-13

46. Rudich R, Santilli J, Rockwell WJ. Indoor mold exposure: a possible factor in the etiology of multifocal choroiditis. *Am J Ophthalmol*. 2003,135(3):402–404

47. Dearborn DG, Smith PG, Dahms BB, et al. Clinical profile of 30 infants with acute pulmonary hemorrhage in Cleveland. *Pediatrics*. 2002;110(3):627–637

48. Montaña E, Etzel RA, Allan T, Horgan TE, Dearborn DG. Environmental risk factors associated with pediatric idiopathic pulmonary hemorrhage and hemosiderosis in a Cleveland community. *Pediatrics*. 1997;99(1):E5

49. Etzel RA, Montaña E, Sorenson WG, et al. Acute pulmonary hemorrhage in infants associated with exposure to *Stachybotrys atra* and other fungi. *Arch Pediatr Adolesc Med*. 1998;152(8):757–762

50. Centers for Disease Control and Prevention. Update: pulmonary hemorrhage/hemosiderosis among infants—Cleveland, Ohio, 1993–1996. *MMWR Morb Mortal Wkly Rep*. 2000;49(9):180–184

51. Jarvis BB, Sorenson WG, Hintikka EL, et al. Study of toxin production by isolates of *Stachybotrys chartarum* and *Memnoniella echinata* isolated during a study of pulmonary hemosiderosis in infants. *Appl Environ Microbiol*. 1998;64(10):3620–3625

52. Flappan SM, Portnoy J, Jones P, Barnes C. Infant pulmonary hemorrhage in a suburban home with water damage and mold (*Stachybotrys atra*). *Environ Health Perspect*. 1999;107(11):927–930

53. Weiss A, Chidekel AS. Acute pulmonary hemorrhage in a Delaware infant after exposure to *Stachybotrys atra*. *Del Med J*. 2002;74(9):363–368

54. Habiba A. Acute idiopathic pulmonary haemorrhage in infancy: case report and review of the literature. *J Paediatr Child Health*. 2005;41(9-10):532–533

55. Novotny WE, Dixit A. Pulmonary hemorrhage in an infant following two weeks of fungal exposure. *Arch Pediatr Adolesc Med*. 2000;154(3):271–275

56. Thrasher JD, Hooper DH, Taber J. Family of 6, their health and the death of a 16 month old male from pulmonary hemorrhage: identification of mycotoxins and mold in the home and lungs, liver and brain of deceased infant. *Int J Clin Toxicol.* 2014;2:00-00

57. Yike I, Rand T, Dearborn DG. The role of fungal proteinases in pathophysiology of *Stachybotrys chartarum. Mycopathologia.* 2007;164(4):171–181

58. McCrae KC, Rand TG, Shaw RA, et al. DNA fragmentation in developing lung fibroblasts exposed to *Stachybotrys chartarum (atra)* toxins. *Pediatr Pulmonol.* 2007;42(7):592–599

59. Kováciková Z, Tátrai E, Piecková E, et al. An in vitro study of the toxic effects of *Stachybotrys chartarum* metabolites on lung cells. *Altern Lab Anim.* 2007;35(1):47–52

60. Pieckova E, Hurbankova M, Cerna S, Pivovarova Z, Kovacikova Z. Pulmonary cytotoxicity of secondary metabolites of *Stachybotrys chartarum (Ehrenb) Hughes. Ann Agric Environ Med.* 2006;13(2):259–262

61. Rotter BA, Prelusky DB, Pestka JJ. Toxicology of deoxynivalenol (vomitoxin). *J Toxicol Environ Health.* 1996;48(1):1–34

62. Belmadani A, Steyn PS, Tramu G, Betbeder AM, Baudrimont I, Creppy EE. Selective toxicity of ochratoxin A in primary cultures from different brain regions. *Arch Toxicol.* 1999;73(2):108–114

63. Kwon OS, Slikker W Jr, Davies DL. Biochemical and morphological effects of fumonisin B1 on primary cultures of rat cerebrum. *Neurotoxicol Teratol.* 2000;22(4):565–572

64. Islam Z, Harkema JR, Pestka JJ. Satratoxin G from the black mold *Stachybotrys chartarum* evokes olfactory sensory neuron loss and inflammation in the murine nose and brain. *Environ Health Perspect.* 2006;114(7):1099–1107

65. Islam Z, Hegg CC, Bae HK, Pestka JJ. Satratoxin G-induced apoptosis in PC-12 neuronal cells is mediated by PKR and caspase independent. *Toxicol Sci.* 2008;105(1):142–152

66. Stockmann-Juvala H, Savolainen K. A review of the toxic effects and mechanisms of action of fumonisin B1. *Hum Exp Toxicol.* 2008;27(11):799–809

67. Jedrychowski W, Maugeri U, Perera F, et al. Cognitive function of 6-year-old children exposed to mold-contaminated homes in early postnatal period: prospective birth cohort study in Poland. *Physiol Behav.* 2011;104(5):989–995

68. Etzel RA. What the primary care pediatrician should know about syndromes associated with exposures to mycotoxins. *Curr Probl Pediatr Adolesc Health Care.* 2006;36(8):282–305

69. Storey E, Dangman KH, Schenck P, et al. *Guidance for Clinicians on the Recognition and Management of Health Effects Related to Mold Exposure and Moisture Indoors.* Farmington, CT: University of Connecticut; 2004. http://health.uconn.edu/occupational-environmental/wp-content/uploads/sites/25/2015/12/mold_guide.pdf. Accessed February 27, 2018

70. Rossman MD, Thompson B, Frederick M, et al. HLA and environmental interactions in sarcoidosis. *Sarcoidosis Vasc Diffuse Lung Dis.* 2008;25(2):125–132

71. Taskar V, Coultas D. Exposures and idiopathic lung disease. *Semin Respir Crit Care Med.* 2008;29(6):670–679

72. American Industrial Hygiene Association. *Recognition, Evaluation, and Control of Indoor Mold.* Prezant B, Weekes DM, Miller DM, eds. Fairfax, VA: American Industrial Hygiene Association; 2008

73. Government Accountability Office. *Indoor Mold.* September 2008. https://www.gao.gov/new.items/d08980.pdf. Accessed February 27, 2018

74. Platt SD, Martin CJ, Hunt SM, Lewis CW. Damp housing, mould growth, and symptomatic health state. *BMJ.* 1989;298(6689):1673–1678

75. Tovey ER, Green BJ. Measuring environmental fungal exposure. *Med Mycol.* 2005;43(Suppl 1):567–570

76. Yike I, Distler AM, Ziady AG, Dearborn DG. Mycotoxin adducts on human serum albumin: biomarkers of exposure to *Stachybotrys chartarum*. *Environ Health Perspect*. 2006;114(8):1221–1226

77. Hooper DG, Bolton VE, Guilford FT, Straus DS. Mycotoxin detection in human samples from patients exposed to environmental molds. *Int J Mol Sci*. 2009;10(4):1465–1475

78. Jones R, Recer GM, Hwang SA, Lin S. Association between indoor mold and asthma among children in Buffalo, New York. *Indoor Air*. 2011;21(2):156–164

79. Tischer CG, Heinrich J. Exposure assessment of residential mould, fungi and microbial components in relation to children's health: achievements and challenges. *Int J Hygiene Envir Health*. 2013;216(2):109–114

80. Kercsmar CM, Dearborn DG, Schluchter M, et al. Reduction in asthma morbidity in children as a result of home remediation aimed at moisture sources. *Environ Health Perspect*. 2006;114(10):1574–1580

81. Butz AM, Matsui EC, Breysse P, et al. A randomized trial of air cleaners and a health coach to improve indoor air quality for inner-city children with asthma and secondhand smoke exposure. *Arch Pediatr Adolesc Med*. 2011;165(8):741–748

82. Lanphear BP, Hornung RW, Khoury J, Yolton K, Lieri M, Kalkbrenner A. Effects of HEPA air cleaners on unscheduled asthma visits and asthma symptoms for children exposed to secondhand tobacco smoke. *Pediatrics*. 2011;127(1):93–101

83. Abanses JC, Arima S, Rubin BK. Vicks VapoRub induces mucin secretion, decreases ciliary beat frequency, and increases tracheal mucus transport in the ferret trachea. *Chest*. 2009;135(1):143–148

Chapter 21

# Air Pollutants, Outdoor

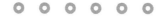

## KEY POINTS

- Outdoor air pollution continues to be a serious problem affecting the health of children.
- The detrimental effects of outdoor air pollution start at the preconception stage and can be manifested during the newborn period and childhood, continuing into adulthood.
- Exposure to air pollution can cause asthma and other respiratory conditions. Air pollution can affect multiple body systems, causes neurodevelopmental problems, and has been associated with the occurrence of malignancy.

## INTRODUCTION

In 2012, exposure to air pollution was linked to 1 out of every 8 deaths globally, or around 7 million premature deaths. Of these deaths, about 3.7 million were related to outdoor air pollution.[1] The United Nations Children's Fund report "Clear the Air for Children" in 2016 estimated that about 300 million children were living in areas where outdoor air pollution exceeded international guidelines by at least 6 times.[2] Outdoor air pollution consists of a complex mixture of pollutants found in ambient (outdoor) air that affect the health of individuals in all age groups.[3,4] Outdoor air pollutants come from many sources, including large industrial facilities; smaller operations, such as dry cleaners and gas stations; natural sources, such as wildfires; highway vehicles; and other sources such as aircraft, locomotives, and lawn mowers. The relative importance of these different sources varies from one community to another, depending on regional and nearby sources of pollution, time of day, and weather conditions. The potential for health risks posed by outdoor air pollution depends on the concentration and composition of the mixture, the duration of exposures, and the age, health status, and genetic makeup of exposed individuals.

The US Environmental Protection Agency (EPA) monitors air pollutants in 3 categories: (1) criteria pollutants (ie, ozone, respirable particulate matter, lead, sulfur dioxide, carbon monoxide, nitrogen oxides); (2) toxic chemicals, or hazardous air pollutants, released by motor vehicles, industrial facilities, wood combustion, agricultural activities, and other sources; and (3) greenhouse gases (GHG), generated from burning of fossil fuels and other activities, and responsible for climate change. Table 21-1 summarizes US EPA-monitored air pollutants, their sources, and the most common health effects described.

In the United States, a national monitoring network has been established to monitor levels of criteria pollutants and hazardous air pollutants.[5,6] Greenhouse gas emissions have been monitored since 2011 via a mandatory reporting program. With the implementation of the Clean Air Act and the National Ambient Air Quality Standards (NAAQS), steady improvement in air quality has been achieved in the United States. Between 1970 and 2017, total

## Table 21-1. Air Pollutants Monitored by the US Environmental Protection Agency

| POLLUTANT | SOURCE | HEALTH EFFECTS |
|---|---|---|
| Criteria pollutants | Power plants, motor vehicle emissions, industrial operations, combustion of organic material, coal-fired power plants, smelters, pulp and paper mills | Low birth weight, prematurity, stillbirths, respiratory and cardiovascular effects, immune abnormalities |
| Toxic chemicals (hazardous air pollutants) | Motor vehicle emissions, stationary industrial facilities and smaller area sources (such as dry cleaners), indoor sources, volcanic eruptions, forest fires | Known or suspected to cause cancer, reproductive effects or birth defects, or adverse environmental effects among others |
| Greenhouse gases | Heat-trapping gases released into the atmosphere primarily from burning of fossil fuels and responsible for climate change | |

emissions of the 6 principal air pollutants dropped by 73%.[7] In addition, the emissions of air toxics declined by 68% from 1990 to 2011.[8] However, air quality in some areas of the United States actually declined in recent years, and recent research suggests health effects at levels of some pollutants previously considered to be safe.[4]

## SPECIFIC AIR POLLUTANT GROUPS

## Criteria Pollutants

The US EPA has established NAAQS for 6 principal pollutants, referred to as criteria pollutants (eg, ozone, respirable particulate matter, lead, sulfur dioxide, carbon monoxide, nitrogen oxides). These standards have been set taking into consideration their effects on human health (primary standards) and the environment (secondary standards).

### Ozone

Ozone ($O_3$), the principal component of urban smog, is a secondary pollutant formed in the atmosphere from a photochemical reaction between volatile organic compounds and nitrogen oxides in the presence of sunlight[9] (Figure 21-1).

   The primary sources of these precursor compounds include motor vehicle exhaust and power plants, although hydrocarbon emissions from chemical plants and refineries and evaporative emissions from gasoline and natural sources also can contribute to their formation. Atmospheric movement of these precursor pollutants may produce ozone hundreds of miles downwind from the sources of these pollutants. Concentrations of ozone generally are

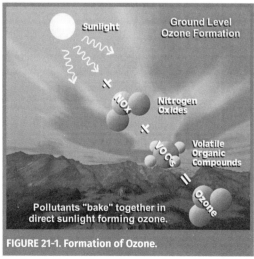

**FIGURE 21-1. Formation of Ozone.**

Source: From NASA. https://aura.gsfc.nasa.gov/outreach/garden_faq.html

highest on hot, dry, stagnant summer days and increase to maximum concentrations in the late afternoon. Changes in weather patterns can contribute to differences in ozone concentrations from year to year. Most personal exposure occurs in outdoor settings. In 2015, the US EPA revised the primary and secondary ozone standard levels to 0.070 parts per million (ppm) from the 0.075 ppm level established in 2008.[10]

### Particulate Matter

Particulate matter (PM) is a general term that refers to an airborne mixture of solid particles and liquid droplets. The term is applied to pollutants of varying chemical composition and physical properties. Particle size is the primary determinant of whether the particles will be deposited in the lower respiratory system. Particles larger than 10 mcm in aerodynamic diameter are too large to be inhaled beyond the nasal passages. Children, however, frequently breathe through their mouths, thus bypassing the nasal clearance mechanism.

All particulate matter less than 10 mcm in aerodynamic diameter is known as $PM_{10}$. These particles cannot be seen with the naked eye, but their presence in the atmosphere is seen as sooty clouds or general haze that impairs visibility. Fine particles are smaller than 2.5 mcm in aerodynamic diameter and are referred to as $PM_{2.5}$. Fine particles result from the combustion of fuels used in motor vehicles, power plants, and industrial operations as well as the combustion of organic material in fireplaces and wood stoves. Particles between 2.5 mcm and 10 mcm in aerodynamic diameter (or even larger) are referred to as coarse particles. Coarse particles include dusts generated from the mechanical breakdown of solid matter (eg, rocks, soil, dust) and windblown dust. Compared with coarse particles, fine particles can remain suspended in the atmosphere for longer periods and be transported over longer distances. As a result, the concentration of fine particles tends to be more uniformly distributed over large urban areas, whereas the concentration of coarse particles tends to be more localized near particular sources. Although fine and coarse particles have been linked with adverse health effects, fine particles may have stronger respiratory effects in children than do coarse particles.[11] Particulate matter easily moves from outdoors to indoors, and ambient measurements are good proxies for overall personal exposure.

Although air quality standards have been established for $PM_{2.5}$ and $PM_{10}$ particles, the possibility of establishing standards for ultrafine particles (aerodynamic diameter of 100 nanometers) is under consideration because of the increasing evidence of the role of these particles in inflammatory conditions, including respiratory and cardiovascular disease.[12] Major sources of ultrafine particles include motor vehicle exhaust (especially diesel), power plants, fires, and wood stoves.

## Lead

Before the introduction of unleaded gasoline in the United States, leaded gasoline in motor vehicles was an important source of lead exposure for children. Today, paint and soil generally are the most common sources of lead exposure for US children (see Chapter 32); however, industrial operations, such as ferrous and nonferrous smelters, battery manufacturers, and other sources of lead emissions, can generate air emissions of lead that are potentially harmful for nearby communities. In a few countries, use of leaded gasoline continues (see Chapter 14).

## Sulfur Compounds

Sulfur-containing compounds include sulfur dioxide, sulfuric acid ($H_2SO_4$) aerosol, and sulfate particles. The primary source of sulfur dioxide is from the burning of coal and sulfur-containing oil; thus, major emitters of sulfur dioxide include coal-fired power plants, smelters, and pulp and paper mills. Sulfuric acid aerosol is formed in the atmosphere from the oxidation of sulfur dioxide in the presence of moisture. Facilities that either manufacture or use acids also can emit sulfuric acid aerosol. Sulfate particles are formed in the atmosphere from the chemical reaction of sulfuric acid with ammonia and may be measured as part of the fine particle fraction ($PM_{2.5}$ sulfate). In addition to adverse short- and long-term health effects on the respiratory system, sulfur dioxide contributes to the formation of acid rain.

## Carbon Monoxide and Nitrogen Dioxide

In addition to fine particles and photochemical pollution, motor vehicle emissions also contribute to outdoor levels of carbon monoxide and nitrogen dioxide. Another important source of nitrogen oxides is fuel combustion from power plants. The emissions of nitrogen oxides that lead to nitrogen dioxide also contribute to the formation of ozone and nitrogen-bearing particles (nitrates and nitric acid). Outdoors, carbon monoxide occurs in areas of heavy traffic and is primarily a problem in cold weather because people idle their cars and temperature inversions trap the pollutants near the ground. Indoor sources of nitrogen dioxide and carbon monoxide can generate higher levels indoors than those typically measured outdoors (see Chapters 20 and 25).

## TOXIC AIR POLLUTANTS

Toxic air pollutants, also known as air toxics or hazardous air pollutants, represent a large group of substances, including volatile organic compounds, metals such as mercury, solvents, and combustion byproducts (eg, dioxin). These substances are known or suspected to cause cancer, affect reproductive health, cause birth defects, exacerbate respiratory diseases, and cause other serious health effects. Currently, 187 substances are included on the list of hazardous air pollutants subject to emission regulations under the Clean Air Act, 30 of which pose major health threats in urban areas.[10] Most exposure to volatile organic compounds occurs indoors and some compounds, such as benzene, 1,3-butadiene, and diesel exhaust, are emitted primarily from mobile sources, such as cars and trucks. Other toxic air pollutants come primarily from large, stationary industrial facilities. Smaller area sources (eg, dry cleaners), indoor sources, volcanic eruptions, and forest fires also can release toxic air pollutants. Industrial sources (eg, chemical plants) contribute a relatively small proportion to the average person's total exposure to many of these substances (see Chapter 20).

## GREENHOUSE GASES

Greenhouse gases (GHG), responsible for climate change, are heat-trapping gases released into the atmosphere primarily from the burning of fossil fuels and to a lesser extent from industrial activities, deforestation, and some agricultural practices. Of the vulnerable groups, children are particularly susceptible to the detrimental effects of the changing climate.[13] Because GHGs have an indirect but significant effect on human health, regulation of GHG production for large stationary sources under the US Clean Air Act began in January 2011.[14] Under this and other subsequent directives, production of the most abundant, long-lived GHGs (eg, carbon dioxide, methane, nitrous oxide, hydrofluorocarbons, perfluorocarbons, sulfur hexafluoride, and nitrogen trifluoride) is regulated because they endanger public health and welfare. More information on the harmful effects of GHGs on human health can be found in Chapter 58.

## OTHER AIR POLLUTANTS

### Traffic-related Air Pollutants and Diesel Exhaust

In most urban areas, traffic-related emissions are a major source of air pollution. Concentrations of traffic-related pollutants and diesel exhaust are highest near and downwind of busy roads.[15] Because traffic pollution is a complex mixture, the components that have the strongest associations with health effects are not entirely clear. Traffic emissions contain numerous respiratory irritants and carcinogens, and laboratory and clinical studies have shown that constituents of traffic pollution can induce airway and systemic inflammation and increased airway responsiveness.[16] In 2012, the International Agency for Research on Cancer (IARC) declared diesel exhaust a carcinogen.[17] Over the last decade, numerous epidemiologic studies in the United States and Europe have found links between living near areas of high traffic density and increased respiratory symptoms (eg, wheezing, bronchitis), asthma symptoms, and asthma hospitalizations.[18–20] In addition, longitudinal studies of children's respiratory health have shown that children living near high-traffic roads had higher deficits in lung function and may have an increased risk for developing asthma compared with those children living farther away from traffic.[21,22]

Several epidemiologic studies suggest that diesel exhaust may be particularly harmful to children.[19] Diesel exhaust particles may enhance allergic and inflammatory responses to antigen challenge and may facilitate the development of new allergies and allergic asthma.[23,24]

Because most US school buses run on diesel fuel, a child riding in a school bus may be exposed to as much as 4 times the level of diesel exhaust as one riding in a car.[25] The US EPA Clean School Bus Program (www.epa.gov/cleanschoolbus) encourages policies to eliminate idling and includes grants to local school districts for retrofitting and replacing buses to reduce pollution.

## Odors

The chemical identity of odors can sometimes be difficult to determine. Some common sources of odorous air pollution include sewage treatment plants, landfills, livestock feed lots, composts, pulp mills, geothermal plants, waste lagoons, tanneries, and petroleum refineries, among others. The odor of some compounds can be detected at levels below those generally recognized as posing a significant health risk. However, odors can negatively affect a person's quality of life and can exacerbate health problems among people who are particularly sensitive to odors.[26] Hydrogen sulfide, a prevalent odorous air pollutant, is emitted as part of a variety of industrial processes, including oil refining, wood pulp production, and wastewater treatment as well as from concentrated animal feeding operations, geothermal plants, and landfills. Hydrogen sulfide, also known as sewer gas, has an odor similar to that of rotten eggs.

## Hydraulic Fracturing or Fracking-related Air Pollution

Hydraulic fracturing or fracking is the high-pressure injection of water, proppants, and chemicals into the shale layer to create fractures in rock formations that stimulate the flow of natural gas or oil.[26] From well-site preparation to production, processing, and storage, the process of fracking generates a combination of criteria pollutants, hazardous air pollutants, diesel exhaust, and GHGs known to cause airway irritation, exacerbation of respiratory conditions, central nervous system damage, birth defects, premature death, and malignancy.[27] More information on the harmful effects of fracking on human health can be found in Chapter 57.

## ROUTES OF EXPOSURE

The primary route of exposure to air pollution is through inhalation. Substances released into the atmosphere, however, can enter the hydrologic cycle as a result of atmospheric dispersion and precipitation, thus contaminating aquatic ecosystems. Similarly, deposition of suspended particulate matter occurs in soil. Material that was originally released into the atmosphere can be ingested as a result of the subsequent contamination of water, soil, or vegetation, or the consumption of fish from contaminated waters. Some toxic air pollutants (eg, mercury, lead, polychlorinated biphenyls, dioxins) degrade very slowly or not at all and can persist or accumulate in soil and the sediments of lakes and streams (see Chapters 17 and 18).

## SYSTEMS AFFECTED

Most of the common outdoor air pollutants are recognized irritants to the respiratory system, with ozone being the most potent irritant. Other adverse effects of air pollution include low birth weight, preterm birth, immune alterations, increased frequency of infections, neurodevelopmental abnormalities, and malignancies.[28-33] Some toxic air pollutants have other systemic effects (eg, cancer, impaired neurologic development). The specific health risks from many of these toxic compounds (lead, mercury, carbon monoxide, dioxins, volatile organic compounds) are addressed in other chapters.

## CLINICAL EFFECTS

The damaging health effects of air pollution start during the preconception period and continue throughout childhood and into adulthood. Children are considered especially vulnerable to outdoor air pollution because they spend more time outside compared with adults, often while being physically active. These circumstances create a greater opportunity for exposure to pollutants. While playing or at rest, children breathe more rapidly and inhale more pollutants per kilogram of body weight than do adults. In addition, because airway passages in children are narrower than those in adults, inflammation caused by air pollution can result in proportionally greater airway obstruction. Unlike most adults, children may not cease vigorous outdoor activities when bronchospasm occurs.

From the viewpoint of toxicity, the key distinguishing features of outdoor air pollutants are their chemical and physical characteristics and concentration. Air pollutants may occur together; for example, on days when ozone levels are high, outdoor air levels of fine particles and acid aerosols also may be high. Epidemiologic methods can be applied to attempt to determine the relative contribution of the different pollutants. The combined effects of multiple pollutants are not completely understood but could be synergistic.

Exposure to air pollution during pregnancy has been associated with adverse outcomes, such as low birth weight, small for gestational age, and preterm birth.[28,34-38] A relationship between chronic and acute exposure to ozone and risk of stillbirth has been described.[39] In older children, the health effects associated with outdoor air pollution are primarily related to increased respiratory symptoms, such as asthma exacerbations, wheezing and cough, transient decrements in lung function, and upper airway infections.[31] In

2008, asthma accounted for an estimated 14.4 million lost school days among children nationally.[40]

Because children with asthma have increased airway reactivity, the effects of air pollution on the respiratory system can be more serious. Increases in the number of hospital emergency department admissions have been observed when air pollution levels are elevated, which commonly occurs in major urban areas.[41] Compared with adults, children with asthma are more susceptible to severe exacerbations and intensive care unit admissions after exposure to high levels of air pollutants, such as fine particulate matter and ozone.[42] Children with poorly controlled asthma may be more susceptible to asthma exacerbations on days of poor air quality. Most of the acute respiratory effects of outdoor air pollution, such as symptoms of cough, shortness of breath, or decrements in lung function, are thought to be reversible, but studies indicate that long-term exposure to outdoor air pollution (particulates and related co-pollutants and possibly ozone) has been associated with decrements in lung function among children.[43] Emerging evidence links early exposure to air pollution with the development of asthma.[44,45] Some of the increases in the prevalence of chronic obstructive lung disease in adults who live in more polluted areas may be the result of exposures that occurred during childhood. Exposure to high levels of $PM_{2.5}$ and ozone among patients with asthma has been associated with a higher risk for the development of chronic obstructive pulmonary disease (COPD). When a person has both asthma and COPD, it is known as the asthma–COPD overlap syndrome.[46–48]

Other adverse events may occur and certain patient populations can be adversely affected by exposure to air pollution. Among patients with cystic fibrosis, air pollution exposure has been associated with lung function decline and increased pulmonary exacerbations.[49] The mean annual concentration of $PM_{2.5}$ in the calendar year prior to birth is an independent risk factor for methicillin-resistant *Staphylococcus aureus* and *Pseudomonas* acquisition.[50,51] Exposure to ozone, nitrogen oxides, sulfur oxides, and particulate matter have all been associated with increased morbidity in patients with sickle cell disease.[52]

In 2013, the IARC classified air pollution as a human carcinogen.[53] To this effect, exposure to traffic pollution, particularly benzene, has been associated with leukemia in the pediatric population.[30] The effect of air pollution on neurodevelopmental conditions is of great concern for pediatric populations because it causes neuroinflammation. In addition, tissue changes seen in the early stages of Alzheimer and Parkinson disease have been noted in children who have been highly exposed to air pollution.[32] Exposure to high levels of $PM_{2.5}$ during the third trimester of pregnancy has been related to a higher risk of autistic spectrum disorder in children.[29]

The mechanisms by which air pollution can cause adverse effects are complex; gene-environment interactions are likely to be important. Ozone and ambient particulate matter are highly reactive oxidants, and there is emerging evidence that variants in genes that control the inflammatory and antioxidant response systems, as well as the changes in inflammatory markers result-ing from these exposures, may increase a child's susceptibility to the adverse effects of air pollution.[54,55]

Mechanistic, clinical, and epidemiologic studies suggest that antioxidants and nutritional status may modify the effect of air pollution on respiratory health.[56] Further studies are needed to address the role of supplementation strategies in the prevention of air pollution-related effects in children living in areas with high ambient air pollution.

## PREVENTION OF EXPOSURE

Under the Clean Air Act, the US EPA has the authority to set standards for air pollutants that protect the health of people with specific sensitivities, includ-ing children and those with asthma (see Table 21-2).[57] Current US NAAQS are

## Table 21-2. Clean Air Act Amendments

**Setting Guidelines for Criteria Air Pollutants**
A few common air pollutants are regulated by first developing health-based criteria (science-based guidelines) as the basis for setting permissible levels. One set of limits (primary standard) protects health; another set of limits (secondary standard) is intended to prevent environmental and property damage. The criteria air pollutants are ozone, carbon monoxide, particulate matter, sulfur dioxide, lead, and nitrogen dioxide.

**Regulation of Nonattainment Areas**
A nonattainment area is a geographic area whose air quality does not meet federal air quality standards designed to protect public health. Nonattainment areas are classified according to the severity of the area's air pollution problem. For ozone, these classifications are "marginal," "moderate," "serious," "severe," and "extreme." The EPA assigns each nonattainment area to 1 of these categories, thus triggering varying requirements the area must comply with to meet the ozone standard. Similar programs exist for areas that do not meet the federal health standards for carbon monoxide and particulate matter.

**Regulation of Mobile Sources**
Cars and trucks are the sources for more than half of the pollutants that contribute to ozone and up to 90% of carbon monoxide emissions in urban areas. Tighter standards were established to reduce tail-pipe emissions and control fuel quality. Reformulated gasoline was required in the cities with the worst ozone problems, and oxygenated fuel was introduced in the winter months in areas that exceeded the carbon monoxide standard.

**Reduction of Toxic Air Pollutants**
Toxic air pollutants are those that are hazardous to human health or the environment but are not specifically covered under another portion of the Clean Air Act. Emissions of toxic air pollutants are to be reduced through "maximum achievable control technology" standards for each major category of emissions sources.

**Regulation of Greenhouse Gases**
Under the Clean Air Act, regulation of greenhouse gases emissions from mobile and stationary sources began in 2011.

shown in Table 21-3.[58] Although ambient concentrations of these 6 pollutants have decreased over the past decade, large numbers of people are still exposed to potentially unhealthful levels of these pollutants.

## Table 21-3. National Ambient Air Quality Standards

| POLLUTANT | | PRIMARY/ SECONDARY | AVERAGING TIME | LEVEL | FORM |
|---|---|---|---|---|---|
| Carbon monoxide (CO) | | Primary | 8 h | 9 ppm | Not to be exceeded more than once per yr |
| | | | 1 h | 35 ppm | |
| Lead (Pb) | | Primary and secondary | Rolling 3 mo average | 0.15 mcg/m$^3$ | Not to be exceeded |
| Nitrogen dioxide (NO$_2$) | | Primary | 1 h | 100 ppb | 98th percentile of 1-h daily maximum concentrations, averaged over 3 yr |
| | | Primary and secondary | 1 yr | 53 ppb | Annual mean |
| Ozone | | Primary and secondary | 8 h | 0.07 ppm | Annual fourth-highest daily maximum 8-hour concentration, averaged over 3 yr |
| Particulate matter (PM) | PM$_{2.5}$[a] | Primary | 1 yr | 12 mcg/m$^3$ | Annual mean, averaged over 3 yr |
| | | Secondary | 1 yr | 15 mcg/m$^3$ | Annual mean, averaged over 3 yr |
| | | Primary and secondary | 24 h | 35 mcg/m$^3$ | 98th percentile, averaged over 3 yr |
| | PM$_{10}$[b] | Primary and secondary | 24 h | 150 mcg/m$^3$ | Not to be exceeded more than once per year on average over 3 yr |
| Sulfur dioxide (SO$_2$) | | Primary | 1 h | 75 ppb | 99th percentile of 1-hr daily maximum concentration, averaged over 3 yr |
| | | Secondary | 3 h | 0.5 ppm | Not to be exceeded more than once per year |

Source: https://www.epa.gov/criteria-air-pollutants/naaqs-table
Abbreviations: ppb, parts per billion; ppm, parts per million.
[a] Particles up to 2.5 mcm in aerodynamic diameter.
[b] Particles up to 10 mcm in aerodynamic diameter.

The US EPA established the revised NAAQS for particulate matter and ozone in 2006 and 2015, respectively. For particulate matter, the new standards retain the current annual $PM_{10}$ standard of 150 mcg/m$^3$ but establish a new primary annual standard for $PM_{2.5}$ of 12 mcg/m$^3$ and a new 24-hour standard (air measurement made for 24 hours) for $PM_{2.5}$ of 35 mcg/m$^3$. For ozone, a new 8-hour standard of 0.070 ppm was adopted in 2015. It should be noted that there are different averaging times used for each pollutant. The US Supreme Court upheld the scientific basis for the revised standards.

The Clean Air Act Amendments also give the US EPA the authority to develop technology-based emission standards for 187 hazardous air pollutants. Although these standards are designed to protect public health, they are based on the available technology to control emissions.

## Air Quality Index

Most large metropolitan areas are required to regularly monitor air quality for one or more of the NAAQS. The result of air quality monitoring is expressed as the Pollutant Standards Index, which also is commonly known as the Air Quality Index. The Air Quality Index converts the concentrations of 5 specific pollutants (ozone, carbon monoxide, nitrogen dioxide, sulfur dioxide, particulate matter) into one number, scaled from 0 to 500. An Air Quality Index value of 100 corresponds to the short-term national ambient air quality standard; thus, an Air Quality Index value greater than 100 indicates that the concentration of one or more pollutants exceeds its national standard. The descriptor terms associated with different Air Quality Index values are as follows: 0 to 50 = good; 51 to 100 = moderate; 101 to 150 = unhealthy for sensitive groups; 151 to 200 = unhealthy; 201 to 300 = very unhealthy; and 301 to 500 = hazardous. Table 21-4 gives additional information about the Air Quality Index.[59]

During periods of poor air quality, children's outdoor physical activity should be curtailed according to the guidelines provided in the Air Quality Index Table (See Table 21-4) (www.airnow.gov).

Finally, prevention of exposures to air pollution is an environmental justice issue. Children living near busy roads and industrial sources of pollution are more likely to be socially and economically disadvantaged.

## Table 21-4. Air Quality Index (AQI) and Associated General Health Effects and Cautionary Statements

| INDEX VALUE | AQI DESCRIPTOR | GENERAL HEALTH EFFECTS | GENERAL CAUTIONARY STATEMENTS |
|---|---|---|---|
| 0–50 | Good | None for the general population. | None required. |
| 51–100 | Moderate | Few or none for the general population. Possibility of aggravation of heart or lung disease among persons with cardiopulmonary disease and the elderly with elevations of $PM_{2.5}$.[a] | Unusually sensitive people should consider limiting prolonged outdoor exertion. |
| 101–150 | Unhealthy for sensitive groups | Mild aggravation of respiratory symptoms among susceptible people. | Active children and adults and people with respiratory disease (eg, asthma) and cardiopulmonary disease should avoid prolonged outdoor exertion. |
| 151–200 | Unhealthy | Significant aggravation of symptoms and decreased exercise tolerance in persons with heart or lung disease. Possible respiratory effects in the general population. | Active children and adults and people with respiratory and cardiovascular disease should avoid prolonged outdoor exertion. Everyone else, especially children, should limit prolonged outdoor exertion. |
| 201–300 | Very unhealthy | Increasingly severe symptoms and impaired breathing likely in sensitive groups. Increasing likelihood of respiratory effects in the general population. | Active children and adults and people with respiratory and cardiovascular disease should avoid all outdoor exertion. All others should limit outdoor exertion. |
| 301–500 | Hazardous | Severe respiratory effects and impaired breathing in sensitive groups, with serious risk of premature mortality in persons with cardiopulmonary disease and the elderly. Increasingly severe respiratory effects in the general population. | Elderly and persons with existing respiratory and cardiovascular diseases should stay indoors with the windows closed. Everyone should avoid outside physical exertion. |

[a] Particles up to 2.5 mcm in aerodynamic diameter.

## Frequently Asked Questions

Q   *How can I find out about the levels of air pollution in my community?*

A   Information about the air quality in a community is often found on the
Weather page of the local newspaper and is also available through www.
airnow.gov.

Q   *What can be done to protect my children from outdoor air pollution when they
want and need to be able to play outdoors?*

A   The potential harm posed by outdoor air pollution depends on the concentration of pollutants, which can vary from day to day, and even during the
course of a day. Although exposure to outdoor air pollutants cannot be
entirely prevented, it can be reduced by restricting the amount of time that
children spend outdoors during periods of poor air quality, especially time
spent engaged in strenuous physical activity. For example, ozone levels
during the summer tend to be highest in the middle to late afternoon. On
days when ozone levels are expected or reported to be high, outdoor activities could be restricted during the afternoon or rescheduled to the morning,
particularly for children who have exhibited sensitivity to high levels of air
pollution. In many areas, local radio stations, television news programs, and
newspapers regularly provide information about air quality conditions.

Q   *The recommendation to exercise in the early morning often conflicts with the
reality of children's sports activity schedules. Should organized sports activities
be canceled on days when air quality is poor?*

A   Children should be encouraged to participate in physical activities because
of the many health benefits associated with exercise. In most instances, the
health benefits of physical activity likely outweigh the potential harm posed
by intermittent or moderate levels of air pollution. However, on hot summer
days when temperatures as well as smog levels are high, this balance could
shift, and it may be advisable to shorten or cancel outdoor physical activities, especially for young children. When children have asthma, physicians
and parents aim for optimal asthma control so that children can participate
in normal outdoor sports activities, even on days with poor air quality. When
asthma is unstable, children need to curtail their physical activities until
their asthma becomes controlled again. Evidence suggests that children who
exercise heavily (participating in 3 or more sports) and who live in communities with high levels of ozone pollution may experience a higher risk for the
development of asthma compared with children who do not play sports.[60]

Q   *My family lives in an area that places them at risk of exposure to increased
levels of outdoor air pollution. How can I help my child with asthma?*

A   It is very appropriate for parents to discuss their concerns about air pollution and other possible asthma triggers with their child's physician. A
child's entire environment, including the home, school, and playground,

should be reviewed for possible asthma triggers. Improved medical management of the child's asthma and control of exposure to allergens and irritants in the child's home may be very effective in preventing asthma exacerbations. If a parent or a physician believes that emissions from a particular facility are harmful to a child with asthma, this information should be shared with the local or state environmental agencies that have authority over operating permits and enforcement actions.

Q *Would face dust masks be effective for protecting my children when air pollution levels are high?*

A Dust masks and other forms of respiratory protection, which are sized for adults and not children, are not recommended to protect against outdoor air pollution. Not only do poor fit and uncertain compliance limit any potential benefits, but most simple dust masks do not include the materials needed to filter out harmful volatile organic compounds or ozone.

Q *What is the relationship between ozone in urban smog and stratospheric ozone?*

A These issues are unrelated. Ozone in the troposphere, or ground level, is a major component of urban smog and a respiratory health hazard. The formation of ground-level ozone is independent of ozone in the upper atmosphere (the stratosphere). Stratospheric ozone provides a protective shield absorbing harmful ultraviolet radiation. Too little stratospheric ozone increases the risk of skin cancer and eye damage from ultraviolet rays.

Q *Why is asthma on the increase?*

A Scientists and public health officials are concerned by the apparent increase in the prevalence of asthma. The explanation for the increase has not been found but seems most likely to be related to a complex combination of factors, including increased exposure to environmental allergens and irritants indoors; increased exposure to complex environmental pollutants, such as secondhand tobacco smoke, diesel exhaust, and irritant gases during the early postnatal period of life; genetic susceptibility; delayed maturation of immune responses because of changes in exposure to infection and infectious products; dietary factors; and psychosocial factors, such as stress and poverty.[31,32] Emerging evidence from scientific studies suggests that long-term exposures to air pollution and proximity to traffic may cause some cases of asthma, especially in those people with genetic susceptibility.[22,41,54,55]

Q *Are odors from hog farms harmful to children?*

A Odors are an indicator of the presence of chemical emissions. Emissions from hog farms include volatile organic compounds, hydrogen sulfide, ammonia, endotoxins, and organic dusts. At sufficient concentrations over extended periods, there is ample evidence that these chemicals can cause disease. Whether the level and duration of exposures from emissions from hog farms is sufficient to cause harm to children through classic toxicological mechanisms is not known.[42] However, it is known that odors can affect people through psychophysiological mechanisms, resulting in increased respiratory symptoms and other indicators of reduced quality of life.[21]

Q   *If I live in an area with good air quality, is living next to a freeway still a concern? If so, what can I do to reduce my child's overall exposure to traffic pollution?*

A   Levels of traffic pollution are highest when driving on a high traffic road, especially when there is stop-and-go traffic. Even if you live in an area with good regional air quality, pollution levels can be very high near a busy freeway, and high levels have been associated with increased risk of respiratory symptoms, including asthma.[13–16] A multifaceted approach is needed to reduce children's overall exposures. Avoid standing near idling motor vehicles when possible. When walking or playing, choose areas away from traffic; even a distance of 300 to 600 feet (100 to 200 meters) will make a difference. Close windows and doors during peak traffic hours and place the air conditioner setting on recirculate. Encourage schools to enforce no idling rules at school pickup areas and advocate for switching school bus fleets to non-diesel fuel. Support federal and state efforts to reduce motor vehicle emissions. Some state and local governments have adopted laws to limit or require reduction strategies if schools or new residences are built close to busy roads. For other strategies, see traffic fact sheets at: www.oehha.ca.gov/public_info/public/kids/airkidshome.html.

## Resources

**Air Quality Index**
Web site: https://airnow.gov/index.cfm?action=aqibasics.aqi

**American Lung Association**
Phone: 1-800-LUNGUSA or 1-800-548-8252
e-mail: info@lung.org
Web site: www.lungusa.org

**EPA environmental justice screening and mapping tool**
Web site: https://www.epa.gov/ejscreen

**EPA MyEnvironment**
Web site: https://www3.epa.gov/enviro/myenviro/

**Health Effects Institute**
Phone: 1-617-488-2300
e-mail: webmaster@healtheffects.org
Web site: www.healtheffects.org

**Toxics Release Inventory (TRI) scorecard**
Web site: http://scorecard.goodguide.com/

**US Environmental Protection Agency, Office of Air Quality Planning and Standards**
Web site: http://airnow.gov

# References

1. World Health Organization. 7 million premature deaths annually linked to air pollution. http://www.who.int/mediacentre/news/releases/2014/air-pollution/en/. Published March 25, 2014. Accessed January 16, 2018

2. United Nations Children's Fund. *Clean the Air for Children.* New York, NY: United Nations Children's Fund; 2016. https://www.unicef.org/publications/files/UNICEF_Clear_the_Air_for_Children_30_Oct_2016.pdf. Accessed January 16, 2018

3. US Environmental Protection Agency. Office of Air Quality Planning and Standards. *National Air Quality- Status and Trends through 2007.* Washington, DC: US Environmental Protection Agency; 2008. EPA Publication No. 454/R-08-006. https://www.epa.gov/sites/production/files/2017-11/documents/trends_brochure_2007.pdf. Accessed March 6, 2018

4. Nadadur SS, Miller CA, Hopke PK, et al. The complexities of air pollution regulation: the need for an integrated research and regulatory perspective. *Toxicol Sci.* 2007;100(2):318–327

5. US Environmental Protection Agency. Air pollution monitoring. https://www3.epa.gov/airquality/montring.html. Updated June 8, 2016. Accessed January 16, 2018

6. US Environmental Protection Agency. National Air Toxics Trends Stations Work Plan Template. https://www3.epa.gov/ttnamti1/files/ambient/airtox/nattsworkplantemplate.pdf. Revised March 2015. Accessed January 16, 2018

7. US Environmental Protection Agency. Historical Rulemakings. Greenhouse Gas Reporting Program (GHGRP). https://www.epa.gov/ghgreporting. Accessed January 16, 2018

8. US Environmental Protection Agency. Our Nation's Air. 2018. https://gispub.epa.gov/air/trendsreport/2018. Accessed August 6, 2018

9. US Environmental Protection Agency. Air emissions sources. https://www.epa.gov/air-emissions-inventories/air-pollutant-emissions-trends-data. Accessed August 6, 2018

10. US Environmental Protection Agency. Urban air toxic pollutants. https://www.epa.gov/urban-air-toxics/urban-air-toxic-pollutants. Accessed January 16, 2018

11. Schwartz J, Neas LM. Fine particles are more strongly associated than coarse particles with acute respiratory health effects in school children. *Epidemiology.* 2000;11(1):6–10

12. Li N, Georas S, Alexis N, et al. A work group report on ultrafine particles (American Academy of Allergy, Asthma & Immunology): why ambient ultrafine and engineered nanoparticles should receive special attention for possible adverse health outcomes in human subjects. *J Allergy Clin Immunol.* 2016;138(2):386–396

13. Ahdoot S, Pacheco SE, American Academy of Pediatrics Council on Environmental Health. Global climate change and children's health. *Pediatrics.* 2015;136(5):e1468–e1584

14. US Environmental Protection Agency. Clean Air Act permitting for greenhouse gases: guidance and technical information. Fact sheet. https://www.epa.gov/sites/production/files/2015-12/documents/ghgpermittingtoolsfs.pdf. Accessed January 16, 2018

15. Zhu Y, Hinds WC, Kim S, Sioutas C. Concentrations and size distribution of ultrafine particles near a major highway. *J Air Waste Manag Assoc.* 2002;52(9):1032–1042

16. Gilmour MI, Jaakkola MS, London SJ, Nel AE, Rogers CA. How exposure to environmental tobacco smoke, outdoor air pollutants, and increased pollen burdens influences the incidence of asthma. *Environ Health Perspect.* 2006;114(4):627–633

17. World Health Organization, International Agency for Research on Cancer. IARC: Diesel engine exhaust carcinogenic. https://www.iarc.fr/en/media-centre/pr/2012/pdfs/pr213_E.pdf. Accessed January 16, 2018

18. Delfino RJ. Epidemiologic evidence for asthma and exposure to air toxics: linkages between occupational, indoor, and community air pollution research. *Environ Health Perspect.* 2002;110(Suppl 4):573–589

19. Brunekreef B, Janssen NA, de Hartog J, Harssema H, Knape M, van Vliet P. Air pollution from truck traffic and lung function in children living near motorways. *Epidemiology.* 1997;8(3):298–303

20. Kim JJ, Huen K, Adams S, et al. Residential traffic and children's respiratory health. *Environ Health Perspect.* 2008;116(9):1274–1279

21. Gauderman WJ, Vora H, McConnell R, et al. Effect of exposure to traffic on lung development from 10 to 18 years of age: a cohort study. *Lancet.* 2007;369(9561):571–577

22. McConnell R, Berhane K, Yao L, et al. Traffic, susceptibility, and childhood asthma. *Environ Health Perspect.* 2006;114(5):766–772

23. Diaz-Sanchez D, Garcia MP, Wang M, Jyrala M, Saxon A. Nasal challenge with diesel exhaust particles can induce sensitization to a neoallergen in the human mucosa. *J Allergy Clin Immunol.* 1999;104(6):1183–1188

24. Brandt EB, Biagini Myers JM, Acciani TH, et al. Exposure to allergen and diesel exhaust particles potentiates secondary allergen-specific memory responses, promoting asthma susceptibility. *J Allergy Clin Immunol.* 2015;136(2):295–303

25. Natural Resources Defense Council. *No breathing in the aisles: diesel exhaust inside school buses.* 2001. https://www.nrdc.org/sites/default/files/schoolbus.pdf. Accessed January 14, 2018

26. US Environmental Protection Agency. The process of hydraulic fracturing. https://www.epa.gov/hydraulicfracturing/process-hydraulic-fracturing. Accessed January 16, 2018

27. National Resources Defense Council. Fracking fumes: air pollution from hydraulic fracturing threatens public health and communities. https://www.nrdc.org/sites/default/files/fracking-air-pollution-IB.pdf. Accessed January 16, 2018

28. Mendola P, Wallace M, Hwang BS, et al. Preterm birth and air pollution: critical windows of exposure for women with asthma. *J Allergy Clin Immunol.* 2016;138(2):432–440.e5

29. Raz R, Roberts AL, Lyall K, et al. Autism spectrum disorder and particulate matter air pollution before, during, and after pregnancy: a nested case–control analysis within the Nurses' Health Study II Cohort. *Environ Health Perspect.* 2015;123(3):264–270

30. Filippini T, Heck JE, Malagoli C, Del Giovane C, Vinceti M. A review and meta-analysis of outdoor air pollution and risk of childhood leukemia. *J Environ Sci Health C Environ Carcinog Ecotoxicol Rev.* 2015;33(1):36–66

31. MacIntyre EA, Gehring U, Mölter A, et al. Air pollution and respiratory infections during early childhood: an analysis of 10 European birth cohorts within the ESCAPE Project. *Environ Health Perspect.* 2014;122(1):107–113

32. Calderón-Garcidueñas L, Torres-Jardón R. The impact of air pollutants on the brain. *JAMA Psychiatry*. 2015;72(6):529–530

33. Gruzieva O, Merid SK, Gref A, et al. Exposure to traffic-related air pollution and serum inflammatory cytokines in children. *Environ Health Perspect*. 2017;125(6):067007

34. Stieb DM, Chen L, Hystad P, et al. A national study of the association between traffic-related air pollution and adverse pregnancy outcomes in Canada, 1999-2008. *Environ Res*. 2016;148: 513–526

35. van den Hooven EH, Pierik FH, de Kluizenaar Y, et al. Air pollution exposure during pregnancy, ultrasound measures of fetal growth, and adverse birth outcomes: a prospective cohort study. *Environ Health Perspect*. 2012;120(1):150–156

36. Hyder A, Lee HJ, Ebisu K, Koutrakis P, Belanger K, Bell ML. PM2.5 exposure and birth outcomes: use of satellite- and monitor-based data. *Epidemiology*. 2014;25(1):58–67

37. DeFranco E, Moravec W, Xu F, et al. Exposure to airborne particulate matter during pregnancy is associated with preterm birth: a population-based cohort study. *Environ Health*. 2016;15:6

38. Vinikoor-Imler LC, Davis JA, Meyer RE, Messer LC, Luben TJ. Associations between prenatal exposure to air pollution, small for gestational age, and term low birthweight in a state-wide birth cohort. *Environ Res*. 2014;132:132–139

39. Mendola P, Ha S, Pollack AZ, et al. Chronic and acute ozone exposure in the week prior to delivery is associated with the risk of stillbirth. *Int J Environ Res Public Health*. 2017;14(7)

40. Centers for Disease Control and Prevention. Asthma-related school absenteeism and school concentration of low-income students in California. https://www.cdc.gov/pcd/issues/2012/11_0312.htm. Accessed January 16, 2018

41. Tolbert PE, Mulholland JA, MacIntosh DL, et al. Air quality and pediatric emergency room visits for asthma in Atlanta, Georgia USA. *Am J Epidemiol*. 2000;151(8):798–810

42. Silverman RA, Ito K. Age-related association of fines particles and ozone with severe acute asthma in New York City. *J Allergy Clin Immunol*. 2010;125(2):367–373

43. Urman R, McConnell R, Islam T, et al. Associations of children's lung function with ambient air pollution: joint effects of regional and near-roadway pollutants. *Thorax*. 2014;69(6): 540–547

44. Gehring U, Wijga AH, Hoek G, et al. Exposure to air pollution and development of asthma and rhinoconjunctivitis throughout childhood and adolescence: a population-based birth cohort study. *Lancet Respir Med*. 2015;3(12):933–942

45. Sbihi H, Tamburic L, Koehoorn M, Brauer M. Perinatal air pollution exposure and development of asthma from birth to age 10 years. *Eur Respir J*. 2016;47(4):1062–1071

46. To T, Zhu J, Larsen K, et al. Progression from asthma to chronic obstructive pulmonary disease. Is air pollution a risk factor? *Am J Respir Crit Care Med*. 2016;194(4):429–438

47. Stocks J, Sonnappa S. Early life influences on the development of chronic obstructive pulmonary disease. *Ther Adv Resp Dis*. 2013;7(3):161–173

48. Grigg J. Particulate matter exposure in children: relevance to chronic obstructive pulmonary disease. *Proc Am Thorac Soc*. 2009;6(7):564–569

49. Goss CH, Newsom SA, Schildcrout JS, Sheppard L, Kaufman JD. Effect of ambient air pollution on pulmonary exacerbations and lung function in cystic fibrosis. *Am J Respir Crit Care Med*. 2004;169:816–821

50. Psoter KJ, De Roos AJ, Wakefield J, Mayer JD, Rosenfeld M. Air pollution exposure is associated with MRSA acquisition in young U.S. children with cystic fibrosis. *BMC Pulm Med*. 2017;17(1):106

51. Psoter KJ, De Roos AJ, Mayer JD, Kaufman JD, Wakefield J, Rosenfeld M. Fine particulate matter exposure and initial Pseudomonas aeruginosa acquisition in cystic fibrosis. *Ann Am Thorac Soc*. 2015;12(3):385–391

52. Piel FB, Steinberg MH, Rees DC. Sickle cell disease. *N Engl J Med*. 2017;376(16):1561–1573

53. World Health Organization. IARC: outdoor air pollution a leading environmental cause of cancer deaths. https://www.iarc.fr/en/media-centre/iarcnews/pdf/pr221_E.pdf. Accessed January 16, 2018

54. London SJ. Gene-air pollution interactions in asthma. *Proc Am Thorac Soc*. 2007;4(3):217–220

55. Salam MT, Gauderman WJ, McConnell R, Lin PC, Gilliland FD. Transforming growth factor- 1 C-509T polymorphism, oxidant stress, and early-onset childhood asthma. *Am J Respir Crit Care Med*. 2007;176(12):1192–1199

56. Romieu I, Castro-Giner F, Kunzli N, Sunyer J. Air pollution, oxidative stress and dietary supplementation: a review. *Eur Respir J*. 2008;31(1):179–197

57. US Environmental Protection Agency. Office of Air Quality Planning and Standards. *The plain English guide to the clean air act*. Washington, DC: US Environmental Protection Agency. 2007. Publication No. EPA-456/K-07-001. https://www.epa.gov/clean-air-act-overview/plain-english-guide-clean-air-act. Accessed March 6, 2018

58. US Environmental Protection Agency. NAAQS table. https://www.epa.gov/criteria-air-pollutants/naaqs-table. Accessed January 16, 2018

59. US Environmental Protection Agency. *Air Quality Index: A Guide to Air Quality and Your Health*. Washington, DC: Environmental Protection Agency. 2003. https://www3.epa.gov/airnow/aqi_brochure_02_14.pdf. Accessed March 6, 2018

60. Merchant JA, Kline J, Donham KJ, Bundy DS, Hodne CJ. Human health effects. In: *Iowa Concentrated Animal Feeding Operation Air Quality Study, Final Report*. Ames, IA: Iowa State University and the University of Iowa Study Group; 2002:121–145. http://www.public-health.uiowa.edu/ehsrc/CAFOstudy.htm. Accessed January 16, 2018

Chapter 22

# Arsenic

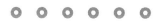

## KEY POINTS

- Arsenic is a metal-like element with widespread presence from natural and industrial sources.
- Exposure occurs through ingestion, inhalation, and through the placenta.
- Arsenic is a carcinogen; chronic exposure raises the risk of bladder, lung, and skin cancers.
- Public health policies focus mainly on arsenic in water; standards have been set.
- There is concern about arsenic in rice and apple products often consumed by infants and children.

## INTRODUCTION

Arsenic (As) is the 20th most abundant element in the earth's crust. This metal-like element has been recognized for centuries both as a valuable substance with many potential uses as well as a highly effective poison that is toxic to virtually all members of the animal kingdom, from insects to humans. In recent years, the scope of human exposure (and associated health consequences) has led to the passage of federal laws designed to protect the public from excessive exposure to arsenic.

Children may have greater exposure to arsenic than adults because of their smaller size and hand-to-mouth activities. Because many aspects of organogenesis and organ maturity take place during early life, exposure to arsenic, which has antimetabolic and carcinogenic properties, may have a greater impact on children.

Arsenic exists naturally in inorganic and organic forms. Inorganic arsenic is found in trivalent (arsenite) and pentavalent (arsenate) forms. Trivalent arsenic is substantially more toxic and carcinogenic than pentavalent. Most industrial uses of arsenic employ the trivalent form.

Organic arsenic exists in several forms, including methylarsonic and dimethylarsinic acids.[1] Naturally occurring forms of organic arsenic are considered nontoxic, although organic arsenicals that have been developed as pesticides (eg, dimethylarsinic acid) are very toxic.

## ROUTES OF EXPOSURE

Routes of exposure for arsenic include ingestion or inhalation. Arsenic also can be transmitted across the placenta. No significant exposure occurs when arsenic meets with intact skin.

## SOURCES OF EXPOSURE

### Natural

Arsenic is distributed in the earth in discrete locations or "veins." In the United States, higher concentrations are found in the southwestern states, eastern Michigan, and parts of New England.[2] Large veins of arsenic in bedrock can create contaminated earth adjacent to areas with little to no arsenic. Significant concentrations of arsenic can develop in groundwater that comes into contact with this earth, leading to contamination of well water. Arsenic in the earth's crust also leaches into ocean water where it is ingested by marine life, thus entering the food chain (in the form of relatively nontoxic organoarsenicals).

### Anthropogenic

Arsenic has been used industrially for many purposes, including pest control, and in the semiconductor, petroleum refining, and mining/smelting industries.[2] The reliable toxicity of arsenic contributed to its widespread use as a pesticide and antimicrobial agent. Before safer alternatives were found, arsenic was commonly administered to humans for treatment of syphilis, trypanosomiasis, and other infections, as well as for skin conditions (for which it was known as Fowler solution).[3] As a pesticide for home use, arsenic was used broadly until the US Environmental Protection Agency (US EPA) banned most arsenical pesticides in 1991. Until that year, sodium arsenate (Terro) was a common ant killer for home use. Of note, one arsenic-based pesticide that was exempt from this ban was chromated copper arsenate (CCA), a wood preservative used to impregnate pressure-treated wood and prevent termites and other pests from accelerating the decomposition of wood. CCA contains 22% arsenic by weight; a 12-foot section of pressure-treated wood contains approximately 1 ounce (28 g) of arsenic.[4] Use of CCA was discontinued in 2003. Gallium arsenide, another form of arsenic, is a semiconductor that is used often in place of silicon.[1] Arsenic also may be found in alternative medicines, including Chinese proprietary medications and herbal remedies.[5]

As a result of anthropogenic use, arsenic is widely distributed in the environment. For example, the Agency for Toxic Substances and Disease Registry and the US EPA have identified it at 1,014 of the 1,598 National Priorities List sites.[6]

Because of widespread presence of arsenic in nature, along with extensive industrial uses, human exposure can be extensive. Industrial emissions, including incineration, can release arsenic into the atmosphere. Water, particularly unprocessed well water, may have significant inorganic arsenic contamination.[7] Many small water systems and private wells do not have arsenic treatment systems installed. Even treated water may be left with residual concentrations of arsenic, depending on the efficacy of the purification technique.

Foods, particularly seafood, can contain large quantities of organic arsenic; shellfish (eg, oysters, lobster) can have extremely large concentrations (as much as 120 parts per million [ppm] versus 2 to 8 ppm in fish).[3] This form of arsenic, however, is relatively nontoxic so there is little concern about eating these foods. It is important to note that organoarsenicals will contribute to total arsenic in screening assays.

Although arsenic pesticides have been almost completely banned, foods can still be contaminated with arsenic from past use, inadvertent use, or misuse of pesticides. In addition, inorganic arsenical pesticides are still used occasionally in agriculture. For example, chickens may have small amounts of inorganic pesticide added to their feed as an anthelmintic. Foods containing inorganic arsenical pesticides can be very toxic and could be unsafe for consumption, especially by children. The US Food and Drug Administration (FDA) estimates that a 6-year-old child consumes an average of 4.6 mcg of inorganic arsenic daily in food. Exposure to inorganic arsenic in water, although highly variable, is estimated to be up to 4.5 mcg daily.[4]

Soil contamination by arsenic (eg, from nearby mining, hazardous waste sites, agricultural use) can expose children playing nearby and can contaminate clothes and be brought into the home. Sawing or burning wood treated with CCA can expose children to arsenic. As noted in a case report, mild arsenic poisoning occurred in a family of 8 who were exposed to fumes from the burning of CCA-treated wood.[8]

## TOXICOKINETICS, BIOLOGICAL FATE

Arsenic is well absorbed after its inhalation or ingestion. In animal models, gastrointestinal absorption of arsenic is increased in the presence of iron deficiency. Once absorbed, the half-life of arsenic in blood is 10 hours.

Circulating arsenic crosses the placenta and can result in elevated arsenic concentrations in the newborn, and even fetal demise.[1] The human body is able to detoxify small amounts of absorbed inorganic arsenic by transforming it to organic species, including monomethylarsenate, dimethylarsenate, or trimethylarsenate forms. Children usually are less able than adults to detoxify forms of methylated arsenic and, consequently, children's bodies have more persistent concentrations of the toxic inorganic metal.[4] One recent study, however, suggests that some children can detoxify methylated arsenic more efficiently than their mothers.[9]

Elimination of arsenic is almost exclusively renal; only 10% is excreted in bile. The average concentration of arsenic in urine is less than 25 mcg/L. Within 2 to 4 weeks after exposure, the remaining body burden of arsenic is found in hair, skin, and nails.[1]

## SYSTEMS AFFECTED

Arsenic affects every organ in the body. Its primary action is as an antimetabolite. The mechanism of arsenic toxicity includes its replacement of phosphate molecules in adenosine triphosphate (arsenolysis), as well as potent inhibitory effects on key enzymes, including thiamine pyrophosphate. Arsenic has been shown to have endocrine-disrupting effects, inhibiting glucocorticoid-mediated transcription.[10] The clinical significance of this finding is unknown. Primary target organs for arsenic effects are the gastrointestinal tract and skin because these are the most metabolically active tissues in the body. Arsenic exposure is associated with an increased risk of diabetes mellitus.[10]

## CLINICAL EFFECTS

The characteristics of arsenic toxicity are different for acute versus chronic exposures. Acute, high-dose exposure to inorganic arsenic (greater than 3 to 5 mg/kg) affects all major organs, including the gastrointestinal tract, brain, heart, kidneys, liver, bone marrow, skin, and peripheral nervous system. Within 30 minutes of severe ingestions, gastrointestinal injury can occur, manifested by nausea, vomiting, hematemesis, diarrhea, and abdominal cramping. Intractable shock can ensue.[11] Lower-dose exposures result in a more protracted course consisting of initial signs of gastrointestinal upset, followed by bone-marrow suppression with pancytopenia, hepatic dysfunction, myocardial depression with cardiac conduction disturbances, and peripheral neuropathy.[12] The peripheral neuropathy of arsenic is of the sensorimotor type, typically involving the lower extremities more than the upper extremities, and generally is stocking-glove in distribution. Because an early sign of exposure consists of ascending paresthesias, quickly followed by loss of proprioception, anesthesia, and weakness, the clinical picture mimics Guillain-Barré syndrome. Severe central nervous system dysfunction is uncommon. Many of these effects can be permanent. A characteristic feature of acute arsenic exposure is the appearance of Mees' lines (white, transverse creases across the fingernails that typically appear a few weeks after the poisoning event).

Chronic exposure may produce generalized fatigue and malaise. Bone marrow depression, if present, is low grade. Other complications include malnutrition, inanition, and increased risk of infections, particularly pneumonia.

Fetal and early childhood exposure to arsenic has been linked to bronchiectasis in early adulthood. Analysis of data from a historical cohort study conducted in Antofagasta, Chile, where arsenic-contaminated water was introduced into the municipal water supply as the population grew, revealed that birth cohorts with fetal and early childhood exposure to arsenic had dramatically increased standardized mortality ratios (the ratio of observed deaths to expected deaths) for lung cancer (6.1) and especially bronchiectasis (46.2) during adulthood (ages 30–49 years).[13]

In utero arsenic exposure also appears to predict the risk of infections during the first year of life, presenting as respiratory symptoms and diarrhea.[14,15] In children, arsenic can affect intellectual function, hepatic function, and skin.[16,17] Skin changes of arsenic poisoning include eczematoid eruptions, hyperkeratosis, and dyspigmentation. Alopecia also may occur.[1,3,6,12]

Arsenic is classified as a known human carcinogen by the National Toxicology Program and the International Agency for Research on Cancer.[18,19] In a dose-response relationship, chronic exposure is associated with an increased risk of bladder, lung, and skin cancers.[18] Exposure to arsenic in drinking water during early childhood or in utero greatly increases subsequent mortality in young adults from lung cancer.[20] Arsenic also has been associated with a higher risk of acute myelogenous leukemia, aplastic anemia, and cancers of the kidney and liver.[21] The chronic consumption of water contaminated with arsenic in a concentration of 500 ppm (1 ppm = 1 mg/L) is associated with an estimated risk of 1 in 10 people developing lung, bladder, or skin cancer. At a concentration of 50 parts per billion (ppb) (1 ppb = 1 mcg/L), cancer mortality is estimated to be in the range of 0.6 to 1.5 per 100, or approximately 1 in 100 people.[22] At 10 ppb, the US EPA drinking water standard since 2006, the risk of bladder or lung cancer is 1 to 3 per 1,000 people. Even at arsenic concentrations of 3 ppb, the lifetime risk for bladder and lung cancer is 4 to 10 per 10,000 people.[18] Given that federal standards for environmental carcinogens historically have been set at concentrations that produce a cancer risk in the range of 1 in 1 million, the allowable amount of arsenic in drinking water confers an unusually high risk.

Because of transplacental transmission of arsenic, women chronically exposed to arsenic-contaminated water are at increased risk for spontaneous abortion, stillbirth, and preterm birth.[23] Although inorganic arsenic is teratogenic in animals, it has not been shown clearly to have teratogenicity in humans.[1]

## DIAGNOSTIC METHODS

Because most arsenic is excreted in urine, the diagnostic test of choice is a urine collection.[12] In adult patients, the concentration of arsenic in a single urine specimen is commonly measured, adjusting the concentration to the concentration of urinary creatinine. Such spot urine tests for arsenic have not been well validated in children and generally are not recommended. The preferred method is a timed urinary collection for 8 to 24 hours. The method most commonly used for arsenic measurement in urine does not distinguish the organic form from the more toxic inorganic forms. Therefore, in circumstances in which it is important to determine the form of arsenic, the pediatrician should request that the urinary arsenic be speciated (see Chapter 6). Alternatively, to establish a diagnosis of intoxication by inorganic arsenic, patients should abstain from ingestion of all seafood for at least 5 days prior to conducting the urine collection. Because the half-life of arsenic in blood is short, its measurement in blood is not recommended.

Hair and fingernail analyses have been used for the diagnosis of arsenic exposure. However, like hair analysis for most other environmental agents, the validity of this test has not been established.[12] Although techniques including segmental analysis and use of pubic hair may improve the reliability of hair analysis, hair should not be the sole specimen analyzed for the diagnosis of arsenic poisoning. Similarly, fingernail analysis is not sufficiently sensitive to establish the diagnosis of arsenic poisoning. Therefore, neither hair nor nail analysis is recommended.[1,24]

## TREATMENT

If a diagnosis of significant arsenic exposure is established, chelation therapy may be indicated. Chelators demonstrated to be effective in accelerating arsenic clearance are dimercaprol, d-penicillamine, and succimer.[7] As with all metal intoxications, chelation therapy should be undertaken only in consultation with a medical toxicologist.

## PREVENTION OF EXPOSURE

Public health policies primarily have focused on control of arsenic in water. The US EPA, through the Safe Drinking Water Act, is required to regulate the concentration of water contaminants, including arsenic. Since 1947, the maximum contaminant level of arsenic in water has been 50 ppb. In 2001, the US EPA adopted a lower standard for arsenic in drinking water of 10 ppb.[25]

Further recommendations have been made to reduce the standard to 3 ppb because even at this concentration, cancer mortality risk exceeds 1 in 10,000.[22] However, municipal systems and existing technology cannot achieve—at a reasonable cost—concentrations of arsenic in water lower than 3 ppb.

The World Health Organization recommends a water standard of 10 ppb.[2] Other guidelines for the public include the recommendation that all drinking water wells be tested for arsenic.[7] In areas with large water systems, water is tested for arsenic by the water company or provider. Water providers are required to inform consumers when water fails to meet drinking water standards. In areas with elevated levels of arsenic in drinking water, home water treatment devices are available; however, these have varying efficacy at removing arsenic. Using bottled water is an option. Boiling water and filtering water through charcoal filters will not remove arsenic.

In 2012, the nonprofit Consumers Union published the results of 2 studies of arsenic in food products. The first study revealed elevated concentrations of arsenic in various apple and grape juices; the second found elevated levels of arsenic in over 200 rice-containing products, including rice cereal, a significant source of arsenic exposure in infants.[26,27] The results, published in the organization's *Consumer Reports*, called for federal regulation of arsenic in these products. In 2016, the FDA proposed draft guidance to industry to limit inorganic arsenic to 100 ppb in infant rice cereal.[28]

In 2003, as a result of an agreement between the EPA and manufacturers of pressure-treated wood, residential use of CCA ended in the United States. However, existing structures continue to be potential sources of concern.

## Frequently Asked Questions

Q  *What precautions should I take about my young children's exposure to the pressure-treated wood on my deck and playground structure?*

A  Chromated copper arsenate (CCA) is a pesticide used in pressure-treated wood to prolong its useful life. Treated wood commonly is used for decking, poles that are sunk in the ground, raised beds for gardens, and playground play structures. With aging of the wood and exposure to water, arsenic may leach out and be present on the wood surface and in soil under decks or in garden beds made of CCA-treated lumber. Touching treated wood or contaminated soils and then engaging in hand-to-mouth activities may result in children having significant exposure to arsenic, a known human carcinogen.[29,30] In several countries that have banned or severely restricted the use of CCA, alternative treatments are available. Currently, there is limited availability of lumber treated with these chemicals in the United States.[31] Coating treated wood with a sealant at least every year (in accordance with wood manufacturers' recommendations) will reduce arsenic leaching.[32] Steps to reduce children's exposure include:

1.  When possible, use alternatives to CCA-treated wood for new outdoor structures, including rot-resistant woods.

2. Keep children and pets out from under deck areas where arsenic may have leached.

3. Do not use CCA-treated wood for raised gardens, and do not grow vegetables near CCA-treated decks.

4. Never burn CCA-treated wood.

5. Make sure that children wash their hands after playing on CCA-treated surfaces, particularly before eating.

6. Cover picnic tables that are made with treated wood with a plastic cover before placing food on the table.

Q  *What types of coatings are most effective to reduce leaching of arsenic from CCA-treated wood?*

A  Some studies suggest that applying certain penetrating coatings (eg, oil-based, semitransparent stains) on a regular basis (once per year or every other year, depending on wear and weathering) may reduce the migration of wood preservative chemicals from CCA-treated wood. In selecting a finish, consumers should be aware that, in some cases, film-forming, non-penetrating stains (eg, latex semitransparent, latex opaque, oil-based opaque stains) on outdoor surfaces, such as decks and fences, are not recommended because they are less durable. Talk with someone at a hardware or paint store about appropriate coatings in your area.

Q  *My child's child care center, which has a large play structure built from pressure-treated wood, was recently found to have soil arsenic concentrations of 80 ppm. Should I be concerned?*

A  Cleanup standards for arsenic in soil are established by federal (US EPA) and state guidelines. State guidelines are highly variable, depending on background concentrations of arsenic in soil, and range from 10 to 1,000 ppm. On the basis of conservative risk estimates, remediation should be considered when the soil arsenic concentration exceeds 20 to 40 ppm in areas where children routinely play. Options, depending on concentration, include placement of a ground cover (eg, additional soil) or removal. If the source of arsenic is determined to be the structure and not background activity, the child care center also should develop a plan for frequent application of a wood sealant or other barrier while removal plans for the structure are developed.

Q  *Do I need to limit my child's seafood consumption because of possible arsenic contamination? Are there ever fish advisories about arsenic like there are for mercury and polychlorinated biphenyls?*

A  The arsenic in seafood is organic, a form that has not been associated with toxicity. Therefore, there is no reason to limit your child's consumption of seafood as an arsenic avoidance measure.

Q  *I am worried about arsenic in food products. Do I need to limit the amount of apple juice or rice cereal that I give to my child?*

A  Elevated concentrations of arsenic have been detected in studies of juices—including grape and apple—and rice products. As of 2016, the FDA has proposed an action level of 10 ppb for inorganic arsenic in juice, identical to the US EPA's 2001 limit for drinking water, and 100 ppb for infant rice cereal. Until these limits are finalized, it makes sense to vary the source of children's juice and cereal.

Rice cereal is traditionally given to infants as their first solid food, but other first foods include cereals made from other grains such as oatmeal or barley. In addition to containing less arsenic, these other cereals are less likely to cause constipation. Finely chopped or pureed meat (which has iron) and pureed vegetables may also be used as first foods. In addition, rice milk is not recommended for infants.

Q  *What other steps can I take to limit my family's exposure to arsenic in foods?*

A  A well-balanced diet contains a variety of grains other than rice, such as wheat, barley, oats, and quinoa. To decrease the amount of arsenic when eating rice, rinse it before cooking and cook the rice in plenty of water, as you would cook pasta. Look for rice syrup on food labels and avoid buying products made with rice syrup.

Q  *Our family uses a private well for our drinking water. Should the water be tested for arsenic?*

A  If your well is a new well, the water should be tested for arsenic and other contaminants. It is recommended that previously tested well water be retested for arsenic every 3 to 5 years, unless there are special circumstances warranting more frequent testing.

## References

1. Dart R. Arsenic. In: Sullivan J, Krieger G, eds. *Hazardous Materials Toxicology: Clinical Principles of Environmental Health.* Baltimore, MD: Williams & Wilkins Co; 1992:818–824

2. Breslin K. Safer sips: removing arsenic from drinking water. *Environ Health Perspect.* 1998;106(11):A548–A550

3. Malachowski ME. An update on arsenic. *Clin Lab Med.* 1990;10(3):459–472

4. Environmental Working Group. *Poisoned Playgrounds.* Washington, DC: Environmental Working Group; 2001. https://www.ewg.org/research/poisoned-playgrounds. Accessed January 20, 2018

5. Espinoza EO, Mann MJ, Bleasdell B. Arsenic and mercury in traditional Chinese herbal balls. *N Engl J Med.* 1995;333(12):803–804

6. Agency for Toxic Substances and Disease Registry. *Arsenic.* Atlanta, GA: Agency for Toxic Substances and Disease Registry; 2001. https://www.atsdr.cdc.gov/toxprofiles/tp.asp?id=22&tid=3. Accessed August 27, 2018

7. Franzblau A, Lilis R. Acute arsenic intoxication from environmental arsenic exposure. *Arch Environ Health.* 1989;44(6):385–390

8. Peters HA, Croft WA, Woolson EA, Darcey BA, Olson MA. Seasonal arsenic exposure from burning chromium-copper-arsenate-treated wood. *JAMA.* 1984;251(18):2393–2396

9. Skröder Löveborn H, Kippler M, Lu Y, et al. Arsenic metabolism in children differs from that in adults. *Toxicol Sci* 2016;152(1):29–39

10. Kaltreider RC, Davis AM, Lariviere JP, Hamilton JW. Arsenic alters the function of the glucocorticoid receptor as a transcription factor. *Environ Health Perspect.* 2001;109(3): 245–251

11. Levin-Scherz JK, Patrick JD, Weber FH, Garabedian C Jr. Acute arsenic ingestion. *Ann Emerg Med.* 1987;16(6):702–704

12. Landrigan PJ. Arsenic—state of the art. *Am J Ind Med.* 1981;2(1):5–14

13. Smith AH, Marshall G, Yuan Y, et al. Increased mortality from lung cancer and bronchiectasis in young adults after exposure to arsenic in utero and in early childhood. *Environ Health Perspect.* 2006;114(8):1293–1296

14. Farzan SF, Korrick S, Li Z, et al. In utero arsenic exposure and infant infection in a United States cohort: a prospective study. *Environ Res.* 2013;126:24–30

15. Farzan SF, Li Z, Korrick SA, et al. Infant infections and respiratory symptoms in relation to in utero arsenic exposure in a U.S. cohort. *Environ Health Perspect.* 2016;124(6):840–847

16. von Ehrenstein OS, Poddar S, Yuan Y, et al. Children's intellectual function in relation to arsenic exposure. *Epidemiology.* 2007;18(1):44–51

17. Wang SX, Wang ZH, Cheng XT, et al. Arsenic and fluoride exposure in drinking water: children's IQ and growth in Shanyin county, Shanxi province, China. *Environ Health Perspect.* 2007;115(4):643–647

18. National Toxicology Program. *14th Report on Carcinogens.* Research Triangle Park, NC: National Toxicology Program; 2016. https://ntp.niehs.nih.gov/pubhealth/roc/index-1.html. Accessed March 6, 2018

19. International Agency for Research on Cancer. Overall evaluations of carcinogenicity: an updating of IARC monographs volumes 1 to 42. *IARC Monogr Eval Carcinog Risks Hum Suppl.* 1987;7:1–440. http://monographs.iarc.fr/ENG/Monographs/suppl7/index.php. Accessed August 27, 2018

20. Liaw J, Marshall G, Yuan Y, Ferreccio C, Steinmaus C, Smith AH. Increased childhood liver cancer mortality and arsenic in drinking water in northern Chile. *Cancer Epidemiol Biomarkers Prev.* 2008;17(8):1982–1987

21. Khan MM, Sakauchi F, Sonoda T, Washio M, Mori M. Magnitude of arsenic toxicity in tube-well drinking water in Bangladesh and its adverse effects on human health including cancer: evidence from a review of the literature. *Asian Pac J Cancer Prev.* 2003;4(1):7–14

22. National Research Council. *Arsenic in Drinking Water: 2001 Update.* National Academies Press; 2001. http://www.nap.edu/books/0309076293/html/. Accessed January 14, 2018

23. Ahmad SA, Sayed MH, Barua S, et al. Arsenic in drinking water and pregnancy outcomes. *Environ Health Perspect.* 2001;109(6):629–631

24. Hall A. Arsenic and arsine. In: Shannon MW, Borron SW, Burns M, eds. *Haddad and Winchester's Clinical Management of Poisoning and Drug Overdose.* New York, NY: Elsevier Inc; 2007:1024–1027

25. US Environmental Protection Agency. Chemical contaminant rules. https://www.epa.gov/dwreginfo/chemical-contaminant-rules. Accessed January 14, 2018.

26. Consumer Reports. Arsenic in your juice: how much is too much? Federal limits don't exist. *Consum Rep.* 2012;77(1):22–27. http://www.consumerreports.org/cro/magazine/2012/01/arsenic-in-your-juice/index.htm. Accessed January 14, 2018

27. Consumer Reports. Arsenic in your food: our findings show a real need for federal standards for this toxin. *Consum Rep.* 2012;77(11):22–27. http://www.consumerreports.org/cro/magazine/2012/11/arsenic-in-your-food/index.htm. Accessed January 14, 2018

28. Food and Drug Administration. FDA proposes limit for inorganic arsenic in infant rice cereal. April 1, 2016. http://www.fda.gov/NewsEvents/Newsroom/PressAnnouncements/ucm493740.htm. Accessed January 14, 2018

29. California Department of Health Services. *Evaluation of Hazards Posed by the Use of Wood Preservatives on Playground Equipment.* Sacramento, CA: Office of Environmental Health Hazard Assessment; 1987

30. Stilwell DE, Gorny KD. Contamination of soil with copper, chromium, and arsenic under decks built from pressure treated wood. *Bull Environ Contam Toxicol.* 1997;58(1):22–29

31. Fields S. Caution—children at play: how dangerous is CCA? *Environ Health Perspect.* 2001;109(6):A262–A269

32. Consumer Reports. Exterior deck treatments test: all decked out. *Consum Rep.* 1998;63:32–34

Chapter 23

# Asbestos

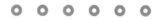

## KEY POINTS

- Asbestos is a virtually indestructible mineral that resists heat, fire, and acid and has been used in a wide range of manufactured goods since the turn of the 20th century.
- Although asbestos use has been severely curtailed in the United States since the 1970s, it has never been legally banned and remains present in homes, schools, and other buildings to this day.
- Disruption of asbestos-containing materials during construction or renovation liberates asbestos fibers into the air that pose a health risk to residents, workers, household contacts of workers, school children, and community members.
- Any level of asbestos exposure carries some health risk, including mesothelioma and lung cancer.
- In persons exposed to asbestos, smoking amplifies the risk of lung cancer 10-fold; therefore, pediatricians should emphasize the importance of not smoking when counseling families with a history of possible asbestos exposure.

## INTRODUCTION

Asbestos is a fibrous mineral product and includes 6 minerals: amosite, chrysotile, crocidolite, and the fibrous varieties of tremolite, actinolite, and anthophyllite. Asbestos occurs naturally in rock formations in certain areas of the world and is mined and refined for commercial use. It can also be found in small amounts in other rock formations, including marble and vermiculite ore, which are mined and processed for other purposes. Asbestos fibers vary in length; they may be straight or curled; they can be carded, woven, and spun into cloth; and they can be used in bulk or mixed with materials such as asphalt or cement.

Asbestos is virtually indestructible. It resists heat, fire, and acid. Because of these properties, asbestos has been used in a wide range of manufactured goods, including insulation; roofing shingles; ceiling and floor tiles; paper products; asbestos cement; clutches, brakes, and transmission parts; textiles; packaging; gaskets; and coatings. Between the 1920s and the early 1970s, millions of tons of asbestos were used in the construction of homes, schools, and public buildings in the United States, mainly for insulation and fireproofing.

Products contaminated with asbestos can be found in many settings. Today in the United States, use of asbestos in new construction has come to almost a complete halt. However, large amounts of asbestos remain in place in older buildings, especially in schools, posing a potential hazard to children, adolescents, and adults now and in the future. Large amounts of asbestos are still used in new construction in other nations, especially in certain low- and middle-income countries. In addition, children may be exposed paraoccupationally (eg, from fibers brought home on the clothes of a parent who works in an asbestos industry), or environmentally in communities where mining or manufacturing of asbestos-containing materials takes place. These routes of exposure have been linked to both noncancerous and malignant disease in adults with a history of childhood exposure. A major challenge to pediatricians, public health officials, and school authorities in the United States has been to develop a systematic and rational approach to dealing with asbestos in schools and other buildings to protect the health of children.

In 1980 (the last time that national statistics were compiled), the US Environmental Protection Agency (EPA) estimated that more than 8,500 schools nationwide contained deteriorated asbestos and approximately 3 million students (as well as more than 250,000 teachers, personnel, and staff) were at risk of exposure.[1] Subsequent field studies have found that approximately 10% of the asbestos in schools is deteriorating and/or accessible to children and, thus, poses an immediate threat to health. The remaining 90% is not deteriorating or accessible to children and, therefore, does not pose an immediate hazard.[2]

## ROUTES OF EXPOSURE

Inhalation of microscopic airborne asbestos fibers is the most concerning route of exposure. Asbestos becomes a health hazard when fibers become airborne.[3] Asbestos that is tightly contained within building materials (eg, insulation, ceiling tiles) or behind barriers poses no immediate hazard. However, when asbestos fibers are liberated into the air through deterioration, destruction, repair, or renovation of asbestos-containing materials or from hobbyist activities such as the carving of marble or soapstone that may contain asbestos, children and adults are at risk of inhaling airborne fibers.

Children can be exposed to asbestos if they live in areas where mining or refining of asbestos-containing ore occurs. From 1924 through 1990, vermiculite ore was mined and milled from Zonolite Mountain in Libby, Montana. The vermiculite was used widely in the community at residential and commercial locations. It was also disbursed across the country to as many as 245 processing sites. The ore from Libby was contaminated with asbestos, and radiologic evidence of adverse health effects has been noted in workers employed in Libby at the mine, mill, and refining plant. Workers in the mine and their families have experienced increased rates of asbestos-related diseases, including mesothelioma.[4,5] In 2002, the Agency for Toxic Substances and Disease Registry reported that asbestosis mortality rates in the Libby community were 40 to 80 times higher than expected and lung cancer mortality was 20% to 30% higher than expected.[6] Most of these cases were in workers or their household contacts. Children also can be exposed to asbestos from living in homes where Libby asbestos-contaminated vermiculite was applied to the outdoor soil and in areas where there are naturally occurring deposits of ore that contain asbestos. The US EPA preremediation Contaminant Screening Survey in Libby revealed that in the 44% of homes with visible exterior vermiculite, airborne concentrations of asbestos during digging and gardening activities were 3 to 15 times higher than that in homes without visible exterior vermiculite. In addition, 73% of inhabitants reported participating in these outdoor activities before the age of 6 years old.[7] A case-control study in California found that residential proximity to naturally occurring asbestos showed a dose-response association with mesothelioma, independent of occupational asbestos exposure.[8] A cross-sectional study of mesothelioma cases in Italy between 1993 and 2008 associated 8.8% of cases with nonoccupational exposures; 4.4% of cases resulted from living with an occupationally exposed cohabitant, and 4.3% of cases occurred in persons having no occupational exposure but who were living near a source of asbestos pollution. Clusters of environmental exposure-related cases were mainly related to asbestos-cement industry plants, ship building and repair activities, and soil contamination.[9,10]

Gastrointestinal exposure to asbestos occurs rarely, usually in circumstances in which drinking water is transferred through deteriorating asbestos-containing concrete pipes. Asbestos fibers also can enter drinking water that passes through rock formations that contain naturally occurring asbestiform fibers.

## SYSTEMS AFFECTED

Asbestos can cause cancer in the lungs, throat, larynx, and ovaries and probably in the gastrointestinal tract. Malignancies caused by asbestos also are seen in the pleura, pericardium, and peritoneum. High-dose occupational exposure (an unlikely exposure situation in children) can cause asbestosis, a fibrotic disease of the lungs and/or pleura.

## CLINICAL EFFECTS

Asbestos produces no acute toxicity. Asbestosis, sometimes referred to as white lung disease, may develop in workers who have been heavily exposed to asbestos in industry. The effects of long-term exposure to asbestos typically do not manifest until at least 20 years after the initial exposure. In its earlier stages, asbestosis neither causes symptoms nor impairs lung function. In later stages, asbestosis presents with a cough and exertional dyspnea. Data on non-cancer symptoms related to environmental exposure during childhood are sparse. An analysis was conducted on respiratory symptom data collected from persons aged 10 to 29 years who had lived in Libby, Montana and who were younger than 18 years old when the vermiculite mine closed in 1990. The analysis revealed an increased prevalence of cough (10.8%) and shortness of breath with exertion (14.5%). These symptoms were positively associated with frequent handling of vermiculate insulation.[11] Extensive pulmonary fibrosis generally develops in patients with advanced disease. Asbestosis is not seen in children because of their much lower levels of exposure.

The main risk of asbestos to children lies in its capacity to cause cancer many years after exposure. The two most important cancers caused by asbestos are lung cancer and malignant mesothelioma, a cancer that can occur in the pleura, pericardium, or peritoneum. Symptoms of mesothelioma include chest pain under the rib cage, painful coughing, shortness of breath, and unexplained weight loss. Asbestos also has been observed to cause cancer of the throat, larynx, and gastrointestinal tract among adults heavily exposed in industry. A link has been noted between low-level exposure to asbestos in the community and cancer of the ovary.[12]

The relationship between asbestos and cancer was first recognized among workers exposed occupationally as miners, shipbuilders, and insulation workers.[13] Thousands of cases of mesothelioma and lung cancer have occurred in these men and women, and cases resulting from past exposures will continue to develop for many years to come. An estimated 300,000 US workers will eventually die of asbestos-related diseases, and it is projected that 250,000 workers will die over the next 35 years in western Europe because the adoption of protective measures was delayed.[14,15] Mesothelioma cases in the

United States peaked in men in the mid-1990s and were predicted to slowly decline, although deaths were not expected to come down to background rates until 2055, 80 years after widespread use in the United States ceased.[16] In 2017, the Centers for Disease Control and Prevention reported that the annual number of mesothelioma deaths increased 4.8% from 2,479 to 2,579 between 1999 and 2015, particularly in individuals older than 85 years, although the age-adjusted death rate decreased 21.7% in the same period from 13.96 deaths to 10.93 deaths per million people. This rise in total mesothelioma deaths defies earlier predictions and may be the result of ongoing exposure from environmental sources and the liberation of asbestos fibers from renovation and construction activities despite Occupational Safety and Health Administration regulations aimed at protecting workers, their families, and members of the surrounding community.[17] Ongoing exposures in low- and middle-income nations will produce a further toll of disease and death that has not been well described.

## Lung Cancer

Asbestos exposure can, by itself, cause lung cancer. In addition, a strongly synergistic interaction has been found between asbestos and cigarette smoking, resulting in lung cancer.[18] Adults who are exposed to asbestos but who do not smoke have 5 times the background rate of lung cancer. In contrast, adults who are exposed to asbestos and who also smoke have more than 50 times the background rate of lung cancer. This powerful synergistic association is one more reason why pediatricians should urge parents, children, and adolescents not to smoke.

## Mesothelioma

Malignant mesothelioma appears to occur solely as a result of exposure to asbestos. No interaction is evident between asbestos and smoking in the causation of mesothelioma. Mesothelioma is the form of cancer that is of greatest concern for children exposed to asbestos in homes and schools because it can be caused by low levels of exposure and can appear as late as 5 decades after exposure. Women in a community in Australia who were former residents of an asbestos mining and milling town who did not work in the asbestos industry but were exposed to asbestos in their environment or in their home were found to have excess cancer mortality.[12]

## DOSE-RESPONSE

The degree of cancer risk associated with asbestos is dose-related, and the greater the cumulative exposure, the greater the risk.[19] Families with children with brief, low-level exposures to airborne asbestos should be reassured that the risk of cancer resulting from the asbestos exposure is very low. However, any exposure to asbestos involves some risk of cancer; no safe threshold level of exposure has been established. For example, mesotheliomas have been observed decades after exposure among the spouses and children of asbestos workers who brought asbestos fibers home on their work clothing, among nonsmoking women who were never employed in the asbestos industry but lived their entire lives in the asbestos mining area of Quebec, and among people who lived in a town near an asbestos-cement factory in Italy.[20,21]

Some scientists and industry representatives have claimed that the form of asbestos used most commonly in buildings in North America (Canadian chrysotile) is harmless. Extensive clinical, epidemiologic, and toxicologic data have, however, consistently documented that chrysotile asbestos is carcinogenic in experimental animals and can cause lung cancer and mesothelioma in humans.[22] All forms of asbestos are hazardous and carcinogenic. Exposure to all forms of asbestos must be kept to a minimum.[23]

## DIAGNOSTIC METHODS

There is no reliable method of detecting past asbestos exposure except through obtaining a history of exposure. Chest x-rays are not indicated for children exposed or potentially exposed to asbestos because acute radiographs provide no information about whether exposure has occurred and the children are unnecessarily exposed to ionizing radiation. The radiographic findings of pleural or pericardial plaques—raised fibrous plaques that are sometimes calcified—that occur within the pleura or pericardium are evidence of past exposure to asbestos. The latency period from first exposure to the development of pleural or pericardial plaques ranges from 10 years to more than 40 years in heavily occupationally exposed adults.[24] Such plaques were seen in 6.4% of US men and 1.7% of US women aged 35 to 74 years who were examined between 1976 and 1980 in the second National Health and Nutrition Examination Survey. No comparable data are available for children.[25]

To determine whether children are at risk of asbestos exposure or have been exposed, an environmental inspection in schools and other buildings where children live, work, and play may be undertaken by a properly certified inspector. Bulk samples of insulation or other suspicious materials should be obtained and examined by electron microscopy in a certified laboratory. Children may be at risk of exposure if asbestos in a building is deteriorating or it is within reach or renovations are taking place. Air sampling is of little value in assessing a potential asbestos hazard to children in a school because airborne releases of asbestos fibers are typically intermittent and likely to be missed.

## TREATMENT

Because asbestos exposure does not produce acute symptoms, there is no treatment for acute exposure. In addition, no treatment removes asbestos fibers from the lungs once they are inhaled. It is important to discuss the risk of developing health problems if there has been asbestos exposure (see Chapter 49). Although no exposure is completely free of risk, parents and exposed children may be assured that the risk associated with brief, low-level exposure to asbestos is minimal.[26] The context of such a discussion provides an important teachable moment in which a pediatrician can reinforce information about the need to avoid tobacco smoking. Cigarette smoking causes more than 480,000 deaths in the United States every year (see Chapter 43).

## PREVENTION OF EXPOSURE

The best way to prevent asbestos exposure is to use less hazardous materials in building construction and renovation. This approach is now followed almost universally in the United States, Canada, and western Europe, where the use of asbestos in new construction is severely restricted. The Collegium Ramazzini, an independent group of experts in environmental and occupational medicine, has issued repeated calls for an international ban on all new uses of asbestos, especially in low- and middle-income nations where asbestos is still widely used.[27,28]

The removal or renovation of existing structural asbestos may aerosolize fibers and significantly increase its hazard to health. Small areas of fraying asbestos insulation can be contained by carefully wrapping it in duct tape. Loose vermiculite attic insulation is a pebble-like, lightweight, brown or gold colored product that can contain varying amounts of asbestos and should not be disturbed. If more than minor repairs are needed or if asbestos is to be removed, a certified asbestos contractor always should be hired and full US EPA and state regulations should be obeyed. Because asbestos may not be obvious in the home, families considering remodeling should educate themselves about items that may contain asbestos that could be liberated by renovation work. Do-it-yourself removal of asbestos is never recommended.

In schools, preventing asbestos exposure requires full compliance with the provisions of the federal Asbestos Hazard Emergency Response Act (AHERA) of 1986. This act requires periodic inspection of every school—public, private, and parochial—by a certified inspector, and it establishes criteria specifying when asbestos must be removed and when it can be safely managed in place. Removal, when needed, must proceed in full compliance with state and federal laws. The results of all inspections conducted under AHERA must be made available to the public by school authorities (see Chapter 11).

## Frequently Asked Questions

Q   *How will I know if there are asbestos materials in my house?*

A   Asbestos is not found as commonly in private homes in the United States as in schools, apartment buildings, and public buildings. Nevertheless, asbestos is present in many homes, especially those built prior to the 1970s.

The following are locations in homes where asbestos may be found:
— Insulation around pipes, stoves, and furnaces (the most common locations)
— Insulation in walls and ceilings, such as sprayed-on or troweled-on material or vermiculite attic insulation (see www.epa.gov/asbestos/pubs/insulation.html)
— Patching and spackling compounds and textured paint
— Roofing shingles and siding
— Older appliances, such as washers and dryers
— Older asbestos-containing floor tiles

To determine whether your home contains asbestos, you can take the following steps:
— Evaluate appliances and other consumer products by examining the label or the invoices to obtain the product name, model number, and year of manufacture. If this information is available, the manufacturer can supply information about asbestos content.
— Evaluate building materials. A professional asbestos manager with qualifications similar to those of managers employed in school districts may be hired. This person can inspect your home to determine whether asbestos is present and give advice on its proper management.
— Test for asbestos. State and local health departments as well as regional US EPA offices have lists of individuals and laboratories certified to analyze a home for asbestos and test samples for the presence of asbestos (see Resources at the end of the chapter).

Q   *If there is asbestos in my home, what should I do?*

A   If asbestos-containing materials are found in your home, the same options exist for dealing with these materials as in a school. In most cases, asbestos-containing materials in a home are best left alone. If materials such as insulation, tiling, and flooring are in good condition and out of the reach of children, there is no need to worry. However, if materials containing asbestos are deteriorating or if you are planning renovations and the materials will be disturbed, it is best to find out whether the materials contain asbestos before renovations begin and, if necessary, have the materials properly removed. Improper removal of asbestos may cause serious contamination by dispersing fibers throughout the area. Any asbestos removal in a home must be performed by properly accredited and certified contractors. A listing of certified contractors in your area may be obtained from state or local health departments or from the regional office of the US EPA (see Resources at the end of the chapter). Many contractors who advertise themselves as asbestos experts have not been trained properly. Only contractors who have been certified by the US EPA or by a state-approved training school should be hired. The contractor should provide written proof of up-to-date certification.

Children should not be permitted to play in areas where there are friable asbestos-containing materials.

To obtain additional information about asbestos in the home, you can read more on the US EPA Web site (www.epa.gov/asbestos/pubs/ashome.html). Information can also be found on the US EPA Hotline Web site at www.epa.gov/home/epa-hotlines. State or local health departments will have additional information about asbestos (see Resources at the end of the chapter).

Q   *I had my home's air tested and the report shows asbestos fibers. What should I do?*

A   Several different methods of testing for asbestos fibers in air are available and interpretation is complex. Air testing is generally only performed if there is a known asbestos hazard identified from inspection or bulk material testing. Because of the complexity of testing and interpretation, families should consult with one of the Pediatric Environmental Health Specialty Units (www.pehsu.net) or the local Department of Health.

Q   *Is there asbestos in hair dryers?*

A   In the past, asbestos was used in some electrical appliances, including hair dryers. However, hair dryers containing asbestos were recalled by the US Consumer Product Safety Commission (CPSC) in 1980, and currently, manufacturers of household appliances in the United States are not allowed to use asbestos.

Q   *Is there asbestos in talc?*

A   Talc, like asbestos, is a mineral product. Talc from some mines contains asbestos-like fibers, and these fibers are present in talcum powder made from that talc. Because talcum powder is not required to carry a label indicating whether it contains asbestos-like fibers, parents should not use talc-containing products for infant and child care. A further reason to avoid talcum powder in the nursery is to prevent talc pneumoconiosis, which can result from accidental inhalation of bulk powder if a can should tip over into a baby's face. Talc pneumoconiosis has been associated with several infant fatalities. Women should avoid exposure because genital use of talc has been associated with ovarian cancer and has been classified as possibly carcinogenic (group 2B) by the International Agency for Research on Cancer.[29]

*Q*  *Is silica the same as asbestos?*

A  No. Silica, or silica dioxide, is a mineral most commonly called quartz and makes up most of the sand in the world. Inhalation of very fine silica particles can cause an inflammatory lung disease that can be both acute and chronic and can lead to lung fibrosis. Silicosis is almost exclusively an occupational disease described in workers without adequate respiratory protection who are engaged in mining, sandblasting, or other work that can generate large amounts of crystalline silica dust. Children can be at risk if they are engaged as child laborers in such settings. Typical sand on the beach has much larger particles and does not pose a risk of silicosis.[30]

*Q*  *Is there asbestos in play sand?*

A  Play sand that comes from naturally occurring sand deposits, such as sand dunes or beaches, generally does not contain asbestos. However, some commercially available play sand is produced by crushing quarried rock, and this sand has been shown to contain asbestos-like fibers. The CPSC does not require that the label on play sand indicate the source of the sand. The label on sand is not required to carry any information on whether it contains asbestos-like fibers. For these reasons, pediatricians are advised to warn parents against the use of play sand unless the source of the sand can be verified or the sand is certified as being free of asbestos.

*Q*  *My spouse works with asbestos. Is there danger to my child?*

A  Any family member who works in an occupation potentially involving contact with asbestos (or similar fibers such as fiberglass or reactive ceramic fibers) may bring home fibers on clothing, shoes, hair, skin, and in the car. These fibers can contaminate the home environment and become a source of exposure to children.[31]

Studies conducted in the homes of asbestos workers have shown that the dust in these homes can be heavily contaminated by asbestos fibers. Mesothelioma, lung cancer, and asbestosis all have been observed in the family members of asbestos workers. In many cases, these diseases occurred years or even decades after the exposure.

Preventing household exposure is essential. People who work with asbestos (eg, construction and demolition workers, workers who repair brakes) must scrupulously shower, change clothing, and change shoes before getting into a car and returning home. These procedures are mandated by the federal Occupational Safety and Health Act but often are not enforced. Workers often are not aware of their exposure. Exposure is prevented only if employees leave contaminated shoes and clothing at the workplace.

Many jobs involve potential occupational exposure to asbestos. These include:

- Asbestos mining and milling
- Asbestos product manufacture
- Construction trades, including sheet metal work, carpentry, plumbing, insulation work, air conditioning, rewiring, cable installation, spackling, drywall work, and demolition work
- Shipyard work
- Asbestos removal
- Fire fighting
- Custodial and janitorial work
- Brake repair

Q   *Was there a risk of asbestos exposure from the events of September 11, 2001?*

A   The risk to children associated with low levels of exposure to asbestos or with brief encounters lasting only a few days or weeks such as occurred in September 2001 in communities near the World Trade Center in New York City is not nil. However, the risk associated with such exposure is certainly much lower than the risk that results from continuing exposure, such as occurs among adults in industry who have been exposed for many years.[32]

## Resources

**Agency for Toxic Substances and Disease Registry**
Phone: 888-422-8737
Web site: www.atsdr.cdc.gov/Asbestos

**United States Consumer Product Safety Commission**
Phone: 800-638-2772
Web site: https://www.cpsc.gov/safety-education/safety-guides/home/asbestos-home

**US Environmental Protection Agency**
Phone: 202-272-0167
Web site: www.epa.gov/asbestos/index.html

**State and local health departments also can provide information about asbestos.**

# References

1. American Academy of Pediatrics, Committee on Environmental Hazards. Asbestos exposure in schools. *Pediatrics.* 1987;7(2):301–305

2. US Environmental Protection Agency. Asbestos-containing materials in schools: final rule and notice. *Fed Regist.* 1987;52:41826–41903

3. American Academy of Pediatrics, Committee on Injury and Poison Prevention. *Handbook of Common Poisonings in Children.* Rodgers GC Jr, ed. 3rd ed. Elk Grove Village, IL: American Academy of Pediatrics; 1994

4. Agency for Toxic Substances and Disease Registry. *Asbestos Exposure in Libby, Montana, Medical Testing and Results.* Atlanta, GA: Agency for Toxic Substances and Disease Registry. https://www.atsdr.cdc.gov/news/libby-pha.pdf. Accessed January 20, 2018

5. Sullivan PA. Vermiculite, respiratory disease, and asbestos exposure in Libby, Montana: update of a cohort mortality study. *Environ Health Perspect.* 2007;115(4):579–585

6. Agency for Toxic Substances and Disease Registry. *Summary Report: Exposure to Asbestos-Containing Vermiculite from Libby, Montana, at 28 Processing Sites in the United States.* http://www.atsdr.cdc.gov/asbestos/sites/national_map/Summary_Report_102908.pdf. Accessed January 14, 2018

7. Ryan PH, LeMasters GK, Burkle J, Lockey JE, Black B, Rice C. Childhood exposure to Libby amphibole during outdoor activities. *J Expo Sci Environ Epidemiol.* 2015;25(1):4–11

8. Pan XL, Day HW, Wang W, Beckett LA, Schenker MB. Residential proximity to naturally occurring asbestos and mesothelioma risk in California. *Am J Respir Crit Care Med.* 2005;172(8):1019–1025

9. Corfiati M, Scarselli A, Binazzi A, et al. Epidemiological patterns of asbestos exposure and spatial clusters of incident cases of malignant mesothelioma from the Italian national registry. *BMC Cancer.* 2015;15:286

10. Marinaccio A, Binazzi A, Bonafede M, et al. Malignant mesothelioma due to non-occupational asbestos exposure from the Italian national surveillance system (ReNaM): epidemiology and public health issues. *Occup Environ Med.* 2015;72(9):648–655

11. Vinikoor LC, Larson TC, Bateson TF, Birnbaum L. Exposure to asbestos-containing vermiculite ore and respiratory symptoms among individuals who were children while the mine was active in Libby, Montana. *Environ Health Perspect.* 2010;118(7):1033–1128

12. Reid A, Heyworth J, de Klerk N, Musk AW. The mortality of women exposed environmentally and domestically to blue asbestos at Wittenoom, Western Australia. *Occup Environ Med.* 2008;65(11):743–749

13. Selikoff IJ, Churg J, Hammond EC. Asbestos exposure and neoplasia. *JAMA.* 1964;188:22–26

14. Nicholson WJ, Perkel G, Selikoff IJ. Occupational exposure to asbestos: population at risk and projected mortality—1980-2030. *Am J Ind Med.* 1982;3(3):259–311

15. Peto J, Decarli A, LaVecchia C, Levi F, Negri E. The European mesothelioma epidemic. *Br J Cancer.* 1999;79(3-4):666–672

16. Price B, Ware A. Mesothelioma trends in the United States: an update based on surveillance, epidemiology, and end results program data for 1973 through 2003. *Am J Epidemiol.* 2004;159(2):107–112

17. Mazurek JM, Syamlal G, Wood JM, Hendricks SA, Weston A. Malignant Mesothelioma Mortality - United States, 1999-2015. *MMWR Morb Mortal Wkly Rep.* 2017;66(8):214–218

18. Selikoff IJ, Hammond EC, Churg J. Asbestos exposure, smoking and neoplasia. *JAMA.* 1968;204(2):106–112

19. Agency for Toxic Substances and Disease Registry. *Toxicological Profile on Asbestos.* 2001. https://www.atsdr.cdc.gov/toxprofiles/tp61.pdf. Accessed January 14, 2018

20. Camus M, Siemiatycki J, Meek B. Nonoccupational exposure to chrysotile asbestos and the risk of lung cancer. *N Engl J Med*. 1998;338(22):1565–1571

21. Magnani C, Dalmasso P, Biggeri A, Ivaldi C, Mirabelli D, Terracini B. Increased risk of malignant mesothelioma of the pleura after residential or domestic exposure to asbestos: a case-control study in Casale Monferrato, Italy. *Environ Health Perspect*. 2001;109(9):915–919

22. International Agency for Research on Cancer. IARC Working Group on the Evaluation of Carcinogenic Risks to Humans. IARC Monographs. Lyon, France: International Agency for Research on Cancer. 1987;Suppl 7:106–116. http://monographs.iarc.fr/ENG/Monographs/suppl7/index.php. Accessed January 14, 2018

23. Landrigan PJ. Asbestos—still a carcinogen. *N Engl J Med*. 1998;338(22):1618–1619

24. Epler GR, McLoud TC, Gaensler EA. Prevalence and incidence of benign asbestos pleural effusion in a working population. *JAMA*. 1982;247(5):617–622

25. Rogan WJ, Ragan NB, Dinse GE. X-ray evidence of increased asbestos exposure in the US population from NHANES I and NHANES II 1973–1978. National Health Examination Survey. *Cancer Causes Control*. 2000;11(5):441–449

26. Needleman HL, Landrigan PJ. *Raising Children Toxic Free: How to Keep Your Child Safe From Lead, Asbestos, Pesticides, and Other Environmental Hazards*. New York, NY: Farrar, Straus and Giroux; 1994

27. Landrigan PJ, Soffritti M. Collegium Ramazzini call for an international ban on asbestos. *Am J Ind Med*. 2005;47(6):471–474

28. Ramazzini C. Asbestos is still with us: repeat call for a universal ban. *Odontology*. 2010;98(2):97–101

29. World Health Organization. Talc Not Containing Asbestiform Fibres. In: *IARC Monographs on the Evaluation of Carcinogenic Risks to Humans*. Volume 93: Carbon Black, Titanium Dioxide, and Talc. 2010:277–412

30. Centers for Disease Control and Prevention. Preventing Silicosis. National Institute of Occupational Safety and Health (NIOSH). 10/31/1996. US Department of Labor. https://www.cdc.gov/features/preventing-silicosis/index.html. Accessed January 20, 2018

31. Chisolm JJ Jr. Fouling one's own nest. *Pediatrics*. 1978;62(4):614–617

32. Landrigan PJ, Lioy PJ, Thurston G, et al. Health and environmental consequences of the world trade center disaster. *Environ Health Perspect*. 2004;112(6):731–739

Chapter 24

# Cadmium, Chromium, Manganese, and Nickel

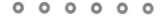

## KEY POINTS

- Cadmium has been used in imported jewelry and children's toys. The most common source is from tobacco smoke.
- Hexavalent chromium, a known carcinogen, is the most toxic form of chromium. The most likely source for children is well water; well water should be tested if this is a primary water source.
- Manganese has increasingly been found to have associations with neurotoxicity at concentrations above the adequate intake recommended.
- Allergic reactions to nickel (as contact dermatitis) are common in exposed children, and in children with orthopedic implants in whom the reaction may be mistaken for postoperative infection.

This chapter discusses cadmium, chromium, manganese, and nickel, metallic elements whose health effects are increasingly being understood (see Table 24-1).

## CADMIUM

Cadmium (Cd) is a heavy metal found in the earth's crust and is commonly associated with other metals such as lead, zinc, and copper. Thus, it is usually extracted as a byproduct when other metals are produced. It is disseminated in the environment by natural processes (erosion of rocks, forest fires, eruption

## Table 24-1. Sources, Health Effects, and Diagnosis of Exposure to Cadmium, Chromium, Manganese, and Nickel

| METAL | SOURCES | ACUTE EXPOSURE | CHRONIC EXPOSURE | DIAGNOSIS |
|---|---|---|---|---|
| Cadmium | ■ Extracted as a byproduct with other metals<br>■ Industry such as mining, smelting, battery manufacturing, coatings and platings, plastics<br>■ Gold and silver solder for jewelry<br>■ Cigarette smoke<br>■ Foods (leafy vegetables, potatoes, grains including rice, meat) | Inhalation<br>■ Severe pneumonitis (cadmium fume fever)<br>Oral (large doses)<br>■ Hemorrhagic vomiting and diarrhea with abdominal pain<br>■ Renal failure<br>■ Death | Inhalation<br>■ Renal toxicity with microproteinuria<br>■ Decreased bone mass/osteoporosis<br>■ Lung cancer<br>Oral<br>■ Itai-itai disease (syndrome of renal disease coupled with brittle bones) after eating contaminated rice<br>Children<br>■ Learning disabilities associated with higher levels (poor evidence) | ■ Urine cadmium by 24-hour collection is gold standard<br>■ Microproteinuria is the first sign of renal toxicity |
| Chromium (Hexavalent) | ■ Tanned leather<br>■ Chromated copper arsenate (CCA) lumber<br>■ Stainless steel and tin-free steel products<br>■ Chrome plating<br>■ Pigments<br>■ Cigarette smoke<br>■ Foods (meat, cheese, whole grains, eggs, fruits and vegetables)<br>■ Contaminated water | Dermal<br>■ Allergic contact dermatitis<br>■ Eczematous dermatitis (Blackjack disease)<br>Oral (large doses)<br>■ Renal failure<br>Inhalation<br>■ Acute pneumonitis<br>■ Nasal mucosal irritation, runny nose, sneezing, nosebleeds, and nasal septum ulcers | Inhalation<br>■ Nasal and lung cancers<br>■ Chronic lung disease (pneumoconiosis)<br>Dermal<br>■ Type IV hypersensitivity<br>Reproductive<br>■ Decreased fertility<br>■ Increased loss of pregnancy<br>■ Reproductive organ disease<br>■ Low birth weight infants | ■ Urine chromium reflects acute exposure (1–3 days)<br>■ Largely based on historical evidence and environmental documentation |

| | | | | |
|---|---|---|---|---|
| Manganese | ■ Foods and beverages (whole barley, rye, wheat, pecans, almonds, leafy green vegetables, tea)<br>■ Production of steel alloys, batteries, glass and ceramics<br>■ Metal cleaning, bleaching, flower preservation, and photography (permanganates)<br>■ Gasoline (organic manganese)<br>■ Air, soil, and water contamination | Inhalation<br>■ "Metal fume fever" or manganese pneumonitis<br>Dermal<br>■ Corrosive injury (permanganate solutions) | Inhalation<br>■ "Manganese madness" (emotional lability, hallucinations, asthenia, irritability, and insomnia)<br>■ Parkinson-like disease (masklike facies, cogwheel rigidity, tremor, and clumsiness)<br>■ Cognitive impairments with poor memory and attention (long-term exposures in children)<br>Reproductive<br>■ Decreased spermatogenesis (occupational exposure)<br>■ Birth defects such as still births, cleft lip, imperforate anus, cardiac defects, deafness (reproductive exposures) | ■ Whole blood analysis (normal levels found to be 4 to 15 mcg/L)<br>■ Serum concentrations and urine analysis are of limited value |
| Nickel | ■ Used in alloys with copper, chromium, iron, and zinc<br>■ Used to manufacture stainless steel<br>■ Tobacco smoke (nickel carbonyl)<br>■ Emissions from mining and recycling, steel production, and municipal incineration<br>■ Power plants fueled by peat, coal, natural gas, and oil<br>■ Industrial waste<br>■ Food and contaminated water (cocoa, nuts, soybeans, oatmeal, vegetables, fish)<br>■ Iatrogenic exposures (dialysis, dental and surgical prostheses) | Dermal<br>■ Allergic contact dermatitis | Inhalation<br>■ Respiratory cancers of lung, larynx, and nasopharyngeal passages<br>■ Adrenal, hepatic and renal failure leading to death (nickel carbonyl)<br>■ Atopic dermatitis (nickel sulfate)<br>■ Endocrinopathies<br>■ Cardiovascular illness | ■ Urine concentrations (5 mcg/L upper limit of normal) |

of volcanoes) and by human activities (mining; smelting; disposal of products containing cadmium, such as batteries; waste incineration).[1] Cadmium can be taken up by plants (in particular, "root" plants, such as potatoes or onions) or animals (in particular, in the liver and kidneys), thereby entering the food chain. Airborne cadmium pollution from hazardous waste sites and/or industry may create inhalational exposures. Cadmium is a common industrial chemical used in the production of batteries (primary), pigments, coatings and platings, and as a stabilizer for plastics. Its fume is generated by use of gold and silver solder during jewelry fabrication. Cigarette smoke is a well-known source of cadmium because tobacco plants take up cadmium found in soil. The nicotine liquids used in electronic cigarettes and "vaping" solutions do not contain cadmium. Cadmium has been found in children's jewelry.[2]

## Routes of Exposure

Cadmium can be ingested or inhaled. The primary route of exposure in children is via ingestion of food contaminated with cadmium in the soil. A child may be exposed after swallowing cadmium-containing jewelry. Exposure may also occur from biting, sucking, or mouthing cadmium-containing jewelry or from hand-to-mouth contact after handling a jewelry piece.[2] Cadmium may be inhaled through exposure to secondhand tobacco smoke (SHS). Dermal absorption is negligible.

## Sources of Exposure

Significant potential sources of cadmium exposure for humans include foods (leafy vegetables, potatoes, grains [rice], liver/kidney meats), tobacco smoke, and occupational exposures. Areas with very high levels of cadmium in the soil can lead to significant exposure through locally grown food.[3,4]

## Biological Fate

Absorption of cadmium depends on the route of exposure. After inhalation, cadmium is well absorbed from the lungs. Nearly 50% of inhaled cadmium is absorbed from the lungs into the systemic circulation during active smoking.[1,5,6] Smokers typically have cadmium blood concentrations that are much higher than those of nonsmokers.[4] Smokers (and children exposed to SHS) also have higher urinary cadmium concentrations.[7] Gastrointestinal tract absorption is less efficient, and adults absorb approximately 1% to 10% of ingested cadmium.[1,8] Nutritional deficiencies, such as iron deficiency, will increase cadmium absorption.[9] Dermal absorption is slow and would not result in significant toxicity unless the cadmium were in a concentrated solution in contact with skin for a prolonged time (eg, hours).[10]

Cadmium bioaccumulates in the liver and kidneys, with approximately 50% of total cadmium body stores found in these 2 organs. Bone is a third depot for cadmium, and bone toxicity can be direct (through incorporation into the bone matrix) and indirect (via renal disease and subsequent disturbances in calcium excretion and vitamin D metabolism). The elimination half-life of cadmium in the liver and kidney ranges from 10 to 40 years with most of the body burden in the kidney. The primary route of elimination is through the urine. The rate of excretion is low, in part because cadmium binds tightly to metallothionein, a transport and storage protein synthesized in response to cadmium and zinc exposure, preventing excretion into the tubules. In addition, most filtered cadmium is reabsorbed in the renal tubules. Cadmium concentration in blood reflects recent exposure; urinary cadmium concentration more closely reflects total body burden. However, the kidney also is a prime target of cadmium toxicity, and if renal damage from cadmium exposure occurs, the excretion rate may increase sharply, and urinary cadmium concentrations will no longer reflect the body burden.[11]

## Systems Affected

Exposure to cadmium may affect organs including the lungs, nervous system, bones, and kidneys. The route of exposure in some cases may determine the site of toxicity (ie, inhalation and lung toxicity). The property of bioaccumulation tends to increase the risks from chronic toxicity.

## Clinical Effects

### Acute and Short-term Effects

Acute exposure via inhalation can lead to severe pneumonitis (cadmium fume fever). In humans, several fatal inhalation exposures have occurred through occupational accidents. High-dose inhaled cadmium is particularly toxic to the lungs and produces a well-described pneumonitis with fever and significant radiographic changes. During the acute inhalation, symptoms are relatively mild, but within a few days following exposure, severe pulmonary edema and chemical pneumonitis develop, sometimes causing death because of respiratory failure. Exposures to environmental contaminants (eg, cadmium in secondhand smoke) have little acute toxicity, but bioaccumulation of cadmium is a concern for chronic health effects because of cadmium's very long elimination half-life.

Large oral exposure can produce vomiting, diarrhea (which can be hemorrhagic), and abdominal pain. This can progress to renal failure and death.

Silver et al,[12] using data from the National Health and Nutrition Examination Survey (NHANES), reported higher serum cadmium levels associated with iron deficiency and iron-deficiency anemia. Although the cadmium exposures may have decreased iron absorption leading to anemia, it is also possible that the iron deficiency increased the absorption of cadmium.

## Chronic Toxicity

Cadmium is well recognized as a toxicant in occupational exposures. Chronic occupational exposures most commonly produce renal toxicity; micropro-teinuria is one of the earliest signs. Chronic exposure effects also include decreased bone mass/osteoporosis and lung cancer.[13,14] A tragic episode of industrial dumping of cadmium into the environment occurred in the Jinzu and Kakehashi river basins in Japan, leading to contamination of locally grown rice. This event produced widespread human exposure and a syndrome of renal disease coupled with brittle bones referred to as "Itai-itai" (ouch-ouch) disease.[15] The disease was particularly common among women, perhaps because of their higher prevalence of iron deficiency and, therefore, greater cadmium absorption.[9]

The US Environmental Protection Agency (EPA) has classified cadmium as a group B1 or "probable" human carcinogen; the International Agency for Research on Cancer (IARC) and the US National Toxicology Program have classified cadmium as a known human carcinogen.[13]

Some epidemiologic studies have suggested that cadmium exposure may be associated with adverse neurodevelopmental outcomes in children. Nationally representative data from NHANES for children 6 years and older showed that higher urinary cadmium concentrations were associated with a higher risk for the development of learning disabilities and the need for special educa-tion; there was no association found for a higher risk of attention-deficit/hyperactivity disorder (ADHD).[16] It is possible that cadmium exposure contributes to these neurobehavioral effects. The study authors acknowledge that it is also possible that children with neurobehavioral effects have behaviors and activities that result in higher cadmium exposure.

ADHD has not been associated with higher urinary cadmium concentra-tions.[14] This finding was confirmed in a subsequent case-control study in which postnatal lead exposure was associated with ADHD, but no association was found with postnatal exposures to mercury or cadmium.[16,17] Poverty also has been associated with higher cadmium urine concentrations.[14]

## Diagnosis

Cadmium can be measured in whole blood or urine. Urinary cadmium concentrations are considered to be the gold standard measure of cumulative exposure because cadmium accumulates in the kidney; urine concentrations, thus, reflect long-term exposure. Twenty-four–hour urine collections are often desirable, but spot urine measures in conjunction with urinary creatinine to adjust for urine volume have been used to assess exposure.[1] Young children, however, typically have lower urine creatinine concentrations, and adjusting the measured cadmium concentration by creatinine can inflate the adjusted value (see Chapter 6). Twenty-four–hour urinary excretion in adults should be less than 10 mcg/g of creatinine; there is no child-specific standard to determine cadmium toxicity.

Background urine and blood concentrations in American children have been measured as part of the NHANES. Data from 2013 to 2014 indicated that fewer than 30% of children aged 1 to 12 years had blood cadmium concentrations above the detection limit of 0.1 mcg/L. The 75th percentile for children aged 1 to 5 years was 0.10 mcg/L, and for children aged 6 to 11 years was 0.12 mcg/L. Urine cadmium also was not detectable above 0.036 mcg/L in most children aged 6 to 11 years, but the 75th percentile was 0.05 mcg/L (0.086 mcg/g creatinine). In the same time period, children aged 12 to 19 years had a geometric mean urine cadmium concentration of 0.064 mcg/L (0.058 mcg/g creatinine) and adults older than 19 years had a geometric mean of 0.156 mcg/L (0.182 mcg/g creatinine).[18]

Among adults with low levels of environmental exposure, urine concentrations as low as 1 mcg/g creatinine have been associated with an increased likelihood of microproteinuria and renal markers of adverse kidney effects, including N-acetyl-β-glucosaminidase.[19] The earliest signs of renal abnormalities in adult workers typically occur at 2 mcg/g creatinine and include microscopic proteinuria—in particular, $\beta_2$-microglobulin and $\alpha_1$-microglobulin are spilled. Each of these can also be measured directly. At urinary cadmium concentrations of 4 mcg/g of creatinine, enzymes such as N-acetyl-β-glucosaminidase are found in urine; signs of more significant glomerular damage (eg, albumin in the urine, decreases in the glomerular filtration rate) are seen. In the final stages of cadmium nephropathy, glycosuria, wasting of calcium and phosphate, and altered calcium metabolism with secondary effects on the skeleton (osteoporosis and osteomalacia) are seen, in part resulting from the effects on the kidneys and bone.[20]

## Treatment

No effective treatment exists for cadmium toxicity. Chelation therapy mobilizes tissue cadmium and increases renal cadmium concentrations, increasing renal toxicity.

## Prevention of Exposure

Because there is no effective treatment for cadmium toxicity or exposure, prevention is key. Children younger than 6 years should not be given or allowed to play with inexpensive metal jewelry.[2] Cadmium should not be used in consumer products unless absolutely necessary, particularly in products designed to be used by or with children. Cadmium is not allowed to be used in children's jewelry manufactured in the United States. Reducing children's exposure to secondhand smoke has obvious health benefits beyond reducing cadmium exposure. Consumption of the liver and kidney from exposed animals are potential sources of cadmium in the diet. Exposure to environmental cadmium can be prevented by reducing environmental levels in soil, in water used to irrigate food crops, and by reducing drinking water levels of cadmium. Cadmium concentrations in drinking water supplies are typically less than 1 mcg/L (1 part per billion [ppb, equivalent to mcg/L]). The US EPA established a no-observed-adverse-effect level (NOAEL) of 0.01 mg/kg/day in water and set the maximum contaminant level (MCL) for cadmium in water at 0.005 mg/L or 5 ppb.[1]

## CHROMIUM

Chromium (Cr) is a metal found in the earth, in plants, and in animals, including humans. The most common forms are elemental (metallic) chromium (0), trivalent chromium (III), and hexavalent chromium (VI).[21] Chromium (III), the naturally occurring form, is an essential nutrient. Chromium stimulates fatty acid and cholesterol synthesis and is important in insulin metabolism.[22] Hexavalent chromium (chromate) is derived mainly by industrial processes but can occur by the oxidation of trivalent chromium. Hexavalent is a toxic form of chromium.

Chromium can be found in many consumer products including leather tanned with chromic sulfate and stainless-steel cookware. Chromated copper arsenate (CCA) was used in the past as a wood preservative. Pressure-treated lumber containing CCA may still be present in outdoor playgrounds and other structures (see Chapter 22). Some wood is now treated with copper dichromate. Children have higher chromium levels on their hands when playing in playgrounds treated with CCA compared with playgrounds treated without the arsenic component; this implies that the arsenic-bound chromium is released more readily than chromium alone.[23] Chromium, in its elemental form, is a component of iron-based alloys such as stainless steel and tin-free steel. During the production of steel, chromium and its oxides can be released into the environment intentionally or unintentionally.[24] Chromium is present in tobacco smoke.[21]

### Routes of Exposure

Chromium can be ingested, inhaled, and absorbed through the skin. Hexavalent chromium crosses the placenta and passes into human milk.

### Sources of Exposure

Chromium is naturally found in many foods and beverages (eg, meat, cheese, whole grains, eggs, some fruits and vegetables). The Adequate Intake (AI [a dietary recommendation made by the Food and Nutrition Board of the

Institute of Medicine]) for chromium ranges from 0.2 mcg/day for infants to 35 mcg/day for adolescent males to 45 mcg/day for lactating women.[22]

Chromium enters the soil, air, and water primarily as a result of industrial emissions of the trivalent and hexavalent forms. Typical chromium concentrations in soil are 37 parts per million (ppm [equivalent to mg/kg]) but can range from 1 to 2,000 ppm.[21] Chromium is a contaminant found in approximately 50 National Priorities List Superfund hazardous waste sites and in many landfills. Chromium in air is found as fine dust particles that can settle in soil and water.[24] Most atmospheric chromium results from anthropogenic sources including fossil fuel combustion and steel production. Chromium concentrations in the atmosphere are estimated at 0.01 mcg/m$^3$ in rural areas and 0.01 to 0.03 mcg/m$^3$ in urban areas.[21] Chromium is not a regulated air contaminant.

The amount of chromium in uncontaminated water is low. Historically, chromium contamination of water could be extensive with groundwater exceedances found from naturally occurring and industrial releases into groundwater aquifers where chromium can move to areas distant from the original site of contamination.[25] Typical concentrations of chromium in tap water are 0.4 to 8.0 ppb and concentrations in rivers and lakes typically are between 1 and 30 ppb.[21] Ground water contamination has occurred. Between 1952 and 1966, the Pacific Gas and Electric Company dumped millions of gallons of chromium-containing waste water in areas around Hinkley, California. Concentrations of hexavalent chromium in water were 580 ppb in ground and well-water, far in excess of the state limit of 50 ppb.[25]

Children's exposure to hexavalent chromium most commonly occurs via ingestion of contaminated water or play near a hazardous waste site.[21] Chromium-laden dust can be found in house dust in areas where there is significant local contamination. Adults who work in industries using chromium can bring significant amounts into the home on clothing and shoes. When children play on structures made of wood preserved with CCA, chromium and arsenic are detectable on their hands.[23] There are no current data to indicate that chromium from CCA is absorbed and enters the blood. Exposure to chromium from burning or demolition of wood treated with CCA appears to be small.[26]

## Biological Fate

Absorption of chromium depends on the route of exposure and the form of the element. After inhalation, elemental and trivalent chromium are poorly absorbed; in contrast, the hexavalent form, because it is more water soluble, is well absorbed from the lungs. After ingestion, trivalent chromium salts are poorly absorbed (less than 2%), but up to 50% of the hexavalent form can be absorbed from the gastrointestinal tract.[27] A significant proportion of ingested hexavalent chromium, however, is converted to the less soluble trivalent form in the gut, considerably limiting its absorption. Hexavalent chromium in the blood also is converted rapidly to the less toxic trivalent chromium by erythrocytes. After dermal contact, chromium (III) and (VI) are both absorbed; the amount depends on the condition of the skin and the particular compound.[21,28]

Chromium is stored in all body tissues although retention does not seem to be prolonged; the kidneys excrete approximately 60% of a chromium dose within 8 hours of ingestion.[21] An estimated 80% of chromium is excreted by the kidneys; bile and sweat are minor routes of excretion.

## Systems Affected

Acute exposure to chromium may affect organs including the skin, gastrointestinal tract, kidneys, and lungs.

## Clinical Effects

### Acute and Short-term Effects

Hexavalent chromium, the most toxic of the three forms of chromium, can have immediate and long-term effects. Even short-term skin exposure can result in significant irritation and sensitization, producing allergic contact dermatitis with subsequent exposures. Chromium is considered second only to nickel in being the most allergenic metal to which humans are regularly exposed.[21] Once found in significant concentration in detergents and bleaches, chromium was thought to be the cause of the once common "housewives' eczema."[29] "Blackjack disease" was a term describing eczematous dermatitis found in card players exposed to chromium in felt. Ingestion of high-dose hexavalent chromium produces gastrointestinal symptoms (ie, nausea, vomiting, hematemesis), which can be severe. Large ingestions can produce acute renal failure. High-dose inhalation can produce acute pneumonitis. Other acute toxicities include effects on the nasal mucosa, with runny nose, sneezing, nosebleeds, and with repeated exposures, nasal septum ulcers.[21]

### Chronic/Long-term Effects

Chronic inhalation of hexavalent chromium is associated with increased risks of nasal and lung cancers in adults, including people who work in industries using chromium.[21,24,28] The IARC, the US National Toxicology Program, the World Health Organization (WHO), and the US EPA have concluded that hexavalent chromium is a human carcinogen.[19] The risk of lung cancer increases with the duration of exposure, with latency periods ranging from 13 to 30 years (although cases have appeared following as few as 5 years of exposure).[21,30] Declines in the incidence of cancer as exposures fall among chromium workers suggest a threshold effect for the carcinogenic potential of hexavalent chromium. Carcinogenicity has not been observed from exposure to elemental or trivalent chromium salts, but DNA adducts formed from intermediates during the intracellular reduction of hexavalent chromium to trivalent chromium have been suggested as a mechanism.[30] Data suggest that hexavalent chromium increases the risk of other cancers (bone, stomach, prostate cancers; lymphoma, leukemia) in adults.

Hexavalent chromium has other toxicities. Low birth weight, birth defects, and other reproductive toxicities have been observed in experimental animal models of chronic hexavalent chromium exposure.[21] Epidemiologic studies in humans have documented decreased fertility, increased pregnancy losses, and reproductive organ diseases and neoplasms with ongoing exposure to hexavalent chromium in nonindustrial settings.[31] Pregnant women with increased urinary concentrations of hexavalent chromium were found to have an increased risk of having low birth weight infants.[32]

Type IV hypersensitivity skin reactions with contact dermatitis or eczema are common consequences of long-term dermal exposure in which eczema develops on the hands in approximately 20% of workers who perform wet work. Dermatitis from chromium has decreased over time because of regulatory efforts.[29] Chronic inhalational exposure can produce chronic lung disease (pneumoconiosis).

## Diagnosis

Chromium can be measured in serum or urine; however, blood can be contaminated with chromium that is a component of the stainless-steel needle used in the specimen collection. In a representative sample of adults in the United States who had blood chromium measured in 2015 to 2016, only about 10% had concentrations above 0.41 mcg/L, the limit of detection; the 95th percentile was 1.08 mcg/L.[18] Total serum concentrations have been reported as ranging from 0.052 to 0.156 mcg/L. Urine measurement of chromium generally reflects absorption over the previous 1 to 3 days; the typical range of concentration in urine is 0 to 40 mcg/L.[33] Samples of human milk may have an average concentration of 0.3 ppb of chromium. These analyses are not useful in the clinical setting. Because of species interconversion, no biological specimen has sufficient sensitivity to identify exposure to one particular form (eg, hexavalent).[21] Diagnosis of toxicity, therefore, relies largely on historical evidence and environmental documentation of exposure, supplemented by biological monitoring.

## Treatment

Any treatment of chromium (as well as manganese and nickel) exposure should be conducted in consultation with an expert in pediatric environmental health and/or occupational health. No known chelators of chromium are available. Given its rapid and apparently complete elimination, however, chelation should not be needed. Ascorbic acid (vitamin C) is considered a valuable treatment after hexavalent chromium ingestion because of its ability to reduce hexavalent chromium to the less soluble trivalent chromium.

## Prevention of Exposure

Exposure to chromium can be prevented by fencing hazardous land sites and prohibiting children from playing in soils near sites where chromium may have been discarded. Because of possible chromium contamination of well water, analysis for chromium in well water should be considered before that water is consumed. The US EPA has set a limit of 100 ppb total chromium (not hexavalent specifically) in water.[34] Chromium concentrations in air are not regulated, although control measures are being enacted; environmental rules that help to reduce exposure from ambient atmospheric pollution are needed.

Ingestions of chromium also should be minimized. Reference (maximum recommended) doses for chromium are 1 mg/kg per day for trivalent chromium and 5 mcg/kg per day for hexavalent chromium.[21]

## MANGANESE

Manganese (Mn) is a metal known for its light weight and durability. Uses of inorganic manganese include production of steel alloys, batteries, glass and ceramics, incendiaries, fungicides, and as a catalyst for the chlorination of organic compounds. Permanganates (manganese oxides) are used as disinfectants and in metal cleaning, bleaching, flower preservation, and photography. Organic manganese compounds are used as gasoline and fuel oil additives and as fungicides.[35] Manganese is an essential human nutrient involved in the formation of bone and in the metabolism of amino acids, lipids, and carbohydrates. Manganese is required in several enzymes: hexokinase, xanthine oxidase, pyruvate carboxylase, arginase, manganese superoxide dismutase, and the neuron-specific enzyme glutamine synthetase.[22]

Manganese is present in the environment in inorganic and organic forms. There are 7 species of inorganic forms, ranging in valence from 0 to $7^+$; heptavalent manganese includes the permanganates, which are potent oxidizing agents. The primary organomanganese compound of concern is methylcyclopentadienyl manganese tricarbonyl (MMT), an antiknock gasoline additive.[35]

### Routes of Exposure

Manganese can be ingested and inhaled. Manganese crosses the placenta and passes into human milk.

### Sources of Exposure

Foods and beverages are significant sources of manganese. Foods high in manganese include whole barley, rye, and wheat; pecans; almonds; and leafy green vegetables. The highest amounts are found in nuts. Tea is a high-source beverage. Foods and beverages provide mean daily intakes of 2.7 and 3.4 mg in women and men, respectively. Dietary intake is much higher among vegetarians, approaching 10 mg daily.[22] Higher blood manganese levels have been observed in pregnant women, suggesting that gender and reproductive status should be considered when assessing for manganese toxicity.[36]

The AI for manganese varies. Infants younger than age 6 months have an AI of 0.003 mg/day whereas those between age 6 and 12 months should receive 0.6 mg/day. Children older than 1 year can receive between 1.2 and 2.2 mg/day depending on their age. The requirement is higher in pregnant and breast feeding women (2 and 2.6 mg/day, respectively).[22] Manganese concentration in human milk is very low (4 to 8 mcg/L) and varies with month of lactation. In addition, elevated manganese levels in mothers do not correlate with levels in human milk.[37] Cow milk and cow milk-based formulas have concentrations of 15 to 25 mcg/L, and soy formulas have concentrations 50 to 75 times higher than human milk. Absorption is greater from human milk. Soy and rice "milks" that are not formulas and not intended to be ingested by infants may contain even more manganese and result in intakes that exceed the upper limit for children aged 1 to 3 years.[38] Dietary supplements and alternative medicines can contain significant amounts of manganese; cases of manganese toxicity from the use of a Chinese herbal remedy have been reported.[22]

Diet (ie, food and formula for children) is the primary source of manganese which, alone, may result in elevated levels. The Tolerable Upper Level of Intake (UL) has been assessed with a dose of 11 mg/day as the NOAEL in adults. Further studies have determined the Lowest Observable Adverse Effect Level (LOAEL) to be 15 mg/day in adults. Data are inadequate regarding risks to children. Thus, the UL for children is extrapolated using reference body weights within assigned age groups. The UL has not been established for children younger than 1 year. The UL's for children older than 1 year range from 2 mg to 6 mg/day depending on the age of the child. No adjustments for pregnant or lactating women have been made.[22]

Major sources of nondietary manganese exposure for children include air, water, and soil pollution.[35] Average levels of manganese in outdoor air are generally higher in urban areas and have decreased over time.[39] Sources of atmospheric manganese include combustion of fossil fuels (20%) and industrial emissions (80%). In 2015, manganese accounted for 7% of total releases from facilities reporting to the US EPA. Over 223 million pounds were released into air (1%), water (3%), land (66%), or offsite disposal sites (31%).[40]

Methylcyclopentadienyl manganese tricarbonyl (25.2% manganese) was introduced into gasoline in the 1970s, replacing lead as an antiknock compound. An initial ban of MMT in the late 1970s was lifted in 1995, but

MMT is rarely used today in the United States. It continues to be used in other countries (see Chapter 30).

Water contamination is another potential source of excess manganese. Freshwater typically contains manganese in a range of 1 to 200 mcg/L. Well water contamination from natural and anthropogenic sources is relatively common, with concentrations up to an order of magnitude greater (up to 2,000 mcg/L).

Soil can contain high manganese concentrations occurring naturally and from surface pollution. Concentrations of manganese in soil range from 40 to 900 ppm, with an average of 330 ppm; concentrations near industry can approach 4,600 ppm.[41] This may also impact levels of manganese in indoor dust samples which are higher in homes in closer proximity to industry. Dust samples in homes near agricultural areas using manganese-containing fungicides were also found to have higher levels of manganese depending on housekeeping practices and soil types.[41,42] In a pattern similar to that observed when lead was added to gasoline, manganese concentrations in soil decrease as distances from heavily traveled roads increase.[35]

## Biological Fate

Manganese, an essential constituent of several metalloenzymes, is associated with bone and connective tissue formation, reproduction, and metabolism. Absorption from the gut is highly regulated via homeostatic mechanisms. Iron and manganese share the same mucosal transport system. Very little manganese is absorbed from the gastrointestinal tract; the average absorption of dietary manganese averages 3% to 5%.[22,35] Children have less well developed homeostatic mechanisms for regulating manganese absorption and elimination. Iron deficiency and low protein intake are associated with increased oral manganese absorption, and high dietary calcium or phosphate decrease its absorption. There appears to be extensive genetic modulation of manganese absorption from the gut, mediated by the highly prevalent hemochromatosis gene. Women typically absorb more manganese than men, presumably because of their lower iron stores. During pregnancy, levels of maternal and fetal manganese biomarkers change; maternal levels of manganese do not appear to be strongly related to fetal levels.[43] Once absorbed, manganese is transported by plasma proteins (including the β-1 globulin transmanganin) and within erythrocytes, and then is distributed to the tissues.[44] Plasma protein transferrin also is important in manganese transport. The biological half-life of manganese is approximately 40 days in blood but may be longer with chronic exposures and accumulation in deep compartments. Elimination is primarily via feces, and to a minor extent, via urine.

In animals, manganese was eliminated from the brain at a slower rate compared with the liver and kidney. Studies in rats suggest that bone accumulation can occur and may account for continued increase of manganese concentrations in the central nervous system (CNS) after exposure has ended.[44]

Unlike ingested manganese, inhaled manganese is completely absorbed; through this route, it can be transported directly to the CNS via nasal mucosa and the lungs.[35]

## Systems Affected

Acute exposure to manganese can affect the lungs and skin. Chronic exposure may result in neurotoxicity, pulmonary disease, and reproductive toxicity.

## Clinical Effects

### Acute Effects

Acute exposure to manganese oxides can produce a syndrome known as "metal fume fever" or manganese pneumonitis.[35] This syndrome includes flulike symptoms, such as fever, cough, congestion, and malaise. This illness most commonly occurs in the industrial setting with processes such as welding or metal cutting. Permanganate solutions can be extremely corrosive.[45] CNS toxicity from manganese has only been reported following long-term or chronic exposure.

### Chronic/Long-term Effects

Central nervous system effects of manganese were first described in the 1800s, when the term "manganese madness" was first coined in workers.[35] Initial symptoms of manganese toxicity are psychiatric, characterized by emotional lability, hallucinations, asthenia, irritability, and insomnia. Chronic manganese intoxication (manganism) is best known for inducing neurological injury that mimics Parkinson disease, with masklike facies, cogwheel rigidity, tremor, and clumsiness. This syndrome typically appears after 2 to 25 years of excess manganese exposure but also has been observed within several months of heavy exposure.[35] Manganese-induced neurotoxicity can be progressive and can worsen after exposure has ended. Decreased verbal and visual memory was reported in a 10-year-old child who was chronically exposed by drinking well water with high manganese levels.[46]

Multiple mechanisms for neurotoxicity have been proposed. Manganese can displace iron from transferrin; the neurotoxicity of manganese may, therefore, be related to increases in iron-induced oxidative injury to neurons.[47] Experimental studies in animals suggest that neonates have greater transport of manganese into the CNS, a lower threshold for manganese-induced neurotoxicity, and greater retention of manganese in the brain compared with older animals.[48] Iron deficiency is associated with increased CNS concentrations of manganese because of upregulation of divalent metal transporters in the

CNS.[47] Therefore, infants, children, and menstruating women are at greater risk of manganese neurotoxicity. Iron excess also increases the risk of manganese neurotoxicity. Pathologic changes include deterioration of the globus pallidus and corpus striatum as well as decreased activity of catecholamines (particularly dopamine) and serotonin in the corpus striatum.[47] Unlike Parkinson disease, manganese toxicity is associated with preservation of nigro-striatal dopaminergic pathways.[48] Liver failure-associated encephalopathy has also been associated with increased manganese levels suggesting that decreased clearance can result in accumulation and toxicity. Manganese may interact with copper for its transport; low CNS copper levels have been found after manganese exposures.[49]

Although manganese-induced neurotoxicity is most commonly found after chronic inhalation, ingestion of manganese-contaminated water also has been associated with neurotoxicity. Children with environmental exposure to manganese in drinking water and associated elevated blood manganese levels had lower scores on neuropsychological tests, with more pronounced effects in rural children.[50] A review of studies found evidence for cognitive impairments associated with manganese exposures, although limitations existed because co-exposures were not assessed.[51] Children with chronic exposures (greater than 3 years) of high levels of manganese in drinking water were found to have poorer memory and attention, but no association with hyperactivity was found.[52] Chronic inhalation of manganese dust can lead to pulmonary disease, manifested by chronic respiratory tract inflammation.[35]

Prenatal and early life exposures to higher levels of manganese have been associated with adverse neuromotor function in adolescents.[53] Similarly, maternal blood manganese levels at the time of delivery were negatively associated with neurodevelopmental outcomes in childhood. A review of perinatal exposures to metals and mixtures found that early life exposures to manganese were consistently associated with cognitive and behavioral impairments in children. There is a strong recognition that exposures to metal mixtures have a more pronounced impact on neurodevelopment than exposures to manganese alone.[54] Reproductive toxicities in males can occur with chronic manganese exposure. Decreased spermatogenesis occurs in animals; epidemiologic studies have shown a significant decrease in the number of children born to workers exposed to manganese dust.[55] Stillbirths and birth defects, including cleft lip, imperforate anus, cardiac defects, and deafness, have been reported in populations chronically exposed to excessive manganese.[35]

## Diagnosis

Normal ranges of manganese concentrations are approximately 4 to 15 mcg/L in blood, 1 to 8 mcg/L in urine, and 0.4 to 0.85 mcg/L in serum. Manganese is bound to red blood cells, making serum concentrations very low and subject to contamination by hemolysis. The NHANES has been measuring whole blood and urine manganese in a representative sample of the US population since 2011. In the 2011 to 2012 and 2013 to 2014 survey periods, the geometric mean whole blood manganese for children aged 1 to 5 years was 10.7 and 10.9 mcg/L and the 95th percentile was 18.2 and 18.3 mcg/L, respectively. Children aged 6 to 11 years had similar whole blood concentrations.[56] Urinary measurements are of limited value to evaluate manganese exposure most likely because urine is a minor route for manganese elimination. In the 2011 to 2012 NHANES survey period, the geometric mean urinary manganese for the total population was 0.123 mcg/L, and for children aged 6 to 11 years, was 0.143 mcg/L.[18] Human milk concentrations of manganese vary widely (6.2 mcg/L to 17.6 mcg/L) depending on when the sample is taken after birth and, presumably other factors.[35]

## Treatment

Treatment of excess manganese exposure may include chelation therapy, but it has not been documented to be effective for toxic manganese exposures.[57] However, one case report documents a young child with neurological deficits and significantly elevated manganese levels who was prescribed a manganese-free diet and underwent chelation with calcium disodium edetate (CaNa$_2$EDTA) 4 months after her initial presentation. By report, she had mild improvement of acute symptoms but residual gait abnormalities.[58] Thus, CaNa$_2$EDTA may increase urinary excretion and result in clinical improvement in selected cases of severe acute manganese intoxication. It should not, however, be routinely recommended. Hemodialysis is ineffective.[59]

## Prevention of Exposure

Prevention of manganese exposure includes taking environmental actions to reduce outdoor air pollution and ensuring that water supplies, particularly well water, are closely monitored. The US EPA has calculated a reference ambient air concentration (an estimate of a continuous inhalation exposure to humans [including sensitive subgroups] that is likely to be without an appreciable risk of deleterious effects during a lifetime) of manganese on the basis of changes in neuropsychological function in adults, to equal 0.05 mcg/m$^3$.[60] This reference dose was last updated in 1993. It has not been updated since; therefore, information from current literature has not been taken into account. The US EPA limit for manganese in water is 50 mcg/L. Because this is not a health-based standard and is set for aesthetic or cosmetic reasons to avoid stains on plumbing and laundered clothes, all efforts should be made to ensure that concentrations of manganese in drinking water remain below this concentration. Methylcyclopentadienyl manganese tricarbonyl should not be used in gasoline.

## NICKEL

Nickel (Ni) is a white magnetic metal commonly used in alloys with copper, chromium, iron, and zinc. These alloys are used in fuel production, making jewelry, clothing fasteners, metallic coins, domestic utensils, medical prostheses, heat exchangers, valves, and magnets. Most is used to manufacture stainless steel. Nickel salts are used in electroplating, pigments, ceramics, and batteries, and serve as a catalyst in food production. Nickel compounds, especially nickel carbonyl ($Ni[CO]_4$), a potent carcinogen, are present in tobacco smoke.[61]

Nickel occurs naturally in the earth's crust and may be emitted from volcanoes and in rock dust. It is a natural constituent of soil and is transported in streams and waterways.[61] Anthropogenic emissions include industrial sources from mining and recycling, steel production, and municipal incineration.[62] Power plants fueled by peat, coal, natural gas, and oil are sources of nickel compound emissions.[63] Nickel accumulates along roadways from abrasion of metal parts of vehicles and the use of gasoline containing nickel. Industrial waste has been disposed of by land spreading, land filling, ocean dumping, and incineration. Emissions by aerosols can be transported far from the source.[61]

### Routes of Exposure

Nickel can enter the body through inhalation, ingestion, or the skin.

### Sources of Exposure

Food is the most common source of nickel, but other sources may result in exposure. Children are exposed to nickel through air, especially when it contains tobacco smoke. Food and contaminated drinking water are other potential sources. Dermal absorption can occur when skin is abraded or otherwise not intact. Iatrogenic exposure potentially occurs through dialysis and through dental and surgical prostheses.[64] Significant amounts of nickel have been found after minimally invasive repair of pectus excavatum, resulting in allergic reactions that may mimic infection.[65] Nickel has been found to leach from stainless-steel cookware, especially in mildly acidic conditions at boiling temperatures.[66]

Natural food sources of nickel include cocoa, nuts, soybean, and oatmeal. Oysters and salmon may accumulate high levels when fished from water with increased concentrations of nickel. Nickel may be present in higher concentrations in vegetables such as peas, beans, cabbage, spinach, and lettuce. Certain plants and bacteria carry nickel-containing enzymes. Nickel, however, has not been shown to be an essential nutrient in humans.[61] Nickel deficiency has been induced in rats, chicks, cows, and goats. Decreasing growth and abnormal morphology and oxidative metabolisms in the liver have been noted in these animals. Nickel may act as a ligand cofactor facilitating the gastrointestinal absorption of ferric irons.[67]

## Biological Fate

After nickel enters the body, soluble ions of nickel may be absorbed directly, whereas insoluble compounds may be phagocytosed. Nickel bisulfide ($Ni_3S_2$) and nickel oxide (NiO) are relatively insoluble; however, these compounds may contribute to carcinogenesis by increasing apoptosis and DNA histone methylation when phagocytosed by cells lining the respiratory tract.[68,69] Soluble nickel compounds may be absorbed through the gastrointestinal tract from water and food but a large percentage of this nickel is excreted in feces. Soluble nickel that enters the bloodstream may accumulate in the kidneys and be excreted in the urine.[61] Some nickel salts may be absorbed through intact skin.

## Clinical Effects

Workers in nickel refinery and processing industries exposed by inhalation have a higher incidence of respiratory cancers of the lung, larynx, and nasopharyngeal passages.[61,68] Nickel carbonyl inhalation in workers has been described to cause adrenal, hepatic, and renal damage leading to death. Inhaled nickel sulfate has been associated with atopic dermatitis.[70] Occupational exposure is associated with a higher incidence of endocrinopathies, adverse cardiovascular outcomes, and histone methylation.[71–75]

The most common adverse health effect in children from nickel is the development of allergic contact dermatitis. A significant number of these children will have an allergy to nickel diagnosed by patch testing.[76] A recent review places nickel among the 10 most common allergens with a frequency ranging from 7.76% to 46% of persons affected.[77] Nickel is one of the most common causes of contact dermatitis from jewelry, white gold, wrist watches, metal clothing fasteners, and dental prostheses. A nickel allergy may be induced on the ears by ear piercing, on the abdomen from snaps in the waistband of pants in which the component of a snap in the waistband of pants rubs against the skin, and on wrists and necks by jewelry.[61,70,78] Nickel allergy has developed in children with orthodontic and surgical hardware that results in inflammation around the sites of implantation, possibly promoting confusion in the diagnosis.[65,79,80] Nickel dermatitis has been described in infants.[81]

## Diagnosis

A urine nickel concentration of 5 mcg/dL in a person with acute exposure is considered to be at the upper limit of normal. Acute poisoning is diagnosed at higher concentrations.[61]

## Treatment

Acute toxicity may be treated with chelating agents, especially diethyl-dithiocarbamate, but even one dose given immediately after exposure increases CNS uptake.[82] Disulphiram, which is metabolized to diethyl-dithiocarbamate, may be effective. Penicillamine has been used in treating acute toxic effects of nickel compounds.[61]

## Regulations

The US EPA has designated nickel and its compounds as toxic pollutants and recommends that drinking water should contain no more than 0.1 mg/L.

The WHO has classified nickel compounds as group I carcinogens (human carcinogens) and metallic nickel as a group IIB carcinogen (possible human carcinogen).[61] In 1996, the European Union (EU) announced a directive to restrict the use of nickel to reduce the prevalence of nickel allergy. The directive prohibits the use of nickel in jewelry, especially earrings, for pierced ears, wristwatches, and clothing that may be in direct contact with the skin for prolonged periods.[83] This has led to a significant decrease in nickel allergies in adults within the EU.[84]

## Prevention of Exposure

Because the incidence of nickel dermatitis is high and sensitization to nickel develops in many people, it is prudent to educate the public about its widespread use in jewelry and clothes fasteners and to alert people with sensitivity to avoid exposing their skin to nickel. People who are sensitive to nickel and those who have atopic tendencies may also want to avoid nickel-containing stainless-steel cookware.

## SUMMARY

Although each of these metals is listed separately, exposures do not occur in isolation. With some exceptions, most exposures to heavy metals occur as mixtures when children contact two or more metals used concomitantly in manufacturing or disposal. For example, recycling of electronic waste (e-waste) is poorly regulated, resulting in a global environmental health issue because chemicals escape into the environment through manual dismantling, open burning, or open dumping.[85] Residual metals enter the soil, water, and air, resulting in exposures. E-waste may contain lead, cadmium, chromium, manganese, nickel, mercury, arsenic, copper, zinc, aluminum, and cobalt, with each metal contributing to possible adverse effects among those exposed.

Unfortunately, research studies and regulations continue to focus on individual metals or contaminants rather than assessing the effects of mixtures and their effects on human health. The extent to which mixtures have synergistic or additive effects on a person's health is unknown. Pediatricians should be mindful of the limitations of studies and recognize that children have multiple exposures that we are currently not able to fully measure.

## Frequently Asked Questions

Q   *Should I worry about the nickel in coins, cookware, jewelry, and clothes fasteners? Can my child develop cancer from nickel?*

A   Metallic nickel has not been shown to produce cancer in children. Contact with metallic nickel can cause allergic dermatitis, generally if the metal is in contact with the skin for prolonged periods. Workers in nickel refineries who inhaled large quantities of nickel salts were found to have a higher risk of cancers of the nasopharynx and lungs. Children are generally not exposed to such high levels from nickel in the outdoor air.

Q   *My child is overweight and has acanthosis nigricans with marked elevation in her serum insulin. Do you think she is deficient in chromium? Should her level be measured?*

A   There is no known correlation between chromium deficiency and insulin resistance; therefore, obtaining a chromium level in blood or urine would not be helpful. In addition, it is difficult to collect a blood specimen without some chromium contamination from the stainless-steel needle used to obtain the blood specimen.

Q   *A rash developed on my child's hands and back. I found him sleeping on his iPad, and I wonder if he has an allergy to metal in his iPad.*

A   Allergic contact dermatitis has been known to occur from the use of handheld devices.[86] This is usually caused by a nickel allergy, but other metals may be implicated. With the increasing prevalence of nickel allergy in the United States, parents should be aware of the presence of this metal in these devices. Nickel-free cases are available. Using a cover regularly in this situation is recommended.

Q   *I have heard that laboratories can measure many harmful chemicals in my child's blood. Can you order all the possible tests for her?*

A.   It is not good clinical practice to order such tests because we do not yet know what every result means. For many chemicals, interpreting the results is not always possible because we do not have information on what range of values (also known as "reference values") are found in "healthy persons." In the same context, we also do not have information on what values cause harm. Therefore, very few chemicals can be measured and interpreted accurately.

# References

1. U.S. Department of Health and Human Services, Public Health Service. Agency for Toxic Substances and Disease Registry. *Toxicological Profile for Cadmium. September 2012.* https://www.atsdr.cdc.gov/toxprofiles/tp5.pdf. Accessed March 1, 2018

2. New York State Department of Health. *Cadmium in Children's Jewelry.* http://www.health.state.ny.us/environmental/chemicals/cadmium/cadmium_jewelry.htm. Accessed March 1, 2018

3. Zhang Y, Liu P, Wang C, Wu Y. Human health risk assessment of cadmium via dietary intake by children in Jiangsu Province, China. *Environ Geochem Health.* 2017;39(1):29–41

4. Jean J, Sirot V, Vasseur P, et al. Impact of a modification of food regulation on cadmium exposure. *Regul Toxicol Pharmacol.* 2015;73(1):478–483

5. Satarug S, Moore M. Adverse health effects of chronic exposure to low-level cadmium in foodstuffs and cigarette smoke. *Environ Health Perspect.* 2004;121(10):1099–1103

6. Hecht EM, Arheart K, Lee DJ, Hennekens CH, Hlaing WM. A cross-sectional survey of cadmium biomarkers and cigarette smoking. *Biomarkers.* 2016;21(5):429–435

7. Berglund M, Larsson K, Grander M, et al. Exposure determinants of cadmium in European mothers and their children. *Environ Res.* 2015;141:69–76

8. Reeves PG, Chaney RL. Bioavailability as an issue in risk assessment and management of food cadmium: a review. *Sci Total Environ.* 2008;398(1-3):13–19

9. Suh YJ, Lee JE, Lee DH, et al. Prevalence and relationships of iron deficiency anemia with blood cadmium and vitamin D levels in Korean women. *J Korean Med Sci.* 2016;31(1):25–32

10. Lansdown AB, Sampson B. Dermal toxicity and percutaneous absorption of cadmium in rats and mice. *Lab Anim Sci.* 1996;46(5):549–554

11. Rani A, Kumar A, Lal A, Pant M. Cellular mechanisms of cadmium induced toxicity: a review. *Int J Environ Health Res.* 2014;24(4):378–399

12. Silver MK, Lozoff B, Meeker JD. Blood cadmium is elevated in iron deficient U.S. children: a cross-sectional study. *Environmental Health.* 2013;12:117

13. Chen P, Duan X, Li M, et al. Systematic network assessment of the carcinogenic activities of cadmium. *Toxicol Appl Pharmacol.* 2016;310:150–158

14. Åkesson A, Barregard L, Bergdahl IA, Nordberg GF, Nordberg M, Skerfving S. Non-renal effects and the risk assessment of environmental cadmium exposure. *Environ Health Perspect.* 2014;122(5):431–438

15. Ogawa T, Kobayashi E, Okubo Y, Suwazono Y, Kido T, Nogawa K. Relationship among prevalence of patients with Itai-itai disease, prevalence of abnormal urinary findings, and cadmium concentrations in rice of individual hamlets in the Jinzu River basin, Toyama prefecture of Japan. *Int J Environ Health Res.* 2004;14(4):243–252

16. Ciesielski T, Weuve J, Bellinger DC, Schwartz J, Lanphear B, Wright RO. Cadmium exposure and neurodevelopmental outcomes in U.S. children. *Environ Health Perspect.* 2012;120(5):758–763

17. Kim S, Arora M, Fernandez C, Landero J, Caruso J, Chen A. Lead, mercury, and cadmium exposure and attention deficit hyperactivity disorder in children. *Environ Res.* 2013;126:105–110

18. Centers for Disease Control and Prevention. Fourth National Exposure Report, Updated Tables, January 2018. https://www.cdc.gov/exposurereport/index.html. Accessed March 1, 2018

19. Akesson A, Lundh T, Vahter M, et al. Tubular and glomerular kidney effects in Swedish women with low environmental cadmium exposure. *Environ Health Perspect.* 2005;113(11):1627–1631

20. Roels HA, Hoet P, Lison D. Usefulness of biomarkers of exposure to inorganic mercury, lead, or cadmium in controlling occupation and environmental risks of nephrotoxicity. *Ren Fail.* 1999;21(3-4):251–262

21. Agency for Toxic Substances and Disease Registry. *Toxicological Profile for Chromium.* 2012. http://www.atsdr.cdc.gov/ToxProfiles/tp7.pdf. Accessed March 1, 2018

22. Institute of Medicine, Food and Nutrition Board. *Dietary Reference Intakes for Vitamin A, Vitamin K, Arsenic, Boron, Chromium, Copper, Iodine, Iron, Manganese, Molybdenum, Nickel, Silicon, Vanadium, and Zinc.* Washington, DC: National Academies Press; 2002. http://www.nap.edu/catalog.php?record_id=10026. Accessed March 1, 2018

23. Hamula C, Wang Z, Zhang H, et al. Chromium on the hands of children after playing in playgrounds from chromated copper arsenate (CCA)-treated wood. *Environ Health Perspect.* 2006;114(3):460–465

24. Vimercati L, Gatti MF, Gagliardi T, et al. Environmental exposure to arsenic and chromium in an industrial area. *Environ Sci Pollut Res.* 2017;24(12):11528–11535

25. Biomonitoring California. Chromium. Potential Designated Chemical. https://www.biomonitoring.ca.gov/sites/default/files/downloads/PotenDesigChromium032714.pdf. Accessed March 1, 2018

26. Wasson SJ, Linak WP, Gullett BK, et al. Emissions of chromium, copper, arsenic, and PCDDs/Fs from open burning of CCA-treated wood. *Environ Sci Technol.* 2005;39(22):8865–8876

27. Sun H, Brocato J, Costa M. Oral chromium exposure and toxicity. *Curr Environ Health Rep.* 2015;2(3):295–303

28. Pellerin C, Booker SM. Reflections on hexavalent chromium: health hazards of an industrial heavyweight. *Environ Health Perspect.* 2000;108(9):A402–A407

29. Holness DL. Recent advances in occupational dermatitis. *Curr Opin Allergy Clin Immunol.* 2013;13(2):145–150

30. Sedman RM, Beaumont J, McDonald TA, Reynolds S, Krowech G, Howd R. Review of the evidence regarding the carcinogenicity of hexavalent chromium in drinking water. *J Environ Sci Health C Environ Carcinog Ecotoxicol Rev.* 2006;24(1):155–182

31. Remy LL, Byers V, Clay T. Reproductive outcomes after non-occupational exposure to hexavalent chromium, Willits California, 1983–2014. *Environmental Health.* 2017;16:18

32. Xia W, Hu J, Zhang B, et al. A case-control study of maternal exposure to chromium and infant low birth weight in China. *Chemosphere.* 2016;144:1484–1489

33. Li P, Li Y, Zhang J, Yu SF, Wang ZL, Jia G. Establishment of a reference value for chromium in the blood for biological monitoring among occupational chromium workers. *Toxicol Ind Health.* 2016;32(10):1737–1744

34. US Environmental Protection Agency. Drinking Water Contaminants – Standards and Regulations. https://www.epa.gov/dwstandardsregulations. Accessed March 1, 2018

35. Agency for Toxic Substances and Disease Registry. *Toxicological Profile for Manganese.* Washington, DC: US Department of Health and Human Services, Public Health Service; 2012. https://www.atsdr.cdc.gov/toxprofiles/tp151.pdf. Accessed March 1, 2018

36. Oulhote Y, Mergler D, Bouchard MF. Sex- and age-differences in blood manganese levels in the U.S. general population: national health and nutrition examination survey 2011–2012. *Environ Health.* 2014;13:87

37. Ljung KS, Kippler MJ, Goessler W, Grandér GM, Nermell BM, Vahter ME. Maternal and early life exposure to manganese in rural Bangladesh. *Environ Sci Technol.* 2009;43(7):2595–2601

38. American Academy of Pediatrics, Committee on Nutrition. *Pediatric Nutrition Handbook.* Kleinman RE, ed. Elk Grove Village, IL: American Academy of Pediatrics; 2018

39. National Air Toxics Assessment. 2011 NATA: Assessment Results. https://www.epa.gov/national-air-toxics-assessment/2011-nata-assessment-results#pollutant. Accessed March 1, 2018

40. US Environmental Protection Agency. Toxics Release Inventory. TRI National Analysis. Releases of Chemicals in the 2015 TRI National Analysis. https://www.epa.gov/trinationalanalysis/releases-chemicals-2015-tri-national-analysis. Accessed March 1, 2018

41. Pavilonis BT, Lioy PJ, Guazzetti S, et al. Manganese concentrations in soil and settled dust in an area with historic ferroalloy production. *J Expo Sci Environ Epidemiol.* 2015;25(4):443–450

42. Gunier RB, Jerrett M, Smith DR, et al. Determinants of manganese levels in house dust samples from the CHAMACOS cohort. *Sci Total Environ.* 2014;497–498:360–368

43. Gunier RB, Mora AM, Smith D, et al. Biomarkers of manganese exposure in pregnant women and children living in an agricultural community in California. *Environ Sci Technol.* 2014;48(24):14695–14702

44. O'Neal SL, Zheng W. Manganese toxicity upon overexposure: a decade in review. *Curr Environ Health Rep.* 2015;2(3):315–328

45. Willhite CC, Bhat VS, Ball GL, McLellan CJ. Emergency do not consume/do not use concentrations for potassium permanganate in drinking water. *Hum Exp Toxicol.* 2013;32(3):275–298

46. Woolf A, Wright R, Amarasiriwardena C, Bellinger D. A child with chronic manganese exposure from drinking water. *Environ Health Perspect.* 2002;110(6):613–616

47. Verity MA. Manganese neurotoxicity: a mechanistic hypothesis. *Neurotoxicology.* 1999;20 (2-3):489–497

48. Aschner M. Manganese: brain transport and emerging research needs. *Environ Health Perspect.* 2000;108(Suppl 3):429–432

49. Neal AP, Guilarte TR. Mechanisms of lead and manganese neurotoxicity. *Toxicol Res (Camb).* 2013;2(2):99–114

50. Nascimento S, Baierle M, Goethel G, et al. Associations among environmental exposure to manganese neuropsychological performance, oxidative damage and kidney biomarkers in children. *Environ Res.* 2016;147:32–43

51. Zoni S, Lucchini RG. Manganese exposure: cognitive, motor and behavioral effects on children: a review of recent findings. *Curr Opin Pediatr.* 2013;25(2):255–260

52. Oulhote Y, Mergler D, Barbeau B, et al. Neurobehavioral function in school-age children exposed to manganese in drinking water. *Environ Health Perspect.* 2014;122(12):1343–1350

53. Chiu YM, Claus Henn B, Hsu HL, et al. Sex differences in sensitivity to prenatal and early childhood manganese exposure on neuromotor function in adolescents. *Environ Res.* 2017;159:458–465

54. Sanders AP, Claus Henn B, Wright RO. Perinatal and childhood exposure to cadmium, manganese, and metal mixtures and effects on cognition and behavior: a review of recent literature. *Curr Environ Health Rep.* 2015;2(3):284–294

55. Lauwerys R, Roels H, Genet P, Toussaint G, Bouckaert A, De Cooman S. Fertility of male workers exposed to mercury vapor or to manganese dust: a questionnaire study. *Am J Ind Med.* 1985;7(2):171–176

56. Claus Henn B, Bellinger DC, Hopkins MR, et al. Maternal and cord manganese concentrations and early childhood neurodevelopment among residents near a mining-impacted superfund site. *Environ Health Perspect.* 2017;125(6):067020

57. Taba P. Metals and movement disorders. *Curr Opin Neurol.* 2013;26(4):435–441

58. Brna P, Gordon K, Dooley JM, Price V. Manganese toxicity in a child with iron deficiency and polycythemia. *J Child Neurol.* 2011;26(7):891–894

59. Hines EQ, Soomro I, Howland MA, Hoffman RS, Smith SW. Massive intravenous manganese overdose due to compounding error: minimal role for hemodialysis. *Clin Toxicol (Phila)*. 2016;54(6):523–525

60. US Environmental Protection Agency. Manganese. Integrated Risk Information System IRIS. http://www.epa.gov/iris/subst/0373.htm. Accessed March 1, 2018

61. Agency for Toxic Substances and Disease Registry. *Toxicological Profile for Nickel (update)*. Washington, DC: US Department of Health and Human Services, Public Health Service; 2005

62. Ngole-Jeme VM, Fantke P. Ecological and human health risks associated with abandoned gold mine tailings contaminated soil. *PLoS One*. 2017;12(2):e0172517

63. Harari R, Harari F, Forastiere F. Environmental nickel exposure from oil refinery emissions: a case study in Ecuador. *Ann Ist Super Sanita*. 2016;52(4):495–499

64. Gomez de Ona C, Martinez-Morillo E, Gago Gonzalez E, et al. Variation of trace element concentrations in patients undergoing hemodialysis in the north of Spain. *Scand J Clin Lab Investigation*. 2016;76(6):492–499

65. Fortmann C, Goen T, Kruger M, Ure BM, Petersen C, Kubler JF. Trace metal release after minimally-invasive repair of pectus excavatum. *PLoS One*. 2017;12(10):e01866323

66. Guarneri F, Costa C, Cannavò SP, et al.Release of nickel and chromium in common foods during cooking in 18/10 (grade 316) stainless steel pots. *Contact Dermatitis*. 2017;76(1):40–48

67. Nielsen FH, Shuler TR, McLeod TG, Zimmerman TJ. Nickel influences iron metabolism through physiologic, pharmacologic and toxicologic mechanisms in the rat. *J Nutr*. 1984;114(7):1280–1288

68. Casey SC, Vaccari M, Al-Mulla F, et al. The effect of environmental chemicals on the tumor microenvironment. *Carcinogenesis*. 2015;36(Suppl 1):S160–S183

69. Brocato J, Costa M. Basic mechanics of DNA methylation and the unique landscape of DNA methylome in metal-induced carcinogenesis. *Crit Rev Toxicol*. 2013;43(6):493–514

70. Isaksson M, Olhardt S, Radehed J, Svensson A. Children with atopic dermatitis should always be patch-tested if they have hand or foot dermatitis. *Acta Derm Venereol*. 2015;95(5):583–586

71. Yang AM, Cheng N, Pu HQ, et al. Metal exposure and risk of diabetes and prediabetes among Chinese occupational workers. *Biomed Environ Sci*. 2015;28(12):875–883

72. Yang AM, Bai YN, Pu HQ, et al. Prevalence of metabolic syndrome in Chinese nickel-exposed workers. *Biomed Environ Sci*. 2014;27(6):475–477

73. Wong JY, Fang SC, Grashow R, Fan T, Christiani DC. The relationship between occupational metal exposure and arterial compliance. *J Occup Environ Med*. 2015;57(4):355–360

74. Bai YN, Yang AM, Pu HQ, et al. Nickel-exposed workers in China: a cohort study. *Biomed Environ Sci*. 2014;27(3):208–211

75. Ma L, Bai Y, Pu H, et al. Histone methylation in nickel-smelting industrial workers. *PLoS One*. 2015;10(10):e0140339

76. Gumulka M, Matura M, Liden C, Kettelarij JA, Julander A. Nickel exposure when working out in the gym. *Acta Derm Venereol*. 2015;95(2):247–249

77. Rodrigues DF, Goulart EM. Patch-test results in children and adolescents: systemic review of a 15-year period. *An Bras Dermatol*. 2016;91(1):64–72

78. Goldenberg A, Admani S, Pelletier JL, Jacob SE. Belt buckles – Increasing awareness of nickel exposure in children: a case report. *Pediatrics*. 2015;136(3):e691–e693

79. Pazzini CA, Pereira LJ, Marques JL, Ramos-Jorge J, Aparecida da Sliva T, Paiva SM. Nickel-free vs conventional braces for patients allergic to nickel: gingival and blood parameters during and after treatment. *Am J Orthod Dentofacial Orthop*. 2016;150(6):1014–1019

80. Warshaw EM, Kinglsey-Loso JL, DeKoven JG, et al. Body piercing and metal allergic contact sensitivity: North American contact dermatitis group data from 2007 to 2010. *Dermatitis*. 2014;25(5):255–264

81. Ho VC, Johnston MM. Nickel dermatitis in infants. *Contact Dermatitis.* 1986;15(5):270–273

82. Andersen O, Aaseth J. A review of pitfalls and progress in chelation treatment of metal poisonings. *J Trace Elem Med Biol.* 2016;38:74–80

83. Delescluse J, Dinet Y. Nickel allergy in Europe: the new European legislation. *Dermatology.* 1994;189(Suppl 2):56–57

84. Garg S, Thyssen JP, Uter W, et al. *Br J Dermatol.* 2013;169(4):854–858

85. Zeng X, Xu X, Boezen HM, Huo X. Children with health impairments by heavy metals in an e-waste recycling area. *Chemosphere.* 2016;148:408–415

86. Jacob SE, Admani S. iPad: increasing nickel exposure in children. *Pediatrics.* 2014;134(2): e580–e582

Chapter 25

# Carbon Monoxide

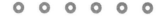

## KEY POINTS

- Carbon monoxide (CO) in the bloodstream causes a leftward shift of the oxyhemoglobin dissociation curve, resulting in decreased oxygen delivery to the tissues.
- Symptoms of CO poisoning are nonspecific; symptoms include headache, dizziness, fatigue, lethargy, weakness, drowsiness, confusion, irritability, loss of consciousness, and coma, and are not well correlated with the level of exposure.
- Administering 100% oxygen as the antidote will effectively reduce the elimination half-life of carboxyhemoglobin (COHb) to approximately 1 hour.
- Hyperbaric oxygen therapy has been used although there is insufficient evidence that it prevents neuropsychological sequelae.
- Primary prevention of CO poisoning requires limiting exposure to known sources.

## INTRODUCTION

Carbon monoxide (CO) is a colorless, odorless, tasteless toxic gas that is a product of the incomplete combustion of carbon-based fuels. Carbon monoxide has a vapor density slightly less than that of air. The health effects from acute CO exposure range from nonspecific flulike symptoms, such as headache, dizziness, nausea, vomiting, weakness, and confusion, to coma and death from prolonged or intense exposure. Fetuses, infants, pregnant women, elderly people, and people with anemia or with a history of cardiac or respiratory disease may be particularly sensitive to CO. Evidence of delayed neuropsychological health effects and slow resolution of these sequelae from CO exposures are documented in the literature, although no definitive diagnostic or therapeutic approaches have been established. The effects of long-term, low-level exposure is another area of CO poisoning that lacks a definitive approach for diagnosis and treatment.[1,2]

Unintentional CO poisonings accounted for approximately 440 deaths (all ages) and approximately 21,000 emergency department visits in the United States annually between 1999 and 2012.[3-6] From 2000 to 2009, approximately 6,800 calls per year were made to poison control centers about CO exposure.[5] From the most recently available data, it is estimated that there are 2,300 hospital discharges annually for CO-related conditions.[5] In a study of 3,034 poisoning deaths among persons aged 10 to 19 years, 38.2% were attributable to CO inhalation, of which 65.1% were categorized as suicide and 34.9% as unintentional. Motor vehicle exhaust accounted for 84.4% of the CO-related suicides and 65.6% of the unintentional fatal CO poisonings.[7]

The clinical presentation of mild and severe CO poisoning is nonspecific, thus creating a diagnostic challenge as well as making it difficult to estimate the prevalence of unintentional encounters.[2,8-11] Often, the clinical presentation can mimic influenza. In a study of 46 children presenting during winter months to the emergency department for flu-like symptoms, more than half had COHb concentrations that exceeded 2%, and 6 of these children had COHb concentrations that exceeded 10%.[8]

## ROUTE AND SOURCES OF EXPOSURE

The route of exposure to CO is through inhalation. Unintentional exposure to CO can be largely attributed to smoke inhalation from fires, motor vehicle exhaust, faulty or improperly vented gas-fueled (natural or liquified petroleum) appliances (including heating appliances), solid fuel appliances (eg, wood burning stoves), and tobacco smoke. Confined, poorly ventilated spaces such as garages, campers, tents, and boats also are susceptible to elevated, often lethal, levels of CO.[1] Common sources of CO exposure are listed in Table 25-1. Exposure to CO may occur in and around motor vehicles when there is inadequate combustion resulting from substandard vehicle maintenance and poor ventilation. Exposure also may occur when gasoline-powered equipment, such as generators, lawn mowers, snow blowers, leaf blowers, and ice rink resurfacing machines, are used in poorly ventilated spaces.[1,7,12]

The risk from CO poisoning increases after natural or manmade disasters, when gasoline-powered generators may be more frequently used to supply power. After Hurricane Ike, generators were used to supply electricity used to watch television or power video games, resulting in the CO poisoning death of one child and the poisoning injuries of 15 other children.[13]

| Table 25-1. Sources of Carbon Monoxide Exposure |
| --- |
| ■ Motor vehicle exhaust |
| ■ Motorboats |
| ■ Unvented kerosene and propane gas space heaters |
| ■ Leaking chimneys and furnaces |
| ■ Backdrafting from furnaces |
| ■ Woodstoves and fireplaces |
| ■ Charcoal or propane grills |
| ■ Gas appliances: stoves, dryers, water heaters |
| ■ Gasoline-powered generators |
| ■ Gasoline-powered equipment: ice rink resurfacers, lawn mowers, leaf blowers, floor polishers, snow blowers, pressure washers |
| ■ Tobacco smoke |

## SYSTEMS AFFECTED

CO is inhaled, diffuses across the alveolar-capillary membrane, and is measurable in the bloodstream as COHb. The relative affinity of CO for hemoglobin is approximately 240 to 270 times greater than that of oxygen, resulting in decreased oxygen-carrying capacity of the blood when CO concentrations are elevated. CO in the bloodstream causes a leftward shift of the oxyhemoglobin dissociation curve, resulting in decreased oxygen delivery to the tissues. Removal from the source of CO exposure leads to dissociation of the COHb complex, resulting in excretion of CO by the lungs.[14,15]

Infants and children have an increased susceptibility to CO toxicity because of their higher metabolic rates. Fetuses are especially vulnerable. Maternal CO diffuses across the placenta and increases the levels of CO in the fetus. Fetal hemoglobin has an even higher affinity for CO than does adult hemoglobin. The elimination half-life of COHb is also longer in the fetus than in the adult. The leftward shift in the normal oxyhemoglobin dissociation curve caused by CO results in a substantial decrease in oxygen delivery to the placenta and ultimately to fetal tissues.[16,17] Children with existing pulmonary, cardiac, or hematologic illness (eg, anemia) that compromises oxygen delivery also are more susceptible to adverse effects at lower levels of CO exposures than are healthy individuals.[1]

Carbon monoxide poisoning results in tissue hypoxia, which has an adverse effect on multiple organ systems. Systems with high metabolic rates and high oxygen demand are preferentially affected, with the central nervous and cardiovascular systems being the primary targets.[1,2,18] Typical pathologic changes found on neuroimaging studies, when present, include bilateral necrosis in the basal ganglia, including the caudate, globus pallidus, and putamen. Imaging can also demonstrate diffuse homogenous demyelination of the white matter of the cerebral hemispheres.[19,20] Cardiac toxicity can be manifested by ischemia on electrocardiography, arrhythmia, and infarction.[18]

Recent research has focused on investigating the possible mechanisms of toxicity from CO. One primary mechanism is tissue hypoxia, attributable to decreased oxygen-carrying capacity but also attributable to decreased cardiac output secondary to myocardial dysfunction. Other mechanisms of interest that are being investigated include the production of hydroxyl radicals and nitric oxide radicals.[2]

## CLINICAL EFFECTS

The clinical presentation of CO poisoning is highly variable, and the severity of the symptoms does not correlate well with the level of exposure (parts per million [ppm] of CO over time) and clinical laboratory determination of poisoning (blood COHb concentrations). This important phenomenon is explained in part by the fact that within the body, CO can be found in 4 distinct states. In addition to binding to hemoglobin, CO binds to both myoglobin and the cytochrome p450 system and exists in its free state in the plasma at a low concentration. It is the free state CO that is thought to play an important role in clinical toxicity. This is illustrated by animal studies that showed no clinical symptoms in animals transfused with blood containing highly saturated COHb but minimal free CO. Low concentrations of COHb may be present in cases of severe poisoning.[2,8,10,14]

Symptoms of CO poisoning include headache, dizziness, fatigue, lethargy, weakness, drowsiness, nausea, vomiting, skin pallor, dyspnea on exertion, palpitations, confusion, irritability, irrational behavior, loss of consciousness, coma, and death. Severity of symptoms ranges from mild to very severe (coma, respiratory depression) and is not correlated with the magnitude of COHb concentrations.[18] In a series of pediatric patients treated for CO poisoning, lethargy and syncope were reported more frequently than in an adult series. These symptoms also occurred at lower COHb concentrations than usually reported for adults.[10] Delayed neuropsychological sequelae following CO exposure have been reported in adults and children. Sequelae can occur as early as 24 hours after exposure, with impairment in memory, attention, and executive functioning.[21] Other impairments can include cognitive and personality changes, parkinsonism, dementia, and psychosis.[10,16,18,22] The incidence of delayed neuropsychiatric sequelae varies widely but has been estimated to occur in 10% to 30% of patients.[18] Neuropsychiatric testing is only completed on a small proportion of patients being treated for CO poisoning.[22]

## DIAGNOSIS

A thorough history and physical examination and a high index of clinical suspicion are necessary to diagnose CO poisoning. Physicians should consider CO exposure when members of the same household present with similar nonspecific symptoms. Clinical examination is often without findings suggestive of CO poisoning, other than the nonspecific signs and symptoms described in the previous section.

Measurement of oxygen saturation by pulse oximetry and arterial blood gas determination are not helpful in the diagnosis of CO poisoning. The pulse oximeter typically misinterprets COHb as oxyhemoglobin, resulting in an elevated oxygen saturation reading by this device.[23] Arterial oxygen tension ($PaO_2$) is typically normal in CO poisoning because $PaO_2$ measures the amount of oxygen dissolved in plasma, which is unaffected in this condition. However, the blood gas determination will demonstrate metabolic acidosis in significant CO poisoning.

The measurement of blood COHb may help to establish whether exposure to CO has occurred. An elevated concentration confirms the diagnosis of CO poisoning. Low and moderately increased concentrations must be interpreted with caution because the COHb concentration does not indicate severity of illness. Delay between exposure and laboratory measurement, treatment with oxygen, and complicating factors, such as exposure to tobacco smoke, should be considered when interpreting COHb results. Background concentrations of COHb range from 1% to 3% in nonsmokers.[18] Baseline COHb concentrations in smokers typically range from 3% to 8%, although higher values have been reported.[18,24,25]

## TREATMENT

Patients who have been exposed to CO should be removed from the source immediately. Therapy consists of supplemental oxygen, ventilatory support, and monitoring for cardiac dysrhythmias. The elimination half-life of COHb is approximately 4 hours in room air. Administering 100% oxygen as the antidote will effectively reduce the elimination half-life of COHb to approximately 1 hour. Administration of hyperbaric oxygen (HBO) decreases the half-life to approximately 20 to 30 minutes.[14,15,18]

The use of HBO remains controversial.[26–30] Although the half-life of COHb with HOB administration has been demonstrated to be less than the half-life of COHb when 100% oxygen is used, the primary outcome of interest, preventing neurological sequelae, has proven to be more elusive.

Several recent retrospective case series have suggested a benefit of HBO therapy; however, the nature of the design and a lack of randomization do not change the level of recommendation from past Cochrane Reviews that analyzed the available randomized controlled studies of HBO therapy. Other reviews have been conducted, including a systematic review in 2005, an update of a Cochrane Database of Systematic Reviews published in 2011, and a policy statement from the American College of Emergency Physicians.[27,29,31] The findings from these reviews state that the evidence continues to be insufficient to support the use of HBO therapy for patients with CO poisoning. The authors identified 7 randomized controlled trials (RCTs); however, one was excluded because it did not identify any clinical outcome. Of the remaining 6 trials, 2 reported a beneficial effect of HBO as indicated by reduced neurological sequelae at 1 month, and 4 others did not report any beneficial effects.[27,29]

When data from all 6 RCTs were pooled, there were 1,997 patients, of which 1,335 were randomized to either HBO or normobaric oxygen. The pooled analysis did not demonstrate a statistically significant improvement in the prevention of neurologic sequelae (OR = 0.78 [95% CI, 0.54–1.12]). It should also be noted that there was a large degree of variation between the treatment regimens, severity of poisoning, and outcome assessments.[27]

A few RCTs have used a blinded control with a sham treatment in the HBO chamber. In one trial of patients aged 16 years and older who had CO poisoning, the patients showed fewer cognitive sequelae following 3 HBO treatments within a 24-hour period.[28] Because this RCT did not enroll children younger than 16 years, it is not known whether the results can be generalized to children. The other RCT failed to show benefit from this intervention.[26] In the most recent RCT no effect was shown.[32] Most notably, the authors only allowed randomization to patients who were less severely poisoned.[32] Despite the lack of supporting evidence, it appears that the use of HBO for the treatment of CO poisoning in the United States has remained the same since 1992.[4]

If HBO therapy is being considered, the following have been used as criteria: (1) COHb concentration of 25% or greater; (2) anginal pain or ischemia on electrocardiogram; or (3) measurable neurologic impairment.[15] The choice of treatment modalities is tailored to the patient on the basis of the severity of the poisoning, as determined by the observed clinical manifestations. An additional consideration for using HBO therapy should be the location of the nearest center with a hyperbaric chamber and whether such a transfer may delay treatment. When the patient with CO poisoning is cared for, consultation with a pediatric critical care specialist familiar with treatment options, including HBO therapy, is suggested. In addition, because treatment with HBO needs to be individualized, providers should also consult with the poison control center or the Divers Alert Network (www.diversalertnetwork.org).

## PREVENTION OF EXPOSURE

Primary prevention of CO poisoning requires limiting exposure to known sources. Proper installation, maintenance, and use of combustion appliances can help to reduce excessive CO emissions. Table 25-2 provides suggestions to prevent CO poisoning.[12]

## Table 25-2. Preventing Problems With CO in the Home and Other Environments

**Fuel-burning Appliances**

- Forced-air furnaces should be checked by a professional once a year or as recommended by the manufacturer. Pilot lights can produce CO and should be kept in good working order.

- All fuel-burning appliances (eg, gas water heaters, gas stoves, gas clothes dryers) should be checked professionally once a year or as recommended by the manufacturer.

- Gas cooking stove tops and ovens should not be used for supplemental heat.

**Fireplaces and Woodstoves**

- Fireplaces and woodstoves should be checked professionally once a year or as recommended by the manufacturer. Check to ensure the flue is open during operation. Proper use, inspection, and maintenance of vent-free fireplaces (and space heaters) are recommended.

**Space Heaters**

- Fuel-burning space heaters should be checked professionally once a year or as recommended by the manufacturer.

- Space heaters should be properly vented during use, according to the manufacturer's specifications.

**Barbecue Grills/Hibachis**

- Barbecue grills and hibachis should never be used indoors.

- Barbecue grills and hibachis should never be used in poorly ventilated spaces such as garages, campers, and tents.

**Automobiles/Other Motor Vehicles**

- Regular inspection and maintenance of the vehicle exhaust system are recommended. Many states have vehicle inspection programs to ensure this practice.

- Never leave an automobile running in the garage or other enclosed space; CO can accumulate even when a garage door is open.

**Generators/Other Fuel-powered Equipment**

- Follow the manufacturer's recommendations when operating generators and other fuel-powered equipment.

- Never operate a generator indoors.

**Boats**

- Be aware that carbon monoxide poisoning can mimic symptoms of sea sickness.

- Schedule regular engine and exhaust system maintenance.

- Consider installing a CO detector in the accommodation space on the boat.

- Never swim under the back deck or swim platform because carbon monoxide builds up near exhaust vents.

The US Environmental Protection Agency (EPA) has set significant harm levels of 50 parts per million (ppm) (8-hour average), 75 ppm (4-hour average), and 125 ppm (1-hour average). Exposure under these conditions could result in COHb concentrations of 5% to 10% and may cause significant health effects in sensitive individuals. COHb concentrations, however, do not necessarily correlate with the degree of toxicity. The current ambient (outdoor) air quality standards for CO (9 ppm for 8 hours and 35 ppm for 1 hour) are intended to keep COHb concentrations below 2.1% to protect the most sensitive members of the general population (ie, individuals with coronary artery disease).[1]

Smoke detectors and CO detectors, when used properly, may provide early detection and warning and may prevent unintentional CO-related deaths. In a review of patient data from August 2008 through January 2010 for patients treated in the United States (864 patients), it was noted that only 10% of patients had a CO detector at the location where they were exposed.[33] CO detectors are designed to sound an alarm before potentially life-threatening levels of CO are reached. CO detectors measure the amount of CO (ppm) that has accumulated over time and should sound an alarm within 189 minutes when CO in the air reaches 70 ppm, corresponding to a concentration of approximately 5% COHb in the blood.[34] This is based on relationships between CO levels measured in air and corresponding blood COHb concentrations in adults. Significant exposure to children may have occurred before the CO alarm sounds.[34]

The US Consumer Product Safety Commission recommends installation of a CO detector in the hallway near every separate sleeping area of the home. A residential CO detector should meet the requirements of the most recent revision of Underwriters Laboratories Standard 2034.[35] Because electric heating and cooking appliances shut down during a power failure, battery-operated detectors are recommended when gas appliances or auxiliary heating sources (eg, fireplaces) are used during periods when electrical service is disrupted. The effectiveness of CO detectors in preventing CO poisoning has not been evaluated.

## Frequently Asked Questions

Q  *What things can I do to help limit my family's exposure to CO?*

A  Table 25-2 lists recommendations for preventing CO problems in the home and other environments.[12]

Q  *Is using a CO detector a good way to prevent CO poisoning?*

A  Carbon monoxide detectors are widely available in stores, and consumers may want to consider buying one as a backup but not as a replacement for the proper use and maintenance of fuel-burning appliances (see Table 25-2). The technology of CO detectors is still developing. Several types are on the market, and they are not generally considered to be as reliable as the smoke detectors found in homes today. Some CO detectors have been laboratory tested, and their performance varied. Some performed well, others failed to alarm even at very high CO levels, and still others alarmed at very low levels that do not pose any immediate health risk. With smoke detectors, you can easily confirm the cause of the alarm, but because CO is invisible and odorless, it is more difficult to determine whether an alarm is false or a real emergency.

Organizations such as Consumers Union (publisher of *Consumer Reports*), the American Gas Association, and Underwriters Laboratories have published guidance for consumers. Look for Underwriters Laboratories certification on any CO detector. CO detectors always have been and still are designed to sound an alarm before potentially life-threatening levels of CO are reached. The Underwriters Laboratories Standard 2034 has strict requirements that the detector and alarm must meet before it can sound. As a result, the possibility of nuisance alarms is decreased.

Q   *Should I purchase a CO detector for my motor home or other recreational vehicles?*

A   The US Consumer Product Safety Commission notes that CO detectors are available for boats and recreational vehicles and that they should be used, and that the Recreational Vehicle Industry Association requires CO detectors in motor homes and in towable recreational vehicles that have a generator or are prepped for a generator.

Q   *What do I do if my CO detector sounds an alarm?*

A   Never ignore a CO detector alarm. If the CO detector goes off:
   — Make sure it is your CO detector and not your smoke detector.
   — Check to see if any member of the household is experiencing symptoms of poisoning.
   — If they are, get them out of the house immediately and call 911. Seek medical attention at an emergency department. Tell the doctor that you suspect CO poisoning.
   — If no one is feeling symptoms, ventilate the home with fresh air, turn off all potential sources of CO including oil or gas furnace, gas water heater, gas range, oven, gas dryer, gas or kerosene space heater, and any vehicle or small engine.
   — Have a qualified technician inspect your fuel-burning appliances and chimneys to make sure they are operating correctly and that there is nothing blocking the fumes from being vented out of the house. Checking appliances and other possible CO sources should be done before they are turned back on.

Q  *I recently found out that my furnace has been leaking CO, even though I feel fine. Are there any long-term effects?*

A  No data are available that show chronic CO exposure produces any long-term sequelae. The long-term effects, such as the neuropsychiatric sequelae, only have been described in patients who have had documented evidence of a severe, acute CO poisoning. Even though you feel fine, it is imperative that you and your family vacate the premises and have the furnace problem evaluated and fixed immediately. Ignoring this problem could prove fatal to you and your family.

Q  *Are carbon monoxide detectors required in my home?*

A  Many states or municipalities have enacted laws requiring the use of CO detectors in rental units and other residences. The specific requirements vary by state and town.

## Resources

**Divers Alert Network**
Web site: www.diversalertnetwork.org

**Undersea and Hyperbaric Medical Society**
Phone: 301-942-2980
Web site: http://uhms.org

**Underwriters Laboratories**
Phone: 847-272-8800
Web site: www.ul.com

**US Consumer Product Safety Commission**
Phone: 800-638-2772
Web site: www.cpsc.gov

**US Environmental Protection Agency Indoor Air Quality Information Clearinghouse**
Phone: 800-438-4318
Web site: www.epa.gov/iaq/iaqinfo.html

## References

1. US Environmental Protection Agency. Integrated Science Assessment for Carbon Monoxide (Final Report, Jan 2010). EPA/600/R-09/019F, 2010. https://cfpub.epa.gov/ncea/risk/recordisplay.cfm?deid=218686&CFID=78776911&CFTOKEN=81884369. Accessed January 14, 2018

2. Raub JA, Mathieu-Nolf M, Hampson NB, Thom SR. Carbon monoxide poisoning—a public health perspective. *Toxicology.* 2000;145(1):1–14

3. Centers for Disease Control and Prevention. Carbon monoxide-related deaths—United States, 1999-2004. *MMWR Morb Mortal Wkly Rep.* 2007;56(50):1309–1312

4. Hampson NB. U.S. mortality due to carbon monoxide poisoning, 1999—2104. Accidental and intentional deaths. *Ann Am Thoracic Society.* 2016;13(10):1768–1774

5. Iqbal S, Clower JH, King M, Bell J, Yip FY. National carbon monoxide poisoning surveillance framework and recent estimates. *Public Health Rep.* 2012;127(5):486–496

6. Sircar K, Clower J, Shin MK, Bailey C, King M, Yip F. Carbon monoxide poisoning deaths in the United States, 1999 to 2012. *Am J Emerg Med.* 2015;33(9):1140–1145

7. Shepherd G, Klein-Schwartz W. Accidental and suicidal adolescent poisoning deaths in the United States, 1979 -1994. *Arch Pediatr Adolesc Med.* 1998;152(12):1181–1185

8. Baker MD, Henretig FM, Ludwig S. Carboxyhemoglobin levels in children with nonspecific flu-like symptoms. *J Pediatr.* 1988;113(3):501–504

9. Heckerling PS, Leikin JB, Terzian CG, Maturen A. Occult carbon monoxide poisoning in patients with neurologic illness. *J Toxicol Clin Toxicol.* 1990;28(1):29–44

10. Crocker PJ, Walker JS. Pediatric carbon monoxide toxicity. *J Emerg Med.* 1985;3(6):443–448

11. Weaver LK. Carbon monoxide poisoning. *N Engl J Med.* 2009;360(12):1217–1225

12. American Thoracic Society. Environmental controls and lung disease. *Am Rev Respir Dis.* 1990;142(4):915–939

13. Fife CE, Smith LA, Maus EA, et al. Dying to play video games: carbon monoxide poisoning from electrical generators used after Hurricane Ike. *Pediatrics.* 2009;123(6):e1035–e1038

14. Vreman HJ, Mahoney JJ, Stevenson DK. Carbon monoxide and carboxyhemoglobin. *Adv Pediatr.* 1995;42:303–334

15. Piantadosi CA. Diagnosis and treatment of carbon monoxide poisoning. *Respir Care Clin North Am.* 1999;5(2):183–202

16. Koren G, Sharev T, Pastuszak A, et al. A multicenter prospective study of fetal outcome following accidental carbon monoxide poisoning in pregnancy. *Reprod Toxicol.* 1991;5(5):397–403

17. Kopelman AE, Plaut TA. Fetal compromise caused by maternal carbon monoxide poisoning. *J Perinatol.* 1998;18(1):74–77

18. Ernst A, Zibrak JD. Carbon monoxide poisoning. *N Engl J Med.* 1998;339(22):1603–1608

19. Bianco F, Floris R. MRI appearances consistent with haemorrhagic infarction as an early manifestation of carbon monoxide poisoning. *Neuroradiology.* 1996;38(Suppl 1):S70–S72

20. Hopkins RO, Fearing MA, Weaver LK, Foley JF. Basal ganglia lesions following carbon monoxide poisoning. *Brain Injury.* 2006;20(3):273–281

21. Porter SS, Hopkins RO, Weaver LK, Bigler ED, Blatter DD. Corpus callosum atrophy and neuropsychological outcome following carbon monoxide poisoning. *Arch Clin Neuropsychol.* 2002;17(2):195–204

22. Seger D, Welch L. Carbon monoxide controversies: neuropsychologic testing, mechanism of toxicity, and hyperbaric oxygen. *Ann Emerg Med.* 1994;24(2):242–248

23. Buckley RG, Aks SE, Eshom JL, Rydman R, Schaider J, Shayne P. The pulse oximetry gap in carbon monoxide intoxication. *Ann Emerg Med.* 1994;24(2):252–255

24. Hausberg M, Somers VK. Neural circulatory responses to carbon monoxide in healthy humans. *Hypertension.* 1997;29(5):1114–1118

25. Hee J, Callais F, Momas I, et al. Smokers' behaviour and exposure according to cigarette yield and smoking experience. *Pharmacol Biochem Behav.* 1995;52(1):195–203

26. Scheinkestel CD, Bailey M, Myles PS, et al. Hyperbaric or normobaric oxygen for acute carbon monoxide poisoning: a randomized controlled clinical trial. *Med J Aust.* 1999;170(5):203–210

27. Buckley NA, Juurlink DN, Isbister G, Bennett MH, Lavonas EJ. Hyperbaric oxygen for carbon monoxide poisoning. *Cochrane Database Syst Rev.* 2011;(4):CD002041

28. Weaver LK, Hopkins RO, Chan KJ, et al. Hyperbaric oxygen for acute carbon monoxide poisoning. *N Engl J Med.* 2002;347(14):1057–1067

29. Wolf FJ, Lavonas EJ, Sloan EP, Jagoda AS, American College of Emergency Physicians. Clinical policy: critical issues in the management of adult patients presenting to the emergency department with acute carbon monoxide poisoning. *Ann Emerg Med.* 2008;51:138–152

30. Hampson NB, Piantadosi CA, Thom SR, Weaver LK. Practice recommendations in the diagnosis, management, and prevention of carbon monoxide poisoning. *J Resp Crit Care Med.* 2012;186(11):1095–1101

31. Buckley NA, Isbister GK, Stokes B, Juurlink DN. Hyperbaric oxygen for carbon monoxide poisoning: a systematic review and critical analysis of the evidence. *Toxicol Rev.* 2005;24(2): 75–92

32. Annane D, Chadda K, Gajdos P, Jars-Guincestre MC, Chevret S, Raphael JC. *Intensive Care Med.* 2011;37(3):486–492

33. Clower JH, Hampson NB, Iqbal S, Yip FY. Recipients of hyperbaric oxygen treatment for carbon monoxide poisoning and exposure circumstances. *Am J Emer Med.* 2012;30(6):846–851

34. Etzel RA. Indoor air pollutants in homes and schools. *Pediatr Clin North Am.* 2001;48(5): 1153–1165

35. Underwriters Laboratories. *UL2034: Standard for Single and Multiple Station Carbon Monoxide Detectors.* 1992. Revised Standard 2034. http://ulstandards.ul.com/ standard/?id=2034. Accessed January 14, 2018

Chapter 26

# Cold and Heat

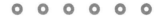

## KEY POINTS

- Children spend more time outdoors than adults, particularly during the summer months, as well as during play and sports. This places them at risk of heat-related injury. Exertional heatstroke is the leading cause of preventable death in youth sports.
- Keys for safe activity in the heat include being appropriately acclimatized, avoiding excessive activity following a recent illness, and maintaining adequate hydration.
- Children may be more susceptible to hypothermia than adults because of their large body surface area-to-mass ratio, which predisposes them to rapid heat loss. Newborn infants are highly prone to hypothermia because of their large body surface area, small amount of subcutaneous fat, and decreased ability to shiver.
- An associated hazard resulting from exposure to extreme cold is the use of potentially dangerous heating sources.

## INTRODUCTION

Heat and cold stress are environmental hazards. Optimal human body function requires a body temperature of approximately 98.6°F (37°C). As homeotherms (organisms that generate heat to maintain body temperature, typically above the temperature of surroundings [also known as endotherms]), humans have several mechanisms for maintaining body temperature in a narrow range. These mechanisms, which emanate from the hypothalamic temperature-regulating center, include vasodilation and sweating (with heat stress) and piloerection and shivering (with cold stress). Aside from the automated temperature control mechanisms mentioned, behaviors that may not occur at a conscious level (eg, the decision to wear appropriate cool or warm clothing) can impact the body's ability to maintain optimal temperature control.[1]

Children and adults use the same mechanisms to cope with heat or cold stress (see Cold section and Tables 26-1 and 26-2 for more information).[2] Limited evidence suggests that older children and adolescents may have equivalent heat-dissipating capacity as adults.[3] Recent studies compared the heat tolerance between prepubertal children and adults of the same gender.[4-6] Little research addresses the capacity of younger children, especially toddlers and infants, to dissipate heat, although available evidence suggests that they may have a lesser ability to do so.[7]

The keys for safe activity in the heat include having the child be appropriately acclimatized, avoiding excessive activity following a recent illness, and maintaining hydration.[3]

Four physical properties—convection, conduction, radiation, and evaporation—determine the interaction between ambient and body temperatures. Convection is a mechanism of heat exchange through a medium such as air or water. Air is a relatively inefficient medium; exposure to cold air must take place over several hours for hypothermia to develop in a human. Water is a medium that transmits energy more efficiently; cold-water immersion can change body temperature in minutes. Conduction is the transfer of heat between 2 bodies in contact (eg, skin-to-skin contact). Radiation is the process by which the body gains heat from surrounding hot objects, such as hot pipes, and loses heat to cold objects, such as chilled metallic surfaces, without any direct contact. Evaporation is the cooling mechanism of the human body via perspiration.

Environmental temperature extremes result from a significant increase or decrease in ambient temperatures. Extremely warm or cold ambient temperature, winter storms, inadequate home heating or cooling, extended exposure to temperature extremes without proper clothing, and overheated indoor environments, such as motor vehicles, can be among the causes of environmental temperature extremes.

The public health consequences of cold and heat extremes are substantial. With climate change, extreme heat events have become more frequent and prolonged in many regions of the United States.[8] This places more people at risk from heat-related illness.[9-11] In the past decade, numerous extreme heat events have occurred worldwide, causing severe impacts on society and resulting in many heat-related deaths.[11] The European summer heat wave of 2003 killed an estimated 15,000 to 30,000 people and more than 650 people died in Chicago's 1995 heat wave.[9,12] Extreme heat events are likely to increase.[9,13] Conversely, the number of extreme cold waves in the United States in recent years has been the lowest since record keeping began.[8]

## Table 26-1. Physiologic Effects of Extreme Cold and Heat

| BODY SYSTEM | COLD | HEAT |
|---|---|---|
| Neurologic | Delirium<br>Central nervous system depression | Coma<br>Seizures |
| Cardiovascular | Bradycardia<br>Cardiac arrest | Tachycardia<br>Cardiovascular collapse |
| Musculoskeletal | Shivering | Rhabdomyolysis |
| Metabolic | Hyperglycemia | Metabolic acidosis |
| Respiratory | Depressed respirations | Tachypnea |

## COLD

Humans are less able to compensate for cold stress compared with heat stress.[14] Cold injury can be systemic, such as hypothermia, (defined as a core body temperature less than 95°F [35°C]) or local, such as cold injuries to various body parts ( frostnip and frostbite). Children may be more susceptible to hypothermia than adults because of their large body surface area-to-mass ratio, which predisposes them to rapid heat loss.[15] Newborn infants are especially prone to hypothermia because of their large body surface area, less subcutaneous fat, and decreased ability to shiver. Additional risk factors for the development of hypothermia in children include hypothyroidism, hypoglycemia, and ingestion of ethanol or certain medications (eg, opioids, phenothiazines). Hypothermia is classified as mild, moderate, or severe (Table 26-2).

## Table 26-2. Physiologic Effects and Clinical Manifestations of Cold

| CORE BODY TEMPERATURE | PHYSIOLOGIC RESPONSE |
|---|---|
| **Mild**<br>(90° F–95° F; 32° C–35° C) | Shivering<br>Tachycardia or bradycardia<br>Confusion |
| **Moderate**<br>(82.4° F–90° F; 28° C–32° C) | Loss of shivering<br>Loss of deep tendon reflexes; peripheral anesthesia<br>Bradycardia, hypotension<br>Central nervous system depression |
| **Severe**<br>(<82.4° F; <28° C) | Severe bradycardia<br>Cardiac arrhythmias<br>Coma |

Several causes of cold exposure can be identified. Winter storms can occur unpredictably, leading to sudden and prolonged periods of cold temperatures. If the storm produces a power failure, the interior of a home can become dangerously cold. Direct contact with water is another important cause of cold exposure; cold-water immersion can produce hypothermia in minutes because of water's efficient conductive ability. Wet clothing can increase heat loss fivefold.[15]

An associated hazard resulting from cold extremes is the use of potentially dangerous heating sources. Families may use gas stoves, fireplaces, wood stoves, space heaters, and propane heaters as supplements or alternatives to home heating or during power outages. These heat sources carry the threat of fire hazard, production of indoor air pollutants (in the case of poorly maintained fireplaces and wood stoves), and carbon monoxide poisoning (with improper use of propane heaters and generators [see Chapter 25]).

Children and adults respond physiologically to cold extremes in the same way (see Tables 26-1 and 26-2).[2] As core body temperature falls, the metabolic rate increases to create more heat. At body temperatures of 90°F to 95°F (32°C–35°C), patients experience shivering, "goose bumps," lethargy, and bradycardia. With moderate hypothermia (82.4°F–90°F [28°C–32°C]), shivering ends; disorientation and stupor occur. Severe hypothermia (<82.4°F [<28°C]) produces profound bradycardia and cardiac arrhythmias. Slowed nerve conduction velocity contributes to the development of numbness (anesthesia). Disorientation can occur. An electrocardiogram will display a J-wave (Osborn wave), characteristic of severe hypothermia.

An unusual compensatory mechanism for extreme cold is known as the diving reflex. When the body is immersed in cold water, which produces rapid hypothermia, it begins to preferentially divert blood from organs, including the gastrointestinal tract and kidneys, to the brain and heart. As a result, there is remarkable preservation of the central nervous system for extended periods of oxygen deprivation.

Cold injuries can be mild or severe and the effects may be transient or permanent. Hypothermia can be mild, moderate, or severe, depending on the core body temperature. Mild hypothermia can consist of pain and pallor of the cold-exposed area, shivering, and social withdrawal. It is commonly found among skiers, sledders, skaters, and other outdoor sports enthusiasts.[14,15] Moderate to severe hypothermia (core temperature between 82°F and 90°F; 28°C to 32°C) may result in loss of shivering, confusion, and cardiac arrhythmias.[15] Chronic cold injury, just above freezing, can produce an uncommon condition called chilblain, also known as perniosis (an area of localized cutaneous inflammation that is often mistaken for Raynaud phenomenon). The lesions are purplish-red, painful, and pruritic.[16] Exposure to a cold and wet environment can result in trench foot, also known as immersion foot. Recovery from hypothermia is usually complete. Frostbite, on the other hand, is a severe form of cold injury and results in permanent tissue damage, particularly the digits, ears, and nose. Therefore, recovery from frostbite can be incomplete.[15]

Children with significant cold injury should be evaluated by a pediatrician or in an emergency department, particularly if they have a significant change in behavior or a body part that appears cold, stiff, or pale. Treatment of cold injury consists of rewarming the affected area. Rewarming should only be initiated when no chance of additional cold exposure exists because rewarming of injured tissue followed by additional cold exposure can produce greater injury to the affected body part (re-freezing injury).[15] The child's affected body part should be placed against another person's body part. If hands are involved, the affected person may place the hands in his or her axillae. If that is not possible, the exposed body part can be placed near a heat source or in warm water as soon as possible. Care should be taken to avoid burning the area. It is also important not to rub the affected area; rather, the affected area (such as hands) should be placed under water and soaked, not rubbed together. In moderate to severe cases of hypothermia, more aggressive forms of active rewarming may be required, particularly if the patient is unresponsive. Advanced life support measures, notably defibrillation, are not as effective when the core body temperature is less than 86°F (30°C), so if initially unsuccessful, defibrillation should be attempted again after rewarming.[15]

## Prevention

Preventing injury from cold extremes consists of several interventions:
- Wearing proper cold-weather gear;
- Carefully selecting and limiting time periods of cold exposure;
- Avoiding severe cold;
- Finding alternate shelter if the home or residence has lost its heat; and
- Using safe indoor heating sources.

## HEAT

As with cold extremes, heat extremes have changed in pattern and prevalence over recent years. This has been associated in part with climate change, particularly the greenhouse effect.[10] Carbon dioxide, produced primarily by fuel combustion, creates an atmospheric blanket that traps solar energy that is naturally reflected from the earth's surface (see Chapter 58).

Over the last decade, extreme heat events have increased in prevalence around the globe, and these are expected to increase with rising average global temperature. By the end of the 21st century, it is likely that average summer temperatures will exceed the most extreme temperatures recorded in many regions of the world.[17] An important secondary consequence of heat extremes is the increased production of smog and other ambient pollutants and the development of wildfires and power failures.[9]

Children spend more time outdoors than adults, particularly during the summer months, during play, sports, and work activities, placing children at risk of heat injury. Exertional heatstroke is the leading cause of preventable death in youth sports.[18,19] Adolescents may spend extended periods outdoors working in landscaping or agriculture. An estimated 120,000 children work as farm laborers in the United States.[20] Outdoor workers are at risk for the development of severe or even fatal heat-related injuries.[21]

The human body has several mechanisms, including vasodilation and sweating, to maintain normal temperature across a wide range of ambient temperatures.[1] Vasodilation results in simple radiant loss from hot skin; this can account for up to 60% of the body's cooling ability. Sweating and its evaporation account for 25% of heat-reducing capacity.[9] High humidity prevents evaporative loss, leading to decreased cooling ability and a greater risk of hyperthermia.[1] Children aged 9 to 12 years have equivalent exercise tolerance when compared with similarly fit and acclimatized adults.[3-6] Research documents that the skin and rectal temperatures, exercise tolerance time, and heart rate were all similar between the children and an adult comparison group.[3-6]

Other risk factors for heat-associated illness in children include chronic diseases (eg, diabetes mellitus, obesity, cystic fibrosis), medications (eg, anticholinergics, stimulant medications, opioids, phenothiazines), and reduced ability to seek protection or communicate needs (infants and children with physical disabilities). A current or recent illness, particularly gastroenteritis, may produce residual effects of fluid loss. Sickle cell trait also increases the risk of complications associated with strenuous exercise in the heat.[3]

Heat extremes can produce several health effects in children, the most common of which is dehydration, while the most severe include rhabdomyolysis, exercise-associated collapse, and death. Dehydration occurs from the combination of insensible water losses through exhaled air and sweating. Children generally sweat at a rate of 1 L/hour/m$^2$. In unacclimatized adolescents, 1 to 4 L of fluid can be lost in a single hour of exertion, accompanied by the loss of several grams of salt.

When the body is no longer able to compensate for temperature extremes, the core temperature rises and produces pyrexia (fever). Core body temperatures of 100°F to 106°F (37.8°C–41.1°C) can lead to sweating, tachycardia, and disorientation. Body temperatures greater than 106°F (41.1°C) are associated with agitation, seizures, tachycardia, ventricular irritability, and metabolic acidosis. Body temperatures greater than 110°F (43.3°C) can quickly lead to cardiovascular collapse.

## Types of Heat Injury

Injuries resulting from heat extremes include heat exhaustion, heat cramps, and heat stroke. These often occur in a continuum when early signs of heat injury are not addressed.[22]

Heat exhaustion typically results from the combination of sustained heat and dehydration. Children can develop faintness, extreme tiredness, and headache; there may be fever and intense thirst.[22] Other signs and symptoms include nausea, vomiting, hyperventilation, and paresthesias. Heat exhaustion is treated with rest, fluids, and hydration with electrolyte-containing drinks.

Heat cramps most commonly occur in children who are participating in outdoor sports, work, or play. Therefore, heat cramps typically occur in conditioned children who have been drinking water but have not been adequately replacing electrolyte losses. Heat cramps usually start during relaxation and can be triggered by cold.[1] Children complain of muscle aches with the lower extremities more commonly affected than the upper extremities. Pain may be severe and may result from muscle spasms. The cause of the pain of heat cramps is unclear but has been attributed in part to electrolyte disturbances and accumulation of lactic acid in muscles. The treatment for heat cramps is rest, cooling, and hydration with electrolyte-containing drinks. Although the loss of electrolytes appears to be a risk factor, there is no role for salt tablets.

Heat stroke, the most extreme form of heat-related illness, is an emergency that occurs independently of hydration. Heat stroke occurs with a core body temperature (via rectal temperature shortly after collapse) of greater than 104°F to 105°F (40°C–40.5°C), along with signs of central nervous system dysfunction.[19] It is typically categorized as exertional and nonexertional. Exertional heat stroke tends to occur in athletes, soldiers, and laborers; it remains one of the most common causes of death and disability among US high school athletes, with more than 9,000 illnesses per year.[1,19,22,23] Nonexertional heat stroke occurs in the absence of physical activity. In children, nonexertional heat stroke is most often the result of being left unattended in vehicles because the temperature inside a car rapidly rises above the ambient temperature.[22,24] In children with heat stroke, stupor or coma, tachycardia, hypertension, or hypotension develop. Severe rhabdomyolysis can occur, resulting in myoglobinuria and acute renal failure, complications that are often fatal.

Victims of classical heat stroke have, by definition, lost the ability to sweat. It is important to note, however, that athletes with exertional heat stroke will have hot sweaty skin.[19] Sweating is the primary mechanism for body cooling; without sweating, the core body temperature of heat stroke victims can increase to more than 115°F (46°C).

Patients with evidence of heat stroke should immediately be taken to a hospital where aggressive cooling techniques can be initiated to bring the temperature back to normal. In situations of exertional heat stroke in athletes, cooling should immediately begin on the sidelines because this may be lifesaving. In addition, if a rectal temperature is not available or is not feasible in the event of school policy/legal issues, the physician should rely on the presence of abnormal neurologic signs and symptoms and the circumstances surrounding the collapse and begin treatment without delay. Cold water immersion is the best method for cooling and should begin before the athlete gets to the hospital.[3,19] Intravenous hydration and fluid monitoring are needed. Antipyretics, such as acetaminophen or ibuprofen, should play no role in pyrexia caused by heat exposure. All school sports teams should have an emergency action plan in place, with certified athletic trainers on site to begin management of such an emergency.[3,19]

## Prevention

Preventive measures include:

1. Families without reliable access to air conditioning should make plans for home cooling, such as fans, water, wet towels, or alternate shelters in the event of a heat wave.

2. Parents and caregivers should never leave children unattended in vehicles, particularly on hot days. The interior of automobiles can reach temperatures greater than 158°F (70°C). The temperature increase reaches 80% of its peak within 30 minutes; cracking the window open does not significantly change the rate of increase.[24]

3. A well-outlined program of conditioning for athletes that includes acclimatization, adequate access to water, and periods of rest/recovery should be available. The recovery time period should also be increased during times of high heat. Athletes should maintain adequate hydration, and can be taught to monitor their urine color, which should be a light yellow.[19]

4. An emergency action plan should be available for all school and other youth-related sports and activity programs to include the management of exertional heat stroke.[3]

5. For adolescents who work outdoors, heat-stress management programs should be created by the employer.[10] These should provide:

    a. training of supervisors and employees in the prevention, recognition, and treatment of heat illness;

    b. creation and implementation of a heat-acclimatization program;

    c. availability of proper amounts and types of fluids;

    d. creation of work/rest schedules appropriate for the heat index;

    e. access to shade or cooling areas;

    f. monitoring of the environment and of workers during hot conditions; and

    g. prompt medical attention to workers who show signs of heat illness.

    Similar recommendations from the American Academy of Pediatrics have been created for team sports during heat extremes (Table 26-3).[3] Athletes

## Table 26-3. Key Exertional Heat-illness Risk Factors During Exercise, Sports, and Other Physical Activities and Recommended Responses (Actions) for Reducing Physiologic Strain and Improving Activity Tolerance and Safety

Risk factors[a]

- Hot and/or humid weather
  - Poor preparation
  - Not heat-acclimatized
  - Inadequate prehydration
  - Little sleep/rest
  - Poor fitness
- Excessive physical exertion
  - Insufficient rest/recovery time between repeat bouts of high-intensity exercise (eg, repeat sprints)
- Insufficient access to fluids and opportunities to rehydrate
- Multiple same-day sessions
  - Insufficient rest/recovery time between practices, games, or matches
- Overweight/obese (BMI ≥85th percentile for age) and other clinical conditions (eg, diabetes) or medications (eg, attention-deficit/hyperactivity disorder medications)
- Current or recent illness (especially if it involves/involved gastrointestinal distress or fever)
- Clothing, uniforms, or protective equipment that contribute to excessive heat retention

Actions[b]

- Provide and promote consumption of readily accessible fluids at regular intervals before, during, and after activity
- Allow gradual introduction and adaptation to the climate, intensity, and duration of activities and uniform/protective gear
- Physical activity should be modified
  - Decrease duration and/or intensity
  - Increase frequency and duration of breaks (preferably in the shade)
  - Cancel or reschedule to cooler time
- Provide longer rest/recovery time between same-day sessions, games, or matches
- Avoid/limit participation if child or adolescent is currently or was recently ill
- Closely monitor participants for signs and symptoms of developing heat illness
- Ensure that personnel and facilities for effectively treating heat illness are readily available onsite
- In response to an affected (moderate or severe heat stress) child or adolescent, promptly activate emergency medical services and rapidly cool the victim

[a] With the presence of any of these risk factors or other medical conditions adversely affecting exercise-heat safety, some or all of the actions listed may be appropriate responses to reduce the risk of exertional heat illness and improve well-being.
[b] As environmental conditions become more challenging (heat and humidity increase) and as additional other listed risk factors are present, the possible actions to improve safety become more urgent. Note that each listed action does not necessarily correspond or apply to any particular or every listed risk factor.
Table reproduced from American Academy of Pediatrics, Council on Sports Medicine and Fitness and Council on School Health. "Climatic Heat Stress and Exercising Children and Adolescents." 2011[3]

should wear light clothing. Garments that restrict sweat loss (eg, waterproof outfits) are extremely dangerous and should never be used in hot environments.[22] Ensuring adequate hydration for the athlete is a must. Likewise, the athlete should not participate if he or she has been recently ill, particularly with a gastrointestinal illness, thus reducing overall hydration status.[3]

Communities should have established plans for heat waves. Campaigns should be initiated every summer to advise citizens of plans for management of heat extremes.[9] Warning systems for heat avoidance should be established. Such recommendations may differ for artificial turf and natural grass surfaces because artificial turf absorbs heat, making those surfaces hotter than natural grass surfaces when subject to the same environmental conditions.[25] Finally, local public health authorities should develop a system for identifying and contacting high-risk individuals; this is best coordinated with social services, visiting nurses, and volunteer agencies.[9]

## Frequently Asked Questions

Q   *What are the recommendations for hydration in excessive heat?*

A   Recommendations for athletic activities during heat have been published by the American Academy of Pediatrics.[3] During the activity, periodic drinking should be enforced. For children aged 9 to 12 years, 100 mL to 250 mL of fluids every 20 minutes is recommended. For adolescents, 1.0 to 1.5 L every hour is recommended. Generally, water is sufficient to maintain hydration. However, if the exercise is strenuous or lasts longer than 1 hour, an electrolyte-supplemented beverage should be used.

Q   *Is there a certain temperature at which I should not let my child play outdoors?*

A   Heat indices have been created to identify the health threats arising from the combined influence of temperature and humidity. Air quality indices may be included in the determination of whether to avoid outdoor play (see Chapter 21). These are available at https://airnow.gov/, and are also typically printed in newspapers and broadcast on television and radio. Along similar lines, cold indices typically combine multiple factors, including ambient temperature and wind chill factor; these can be obtained from local weather sources. The Centers for Disease Control and Prevention extreme heat guidebook is available at www.cdc.gov/climateandhealth/pubs/extreme-heat-guidebook.pdf.

## Resources

### Centers for Disease Control and Prevention

Heat-related Illness Web site:
www.cdc.gov/disasters/extremeheat/children.html
Hypothermia Web site:
www.cdc.gov/disasters/winter/staysafe/hypothermia.html

# References

1. Ewald MB, Baum CR. Environmental emergencies. In: Fleisher GR, Ludwig S, eds. *Textbook of Pediatric Emergency Medicine*. Philadelphia, PA: Lippincott Williams & Wilkins; 2010:1017–1021

2. Centers for Disease Control and Prevention. Winter Weather: Hypothermia. https://www.cdc.gov/disasters/winter/staysafe/hypothermia.html. Accessed March 3, 2018

3. American Academy of Pediatrics, Council On Sports Medicine and Fitness and Council on School Health. Climatic Heat Stress and Exercising Children and Adolescents. *Pediatrics*. 2011;128(3):e1539

4. Inbar O, Morris N, Epstein Y, Gass G. Comparison of thermoregulatory responses to exercise in dry heat among prepubertal boys, young adults and older males. *Exp Physiol*. 2004;89(6):691–700

5. Rivera-Brown AM, Rowland TW, Ramirez-Marrero GA, Santacana G, Vann A. Exercise tolerance in a hot and humid climate in heat-acclimatized girls and women. *Int J Sports Med*. 2006;27(12):943–950

6. Rowland T, Garrison A, Pober D. Determinants of endurance exercise capacity in the heat in prepubertal boys. *Int J Sports Med*. 2007;28(1):26–32

7. Sinclair WH, Crowe MJ, Spinks WL, Leicht AS. Pre-pubertal children and exercise in hot and humid environments: a brief review. *J Sports Sci Med*. 2007;6(4):385–392

8. Melillo JM, Richmond TC, Yohe GW. Climate Change Impacts in the United States: The Third National Climate Assessment. Washington, DC: US Global Change Research Program; 2014

9. Kovats RS, Hajat S. Heat stress and public health: a critical review. *Annu Rev Public Health*. 2008;29:41–55

10. American Academy of Pediatrics Committee on Environmental Health. Global climate change and children's health. *Pediatrics*. 2015;136:992–997

11. Coumou D, Robinson A, Rahmstorf S. Global increase in record-breaking monthly-mean temperatures. *Climatic Change*. 2013;118:771–782

12. Bouchama A. The 2003 European heat wave. *Intensive Care Med*. 2004;30(1):1–3

13. O'Neill MS, Ebi KL. Temperature extremes and health: impacts of climate variability and change in the United States. *J Occup Environ Med*. 2009;51(1):13–25

14. Jurkovich GJ. Environmental cold-induced injury. *Surg Clin North Am*. 2007;87(1):247–267

15. Fudge J. Preventing and managing hypothermia and frostbite injury. *Sports Health*. 2016;8(2):133–139

16. Simon TD, Soep JB, Hollister JR. Pernio in pediatrics. *Pediatrics*. 2005;116(3):e472–e475

17. Battisti DS, Naylor RL. Historical warnings of future food insecurity with unprecedented seasonal heat. *Science*. 2009;323(5911):240–244

18. Bergeron MF. Reducing sports heat illness risk. *Pediatrics Rev*. 2013;34(6):270–279

19. Casa DJ, Guskiewicz KM, Anderson SA, et al. National athletic trainers' association position statement: preventing sudden death in sports. *J Athl Train*. 2012;247(1):96–118

20. Bureau of Labor Statistics. Youth employment in agriculture. In: Report on the Youth Labor Force. Vol RYLF 2000. Washington, DC: US Department of Labor; 2000:52

21. Centers for Disease Control and Prevention. Heat-related deaths among crop workers—United States, 1992-2006. *MMWR Morb Mortal Wkly Rep*. 2008;57(24):649–653

22. Jardine D. Heat illness and heat stroke. *Pediatr Rev*. 2007;28(7):249–258

23. Centers for Disease Control and Prevention. Heat illness among high school athletes: United States, 2005–2009. *MMWR Morb Mortal Wkly Rep*. 2010;59(32):1009–1010

24. McLaren C, Null J, Quinn J. Heat stress from enclosed vehicles: moderate ambient temperatures cause significant temperature rise in enclosed vehicles. *Pediatrics*. 2003;116(1):e109–e112

25. Claudio L. Synthetic turf: health debate takes root. *Environ Health Perspect*. 2008;116(3):A116–A122

Chapter 27

# Electric and Magnetic Fields

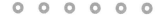

## KEY POINTS

- Magnetic field levels are reduced dramatically by increasing distance from the source, with levels reduced to background levels at distances as short as a few feet from most electrical appliances.
- The dominant sources of radio-frequency exposure in the general population are from wireless communication, especially the use of handheld devices that include mobile phones and cordless phones. Exposure decreases rapidly with increasing distance from the exposure source. Therefore, cell phone radiation exposures can be reduced by encouraging children to use text messaging when possible, make only short and essential calls on cell phones, use hands-free kits and wired headsets, and maintain the cell phone an inch or more away from the head.
- Modern children will likely experience a longer period of exposure to radio-frequency fields from cell phone use than will adults because many will have started using cell phones at earlier ages, resulting in a longer lifetime exposure.

## INTRODUCTION

Electric and magnetic fields (EMFs) are invisible lines of force created by electric charges that surround power lines, electrical appliances, and other electrical equipment. Humans also are exposed to electric and magnetic fields from natural sources, including the earth's magnetic field.[1] Electric and magnetic fields also are emitted by living organisms, including humans. The widespread use of electricity began in the late 1800s and led to expanding usage for heating, lighting, communications, and other uses.[1]

The most common form of electricity is alternating current (AC), which reverses direction 60 times per second in the United States.[2] The unit that denotes the frequency of alternation is called a hertz (Hz). Electrical charges create electric fields when the charges stand still and magnetic fields when the charges are in motion. The strength or intensity of magnetic fields is commonly measured in units called gauss (1 gauss = 1,000 milligauss) or tesla. One tesla equals 1 million microtesla; 1 milligauss is the same as 0.1 microtesla.

The electric and magnetic fields associated with electric power are extremely low-frequency or power-frequency (50 Hz or 60 Hz, respectively) field levels. Cellular telephones (commonly known as cell phones) and towers emit and receive radio-frequency and microwave-frequency electric and magnetic fields, involving a much higher frequency range (800–900 and 1,800–1,900 megahertz [MHz; 1 MHz = 1 million Hz]) than power lines or many electrical appliances.[2]

## SOURCES OF EXPOSURE

### Extremely Low-frequency Magnetic Field Exposures

Electricity produced from coal or other sources at power plants is sent through long-distance high-power transmission lines to substations, where the current is stepped down.[2] The lower levels of electrical current are then transmitted to homes, schools, workplaces, and other locations via distribution lines. It is estimated that only approximately 1% of children reside near high-voltage power lines.[3] Approximately 1% to 10% of the US population has average residential exposures exceeding 0.2 microtesla, whereas the prevalence of exposures greater than 0.5 microtesla is less than 1%.[4] The primary sources of extremely low-frequency exposure for children are from home electrical wiring and appliances held close to the body (including hair dryers, heating pads, and electric blankets) and other devices to which children are exposed at varying distances (including televisions and computer monitors).[2,5] Children are also exposed at varying levels at school and during transportation to and from activities. In a study conducted in the 1990s of children who carried computerized meters that took measurements every 30 seconds while at home or away from home over the course of 24 hours, median magnetic fields in homes measured between 0.05 and 0.1 microtesla.[6]

Magnetic field levels are reduced dramatically by increasing distance from the source, with levels reduced to background levels at distances as short as a few feet from most electrical appliances (Table 27-1), approximately 100 ft from a distribution line, and 300 ft to 500 ft from a transmission line.[2] Over the past few decades, the change in power regulation of electrical equipment from

## Table 27-1. Median 60-Hz Magnetic Field Exposure Level (in Microtesla) From Household Appliances According to Distance from the Appliance

| MAJOR CATEGORY | SPECIFIC TYPE | DISTANCE | | | |
| --- | --- | --- | --- | --- | --- |
| | | 6 in | 1 ft | 2 ft | 4 ft |
| Bathroom | Hair dryer | 30 | 0.1 | — | — |
| | Electric shaver | 10 | 2 | — | — |
| Kitchen | Blender | 7 | 1 | 0.2 | — |
| | Can opener | 60 | 15 | 2 | 0.2 |
| | Coffee maker | 0.7 | — | — | — |
| | Dishwasher | 2 | 1 | 0.4 | — |
| | Food processor | 3 | 0.6 | 0.2 | — |
| | Microwave oven[a] | 20 | 0.4 | 1 | 0.2 |
| | Mixer | 10 | 1 | 0.1 | — |
| | Electric oven[a] | 0.9 | 0.4 | — | — |
| | Refrigerator | 0.2 | 0.2 | 0.1 | — |
| | Toaster | 1 | 0.3 | — | — |
| Living/family room | Ceiling fan | NM | 0.3 | — | — |
| | Window air conditioner | NM | 0.3 | 0.1 | — |
| | Color TV | NM | 0.7 | 0.2 | — |
| Laundry/utility room | Electric dryer | 0.3 | 0.2 | — | — |
| | Washing machine | 2 | 0.7 | 0.1 | — |
| | Iron | 0.8 | 0.1 | — | — |
| | Vacuum cleaner | 30 | 6 | 1 | 0.1 |
| Bedroom | Digital clock | NM | 0.1 | — | — |
| | Analogue (dial-face) clock | NM | 1.5 | 0.2 | — |
| | Baby monitor | 0.6 | 0.1 | — | — |

*(continued)*

## Table 27-1. Median 60-Hz Magnetic Field Exposure Level (in Microtesla) From Household Appliances According to Distance from the Appliance (*continued*)

| MAJOR CATEGORY | SPECIFIC TYPE | DISTANCE | | | |
|---|---|---|---|---|---|
| | | 6 in | 1 ft | 2 ft | 4 ft |
| Workshop | Battery charger | 3 | 0.3 | — | — |
| | Drill | 15 | 3 | 0.4 | — |
| | Power saw | 20 | 4 | 0.5 | — |
| Office | Video display terminal (color monitor) | 1.4 | 0.5 | 0.2 | — |
| | Electric pencil sharpener | 20 | 7 | 2 | 0.2 |
| | Fluorescent lights | 4 | 0.6 | 0.2 | — |
| | Fax machine | 0.6 | — | — | — |
| | Copy machine | 9 | 2 | 0.7 | 0.1 |
| | Air cleaner | 18 | 3.5 | 0.5 | 0.1 |

[a] For microwave ovens, the range of 60-Hz magnetic field levels (in microtesla) according to distance are: at 6 in: 10–30; at 1 ft: 0.1–20; at 2 ft: 0.1–3; and at 4 ft: 0–2.
Abbreviations: —, indicates magnetic field levels at background level or lower; NM, not measured.

transformers to electronics (eg, switched power supplies to laptops, cell phone chargers) has changed the frequency of magnetic field exposure with 150 Hz becoming a dominating frequency.[7]

## Radio-frequency Exposures

The dominant sources of radio-frequency exposure in the general population are from wireless communication, especially the use of handheld devices that include mobile phones and cordless phones.[8] Exposure decreases rapidly with increasing distance from the exposure source, and use of a wired hands-free device can reduce exposure to the head by approximately 90%. The first handheld mobile phones used the analogue system, which had more than three times the maximum average radiated power than the digital phones that replaced them in the early 1990s.[8] The primary sources of radio-frequency and microwave-frequency exposures to children were typically from microwave ovens and handheld cell phones.[8,9] These exposures have significantly changed with the advent of wireless in-house communications, such as wireless monitors used in or near cribs/beds, cordless phones, wireless computer technology, and cell phone use by someone in close proximity to children and by children themselves.[3] At present, radio-frequency exposures have been less well-characterized than the extremely low-frequency magnetic fields associated with household appliances. The rapid evolution of these technologies and difficulties in measuring radio-frequency exposures contribute to the challenges in studying these exposures and child health.[10]

It is important to note that modern children will likely experience a longer period of exposure to radio-frequency fields from cell phone use than will adults because many will have started using cell phones at earlier ages, resulting in a longer lifetime exposure. Furthermore, cell phone use by children can result in approximately two times higher average radio-frequency energy deposition in the brain and up to 10 times higher exposure to the bone marrow because of the different shape of their head, thinner skulls, higher fluid content of their brains, and high conductivity of their bone marrow.[8,11]

## EFFECTS OF EXPOSURE TO ELECTRIC AND MAGNETIC FIELDS

### Extremely Low-frequency Magnetic Field Exposures

The 60-Hz extremely low-frequency fields deliver low "packets" of energy not strong enough to break chemical bonds to cause irreversible changes to molecules, such as DNA, or to body tissue.[2] Epidemiologic studies suggesting an association between residential magnetic field exposures and childhood leukemia estimated exposure in a variety of ways, including (1) distance of residences from power lines; (2) "wire codes," a system of classification based on type of power line (transmission lines or distribution lines) and distance from the lines; (3) measurements (including spot or 30-second measurements, 24- and 48-hour residential measurements, and personal measurements) of children's estimated exposure to the magnetic field obtained after diagnosis; and (4) estimates of the magnetic field around the time of diagnosis on the basis of historical records of current flows and the distance of the lines from the home.[1,8]

### Radio-frequency Exposures

The low-energy packets from microwaves cannot break up DNA, but the electric charges on water molecules "wiggle" in response to the oscillations of the microwaves.[8,9] The friction generated by the wiggling generates heat by the same basic principle that allows microwave ovens to heat food. Radio-frequency fields from radio and television transmitters or cell phones alternate millions of times per second, compared with extremely low-frequency or power-frequency fields that alternate only 60 times per second.[1,8,9] At high power levels, microwave- or radio-frequency radiation can heat body tissues or create electric currents that might interfere with a cardiac pacemaker or the normal cardiac conduction system when a person is very near the source. Suggested exposure limits have been derived to avoid these adverse biological effects at high power levels. Interference with cardiac pacemakers and implantable defibrillators from sources producing lower-frequency exposures (such as power lines, rail transportation, and welding equipment), as well as higher-frequency sources (such as cell phones, paging transmitters, citizen band radios, wireless computer links, microwave signals, and radio and television transmitters) is currently an area of active research. Although a federal radio-frequency protection guide for workers was issued in 1971, it was advisory and not regulatory. The radio-frequency exposure safety limits adopted by the Federal Communications Commission in 1996 are based on criteria quantified according to the specific absorption rate, a measure of the rate at which the body absorbs radio-frequency energy.[9]

Power levels associated with handheld cell phones are low, and it is unlikely that such exposures cause consequential heating of brain tissue.[10,12] Similarly, the exposure to the general public from radio waves emanating from cellular transmitting towers is very low at distances greater than several meters from the antenna.[9]

## EPIDEMIOLOGIC STUDIES OF EXPOSURE

### Extremely Low-frequency Magnetic Field Exposures

Extremely low-frequency magnetic fields have been studied as a risk factor for childhood leukemia since the late 1970s. On the basis of more than 20 epidemiologic studies published before 2001, the International Agency for Research on Cancer (IARC) classified extremely low-frequency magnetic fields as a possible carcinogen.[13] This classification was based on limited evidence from epidemiologic studies of childhood leukemia and inadequate evidence from experimental animals.[13,14] This assessment was confirmed by the World Health Organization (WHO) in their review of more recent studies.[15] In their most recent update in 2015, the European Commission's Scientific Committee on Emerging and Newly Identified Health Risks (EU SCENIHR) also confirmed that the evidence of possible carcinogenicity remains unchanged.[7] The strongest evidence in the original IARC and more recent WHO and SCENIHR reviews came from the pooled analyses of the original studies. Greenland et al[16] found a combined relative risk estimate of 1.7 (CI 1.2–2.3) in children exposed to average magnetic fields of greater than 0.3 microtesla compared with those exposed to 0.1 microtesla or less. A pooled analysis by Ahlbom et al[17] used long-term measurements or calculated fields and found a relative risk of 2.0 (CI 1.3–3.1) for exposures of 0.4 microtesla or greater compared with exposures of less than 0.1 microtesla. Kheifets et al[18] conducted a similar analysis to that of Ahlbom et al[17] for the more recent studies and found similar modest increases in leukemia risk. The number of exposed children in these pooled datasets was small; only 125 of 13,474 leukemia cases (0.9%) had exposures of greater than 0.3 microtesla.

In a recent pooled study by Schuz et al[19] of survival from childhood acute lymphoblastic leukemia, the authors did not find an association with extremely low-frequency magnetic field exposure. A meta-analysis of paternal occupational exposure to extremely low-frequency magnetic fields and childhood leukemia risk was not conclusive. An increased risk of 35% was shown but there was some evidence of publication bias (studies showing no association were less likely to be published).[20]

The studies of extremely low-frequency magnetic fields have been predominately retrospective and are limited by challenges in measuring actual exposure and selection and recall bias. It is important to note, however, that studies based on calculated magnetic fields that were not affected by selection or recall bias have also shown a modest positive association with leukemia risk. Other factors, such as traffic density and pesticide use near power lines can be correlated with extremely low-frequency magnetic fields and may be risk factors for leukemia. No potential confounding exposure that might explain the association with childhood leukemia has been identified, however.[14]

Little evidence has been shown of an association of residential magnetic field exposures and other childhood cancers. Childhood brain tumors have been the most well studied. In a meta-analysis of studies on magnetic field exposure and childhood brain tumors, 13 studies were analyzed separately based on their exposure assessment method including estimates based on distance, wire codes, calculated fields, and measurements; no evidence was found of an increased risk for exposures of 0.2 microtesla or greater compared with less than 0.2 microtesla.[21] A 2010 pooling study of the original data from 10 studies from Europe, Japan, and the United States found no increased risk of childhood brain tumors for extremely low-frequency magnetic field exposures of 0.4 microtesla or greater compared with less than 0.1 microtesla.[22]

The few studies of childhood leukemia and brain and nervous system tumors evaluating use of electrical appliances have observed small increases in the risk of childhood leukemia linked with prenatal and postnatal use of electric blankets, hair dryers, and televisions.[1,23] An extensive body of literature evaluating adult occupational (but not residential) exposures to extremely low-frequency magnetic field exposures suggests that there may be modest increases in the risk of brain tumors and chronic lymphocytic leukemia.[1,23] Some epidemiologic evidence has suggested that male, and to a lesser extent female, breast cancer may be linked with occupational (but not residential) exposure to extremely low-frequency electric and magnetic fields, but the evidence is inconsistent.[1,23] Several studies have evaluated the relationship of residential electric and magnetic field exposures and occurrence of adult brain tumors, leukemia, and breast cancer; there is no consistent evidence of association.[1,23]

In summary, a twofold excess risk of childhood leukemia is associated with residential magnetic field exposures of 0.4 microtesla or higher, but risks of childhood leukemia are not increased with lower magnetic field levels. No consistent dose-response relationship exists, and animal studies do not support a relationship. Risks of pediatric brain tumors are not linked with residential magnetic fields on the basis of results of a pooled analysis of major studies. Reasons are unknown for the elevated risk of childhood leukemia in relation to high residential magnetic field exposures, but biases have been suggested as a partial explanation.[24,25] Findings have been inconsistent for childhood leukemia and brain tumors in relation to prenatal or postnatal exposures to electrical appliances.

### Radio-frequency and Microwave-frequency Exposures

The health effects from radio-frequency and microwave-frequency exposures have been recently reviewed by the IARC, the EU SCENIHR, and the Independent Advisory Group on Non-Ionizing Radiation (AGNIR) of Public Health England.[7,8,26] In 2011, the IARC classified radio-frequency fields as possibly carcinogenic to humans, based on epidemiological case-control studies of adult brain cancer and mobile phone use.[8] At that time, the largest of the epidemiologic studies was the INTERPHONE study of adult brain and head and neck tumors in Australia, Canada, Denmark, Finland, France, Germany, Israel, Italy, Japan, New Zealand, Norway, Sweden, and the United Kingdom. Results from that study showed no association of cell phone use and glioma or meningioma over all exposure levels; however, those persons whose usage was in the highest 10% level of total time of cell phone calls had an increased risk of glioma.[27] In 2012, the AGNIR concluded that the "accumulating evidence on adult cancer risks. . . . is increasingly in the direction of no material effect of exposure," based on the epidemiologic studies of mobile phone use and adult brain cancer together with analyses of cancer incidence trends.[26] Based on the most recent data, the SCENIHR review concluded that the evidence for an effect on adult glioma has become weaker since the IARC evaluation.[7] It was noted in all the assessments that conclusions could not be drawn about latency periods longer than 15 years since first mobile phone use because of limited numbers of patients with brain tumors in the epidemiologic studies reporting long-term use, and thus, limited statistical power.

The first published analysis of cell phone use and childhood brain tumors was a large case-control study conducted in Denmark, Sweden, Norway, and Switzerland (the CEFALO study), which included children and adolescents who were diagnosed with brain tumors between 2004 and 2008, at ages from 7 to 19 years. It found no association between cell phone use and brain tumor risk either by time since initiation of use, amount of use, or by the location of the tumor.[28] Another large international case-control study of childhood and young adult brain tumors (ages 10 to 24) and cell phone use is underway in Europe and results are expected soon.[29]

The evidence for other health outcomes in children in relation to cell phone use is inconclusive. Cell phone use by mothers was studied in the Danish National Birth Cohort, which enrolled mothers whose children were born between 1996 and 2002. A questionnaire was administered when the children reached age 7 years and included questions on behavior and pre- and postnatal cell phone use. A higher overall risk of behavioral problems was found in the children with the highest exposure to pre- and postnatal maternal cell phone use.[30] However, the authors urged caution in the interpretation of their results because there is no known biological mechanism to explain these results. They also noted that the findings may not be causal because of unmeasured confounding factors. A later analysis of behavioral problems in the Danish cohort included children who were 7 years old and born between 1998 and 2002; the analysis evaluated questionnaire responses from the children about cell phone use.[31] A weaker positive association with cell phone use was found, which was strongest in children born in earlier birth cohorts. Information on developmental milestones among infants in the cohort was collected by phone interviews when the children were 6 and 18 months old.[32] Maternal cell phone use during the pregnancy was not related to motor or cognitive and language developmental delays.

## LABORATORY STUDIES

### Extremely Low-frequency Magnetic Field Exposures

Because the 60-Hz and radio-frequency fields usually present in the environment do not ionize molecules or heat tissues, it was believed that they have no effect on biological systems.[12,33] During the mid-1970s a variety of laboratory studies on cell cultures and animals demonstrated that biological changes could be produced by these fields when applied in intensities of hundreds or thousands of microtesla. A series of comprehensive studies reported during 1997 to 2001 showed no consistent evidence of an association between extremely low-frequency magnetic field exposures and the risk of leukemia or lymphoma in rodents on the basis of long-term bioassays (up to 2.5 years), initiation/promotion studies, investigations in transgenic models, and tumor growth studies. Three large-scale chronic bioassays of carcinogenesis in rats or mice exposed to magnetic fields for 2 years revealed no increase in mammary cancer, resulting in a general consensus that power-frequency magnetic fields do not act as a complete carcinogen in the rodent.[33,34]

Inconsistent findings from one laboratory suggesting that magnetic fields may stimulate mammary carcinogenesis in rats treated with a chemical carcinogen could not be replicated in 2 other laboratories.[33,34] A specific concern in relation to breast cancer was that extremely low-frequency magnetic field exposures might mediate occurrence of breast cancer through the melatonin pathway.[35,36] To date, the experimental literature has shown relatively little support for this hypothesis.[35,36] In studies undertaken to investigate alterations in cellular processes associated with magnetic field exposures that were previously reported in the literature, regional electric and magnetic field exposure facilities were established and provided with experimental protocols, cell lines, and relevant experiment details. In general, these studies found no effects of magnetic fields on: (1) gene expression, particularly those genes that may be involved in cancer; (2) killing of cells cultured from patients with ataxia-telangiectasia, which are highly sensitive to genotoxic chemicals; (3) gap junction intercellular communication; (4) the influx of calcium ions across the plasma membrane of cells or the intracellular calcium concentration; (5) activity of ornithine decarboxylase (an enzyme implicated in tumor promotion); or (6) other in vitro processes that may be related to carcinogenesis.[33,34] In a review of 63 laboratory-based studies published between 1990 and 2003, the conclusions from 29 investigations did not identify increased cytogenetic damage following electric and magnetic field exposure, whereas 14 studies suggested a genotoxic potential of electric and magnetic field exposure. The observations in 20 other reports were inconclusive.[35,37] Therefore, the preponderance of the evidence suggests that electric and magnetic fields are not genotoxic or carcinogenic.[13,33–35,37]

## Radio-frequency and Microwave-frequency Exposures

Although some experimental studies suggest that radio-frequency fields may accelerate the development of certain tumors, including one demonstrating an increase in lymphoma incidence in transgenic mice, overall data from more than 100 studies conducted in frequency ranges from 800 to 3,000 MHz indicate that these exposures are not directly mutagenic, nor do they act as cancer initiators.[8,38] Adverse effects from exposure of organisms to high radio-frequency exposure levels are predominantly the result of hyperthermia, although some studies suggest an effect on intracellular levels of ornithine decarboxylase.[37–40] The 2011 IARC monograph review of data to evaluate the mechanisms by which radio-frequency radiation may cause or enhance carcinogenesis concluded that there was only weak evidence for genotoxicity, changes in proteins and cellular signaling, oxidative stress, and changes in neural functions in the brain.[8] Currently, the National Institutes of Health's National Toxicology Program (NTP) is conducting studies in rats and mice on cell phone radio-frequency radiation using frequencies and modulations currently used in the United States. The NTP found a statistically significant increase in the incidence of heart schwannomas in treated male rats at the highest dose (50 volts per meter [V/m]). They also found an increase in the incidence of malignant glial tumors in treated female rats at the highest dose (50 V/m), although this did not reach statistical significance. These tumors were of the same histotype as those observed in some epidemiologic studies of cell phone users.[41]

## Frequently Asked Questions

*Q   I am about to buy a house, but there is a power line (or transformer) near the home. Should I buy it?*

A   This is a decision only a parent can make. It is important to consider that there remains a small degree of uncertainty in the literature on electric and magnetic field exposure and cancer risk. This uncertainty should be considered in the context of the low individual risk and the comparable environmental risks (eg, traffic hazards) in other locations. Obtaining magnetic field measurements in the home sometimes will show that field levels are at approximately the average level despite proximity to the power line.

*Q   Our child has leukemia and was exposed to power lines or an electric appliance. Could this have caused the leukemia?*

A   From an objective viewpoint, pinpointing the cause of your child's leukemia is currently beyond the ability of science. Even when there is scientific consensus that a factor, such as ionizing radiation, can cause childhood leukemia, it is impossible to be certain whether a particular case of leukemia was caused by radiation. It is even more problematic for electric and magnetic fields, for which evidence of an association is weak.

*Q   Have any states or countries set standards for electric and magnetic fields?*

A   Lack of knowledge has prevented scientists from strongly recommending any health-based regulations. The International Agency for Research on Cancer recommends that policy makers establish guidelines for electric and magnetic field exposures for both the general public and workers and that low-cost measures of reducing exposure be considered. Several states have adopted regulations governing transmission line-generated 60-Hz fields. The initial concern was the risk of electric shock from strong electric fields (measured in kilovolts [kV] per meter). Some states, such as Florida and New York, have adopted regulations that preclude new lines from exceeding the fields at the edge of the current right-of-way. These standards are in the hundreds of milligauss. The California Department of Education requires that new schools be built at certain distances from transmission lines. These distances, 100 ft for 100-kV lines and 250 ft for 345-kV power lines, were chosen on the basis of the estimate that electric fields would have reached the background level at these distances. All of the current regulations relate to transmission lines, and no state has adopted regulations that govern distribution lines, substations, appliances, or other sources of electric and magnetic fields.

Q   *Is it all right for my child or teenager to use a cell phone?*

A   Epidemiologic studies to assess the risk of cell phone use by children, adolescents, and young adults are ongoing. The level of energy absorption in children while using cell phones is comparable to the levels in adults; however, because of the larger number of ions contained in the tissue of children, the specific tissue absorption rate may be higher. Experts in some countries have suggested that widespread use of cell phones by children be discouraged.[3,42] The American Academy of Pediatrics has recently issued recommendations on reducing exposure among children.[43] Because modern children will experience a longer period of exposure to cell phones than current adults, additional research in this area is needed. In the interim, exposures can be reduced by encouraging children to use text messaging when possible, make only short and essential calls on cell phones, use hands-free kits and wired headsets, and maintain the cell phone an inch or more away from the head. Talking on a cell phone while driving or texting while driving results in distraction and increases the risk of automobile crashes with resulting injuries and fatalities. Teenagers and others should not talk on the phone or text while driving.

Q   *How can I limit cell phone radiation exposure to myself and my children?*

A   The American Academy of Pediatrics reminds parents that cell phones are not toys and it is not recommended for infants and toddlers to play with them. Some cell phone safety tips for families are listed below. Additional information can be found at: https://www.healthychildren.org/English/safety-prevention/all-around/Pages/Cell-Phone-Radiation-Childrens-Health.aspx

—   Use text messaging when possible and use cell phones in speaker mode or with the use of hands-free kits.

—   When talking on the cell phone, try holding it an inch or more away from your head.

—   Make only short or essential calls on cell phones.

—   Avoid carrying your phone against the body like in a pocket, sock, or bra. Cell phone manufacturers cannot guarantee that the amount of radiation you are absorbing will be at a safe level.

—   Keep an eye on your signal strength (ie, how many bars you have). The weaker your cell signal, the harder your phone has to work and the more radiation it gives off. It is better to wait until you have a stronger signal before using your device. Avoid making calls in cars, elevators, trains, and buses. The cell phone works harder to get a signal through metal, so the power level increases.

— If you plan to watch a movie on your device, download it first, then switch to airplane mode while you watch to avoid unnecessary radiation exposure.

Q   *What exposures occur from Wi-Fi networks at home and in schools?*

A   Wireless local area networks, or Wi-Fi, use radio waves to connect Wi-Fi–enabled devices to an access point that is connected to the Internet. Most Wi-Fi devices operate at radio-frequencies that are similar to cell phones, typically 2.4 to 2.5 GHz, although more recently there are Wi-Fi devices that operate at somewhat higher frequencies (5, 5.3, or 5.8 GHz). Radio-frequency radiation exposure from Wi-Fi devices is considerably lower than that from cell phones. The UK Health Protection Agency (now part of Public Health England) conducted a measurement study to assess children's exposures to radio-frequency exposures from Wi-Fi and concluded that exposures were well below recommended maximum levels and there was "no reason why Wi-Fi should not continue to be used in schools and other places."[44]

Q   *I understand the uncertainty in the science, but I believe that it is prudent to avoid magnetic fields when possible. What low- and no-cost measures of avoidance can I take?*

A   For most people, their highest magnetic field exposures come from using household appliances with motors, transformers, or heaters. The easily avoidable exposures would come from these appliances. If a parent is concerned about electric and magnetic field exposure from appliances, the major sources of exposure could be identified and the parent could limit the child's time near such appliances.[2] Manufacturers have reduced magnetic field exposures from electric blankets (since 1990) and from computers (since the early 1990s). Because magnetic fields decline rapidly with increasing distance, an easy measure is to increase the distance between the child and the appliance.

Q   *What are the concerns about cell phone use among pregnant women?*

A   Three studies on this topic from the Danish National Birth Cohort have been published. Two studies demonstrated that cell phone use prenatally was associated with behavioral difficulties, such as emotional and hyper-activity problems, around the age of school entry.[30,31] A third study of cell phone use during pregnancy did not identify delays in developmental milestones among offspring up to 18 months of age.[32] Additional research from other populations is needed to clarify this issue.

## Resources

**American Academy of Pediatrics**

Healthy Children.org

Cell Phone Radiation & Children's Health: What Parents Need to Know
https://www.healthychildren.org/English/safety-prevention/all-around/
Pages/Cell-Phone-Radiation-Childrens-Health.aspxDocument4

https://www.healthychildren.org/English/family-life/Media/Pages/
Cell-Phones-Whats-the-Right-Age-to-Start.aspx

https://www.healthychildren.org/English/safety-prevention/all-around/
Pages/Cell-Phone-Radiation-Childrens-Health.aspx

**National Cancer Institute**

Fact Sheets:

Electromagnetic Fields and Cancer. https://www.cancer.gov/about-cancer/
causes-prevention/risk/radiation/electromagnetic-fields-fact-sheet

Cell Phones and Cancer Risk. https://www.cancer.gov/about-cancer/
causes-prevention/risk/radiation/cell-phones-fact-sheet

**National Institute of Environmental Health Sciences**

Phone: 919-541-3345

Web site: www.niehs.nih.gov

Electric & Magnetic Fields. http://www.niehs.nih.gov/health/topics/
agents/emf/

**National Research Council**

Possible Health Effects of Exposure to Residential Electric and Magnetic
Fields. https://www.nap.edu/catalog/5155/possible-health-effects-of-
exposure-to-residential-electric-and-magnetic-fields

**US Federal Communications Commission (FCC)**

The FCC licenses communications systems that use radio-frequency
and microwave-frequency EMF. https://transition.fcc.gov/bureaus/oet/
info/documents/bulletins/oet56/oet56e4.pdf

Fact sheet on Wireless devices and health concerns. https://www.fcc.gov/
consumers/guides/wireless-devices-and-health-concerns

Safety information on radiofrequency and microwave emissions from
devices regulated by the FCC.

https://www.fcc.gov/engineering-technology/electromagnetic-
compatibility-division/radio-frequency-safety/faq/rf-safety

## US Food and Drug Administration (FDA)

Phone: 888-INFO-FDA (888-463-6332)

Information about cellular telephones. www.fda.gov/Radiation-
EmittingProducts/RadiationEmittingProductsandProcedures/
HomeBusinessandEntertainment/CellPhones/

## World Health Organization

Monograph No. 238, and Fact Sheet Nos. 193 and 304. www.who.int/peh-emf/
en and https://www.iarc.fr/en/media-centre/iarcnews/2011/IARC_
Mobiles_QA.pdf www.who.int/peh-emf/publications/facts/fs304/en/

## REFERENCES

1.  Feychting M, Ahlbom A, Kheifets L. EMF and health. *Annu Rev Public Health*. 2005;26:165–189
2.  EMF RAPID Program. Electric and Magnetic Fields Associated with the Use of Electric
    Power. Research Triangle Park, NC: National Institute of Environmental Health Sciences,
    National Institutes of Health; 2002. http://www.niehs.nih.gov/health/materials/electric_and_
    magnetic_fields_associated_with_the_use_of_electric_power_questions_and_answers_
    english_508.pdf. Accessed March 4, 2018
3.  Kheifets L, Repacholi M, Saunders R, van Deventer E. The sensitivity of children to
    electromagnetic fields. *Pediatrics*. 2005;116(2):e303–e313
4.  Maslanyj M, Simpson J, Roman E, Schuz J. Power frequency magnetic fields and risk of
    childhood leukaemia: misclassification of exposure from the use of the 'distance from power
    line' exposure surrogate. *Bioelectromagnetics*. 2009;30(3):183–188
5.  Zaffanella L. Survey of Residential Magnetic Field Sources: Volumes 1 and 2. Palo Alto,
    CA: Electric Power Research Institute; 1993. http://www.epri.com/abstracts/Pages/
    ProductAbstract.aspx?ProductId=TR-102759-V1. Accessed March 4, 2018
6.  Friedman DR, Hatch EE, Tarone R, et al. Childhood exposure to magnetic fields: residential
    area measurements compared to personal dosimetry. *Epidemiology*. 1996;7(2):151–155
7.  SCENIHR. 2015. Scientific Committee on Emerging and Newly Identified Health Risks:
    Potential health effects of exposure to electromagnetic fields (EMF). http://ec.europa.eu/
    health/scientific_committees/emerging/docs/scenihr_o_041.pdf. Accessed March 4, 2018
8.  International Agency for Research on Cancer. IARC Monographs on the Evaluation of
    Carcinogenic Risks to Humans. Non-ionizing radiation. Vol 102, Part 2, Radiofrequency
    electromagnetic fields. Lyon, France: International Agency for Research on Cancer; 2013
9.  Cleveland RF Jr, Ulcek JL. Questions and Answers About Biological Effects and Potential
    Hazards of Radiofrequency Electromagnetic Fields. 4th ed. Washington, DC: Federal
    Communications Commission; 1999. OET Bulletin No. 56. https://transition.fcc.gov/bureaus/
    oet/info/documents/bulletins/oet56/oet56e4.pdf. Accessed March 4, 2018
10. International Commission on Non-Ionizing Radiation Protection. ICNIRP statement on EMF-
    emitting new technologies. *Health Phys*. 2008;94(4):376–392
11. Christ A, Gosselin MC, Christopoulou M, Kühn S, Kuster N. Age-dependent tissue-specific
    exposure of cell phone users. *Phys Med Biol*. 2010;55(7):1767–1783
12. Dimbylow PJ, Mann SM. SAR calculations in an anatomically realistic model of the head for
    mobile communication transceivers at 900 MHz and 1.8 GHz. *Phys Med Biol*. 1994;39(10):
    1537–1553

13. International Agency for Research on Cancer. IARC Monographs on the Evaluation of Carcinogenic Risks to Humans. Volume 80. Non-Ionizing Radiation, Part 1: Static and Extremely Low-Frequency (ELF) Electric and Magnetic Fields. Lyon, France: International Agency for Research on Cancer; 2002

14. Schuz J. Implications from epidemiologic studies on magnetic fields and the risk of childhood leukemia on protection guidelines. *Health Phys.* 2007;92(6):642–648

15. World Health Organization. 2007. Environmental Health Criteria Document on ELF Fields, Doc No. 238, downloadable from the WHO EMF Project. www.who.int/emf. Accessed March 4, 2018

16. Greenland S, Sheppard AR, Kaune WT, Poole C, Kelsh MA. A pooled analysis of magnetic fields, wire codes, and childhood leukemia. Childhood Leukemia-EMF Study Group. *Epidemiology.* 2000;11(6):624–634

17. Ahlbom A, Day N, Feychting M, et al. A pooled analysis of magnetic fields and childhood leukaemia. *Br J Cancer.* 2000;83(5):692–698

18. Kheifets L, Ahlbom A, Crespi CM, et al. Pooled analysis of recent studies on magnetic fields and childhood leukaemia. *Br J Cancer.* 2010;103(7):1128–1135

19. Schuz J, Grell K, Kinsey S, et al. Extremely low-frequency magnetic fields and survival from childhood acute lymphoblastic leukemia: an international follow-up study. *Blood Cancer J.* 2012;2:e98

20. Su L, Fei Y, Wei X, et al. Associations of parental occupational exposure to extremely low-frequency magnetic fields with childhood leukemia risk. *Leuk Lymphoma.* 2016;57(12): 2855–2862

21. Mezei G, Gadallah M, Kheifets L. Residential magnetic field exposure and childhood brain cancer: a meta-analysis. *Epidemiology.* 2008;19(3):424–430

22. Kheifets L, Ahlbom A, Crespi CM, et al. A pooled analysis of extremely low-frequency magnetic fields and childhood brain tumors. *Am J Epidemiol.* 2010;172(7):752–761

23. Ahlbom IC, Cardis E, Green A, Linet M, Savitz D, Swerdlow A. Review of the epidemiologic literature on EMF and health. *Environ Health Perspect.* 2001;109(Suppl 6):911–933

24. Kheifets L, Shimkhada R. Childhood leukemia and EMF: review of the epidemiologic evidence. *Bioelectromagnetics.* 2005;(Suppl 7):S51–S59

25. Hatch EE, Kleinerman RA, Linet MS, et al. Do confounding or selection factors of residential wiring codes and magnetic fields distort finding of electromagnetic fields studies? *Epidemiology.* 2000;11(2):189–198

26. AGNIR. 2012. Health effects from radiofrequency electromagnetic fields. Report from the Independent Advisory Group on Non-Ionising Radiation. In: Documents of the Health Protection Agency R, Chemical and Environmental Hazards. RCE 20, Health Protection Agency, UK, ed.

27. INTERPHONE Study Group. Brain tumour risk in relation to mobile telephone use: results of the INTERPHONE international case-control study. *Int J Epidemiol.* 2010;39(3):675–694

28. Aydin D, Feychting M, Schüz J, et al. Mobile phone use and brain tumors in children and adolescents: a multicenter case-control study. *J Natl Cancer Inst.* 2011;103(16):1264–1276

29. Sadetzki S, Eastman Langer C, Bruchim R, et al. The MOBI-Kids study protocol: challenges in assessing childhood and adolescent exposure to electromagnetic fields from wireless telecommunication technologies and possible association with brain tumor risk. *Front Public Health.* 2014;2:124.

30. Divan HA, Kheifets L, Obel C, Olsen J. Prenatal and postnatal exposure to cell phone use and behavioral problems in children. *Epidemiology.* 2008;19(4):523–552

31. Divan HA, Kheifets L, Obel C, Olsen J. Cell phone use and behavioural problems in young children. *J Epidemiol Community Health.* 2012;66(6):524–529

32. Divan HA, Kheifets L, Olsen J. Prenatal cell phone use and developmental milestone delays among infants. *Scand J Work Environ Health*. 2011;37(4):341–348

33. American Physical Society. APS council adopts statement on EMFs and public health. APS News Online. 1995;4(7). Reaffirmed 2008. http://www.aps.org/publications/apsnews/199507/council.cfm. Accessed March 4, 2018

34. Moulder JE. The electric and magnetic fields research and public information dissemination (EMF-RAPID) program. *Radiat Res*. 2000;153(5 Pt 2):613–616

35. Brainard GC, Kavet R, Kheifets LI. The relationship between electromagnetic field and light exposures to melatonin and breast cancer risk: a review of the relevant literature. *J Pineal Res*. 1999;26(2):65–100

36. Davis S, Mirick DK, Stevens RG. Residential magnetic fields and the risk of breast cancer. *Am J Epidemiol*. 2002;155(5):446–454

37. Vijayalaxmi, Obe G. Controversial cytogenetic observations in mammalian somatic cells exposed to extremely low frequency electromagnetic radiation: a review and future research recommendations. *Bioelectromagnetics*. 2005;26(5):412–430

38. Repacholi MH, Basten A, Gebski V, Noonan D, Finnie J, Harris AW. Lymphomas in E mu-Pim1 transgenic mice exposed to pulsed 900 MHZ electromagnetic fields. *Radiat Res*. 1997;147(5):631–640

39. Brusick D, Albertini R, McRee D, et al. Genotoxicity of radiofrequency radiation. DNA/Genetox Expert Panel. *Environ Mol Mutagen*. 1998;32(1):1–16

40. Repacholi MH. Health risks from the use of mobile phones. *Toxicol Lett*. 2001;120(1-3):323–331

41. Falcioni L, Bua L, Tibaldi E, et al. Report of final results regarding brain and heart tumors in Sprague-Dawley rats exposed from prenatal life until natural death to mobile phone radiofrequency field representative of a 1.8 GHz GSM base station environmental emission. *Environ Res*. 2018;165:496–503

42. Independent Expert Group on Mobile Phones. Mobile Phones and Health. http://webarchive.nationalarchives.gov.uk/20100221114405/http://www.iegmp.org.uk/. Accessed March 4, 2018

43. American Academy of Pediatrics Healthy Children.org Cell Phone Radiation & Children's Health: What Parents Need to Know. https://www.healthychildren.org/English/safety-prevention/all-around/Pages/Cell-Phone-Radiation-Childrens-Health.aspx. Accessed March 4, 2018

44. Public Health England. Wireless networks (wi-fi): radio waves and health. Guidance. Published November 1, 2013. https://www.gov.uk/government/publications/wireless-networks-wi-fi-radio-waves-and-health/wi-fi-radio-waves-and-health. Accessed March 4, 2018

Chapter 28

# Electronic Nicotine Delivery Systems and Other Alternative Nicotine Products

○ ○ ○ ○ ○ ○

## KEY POINTS

- Electronic nicotine delivery systems (ENDS), such as electronic cigarettes, are rapidly rising in popularity among youth, thereby raising concerns about addicting a new generation to nicotine and tobacco.
- Nicotine, a main ingredient in most of these products, is a highly addictive and toxic component with neurotoxic effects on developing brains, including the adolescent brain.
- Other chemicals in ENDS, such as flavorings considered safe when ingested, have not been tested for safety when they are inhaled.
- Youth who start with the use of ENDS are more likely to go on to use other forms of tobacco, including combustible tobacco, and are less likely to stop tobacco use.
- The aerosol inhaled from ENDS can contain harmful and potentially harmful ingredients; the aerosol can affect non-users through secondhand and thirdhand exposure.
- The concentrated nicotine solution used in ENDS devices is a poisoning risk to children.

■ Clinicians should ask patients about the use of ENDS and other tobacco products, counsel users to quit, and offer anticipatory guidance to prevent initiation of tobacco and nicotine product use.

■ Effective public policies to protect youth from ENDS and other tobacco products are needed.

Tobacco use remains the leading cause of preventable morbidity and mortality in the world, including in the United States.[1–4] Cigarette consumption in US adults, however, declined from nearly 21 of every 100 adults (20.9%) in 2005 to more than 15 of every 100 adults (15.5%) in 2016.[5] As cigarettes decline in popularity, there has been a surge in the use of alternative nicotine products, providing other ways to consume tobacco or nicotine. For example, the use of non-cigarette combustible tobacco, such as hookah, has increased by 96.9%.[6] Alternative nicotine products are a mix of old and new, encompassing forms of smoking that pre-date commercial cigarettes, such as cigars and chewing tobacco, new products introduced in the current century such as dissolvable tobacco and electronic cigarettes ("e-cigarettes"), and new interest in traditional smoking methods, such as hookah.

## ELECTRONIC NICOTINE DELIVERY SYSTEMS

Electronic nicotine delivery systems (ENDS) can be referred to by many terms, including electronic cigarettes, e-cigarettes, e-cigars, vape pens, vapes, e-hookah, JUUL, mechanical mods, and others. The term "ENDS" is not entirely accurate because these devices deliver more than nicotine. The best-known example of an ENDS product is the e-cigarette. ENDS are handheld devices that produce an aerosol for inhalation from a solution that typically contains nicotine, flavoring chemicals, and carrier solvents. Other toxicants and carcinogens, such as tobacco-specific nitrosamines, can be present as contaminants and may be generated by heating the solution. Wide variability exists in product design and engineering.[7] Some devices resemble a conventional cigarette. Others may bear a closer resemblance to a pen, a crayon, or even a flash drive for a computer. Using e-cigarettes is often referred to as "vaping."

No regulations on content, design, or even manufacturing standards exist in the United States at present. Other substances of abuse, such as marijuana and hashish, can be delivered via ENDS devices. Some ENDS devices appear to be designed and/or marketed specifically for delivery of these substances (often referred to as "Herb" on their marketing materials).

In addition to nicotine, toxicants in ENDS products include ultrafine particulates, volatile organic compounds, metallic nanoparticles (ie, nickel, tin, cadmium, lead) and tobacco-related carcinogens including nitrosamines and polycyclic aromatic hydrocarbons. Products come in different strengths of nicotine. More than 7,000 flavors are available commercially (popular flavors include candy, desserts, fruits, and mint)[8,9] and flavoring chemicals have been found in more than 90% of e-cigarette samples tested.[10] Flavorings that may be safe to eat may be toxic when inhaled. The flavors used in ENDS products have only been evaluated for safety via ingestion; little scientific information has been reported about the effect of inhaling particular flavors. Many flavoring agents used are known pulmonary irritants. Others, such as diacetyl, can cause pulmonary fibrosis and bronchiolitis obliterans. Many have been shown to injure airway cells in vitro.[11,12]

The amount of nicotine, flavorings, and other constituents in ENDS varies widely. Contaminants or adulterants may not be disclosed. Heating produces additional toxicants that can present health risks.[13]

Nonusers can be exposed to the aerosol coming directly from a device and from aerosol exhaled by the user; these are termed secondhand emissions. Metabolites of 5 carcinogens (acrylamide, acrolein, crotonaldehyde, acrylonitrile, and propylene oxide) were found to be significantly higher in the urine of adolescents who were ENDS-only users compared with nonusers.[14] Thirdhand ENDS emissions, similar to thirdhand emissions of tobacco smoke, remain in dust and on surfaces after ENDS use. ENDS toxicants can then be re-volatilized or re-suspended to produce secondary pollutants.

## History of Electronic Nicotine Delivery Systems

The Chinese pharmacist Hon Lik developed the e-cigarette in 2003. These products entered the US marketplace in approximately 2007. The US Food and Drug Administration (FDA) initially attempted to keep the product off the US market, claiming it was a combination drug device product under the Federal Food, Drug, and Cosmetic Act. The industry sued the FDA and won, claiming it was a tobacco product and not a drug for tobacco dependence treatment. In 2016, the FDA issued a "deeming rule" that would have extended its authority to regulate ENDS products to protect public health under the authority of the Family Smoking Prevention and Tobacco Control Act, and require pre-market review of new tobacco products (ie, those not on the market on February 15, 2007.) The FDA, however, deferred its responsibilities for pre-market review of ENDS products. In April 2018, the FDA announced new enforcement actions against retailers of JUUL electronic cigarettes who market their products to youth. In addition, a Youth Tobacco Prevention Plan was announced to examine the appeal to youth of these products and to limit access of products to minors.[15]

## Electronic Nicotine Delivery Systems and Children

A dramatic rise in e-cigarette use among American youth has occurred in recent years. Use of e-cigarettes increased from 1.4% in 2011 to 4.3% in 2016 among middle school students, and from 4.7% in 2011 to 11.3% in 2016 among high school students.[13,16] The 2017 Monitoring the Future survey revealed even higher use with 19% of 12th graders reporting vaping nicotine in the past year and annual prevalence levels of 8% and 16% for 8th and 10th graders, respectively.[17]

ENDS appeal to youth who would not otherwise be attracted to tobacco products.[18] Flavoring agents, appealing and discreet designs, promotion on broadcast media, print media, social media, promotional activities (ie, vaping cloud competitions, vape tricks), point of sale advertising, and use of celebrity role models have contributed to the rapid rise in ENDS use among youth. Marketing themes mirror those found to appeal to youth in conventional cigarette advertising. The most common reasons that young people give for using e-cigarettes are curiosity, flavoring/taste, and low perceived harm.[13] The JUUL product, an ENDS device designed to look like a flash drive, is popular among high school students because it is discreet enough to be used where e-cigarette use is prohibited and may not be recognized as an ENDS device by school personnel.[19] Youth may refer to ENDS product use as "vaping" or "Juuling."

Youth who use ENDS are more likely to initiate use of combustible tobacco and less likely to stop use of combustible tobacco.[20,21] Two thirds of middle and high school students who use e-cigarettes also report use of other tobacco products.[13] The evidence to date suggests that ENDS are addicting a new generation to nicotine and tobacco.[21]

Concern has been raised that ENDS use may be a "gateway" that facilitates abuse of other drugs. Nicotine has been shown to function as a gateway drug in animal models and human observational studies. In laboratory animal studies, priming with nicotine increases the rewarding properties of cocaine.[22] In persons aged 12 to 17 years, use of illicit drugs is much more common among current smokers than nonsmokers (55% versus 6%).[23]

## OTHER ALTERNATIVE TOBACCO PRODUCTS

Hookahs, also known as waterpipes or narghiles, are smoking instruments that pass tobacco smoke though water before inhalation. Their key pieces include a head, water bowl, and hoses. The head is commonly filled with shisha, which is moist tobacco or other combustible vegetative matter, often combined with sweetener and flavorings, then covered with a perforated piece of aluminum foil on top of which a lit charcoal is placed. The lit charcoal heats the shisha below as a smoker inhales through the hose to bubble the smoke of the tobacco and charcoal through the water bowl.[24] Hookah use often is a social activity, with one or multiple hoses connected to one bowl. Hookah use among children and adults has rapidly increased in recent years, resulting in a global epidemic.[25] In the span of 5 years (2011 to 2016), hookah use among adolescents increased by 17%,[6] and more than 12% of US adults have used the product.[26] Bidis are tobacco wrapped in a tendu leaf. Kreteks are tobacco flavored with cloves.

## Non-cigarette Combustible Tobacco

Because of differing taxation rates and regulations of flavorings, cigars, cigarillos, pipe tobacco, and roll-your-own tobacco have become more popular. Recent changes to federal excise taxes made pipe tobacco a much cheaper alternative to roll-your-own; between 2008 and 2011, sales of roll-your-own tobacco decreased by 75.7% and sales of pipe tobacco increased by 573.1%. Similar changes in taxation policy between large and small cigars led manufacturers to slightly modify their products to fall into the more favorable large cigar taxation group, resulting in more than doubling of large cigar consumption between 2008 and 2011.[6] Cigars and cigarillos are legally differentiated from cigarettes by containing tobacco in the wrapper; manufacturers, however, have made cigars and cigarettes so similar in appearance that when smokers were shown pictures of these products, more than 40% misidentified one brand of cigar as a cigarette.[27] Although flavorings in cigarettes (other than menthol) were banned in the United States in 2009, other tobacco products were not similarly regulated and all the previously mentioned combustible tobacco products are available in a wide range of flavors, which can appeal to children.[28]

Although not currently available in the United States, "heat-not-burn" is the latest tobacco product that has entered the marketplace. It uses disposable tobacco sticks soaked in propylene glycol that are inserted into a holder that heats the product to create an emission. These devices produce the same toxicants and carcinogens as conventional cigarettes, although, according to some studies, the toxicants are present in lower quantities. Although the industry claims that these devices are harm reduction products, the evidence is not sufficient to support their claim. As with ENDS, there is concern that these devices may serve as an introductory product for youth. In Japan, where the product has been released and promoted, 20% of persons aged 15 to 19 years reported trying the product.[29,30]

## Smokeless Tobacco Products

Several forms of smokeless tobacco are on the market, many of which have been introduced recently. Traditional forms of smokeless tobacco include chewing tobacco, dip, and dry snuff. Chewing tobacco is chewed on and the juices spit out. Dip tobacco (also called moist snuff) is placed between the lower lip and teeth and sucked on, and the resulting juices also are spit out. Dry snuff, of anatomical snuff box fame (because snuff could be placed there and then inhaled), can be inhaled through the nose ("snorted"), or used orally.[31] New products termed "dissolvable tobacco products" (DTPs) also have come to market. DTPs were first introduced to the United States in 2001 by Avira, and in 2009 Camel released an expanded line in the form of orbs, sticks, and strips similar in appearance and size to small candies, toothpicks, and breath strips. These DTPs consist of finely milled tobacco mixed with flavorings. Snus (rhymes with goose), a small pouch similar to a tea bag, is filled with tobacco and placed under the upper lip.[32] Because of their discrete use and lack of spitting, snus and DTPs have been widely marketed as alternatives or accompaniments to cigarette smoking in places such as airports, where smoking is prohibited.[33] More than 1 million students—5.8% of high school students and 2.2% of middle school students—used smokeless tobacco in 2016.[16]

Hookah, smokeless tobacco, and cigars are popular among youth, with use reported by 5% to 8% of high school students in the United States. These products are available with flavors such as fruit, candy, and mint. Close to one half of adolescents who use tobacco use 2 or more types of tobacco products.[34,35]

Table 28-1 lists traditional and alternative tobacco and nicotine products.

## ROUTES OF EXPOSURE

The route of exposure to alterative nicotine products depends on the type of product. For users of electronic cigarettes, hookah, cigars, and other non-cigarette combustible tobacco, exposure occurs by direct inhalation. Children and others can be exposed to the secondhand aerosol and particulates emanating from these products. Children can be exposed to smokeless tobacco products by intentional use or unintentionally consuming them if products are confused with candy.[36] Exposure to nicotine-containing e-liquid used to fill e-cigarettes can occur unintentionally, or by intentional ingestion, dermal contact, or intravenous injection.[37–39] Exposure to smokeless tobacco products occurs through ingestion.

### Systems Affected

Nicotine affects the brain, including the developing brain. In acute toxicity, nicotine binds to nicotinic cholinergic receptors leading to sympathetic nervous stimulation, parasympathetic stimulation, and neuromuscular blockade.

Chronic effects arise from nicotine addiction. Nicotine, the primary psychoactive and addictive constituent of tobacco and alternative tobacco products, changes brain structure and chemistry leading to an addiction that is often severe. More than two thirds of people who have tried 1 cigarette go on to become daily smokers.[40] One study found that almost one third of nonsmoking individuals who have tried an e-cigarette go on to initiate conventional cigarette smoking.[21] Children and adolescents are particularly vulnerable to the development of nicotine addiction.[13]

Exposure to nicotine can affect the fetus. The 2014 Report of the US Surgeon General on the health consequences of smoking concluded, "The evidence is sufficient to infer that nicotine exposure during fetal development, a critical window for brain development, has lasting adverse consequences for brain development."[4] The 2016 Report of the US Surgeon General concluded, "Nicotine delivered by e-cigarettes during pregnancy can result in multiple adverse consequences, including sudden infant death syndrome, and could result in altered corpus callosum, deficits in auditory processing, and obesity."[13]

Nicotine exposure during gestation can have an impact on fetal lung development. Tobacco product use by pregnant women increases the risk for wheezing in their children. Laboratory animal models show changes in lung development specifically caused by the actions of nicotine at the alpha-7 nicotinic cholinergic receptor.[41,42]

Studies in laboratory animal models demonstrate that inhalation of nicotine-containing e-cigarettes leads to changes in the lungs associated with the development of chronic obstructive pulmonary disease.[43] Although many carcinogens are present in the emission of tobacco products, emerging research suggests that nicotine itself can promote a cancer-supporting microenvironment by a number of mechanisms including suppressing apoptosis of precancerous cells, damage to the genome, disruption of cellular metabolic processes, amplification of oncogenes, and inactivation of tumor suppressor genes.[44,45] Emerging research suggests that e-cigarette emissions alter innate immunity of the lungs, predisposing persons to infection and lung damage.[46,47]

## Toxicity of Other Constituents

Flavoring agents in ENDS and other tobacco products can cause irritation leading to cough, bronchitis, and asthma. Some components (ie, cinnamaldehyde) may have cytotoxic effects. Commonly used flavoring agents (ie, diacetyl) are linked to airway epithelial damage and to bronchiolitis obliterans. Heating of the liquid to create the aerosol can generate additional toxicants and carcinogens including formaldehyde, acetaldehyde, and acrolein.[48] Metallic nanoparticles, including tin, lead, nickel, and cadmium, have been found in ENDS aerosols,[49] believed to be generated from the heating elements and atomizer. Chemicals used for flavoring may not be disclosed correctly on product labels. Because the nicotine for ENDS is extracted from tobacco, the ENDS solutions are commonly contaminated with tobacco-related toxins and carcinogens and the solvents used for nicotine extraction.[13]

## Clinical Effects

### Nicotine Toxicity

The early symptoms of acute nicotine toxicity include tremor, nausea, tachycardia, increased blood pressure, salivation, sweating, vomiting, cardiac arrhythmias, and seizures. Late symptoms (0.5 to 4 hours) include hypotension, bradycardia,

## Table 28-1. Tobacco Products

| PRODUCT | DESCRIPTION | COMMENTS |
|---|---|---|
| Cigarette | A small roll of paper filled with cut tobacco and smoked | Cigarettes are still the most common form of tobacco used by youth. |
| Cigars and little cigars | A cigar is a tightly-rolled bundle of dried and fermented tobacco, wrapped in a tobacco leaf. Cigars come in flavors including "cherry," "peach," and "grape." Little cigars are similar to regular cigarettes, except that their wrapping is tobacco leaf rather than paper. | In the United States, cigars are exempt from many of the marketing regulations that govern cigarettes; cigars are taxed at a far lower rate than cigarettes. Flavors and lower cost appeal to children. |
| Pipe | A tube with a small bowl at one end; used for smoking tobacco | Pipes use black (air cured) tobacco, which carries a higher risk of esophageal cancer. |
| Hookah or Narghile | A single or multi-stemmed instrument for smoking in which the smoke is cooled by passing through water. A hookah uses moist tobacco ("shisha") that is often combined with sweeteners and flavorings. A piece of charcoal placed on top of the shisha heats it as the smoker inhales. | Longer duration of a smoking session and deeper inhalation lead to much higher smoke intake than cigarette smoking. |
| Bidi or Beedi | A thin, South Asian cigarette filled with tobacco flake and wrapped in a tendu leaf tied with a string at one end. | Bidis must be puffed more rapidly than regular cigarettes to remain lit. Bidis contain more tar, nicotine, and carbon monoxide than the typical cigarette. |
| Kretek | Cigarettes made with a blend of tobacco, cloves, and other flavors. The word 'kretek' is an onomatopoetic term for the crackling sound of burning cloves. | Cloves contain eugenol, whose local anesthetic effect allows deeper inhalation. |

| Product | Description | |
|---|---|---|
| Chewing tobacco | Loose leaves, plugs, or twists of tobacco placed between the cheek and gum | |
| Snuff | Finely ground tobacco packaged in cans or pouches, which can be sold dry (powdered form that is sniffed) or moist (placed between the lower lip or cheek and gum) | |
| Snus | A moist powder tobacco product originating from a variant of dry snuff. It is usually not fermented. | |
| Dissolvable tobacco | Finely milled tobacco mixed with flavorings. Unlike ordinary chewing tobacco, it dissolves in the mouth. Orbs or pellets look similar to small breath mints. Sticks similar to toothpicks are for insertion between the upper lip and gum. Strips administer nicotine through thin film drug delivery technology and look similar to breath-freshening strips. | Discreet form, candy-like appearance, and added flavorings that make them attractive to young children |
| Electronic nicotine delivery systems (ENDS) termed e-cigarettes, e-cigs, hookah sticks, e-hookahs, vape pens, JUUL, others | Battery-powered devices heat a solution to create a vapor. There is no regulation on content. Devices usually contain nicotine, propylene glycol, glycerin, and flavoring agents. Heating the mixture creates other toxicants. | Flavors and promotion increase appeal to youth. |
| Heat-not-burn tobacco | Disposable tobacco sticks soaked in propylene glycol that are inserted into a holder that heats the tobacco | Produces the same toxicants and carcinogens as conventional cigarettes, although in a lower quantity. Not yet on the market in the United States. Has been popular with adolescents where it has been released and promoted. |

(Adapted from Farber HJ, Groner G, Walley S, et al. American Academy of Pediatrics Technical Report: Protecting Children From Tobacco, Nicotine, and Tobacco Smoke. *Pediatrics.* 2015;136(5):e1439–e1467)

lethargy, respiratory failure, and death. The LD$_{50}$ for nicotine is estimated as 0.8 to 13 mg/kg. It is estimated that 2 mL of the concentrated nicotine solution used in some ENDS devices can be sufficient to kill a small child.[7]

### Nicotine Withdrawal Symptoms

Symptoms include irritability, frustration, anger, increased appetite, tremors, depression, insomnia, anxiety, difficulty concentrating, and difficulty feeling pleasure. Nicotine withdrawal is not simply hedonistic craving. When a person is addicted to nicotine, the brain does not work normally without the nicotine.[50]

### Respiratory Irritation From ENDS Use

Propylene glycol and glycerol (the vehicle in ENDS devices) aerosols can cause respiratory irritation and asthma exacerbations.[13]

### Burns and Traumatic Injuries

Failure of the lithium ion battery in ENDS can result in explosion leading to burns and traumatic injuries to the face, bodies, and/or hands, and cause house fires.[7,13]

### Clinical Effects of Other Tobacco Products

Combustible tobacco products harm most organ systems of the body. Tobacco kills people when used as intended. The 2014 Report of the Surgeon General, *The Health Consequences of Smoking: 50 Years of Progress*, describes the diseases that result from cigarette smoking (see Chapter 43).[4]

### Non-cigarette Combustible Tobacco

The clinical effects of non-cigarette combustible tobacco, which includes cigars, cigarillos, pipe tobacco, and loose tobacco for roll-your-own cigarettes, are similar to those from cigarettes. Cigars, cigarillos, and pipe tobacco have dose-response relationships with lung cancer.[51] Cigar smokers with no history of cigarette use have higher rates of oral, esophageal, pancreatic, and laryngeal cancer, coronary heart disease, aortic aneurysm, and all-cause mortality.[52] Cigars and other non-cigarette combustible tobacco products can result in secondhand smoke (SHS) exposure.[53] Large studies of the effects of SHS exposure from non-cigarette combustible tobacco have not yet been completed, but these effects most likely are similar to those resulting from secondhand cigarette smoke exposure given the similarities in combustion method and contents between the two.

### Smokeless Products

The clinical effects of smokeless tobacco products include an increased risk of cancer of the mouth, esophagus, and pancreas,[54] as well as gum disease, tooth loss, tooth decay, leukoplakia, myocardial infarction, stroke, heart disease, and high blood pressure.[54,55] Many studies, however, are limited by the recent introduction of some forms of smokeless tobacco to the market and the poly-use, by some users, of cigarettes and/or alcohol, which are independently associated with cancer.[56,57] Smokeless tobacco can be addictive and expensive, and nicotine can have harmful effects independent of the route of adminis-tration.[58,59] Ingestion of smokeless tobacco products has been of particular concern; new DTPs are shaped and flavored like candy, with concentrations of nicotine high enough to cause symptomatic nausea and vomiting in children after ingestion of only 1 or 2 pieces.[36]

## DIAGNOSTIC METHODS

History is generally the best way to identify tobacco and nicotine use and exposure. Useful questions include the following:

- Do any of your friends use tobacco?
- Have you ever tried a tobacco product?
- How many times have you tried (name of tobacco product)?
- How often do you use (name of tobacco product)?
- Do your friends use e-cigarettes, e-hookah, JUUL, or vape?
- Have you tried an e-cigarette, e-hookah, JUUL, or vape?

Observation of tobacco products, such as a vape pen hanging from a lanyard around the neck, or the impression of a can of smokeless tobacco (dip) in a pocket can be useful diagnostic clues.

## TREATMENT OF CLINICAL SYMPTOMS

### Acute Nicotine Poisoning

Patients with acute nicotine poisoning should be managed with consultation of a medical toxicologist, available through a state or regional poison control center (800-222-1222), or other expert in pediatric poisonings. Supportive care is sufficient for most patients until toxicity resolves.

Muscarinic symptoms (vomiting, diarrhea, bronchorrhea, hypersalivation, and/or wheezing) should be managed with atropine. The dose of atropine should be titrated to dry bronchial secretions without causing significant anticholinergic symptoms (eg, delirium, flushing, elevated temperature).

Nicotinic side effects (eg, seizures, muscle weakness, paralysis) should be managed as follows:

- Treat seizures with benzodiazepines (eg, lorazepam). If seizures persist, phenobarbital should be administered (fosphenytoin and phenytoin are less effective for toxicant-induced seizures).
- Patients with significant muscle weakness and respiratory failure should be intubated and mechanically ventilated.

In patients with severe nicotine poisoning, evaluate serum creatine kinase, urinalysis, and urine myoglobin to monitor for the development of rhabdomyolysis and myoglobinuria.[60]

## Treatment of Tobacco and Nicotine Dependence

Chapter 43 discusses pediatricians' roles in counseling parents and adolescents who use tobacco. Similar strategies can be used for parents and adolescents who use e-cigarettes and other alternative nicotine products. Behaviorally based programs work best for those with mild to moderate degrees of tobacco dependence. The most effective behaviorally based programs focus on problem-solving skills and provide support and encouragement.

Internet-based, telephonic, and smartphone apps to help adolescents stop smoking are available (see Resources). Among adolescents with moderate to severe nicotine dependence, pharmacotherapy for tobacco dependence that has been FDA-approved for use in adults can be an effective adjunct to behavioral therapy. Medications to treat tobacco dependence, however, are not FDA-approved for minors, nonadherence among minors is common, and relapse after stopping therapy is common. Practitioners who choose to recommend the off-label use of pharmacotherapy to adolescent patients should balance the risks of pharmacotherapy against the risks of continued tobacco or ENDS product use. When used, pharmacotherapy for tobacco dependence should be combined with behavioral counseling and close follow up. Psychiatric co-morbidities and other substance abuse may accompany tobacco dependence and make tobacco dependence more difficult to treat. People with psychiatric and other substance abuse co-morbidities should be referred to appropriate mental health professionals.[61]

## PREVENTION OF EXPOSURE

All tobacco and nicotine products should be kept out of reach of children. Concentrated nicotine solutions should have childproof caps and be sold only in quantities that would not be lethal to a child. Labeling, packaging, and product design should avoid appealing to children and youth. National legislation, the Child Nicotine Poisoning Prevention Act, requiring child-safe packaging for all nicotine-containing liquids, was signed into law in January 2016.[62]

Parents and health care providers should counsel children about the importance of not starting tobacco and nicotine product (including ENDS) use. Experimenting with tobacco and nicotine use is not safe. Use of ENDS are not safe, even if the liquid used claims to contain no nicotine. Counseling should start as early as children can understand (usually about age 5 years). Messages should be clear, personally relevant, and age-appropriate.[61]

Nicotine dependence is a fatal disease that is aggressively marketed to young people. Public policies should be put in place to protect youth from tobacco and nicotine product promotion, initiation of usage, and to protect young people from involuntary exposure to emissions from ENDS and other tobacco products. These policies are discussed in detail in the American Academy of Pediatrics policy statements.[7,63]

## FREQUENTLY ASKED QUESTIONS

*Q   Are ENDS effective for stopping smoking?*

A   The research to date suggests that among adults who want to stop smoking, e-cigarettes provide minimal if any benefit over placebo. A meta-analysis of real-world studies suggests that smokers who use e-cigarettes are less likely to stop smoking compared with those individuals who do not use e-cigarettes.[64] Among adolescents, use of e-cigarettes increases the progression of tobacco dependence and decreases the likelihood of stopping smoking.[21]

*Q   Is hookah less harmful than cigarette smoking? Does bubbling the smoke through water remove the toxicants?*

A   Hookah smoking is as harmful—if not more harmful—than cigarette smoking. Passing the smoke through water does not remove the toxicants and carcinogens. The charcoal used to heat the tobacco can raise health risks by producing high levels of carbon monoxide, metals, and cancer-causing chemicals.

Because of the way a hookah is used, smokers may absorb more of the toxic substances also found in cigarette smoke than cigarette smokers do. An hour-long hookah smoking session involves 200 puffs, whereas smoking an average cigarette involves 20 puffs. The amount of smoke inhaled during a typical hookah session is about 90,000 mL, compared with 500 to 600 mL inhaled when smoking a cigarette.[65]

*Q   Are there risks to ENDS that use a solution that does not contain nicotine?*

A   Inaccurate labeling on these products has been identified. ENDS products marketed as being nicotine-free have been found to contain nicotine. ENDS deliver other toxicants in their emissions including metallic nanoparticles, carcinogens, and volatile organic compounds. Many of the flavoring agents used are respiratory irritants and can be damaging to respiratory tissues when inhaled. With or without nicotine, the emissions from ENDS devices are not safe to inhale.

## Resources

**American Academy of Pediatrics Julius B. Richmond Center of Excellence**
Web site: www.aap.org/RichmondCenter

**American College of Chest Physicians Tobacco Dependence Treatment Toolkit, 3rd Edition**
Web site: tobaccodependence.chestnet.org

**American Thoracic Society Fact Sheets on Tobacco, Marijuana, Nicotine, and Other Inhalant Use**
Web site: www.thoracic.org/patients/patient-resources/topic-specific/tobacco-use.php

**Campaign for Tobacco Free Kids**
Web site: www.tobaccofreekids.org

**Reports of the Surgeon General, US Public Health Service**
Web site: www.surgeongeneral.gov/library/reports/index.html

**Smokefree Teen (US Department of Health and Human Services)**
Web site: teen.smokefree.gov/about

## References

1. Samet JM. Tobacco smoking: the leading cause of preventable disease worldwide. *Thorac Surg Clin.* 2013;23(2):103–112
2. Office on Smoking and Health. The Health Consequences of Involuntary Exposure to Tobacco Smoke: A Report of the Surgeon General. Atlanta, GA: Centers for Disease Control and Prevention; 2006. Control of Secondhand Smoke Exposure. http://www.ncbi.nlm.nih.gov/books/NBK44326/. Accessed July 9, 2018
3. Garrett BE, Dube SR, Winder C, Caraballo RS, Centers for Disease Control and Prevention. Cigarette smoking–United States, 2006-2008 and 2009-2010. *MMWR Suppl.* 2013;62(3):81–84
4. US Department of Health and Human Services. *The Health Consequences of Smoking: 50 Years of Progress.* A Report of the Surgeon General. Atlanta, GA: Centers for Disease Control and Prevention, National Center for Chronic Disease Prevention and Health Promotion, Office on Smoking and Health, 2014
5. Centers for Disease Control and Prevention. Current Cigarette Smoking Among Adults in the United States. https://www.cdc.gov/tobacco/data_statistics/fact_sheets/adult_data/cig_smoking/index.htm. Accessed July 9, 2018
6. Centers for Disease Control and Prevention. Consumption of cigarettes and combustible tobacco–United States, 2000-2011. *MMWR. Morb Mortal Wkly Rep.* 2012;61(30):565–569
7. Walley SC, Jenssen BP, American Academy of Pediatrics Section on Tobacco Control. Electronic nicotine delivery systems. *Pediatrics.* 2015;136(5):1018–1026
8. Zhu SH, Sun JY, Bonnevie E, et al. Four hundred and sixty brands of e-cigarettes and counting: implications for product regulation. *Tob Control.* 2014;23(Suppl 3):iii3–iii9

9. Brown CJ, Cheng JM. Electronic cigarettes: product characterisation and design considerations. *Tob Control.* 2014;23(Suppl 2):ii4–ii10

10. Allen JG, Flanigan SS, LeBlanc M, et al. Flavoring chemicals in e-cigarettes: diacetyl, 2, 3-pentanedione, and acetoin in a sample of 51 products, including fruit-, candy-, and cocktail-flavored e-cigarettes. *Environ Health Perspect.* 2016;124(6):733–739

11. Leigh NJ, Lawton RI, Hershberger PA, Goniewicz ML. Flavourings significantly affect inhalation toxicity of aerosol generated from electronic nicotine delivery systems (ENDS). *Tob Control.* 2016;25(Suppl 2):ii81–ii87

12. Tierney PA, Karpinski CD, Brown JE, Luo W, Pankow JF. Flavour chemicals in electronic cigarette fluids. *Tob Control.* 2016;25(e1):e10–e15

13. US Department of Health and Human Services. E-Cigarette Use Among Youth and Young Adults. A Report of the Surgeon General. Atlanta, GA: Centers for Disease Control and Prevention, National Center for Chronic Disease Prevention and Health Promotion, Office on Smoking and Health. 2016

14. Rubinstein ML, Delucchi K, Benowitz NL, Ramo DE. Adolescent exposure to toxic volatile organic chemicals from e-cigarettes. *Pediatrics.* 2018;141(4):e20173557

15. Food and Drug Administration. Statement from FDA Commissioner Scott Gottlieb, M.D., on new enforcement actions and a Youth Tobacco Prevention Plan to stop youth use of, and access to, JUUL and other e-cigarettes. https://www.fda.gov/newsevents/newsroom/pressannouncements/ucm605432.htm. Accessed July 9, 2018

16. Jamal A, Gentzke A, Hu SS, et al. Tobacco use among middle and high school students–United States, 2011-2016. *MMWR Morb Mortal Wkly Rep.* 2017;66(23):597–603

17. Johnston LD, Miech RA, O'Malley PM, Bachman JG, Schulenberg JE, Patrick ME. Monitoring the Future. National Survey Results on Drug Use: 1975-2017. 2017 Overview: Key Findings on Adolescent Drug Use. Ann Arbor, MI: Institute for Social Research, The University of Michigan. http://monitoringthefuture.org/pubs/monographs/mtf-overview2017.pdf. Accessed July 9, 2018

18. Wills TA, Knight R, Williams RJ, Pagano I, Sargent JD. Risk factors for exclusive e-cigarette use and dual e-cigarette use and tobacco use in adolescents. *Pediatrics.* 2015;135(1):e43–e51

19. Chen A. Teenagers Embrace JUUL, Saying It's Discreet Enough To Vape In Class. Health News from NPR. December 4, 2017. https://www.npr.org/sections/health-shots/2017/12/04/568273801/teenagers-embrace-juul-saying-its-discreet-enough-to-vape-in-class. Accessed July 9, 2018

20. Bold KW, Kong G, Camenga DR, et al. Trajectories of e-cigarette and conventional cigarette use among youth. *Pediatrics.* 2018;141(1). pii: e20171832

21. Soneji S, Barrington-Trimis JL, Wills TA, et al. Association between initial use of e-cigarettes and subsequent cigarette smoking among adolescents and young adults: a systematic review and meta-analysis. *JAMA Pediatr.* 2017;171(8):788–797

22. Kandel D, Kandel E. The Gateway Hypothesis of substance abuse: developmental, biological and societal perspectives. *Acta Paediatr.* 2015;104(2):130–137

23. Substance Abuse and Mental Health Services Administration. Results from the 2012 National Survey on Drug Use and Health: Summary of National Findings. NSDUH Series H-46, HHS Publication No. (SMA) 13-4795. Rockville, MD: Substance Abuse and Mental Health Services Administration; 2013. http://www.samhsa.gov/data/sites/default/files/NSDUHnationalfindingresults2012/NSDUHnationalfindingresults2012/NSDUHresults2012.pdf. Accessed July 9, 2018

24. Cobb C, Ward KD, Maziak W, Shihadeh AL, Eissenberg T. Waterpipe tobacco smoking: an emerging health crisis in the United States. *Am J Health Behav.* 2010;34(3):275–285

25. Maziak W. The global epidemic of waterpipe smoking. *Addict Behav.* 2011;36(1-2):1–5

26. Park SH, Duncan DT, El Shahawy O, et al. Analysis of state-specific prevalence, regional differences, and correlates of hookah use in U.S. adults, 2012-2013. *Nicotine Tob Res.* 2017;19(11):1365–1374

27. Casseus M, Garmon J, Hrywna M, Delnevo CD. Cigarette smokers' classification of tobacco products. *Tob Control.* 2016;25(6):628–630

28. Brown JE, Luo W, Isabelle LM, Pankow JF. Candy flavorings in tobacco. *N Engl J Med.* 2014;370(23):2250–2252

29. Tabuchi T, Kiyohara K, Hoshino T, Bekki K, Inaba Y, Kunugita N. Awareness and use of electronic cigarettes and heat-not-burn tobacco products in Japan. *Addiction.* 2016;111(4): 706–713

30. Jenssen BP, Walley SC, McGrath-Morrow SA. Heat-not-burn tobacco products: tobacco industry claims no substitute for science. *Pediatrics.* 2018;141(1). pii: e20172383

31. Melikian AA, Hoffmann D. Smokeless tobacco: a gateway to smoking or a way away from smoking. *Biomarkers.* 2009;14(Suppl 1):85–89

32. Cabrera-Nguyen EP, Cavazos-Rehg P, Krauss M, Kim Y, Emery S. Awareness and use of dissolvable tobacco products in the United States. *Nicotine Tob Res.* 2016;18(5):857–863

33. McMillen R, Maduka J, Winickoff J. Use of emerging tobacco products in the United States. *J Environ Public Health.* 2012;2012:989474

34. Jamal A, Gentzke A, Hu SS, et al. Tobacco use among middle and high school students - United States, 2011-2016. *MMWR Morb Mortal Wkly Rep.* 2017;66(23):597–603

35. Merianos AL, Mancuso TF, Gordon JS, Wood KJ, Cimperman KA, Mahabee-Gittens EM. Dual- and polytobacco/nicotine product use trends in a national sample of high school students. *Am J Health Promot.* 2018;32(5):1280–1290

36. Connolly GN, Richter P, Aleguas A, Pechacek TF, Stanfill SB, Alpert HR. Unintentional child poisonings through ingestion of conventional and novel tobacco products. *Pediatrics.* 2010;125(5):896–899

37. Bassett RA, Osterhoudt K, Brabazon T. Nicotine poisoning in an infant. *N Engl J Med.* 2014;370(23):2249–2250

38. Thornton SL, Oller L, Sawyer T. Fatal intravenous injection of electronic nicotine delivery system refilling solution. *J Med Toxicol.* 2014;10(2):202–204

39. Chen BC, Bright SB, Trivedi AR, Valento M. Death following intentional ingestion of e-liquid. *Clin Toxicol (Phila).* 2015;53(9):914–916

40. Birge M, Duffy S, Miler JA, Hajek P. What proportion of people who try one cigarette become daily smokers? A meta-analysis of representative surveys. *Nicotine Tob Res.* 2017 Nov 4. doi: 10.1093/ntr/ntx243. [Epub ahead of print].

41. Wongtrakool C, Wang N, Hyde DM, Roman J, Spindel ER. Prenatal nicotine exposure alters lung function and airway geometry through α7 nicotinic receptors. *Am J Respir Cell Mol Biol.* 2012;46(5):695–702

42. Farber HJ, Groner J, Walley S, Nelson K; American Academy of Pediatrics Section on Tobacco Control. Protecting children from tobacco, nicotine, and tobacco smoke. *Pediatrics.* 2015;136(5):e1439–e1467

43. Garcia-Arcos I, Geraghty P, Baumlin N, et al. Chronic electronic cigarette exposure in mice induces features of COPD in a nicotine-dependent manner. *Thorax.* 2016;71(12):1119–1129

44. Wang C, Niu W, Chen H, et al. Nicotine suppresses apoptosis by regulating α7nAChR/Prx1 axis in oral precancerous lesions. *Oncotarget.* 2017;8(43):75065–75075

45. Grando SA. Connections of nicotine to cancer. *Nat Rev Cancer.* 2014;14(6):419–429

46. Reidel B, Radicioni G, Clapp P, et al. E-cigarette use causes a unique innate immune response in the lung involving increased neutrophilic activation and altered mucin secretion. *Am J Respir Crit Care Med.* 2018;197(4):492–501

47. Hwang JH, Lyes M, Sladewski K, et al. Electronic cigarette inhalation alters innate immunity and airway cytokines while increasing the virulence of colonizing bacteria. *J Mol Med (Berl)*. 2016;94(6):667–679

48. Klager S, Vallarino J, MacNaughton P, Christiani DC, Lu Q, Allen JG. Flavoring chemicals and aldehydes in e-cigarette emissions. *Environ Sci Technol*. 2017;51(18):10806–10813

49. Olmedo P, Goessler W, Tanda S, et al. Metal concentrations in e-cigarette liquid and aerosol samples: the contribution of metallic coils. *Environ Health Perspect*. 2018;126(2):027010

50. Sachs DPL, Leone F, Farber HJ, et al. *Tobacco Dependence Treatment Toolkit*, 3rd ed. Northbrook, IL: American College of Chest Physicians; 2010. http://tobaccodependence. chestnet.org. Accessed July 9, 2018

51. Boffetta P, Pershagen G, Jöckel KH, et al. Cigar and pipe smoking and lung cancer risk: a multicenter study from Europe. *J Natl Cancer Inst*. 1999;91(8):697–701

52. Chang CM, Corey CG, Rostron BL, Apelberg BJ. Systematic review of cigar smoking and all cause and smoking related mortality. *BMC Public Health*. 2015;15:390

53. Baker F, Ainsworth SR, Dye JT, et al. Health risks associated with cigar smoking. *JAMA*. 2000;284(6):735–740

54. World Health Organization. *IARC Monographs on the Evaluation of Carcinogenic Risks to Humans. Volume 89: Smokeless Tobacco and Some Tobacco-Specific N-Nitrosamines.* Lyon, France: World Health Organization, International Agency for Research on Cancer; 2007

55. Piano MR, Benowitz NL, Fitzgerald GA, et al. Impact of smokeless tobacco products on cardiovascular disease: implications for policy, prevention, and treatment: a policy statement from the American Heart Association. *Circulation*. 2010;122(15):1520–1544

56. Lee PN, Hamling J. Systematic review of the relation between smokeless tobacco and cancer in Europe and North America. *BMC Med*. 2009;7:36

57. Allen NE, Beral V, Casabonne D, et al. Moderate alcohol intake and cancer incidence in women. *J Natl Cancer Inst*. 2009;101(5):296–305

58. Harris AC, Tally L, Schmidt CE, et al. Animal models to assess the abuse liability of tobacco products: effects of smokeless tobacco extracts on intracranial self-stimulation. *Drug Alcohol Depend*. 2015;147:60–67

59. Dwyer JB, McQuown SC, Leslie FM. The dynamic effects of nicotine on the developing brain. *Pharmacol Ther*. 2009;122(2):125–139

60. Bates BA. Toxic plant ingestions and nicotine poisoning in children: management. In: Burns MM, Wiley JF, eds. *UpToDate*. Waltham, MA: UpToDate Inc. http://www.uptodate.com. Accessed July 9, 2018

61. Farber HJ, Walley SC, Groner JA, Nelson KE; American Academy of Pediatrics Section on Tobacco Control. Clinical practice policy to protect children from tobacco, nicotine, and tobacco smoke. *Pediatrics*. 2015;136(5):1008–1017

62. Child Nicotine Poisoning Prevention Act of 2015. https://www.congress.gov/bill/114th-congress/senate-bill/142. Accessed July 9, 2018

63. Farber HJ, Nelson KE, Groner JA, Walley SC; American Academy of Pediatrics Section on Tobacco Control. Public policy to protect children from tobacco, nicotine, and tobacco smoke. *Pediatrics*. 2015;136:998–1007

64. Kalkhoran S, Glantz SA. E-cigarettes and smoking cessation in real-world and clinical settings: a systematic review and meta-analysis. *Lancet Respir Med*. 2016;4(2):116–128

65. Fact Sheet - Hookahs. In: Smoking & Tobacco Use. Centers for Disease Control and Prevention. https://www.cdc.gov/tobacco/data_statistics/fact_sheets/tobacco_industry/hookahs/index.htm. Accessed July 9, 2018

Chapter 29

# Endocrine Disrupting Chemicals

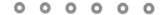

## KEY POINTS

- Endocrine disrupting chemicals are synthetic or natural chemicals that can mimic, block, or alter synthesis, metabolism, or excretion of hormones and thus can disrupt normal hormonal physiology.
- Exposures to endocrine disrupting chemicals are ubiquitous; low doses may be relevant to human health; and exposures can harm offspring.
- Current research on endocrine disrupting chemicals explores effects on neurodevelopment, respiratory diseases, allergies, growth and development, including timing of puberty, and obesity, endometriosis, testicular cancer, and other end points.
- Pediatricians can advise parents about steps they can take to possibly reduce exposures to endocrine disrupting chemicals.

## INTRODUCTION

Endocrine disrupting chemicals (EDCs, also referred to as endocrine disrupters/disruptors) are synthetic or natural chemicals that can mimic, block, or alter synthesis, metabolism, or excretion of hormones and thus can disrupt normal hormonal physiology.[1,2] They also may alter the concentrations of natural hormones. Although initially applied to substances with estrogenic effects, EDCs now refer to chemicals that interfere with other hormones, including thyroid hormones, insulin, and androgens, as well as processes involving multiple hormones, such as growth and development.[1,2]

Chemical endocrine disruption in vertebrates was first identified in the effects of the pesticide dichlorodiphenyltrichloroethane (DDT) on the hatchability of eggs of pelagic (ie, ocean dwelling) birds.[3] DDT and other pesticides, such as methoxychlor and chlordecone,[4] as well as industrial chemicals, such as specific polychlorinated biphenyls (PCBs), can act as estrogens in laboratory assays. Lead, pesticides, phthalates, bisphenol A (BPA), and flame retardants, among other chemicals, have endocrine disrupting properties. Plant-derived estrogens, or phytoestrogens, can also act as estrogens in animals that consume them (see Chapter 16). Table 29-1 lists examples of EDCs.

EDC exposures have been tracked in the US population over the past 20 years through measurements of metabolites in biological samples, such as urine.[5] These data are generally used for research, but can be actionable in certain instances (eg, blood lead levels). Tracking has allowed for the establishment of background EDC exposure levels and facilitates the identification of disparities in exposures by gender, race, ethnicity, or age. Tracking also can demonstrate the effectiveness of federal policies in reducing exposures (eg, declines in exposure to certain chemicals after specific bans, as was seen with lower blood lead levels after lead was removed from gasoline).

### Table 29-1. Examples of Endocrine Disrupting Chemicals

| | |
|---|---|
| **Pesticides** | **Atrazine** (herbicide)<br>**Chlorpyrifos** (pesticide)<br>**Dichlorodiphenyltrichloroethane (DDT)** (organochlorine pesticide)<br>**Dioxin (TCDD)** (byproduct of herbicide production)<br>**Glyphosate** (herbicide) |
| **Food Packaging, Children's Products** | **Bisphenol A (BPA)** (plasticizer)<br>**Phthalates** (plasticizers)<br>**Lead** (in toy jewelry) |
| **Foods** | **Soy isoflavones** (phytoestrogens) |
| **Personal Care Products** | **Phthalates** (plasticizers)<br>**Parabens** (preservative)<br>**Triclosan** (antibacterial agent) |
| **Textiles** | **Perfluorooctanoic Acid (PFOA)** (in outdoor clothing) |
| **Building Materials and Electronics** | **Polybrominated diphenyl ethers (PBDEs)** (flame retardants)<br>**Polychlorinated biphenyls (PCBs)** (dielectric and coolant fluids in electrical apparatus)<br>**Polychlorinated dibenzofurans (PCDFs)** (unwanted by-products in a variety of industrial and thermal processes) |

Adapted from Gore AC, Crews D, Doan LL, La Merrill M, Patisaul H, Zota A. Introduction to Endocrine Disrupting Chemicals: A Guide for Public Interest Organizations and Policymakers. 2014.

Based on population level data, evidence indicating human health impacts from EDCs has grown substantially in recent years. In broad terms, research demonstrates that EDC exposures are ubiquitous; low doses of exposure may be relevant to human health, and EDC exposure can harm offspring.[6] The consequences of exposures to chronic, low dose, and/or combinations of EDCs, especially during potentially critical windows of exposure (eg, *in utero*, infancy, early childhood, adolescence, childbearing years) are largely unknown.

## ROUTES OF EXPOSURE

The primary route of exposure to EDCs is ingestion. For example, foods may be contaminated with phthalates or BPA during food manufacture, or from packaging. Inhalation and dermal absorption are also potential routes of exposure. The fetus may be exposed through the placenta, and infants may be exposed through breastfeeding.

## SYSTEMS AFFECTED AND CLINICAL EFFECTS

### Estrogen Disruption

A wide variety of chemicals have estrogenic activity in biological systems. The most widely used test system is a yeast with a human estrogen receptor and a reporter gene. If the chemical being tested occupies and activates the receptor, then the reporter gene product, usually a phosphorescent protein, is synthesized and can be easily measured. Similar assays exist for other kinds of hormonal activity. A classic example of exogenous estrogen disruption was seen with diethylstilbestrol (DES), a pharmaceutical previously used to prevent miscarriage. It was later found that in the teen and young adult years of some of the daughters of women who took DES while pregnant, clear cell carcinoma of the vagina or cervix developed years after exposure. The development of these usually rare tumors illustrates that endocrine disruption can occur even after a long latency period.

### Androgen Disruption

Dichlorodiphenyldichloroethylene (DDE), a metabolite of DDT commonly found in people worldwide, has repeatedly been shown to be an anti-androgen.[7] When DDE binds with the androgen receptor, it suppresses its normal functions. Such disruption by synthetic chemicals may explain higher rates of testicular cancer seen in recent decades.[8] DDE has also been associated with testicular germ cell cancer in most studies that have looked for an association.[9]

The ratio of male to female births is shifting in industrialized countries, which raises concern that EDC exposures affect sperm.[11] In 1976, an explosion in Seveso, Italy resulted in the population being exposed to large quantities of

2,3,7,8-tetrachlorodibenzo-*p*-dioxin (TCDD), a halogenated hydrocarbon also known as dioxin. Exposed males had changes in sperm counts and motility. The effects were different depending on when in their lives (either infancy, adolescence, or adulthood) the males were exposed.[10] In addition, a clear excess of female births was seen in the Seveso region when the father was exposed.[11] Similarly, a deficiency in male births was seen in a Taiwanese study of people with high exposures to PCBs and polychlorinated dibenzofurans, only when the father was exposed.[12] This finding was reproduced in TCDD-exposed mice.[13]

Anogenital distance (AGD) is a gender-specific trait that is not related to reproductive organs (also known as a sexually dimorphic trait). Anogenital distance is commonly measured in rodents exposed to putative human androgen antagonists. Maternal exposure to phthalates has been associated with changes in AGD in male[14,15] and female[16] children. Researchers suspect that these findings are related to androgen disruption because both human and experimental studies indicate that phthalates reduce testosterone levels.[17,18]

EDCs have been further implicated in disruption of glucose and lipid metabolism, and adipogenesis leading to some being categorized as "obesogens" and "diabetogens." Cross-sectional studies in adults and some children have implicated EDCs in obesity, diabetes mellitus, and cardiovascular disease. Studies of phthalates found associations with obesity among Chinese and non-Hispanic black children but not all studies of phthalates are consistently associated with childhood obesity.[1]

Several agents, including lead and phthalate plasticizers, have been studied for effects on puberty in girls.[1,2,19-23] Phthalate plasticizers have been associated with both early and delayed onset of puberty in numerous human studies. A few studies that examined the relationship between female puberty and exposure to perfluorooctanoic acid (PFOA) (used to make nonstick cookware) found associations between PFOA exposure and delayed puberty.[1,24]

### Thyroid Hormone Disruption

Studies on thyroid disrupting chemicals demonstrated impacts on neurodevelopmental outcomes including IQ and cognition. Some pesticides and PCB congeners can bind to thyroid hormone receptors.[25] In 2 studies of background exposure to PCBs and child development, hypotonia at birth was related to prenatal exposure to PCBs[26] or to a history of consuming PCB-contaminated fish.[27] The finding of hypotonia suggested an effect on thyroid hormone. PCBs were known to be toxic to the developing thyroid gland.[28] Hypotonia has been shown to be accompanied by higher thyroid-stimulating hormone concentrations.[29,30] Although associations between EDCs and a variety of measures of thyroid hormone status have most often been weak, inconsistent, or absent, the capacity of EDCs to act on the thyroid system has a reasonable basis in laboratory evidence and requires further study.

## Neurodevelopment and Behavior

Hormones shape brain development. EDCs may alter brain development through nuclear hormone receptors, steroidogenic enzymes and neurotransmitters, and other pathways.[31] Animal studies demonstrated sex-specific differences in how EDCs affect the brain.[32] Studies in humans have found associations between EDCs and decreased IQ and greater neurodevelopmental problems.[33–35]

## Other Effects

Studies in experimental animals and humans have demonstrated associations between exposure to EDCs (eg, BPA, phthalates) and the development of allergies, wheeze, and asthma through mechanisms yet to be clearly elucidated.[36–38] The prenatal period appears to be a critical window of exposure for offspring in terms of future risk of atopic symptoms.[39–41]

## REGULATION

The Food Quality Protection Act of 1996 requires testing of chemicals that will be released into the environment for their endocrine activity, and the US Environmental Protection Agency (EPA) has developed the Endocrine Disruptor Screening Program of animal and cell-based assays to test for endocrine disruption. Progress toward implementation can be reviewed at the US EPA Endocrine Disruption Web site.[42] Most likely, such testing would serve to select agents for more intense study. It would not replace more traditional tests for general toxicity and carcinogenicity.

Given current standards for testing and disclosure, consumers may be unable to determine whether children's foods, toys, and products contain EDCs. Ultimately, the burden should not be on the consumer to determine which products do or do not contain EDCs. Transparency with respect to labeling, premarket safety testing, third-party certification, and information on alternatives used are needed to shift the burden away from the consumer while ensuring that products are safe before they are placed on the market.

## SUMMARY

Research on EDCs provides evidence to suggest that they may influence human physiology, and that further research must be done to understand their potential harms. Current EDC research explores effects on neurodevelopment, respiratory diseases, allergies, growth and development, including timing of puberty, and obesity, endometriosis, testicular cancer, and other end points.

Available knowledge indicates that substantial harm from EDCs may already be common and that potential harms may be yet more substantial. Further research, public health initiatives, and advocacy are warranted to reduce exposures to EDCs.[1,43]

## Frequently Asked Questions

Q  *My 7-year-old girl is here for her annual physical exam. I have seen news stories about the potential health effects of plasticizers and possible relationship to early puberty. I worry that she uses personal care products including nail polish and lotions with fragrance. Given that she already has early signs of puberty, I would like to know what this means for her health.*

A  It is generally recognized that puberty is occurring earlier in girls. Specifically, the age at onset of breast budding is occurring earlier, although the age at menarche is thought to have remained stable over time. Increasing obesity plays a role in earlier maturation.[44] A variety of EDCs have been shown to either cause delay or promote early development of puberty. Research is ongoing to enhance our understanding of the role of EDCs on growth and development and on puberty because the early onset of puberty is a risk factor for development of breast cancer later in life. Until we know more, it is wise to take a precautionary approach and reduce exposures to EDCs in foods and consumer products.

Q  *I would like to know how my family can avoid exposures to EDCs, such as phthalates and BPA. What can I do?*

A  There are a few simple steps families can take to reduce exposures to phthalates and BPA. They include the following:
- Select fresh foods rather than processed foods.
- Look for children's products that are marked free of phthalates and/or BPA.
- Avoid placing plastics in the dishwasher and microwave because high temperatures may promote leaching of plasticizers such as phthalates and BPA.
- Look to recycling labels in the absence of mandatory labeling.
  — #3 plastics may contain lead and phthalates. #7 plastics may contain BPA.
  — Instead, choose plastics that are labeled #1, 2, 4, and 5.
- Choose stainless steel water bottles rather than plastic. Most stainless steel bottles have no plastic lining.
- Avoid alternatives that contain BPA analogs (eg, bisphenol S or bisphenol F) that also have been found to have endocrine disrupting properties.[45]
- If using formula, choose powdered rather than prepared canned infant formula.

- Consider using glass baby bottles and glass containers for food storage.
- Dust and mop frequently using wet techniques, such as a mop or damp rag, to minimize exposure to phthalates in dust.

Q  *I am concerned that dental sealants contain BPA and am currently debating getting sealants for my twins. What advice do you have about dental sealants?*

A  Dental sealants play an important role in preventing tooth decay and cavities and for this reason, are routinely recommended. Talk to your dentist. Techniques, such as using a pumice stone to wipe off the uncured layer of sealant after applying, along with having children rinse with water and then spit, have been found to reduce BPA exposure during the application process.[46] BPA-free sealants also are available.

## Resources

### Breast Cancer and the Environment Research Program
https://bcerp.org/wp-content/uploads/2017/01/3_BCERP_Outreach_ThePubertyConnection_NEW_508.pdf
https://bcerp.org/health-professionals/endocrine-disrupting-chemicals/

### Endocrine Society 2nd Scientific Statement on EDCs Executive Summary
https://academic.oup.com/edrv/article/36/6/593/2354738/Executive-Summary-to-EDC-2-The-Endocrine-Society-s

### National Institute of Environmental Health Sciences
https://www.niehs.nih.gov/health/topics/agents/endocrine

### Pediatric Environmental Health Specialty Units
www.pehsu.net/_Library/facts/BPAhealthcareproviderfactsheet03-2014.pdf
www.pehsu.net/_Library/facts/BPApatients_factsheet03-2014.pdf
http://tceee.icahn.mssm.edu/wp-content/uploads/sites/11/2015/08/PEHSU-Reg-2-and-10_Dental-Sealants-and-BPA-factsheet.pdf
http://tceee.icahn.mssm.edu/wp-content/uploads/sites/11/2016/08/SealantsBPA.pdf

### United States Environmental Protection Agency
https://www.epa.gov/endocrine-disruption/what-endocrine-disruption

### World Health Organization
www.who.int/ceh/risks/cehemerging2/en/

# References

1. Gore AC, Chappell VA, Fenton SE, et al. EDC-2: The Endocrine Society's Second Scientific Statement on Endocrine-Disrupting Chemicals. *Endocr Rev.* 2015;36(6):E1–E150

2. Gore AC, Crews D, Doan LL, La Merrill M, Patisaul H, Zota A. Introduction to Endocrine Disrupting Chemicals: A Guide for Public Interest Organizations and Policymakers. 2014

3. Fry DM. Reproductive effects in birds exposed to pesticides and industrial chemicals. *Environ Health Perspect.* 1995;103(Suppl 7):165–171

4. Boylan JJ, Egle JL, Guzelian PS. Cholestyramine: use as a new therapeutic approach for chlordecone (kepone) poisoning. *Science.* 1978;199(4331):893–895

5. Centers for Disease Control and Prevention. *Fourth Report on Human Exposure to Environmental Chemicals, 2009.* Department of Health and Human Services. Updated tables March 2018. https://www.cdc.gov/exposurereport/index.html. Accessed July 19, 2018

6. National Institute of Environmental Health Sciences. Endocrine Disruptors. 2010. https://www.niehs.nih.gov/health/materials/endocrine_disruptors_508.pdf. Accessed April 2, 2018

7. Kelce WR, Stone CR, Laws SC, Gray LE, Kemppainen JA, Wilson EM. Persistent DDT metabolite p,p'-DDE is a potent androgen receptor antagonist. *Nature.* 1995;375(6532):581–585

8. Liu S, Semenciw R, Waters C, Wen SW, Mery LS, Mao Y. Clues to the aetiological heterogeneity of testicular seminomas and non-seminomas: time trends and age-period-cohort effects. *Int J Epidemiol.* 2000;29(5):826–831

9. Giannandrea F, Paoli D, Figa-Talamanca I, Lombardo F, Lenzi A, Gandini L. Effect of endogenous and exogenous hormones on testicular cancer: the epidemiological evidence. *Int J Dev Biol.* 2013;57(2-4):255–263

10. Mocarelli P, Gerthoux PM, Patterson DG, et al. Dioxin exposure, from infancy through puberty, produces endocrine disruption and affects human semen quality. *Environ Health Perspect.* 2008;116(1):70–77

11. Davis DL, Gottlieb MB, Stampnitzky JR. Reduced ratio of male to female births in several industrial countries: a sentinel health indicator? *JAMA.* 1998;279(13):1018–1023

12. del Rio Gomez I, Marshall T, Tsai P, Shao YS, Guo YL. Number of boys born to men exposed to polychlorinated byphenyls. *Lancet.* 2002;360(9327):143–144

13. Ishihara K, Warita K, Tanida T, Sugawara T, Kitagawa H, Hoshi N. Does paternal exposure to 2,3,7,8-tetrachlorodibenzo-p-dioxin (TCDD) affect the sex ratio of offspring? *J Vet Med Sci.* 2007;69(4):347–352

14. Swan SH, Main KM, Liu F, et al. Decrease in anogenital distance among male infants with prenatal phthalate exposure. *Environ Health Perspect.* 2005;113(8):1056–1061

15. Suzuki Y, Yoshinaga J, Mizumoto Y, Serizawa S, Shiraishi H. Foetal exposure to phthalate esters and anogenital distance in male newborns. *Int J Androl.* 2012;35(3):236–244

16. Huang PC, Kuo PL, Chou YY, Lin SJ, Lee CC. Association between prenatal exposure to phthalates and the health of newborns. *Environ Int.* 2009;35(1):14–20

17. Lin LC, Wang SL, Chang YC, et al. Associations between maternal phthalate exposure and cord sex hormones in human infants. *Chemosphere.* 2011;83(8):1192–1199

18. Inada H, Chihara K, Yamashita A, et al. Evaluation of ovarian toxicity of mono-(2-ethylhexyl) phthalate (MEHP) using cultured rat ovarian follicles. *J Toxicol Sci.* 2012;37(3):483–490

19. Rogan WJ, Ragan NB. Some evidence of effects of environmental chemicals on the endocrine system in children. *Int J Hyg Environ Health.* 2007;210(5):659–667

20. Breast Cancer and Environment Research Program. Early Puberty and Breast Cancer Risk. https://bcerp.org/health-professionals/early-puberty-and-breast-cancer-risk/. Accessed April 2, 2018

21. Wolff MS, Pajak A, Pinney SM, et al. Associations of urinary phthalate and phenol biomarkers with menarche in a multiethnic cohort of young girls. *Reprod Toxicol.* 2017;67:56–64

22. Wolff MS, Teitelbaum SL, McGovern K, et al. Phthalate exposure and pubertal development in a longitudinal study of US girls. *Hum Reprod.* 2014;29(7):1558–1566

23. Wolff MS, Teitelbaum SL, Pinney SM, et al. Investigation of relationships between urinary biomarkers of phytoestrogens, phthalates, and phenols and pubertal stages in girls. *Environ Health Perspect.* 2010;118(7):1039–1046

24. Lopez-Espinosa MJ, Fletcher T, Armstrong B, et al. Association of perfluorooctanoic acid (PFOA) and perfluorooctane sulfonate (PFOS) with age of puberty among children living near a chemical plant. *Environ Sci Technol.* 2011;45(19):8160–8166

25. Rickenbache U, McKinney JD, Oatley SJ, Blake CC. Structurally specific binding of halogenated biphenyls to thyroxine transport protein. *J Med Chem.* 1986;29(5):641–648

26. Rogan WJ, Gladen BC, McKinney JD, et al. Neonatal effects of transplacental exposure to PCBs and DDE. *J Pediatr.* 1986;109(2):335–341

27. Jacobson JL, Jacobson SW, Fein GG, Schwartz PM, Dowler JK. Prenatal exposure to an environmental toxin: a test of the multiple effects model. *Dev Psychol.* 1984;20:523–532

28. Collins WT, Capen CC. Fine structural lesions and hormonal alterations in thyroid glands of perinatal rats exposed in utero and by the milk to polychlorinated biphenyls. *Am J Pathol.* 1980;99(1):125–142

29. Koopman-Esseboom C, Morse DC, Weisglas-Kuperus N, et al. Effects of dioxins and polychlorinated biphenyls on thyroid hormone status of pregnant women and their infants. *Pediatr Res.* 1994;36(4):468–473

30. Hagmar L. Polychlorinated biphenyls and thyroid status in humans: a review. *Thyroid.* 2003; 13(11):1021–1028

31. Pinson A, Bourguignon JP, Parent AS. Exposure to endocrine disrupting chemicals and neurodevelopmental alterations. *Andrology.* 2016;4(4):706–722

32. Rebuli ME, Patisaul HB. Assessment of sex specific endocrine disrupting effects in the prenatal and pre-pubertal rodent brain. *J Steroid Biochem Mol Biol.* 2016;160:148–159

33. Braun JM. Early-life exposure to EDCs: role in childhood obesity and neurodevelopment. *Nat Rev Endocrinol.* 2017;13(3):161–173

34. Mustieles V, Pérez-Lobato R, Olea N, Fernández MF. Bisphenol A: human exposure and neurobehavior. *Neurotoxicology.* 2015;49:174–184

35. Meeker JD. Exposure to environmental endocrine disruptors and child development. *Arch Pediatr Adolesc Med.* 2012;166:952–958

36. Robinson L, Miller R. The impact of bisphenol A and phthalates on allergy, asthma, and immune function: a review of latest findings. *Curr Environ Health Rep.* 2015;2(4):379–387

37. Spanier AJ, Fiorino EK, Trasande L. Bisphenol A exposure is associated with decreased lung function. *J Pediatr.* 2014;164(6):1403–1408.e1

38. Bornehag CG, Sundell J, Weschler CJ, et al. The association between asthma and allergic symptoms in children and phthalates in house dust: a nested case-control study. *Environ Health Perspect.* 2004;112(14):1393–1397

39. Spanier A, Kahn RS, Kunselman AR, et al. Prenatal exposure to bisphenol A and child wheeze from birth to three years. *Environ Health Perspect.* 2012;120(6):916–920

40. Donohue KM, Miller RL, Perzanowski MS, et al. Prenatal and postnatal bisphenol A exposure and asthma development among inner-city children. *J Allergy Clin Immunol.* 2013;131(3): 736–742

41. Gascon M, Casas M, Morales E, et al. Prenatal exposure to bisphenol A and phthalates and childhood respiratory tract infections and allergy. *J Allergy Clin Immunol.* 2015;135(2):370–378

42. US Environmental Protection Agency. Endocrine Disruption. https://www.epa.gov/endocrine-disruption. Accessed April 2, 2018

43. Attina TM, Hauser R, Sathyanarayana S, et al. Exposure to endocrine-disrupting chemicals in the USA: a population-based disease burden and cost analysis. *Lancet Diabetes Endocrinol.* 2016;4(12):996–1003

44. Golub MS, Collman GW, Foster PM, et al. Public health implications of altered puberty timing. *Pediatrics.* 2008;121(Suppl 3):S218–S230

45. Rochester JR, Bolden AL. Bisphenol S and F: a systematic review and comparison of the hormonal activity of bisphenol A substitutes. *Environ Health Perspect.* 2015;123(7):643–650

46. Fleisch AF, Sheffield PR, Chinn C, Edelstein BL, Landrigan PJ. Bisphenol A and related compounds in dental materials. *Pediatrics.* 2010;126(4):760–768

Chapter 30

# Gasoline and Its Additives

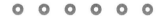

## KEY POINTS

- Gasoline is a complex mixture of hydrocarbons and additives (including lead, manganese, and oxygenates such as methyl tertiary butyl ether [MTBE] and others) that are toxic to children both acutely and with low-dose chronic exposure.
- Children can be exposed via inhalation (intentional or unintentional), ingestion, or through contact with skin.
- Leaking gasoline storage tanks have proven to be a significant source of drinking water contamination.
- Families with drinking water with elevated levels of hydrocarbons or gasoline additives should be advised to use bottled water or install a charcoal filtration system.
- Prevention of exposure to the most toxic additives to gasoline, such as tetraethyl lead, methylcyclopentadienyl manganese tricarbonyl (MMT), MTBE, or benzene, is best achieved by governmental regulation or phasing out of these compounds.

## INTRODUCTION

Gasoline is a complex mixture of volatile hydrocarbons derived by distillation from crude petroleum. Gasoline contains as many as 1,000 different chemical substances, including alkanes, alkenes, and aromatics.[1] The composition of gasoline varies depending on the source of crude oil, refining process, geographic region, season of the year, and performance requirements (octane rating). In 2016, about 143.37 billion gallons (3.421 billion barrels) of finished motor gasoline were consumed in the United States, a new record.[2] In 2012, the United States accounted for approximately 39% of gasoline consumption worldwide.[3,4] Gasoline combustion is an important contributor to ambient air pollution and global climate change.[5] Gasoline frequently contaminates drinking water in the United States.[6] This chapter reviews the health effects of gasoline and its additives. The hazards associated with exposure to automotive exhaust, including diesel exhaust, are considered in Chapter 21.

Toxic and carcinogenic constituents of gasoline include benzene, 1,3-butadiene, 1,2-dibromoethane, toluene, ethyl benzene, antiknock agents, and oxygenates.[1] Benzene, a polycyclic aromatic hydrocarbon, constitutes up to 4% of gasoline by weight, except in Alaska, where it is 5% of gasoline by weight.[7] Benzene is of particular concern because of its ubiquitous presence in gasoline and the strength of scientific evidence showing that it causes cancers including acute myeloid leukemia (AML), acute lymphoblastic leukemia (ALL), chronic lymphocytic leukemia (CLL), multiple myeloma, and lymphoma, among others.[8] Benzene poses this risk not only in occupational settings but also from community exposure to benzene-containing exhaust as illustrated in a French study linking residential proximity to heavy traffic roads to an increased risk of childhood AML.[9]

Tetraethyl lead was the principal antiknock agent used in gasoline in the United States until it was phased out for use in automobile gasoline between 1976 and 1990, resulting in a 90% reduction in children's blood lead concentrations.[10] Tetraethyl lead is used in gasoline in an ever-decreasing number of nations. As of 2017, the United Nations Environment Programme reported that only 3 nations (Algeria, Yemen, and Iraq) were still using leaded gasoline.[11] Average blood lead concentrations among children in nations that use leaded gasoline are 10 to 15 mcg/dL higher than those in US children.[12] Tetraethyl lead is still used in aviation fuel and has been associated with air lead levels above the US Environmental Protection Agency (EPA) National Ambient Air Quality Standard of 0.15 $mcg/m^2$ at 2 of 17 general aviation airports.[13] A 2011 Duke University study found higher blood levels in children who live within 500 meters of these airports.[14] Further discussion of these issues is found in Chapter 32.

Methylcyclopentadienyl manganese tricarbonyl (MMT) has been proposed as a replacement for tetraethyl lead as an antiknock agent.[15] Occupational exposure to manganese is a known cause of parkinsonism.[16] Available data suggest that community exposures to manganese resulting from combustion of MMT in gasoline may be associated with subclinical neurologic impairment.[16-18] A further discussion of MMT and manganese can be found in Chapter 24.

Oxygenates are added to gasoline, especially in the winter months, to reduce carbon monoxide emissions.[19,20] Methyl tertiary butyl ether was the oxygenate most widely used in the United States and was added to gasoline at concentrations up to 15% by volume.[21] Combustion of methyl tertiary butyl ether produces acrid emissions, including formaldehyde, and has been linked to respiratory irritation and asthma attacks in children.[19,22] It has leaked into groundwater in many areas of the United States and is one of the most frequently detected volatile organic compounds found in drinking water sources in the United States.[6] At concentrations as low as 20 parts per billion (ppb), methyl tertiary butyl ether can create an unpleasant taste that can render water undrinkable. In California, a maximum contaminant level of 5 ppb was set for methyl tertiary butyl ether in drinking water based on taste and odor.[23] Methyl tertiary butyl ether was not subjected to toxicologic testing before its commercial introduction.[24] It subsequently has been shown in experimental animal studies to cause lymphatic tumors and testicular cancer.[25] In 1999, in view of these findings, the governor of California issued the first state order in the United States to completely phase out methyl tertiary butyl ether from gasoline by December 31, 2002.[26] As of 2009, 25 states mandated a complete or partial methyl tertiary butyl ether ban.[27]

Ethanol also is used as an oxygenate in the United States and is added at concentrations of up to 10% by volume. People are briefly exposed to low levels of known carcinogens and other potentially toxic compounds while pumping gasoline, regardless of whether the gasoline is oxygenated.[28,29]

## ROUTES AND SOURCES OF EXPOSURE

### Inhalation

Children can inhale volatile gasoline vapors at service stations, along highways, and in communities near petroleum-processing and gasoline-transfer facilities. In addition, children can inhale gasoline engine exhaust. Engine exhaust includes uncombusted gasoline and toxic gasoline combustion products, such as polyaromatic hydrocarbons.[30] If tetraethyl lead or MMT have been added to gasoline, exhaust will contain lead or manganese. Exposure to components of gasoline exhaust, such as carbon monoxide, oxides of nitrogen, and respirable particulates can cause health problems. These issues are considered in detail in Chapter 21 and Chapter 25. Children can be exposed acutely to high doses of gasoline vapor through intentional gasoline sniffing, a form of inhalant abuse.[31,32]

### Dermal Absorption

Gasoline is lipophilic and can be absorbed through the skin.

### Ingestion

Children can inadvertently ingest gasoline. A common scenario is that a child swallows gasoline that has been stored in a container usually containing a food or beverage, such as a soda bottle. Severe toxicity can result. Children can be exposed to certain components of gasoline, such as methyl tertiary butyl ether and benzene, through consumption of contaminated water and through showering. Large ingestions are uncommon in toddlers but may be seen in adolescents. In the 1970s, the practice of gasoline siphoning from parked cars was commonplace and was a potential source of exposure among teenagers. Because gasoline is poorly absorbed via the gastrointestinal tract, toxicity is typically mild if aspiration does not occur.

## SYSTEMS AFFECTED

Ingestion of large amounts of gasoline can result in any or all of 3 acute systemic syndromes: (1) pneumonitis; (2) central nervous system (CNS) toxicity; or (3) visceral involvement, which may include hepatotoxicity, cardiomyopathy, renal toxicity, or hepatosplenomegaly.[33] The widespread contamination of drinking water supplies with low concentrations of gasoline and its additives, such as methyl tertiary butyl ether, raises concern about the potential health effects of chronic low-level exposure. Chronic exposure to gasoline and certain components, such as benzene, may be carcinogenic at high levels of exposure. There are no data in humans about the carcinogenicity of methyl tertiary butyl ether in drinking water or from chronic environmental exposure to methyl tertiary butyl ether in gasoline.

### Lungs

Ingestion of liquid gasoline is followed by chemical pneumonitis.[34,35] Aspiration seems to be the principal route of pulmonary exposure, and therefore, vomiting should not be induced following gasoline ingestion (see the section on Treatment later in the chapter). Symptoms of dyspnea, gagging, and fever may appear within 30 minutes of exposure, but symptoms can be delayed up to 4 hours. Cyanosis appears in 2% to 3% of patients. Symptoms typically worsen over 48 to 72 hours after ingestion but then resolve in 5 days to 1 week. Death occurs in fewer than 2% of cases.

Pathologic changes in the lungs in gasoline pneumonitis include interstitial inflammation, edema, and intra-alveolar hemorrhage. The pathophysiology is incompletely understood but most likely involves direct injury to pulmonary tissue as well as disruption of the surfactant layer.[35] Radiographic changes include increased perihilar markings, basilar infiltrates, and consolidation; these changes appear in 50% to 90% of patients. Radiographs, which may be normal initially, do not correlate well with severity of clinical symptoms or with the clinical examination. Radiographic changes can persist for many weeks after resolution of symptoms. Long-term follow-up of survivors shows occasional cases of bronchiectasis and pulmonary fibrosis and a high prevalence of asymptomatic minor abnormalities (82%) on pulmonary function tests.[36]

### Central Nervous System

The lipophilic nature of gasoline allows it to cross the blood-brain barrier; however, gasoline is poorly absorbed from the gastrointestinal tract, so ingestion does not typically lead to CNS symptoms. Acute inhalational exposure to gasoline vapors in high concentrations is narcotic and can produce dizziness, excitement, anesthesia, and loss of consciousness.[37] Seizures and coma are reported in a small percentage of cases. Dementia and brainstem dysfunction have been documented.[38]

## Cardiovascular System

Sudden sniffing death syndrome, resulting from arrhythmias or cardiac dysfunction, can follow exposure to high concentrations of gasoline vapors for periods as brief as 5 minutes.[32] It is the leading cause of fatality related to inhalant abuse. Cardiomyopathy can occur after chronic gasoline sniffing but is uncommon.

## Liver

High-dose exposure can cause hepatocellular damage and hepatosplenomegaly.[7,23]

## Kidneys

High-dose exposure can cause renal tubular injury.[7,23]

## Carcinogenicity

Chronic occupational exposure to gasoline seems to be associated with renal cell carcinoma and nasal cancer.[1,39] This may be an important public health concern, given the widespread exposure to gasoline vapors in retail service stations and rising rates of kidney cancer in the United States. An association between gasoline exposure and kidney cancer also is seen in animal studies.[1,40] Several components of gasoline are proven or probable carcinogens (Table 30-1).

| Table 30-1. Examples of Human Carcinogens in Gasoline | | |
|---|---|---|
| **CHEMICAL** | **ASSOCIATED CANCERS** | **CLASSIFICATION OF CARCINOGENICITY** |
| Benzene[41] | AML, ALL, multiple myeloma, CLL, non-Hodgkin lymphoma | IARC known/likely human carcinogen<br>EPA human carcinogen |
| 1,3-Butadiene[42] | Lymphoma, leukemia, myeloid metaplasia | IARC known/likely human carcinogen<br>EPA human carcinogen |
| Methyl tertiary butyl ether[43] | Testicular, lymphatic, brain cancers | Not EPA or IARC classified<br>Strongly positive in animal studies; no data in humans |

Abbreviations: ALL, acute lymphoblastic leukemia; AML, acute myeloid leukemia; CLL, chronic lymphocytic leukemia; EPA, Environmental Protection Agency; IARC, International Agency for Research on Cancer.

It is important to note the inherent limitations of epidemiologic studies examining the human carcinogenicity of gasoline and its components. These limitations include (1) the absence of complete information on past exposure levels to gasoline vapor or on concurrent exposures to other substances such as gasoline or diesel engine exhaust; (2) the constantly changing composition of gasoline; and (3) the long latency period, frequently many years, between exposure to a constituent of gasoline and the subsequent appearance of disease. For these reasons, epidemiologic studies tend to underestimate the strength of associations between toxic exposures and disease. Toxicological studies in experimental animals can complement epidemiologic investigations, just as epidemiologic studies complement experimental animal studies.

## DIAGNOSIS

Acute, high-dose exposure to gasoline is diagnosed by history and by detecting the odor of gasoline on exhaled breath. Although methyl tertiary butyl ether and its breakdown product, butyl alcohol, can be measured in exhaled air, blood, and urine, the availability and clinical utility of these measures currently are limited. Benzene can be measured in exhaled air and blood. Certain metabolites of benzene, such as phenol, can be measured in urine. However, this test is not a quantitative indicator of the level of benzene exposure because phenol is present in urine from other sources, such as diet.[44] The tests for the metabolites of methyl tertiary butyl ether and benzene are most appropriately used in the context of epidemiologic studies and are generally not available in clinical settings. Diagnosis is typically made via a history of exposure.

Assessment of levels of exposure to gasoline and its constituents in community air or in groundwater requires expert air or water sampling by a certified environmental scientist or government agency, such as a state or county health department or department of environmental protection. An important source of data on community exposures is the US EPA Toxic Release Inventory (https://www.epa.gov/toxics-release-inventory-tri-program) which can be readily searched through http://scorecard.goodguide.com.

## TREATMENT

Treatment of chemical pneumonitis caused by acute high-dose exposure to gasoline begins with clinical assessment of the severity of illness and evaluation of the amount of gasoline ingested. Many children who ingest a small amount of gasoline never become symptomatic. When such children present for medical evaluation, observation for 4 hours after ingestion can identify those who can be safely discharged. Because most cases involve only small amounts of gasoline, outpatient evaluation with close follow-up (depending on the reliability of the family) is usually sufficient if the child is asymptomatic

4 hours after ingestion. Children who are even mildly symptomatic (ie, with coughing, tachypnea, wheezing, hypoxia) should be admitted for observation because of risk of disease progression. More severe cases require hospital admission, possibly to the pediatric intensive care unit.

Whether to use gastric emptying was the subject of long-standing debate. At present, gastric emptying via ipecac or gastric lavage is contraindicated because of the danger of aspiration.[35,45] Steroids offer little benefit in gasoline pneumonitis. Antibiotics are indicated if bacterial superinfection develops. Debate about whether prophylactic antibiotics are warranted is long-standing and unresolved.

In the most severe cases with advanced respiratory distress, mechanical ventilation may be required. Positive end-expiratory pressure ventilation has been used, as well as high-frequency jet ventilation using very high respiratory rates (220–260 breaths/min). Extracorporeal membrane oxygenation has been used when other options have failed.[35]

## PREVENTION OF EXPOSURE

Exposure of children and adolescents to gasoline and its vapors should be minimized to prevent the occurrence of delayed health consequences, especially cancer. Young children should not pump gasoline or work in retail service stations.

Gasoline should never be stored in a bottle or other container that normally contains a food or beverage and is accessible and attractive to young children. Gasoline should only be stored in a gasoline-labeled container requiring dexterity to open.

Community exposures to gasoline vapors near refineries, transfer stations, and other petroleum-handling facilities may require concerted community action for their amelioration, including the development of partnerships among community residents, pediatricians, and environmental agencies. Prevention of exposures to gasoline and its additives in groundwater requires either installation of activated charcoal filters at the tap or switching to bottled water. Prevention of exposure to the most toxic additives to gasoline, such as tetraethyl lead, MMT, methyl tertiary butyl ether, or benzene, is best achieved by governmental regulation or phasing out of these compounds.[10,26]

## Frequently Asked Questions

Q  *What is the risk to my child of brief exposure to gasoline vapors when she is in the car while I am at a service station filling the tank with gasoline?*

A  The risk is minimal, but exposure should be kept as brief as possible to minimize risk of delayed consequences, especially leukemia caused by inhalation of benzene vapor. Closing the windows is recommended. Adults should not hold infants while fueling vehicles. Some states regulate the age at which children can fuel cars, with age limits typically 16 years of age or older.

Q  *A leaking underground storage tank at a gasoline station has been identified in my neighborhood and I am concerned that it is contaminating my well water. What should I do?*

A  Strong state and federal regulations developed in recent years require monitoring and abatement of leaking underground storage tanks. A parent should inform the state environmental agency and/or US EPA if such a concern is present. Families who may drink water from a gasoline-contaminated source should install activated charcoal filters to their water tap or switch to bottled water. These measures should be taken when there is an unknown source of contamination, when contaminant levels are rising (even though levels still may be below drinking water standards), or when levels of contaminants are steady but higher than drinking water standards (see Chapter 17).

Q  *My family's water supply has measurable amounts of some gasoline components that are below the US EPA standard. The community water authority says that the water meets standards and that for further advice, families should contact their pediatrician. What does this mean for my family's health?*

A  The US EPA sets an enforceable standard or maximum contaminant level based on both their best estimate of health risk and the "ability of public water systems to detect and remove contaminants using suitable treatment technologies."[46] Water that meets US EPA standards is deemed to confer minimal to no health risk. If you are still concerned, activated charcoal filtration will remove benzene and other aromatic components that make up most of gasoline. All filtration systems require care and maintenance. Community water supplies may transiently exceed standards. If the water is in violation of standards, filtration is a short-term solution, but documenting the efficacy of the filter is a problem. A private well that is contaminated with gasoline poses a serious remediation problem because such contamination often represents widespread contamination of groundwater beyond the control of the homeowner. Activated charcoal filtration or a reverse osmosis filtration may be necessary, but it may be difficult or impossible to make the water safe to drink.

Q  *What are the long-term risks of gasoline sniffing to children and adolescents?*

A  Mental deterioration and chronic permanent injury to the nervous system are the principal health dangers of chronic abuse of solvents, including gasoline.[31,47] This leads to trouble with attention, memory, and problem-solving as well as muscle weakness, tremor, and balance problems. The chronic user's mood changes as dementia develops. There are effects on the kidney. Chronic gasoline sniffing also causes certain cancers. Gasoline sniffing is a marker that a child or teenager is at very high risk of trying or already using other drugs.

Q   *Should I be concerned about proposals to add MMT to gasoline as an antiknock agent?*

A   Yes. Manganese is a known neurotoxicant. It is not used currently in US gasoline. MMT use in Canada to improve octane rating and as an antiknock agent began in 1976 but has since been phased out. A few other countries, such as Australia and South Africa, were still permitting the use of MMT as of this writing. Neurotoxic effects have been seen at high- and low-dose exposures and span the range from overt symptomatic parkinsonism at high exposures to subclinical neurobehavioral impairment. Permitting the addition of MMT to the US gasoline supply would not be prudent. This could increase the risk of widespread subclinical neurotoxicity.

Q   *What can I do to reduce gasoline consumption and help combat global climate change?*

A   You can support campaigns to develop safe, efficient mass transportation that will reduce atmospheric emissions and the risk of automotive injury to children. Children should be encouraged, where possible, to walk or bike to school and to play activities, and pediatricians should take the lead in encouraging construction of community walkways and bikeways. Reduction of obesity among children will be an added benefit of this strategy. You can also advocate for land-use planning in your community that results in reduced dependence on driving and that fosters walking, bicycle riding, and use of mass transportation.

## References

1.  Dement JM, Hensley L, Gitelman A. Carcinogenicity of gasoline: a review of epidemiological evidence. *Ann N Y Acad Sci.* 1997;837:53–76

2.  US Energy Information Administration. Petroleum and Other Liquids Data. https://www.eia. gov/dnav/pet/pet_cons_psup_a_EPM0F_VPP_mbbl_a.htm. Accessed January 18, 2018

3.  US Energy Information Administration. Consumption of Motor Gasoline United States. https://www.eia.gov/beta/international/data/browser/#/?pa=0000000001&c=000000000000 0000000000000000000000000000002&ct=0&tl_id=5-A&vs=INTL.62-2-USA-TBPD.A& cy=2012&vo=0&v=H&start=1980&end=2014&showdm=y. Accessed January 18, 2018

4.  United States Energy Information Administration. World Motor Gasoline Consumption by Year. http://www.indexmundi.com/energy/?product=gasoline&. Accessed January 18, 2018

5.  Intergovernmental Panel on Climate Change 5th Assessment. *Climate Change 2014: Synthesis Report.* http://www.ipcc.ch/pdf/assessment-report/ar5/syr/AR5_SYR_FINAL_All_Topics.pdf. Accessed January 18, 2018

6.  Carter JM, Grady SJ, Delzer GC, Koch B, Zogorski JS. Occurrence of MTBE and other gasoline oxygenates in CWS source waters. *American Water Works Association Journal.* 2006;98(4):91

7. Agency for Toxic Substances and Disease Registry. *Toxicological Profile for Benzene, August 2007.* https://www.atsdr.cdc.gov/ToxProfiles/tp.asp?id=40&tid=14. Accessed January 18, 2018

8. Loomis D, Guyton KZ, Grosse Y, et al. Carcinogenicity of benzene. *Lancet Oncol.* 2017;18(12):1574–1575

9. Houot J, Marquant F, Goujon S, et al. Residential proximity to heavy-traffic roads, benzene exposure, and childhood leukemia-The GEOCAP study, 2002-2007. *Am J Epidemiol.* 2015;182(8):685–693

10. Centers for Disease Control and Prevention (CDC). Update: blood lead levels—United States, 1991–1994. *MMWR Morb Mortal Wkly Rep.* 1997;46(7):141–146

11. United Nations Environment Programme. *Leaded Petrol Phase – Out: Global Status as at March 2017.* https://wedocs.unep.org/bitstream/handle/20.500.11822/17542/MapWorldLead_March2017.pdf?sequence=1&isAllowed=y. Accessed July 18, 2018

12. Landrigan PJ, Boffetta P, Apostoli P. The reproductive toxicity and carcinogenicity of lead: a critical review. *Am J Ind Med.* 2000;38(3):231–243

13. United States Environmental Protection Agency. Airport Lead Monitoring through 2013. https://nepis.epa.gov/Exe/ZyPDF.cgi/P100LJDW.PDF?Dockey=P100LJDW.PDF. Accessed January 18, 2018

14. Miranda ML, Anthopolos R, Hastings D. A geospatial analysis of the effects of aviation gasoline on childhood blood lead levels. *Environ Health Perspect.* 2011;119(10):1513–1516

15. Needleman HL, Landrigan PJ. Toxins at the pump. *New York Times.* March 13, 1996:A19

16. Gorell JM, Johnson CC, Rybicki BA, et al. Occupational exposures to metals as risk factors for Parkinson's disease. *Neurology.* 1997;48(3):650–658

17. Mergler D. Neurotoxic effects of low level exposure to manganese in human population. *Environ Res.* 1999;80(2 Pt 1):99–102

18. Mergler D, Baldwin M, Belanger S, et al. Manganese neurotoxicity, a continuum of dysfunction: results from a community based study. *Neurotoxicology.* 1999;20(2-3):327–342

19. Mehlman MA. Dangerous and cancer-causing properties of products and chemicals in the oil refining and petrochemical industry—Part XXII: health hazards from exposure to gasoline containing methyl tertiary butyl ether: study of New Jersey residents. *Toxicol Ind Health.* 1996;12(5):613–627

20. Mannino DM, Etzel RA. Are oxygenated fuels effective? An evaluation of ambient carbon monoxide concentrations in 11 Western states, 1986 to 1992. *J Air Waste Manage Assoc.* 1996;46(1):20–24

21. Ahmed FE. Toxicology and human health effects following exposure to oxygenated or reformulated fuel. *Toxicol Lett.* 2001;123(2-3):89–113

22. Joseph PM, Weiner MG. Visits to physicians after the oxygenation of gasoline in Philadelphia. *Arch Environ Health.* 2002;57(2):137–154

23. Office of Environmental Health Hazard Assessment. Water—Public Health Goal for MTBE in drinking water [memorandum]. Available at: https://oehha.ca.gov/water/public-health-goal/public-health-goal-methyl-tertiary-butyl-ether-drinking-water. Accessed January 19, 2018

24. Mehlman MA. MTBE toxicity. *Environ Health Perspect.* 1996;104(8):808

25. Belpoggi F, Soffritti M, Maltoni C. Methyl-tertiary-butyl ether (MTBE)—a gasoline additive—causes testicular and lymphohaematopoietic cancers in rats. *Toxicol Ind Health.* 1995;11(2):119–149

26. Schremp G. Staff Findings: Timetable for the Phaseout of MTBE From California's Gasoline Supply. California Energy Commission; 1999. https://www.arb.ca.gov/regact/mtberesid/appdxc.pdf. Accessed January 18, 2018

27. US Environmental Protection Agency. *State Actions Banning MTBE (Statewide).* EPA420-B-07-013. August 2007. https://nepis.epa.gov/Exe/ZyNET.exe/P1004KIR.TXT?Zy ActionD=ZyDocument&Client=EPA&Index=2006=Thru=2010&Docs=&Query=&Time= &EndTime=&SearchMethod=1&TocRestrict=n&Toc=&TocEntry=&QField=&QField Year=&QFieldMonth=&QFieldDay=&IntQFieldOp=0&ExtQFieldOp=0&XmlQuery= &File=D%3A%5Czyfiles%5CIndex%20Data%5C06thru10%5CTxt%5C00000009%5CP1004KIR. txt&User=ANONYMOUS&Password=anonymous&SortMethod=h%7C-&Maximum Documents=1&FuzzyDegree=0&ImageQuality=r75g8/r75g8/x150y150g16/i425&Display= hpfr&DefSeekPage=x&SearchBack=ZyActionL&Back=ZyActionS&BackDesc=Results% 20page&MaximumPages=1&ZyEntry=1&SeekPage=x&ZyPURL. Accessed January 18, 2018

28. Backer LC, Egeland GM, Ashley DL, et al. Exposure to regular gasoline and ethanol oxyfuel during refueling in Alaska. *Environ Health Perspect.* 1997;105(8):850–855

29. Moolenaar RL, Hefflin BJ, Ashley DL, Middaugh JP, Etzel RA. Blood benzene concentration in workers exposed to oxygenated fuel in Fairbanks, Alaska. *Int Arch Occup Environ Health.* 1997;69(2):139–143

30. International Agency for Research on Cancer. *Diesel and Gasoline Engine Exhausts and Some Nitroarenes.* IARC Monographs. Vol 46. Lyon, France: International Agency for Research on Cancer; 1989

31. Cairney S, Maruff P, Burns C, Currie B. The neurobehavioural consequences of petrol (gasoline) sniffing. *Neurosci Biobehav Rev.* 2002;26(1):81–89

32. Williams JF, Storck M, American Academy of Pediatrics Committee on Substance Abuse, American Academy of Pediatrics Committee on Native American Child Health. Inhalant abuse. *Pediatrics.* 2007;119(5):1009–1017

33. Reese E, Kimbrough RD. Acute toxicity of gasoline and some additives. *Environ Health Perspect.* 1993;101(Suppl 6):115–131

34. Eade NR, Taussig LM, Marks MI. Hydrocarbon pneumonitis. *Pediatrics.* 1974;54(3):351–357

35. Gummin DD. Hydrocarbons. In: Hoffman RS, Howland MA, Lewin NA, Nelson LS, Goldfrank L, eds. *Goldfrank's Toxicologic Emergencies.* 10th ed. New York, NY: McGraw-Hill Education; 2015

36. Gurwitz D, Kattan M, Levinson H, Culham JA. Pulmonary function abnormalities in asymptomatic children after hydrocarbon pneumonitis. *Pediatrics.* 1978;62(5):789–794

37. Burbacher TM. Neurotoxic effects of gasoline and gasoline constituents. *Environ Health Perspect.* 1993;101(Suppl 6):133–141

38. Ritchie GD, Still KR, Alexander WK, Nordholm AF, Wilson CL, Rossi J 3rd, Mattie DR. A review of the neurotoxicity risk of selected hydrocarbon fuels. *J Toxicol Environ Health B Crit Rev.* 2001;4(3):223–312

39. Lynge E, Andersen A, Nilsson R, et al. Risk of cancer and exposure to gasoline vapors. *Am J Epidemiol.* 1997;145(5):449–458

40. Mehlman MA. Dangerous and cancer-causing properties of products and chemicals in the oil refining and petrochemical industry: part I. Carcinogenicity of motor fuels: gasoline. *Toxicol Ind Health.* 1991;7(5-6):143–152

41. International Agency for Research on Cancer. Benzene. IARC Monographs on the Evaluation of Carcinogenic Risks to Humans. Vol 120 (in press)

42. International Agency for Research on Cancer. 1,3-Butadiene. IARC Monographs on the Evaluation of Carcinogenic Risks to Humans. Vol 100F. 2012. http://monographs.iarc.fr/ENG/Monographs/vol100F/index.php. Accessed January 18, 2018

43. Burns KM, Melnick RL. MTBE: recent carcinogenicity studies. *Int J Occup Environ Health.* 2012;18(1):66–69

44. Agency for Toxic Substances and Disease Registry. *ToxFAQs for Automotive Gasoline.* https://www.atsdr.cdc.gov/toxfaqs/tf.asp?id=467&tid=83. Accessed January 18, 2018

45. Vale JA, Kulig K, American Academy of Clinical Toxicology, European Association of Poisons Centres and Clinical Toxicologists. Position paper: gastric lavage. *J Toxicol Clin Toxicol.* 2004;42(7):933–943

46. US Environmental Protection Agency. *Benzene Hazard Summary.* https://www.epa.gov/sites/production/files/2016-09/documents/benzene.pdf. Accessed January 18, 2018

47. Burns TM, Shneker BF, Juel VC. Gasoline sniffing multifocal neuropathy. *Pediatr Neurol.* 2001;25(5):419–421

# Chapter 31

# Ionizing Radiation (Excluding Radon)

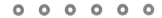

## KEY POINTS

- Radiation exposures are derived from external sources (eg, background radon, cosmic radiation, or medical diagnostic, monitoring, or therapeutic radiation from x-rays) and internal sources (eg, radioactive fallout [ingested in contaminated milk or vegetables, inhaled, or dermally contaminating] or medical radioisotopes [injected or implanted]).
- Children are more vulnerable and at higher risk of deleterious radiation-induced effects compared with adults.
- The risk of cancer associated with most diagnostic radiation is low and use of radiation should not be restricted when clinically indicated. Efforts to encourage carefully considered uses of radiation ("Image Gently") have been published.
- Iodine 131 (I-131) is a radioisotope that may be released after a power plant accident, nuclear weapon detonation, or terrorist event. For those persons exposed, prompt treatment with potassium iodide (KI) can be quite effective in protecting the thyroid.
- KI does not protect against adverse health effects to organs other than the thyroid from I-131, or to any organs from radionuclides other than I-131 that are released in these events.

## INTRODUCTION

Radiation includes energy transmitted by waves through space or some type of medium, such as light seen as colors, infrared rays perceived as heat, and audible radio waves amplified through radio and television. People cannot similarly perceive radiation with shorter wavelengths: ultraviolet rays, x-rays, and gamma rays. Figure 31-1 shows wavelengths for different types of radiation.[1] Ionizing radiation consists of particles generally produced as a result of radioactive decay of unstable nuclei that are characterized by immense energy sufficient to ionize in tissue. This ionization drives outer electrons from their orbits around atoms and can penetrate solid objects. The free electrons created can react with other molecules in living organisms and cause tissue damage.

The dose of absorbed radiation per unit of mass, previously measured as "radiation absorbed dose" (rad) is now measured in Gray (Gy); 1 Gy = 100 rad. One Gy delivers 1 joule (J) of energy per kg of matter. Different types of

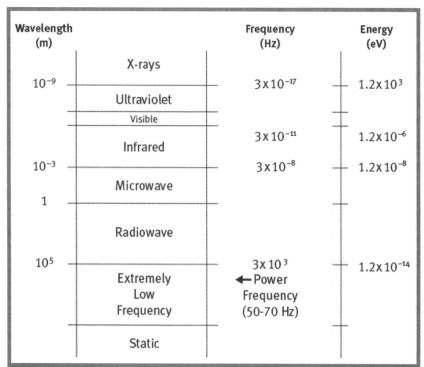

**Figure 31-1. Approximate Range of Wavelength, Frequency, and Energy for Different Types of Electromagnetic Radiation or Fields**

Abbreviations: Hz, Hertz; eV, electronvolts.

radiation differ in their ability to produce effects. Alpha particles consist of helium nuclei that have a very limited ability to penetrate tissue and can barely get through the dead outer layers of skin. Beta particles consist of electrons that can penetrate up to 2 cm of soft tissue. Gamma radiation consists of photons that can penetrate the entire diameter of the body. External exposures derive from proximity to a photon-emitting radiation source, such as an x-ray machine, a nuclear power plant, or a nuclear explosion. Internal exposures occur from intake of radionuclides, such as inhalation or ingestion of fallout, injection of radionuclides for diagnostic purposes, or radionuclides implanted for treatment of cancer.

Different tissues and organs in the body differ in their sensitivity to ionizing radiation and in potential adverse effects. This is why equivalent and effective doses were introduced. Equivalent dose is the product of absorbed dose and a weight factor. The unit of equivalent dose is named the sievert (Sv). The equivalent dose was previously measured as roentgen equivalent man (rem); 1 Sv = 100 rem. Equivalent dose refers to the radiation energy deposited in a specific organ and effective dose corresponds to the sum of the dose to a number of tissues as if the whole body had been exposed. For every tissue, there is a weight factor depending on its sensitivity to radiation-induced effects (Figure 31-2).

## ROUTES OF EXPOSURE

People may be exposed to ionizing radiation externally to any organ including the skin, or internally by inhalation, ingestion, injection (for medical diagnosis or treatment), and implantation (for medical treatment). The fetus may be exposed if the mother is exposed. There may be exposure to radionuclides through human milk.

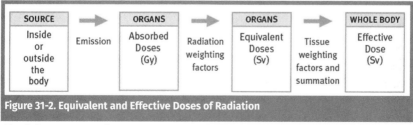

**Figure 31-2. Equivalent and Effective Doses of Radiation**

Abbreviations: Gy, Gray; Sv, sievert.

## SOURCES OF EXPOSURE

Radiation exposures are derived from external sources, such as background cosmic radiation, radon, or medical x-rays, as well as internal sources, such as radioactive fallout (generally ingested in contaminated milk or vegetables) or medical radioisotopes (injected or implanted). These exposures can be from natural or man-made sources. The energy in ionizing radiation is high enough to cause displacement of electrons from atoms and breaks in chemical bonds. This transfer of energy in sufficient doses from the environment to individuals can adversely affect their health.[1,2] X-rays transfer energy along thin paths, whereas neutrons have greater mass and transfer energy along wider paths.

Different ways (ie, direct or indirect) and units are used to measure radiation. An example of a direct measurement is the measurement of radiation on a patient, whereas an example of an indirect measurement is the radiation level emitted by an x-ray machine.

On average, the annual effective dose equivalent of ionizing radiation to the population in the United States is 6 millisieverts (mSv) (0.6 rem), 37% of which is from radon, 13% from other natural sources, 24% from computerized tomography, 12% from nuclear medicine, 7% from interventional fluoroscopy, 5% from medical x-rays, and 2% from other man-made sources.[2]

A fairly recent source of radiation exposure is from large-scale screening of airline passengers by the Transportation Security Administration.[3] The companies that produce airport screening devices indicate that their devices expose people to about half or less of the 0.25 microsievert recommended as a consensus upper limit standard by the American National Standards Institute/Health Physics Society. For comparative purposes, 0.25 microsievert is the same amount of radiation received by flying about a minute and a half because cosmic radiation during commercial flights exposes persons flying to about 10 microsieverts per hour.[4] As another comparison, natural background radiation exposes people to about 0.35 microsievert per hour. Frequent fliers have more exposure because they go through people scanners more often and also receive more exposure to cosmic radiation because they fly more. The consensus standard recommendation is that the total radiation dose limit should be 250 microsieverts per year, equivalent to about 1,000 scans per year. X-ray scanners use a very low-energy and low-intensity radiation, so an embryo or fetus would have minimal exposure to ionizing radiation. The devices used to screen carry-on luggage and other carry-on items are very well shielded so exposures to passengers are very small, and the radiation exposure to the items passing through these devices is too low to affect any items other than certain types of camera film.

Radiation exposure may be instantaneous (atomic bomb), chronic (uranium miners), fractionated (radiotherapy), or partial-body (eg, x-ray or radiotherapy to a specific anatomic site). For a given dose, whole-body exposure is generally more harmful than partial-body exposure. Radioisotopes decay with time into stable elements and have physical half-lives of various lengths, from fractions of a second to millions of years. They also have biological half-lives related to the rate at which they are excreted from the body.

## SYSTEMS AFFECTED AND BIOLOGICAL PROCESSES

Atoms or molecules that become ionized attain stability by forming substances that may alter molecular processes within a cell or its environment. Ionizing radiation, when it collides with a cell, is capable of introducing DNA strand breaks and gene mutations. If this damage is not repaired, the cell may die or be transformed into a malignant cell.

## Acute Effects

Ionizing radiation produces the same reactions regardless of the type of particle or ray emitted. Differences are quantitative, not qualitative. Acute radiation syndrome (ARS) is an acute illness resulting from a substantial exposure (greater than 0.7 Gy or 70 rads) to the entire body delivered in a short time from external, penetrating forms of radiation. Three major categories of adverse physiologic effects have been recognized and, more recently a fourth (cutaneous), as shown in Table 31-1 along with the range of doses at which these effects may occur. The time frame of symptoms and illness has been described as occurring in 4 stages: prodromal (initial symptoms that may include nausea, vomiting, and diarrhea), followed by latent (when the patient may appear and feel healthy), then manifest illness stage (which may last

### Table 31-1. Estimated Whole Body Doses for Effects Following Acute Radiation Exposure[a]

| HEALTH EFFECT | ORGAN | ABSORBED DOSE | |
| --- | --- | --- | --- |
| | | Gy | rad |
| Gastrointestinal syndrome | Gastrointestinal | 6–10 | 600–1,000 |
| Hematopoietic syndrome | Bone marrow | 2–6 | 200–600 |
| Cerebrovascular syndrome | Circulatory system and central nervous system | >20 | >2,000 |
| Cutaneous syndrome | Skin | >2 (to the skin) | >200 |

Abbreviations: Gy, Gray; rad, radiation absorbed dose.
[a] From the National Council on Radiation Protection and Measurements.[5]

from hours to several months), and finally recovery or death. Gastrointestinal syndrome can initially manifest with nausea, vomiting, diarrhea, and anorexia that may occur within minutes to days following exposure. If this syndrome progresses, the patient may experience worsening of these symptoms, mucositis, and parotitis, which may be followed by weight loss, infection, dehydration, electrolyte imbalance, and then, in the absence of recovery, irreparable damage to the gastrointestinal tract. Hematopoietic syndrome may manifest within a few hours with reduced lymphocyte and platelet counts. The absence of blood count recovery is the result of destruction of bone marrow and may lead to fatal hemorrhage and/or infection. Cardiovascular/central nervous system syndrome usually occurs at very high whole-body radiation doses (20 to 50 Gy), with death caused by collapse of the circulatory system, particularly increased pressure in the cranium from increased fluid caused by edema, vasculitis, and meningitis. The cutaneous syndrome results from damage of the basal layer of the skin with subsequent inflammation, erythema, dry or moist desquamation, and epilation from damaged hair follicles. Within a few hours after irradiation, erythema associated with itching may occur and last from days to weeks; progression may involve intense reddening, blistering, and ulceration with subsequent permanent hair loss, damage to sebaceous and sweat glands, skin atrophy, fibrosis, and change in pigmentation and/or necrosis of the tissue.

Most radiation injuries result from high doses of radiation to specific anatomic sites. These high doses can cause a variety of serious localized effects that are associated with the anatomic site of the exposure and can include skin necrosis at the site, permanent damage to localized blood vessels, dental and gum destruction, and loss of function of key organs that can cause hypothyroidism, parathyroid effects, temporary or permanent sterility, or other effects.

## Delayed Effects

In general, the best estimates of dose-related delayed effects of ionizing radiation come from the decades-long studies of the Japanese atomic bomb survivors who in August 1945 experienced a single, instantaneous whole-body exposure; this was possibly complicated by other adverse influences, such as malnutrition in war-torn Japan. Delayed effects largely are attributable to mutagenesis, teratogenesis, and carcinogenesis. The smaller the exposure, the less likely that late effects will be found. A latency period occurs between the exposure to ionizing radiation and its clinical manifestations, especially in the carcinogenic process (see Carcinogenesis, discussed later).

Children are more vulnerable and at a higher risk of deleterious radiation-induced effects than are adults.[6,7] Their tissues are more radiosensitive and children have a longer life expectancy, resulting in a greater potential for manifestation. Female infants have almost double the risk as male infants.[8]

## Mutagenesis

The harmful effects of ionizing radiation are attributable to its ability to induce DNA damage. This results in genotoxicity in the form of DNA strand breaks and whole chromosome breaks. These chromosome breaks in somatic cells (eg, lymphocytes, skin fibroblasts) are detectable decades after exposure[9] and presumably account for the increased rates of cancer observed after exposure in childhood or adulthood. The magnitude of the genotoxic effect depends on the level of exposure and the concentration of ions induced by the absorption of the energy emitted by the ionizing radiation source.

Studies of children conceived after one or both parents were exposed to the atomic bomb have as yet shown no excess of direct genetic effects. The studies started with clinical observations and then included cytogenetic, biochemical, and molecular studies. Scientists evaluated chromosome damage in individuals who were in utero during the atomic bomb detonations in Japan and older than age 40 years at the time of study.[10] They found that the frequency of chromosomal translocations did not increase with the in utero radiation dose. In contrast, children with more prolonged exposure to ionizing radiation after the Chernobyl accident in 1986 were found to have above average levels of genome damage.[11,12]

## Teratogenesis

The effect of a potential teratogen is dependent on the gestational age at the time of exposure as well as the dose absorbed. Much of the information on the effects of acute exposure to ionizing radiation and teratogenesis has been obtained from studies carried out on the survivors of the atomic bomb detonations of Hiroshima and Nagasaki.[13,14] Substantial doses of intrauterine exposure to ionizing radiation were associated with small head size alone or with severe intellectual disability. Susceptibility to radiation-related severe intellectual disability was greatest at 8 to 15 weeks of gestational age, with some occurring during the 16th to 25th week of gestation. The lowest dose that caused severe intellectual disability from atomic bomb exposure was 0.6 Sv. The lowest dose associated with small head size but no intellectual disability was 0.10 to 0.19 Sv among fetuses exposed at 4 to 17 weeks of gestational age. Intellectual disability resulting from radiation exposure may be attributable to interruption in the proliferation and migration of neurons from near the cerebral ventricles to the cortex.

## Carcinogenesis

### Atomic Bomb Exposure

Following the atomic bomb detonations in Hiroshima and Nagasaki, leukemia appeared within a few years and was one of the most striking evident somatic effects of radiation in atomic bomb survivors.[15] In the latest follow-up 55 years after the detonation, radiation-associated excess risks for acute lymphoblastic leukemia and chronic myelogenous leukemia declined dramatically, but elevated risks of acute myeloid leukemia persisted.[16]

After childhood exposure to ionizing radiation, increased incidence and mortality from cancers in adulthood may be observed depending on the radiation dose and whether the study was sufficiently large to observe an increased risk if doses were relatively low. A large study is required to detect increases in risk at low radiation doses. A significant time period of observation is also required to assess effects of childhood radiation exposure and cancer risk. A significant dose response has been observed at doses of 0 to 150 mSv; the dose effect threshold is compatible with zero.[17]

Initial studies of the 807 Japanese atomic bomb survivors exposed in utero suggested that there was no excess of childhood cancer,[14] but a subsequent study of solid cancer incidence in 2,452 adult subjects exposed in utero to the atomic bomb in Japan identified 94 cancers, an increase over the expected number.[18] This effect was identified 50 years after the exposure to the atomic bomb detonation. This study also evaluated 15,388 adult subjects who were younger than age 6 years at the time of the detonation. Dose-related solid cancer risks were increased in adults after both in utero and early childhood exposures. Long-term risks were considerably lower in persons exposed in utero compared with early childhood exposure.[18]

Epidemiologic studies revealed the long-term sequelae of this type of childhood radiation exposure. An excess of thyroid cancer, a very rare childhood cancer, began at age 11 years in children who were exposed to the atomic bomb.[18] Increased rates of breast cancer after childhood exposure were identified at age 30 years (ie, the usual age for early-onset breast cancer in the general population).[19]

### Nuclear Power Plant Accidents

Following a nuclear power plant accident (as occurred in March 2011, when the nuclear power plant near Fukushima, Japan was damaged by a major earthquake and resulting tsunami), individuals, land, and structures in the vicinity of the plant can be exposed to a mixture of radioactive products generated inside the reactor, also known as "nuclear fission products." The main radionuclides representing health risk are radioactive cesium and radioactive iodine. The average lifetime effective doses estimated for adults in Fukushima prefecture and for children aged 1 year were approximately 10 mSv and 20 mSv, respectively. These estimates from the World Health Organization are based on data from a large survey and dose assessments.[20] No overall increases in cancer are expected inside or outside Japan from the Fukushima Daiichi nuclear plant accident. Continued monitoring is needed, however, for the highly contaminated workers and for young children.

The Chernobyl accident in 1986 is the worst nuclear accident to date and there are ongoing studies of the exposed children and the cleanup workers in Ukraine, Belarus, Russia, and other Baltic countries. The populations were exposed to a wide spectrum of radioactive isotopes and in addition to the acute exposure, individuals were further exposed through food, milk, and water supplies. Significantly increased rates of thyroid cancer have been observed among those exposed in childhood or adolescence.[21,22] These persons experienced increases in thyroid cancer as late as 20 years after the initial exposure and there is no evidence of a reduction in risk with greater time since exposure. Increased rates of leukemia following the accident have not been observed in children; however, cleanup workers experienced an increased incidence of chronic lymphocytic leukemia (CLL) and non-CLL leukemia.[23] About 200,000 people from the highly contaminated regions have emigrated to New York City; in 2008, a National Tumor Registry was launched in New York City to follow their health. During the period of 2010 to 2014, 10 adults living in New York City were diagnosed with vitreoretinal lymphoma; investigators found that 6 of the 10 people had lived near Chernobyl, thus suggesting that exposure to the accident also may be a risk factor for the development of this very rare cancer.[24]

### *Diagnostic Radiation*

In the last few decades, radiation exposure from medical diagnostic and therapeutic radiologic procedures has become greater than environmental radiation exposures. It is now estimated that medical radiation accounts for close to half of the total radiation exposure in the United States (Figure 31-3). In 1980, the estimated per capita medical radiation exposure in the United States was 0.54 mSv (mSv = 0.001 Sv). This exposure increased by nearly

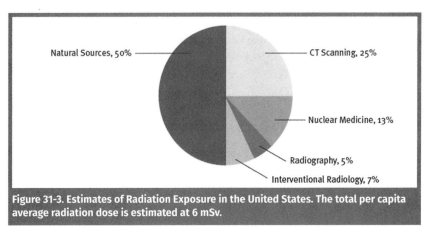

**Figure 31-3. Estimates of Radiation Exposure in the United States. The total per capita average radiation dose is estimated at 6 mSv.**

Natural Sources, 50% — CT Scanning, 25% — Nuclear Medicine, 13% — Radiography, 5% — Interventional Radiology, 7%

The figure and percentages were derived from Mettler et al.[25]
Abbreviation: mSv, millisievert.

600% to 3 mSv between 1982 and 2006 mostly because of a 30-fold increase in the number of computed tomography (CT) scans from 3 to 80 million per year.[25,26] Other increases, although smaller, have occurred from higher dose nuclear medicine and interventional procedures using fluoroscopic guidance. The increases in these 3 categories of procedures have also occurred in other countries, albeit not at the same level as in the United States.[27] Risk projection studies have estimated that the 4 million pediatric CT scans administered annually in the United States could cause up to 4,870 future cancers.[27] The efforts to reduce the dose per procedure to optimize appropriately for the smaller body size and weight of children may reduce the projected numbers of cancers by close to 50%.[28]

The risk factors for most childhood cancers are not known, but radiation exposure is postulated to contribute to childhood cancer risk because of its ability to induce DNA damage (see Chapter 44). Studies that began more than 50 years ago suggested a 1.3-fold excess of leukemia in children aged younger than 10 years after maternal exposure to diagnostic abdominal x-rays during pregnancy.[7] In a meta-analysis of 32 studies, the risk of childhood leukemia was elevated 1.3-fold even after excluding the original study.[29] The concerns raised by these studies led to the near-elimination of diagnostic x-rays during pregnancy.

The potential carcinogenic effects of postnatal conventional diagnostic radiation exposure have been much less studied.[30] Large-scale data collection on pediatric exposure to diagnostic medical radiation began in the mid-1990s. To date, very little evidence indicates that postnatal exposure to conventional diagnostic radiation increases the risk of childhood cancer. A potential exception is the association of an increased breast cancer risk later in life in adolescents who had repeated exposure because of diagnostic examinations for scoliosis.[31,32]

The use of CT scans in pediatric patients for the diagnosis of a variety of conditions has been increasing (see preceding section on Diagnostic Radiation). CT scanning exposes patients to much higher levels of ionizing radiation than conventional radiography.[33,34] Pediatric interventional and fluoroscopic imaging modalities also potentially expose children to high doses of diagnostic radiation. Prompted by concerns about dose levels in children, a number of retrospective cohort studies of pediatric CT scans and cancer were initiated. A large cohort in the United Kingdom found a significant dose-response relationship for leukemia/myelodysplastic syndrome and brain tumors.[35] The UK cohort is one of the centers in the multi-center EPI-CT study,[36] which includes 9 European countries and approximately 1 million children; results are due in the next few years. Recommendations for reducing CT doses for pediatric patients have been published.[37–41]

Data about carcinogenic risks from radiological imaging examinations are based primarily on 2 important sets of follow-up studies. Among children, adolescents, and young women monitored with repeated x-rays for scoliosis, breast cancer was increased.[42] In US and Canadian patients whose tuberculosis was monitored with repeated fluoroscopic examinations decades ago, the risk of breast cancer was also increased.[43,44] In neither population was there evidence of increased risk of leukemia or lung cancer.

### Radiation Therapy

As survival among cancer patients has continued to increase, the risk of treatment-related second cancers has become a growing problem. Efforts have been implemented to reduce radiation exposure of normal tissues surrounding the cancer site, but it has not been totally feasible to prevent such exposures. Because about half of all patients with cancer are treated with radiotherapy as a component of initial treatment, it is important to quantify associated carcinogenicity. Overall, the studies of second cancers suggest a linear dose-response that is observed even for very high fractionated doses to specific organs, although the risks are lower than the risk from the single, acute exposure of the Japanese atomic bomb survivors. Despite the somewhat lower risks, there have been some consistently observed high absolute risks, such as the 30% risk for the development of radiation-associated breast cancer by age 55 among patients with Hodgkin lymphoma treated with 40+ Gy to the chest at age 25. Overall, the risks per Gy have been found to be higher for childhood than for adult exposure.[45]

### Cancer Follow-up Studies

Pediatric cancer patients are frequently followed up during and after treatment with CT or PET examinations. The risks of a second cancer associated with these monitoring examinations have not been evaluated because it would be difficult to disentangle the carcinogenic risks from such examinations from treatment-related, disease-related, or genetic factors.

## SPECIAL SUSCEPTIBILITY AND LATE EFFECTS

### Special Susceptibility

Children with genetic syndromes attributable to defects in DNA repair mechanisms have increased susceptibility to ionizing radiation. Ataxia-telangiectasia (AT) is caused by mutations in the ATM (ataxia-telangiectasia mutated) gene that results in abnormal DNA repair. These patients have severe, progressive ataxia and are prone to the development of lymphoma. When treated with conventional doses of radiotherapy for lymphoma, they suffer an acute radiation reaction that may result in death.[46,47] Multiple mutations have been documented among patients with Fanconi anemia, another inherited DNA repair disorder. These patients are especially sensitive to DNA-damaging agents, including ionizing radiation and chemotherapy.[48]

## Late Effects

Gamma rays (external radiation) and radioisotopes (internal emitters) in fallout have caused delayed radiation effects after in utero or childhood exposure. Developmental effects and cancer were caused by exposure to the atomic bombs; thyroid ablation in 2 infants and thyroid neoplasia in Marshall Islanders were attributable to fallout from nuclear weapons tests;[49] and hundreds of cases of thyroid cancer following childhood or adolescent exposures in Ukraine and Belarus were attributed to fallout from the Chernobyl accident.[21,50]

## DIAGNOSTIC METHODS

Radiation-induced diseases are indistinguishable from their counterparts that occur in the general population. The role of radiation can be implicated only by epidemiologic studies (1) that show a dose-response effect; (2) after alternative explanations have been excluded (eg, cigarette smoking); and (3) that show the link between exposure and the effect is biologically plausible. In clinical practice, if there is suspicion for significant exposure to ionizing radiation (ie, accidental release), biological dosimetry may be conducted through a clinical consultation from a radiation specialist. Biological dosimetry typically does not measure radioactivity directly; it measures clinical or laboratory surrogate endpoints and correlates them with a radiation dose estimated to have produced the effect. Knowing the radiation dose is clinically useful because it can help the clinician select appropriate prophylactic and therapeutic measures; estimate prognosis, which is especially useful in mass casualty situations when resources may be limited; and transfer appropriate patients to facilities with the expertise to manage severe acute radiation syndrome. Biological dosimetry can estimate exposures greater than 0.2 Gy (20 rad) by studies of chromosomal translocations and tests of glycophorin A somatic mutations in red blood cells (the latter is not as well recognized or considered as useful as chromosomal translocations).

## TREATMENT OF CLINICAL SYMPTOMS

The preparedness planning for radiological or nuclear events or other radiation emergencies is the same as for preparedness for all emergency events and can be found on the National Pediatric Readiness Project Web site (https://emscimprovement.center/projects/pediatricreadiness/) and on many American Academy of Pediatrics (AAP) Web pages (https://www.aap.org/en-us/advocacy-and-policy/aap-health-initiatives/Children-and-Disasters/Pages/default.aspx). In addition, recommendations to pediatricians about preparedness planning can be found in the Policy Statement entitled "Pediatric Considerations Before, During and After Radiation/Nuclear Emergencies."[51] Guidance to parents on individual measures immediately following a radiation emergency is spelled out in Table 3 of the Technical Report accompanying the Policy Statement also entitled "Pediatric Considerations Before, During and After Radiation/Nuclear Emergencies."[52] Detailed guidance on the evolving recommendations on the use of potassium iodide (KI) can be found in Table 4 and the accompanying text and references in the same Technical Report. Guidance to professionals on drugs available for treatment of internal contamination is described in Table 5 of the Technical Report along with specific comments about availability and side effects of the available drugs; see text and references in that document.

## PREVENTION

Radioisotopes may be released after a power plant accident, nuclear weapon detonation, or terrorist event. These radioisotopes can be inhaled or ingested. People in exposed areas should avoid drinking fresh milk in particular. Foods are edible if they were harvested or prepared before the fallout occurred and were not exposed to it.

Iodine 131 (I-131 or radioactive iodine) is a radioisotope that would be released after one of these events. Prompt treatment with KI can be quite effective in protecting the thyroid. The Nuclear Regulatory Commission (NRC) recommends that state and local governments provide KI to all citizens living within 10 miles of a nuclear power plant as a supplement to plans for evacuation and sheltering.[53] The American Thyroid Association recommends a 200-mile radius of KI distribution.[54] The US Food and Drug Administration (FDA) and the Centers for Disease Control and Prevention (CDC) have issued guidance aimed at federal agencies and state and local governments responsible for radiation emergencies for the use of KI in radiation emergencies.[55,56] It is based primarily on data accumulated after the accident at the Chernobyl nuclear power plant in 1986. That disaster resulted in the massive release of I-131 and other radioiodines, some with very short half-lives. The short-lived radioiodines are believed to increase the risk of thyroid cancer in children more than that of I-131.

The protective effect of KI lasts about 24 hours and daily dosing provides optimum prophylaxis until a significant risk from inhalation or ingestion no longer exists. Early action is crucial; KI optimally should be administered before exposure, on notification of an emergency.[57] It may also have a protective effect even if taken 3 to 4 hours after exposure.

The FDA issued guidelines and instructions on how to prepare KI tablets as a fluid for infants and children (Tables 31-2 and 31-3).[58] Four KI products are approved by the FDA for over-the-counter use as a thyroid-blocking agent in

## Table 31-2. Guidelines for Potassium Iodide (KI) Administration[a]

| PATIENT | EXPOSURE, Gy (rad) | KI DOSE (mg)[b] |
|---|---|---|
| Age >40 years | >5 (500) | 130 |
| Age 18 through 40 years | ≥0.1 (10) | 130 |
| Adolescents 12 through 17 years[c] | ≥0.05 (5) | 65 |
| Children 4 through 11 years | ≥0.05 (5) | 65 |
| Children 1 month through 3 years[d] | ≥0.05 (5) | 32 |
| Birth through 1 month of age | ≥0.05 (5) | 16 |
| Pregnant or lactating women | ≥0.05 (5) | 130 |

Abbreviation: Gy, Gray; rad, radiation absorbed dose.
[a] From US Food and Drug Administration, Center for Drug Evaluation and Research[55]
[b] KI is useful for exposure to a radioiodine only. KI is given once only to pregnant women and neonates unless other protective measures (evacuation, sheltering, and control of the food supply) are unavailable. Repeat dosing should be on the advice of public health authorities.
[c] Adolescents weighing more than 70 kg should receive the adult dose (130 mg).
[d] KI from tablets or as a freshly saturated solution may be diluted in water and mixed with milk, formula, juice, soda, or syrup. Raspberry syrup best disguises the taste of KI. KI mixed with low-fat chocolate milk, orange juice, or flat soda (eg, cola) has an acceptable taste. Low-fat white milk and water did not hide the salty taste of KI.

radiation emergencies. These are iOSAT tablets (Anbex Inc, www.anbex.com), ThyroSafe tablets (Recipharm, www.thyrosafe.com), ThyroShield oral solution (Arco Pharmaceuticals, www.thyroshield.com), and Potassium Iodide Oral Solution USP (Mission Pharmacal Company, www.liquidki.com). Additional information about radiation disasters can be found in the recent AAP policy statement.[51]

## DIAGNOSTIC RADIATION

The risk of cancer associated with most diagnostic radiation is low and the use of radiation should not be restricted when needed for correct diagnosis or for monitoring patients following treatment, although the types and frequency of radiological imaging examinations should be carefully considered. Any medical procedure has a risk, and diagnostic radiography is no exception. Limitation of radiation; shielding sensitive body parts, such as the thyroid and gonads; and ensuring a non-pregnant state are components of good medical practice.[38] For decades, pediatric radiologists have strongly endorsed the "as low as

## Table 31-3. Guidelines for Home Preparation of Potassium Iodide (KI) Solution[a]

**Tablet size: 130 mg**

- Put one **130 mg** KI tablet in a small bowl and grind into a fine powder with the back of a spoon. The powder should not have any large pieces.
- Add 4 tsp (20 mL) of water to the KI powder. Use a spoon to mix them together until the KI powder is dissolved in the water.
- Add 4 tsp (20 mL) of milk, juice, soda, or syrup (eg, raspberry) to the KI/water mixture. The resulting mixture contains 16.25 mg of KI per teaspoon (5 mL).
- Age-based dosing guidelines
  - Newborn through age 1 month: 1 tsp (5 mL)
  - Age 1 month through 3 years: 2 tsp (10 mL)
  - Age 4 years through 17 years: 4 tsp (20 mL)
    (if child weighs more than 70 kg, give one 130-mg tablet)

**Tablet size: 65 mg**

- Put one **65 mg** KI tablet in a small bowl and grind into a fine powder with the back of a spoon. The powder should not have any large pieces.
- Add 4 tsp (20 mL) of water to the KI powder. Use a spoon to mix them together until the KI powder is dissolved in the water.
- Add 4 tsp (20 mL) of milk, juice, soda, or syrup (eg, raspberry) to the KI/water mixture. The resulting mixture contains 8.125 mg of KI per teaspoon (5 mL)
- Age-based dosing guidelines
  - Newborn through age 1 month: 2 tsp (10 mL)
  - Age 1 month through 3 years: 4 tsp (20 mL)
  - Age 4 years through 17 years: 8 tsp (40 mL) or one 65-mg tablet
    (if child weighs more than 70 kg, give two 65-mg tablets)

**How to store the prepared KI mixture**

- Potassium iodide mixed with any of the recommended liquids will keep for up to 7 days in the refrigerator.
- The US Food and Drug Administration recommends that the KI drink mixtures be prepared fresh weekly; unused portions should be discarded.

[a]Adapted from US Food and Drug Administration, Center for Drug Evaluation and Research[55]

reasonably achievable" (ALARA) principle in diagnostic imaging. In the past several years, ALARA has taken on even greater meaning with the significant increases in use of CT and other diagnostic radiology modalities.[37,39–41] Efforts to encourage judicious uses of radiation ("Image Gently") have been published because of concerns about higher levels of ionizing radiation from sources other than x-rays, and because increased risks of leukemia and brain tumors were found in the first large study of CT scans among children.[35] Table 31-4 shows estimated radiation doses from several procedures.

## Table 31-4. Estimates of Radiation Dose to Children From Diagnostic Radiology[a]

| TYPE OF EXAMINATION | DOSE QUANTITY | DOSE BY AGE AT EXPOSURE | | |
|---|---|---|---|---|
| | | 1 YEAR | 5 YEARS | ADULT |
| **Radiography**[b] | | | | |
| Skull AP | ESD (mSv) | 0.037 | 0.058 | 0.084 |
| Skull LAT | ESD (mSv) | 0.025 | 0.031 | 0.041 |
| Chest PA | ESD (mSv) | 0.024 | 0.037 | 0.051 |
| Abdomen AP | ESD (mSv) | 0.197 | 0.355 | 2.295 |
| Pelvis AP | ESD (mSv) | 0.121 | 0.230 | 1.783 |
| **Dental radiography**[b] | | | | |
| Intraoral | ED (mSv) | | 0.008 | 0.011 |
| Panoramic | ED (mSv) | | 0.015 | 0.015 |
| **Diagnostic fluoroscopy procedures** | | | | |
| Micturating cystourethrography[b] | ED (mSv) | 0.763 | 0.688 | 2.789 |
| Barium swallow[b] | ED (mSv) | 0.589 | 0.303 | 1.632 |
| Cardiac–Atrial septal defect (ASD) occlusion[c] | | | 3.88 | |
| Cardiac–Patent ductus arteriosus (PDA) occlusion[c] | | | 3.21 | |
| Cardiac–Ventricular septal defect (VSD) occlusion[c] | | | 12.1 | |
| **Computed tomography**[d] | | | | |
| Brain | ED (mSv) | 2.2 | 1.9 | 1.9 |
| Facial bone/sinuses | ED (mSv) | 0.5 | 0.5 | 0.9 |
| Chest | ED (mSv) | 2.2 | 2.5 | 5.9 |
| Entire abdomen | ED (mSv) | 4.8 | 5.4 | 10.4 |
| Spine | ED (mSv) | 11.4 | 8 | 10.1 |

## Table 31-4. Estimates of Radiation Dose to Children From Diagnostic Radiology[a] (*continued*)

| TYPE OF EXAMINATION | DOSE QUANTITY | DOSE BY AGE AT EXPOSURE | | |
|---|---|---|---|---|
| | | 1 YEAR | 5 YEARS | ADULT |
| **Diagnostic nuclear medicine[e]** | | | | |
| [123]I sodium iodide (thyroid uptake) | ED (mSv) | 19 | 16 | 7.2 |
| [99]Tcm – DMSA (with normal renal function) | ED (mSv) | 0.7 | 0.8 | 0.8 |

Abbreviations: mGy, milligray (1 mGy = 0.001 Gy); mSv, millisievert.

[a] Dosimetric quantities in the given table are all provided in ED (effective dose); ESD indicates entrance surface dose.

[b] Source: Hart et al.[59]

[c] Source: Onnasch et al.[60] The mean age of patients is 2.5 years.

[d] Source: Galanski et al.[61] Radiation doses to adults are based on data from German studies–results of a nationwide survey on multi-slice CT. Radiation dose in age group category 1 year is dose to pediatric patients (up to 1 year), 5 y (1–5 y), 10 y (6–10 y), and 15 y (11–15 y)

[e] Source: Gadd et al.[62]

Estimates of the radiation dose to the embryo/fetus from maternal diagnostic examinations have been compiled and are quite variable.[63] This is because of differences in the imaging modality, body area evaluated, and gestational age. Because previous studies suggested an increased cancer risk in the offspring of women undergoing diagnostic radiologic procedures during pregnancy, alternative imaging modalities, such as ultrasound, should be considered when clinically feasible. Special populations, such as infants with extremely low birth weight, may undergo multiple radiological examinations during a short period. Fluoroscopy and CT scans should be used sparingly for preterm infants, particularly when other imaging techniques are available. Limiting exposures will keep the cumulative dose low. Pediatricians should make sure that the most conservative procedures are used.

## REGULATIONS

Recommendations concerning radiation protection are made by the National Commission on Radiation Protection and Measurements and the International Commission on Radiological Protection. The Nuclear Regulatory Commission regulates and monitors nuclear facilities and the medical/research uses of radioisotopes.

## FREQUENTLY ASKED QUESTIONS

Q *How many x-rays are safe for my child?*

A The number of x-rays should be as many as your child's physicians think are necessary for diagnosis and follow-up, taking into account the benefit weighed against the (very small) risk. Because the radiation doses from certain diagnostic procedures (eg, CT scans) are high, pediatricians are urged to order radiologic examinations that do not emit ionizing radiation (eg, ultrasound or MRI) if clinically appropriate. Pediatricians should order radiologic examinations emitting ionizing radiation only when necessary and check to ensure that CT operators use settings appropriate for children (see Table 31-4). Although use of gonadal shields during pelvic radiography has been advocated since the 1950s, literature reports show that such shields are frequently not used or used incorrectly. A recent retrospective investigation found that no gonadal shields were used in half of all images of the pelvis in pediatric patients, inadequately protected in one third, and used appropriately in only 17%.[64] The investigators of this report and a 2012 study that found that gonadal shields were placed incorrectly in 91% of girls and 66% of boys,[65] noting that incorrect shield placement could often require repeat exposures and therefore the disadvantages outweighed the benefits.

Q *Will x-ray examinations of my child affect future grandchildren?*

A It is highly unlikely that an individual's x-ray examinations would affect their future children or grandchildren. No genetic effects of radiation from the atomic bombs in Japan have been demonstrated. In evaluating the feasibility of studying the offspring of military veterans exposed to above-ground nuclear tests, an expert committee of the Institute of Medicine noted that exposures of fathers to fallout from weapons tests, as in the South Pacific, seldom exceeded 0.005 rem (0.5 Sv).[66] The committee noted that at anticipated highest risk (0.2% increase in adverse reproductive outcomes), an unrealistically large number of exposed children (212 million) would be needed to detect a statistically significant elevated risk in exposed children compared with unexposed children. It would not be possible to carry out such an enormous study to be able to measure such a very small risk.

Q *Is my child's leukemia attributable to past radiation exposures?*

A There is no way to determine this for an individual patient. Illnesses induced by radiation cannot be distinguished from illnesses in the general population. The relationship can only be established by large epidemiologic studies showing a higher incidence in a radiated group (such as atomic bomb survivors).

*Q   Is there a risk of later recurrence of cancers in children exposed to the Chernobyl accident who have had thyroidectomies for thyroid cancer?*

A   Yes, there is a risk of later recurrence at the same site, similar to the situation in which other types of organs with cancer have been surgically removed (eg, breast cancer, lung cancer, etc). The risk of recurrence of thyroid cancer has been documented particularly in adolescents who have had thyroid cancer. Long-term follow-up is critically important. Young patients who have undergone thyroidectomy should have an ultrasound of the neck, thyroid function tests, and thyroglobulin and anti-thyroglobulin antibodies measured once yearly. If all results are normal after 2 years, less frequent follow-up visits can be scheduled.[67] Patients should be managed in consultation with experts in thyroid cancer.

*Q   We live close to a nuclear power plant. Should I be concerned and take special precautions?*

A   Nuclear power plants are designed and built with public safety as a priority. Emissions from the plant should not require protective actions on your part. However, if you live within 10 miles (16 km) of a nuclear power plant, you may be issued potassium iodide (KI) tablets. In the event of a release of radioactive iodine, these tablets can prevent radioiodine from concentrating in your thyroid. These should be taken only if instructed by local emergency management directors. KI tablets will only protect you from radioactive iodine and not from other radioactive substances.

*Q   What safety measures should be employed for children living in a residence with a person who has undergone treatment with I-131 for thyroid cancer or hyperthyroidism?*

A   The American Thyroid Association Taskforce on Radioiodine Safety has developed recommendations that comply with Nuclear Regulatory Commission regulations and guidelines put forth by the National Council on Radiation Protection and Measurements that provide guidance to physicians and patients for maintaining radiation safety. The recommendations are based on the dose of I-131 administered (see Tables 2A-1 and 2A-2 in The American Thyroid Association Taskforce on Radioiodine Safety).[68] Daytime restrictions are the same for treatment of thyroid cancer and hyperthyroidism, and recommend that the patient should maximize his/ her distance (6 feet, 1.8 meters) from children and women for 1 day, regardless of the dose administered. For nighttime restrictions, the patient should sleep in a separate bed from pregnant partners, children, or infants for 6 to 21 days following treatment for thyroid carcinoma and 15 to 23 days following treatment for hyperthyroidism.

Q   Should women who have been treated with I-131 breastfeed?

A   No, breastfeeding is contraindicated for a woman who is being treated with I-131. Mothers should not resume breastfeeding for the current child after receiving radioiodine treatment but may safely breastfeed babies they may have in the future.[69]

Q   What safety measures should be employed for children living in a residence with a person who has undergone myocardial perfusion treatment with thallium?

A   Limited study of the dosimetry of patients has been conducted and only one research letter published, which indicates that at a distance of 3 feet (0.9 meters) there is no exposure above background levels of radiation.

## Resources

### Centers for Disease Control and Prevention and National Cancer Institute: Radiation Exposure from Iodine 131

Web site: www.atsdr.cdc.gov/hec/csem/iodine/docs/iodine131.pdf

Web site: http://www.cancer.gov/about-cancer/causes-prevention/risk/radiation/i-131

### Environmental Protection Agency, RadTown USA

Web site: www.epa.gov/radtown/index.html

This site has a wide variety of topics related to all types of radiation.

### National Cancer Institute, Pediatric CT scan information

Web site: www.cancer.gov/cancertopics/causes/radiation-risks-pediatric-CT

### National Cancer Institute, Radiation Epidemiology Branch

Web site: http://dceg.cancer.gov/about/organization/programs-ebp/reb

### National Council on Radiation Protection

Web site: www.ncrponline.org

### RadiologyInfo: Radiology information resource for patients

Web site: www.radiologyinfo.org

## REFERENCES

1.  Mettler FA Jr, Upton AC. *Medical Effects of Ionizing Radiation*. 2nd ed. Philadelphia, PA: WB Saunders Co; 1995

2.  Institute of Medicine, Committee to Assess Health Risks from Exposure to Low Levels of Ionizing Radiation. National Research Council. Health Risks from Exposure to Low Levels of Ionizing Radiation: BEIR VII Phase 2. Washington, DC: National Academies Press; 2006

3.  Centers for Disease Control and Prevention. Radiation From Airport Security Screening. https://www.cdc.gov/nceh/radiation/airport_scan.htm. Accessed May 30, 2018

4.  Mehta P, Smith-Bindman R. Airport full body screening: what is the risk? *Arch Intern Med*. 2011;171(12):1112–1115

5.  National Council on Radiation Protection and Measurements. Management of Terrorist Events Involving Radioactive Material. Bethesda, MD: National Council on Radiation Protection and Measurements; 2001. NCRP Report No. 138

6.  Preston RJ. Children as a sensitive subpopulation for the risk assessment process. *Toxicol Appl Pharmacol.* 2004;199(2):132–141

7.  Bithell JF, Stewart AM. Pre-natal irradiation and childhood malignancy: a review of British data from the Oxford Survey. *Br J Cancer.* 1975;31(3):271–287

8.  Delongchamp RR, Mabuchi K, Yoshimoto Y, Preston DL. Cancer mortality among atomic bomb survivors exposed in utero or as young children. *Radiat Res.* 1997;147(3):385–395

9.  Kodama Y, Pawel D, Nakamura N, et al. Stable chromosome aberrations in atomic bomb survivors: results from 25 years of investigation. *Radiat Res.* 2001;156(4):337–346

10. Ohtaki K, Kodama Y, Nakano M, et al. Human fetuses do not register chromosome damage inflicted by radiation exposure in lymphoid precursor cells except for a small but significant effect at low doses. *Radiat Res.* 2004;161(4):373–379

11. Fucic A, Brunborg G, Lasan R, Jezek D, Knudsen LE, Merlo DF. Genomic damage in children accidentally exposed to ionizing radiation: a review of the literature. *Mutat Res.* 2008;658(1-2):111–123

12. Fucic A, Aghajanyan A, Druzhinin V, Minina V, Neronova E. Follow-up studies on genome damage in children after Chernobyl nuclear power plant accident. *Arch Toxicol.* 2016;90(9):2147–2159

13. De Santis M, Di Gianantonio E, Straface G, et al. Ionizing radiations in pregnancy and teratogenesis: a review of literature. *Reprod Toxicol.* 2005;20(3):323–329

14. Miller RW. Discussion: severe mental retardation and cancer among atomic bomb survivors exposed in utero. *Teratology.* 1999;59(4):234–235

15. Ichimaru M, Ishimaru T. Review of thirty years study of Hiroshima and Nagasaki atomic bomb survivors. II. Biological effects. D. Leukemia and related disorders. *J Radiat Res.* 1975;16 Suppl:89–96

16. Hsu WL, Preston DL, Soda M, et al. The incidence of leukemia, lymphoma and multiple myeloma among atomic bomb survivors: 1950-2001. *Radiat Res.* 2013;179(3):361–382

17. Preston DL, Ron E, Tokuoka S, et al. Solid cancer incidence in atomic bomb survivors: 1958-1998. *Radiat Res.* 2007;168(1):1–64

18. Preston DL, Cullings H, Suyama A, et al. Solid cancer incidence in atomic bomb survivors exposed in utero or as young children. *J Natl Cancer Inst.* 2008;100(6):428–436

19. Land CE, Tokunaga M, Koyama K, et al. Incidence of female breast cancer among atomic bomb survivors, Hiroshima and Nagasaki, 1950-1990. *Radiat Res.* 2003;160(6):707–717

20. World Health Organization. Ionizing Radiation. FAQs: Fukushima Five Years On. http://www.who.int/ionizing_radiation/a_e/fukushima/faqs-fukushima/en. Accessed May 31, 2018

21. Brenner AV, Tronko MD, Hatch M, et al. I-131 dose response for incident thyroid cancers in Ukraine related to the Chernobyl accident. *Environ Health Perspect.* 2011;119(7):933–939

22. Zablotska LB, Ron E, Rozhko AV, et al. Thyroid cancer risk in Belarus among children and adolescents exposed to radioiodine after the Chernobyl accident. *Br J Cancer.* 2011;104(1):181–187

23. Zablotska LB, Bazyka D, Lubin JH, et al. Radiation and the risk of chronic lymphocytic and other leukemias among Chernobyl cleanup workers. *Environ Health Perspect.* 2013;121(1):59–65

24. Kempin S, Finger PT, Gale RP, et al. A cluster of vitreoretinal lymphoma in New York with possible link to the Chernobyl disaster. *Leuk Lymphoma.* 2017:1–4

25. Mettler FA Jr, Thomadsen BR, Bhargavan M, et al. Medical radiation exposure in the U.S. in 2006: preliminary results. *Health Phys.* 2008;95(5):502–507

26. Brenner DJ, Hall EJ. Computed tomography: an increasing source of radiation exposure. *N Engl J Med.* 2007;357(22):2277–2284

27. Berrington de González A, Mahesh M, Kim KP, et al. Projected cancer risks from computed tomographic scans performed in the United States in 2007. *Arch Intern Med.* 2009;169(22):2071–2077

28. Lee C, Pearce MS, Salotti JA, et al. Reduction in radiation doses from paediatric CT scans in Great Britain. *Br J Radiol.* 2016;89(1060):20150305

29. Wakeford R. Childhood leukaemia following medical diagnostic exposure to ionizing radiation in utero or after birth. *Radiat Prot Dosimetry.* 2008;132(2):166–174

30. Linet MS, Kim KP, Rajaraman P. Children's exposure to diagnostic medical radiation and cancer risk: epidemiologic and dosimetric considerations. *Pediatr Radiol.* 2009;39(Suppl 1):S4–S26

31. Hoffman DA, Lonstein JE, Morin MM, Visscher W, Harris BS, III, Boice JD Jr. Breast cancer in women with scoliosis exposed to multiple diagnostic x rays. *J Natl Cancer Inst.* 1989;81(17):1307–1312

32. Ronckers CM, Doody MM, Lonstein JE, Stovall M, Land CE. Multiple diagnostic X-rays for spine deformities and risk of breast cancer. *Cancer Epidemiol Biomarkers Prev.* 2008;17(3):605–613

33. Brody AS, Frush DP, Huda W, Brent RL, American Academy of Pediatrics Section on Radiology. Radiation risk to children from computed tomography. *Pediatrics.* 2007;120(3):677–682

34. Applegate KE, Amis ES Jr, Schauer DA. Radiation exposure from medical imaging procedures. *N Engl J Med.* 2009;361(23):2289

35. Pearce MS, Salotti JA, Little MP, et al. Radiation exposure from CT scans in childhood and subsequent risk of leukaemia and brain tumours: a retrospective cohort study. *Lancet.* 2012;380(9840):499–505

36. Bosch de Basea M, Pearce MS, Kesminiene A, et al. EPI-CT: design, challenges and epidemiological methods of an international study on cancer risk after paediatric and young adult CT. *J Radiol Prot.* 2015;35(3):611–628

37. Goske MJ, Applegate KE, Boylan J, et al. The 'Image Gently' campaign: increasing CT radiation dose awareness through a national education and awareness program. *Pediatr Radiol.* 2008;38(3):265–269

38. Strauss KJ, Kaste SC. ALARA in pediatric interventional and fluoroscopic imaging: striving to keep radiation doses as low as possible during fluoroscopy of pediatric patients—a white paper executive summary. *J Am Coll Radiol.* 2006;3(9):686–688

39. Strauss KJ, Goske MJ, Kaste SC, et al. Image gently: ten steps you can take to optimize image quality and lower CT dose for pediatric patients. *AJR Am J Roentgenol.* 2010;194(4):868–873

40. Goske MJ, Applegate KE, Bell C, et al. Image Gently: providing practical educational tools and advocacy to accelerate radiation protection for children worldwide. *Semin Ultrasound CT MR.* 2010;31(1):57–63

41. Bulas DI, Goske MJ, Applegate KE, Wood BP. Image Gently: why we should talk to parents about CT in children. *AJR Am J Roentgenol.* 2009;192(5):1176–1178

42. Ronckers CM, Land CE, Miller JS, Stovall M, Lonstein JE, Doody MM. Cancer mortality among women frequently exposed to radiographic examination for spinal disorders. *Radiat Res.* 2010;174(1):83–90

43. Davis FG, Boice JD Jr, Hrubec Z, Monson RR. Cancer mortality in a radiation-exposed cohort of Massachusetts tuberculosis patients. *Cancer Res.* 1989;49(21):6130–6136

44. Boice JD Jr, Preston D, Davis FG, Monson RR. Frequent chest X-ray fluoroscopy and breast cancer incidence among tuberculosis patients in Massachusetts. *Radiat Res.* 1991;125(2):214–222

45. Berrington de Gonzalez, Gilbert E, Curtis R, et al. Second solid cancers after radiation therapy: a systematic review of the epidemiologic studies of the radiation dose-response relationship. *Int J Radiat Oncol Biol Phys.* 2013;86(2):224–233

46. Perlman S, Becker-Catania S, Gatti RA. Ataxia-telangiectasia: diagnosis and treatment. *Semin Pediatr Neurol.* 2003;10(3):173–182

47. Becker-Catania SG, Gatti RA. Ataxia-telangiectasia. *Adv Exp Med Biol.* 2001;495:191–198

48. Alter BP. Radiosensitivity in Fanconi's anemia patients. *Radiother Oncol.* 2002;62(3):345–347

49. Conard RA, Rall JE, Sutow WW. Thyroid nodules as a late sequela of radioactive fallout, in a Marshall Island population exposed in 1954. *N Engl J Med.* 1966;274(25):1391–1399

50. Tronko MD, Bogdanova TI, Komissarenko IV, et al. Thyroid carcinoma in children and adolescents in Ukraine after the Chernobyl nuclear accident: statistical data and clinicomorphologic characteristics. *Cancer.* 1999;86(1):149–156

51. Paulson JA, American Academy of Pediatrics Council on Environmental Health. Pediatric considerations before, during and after radiological/nuclear emergencies. Policy Statement. *Pediatrics*, in press

52. Linet MS, Kazzi Z, Paulson JA, American Academy of Pediatrics Council on Environmental Health. Pediatric considerations before, during and after radiological /nuclear emergencies. Technical Report. *Pediatrics*, in press

53. US Nuclear Regulatory Commission. Frequently Asked Questions about Potassium Iodide. Washington, DC: US Nuclear Regulatory Commission; 2016. https://www.nrc.gov/about-nrc/emerg-preparedness/about-emerg-preparedness/potassium-iodide/ki-faq.html. Accessed July 1, 2018

54. American Thyroid Association. American Thyroid Association Endorses Potassium Iodide for Radiation Emergencies. Falls Church, VA: American Thyroid Association; 2002. http://www.thyroid.org/ata-endorses-potassium-iodide-for-radiation-emergencies. Accessed May 31, 2018

55. US Food and Drug Administration, Center for Drug Evaluation and Research. Guidance Document Potassium Iodide as a Thyroid Blocking Agent in Radiation Emergencies. Rockville, MD: US Food and Drug Administration; Drug Information Branch; 2001. HFD-210. http://www.fda.gov/downloads/drugs/guidancecomplianceregulatoryinformation/guidances/ucm080542.pdf. Accessed May 31, 2018

56. Centers for Disease Control and Prevention. Emergency Preparedness and Response. Potassium Iodide (KI). https://emergency.cdc.gov/radiation/ki.asp. Accessed May 31, 2018

57. Christodouleas JP, Forrest RD, Ainsley CG, Tochner Z, Hahn SM, Glatstein E. Short-term and long-term health risks of nuclear-power-plant accidents. *N Engl J Med.* 2011;364(24):2334–2341

58. US Food and Drug Administration, Center for Drug Evaluation and Research. Home Preparation Procedure for Emergency Administration of Potassium Iodide Tablets for Infants and Small Children. 2006. https://www.fda.gov/Drugs/EmergencyPreparedness/BioterrorismandDrugPreparedness/ucm072248.htm. Accessed July 1, 2018

59. Hart D, Hillier MC. *Dose to Patients from Medical X-ray Examinations in the UK-2000 Review.* Chilton, UK: National Radiological Protection Board; 2002

60. Onnasch DG, Schroder FK, Fischer G, Kramer HH. Diagnostic reference levels and effective dose in pediatric cardiac catherization. *Br J Radiol.* 2007;80(951):177–185

61. Galanski M, Nagel HD, Stamm G. *Paediatic CT Exposure Practice in the Federal Republic of Germany: Results of a Nation-wide Survey in 2005/06.* Medizinische Hochschule Hannover; 2006

62. Gadd R, Mountford PJ, Oxtoby JW. Effective dose to children and adolescents from radiopharmaceuticals. *Nucl Med Commun.* 1999;20(6):569–573

63. Osei EK, Faulkner K. Fetal doses from radiological examinations. *Br J Radiol.* 1999;72(860):773–780

64. Warlow T, Walker-Birch P, Cosson P. Gonad shielding in paediatric pelvic radiography: effectiveness and practice. *Radiography*. 2014;20(3):178–182

65. Frantzen MJ, Robben S, Postma AA, Zoetelief J, Wildberger JE, Kemerink GJ. Gonad shielding in paediatric pelvic radiography: disadvantages prevail over benefit. *Insights Imaging*. 2012;3(1):23–32

66. Institute of Medicine, Committee to Study the Feasibility of, and Need for, Epidemiologic Studies of Adverse Reproductive Outcomes in Families of Atomic Veterans. Adverse Reproductive Outcomes in Families of Atomic Veterans: The Feasibility of Epidemiologic Studies. Washington, DC: National Academies Press; 1995

67. Tuttle RM, Leboeuf R. Follow up approaches in thyroid cancer: a risk adapted paradigm. *Endocrinol Metab Clin North Am*. 2008;37(2):419–435

68. American Thyroid Association Taskforce on Radioiodine Safety, Sisson JC, Freitas J, et al. Radiation safety in the treatment of patients with thyroid diseases by radioiodine 131I: practice recommendations of the American Thyroid Association. *Thyroid*. 2011;21(4):335–346

69. Society of Nuclear Medicine and Molecular Imaging. Fact Sheet: Guidelines for Patients Receiving Radioiodine I-131 Treatment. http://www.snmmi.org/AboutSNMMI/Content.aspx?ItemNumber=5609. Accessed May 31, 2018

Chapter 32

# Lead

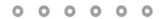

## KEY POINTS

- No safe level of lead has been identified.
- Disparities persist that disproportionately expose certain populations of children and pregnant women to lead.
- The sources for most children with elevated blood lead levels today are lead-laden dust and paint chips from deteriorating lead paint on interior surfaces.

## INTRODUCTION

Childhood lead toxicity has been recognized for more than 100 years. As recently as the 1940s, many people believed that children with lead poisoning who did not die during an acute toxic episode had no residual effects. After it was recognized that learning and behavior disorders occurred in children who recovered from acute toxicity, many believed that only children with frank symptoms suffered neurobehavioral deficits. Starting in the 1970s and continuing today, studies worldwide consistently demonstrated that asymptomatic children with increasing levels of lead had lower IQ scores,[1-3] more language difficulties,[4] attention problems,[5] and behavior disorders.[6,7] With better epidemiological studies, the definition of a harmful level of lead has changed markedly. Abundant scientific evidence now shows that blood lead levels (BLLs) below 10 mcg/dL are associated with adverse cognitive, behavioral, and other effects in infants and children.[3,8,9] Based on this evidence and other important longitudinal prospective studies, in 2012 the Advisory Council on Childhood Lead Poisoning Prevention

convened by the Centers for Disease Control & Prevention (CDC) cited new
scientific data that documents adverse health effects of lead on infants and
children at venous blood concentrations below 10 mcg/dL.[10] In response to
this report, the CDC created a reference value of 5 mcg/dL, based on the 97.5th
percentile of the BLL distribution among children age 1 to 5 years. The CDC
used data generated by the National Health and Nutrition Examination Survey
(NHANES) rather than a health-based action level.[11] The report emphasized
the importance of and focus on primary prevention efforts given the lack of
an identified threshold without deleterious neurodevelopmental effects and
evidence that these effects appear to be irreversible.

It is estimated that 500,000 children (2.5%) younger than 6 years in the United
States have BLLs at or above the current CDC reference level.[12,13] Children living in
3.6 million US households are currently exposed to lead hazards.[12] The continued
exposure of thousands of children to lead-laden dust and paint chips in deteriorating housing mars what would otherwise be a public health triumph. Although
lead levels have decreased in all children tested, environmental health disparities persist that disproportionately affect low-income and minority families and
communities.[14] (See At-risk Populations and Chapter 55).

The CDC emphasizes that the best way to end childhood lead poisoning is
to prevent, control, and eliminate lead exposures. The CDC[11] and the American
Academy of Pediatrics (AAP)[15] currently use the reference value of 5 mcg/dL as
the level that should prompt public health action. The focus has shifted from the
care of symptomatic children toward a primary prevention approach targeting communities most at risk of lead poisoning.[11,16] Reducing or eliminating the
myriad sources of lead before exposures occur is the most reliable and cost-
effective measure to protect children from lead toxicity.[15,17] Because of universal
and targeted blood testing of children for lead exposure, pediatricians commonly
find themselves participating in or even directing these activities.[15]

## ROUTES AND SOURCES OF EXPOSURE

Children may be exposed to lead through the unintentional ingestion of lead-
containing particles, such as dust from paint, soil, or ongoing renovations; or from
contaminated water (Figure 32-1). Lead can be absorbed from the pulmonary tract
if inhaled as fumes or respirable particles. Lead is transmitted in human milk.

Lead (Pb) is a metallic element. In the United States, there have been 2 major
sources of industrially derived lead for children: airborne lead, mostly from the
combustion of gasoline containing tetraethyl lead; and lead-laden dust and
debris, mostly from deteriorating lead-based paint.[11] The largest declines in
BLLs occurred from the 1970s to the 1990s, following the elimination of lead in
motor vehicle gasoline, the ban on lead paint for residential use, removal of lead
from solder in food cans, bans on the use of lead pipes and plumbing fixtures,
and other limitations on the uses of lead[12] (Figure 32-2). Federal legislation in

the 1970s resulted in removal of lead from motor vehicle gasoline and reduced smokestack emissions from smelters and other sources, causing BLLs in children to decrease; lead in aviation gasoline, however, still persists today.[18] The use of heavily leaded paint on interior surfaces ceased in the United States by 1978[15] but there still are significant lead paint hazards in 3.6 million homes inhabited by

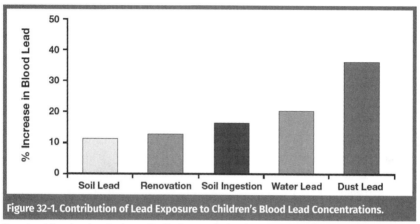

**Figure 32-1. Contribution of Lead Exposure to Children's Blood Lead Concentrations.**

Reproduced from American Academy of Pediatrics Council of Environmental Health[15], adapted from Lanphear et al[19] and Spanier et al.[20]

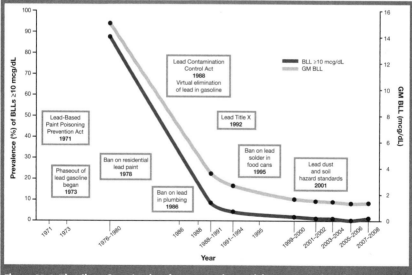

**Figure 32-2. Timeline of Lead Poisoning Prevention Policies and BLLs in Children Aged 1-5 Years, by Year—National Health and Nutrition Examination Survey, United States, 1971-2008.**

Reproduced from American Academy of Pediatrics Council of Environmental Health[15]
Abbreviations: BLL = blood lead level; GM BLL = geometric mean blood lead level

at least 1 child younger than age 6. Exposure is likely in situations where lead-based paint exists in deteriorated conditions.[21,22] Soil contaminated from 'legacy' sources of lead (leaded gasoline and lead-based paint) can recontaminate remediated houses.[23,24] Residual lead in soil in areas heavily affected by airborne lead, such as around smelters, continues to be a problem even decades after the worst sites are closed.[25]

The source for most children with elevated BLLs today is lead-laden dust and paint chips from deteriorating lead paint on interior surfaces. Young children living in homes with deteriorating lead paint can achieve BLLs of at least 20 mcg/dL without frank pica (ingestion of nonfood items).[26] This exposure commonly arises from normal, developmentally appropriate hand-to-mouth behavior in an environment that is contaminated with lead dust. Children with lower BLLs (less than 10 mcg/dL) may have continuous exposures from multiple sources including food, water, soil, and dust.

Lead plumbing (Latin "plumbus" means lead) has contaminated drinking water for centuries, especially if the water has high or low acidity or low mineral content. This was unfortunately exemplified most recently through contaminated drinking water affecting Flint, Michigan. This contamination was the result of several preceding events. The community's water source was changed, resulting in the need to augment disinfection processes. The disinfection processes were done without appropriate corrosion control procedures, leading to an increase in leaching of lead from corroding leaded and galvanized pipes, solder, and plumbing fixtures. Studies of this community identified a statistically significant increased odds of having an elevated BLL in the period following the switch in drinking water source.[27,28] The majority of elevated BLLs tested were in the 5 to 9 mcg/dL range, although few children younger than age 1 were tested.[27]

The US Environmental Protection Agency's (EPA) Lead and Copper Rule is a treatment technique rule to help minimize water contamination in public water systems. This rule employs an action level as a screening tool to determine when certain treatment technique actions are needed. The rule sets a target concentration ("action level") of 0.015 mg/L (15 parts per billion [ppb]) and recommends remediation measures such as corrosion control treatment, source water monitoring, public education, and potentially lead service line replacement if the action level is exceeded in more than 10% of tap water sampled.[12] Notably, the federal government recommends but does not require testing of water in schools or childcare facilities that meet the definition of a public water system. No testing is required for private wells, although private wells account for 10% to 15% of the population's water sources.[29] As suggested by a 2016 National Resources Defense Council report, water violations persist throughout the United States and have for a number of years.[30] In 2015, more than 5,000 community water systems, serving 18 million people, violated the

Lead and Copper Rule.[30] Of these, 1,110 community water systems, serving 3.9 million people, had water lead levels in excess of 15 ppb in at least 10% of homes tested.[30] Infants who consume reconstituted formula, people living in neighborhoods with high levels of socioeconomic disadvantage, and minority populations are at increased risk of lead poisoning from contaminated drinking water.[28] As a result of emerging concerns over lead and water contamination, the US EPA has been working with states, public water systems, and water sector stakeholders to revise existing rules and regulations, identify challenges, and promote best practices.[12] There is no safe level of lead in water; despite this fact, no health-based 'household action level' currently exists.[12] Various regional and state-level resources exist for testing individual drinking water at the tap and mitigating lead contamination in drinking water. Mitigation measures include installing charcoal-based water filters designed to remove lead, using cold water for cooking and formula preparation, allowing water to flush prior to use, and supplying resources to assist school and childcare facilities to minimize water contamination from lead. (See Table 32-1 and Resources).

Children also may be exposed to lead fumes or respirable dust resulting from unsafe remediation practices such as sanding or heating old paint; burning or melting automobile batteries, or melting lead for use in a hobby or craft. Childhood lead poisoning from toy jewelry has occurred including a fatality in a child who ingested a lead charm.[31–33] Lead has been found in older toys made in the United States, imported toys painted with lead-based paint, and plastic toys and vinyl that used lead as a softener.[33,34] Since 2008, the US Consumer Product Safety Commission (CPSC) has set requirements for third-party testing and certification by manufacturers and importers to help reduce the number of non-complying products entering the market.[12] Ongoing CPSC surveillance in partnership with other federal and state agencies demonstrated a reduction in the number of required recalls of these contaminated toys. These agencies collaborate with importers and manufacturers to prevent further importation of products containing unsafe amounts of lead.[12] Although individual children could chew on or ingest these products resulting in lead absorption, the extent to which toys and plastics contribute to lead exposure in most children is not clear. Less common sources of lead include cosmetics, folk remedies, pottery glaze, old or imported cans with soldered seams, and contaminated vitamin supplements.

## AT-RISK POPULATIONS

Disparities persist that disproportionately expose certain subgroups of children and pregnant women to lead exposure based on age, socioeconomic, occupational, developmental, and cultural risk factors. One study identified

| Table 32-1. Risk Factors for Lead Exposure and Prevention Strategies ||
|---|---|
| **RISK FACTOR** | **PREVENTION STRATEGY** |
| **ENVIRONMENTAL** ||
| Paint | Identify, evaluate, and remediate |
| Dust | Control sources |
| Soil | Restrict play in area, plant groundcover |
| Drinking water | Check with local authorities about water testing; morning flush of water from faucet; use cold water for cooking and drinking, especially if tap water is used for preparing formula; implement charcoal filter to reduce contamination<br>Private well water should be tested for lead when the well is new and tested again when a pregnant woman, infant, or child younger than age 18 moves into the home and annually thereafter |
| Folk remedies (examples include Greta and Azarcon, Hispanic traditional medicines; Ghasard, an Indian folk medicine; and Ba-baw-saw, a Chinese herbal remedy) | Avoid use |
| Spices (examples include Southeast Asian spices such as turmeric) and candy from Mexico (ingredient tamarind may contain lead) | Avoid use in young infants, children, and women of reproductive age |
| Cosmetics and religious powders (examples include Swad brand Sindoor, a cosmetic product used in Hinduism; Tiro, an eye cosmetic from Nigeria; Kohl or surma, an eye cosmetic from Southeast Asia) | Avoid use |
| Old ceramic or pewter cookware, old urns/kettles, decorative pottery from Mexico and ceramics from China, or other imported cookware | Avoid use |
| Some imported toys, crayons | Avoid use |

## Table 32-1. Risk Factors for Lead Exposure and Prevention Strategies (*continued*)

| RISK FACTOR | PREVENTION STRATEGY |
|---|---|
| **ENVIRONMENTAL** | |
| Parental occupations (examples include construction and demolition work, lead-paint abatement, pipe fitting and plumbing, battery manufacturing, mining, ship building or other marina work, e-scrap recycling, among others) | Shower and remove work clothing and shoes before leaving work<br>See Occupational Safety and Health Guidance in Resources |
| Hobbies (examples include hobbies involving soldering such as stained glass, jewelry making, pottery glazing, and working with bullets, such as marksmanship at firing ranges, finishing sinkers and certain weights) | Proper use, storage, and ventilation |
| Home renovation | Proper containment, ventilation; pregnant women and young children should vacate premises while work is done and not re-enter until premises certified as lead-safe. Certified lead abatement. |
| Buying or renting a new home | Inquire about lead hazards, look for deteriorated paint before occupancy, hire certified lead risk assessor to evaluate hazard and recommend control options; consult local housing databases of lead hazards as available |
| **HOST** | |
| Hand-to-mouth activity (or pica) | Control sources; frequent hand washing |
| Inadequate nutrition | Screening for iron and vitamin D deficiency. Optimization of iron, calcium, and vitamin D |
| Developmental disabilities | Enrichment programs as available (eg, referral to early intervention (<3 years old) and to public school department for individualized education program (≥3 years old) |

that children—especially those between the ages of 12 to 18 months living in dilapidated pre-World War II housing—experience BLLs 2 to 3 times higher on average than those living in rehabilitated housing.[35] Young children are more likely to have elevated BLLs because of differences in absorption from the gastrointestinal tract and age-appropriate exploration of their environments. They are also more susceptible to the toxic effects of lead compared with adults because of an incomplete blood-brain barrier that more readily permits the entry of lead into the developing nervous system.

National data suggest that disparities exist by race/ethnicity and income. Children living at or below the poverty line who live in older housing are at greatest risk of lead exposure.[14] Children, especially those of low socioeconomic status, are at increased risk of nutritional deficiency, such as iron deficiency. Iron deficiency is associated with a 4- to 5-fold increase in baseline risk of lead exposure because of increased absorption of lead by the divalent metal transporter in the gastrointestinal tract.[36,37]

Other groups of children at increased risk include newly arrived foreign-born families and recent immigrants with young children. These children may have had lead exposure in their native country; for example, approximately 50% of the worldwide burden of lead poisoning occurs in Southeast Asia. It also is possible that their exposure occurred in unsuitable housing once they arrived in the United States.[38–42] A toolkit found on the CDC Web site discusses risks for these children and recommends the following:[14]

1. Blood lead level testing of all refugee children aged 6 months to 16 years upon entry to the United States.

2. Repeat blood lead level testing of all refugee children aged 6 months to 6 years, 3 to 6 months after these children are placed in permanent residences and older children, as warranted, regardless of initial test results.

Children with developmental disorders, such as autism spectrum disorder and other neurological conditions, who have persistent pica behaviors and/or poor cognitive abilities, are at increased risk of lead exposure.[43–48] The increased risk in these children may persist into school age and adolescence, beyond when children are routinely tested for elevated BLLs. Children living in foster care also have an increased risk.[49] Scant guidance exists regarding testing children for elevated lead levels while they are living in foster care.[50] These children have increased susceptibility to adverse effects from lead exposure because they may have other neurodevelopmental comorbidities and often have lived in many different homes. Foster homes are less likely to be assessed for lead hazards before children are placed there. Pediatricians caring for these children therefore should take an environmental history with careful attention to lead exposure.

The National Institute for Occupational Safety and Health (NIOSH) has found that take-home exposure, including lead exposure, is a widespread problem.[51,52] Jobs with lead exposure include but are not limited to: painting, building renovation, demolition, shooting range work, metal scrap cutting and recycling, plumbing, and other industrial fields.[52] A case report demonstrated paraoccupational lead exposures from an e-scrap recycling facility where the father of 2 children worked.[53] Pediatricians should ask about parents' occupations and hobbies that might involve lead.

Table 32-1 includes common sources of lead contamination, risk factors, and prevention strategies. Additional sources of exposure include foreign-purchased cosmetics;[54,55] Southeast Asian spices[56,57] and herbs;[58] dietary supplements;[59] religious powders;[57] ayurvedic[60] or ethnic remedies;[54,57] occupational take-home exposures;[51,53,61] and vocational exposures such as marksmanship.[62,63]

## Table 32-2. Summary of Children's Health Effects by Blood Lead Level

| BLOOD LEAD LEVEL | SUFFICIENT EVIDENCE OR CAUSAL DETERMINATION OF CHILDREN'S HEALTH EFFECTS |
|---|---|
| Below 5 mcg/dL | Nervous System Effects:<br>■ Cognitive function: Decreases in IQ, academic achievement, specific cognitive measures<br>■ Externalizing behaviors: Increased incidence of attention-related and problem behaviors |
| 5–10 mcg/dL | Effects listed above plus<br>Nervous System Effects:<br>■ Auditory Function: decreased hearing<br>Reproductive and Developmental Effects:<br>■ Reduced postnatal growth<br>■ Delayed puberty for girls and boys |
| 10–40 mcg/dL | Effects listed above plus<br>Nervous System Effects:<br>■ Nerve function: slower nerve conduction<br>Blood Effects:<br>■ Decreased hemoglobin, anemia |
| 40–80 mcg/dL | Effects listed above plus<br>Gastrointestinal Effects:<br>■ Abdominal pain, constipation, colic, anorexia, and vomiting |
| Above 80 mcg/dL | Effects listed above plus<br>Nervous System Effects:<br>■ Severe neural effects: convulsions, coma, loss of voluntary muscle control, and death |

Adapted from President's Task Force on Environmental Health Risks and Safety Risks to Children, Key Federal Programs to Reduce Childhood Lead Exposures and Eliminate Associated Health Impacts Report.[12] Based on evidence from references 64–66.

## SYSTEMS AFFECTED

Lead exposure has been linked to many adverse health effects (see Table 32-2).[64–66] Lead acts as a neurotoxicant to the developing brain, resulting in irreversible damage even at relatively low levels of exposure. For lead exposure most commonly identified in the United States, subclinical effects on the central nervous system (CNS) are the most common effects. The best-studied effect is cognitive impairment, measured by IQ tests[3] and poor academic achievement,[10] and externalizing behaviors (problem behaviors directed toward the external environment), such as aggression and disobeying rules.[67,68] Each child with high lead levels in the United States costs approximately $5,600 in medical and special educational services.[14] Cognitive impairment attributable to lead contamination was estimated to cost $50.9 billion annually in lost economic productivity.[22]

A robust literature demonstrated a relationship between BLL at the time of testing and decreased scores on reading and arithmetic tests that is apparent even in children aged 6 to 16, including those whose BLLs by then are less than 5 mcg/dL.[69] Canfield et al[9] reported that among 172 children followed prospectively with measurements of BLLs, 101 had never had a BLL greater than 10 mcg/dL, and there was still a strong negative relationship between BLL and IQ when the children were aged 3 to 5. In most countries, including the United States, BLLs peak at approximately age 2 years because of normal hand-to-mouth exploratory behaviors in this age group, and then decrease without intervention. Although there is some relationship between peak BLL and IQ tested later, it is now clear that contemporaneous blood lead, even though it is lower, is more strongly associated with school-aged IQ.[3,70] Although lead exposure is a risk factor for developmental and behavioral problems, its impact has significant individual variability, which may be modulated by the psychosocial environment and educational experiences of the developing child.[26] Many factors affect cognition and behavior.

Other aspects of CNS function also may be affected by lead, but they are less well documented. Subclinical effects on hearing[71,72] and balance[73] may occur at commonly encountered BLLs. Some studies measured tooth or bone lead levels, which are thought to represent integrated, possibly lifetime, exposure. Teachers reported that students with elevated tooth lead levels were more inattentive, hyperactive, disorganized, and less able to follow directions.[4,74] Further follow-up in 1 of the studies showed higher rates of failure to graduate from high school, reading disabilities, and greater absenteeism in the final year of high school.[75] Elevated bone lead levels were associated with increased attention dysfunction, aggression, and delinquency.[76]

Although there are reasonable animal models of low-dose lead exposure and cognition and behavior,[77] the mechanisms by which lead affects CNS function are not entirely elucidated. Studies examining brain metabolism suggest that these effects may be caused by neuronal dysfunction and alteration in myelin architecture.[78] Lead alters very basic nervous system functions, such as calcium-modulated signaling, at very low concentrations in vitro.[79] The age of 2 years, when lead levels peak, is the same age at which a major reduction in dendrite connections occurs, among other events crucial to development. Thus, it is plausible that lead exposure at that time interferes with a critical development process in the CNS, but what that process is has not been identified. Brain imaging studies in adults with elevated BLLs in childhood have demonstrated region-specific reductions in gray matter volume,[80,81] alterations of white matter microstructure,[82] and a significant impact of lead on brain reorganization associated with language function.[83]

Lead also has important non-neurodevelopmental effects. The kidneys are primary target organs; children exposed to lead are at significantly greater risk of having hypertension as adults. Another renal effect of lead in children is impaired 1-*d*-hydroxylation of vitamin D, a necessary step toward activating this vitamin. A cross-sectional study suggested that environmental exposure to lead may delay growth and pubertal development in black and Mexican-American girls.[84] Episodes of severe lead poisoning can cause growth arrest of long bones, producing "lead lines." Given the advent of more sensitive screening metrics, this is no longer an effective means of diagnosing lead poisoning.

Lead interferes with heme synthesis beginning at BLLs of approximately 25 mcg/dL and after 50 to 70 days or more of exposure.[85] *D*-aminolevulinate dehydratase, an early-step enzyme, and ferrochelatase, which closes the heme ring, are inhibited. Ferrochelatase inhibition is the basis of a formerly used screening test for lead poisoning that measured zinc protoporphyrin and erythrocyte protoporphyrin, the immediate heme precursor. These markers are insensitive measures of lower BLLs and are not specific to elevated BLLs because they also are elevated in the presence of iron deficiency, a common comorbidity among children with elevated BLLs. These markers are used today as a window into the chronicity of ongoing exposure, although it lags behind the BLL.

## CLINICAL EFFECTS

Some children with BLLs greater than 40 mcg/dL may complain of headaches, abdominal pain, loss of appetite, or constipation, or they may be asymptomatic. Children displaying clumsiness, agitation, or decreased activity and somnolence are presenting with premonitory symptoms of CNS involvement that may rapidly proceed to vomiting, stupor, and convulsions.[86] Symptomatic lead poisoning should be treated as an emergency. Although lead can cause peripheral neuropathy and renal disease in adults with occupational exposures, these are rare in children.

## DIAGNOSTIC METHODS

A venous BLL measurement is the gold standard for the diagnosis of lead poisoning. A finger-stick or capillary sample also can be used if care is taken to avoid contamination. Elevated BLLs (5 mcg/dL or greater) found with a capillary test should be confirmed with a timely venous sample and followed by appropriate management of elevated levels based on current guidelines.[10,15,87] Once a child has had an elevated lead level, capillary measurements should no longer be obtained.

### Blood Lead Testing

Until 1997, the AAP and CDC recommended that virtually all children have at least one measurement of blood lead beginning at age 12 months, with a retest at age 24 months, if possible. Because the prevalence of elevated BLLs has decreased substantially, in 1997 the CDC recommended that health departments determine a lead screening strategy for their jurisdictions on the basis of prevalence of housing risks, poverty rates, and children with elevated BLLs. Regardless of local recommendation, however, federal policy requires that all children enrolled in Medicaid receive screening blood lead tests at ages 12 and 24 months and that blood lead testing be performed for children aged 36 to 72 months who have not previously been tested.[10,11] This guidance also recommends that every child who has a developmental delay, behavioral disorder, or speech impairment, or who may have been exposed to lead, should receive a blood lead test.[5] Childhood lead testing is a national quality measure of clinical effectiveness. It is a recognized standard in the Health Effectiveness Data and Information Set (HEDIS), a widely used set of quality of care measures maintained by the National Committee for Quality Assurance for the accreditation of high-functioning managed care organizations and hospitals nationally.[88] Even though this recommendation exists, significant variability remains in lead testing, including for children most at risk who also may be disproportionately affected by gaps in the availability of systematic testing.

Assessments of risks for lead exposures and blood lead testing vary considerably by locale, from universal blood lead testing to targeted blood lead testing determined by risk assessment tools. Clinicians should consult city, county, or state health departments or their regional Pediatric Environmental Health Specialty Unit (www.pehsu.net) to determine the appropriate recommendations for their jurisdiction. This information also is available for most states on the CDC Web site (http://www.cdc.gov/nceh/lead/programs.htm). Children not enrolled in Medicaid and residing in states with no lead testing policy should have blood lead testing in accordance with Medicaid guidelines. The sensitivities of personal risk questionnaires and other substitutes for measuring BLLs vary according to the subgroup assessed and often are unacceptably low. These questionnaires may be more helpful in identifying and mitigating the source of exposure once an elevated BLL is identified.

Because of lead's effects on the developing fetus, the American College of Obstetricians and Gynecologists and some states developed lead screening guidelines for pregnant women.[89] The CDC *Guidelines for the Identification and Management of Lead Exposure in Pregnant and Lactating Women* provides guidance about blood lead testing of pregnant women, medical and environmental management, and follow-up of mothers and infants when maternal lead levels are 10 mcg/dL or greater[88] (http://www.cdc.gov/nceh/lead/publications/leadandpregnancy2010.pdf).[90]

## At-risk Subgroups

Children of all ages who are recent immigrants, refugees, or adoptees have an increased prevalence of elevated—sometimes very elevated—BLLs and should be tested at the earliest opportunity. Those aged 6 months to 6 years and older children, as warranted, should be retested 3 to 6 months after moving into permanent residences[38-42] This guidance refers to recent immigrant populations; there is limited guidance about the frequency of blood lead testing of other high-risk subgroups, such as children in foster care,[49] children with persistent pica behavior secondary to autism spectrum disorders or other neurodevelopmental disorders, or children with paraoccupational exposures.[5,44,48,91]

## Diagnostic Testing

Some experienced clinicians measure the BLL in children with growth retardation, speech or language dysfunction, anemia, attention disorders, or other neurodevelopmental disorders, especially if the parents have a specific interest in the BLL or in health effects from environmental chemicals. The persistent elevation of BLL into school age is unusual, however, even if peak BLL at age 2 years was high and the child's housing has not been abated. Thus, a relatively low BLL in a school-aged child does not rule out earlier lead exposure. If the question of current lead exposure arises, the only reliable way to make a diagnosis is with blood lead measurement. Abdominal radiography can be considered for children who have a history of pica for paint chips or excessive mouthing behaviors or if the BLL is 15 mcg/dL or greater (Table 32-3). Hair, urine, and teeth lead levels or long bone radiographs give no useful clinical information and should not be performed.[92]

No threshold or safe level has been identified for lead exposure. It therefore is critical to have a primary prevention approach to eliminating lead exposure. Targeting elevated BLLs of 5 mcg/dL or greater is efficient for case management purposes and to mitigate continued exposures. This approach is not adequate to prevent unnecessary exposure to 'legacy lead' in vulnerable populations.[15]

## Table 32-3. Recommended Follow-up Actions, According to Blood Lead Level (BLL)[a]

| BLL (mcg/dL) | ACTIONS |
|---|---|
| <5 mcg/dL | 1. Review lab results with family. For reference, the geometric mean blood lead level for children aged 1 to 5 in the United States is less than 2 mcg/dL.<br><br>2. Repeat the blood lead level in 6 to 12 months if the child is at high risk or risk changes during the timeframe. Ensure lead testing is done at age 1 and age 2 and is based on local, state, and federal guidelines.<br><br>3. For children tested at age younger than 12 months, consider retesting in 3 to 6 months because lead exposure may increase as mobility increases.<br><br>4. Perform routine health maintenance including assessment of nutrition, physical and mental development, as well as iron deficiency risk factors as per recommendations in Bright Futures (American Academy of Pediatrics).<br><br>5. Provide anticipatory guidance on common sources of environmental lead exposure: paint in homes built prior to 1978, soil near roadways or other sources of lead, take-home exposures related to adult occupations, imported spices, cosmetics, jewelry, folk remedies, and cookware. |
| 5–14 mcg/dL | 1. Perform steps as described above for levels less than 5 mcg/dL.<br><br>2. Re-test venous blood lead level within 1 to 3 months to ensure that the lead level is not rising. If it is stable or decreasing, retest the blood lead level in 3 months. Refer patient to local health authorities if such resources are available. Most states require elevated blood lead levels be reported to the state health department. Contact the CDC at 800-CDC-INFO (800-232-4636) or the National Lead Information Center at 800-424-LEAD (5323) for resources regarding lead poisoning prevention and local childhood lead poisoning prevention programs.<br><br>3. Take a careful environmental history to identify potential sources of exposures (see #5 above) and provide preliminary advice about reducing/eliminating exposures (eg, washing children's hands/toys frequently, frequent damp mopping of floors, windows, and window sills, leaving shoes at threshold, placing duct tape or contact paper over chipping/peeling paint, ceasing renovations). Consider other children who may be exposed.<br><br>4. Provide nutritional counseling related to calcium and iron. In addition, recommend having a fruit at every meal because iron absorption quadruples when taken with vitamin C-containing foods. Encourage the consumption of iron-enriched foods (eg, cereals, meats). Some children may be eligible for The Special Supplemental Nutrition Program for Women, Infants and Children (WIC) or other nutritional resources. |

## Table 32-3. Recommended Follow-up Actions, According to Blood Lead Level (BLL) (*continued*)

| BLL (mcg/dL) | ACTIONS |
|---|---|
| | 5. Ensure iron sufficiency with adequate laboratory testing (CBC, ferritin, CRP) and treatment per AAP guidelines. Consider starting a multivitamin with iron or iron supplementation as indicated. |
| | 6. Perform structured developmental screening evaluations at child health maintenance visits per recommendations in Bright Futures, and refer to therapeutic programs (eg, Early Intervention Program, Individualized Education Programs) because lead's effect on development may manifest over years. |
| **15–44 mcg/dL** | 1. Perform steps as described above for levels 5–14 mcg/dL. |
| | 2. Determine if there are any overt symptoms. |
| | 3. Confirm blood lead level with venous sample within 1 to 4 weeks. Higher levels require more rapid confirmation. |
| | 4. Arrange for a home investigation to assess for the lead source, if available. If not available, consult with a Pediatric Environmental Health Specialty Unit (PEHSU) regarding other options. |
| | 5. Additional, specific evaluation of the child, such as abdominal radiograph should be considered based on the environmental investigation and history (eg, pica for paint chips, mouthing behaviors). Gut decontamination may be considered if radio-opaque foreign bodies consistent with ingested lead are visualized on radiograph. Any treatment for blood lead levels in this range should be done in consultation with an expert. |
| | 6. Contact PEHSU or poison control center for guidance |
| **>44 mcg/dL** | 1. Follow guidance for BLL 15–44 mcg/dL as listed above. |
| | 2. Confirm the BLL with repeat venous lead level within 48 hours. |
| | 3. Obtain a complete blood count, electrolytes, BUN, creatinine, ALT, and AST in anticipation of chelation therapy. |
| | 4. Abdominal radiograph should be done to look for radio-opaque foreign bodies suggestive of recent ingestion because this finding may change management. |
| | 5. Emergently admit all symptomatic children to a hospital; if there is evidence of significant CNS pathology, consider PICU admission. If asymptomatic, consider hospitalization and/or chelation therapy (managed with the assistance of an expert in lead poisoning) based on status of the home with respect to lead hazards, ability to isolate the lead source, family social situation, and chronicity of the exposure; these are factors that may influence management. |
| | 6. Contact PEHSU or poison control center for assistance. |

[a] Adapted from Pediatric Environmental Health Specialty Unit. Medical Management of Childhood Lead Exposure and Poisoning. http://www.pehsu.net/_Library/facts/medical-mgmnt-childhood-lead-exposure-June-2013.pdf. Accessed April 9, 2018.

## TREATMENT OF CLINICAL SYMPTOMS

A multipronged management approach should be provided to all children with a BLL of 5 mcg/dL or greater[11,15,16] (see Table 32-3). Proper management includes finding and eliminating the source of the lead, instruction in proper hygienic measures (personal and household), optimizing the child's diet and nutritional status, and close follow-up (see Tables 32-3 and 32-4). Because most children with higher BLLs live in or visit regularly a home with deteriorating lead paint, successful therapy depends on eliminating the child's exposure. Any treatment regimen that does not control environmental exposure to lead is considered inadequate. Pediatricians should refer children with elevated BLLs to local public health officials for environmental assessment of the child's residence(s), or other experts in childhood lead exposure, such as the regional Pediatric Environmental Health Specialty Unit (PEHSU). Public health staff should conduct a thorough investigation of the child's environment and family lifestyle for sources of lead. Childhood lead exposure is a multifaceted, complex

| Table 32-4. Clinical Evaluation[a] |
| --- |

**Medical History**
Ask about
- Symptoms
- Developmental history
- Mouthing activities
- Pica
- Previous BLL tests
- Family/maternal history of exposures to lead

**Environmental History**
Paint and soil exposure
- What is the age and general condition of the residence? How long has the family lived at that residence?
- Is there evidence of chewed or peeling paint on woodwork, furniture, or toys?
- Have there been recent renovations or repairs in the house?
- Are there other sites where the child spends significant amounts of time?
- What is the condition of indoor play areas?
- Do outdoor play areas contain bare soil that may be contaminated?
- How does the family attempt to control dust/dirt?

Water exposure
- Does the child's home have leaded pipes or fixtures?
- Has the water been tested at that residence?
- Has the water been tested at other places where the child spends significant amounts of time?

## Table 32-4. Clinical Evaluation (*continued*)

**Relevant Behavioral Characteristics of the Child**
- To what degree does the child exhibit hand-to-mouth activity?
- Does the child exhibit pica?
- Are the child's hands washed before meals and snacks?

**Exposures to and Behaviors of Household Members**
- What are the occupations of adult household members?
- What are the hobbies of household members? (Fishing, working with ceramics or stained glass, and hunting are examples of hobbies that involve risk for lead exposure)
- Are painted materials or unusual materials burned in household fireplaces?

**Miscellaneous Questions**
- Does the home contain vinyl miniblinds made overseas and purchased before 1997?
- Does the child receive or have access to imported food, cosmetics, or folk remedies?
- Is food prepared or stored in imported pottery or metal vessels?

**Nutritional History**
- Take a dietary history
- Evaluate the child's iron status using appropriate laboratory tests
- Ask about history of participation in The Supplemental Nutrition Assistance Program (SNAP), formerly known as The Food Stamp Program, or The Special Supplemental Nutrition Program for Women, Infants, and Children program (WIC)

**Physical Examination**
- Pay particular attention to the neurologic examination and to the child's psychosocial and language development
- Pay particular attention to stigmata of anemia, for example conjunctival pallor and tachycardia

ªAdapted from Centers for Disease Control and Prevention.[11]

condition affecting not only the child's health and well-being, but also the family's housing security, economic status, job security, and stress level.

Deteriorated lead paint is the most common source of exposure, but other sources should be considered (see Table 32-1). BLLs should decrease as the child passes the age of 2 or so, and a stable or increasing BLL past that age is likely to be attributable to ongoing exposure. Among children who have spent prolonged periods in a leaded environment, BLLs will decrease more slowly after exposure ceases,[86] probably because bone stores are greater.

The CDC Advisory Committee on Childhood Lead Poisoning Prevention, the AAP, and the PEHSU network, among other sources, have published potential strategies for a multipronged approach to managing elevated BLLs in children[10,15,87] (see Table 32-3). No studies have identified effective strategies to reduce BLLs of less than 5 mcg/dL.[93] Treatment strategies in the primary care setting include family counseling and education about dietary sources of iron, calcium, vitamin C, vitamin D, and magnesium. Nutritional deficiencies can influence lead absorption and may have their own associations with neurodevelopmental sequelae independent of lead exposures. Specific attention should be paid to identifying and treating iron deficiency and ensuring adequate calcium and zinc intake.

Lead may cause neurotoxic injury known to impair later academic performance and affect life success. At a BLL of 5 mcg/dL or greater, children are 30% more likely to fail third grade reading and math tests and more likely to be non-proficient in math, science, and reading.[94,95] Thus, one of the recommendations for a young child with an elevated BLL is to refer the child to early intervention or a similar educational enrichment program. As of 2013, the majority of states specifically listed elevated BLLs or exposure to toxic substances as eligibility criteria for early intervention services.[96]

Chelation therapy for children with venous BLLs of 20 to 44 mcg/dL can be expected to lower BLLs but has not been shown to reverse or diminish cognitive impairment or other behavioral or neuropsychological effects of lead.[97] Chelation therapy is recommended if the venous BLL is greater than 45 mcg/dL and the exposure has been controlled. A pediatrician experienced in managing children with lead exposure should be consulted—these can be found through the PEHSUs,[87] poison control centers, or through lead programs at state health departments (see Resources). Additional detailed medication treatment guidelines were published by the AAP.[98]

## Prevention of Exposure

The reduction in childhood lead exposure in the United States over the past 4 decades is a testament to the success of a multipronged approach to widespread identification of children with lead exposures, enforcement of the housing code, facilitated residential inspections, careful mitigation and abatement efforts, and educational outreach to the lay public and health care providers by nongovernmental and governmental agencies. There remains the need to address the widespread issue of 'legacy lead': the contamination of housing and continued exposure of children in the United States. Because no safe blood lead level has been identified, in 2012 the CDC and the Advisory Committee on Childhood Lead Poisoning advised that the best way to end the problem is to control, prevent, or eliminate exposures.[10,11]

Primary prevention efforts must focus on removing lead from the environment before a child has a chance to become exposed. Primary prevention efforts contrast to secondary prevention, the identification and management of individual cases after exposure already has caused elevated blood lead with potentially deleterious neurodevelopmental effects.[12] It is of paramount importance to implement primary prevention techniques through ongoing identification of lead-contaminated housing and definitive abatement. It is estimated that each $1 invested in housing abatement of lead hazards results in a return of $17 to $221.[99] The most persistent source of lead in a child's environment—contaminated housing—has been the primary focus of prevention efforts[100]. Individuals who conduct residential abatement (the removal and replacement of lead pipes, enclosure or encapsulation of lead-based paint or lead-contaminated dust or soil) must receive training to minimize further exposure to lead.[24,101] Paint stripping, covering painted areas by sealing or encasement, using high-efficiency particulate air (HEPA) vacuuming and HEPA air filters, and soil and dust removal are all effective methods for lead abatement. Removing all lead from homes and soil in the United States has not, however, been considered as a feasible prevention strategy because of the high cost of abatement.

The costs of remediating residential housing and plumbing are substantial and often pose formidable barriers to compliance by landlords, homeowners, and governmental agencies. Prevention approaches that focus on primary and secondary prevention efforts among high-risk communities are increasingly being used. An approach that incorporates neighborhood-level lead exposure data and census attributes (eg, percent of the population living below the poverty threshold; percent of old housing stock; percent of young children) has the benefit of concentrating the impact of the prevention effort in specific high-risk areas.[15,102–105]

Pediatric health care providers have important roles to play in case finding and managing childhood lead exposure. The testing and subsequent retesting of children with an elevated BLL is paramount in case finding and reducing the chronicity of lead exposure.

## Frequently Asked Questions

Q  *My child was tested and has elevated lead in his blood. How can I eliminate exposure?*

A  In children with elevated blood lead levels, interventions have to be not only effective but also very safe. I am going ask you about potential sources of lead exposure in your home, will test your child for anemia and iron deficiency, and provide iron supplements if needed. We will talk about making sure he has the proper nutrition. I will refer you to our local health department to help identify the lead source and make sure that the source in your home is safely removed. Unsafe renovation practices can further expose children to lead hazards. Having a child with a BLL of 5 to 10 mcg/dL may be a source of concern, but no specific drug therapies have been tested and shown to be safe and effective at these low blood lead levels and are not recommended.

Q   *What about testing for lead in water?*

A   If you are using tap water to give directly to an infant or child, or to reconstitute infant formula or juice or there has been local concern, you may want to have your water tested. To help determine whether your water might contain lead, call the US Environmental Protection Agency's Safe Drinking Water Hotline at 800-426-4791 or your local health department to find out about testing your water. Well water should be tested for lead when the well is new and tested again when a pregnant woman, infant, or child younger than age 18 years moves into the home. For a discussion of well water for infants, see the AAP policy statement on drinking water from private wells.[29] Most water filters, if used correctly, remove lead.

Q   *We have imported cookware and use imported spices, cosmetics, and ayurvedic medicines. Is it safe to use them?*

A   Some imported cookware contains lead. As the dishes wear or become chipped or cracked, lead can leach from the dishes into foods. The US Food and Drug Administration began regulating lead in cookware made in the United States in the 1980s and further strengthened regulations in the 1990s. Dishes made in the United States before these regulations took effect may contain lead. Studies have demonstrated that some imported spices such as turmeric, cosmetics such as kohl and sindoor, and ayurvedic medicines may be contaminated with lead. Because 80% of the spices used in the United States are imported, it is difficult to monitor all spices for contaminants. Although the US Food and Drug Administration is working with other countries to improve the quality of imported spices, cosmetics, and supplements, it always is wise to consider that these products may be sources of lead. When possible, consider using products made in the United States.[54–57]

Q   *Lead was found in my child's school drinking water fountain. Should I have her tested for her blood lead level?*

A   Under the Lead and Copper Rule, there are no special provisions that schools and public early education and childcare facilities that meet the definition of a public water system are required to be included as sampling locations. If an elevated water lead level was reported at your child's school, local resources such as the school, health department, or Pediatric Environmental Health Specialty Unit can be contacted to determine if blood lead level testing is indicated. It is important to take actions to minimize all sources of lead exposure. The primary source of lead exposure for most US children is from contaminated dust and soil. Schools should work with local, state, and regional resources to establish programs to test for lead in drinking water and other media (eg, lead-based paint and soil) and to develop a coordinated health messaging response for families and their communities. The US EPA has developed a 3Ts (Training, Testing, and Telling) toolkit to assist school and childcare facilities to address lead in drinking water in their local communities (see Resources).

Q  *I saw my toddler eating a piece of lead-containing paint. What should I do?*

A  Bring your child to the office so we can test him for lead. He may have ingested similar substances even before you noticed him eating the paint chip. Levels of lead in the blood rise rapidly (within hours to days) and can continue to rise as the paint chip moves through his digestive system. Once the object has been excreted, the blood level will fall to a new level over the next month. If his lead level is 15 mcg/dL or more, we may want to get an abdominal radiograph to see if there is lead there. If that is the case, I will consult with experts in lead exposure to see about next steps. I also will check your child for iron deficiency and treat him with iron if needed.

Your local or state health department may become involved to provide education or visit your home to determine the source of lead exposure. It is important to ask about reliable resources in the community to help to resolve the lead problem, if needed; health departments often are not able to provide this service themselves.

Q  *Is there still lead in canned food?*

A  Cans with soldered seams can add lead to foods. In the United States, soldered cans have been replaced by seamless aluminum containers, but some imported canned products still have lead-soldered seams.

Q  *What are resources for lead?*

A  There are several resources for lead exposure and prevention. Please contact the Pediatric Environmental Health Specialty Unit (PEHSU) network, poison control center, or local public health department's childhood lead poisoning prevention program for further information.

Q  *How can I tell if a toy has lead paint or is made of lead?*

A  Toys are not all routinely tested for lead. Companies that do not uniformly test the toys before selling them import many toys from countries with poorly enforced safety rules. The AAP advises parents to monitor the Consumer Product Safety Commission Web site for notices of recalls and to avoid non-brand toys and toys from discount shops and private vendors. Old and used toys should be examined for damage and clues to the origin of the toy. If the toy is damaged or worn or from a country with a history of poor monitoring of manufacturing practices, the safest action is to not let your child use it. Be particularly attentive to costume jewelry and other small metal pieces that can be swallowed.

## Resources

**Centers for Disease Control and Prevention Childhood Lead Poisoning Prevention Program**
Phone: 1-800-232-4636
Web site: www.cdc.gov/nceh/lead

**Environmental Protection Agency (EPA) Lead Paint Program**
Phone: 1-800-424-5323
Web site: www.epa.gov/lead

**EPA National Lead Information Center**
Phone: 1-800-424-LEAD
Web site: https://www.epa.gov/lead/forms/
lead-hotline-national-lead-information-center

**EPA Office of Children's Health Protection**
Phone: 202-564-2188
Web site: https://www.epa.gov/children

**EPA Safe Drinking Water Hotline**
Phone: 1-800-426-4791

**EPA's 3Ts (Training, Testing, and Telling Approach) for Reducing Lead in Drinking Water in Schools**
Web site: www.epa.gov/dwreginfo/
lead-drinking-water-schools-and-child-care-facilities

**Office of Healthy Homes and Lead Hazard Control, Department of Housing and Urban Development**
Web site: www.hud.gov/offices/lead

**Pediatric Environmental Health Specialty Unit (PEHSU) Network**
Phone: 888-347-2632
Web site: www.pehsu.net

**Poison Control Center (PCC)**
Phone: 1-800-222-1222
Web site: www.aapcc.org/

**President's Task Force on Environmental Health Risks and Safety Risks to Children, Key Federal Programs to Reduce Childhood Lead**
Web site: https://ptfceh.niehs.nih.gov/

# References

1. Schwartz J. Low-level lead exposure and children's IQ: A meta-analysis and search for a threshold. *Environ Res*. 1994;65(1):42–55

2. Pocock SJ, Smith M, Baghurst P. Environmental lead and children's intelligence: a systematic review of the epidemiological evidence. *BMJ*. 1994;309(6963):1189–1197

3. Lanphear BP, Hornung R, Khoury J, et al. Low-level environmental lead exposure and children's intellectual function: an international pooled analysis. *Environ Health Perspect*. 2005;113(7):894–899

4. Needleman HL, Gunnoe C, Leviton A, et al. Deficits in psychologic and classroom performance of children with elevated dentine lead levels. *N Engl J Med*. 1979;300(13):689–695

5. Burke MG, Miller MD. Practical guidelines for evaluating lead exposure in children with mental health conditions: molecular effects and clinical implications. *Postgrad Med*. 2011;123(1):160–168

6. Bellinger D, Needleman HL, Bromfield R, Mintz M. A followup study of the academic attainment and classroom behavior of children with elevated dentine lead levels. *Biol Trace Elem Res*. 1984;6(3):207–223

7. Chen A, Cai B, Dietrich KN, Radcliffe J, Rogan WJ. Lead exposure, IQ, and behavior in urban 5- to 7-year-olds: does lead affect behavior only by lowering IQ? *Pediatrics*. 2007;119(3):e650–e658

8. Nigg JT, Nikolas M, Mark Knottnerus G, Cavanagh K, Friderici K. Confirmation and extension of association of blood lead with attention-deficit/hyperactivity disorder (ADHD) and ADHD symptom domains at population-typical exposure levels. *J Child Psychol Psychiatry*. 2010;51(1):58–65

9. Canfield RL, Henderson CR, Cory-Slechta DA, Cox C, Jusko TA, Lanphear BP. Intellectual impairment in children with blood lead concentrations below 10 microg per deciliter. *N Engl J Med*. 2003;348(16):1517–1526

10. Centers for Disease Control and Prevention. Advisory Committee on Childhood Lead Poisoning Prevention. Low Level Lead Exposure Harms Children: A Renewed Call for Primary Prevention. 2012. http://www.cdc.gov/nceh/lead/ACCLPP/Final_Document_030712.pdf. Accessed April 9, 2018

11. Centers for Disease Control and Prevention. CDC response to Advisory Committee on Childhood Lead Poisoning Prevention recommendations in "low level lead exposure harms children: a renewed call of primary prevention." 2012. http://www.cdc.gov/nceh/lead/acclpp/cdc_response_lead_exposure_recs.pdf. Accessed April 9, 2018

12. President's Task Force on Environmental Health Risks and Safety Risks to Children. Key federal programs to reduce childhood lead exposures and eliminate associated health impacts. 2016. https://ptfceh.niehs.nih.gov/features/assets/files/key_federal_programs_to_reduce_childhood_lead_exposures_and_eliminate_associated_health_impactspresidents_508.pdf. Accessed April 9, 2018

13. Burns MS, Gerstenberger SL. Implications of the new centers for disease control and prevention blood lead reference value. *Am J Public Health*. 2014;104(6):e27–e33

14. Centers for Disease Control and Prevention. At-risk populations. http://www.cdc.gov/nceh/lead/tips/populations.htm. Updated 2015. Accessed April 9, 2018

15. American Academy of Pediatrics Council on Environmental Health. Prevention of childhood lead toxicity. *Pediatrics*. 2016;138(1):10.1542/peds.2016-1493

16. Binns HJ, Campbell C, Brown MJ, Centers for Disease Control and Prevention Advisory Committee on Childhood Lead Poisoning Prevention. Interpreting and managing blood lead levels of less than 10 microg/dL in children and reducing childhood exposure to lead: recommendations of the Centers for Disease Control and Prevention Advisory Committee on Childhood Lead Poisoning Prevention. *Pediatrics*. 2007;120(5):e1285–e1298

17. Nussbaumer-Streit B, Yeoh B, Griebler U, et al. Household interventions for preventing domestic lead exposure in children. *Cochrane Database Syst Rev.* 2016;10:CD006047

18. Miranda ML, Anthopolos R, Hastings D. A geospatial analysis of the effects of aviation gasoline on childhood blood lead levels. *Environ Health Perspect.* 2011;119(10):1513–1516

19. Lanphear BP, Hornung R, Ho M, Howard CR, Eberly S, Knauf K. Environmental lead exposure during early childhood. *J Pediatr.* 2002;140(1):40–47

20. Spanier AJ, Wilson S, Ho M, Hornung R, Lanphear BP. The contribution of housing renovation to children's blood lead levels: a cohort study. *Environ Health.* 2013;12:72

21. Jacobs DE, Clickner RP, Zhou JY, et al. The prevalence of lead-based paint hazards in U.S. housing. *Environ Health Perspect.* 2002;110(10):A599–A606

22. Trasande L, Liu Y. Reducing the staggering costs of environmental disease in children, estimated at $76.6 billion in 2008. *Health Aff (Millwood).* 2011;30(5):863–870

23. Farfel MR, Chisolm JJ, Rohde CA. The longer-term effectiveness of residential lead paint abatement. *Environ Res.* 1994;66(2):217–221

24. Lanphear BP, Matte TD, Rogers J, et al. The contribution of lead-contaminated house dust and residential soil to children's blood lead levels: a pooled analysis of 12 epidemiologic studies. *Environ Res.* 1998;79(1):51–68

25. von Lindern IH, Spalinger SM, Bero BN, Petrosyan V, von Braun MC. The influence of soil remediation on lead in house dust. *Sci Total Environ.* 2003;303(1-2):59–78

26. Charney E, Kessler B, Farfel M, Jackson D. Childhood lead poisoning: a controlled trial of the effect of dust-control measures on blood lead levels. *N Engl J Med.* 1983;309(18):1089–1093

27. Kennedy C, Yard E, Dignam T, et al. Blood lead levels among children aged <6 years - Flint, Michigan, 2013-2016. *MMWR Morb Mortal Wkly Rep.* 2016;65(25):650–654

28. Hanna-Attisha M, LaChance J, Sadler RC, Champney Schnepp A. Elevated blood lead levels in children associated with the Flint drinking water crisis: a spatial analysis of risk and public health response. *Am J Public Health.* 2016;106(2):283–290

29. American Academy of Pediatrics Committee on Environmental Health, Committee on Infectious Diseases, Rogan WJ, Brady MT. Drinking water from private wells and risks to children. *Pediatrics.* 2009;123(6):1599–1605

30. Olson E, Pullen Fedinick K. What's in your water? Flint and beyond. 2016. https://www.nrdc.org/sites/default/files/whats-in-your-water-flint-beyond-report.pdf. Accessed April 9, 2018

31. Centers for Disease Control and Prevention. Death of a child after ingestion of a metallic charm—Minnesota, 2006. *MMWR Morb Mortal Wkly Rep.* 2006;55(12):340–341

32. Centers for Disease Control and Prevention. Lead poisoning of a child associated with use of a cambodian amulet—New York City, 2009. *MMWR Morb Mortal Wkly Rep.* 2011;60(3):69–71

33. Weidenhamer JD, Clement ML. Widespread lead contamination of imported low-cost jewelry in the US. *Chemosphere.* 2007;67(5):961–965

34. Yost JL, Weidenhamer JD. Lead contamination of inexpensive plastic jewelry. *Sci Total Environ.* 2008;393(2-3):348–350

35. Dietrich KN, Ris MD, Succop PA, Berger OG, Bornschein RL. Early exposure to lead and juvenile delinquency. *Neurotoxicol Teratol.* 2001;23(6):511–518

36. Wright RO, Shannon MW, Wright RJ, Hu H. Association between iron deficiency and low-level lead poisoning in an urban primary care clinic. *Am J Public Health.* 1999;89(7):1049–1053

37. Wright RO, Tsaih SW, Schwartz J, Wright RJ, Hu H. Association between iron deficiency and blood lead level in a longitudinal analysis of children followed in an urban primary care clinic. *J Pediatr.* 2003;142(1):9–14

38. Eisenberg KW, van Wijngaarden E, Fisher SG, et al. Blood lead levels of refugee children resettled in Massachusetts, 2000 to 2007. *Am J Public Health.* 2011;101(1):48–54

39. Raymond JS, Kennedy C, Brown MJ. Blood lead level analysis among refugee children resettled in New Hampshire and Rhode Island. *Public Health Nurs.* 2013;30(1):70–79

40. Schmidt CW. Unsafe harbor? elevated blood lead levels in refugee children. *Environ Health Perspect.* 2013;121(6):A190–A195

41. Proue M, Jones-Webb R, Oberg C. Blood lead screening among newly arrived refugees in Minnesota. *Minn Med.* 2010;93(6):42–46

42. Centers for Disease Control and Prevention. Elevated blood lead levels in refugee children—New Hampshire, 2003-2004. *MMWR Morb Mortal Wkly Rep.* 2005;54(2):42–46

43. Accardo P, Whitman B, Caul J, Rolfe U. Autism and plumbism. A possible association. *Clin Pediatr (Phila).* 1988;27(1):41–44

44. Shannon M, Graef JW. Lead intoxication in children with pervasive developmental disorders. *J Toxicol Clin Toxicol.* 1996;34(2):177–181

45. Fitzpatrick M. Autism and environmental toxicity. *Lancet Neurol.* 2007;6(4):297

46. George M, Heeney MM, Woolf AD. Encephalopathy from lead poisoning masquerading as a flu-like syndrome in an autistic child. *Pediatr Emerg Care.* 2010;26(5):370–373

47. Zeager M, Heard T, Woolf AD. Lead poisoning in two children with Landau-Kleffner syndrome. *Clin Toxicol (Phila).* 2012;50(5):448

48. Filipek PA, Accardo PJ, Ashwal S, et al. Practice parameter: screening and diagnosis of autism: report of the quality standards subcommittee of the American Academy of Neurology and the Child Neurology Society. *Neurology.* 2000;55(4):468–479

49. Chung EK, Webb D, Clampet-Lundquist S, Campbell C. A comparison of elevated blood lead levels among children living in foster care, their siblings, and the general population. *Pediatrics.* 2001;107(5):E81

50. Hauptman M, Woolf AD. Lead poisoning and children in foster care: diagnosis and management challenges. *Clin Pediatr (Phila).* 2018;57(8):988–991

51. Roscoe RJ, Gittleman JL, Deddens JA, Petersen MR, Halperin WE. Blood lead levels among children of lead-exposed workers: a meta-analysis. *Am J Ind Med.* 1999;36(4):475–481

52. Centers for Disease Control & Prevention. Report to Congress on the Workers' Home Contamination Study Conducted Under The Workers' Family Protection Act (29 U.S.C. 671a). Cincinnati, OH: US Department of Health and Human Services, CDC, National Institute for Occupational Safety and Health; 1995; DHHS (NIOSH) publication no. 95-123. http://www.cdc.gov/niosh/docs/95-123. Accessed April 9, 2018

53. Newman N, Jones C, Page E, Ceballos D, Oza A. Investigation of childhood lead poisoning from parental take-home exposure from an electronic scrap recycling facility - Ohio, 2012. *MMWR Morb Mortal Wkly Rep.* 2015;64(27):743–745

54. Woolf AD, Hussain J, McCullough L, Petranovic M, Chomchai C. Infantile lead poisoning from an asian tongue powder: A case report & subsequent public health inquiry. *Clin Toxicol (Phila).* 2008;46(9):841–844

55. Nasidi A, Karwowski M, Woolf AD, et al. Infant lead poisoning associated with use of tiro, an eye cosmetic from Nigeria - Boston, Massachusetts; 2011. *MMWR Morb Mortal Wkly Rep.* 2012;61(30):574–576

56. Woolf AD, Woolf NT. Childhood lead poisoning in 2 families associated with spices used in food preparation. *Pediatrics.* 2005;116(2):e314–e318

57. Lin CG, Schaider LA, Brabander DJ, Woolf AD. Pediatric lead exposure from imported indian spices and cultural powders. *Pediatrics.* 2010;125(4):e828–e835

58. Harris ESJ, Cao S, Littlefield BA, et al. Heavy metal and pesticide content in commonly prescribed individual raw Chinese herbal medicines. 2011;409(20):4297–4305

59. Woolf AD, Gardiner P. Use of complementary and alternative therapies in children. *Clin Pharmacol Ther.* 2010;87(2):155–157

60. Meiman J, Thiboldeaux R, Anderson H. Lead poisoning and anemia associated with use of ayurvedic medications purchased on the internet—Wisconsin, 2015. *MMWR Morb Mortal Wkly Rep*. 2015;64(32):883

61. Centers for Disease Control and Prevention. Occupational and take-home lead poisoning associated with restoring chemically stripped furniture—California, 1998. *MMWR Morb Mortal Wkly Rep*. 2001;50(13):246–248

62. Beaucham C, Page E, Alarcon WA, et al. Indoor firing ranges and elevated blood lead levels - United States, 2002-2013. *MMWR Morb Mortal Wkly Rep*. 2014;63(16):347–351

63. Shannon M. Lead poisoning in adolescents who are competitive marksmen. *N Engl J Med*. 1999;341(11):852

64. National Toxicology Program. NTP monograph. Health Effects of Low-Level Lead. NIH Publication No. 12-5996. National Toxicology Program. National Institute of Environmental Health Sciences. U.S. Department of Health & Human Services. 2012. https://ntp.niehs.nih.gov/ntp/ohat/lead/final/monographhealtheffectslowlevellead_newissn_508.pdf. Accessed April 9, 2018

65. US Environmental Protection Agency. Final report: Integrated Science Assessment for Lead. 2013. https://cfpub.epa.gov/ncea/risk/recordisplay.cfm?deid=255721. Accessed April 9, 2018

66. Agency for Toxic Substances and Disease Registry. Toxicological Profile for Lead. Agency for Toxic Substances and Disease Registry. US Department of Health and Human Services. 2007. https://www.atsdr.cdc.gov/toxprofiles/tp13.pdf. Accessed September 12, 2018

67. Lidsky TI, Schneider JS. Adverse effects of childhood lead poisoning: the clinical neuropsychological perspective. *Environ Res*. 2006;100(2):284–293

68. Canfield RL, Gendle MH, Cory-Slechta DA. Impaired neuropsychological functioning in lead-exposed children. *Dev Neuropsychol*. 2004;26(1):513–540

69. Lanphear BP, Dietrich K, Auinger P, Cox C. Cognitive deficits associated with blood lead concentrations. *Public Health Rep*. 2000;115(6):521–529

70. Chen A, Dietrich KN, Ware JH, Radcliffe J, Rogan WJ. IQ and blood lead from 2 to 7 years of age: are the effects in older children the residual of high blood lead concentrations in 2-year-olds? *Environ Health Perspect*. 2005;113(5):597–601

71. Shargorodsky J, Curhan SG, Henderson E, Eavey R, Curhan GC. Heavy metals exposure and hearing loss in US adolescents. *Arch Otolaryngol Head Neck Surg*. 2011;137(12):1183–1189

72. Schwartz J, Otto D. Lead and minor hearing impairment. *Arch Environ Health*. 1991;46(5):300–305

73. Bhattacharya A, Shukla R, Bornschein RL, Dietrich KN, Keith R. Lead effects on postural balance of children. *Environ Health Perspect*. 1990;89:35–42

74. Sciarillo WG, Alexander G, Farrell KP. Lead exposure and child behavior. *Am J Public Health*. 1992;82(10):1356–1360

75. Needleman HL, Schell A, Bellinger D, Leviton A, Allred EN. The long-term effects of exposure to low doses of lead in childhood: an 11-year follow-up report. *N Engl J Med*. 1990;322(2):83–88

76. Needleman HL, Riess JA, Tobin MJ, Biesecker GE, Greenhouse JB. Bone lead levels and delinquent behavior. *JAMA*. 1996;275(5):363–369

77. Rice DC. Behavioral effects of lead: commonalities between experimental and epidemiologic data. *Environ Health Perspect*. 1996;104(Suppl 2):337–351

78. Cecil KM, Dietrich KN, Altaye M, et al. Proton magnetic resonance spectroscopy in adults with childhood lead exposure. *Environ Health Perspect*. 2011;119(3):403–408

79. Markovac J, Goldstein GW. Picomolar concentrations of lead stimulate brain protein kinase C. *Nature*. 1988;334(6177):71–73

80. Cecil KM, Brubaker CJ, Adler CM, et al. Decreased brain volume in adults with childhood lead exposure. *PLoS Med*. 2008;5(5):e112

81. Brubaker CJ, Dietrich KN, Lanphear BP, Cecil KM. The influence of age of lead exposure on adult gray matter volume. *Neurotoxicology.* 2010;31(3):259–266

82. Brubaker CJ, Schmithorst VJ, Haynes EN, et al. Altered myelination and axonal integrity in adults with childhood lead exposure: a diffusion tensor imaging study. *Neurotoxicology.* 2009;30(6):867–875

83. Yuan W, Holland SK, Cecil KM, et al. The impact of early childhood lead exposure on brain organization: a functional magnetic resonance imaging study of language function. *Pediatrics.* 2006;118(3):971–977

84. Selevan SG, Rice DC, Hogan KA, Euling SY, Pfahles-Hutchens A, Bethel J. Blood lead concentration and delayed puberty in girls. *N Engl J Med.* 2003;348(16):1527–1536

85. McIntire MS, Wolf GL, Angle CR. Red cell lead and -amino levulinic acid dehydratase. *Clin Toxicol.* 1973;6(2):183–188

86. Woolf AD, Bellinger D, Goldman R. Clinical approach to childhood lead poisoning. *Pediatr Clin North Am.* 2007;54(2):271–294

87. Newman N, Binns HJ, Karwowski M, Lowry J, and PEHSU Lead Working Group. Recommendations on Medical Management of Childhood Lead Exposure and Poisoning. Pediatric Environmental Health Specialty Unit; 2013. http://www.pehsu.net/_Library/facts/medical-mgmnt-childhood-lead-exposure-June-2013.pdf. Accessed April 9, 2018

88. National Committee for Quality Assurance. Lead screening in children. 2014. http://www.ncqa.org/report-cards/health-plans/state-of-health-care-quality/2016-table-of-contents/lead-screening. Accessed April 9, 2018

89. Committee on Obstetric Practice. Committee opinion no. 533: lead screening during pregnancy and lactation. *Obstet Gynecol.* 2012;120(2 Pt 1):416–420

90. Work Group on Lead and Pregnancy, CDC Advisory Committee on Childhood Lead Poisoning Prevention. Guidelines for the identification and management of lead exposure in pregnant and lactating women. 2010. http://www.cdc.gov/nceh/lead/publications/leadandpregnancy2010.pdf. Accessed April 9, 2018

91. Hussain J, Woolf AD, Sandel M, Shannon MW. Environmental evaluation of a child with developmental disability. *Pediatr Clin North Am.* 2007;54(1):47–62

92. Esteban E, Rubin CH, Jones RL, Noonan G. Hair and blood as substrates for screening children for lead poisoning. *Arch Environ Health.* 1999;54(6):436–440

93. Pfadenhauer LM, Burns J, Rohwer A, Rehfuess EA. Effectiveness of interventions to reduce exposure to lead through consumer products and drinking water: a systematic review. *Environ Res.* 2016;147:525–536

94. Evens A, Hryhorczuk D, Lanphear BP, et al. The impact of low-level lead toxicity on school performance among children in the Chicago public schools: a population-based retrospective cohort study. *Environ Health.* 2015;14:21

95. McLaine P, Navas-Acien A, Lee R, Simon P, Diener-West M, Agnew J. Elevated blood lead levels and reading readiness at the start of kindergarten. *Pediatrics.* 2013;131(6):1081–1089

96. Centers for Disease Control & Prevention. Educational services for children affected by lead expert panel. Atlanta, GA: U.S. Department of Health and Human Services; 2015. http://www.cdc.gov/nceh/lead/publications/Educational_Interventions_Children_Affected_by_Lead.pdf. Accessed April 9, 2018

97. Dietrich KN, Ware JH, Salganik M, et al. Effect of chelation therapy on the neuropsychological and behavioral development of lead-exposed children after school entry. *Pediatrics.* 2004;114(1):19–26

98. American Academy of Pediatrics Committee on Drugs. Treatment guidelines for lead exposure in children. *Pediatrics.* 1995;96(1 Pt 1):155–160

99. Gould E. Childhood lead poisoning: conservative estimates of the social and economic benefits of lead hazard control. *Environ Health Perspect.* 2009;117(7):1162–1167

100. Aschengrau A, Beiser A, Bellinger D, Copenhafer D, Weitzman M. Residential lead-based-paint hazard remediation and soil lead abatement: their impact among children with mildly elevated blood lead levels. *Am J Public Health.* 1997;87(10):1698–1702

101. Brown MJ, Gardner J, Sargent JD, Swartz K, Hu H, Timperi R. The effectiveness of housing policies in reducing children's lead exposure. *Am J Public Health.* 2001;91(4):621–624

102. Vivier PM, Hauptman M, Weitzen SH, Bell S, Quilliam DN, Logan JR. The important health impact of where a child lives: neighborhood characteristics and the burden of lead poisoning. *Matern Child Health J.* 2011;15(8):1195–1202

103. Kennedy C, Lordo R, Sucosky MS, Boehm R, Brown MJ. Evaluating the effectiveness of state specific lead-based paint hazard risk reduction laws in preventing recurring incidences of lead poisoning in children. *Int J Hyg Environ Health.* 2016;219(1):110–117

104. Rosner D. Imagination and public health: the end of lead poisoning in California? *Milbank Q.* 2014;92(3):430–433

105. Lynn J, Oppenheimer S, Zimmer L. Using public policy to improve outcomes for asthmatic children in schools. *J Allergy Clin Immunol.* 2014;134(6):1238–1244

Chapter 33

# Mercury

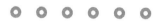

## KEY POINTS

- Signs and symptoms of mercury toxicity depend on the form of mercury. Elemental mercury exposure occurs by inhaling the colorless, odorless vapor. Organic (methylmercury) exposure occurs from consuming certain ocean fish or fish taken from contaminated fresh water lakes or streams.
- Elemental or inorganic mercury exposure typically is diagnosed by increased urine mercury levels.
- Organic (methylmercury) exposure typically is diagnosed by increased blood total mercury levels.
- Autism is not caused by vaccines.
- Thimerosal, containing ethylmercury, has been removed from childhood vaccines and now is only used as a preservative in multi-dose vaccines (eg, influenza, meningococcal B).
- The only proven effective treatment for mercury exposure is to find the source and stop the exposure. Chelation therapy is unproven and may lead to adverse effects.

## INTRODUCTION

Mercury (Hg) occurs in three forms: the metallic element ($Hg^0$, quicksilver or elemental mercury), inorganic salts ($Hg^{1+}$, or mercurous salts, and $Hg^{2+}$, or mercuric salts), and organic compounds (methylmercury, ethylmercury, and phenylmercury) (Table 33-1). Solubility, reactivity, biological effects, and toxicity vary among these forms.

**Table 33-1. Sources and Routes of Exposure for Different Forms of Mercury**

| MERCURY FORM | SOURCE(S) | ROUTE OF EXPOSURE |
|---|---|---|
| Elemental or inorganic | Thermometers, sphygmomanometers, CFL or fluorescent light bulbs; dental amalgams; mercury used in religious or ritual practices; artisanal gold mining | Inhalation of vapor |
| Inorganic salts | Skin lightening creams and soaps; calomel (former use); teething powders (former use) | Ingestion or dermal absorption |
| Methylmercury (organic) | Shark, tuna, tile fish, swordfish; fish taken from mercury-contaminated lakes, rivers, or streams | Ingestion |
| Ethylmercury (thimerosal) | Multi-dose vaccines (meningococcal B and influenza) | Injection |

Abbreviations: CFL, compact fluorescent light

Naturally occurring mercury sources include cinnabar (ore) and fossil fuels, such as coal and petroleum. Environmental contamination has resulted from mining, smelting, and industrial discharges (principally by burning fossil fuels). Atmospheric mercury contributes to local and global contamination. Mercury in lakes and stream sediments can be converted by bacteria into organic mercury compounds, primarily methylmercury, that accumulate in the food chain and progressively bioaccumulate. The result is that certain predator fish from oceans or freshwater may contain higher levels of mercury. Very high exposures to methylmercury in fish in the 1950s following industrial release of mercury into Minamata Bay, Japan, caused serious disturbances in fetal brain development among exposed pregnant women and thousands of cases of acute adult methylmercury toxicity, and an estimated 200,000 individuals had neurologic manifestations of chronic methylmercury exposure.[1] To reduce consumption of the most highly contaminated fish species, states have issued advisories about consumption of locally caught fish, which may vary by fish species or body of water or be applied on a statewide basis. Recommendations on limiting intake of large ocean fish, such as tuna, swordfish, king mackerel, tilefish, and shark, have been issued by the US federal government.[1] Edible seaweed and fish oil supplements have not been found to contain mercury, but there is no ongoing program for sampling these marine-derived foods and supplements.[2,3]

Methylmercury use as a fungicide on seed grains has been banned in the United States since the early 1970s. Consumption of mercury-treated seed grains caused widespread mercury poisoning among people in Iraq and China and has been responsible for neurologic disorders in wildlife.[4] Coal-burning power plants can be a significant source of mercury released into the air, and US regulations have required reductions in these emissions since 2011 (https://www.epa.gov/mats).

Elemental mercury has been used in sphygmomanometers, thermometers, and thermostat switches. Dental amalgams contain 40% to 50% mercury as well as silver and other metals. Fluorescent light bulbs, including tubes and compact bulbs, and disc (button) batteries also contain mercury. Indiscriminate disposal of these items is a source of environmental mercury contamination when they are buried in landfills or burned in waste incinerators rather than recycled. Skin lightening creams and soaps can contain toxic amounts of inorganic mercury.[5] Artisanal gold mining can involve elemental mercury to amalgamate the precious metal, and highly toxic fumes can result when the amalgam is heated to vaporize and remove the mercury. Elemental or inorganic mercury is used in some folk remedies and rituals, including Santeria (a Cuban-based religion), Voodoo (a Haitian-based set of rituals), Espiritismo (a Puerto Rican based spiritual belief system), and Indian Ayurvedic medicine.[6-8]

## ROUTES OF EXPOSURE

### Elemental Mercury and Inorganic Mercury

Elemental mercury is a liquid at room temperature and readily volatilizes to a colorless and odorless vapor. When inhaled, elemental mercury vapor easily passes through pulmonary alveolar membranes and enters the blood, where it distributes primarily into red blood cells and is carried to all tissues of the body, including crossing the blood-brain barrier. Once in a cell, mercury is oxidized to inorganic mercury ($Hg^{2+}$), which hinders its elimination. Approximately 80% of inhaled mercury is absorbed in the body. In contrast, less than 0.1% of elemental mercury is absorbed from the gastrointestinal tract after ingestion, and only minimal absorption occurs with dermal exposure.[9]

### Inorganic Mercury Salts

Inorganic mercury salts are poorly absorbed after ingestion, although mercuric salts tend to be extremely caustic and cause stomach bleeding when ingested. Mercurous salts may be less caustic to the intestinal tract but can result in nephrotoxicity after ingestion or skin application.

### Organic Mercury

Most organic mercury compounds are lipid soluble and are well absorbed from the gastrointestinal tract. Methylmercury is 95% absorbed after ingestion, contributing to concern about consumption of methylmercury-contaminated fish.[10] Methylmercury passes through the placenta, is concentrated in the fetus, and is transferred into human milk. Phenylmercury is well absorbed after ingestion and dermal contact. In contrast to other organic mercury compounds, the carbon-mercury chemical bond of phenylmercury is relatively unstable, resulting in the release of elemental mercury that can be inhaled and absorbed across pulmonary membranes.

Ethylmercury is found in thimerosal, used as an antiseptic and as a preservative for vaccines and other drugs. Prior to 2001, vaccines could contain up to 25 mcg of mercury (as thimerosal) per dose. However, thimerosal use as a vaccine preservative declined as early as 1999, following recommendations to remove mercury from vaccines issued by public health and medical organizations including the American Academy of Pediatrics. Since 2001, no new vaccine licensed by the US Food and Drug Administration (FDA) for use in children has contained thimerosal, despite no evidence of harm caused by the low doses of thimerosal in vaccines. All vaccines routinely recommended for children younger than 6 years of age, except for the influenza vaccine in multi-dose vials, have been thimerosal-free or contain only trace amounts. Meningococcal conjugate vaccine, available as 2 different thimerosal-free products, is the preferred vaccine for children and adolescents; however, multi-dose vials of a third vaccine contain thimerosal. The recombinant meningococcal B vaccines are also thimerosal-free. The FDA publishes a list of thimerosal content of vaccines recommended for children aged 6 years and younger, as well as thimerosal content of other vaccines (https://www.cdc.gov/vaccines/pubs/pinkbook/downloads/appendices/B/excipient-table-2.pdf).

## SYSTEMS AFFECTED AND CLINICAL EFFECTS

### Elemental Mercury

At high concentrations, inhaled mercury vapor produces acute necrotizing bronchitis and pneumonitis, which can lead to death from respiratory failure.[11] Fatalities have resulted from heating elemental mercury in inadequately ventilated areas.[12]

Long-term exposure to mercury vapor primarily affects the central nervous system (CNS). Early nonspecific signs include insomnia, forgetfulness, loss of appetite, and mild tremor and may be misdiagnosed as psychiatric illness. Continued exposure leads to progressive tremor and erethism, characterized by red palms, emotional lability, hypertension, and visual and memory impairments.[13-16] Salivation, excessive sweating, and hemoconcentration are accompanying signs. Mercury also accumulates in kidney tissues. Renal toxicity includes proteinuria or nephrotic syndrome, alone or in addition to other signs of mercury exposure.[17,18] Isolated renal effects may be immunologic in origin.

Mercury exposure from dental amalgams has prompted concerns about subclinical or unusual neurologic effects. A few US state governments have enacted informed consent legislation for dental patients receiving dental restorations.[19] Although dental amalgams are a source of mercury exposure and are associated with slightly higher urinary mercury excretion, there is no scientific evidence for any measurable clinical toxic effects other than rare hypersensitivity reactions.[20,21] Two randomized clinical trials failed to demonstrate neurobehavioral or neuropsychological differences between children with or without dental amalgams.[22–24]

## Inorganic Mercury

Mercuric chloride ($Hg^{2+}$) is well described by its common name, corrosive sublimate. Ingestions usually are inadvertent or with suicidal intent, and gastrointestinal tract ulceration or perforation and hemorrhage are rapidly produced, followed by circulatory collapse. Breakdown of intestinal mucosal barriers leads to extensive mercury absorption and distribution to the kidneys. Acute renal toxic effects include proximal tubular necrosis and anuria.

Acrodynia, or childhood mercury poisoning, was frequently reported in the 1940s among infants exposed to calomel teething powders containing mercurous chloride.[25,26] Cases were reported in infants exposed to phenylmercury used as a fungicidal diaper rinse and in children exposed to phenylmercuric acetate from interior latex paint.[27,28] Susceptibility to the development of acrodynia in children is poorly understood; it is characterized by a maculopapular rash, swollen and painful extremities, peripheral neuropathy, hypertension, and renal tubular dysfunction.[29,30]

## Organic Mercury

Organic mercury toxicity occurs with long-term exposure and affects the CNS. Signs progress from paresthesias to ataxia, followed by generalized weakness, visual and hearing impairment, tremor and muscle spasticity, and finally coma and death. Organic mercury also is a potent teratogen, causing disruption of the normal patterns of neuronal migration and nerve cell histology in the developing brain. In the Minamata Bay disaster with contaminated fish and the Iraq epidemic with contaminated seed grain, mothers who were asymptomatic or showed mild toxic effects gave birth to severely affected infants. Typically, the infants seemed normal at birth, but psychomotor retardation, blindness, deafness, and seizures developed over time.[31]

Because the fetus and infant are more susceptible to the neurotoxic effects of methylmercury, investigators have looked for subclinical effects among children whose mothers' diets included large amounts of fish or marine mammals containing methylmercury and whose blood mercury concentrations were higher than those commonly seen in the United States. Three long-term studies have been conducted: in the Seychelle Islands; the Faroe Islands (between Iceland and Norway); and in New Zealand.[10] Follow-up of children at ages 7, 9, and 14 years showed inconsistent results with regard to motor, attention, and verbal test results.[32,33] A slight decrease in IQ was seen with increasing maternal methylmercury exposure when results from all 3 studies were combined, and this effect was still detected in the children from the Faroe Islands at age 22 years.[34,35] It has been speculated that the beneficial omega-3 fatty acids in the seafoods eaten in the Seychelles may have reduced harmful neurodevelopmental effects of the methylmercury.[36] Therefore, prudence and a desire to avoid unnecessary risk to the developing fetus has prompted recommendations from US federal and state agencies to avoid eating fish likely to have methylmercury contamination.

The US Environmental Protection Agency (EPA) has recommended a daily intake of methylmercury that over a lifetime would not be harmful, even in the developing fetus. This intake of 0.1 mcg/kg body weight/day corresponds approximately to a blood mercury concentration of 5.8 mcg/L.[10] In the United States, more than 90% to 95% of the population have blood mercury concentrations below 5 mcg/L.[37] In 2011 to 2012, less than 2% of US women aged 16 to 44 years had blood methylmercury concentrations higher than 5.8 mcg/L, although more than 15% of Asian women exceeded this value, possibly because of seafood-rich diets.[38]

Ethylmercury may have similar toxicity to methylmercury but has been less well studied. A large number of pharmaceutical products (eg, ear and eye drops, eye ointment, nasal sprays, hemorrhoid relief ointment) may contain thimerosal as a preservative. Very high and repeated exposures to thimerosal-containing products have resulted in toxicity, including acrodynia, chronic mercury toxicity, renal failure, and neuropathy.[39–43] Merthiolate used to irrigate the external auditory canals in a child with tympanostomy tubes caused fatal mercury poisoning.[44] Current formulations of merthiolate may or may not contain thimerosal.

There has been concern that organic mercury exposure from thimerosal-containing vaccines and other sources played a role in the growing incidence of autism. However, numerous scientific studies have failed to support a causal relationship, a federal report that reviewed the science agreed, and the original study suggesting that mercury played a causal role in autism has been retracted and discredited.[45–54] Although some parents still may have concerns, no new evidence shows that thimerosal in vaccines causes autism. In an abundance of caution, thimerosal was removed from all routine childhood vaccines except for some multi-dose influenza vaccines in 2001.

## DIAGNOSTIC METHODS

Diagnosis of mercury poisoning usually is made on the basis of exposure history and physical examination. Urine and blood tests may demonstrate elevated mercury concentrations, depending on the timing of the sample collection relative to when the exposure occurred. For children younger than 12 years, typical background results are blood mercury levels less than 2 mcg/L and single void or spot urine mercury levels less than 4 to 5 mcg/L.[55]

### Elemental Mercury and Inorganic Mercury

Elemental mercury vapor is converted to inorganic mercury in the body, and exposure is best evaluated by measuring urinary mercury. Although a 24-hour urine collection is recommended by some physicians, it may be more feasible in a child to collect a single void or spot urine. Once collected, the urine sample should be frozen, or at least refrigerated until it is shipped to the laboratory. At room temperature, mercury can volatilize from the urine.[56] Some laboratories have specific instructions for sample collection, so it is advisable to contact the laboratory that will do the measurement to ensure that the urine is properly collected and preserved.

Results showing levels greater than 10 to 20 mcg/day in urine are evidence of excessive exposure, and neurologic signs may be present at concentrations greater than 100 mcg/L. The urinary mercury concentration, however, does not necessarily correlate with chronicity or severity of toxic effects, especially if the mercury exposure was intermittent or variable in intensity. Whole blood mercury can be measured, but concentrations tend to return to normal (<0.5–1.0 mcg/L) within 1 to 2 days after an exposure to inorganic mercury ends.

### Organic Mercury

Because organic mercury compounds concentrate in red blood cells, whole blood mercury is measured to diagnose excessive exposure. Blood mercury concentrations rarely exceed 1.5 to 2.0 mcg/L in the unexposed population.[37,38] However, a meal of methylmercury-contaminated fish in the previous 2 to 3 days can transiently elevate blood mercury concentration up to tenfold.[57] Although testing for hair mercury concentration is useful to quantify methylmercury exposure for research studies, this is not recommended in clinical situations. No clinical cut point has been determined to establish toxicity on the basis of a hair mercury concentration. When hair mercury measurement is offered by an outside commercial laboratory, the rationale for measuring exposure is unknown, control for external contamination is usually not considered, and collection and washing protocols are usually not validated.[58]

## TREATMENT

The most important and most effective treatment is to identify the mercury source and end the exposure. Chelating agents, including dimercaprol (BAL in oil) and succimer (DMSA) have been used to enhance inorganic mercury elimination, but whether chelation reduces toxic effects or speeds recovery in people who have been poisoned is unclear.[16,59,60] There is no effective or FDA-approved chelating agent for methylmercury poisoning. Any child with suspected mercury poisoning should be treated in consultation with a physician experienced in managing children with mercury or other poisonings. Children who have had mercury poisoning need periodic follow-up neurologic examinations and developmental assessments by a pediatrician and may need referral for further neurological and developmental evaluations.

Chelation has been proposed by some as a treatment for autism spectrum disorder. However, no evidence documents that mercury contributes to autism. Because chelation can have serious side effects, chelation treatment for autism spectrum disorder is not indicated and may, in fact, be dangerous.[61]

## PREVENTION OF EXPOSURE

Electronic equipment has replaced many mercury-containing oral thermometers and sphygmomanometers in medical settings. Pediatricians who still have mercury-containing devices should safely eliminate their use and may find hospital safety officers to be of assistance; families should be encouraged to do the same. Sources of mercury in school settings should also be catalogued and safely eliminated. Hospitals may offer to dispose of mercury-containing medical devices, and state or local programs for the safe disposal of mercury-containing devices may be available.

Organic mercury fungicides, including methylmercury and phenylmercury (used in latex paints until 1990), are no longer sold or licensed for commercial use in the United States. Newer enclosed methods for preparing mercury amalgams have reduced the likelihood of mercury spillage and exposure during dental amalgam preparation.

The amount of mercury in thermometers and fluorescent and compact fluorescent light (CFL) bulbs is small and usually insufficient to produce clinically significant exposure. If a mercury thermometer or fluorescent or CFL bulb breaks, safe clean up usually can be accomplished by taking care to avoid spreading the mercury (for detailed instructions, see https://www.epa.gov/mercury). To avoid exposure, pregnant women and children should leave the room or area and not help with the cleanup. Vacuuming or sweeping up the breakage should not be done because this may further spread and volatize the mercury. If a thermometer spill occurs on carpeting, the affected carpet area should be carefully removed and discarded because the mercury droplets cannot be removed even if they are no longer visible. Larger spills of elemental mercury of more than 1 pound (approximately equal to 2 tablespoons (30 mL); mercury is very heavy) can pose a significant hazard. The National Response Center (NRC) should be called for assistance. The NRC hotline operates 24 hours a day, 7 days a week: call (800) 424-8802. The poison control center (1-800-222-1222) and local health department also may be able to assist.

The FDA regulations limit methylmercury in commercial fish to 1 part per million (1 mcg/g). Because seafood is an important source of lean protein and beneficial unsaturated fatty acids (eg, omega-3 fatty acids), current recommendations are for pregnant women and young children to eat fish each week and limit consumption of commercial fish likely to be high in mercury or fish that come from local waters under a fish advisory. Specific recommendations summarized here are available from the FDA (http://www.fda.gov/ForConsumers/ConsumerUpdates/ucm397443.htm).

- Eat 8 to 12 ounces (227 to 340 g) of a variety of fish or shellfish each week (2 to 3 servings); children's servings should be the right portion size for the child's age and calorie needs.
- Choose fish lower in mercury, such as salmon, shrimp, pollock, tuna (light canned), tilapia, catfish, and cod.
- Avoid the 4 types of fish highest in mercury: tilefish from the Gulf of Mexico, shark, swordfish, and king mackerel.
- Pay attention to fish advisories when you eat fish caught from streams, rivers, and lakes; if no advice is available, adults should limit such fish to 6 ounces (170 g) a week and young children to 1 to 3 ounces (25 to 85 g) a week, and not eat other fish that week.
- Stay within your calorie needs when adding more fish to your diet.

The federal government does not regulate the levels of mercury in fish caught for sport, but states can issue advisories recommending public limits or avoidance of eating contaminated fish caught from specific freshwater sources. Typically, fish that may have excessive levels of mercury include such species as trout, walleye, pike, muskie, and bass. Current state fish consumption advisories can be found on the US EPA Web site (www.epa.gov/OST/fish ).

## Frequently Asked Questions

Q  *My child swallowed the mercury from an oral thermometer. What do I do?*

A  Elemental mercury in these thermometers is poorly absorbed from the gastrointestinal tract (less than 1% of the amount) and will pass out of the body. No treatment is needed. However, fragments of broken glass are of greater concern for injury.

Q   *Can I throw away CFL or regular fluorescent bulbs?*

A   These light bulbs contain a small amount of mercury, much less than a fever thermometer. When they stop working, they should be taken to a hazardous waste recycler or retailer who can recycle them, typically a store that sells light bulbs. Handle the bulb(s) carefully so they do not break and release the mercury.

Q   *Should pregnant women, lactating women, or women planning pregnancy avoid eating fish?*

A   No known risk outweighs the benefit of eating seafood and fish. Both are sources of high-quality protein and beneficial omega-3 fatty acids. Current recommendations for pregnant women and young children include:

- Eat 8 to 12 ounces (227 to 340 g) (2 to 3 servings) of a variety of fish a week. For young children, the 2 or 3 servings should be the proper portion for age and calorie needs.

- Choose fish lower in mercury, such as salmon, shrimp, pollock, tuna (light, canned), tilapia, catfish, and cod.

- Avoid tilefish from the Gulf of Mexico, shark, swordfish, and king mackerel because they have the highest mercury levels.

- If you eat fish caught from streams, rivers, and lakes, pay attention to fish advisories on those waterbodies.

Scientific studies show that the beneficial effects of breastfeeding outweigh any potential neurotoxic effects on milestone development that could be due to the presence of contaminants (eg, mercury) in human milk.

Q   *Should my child have nonmercury fillings? Or, should mercury fillings be replaced?*

A   Mercury amalgams are a durable material for filling dental caries. There is no scientific evidence that this commonly used dental material causes harm to a child, although a small amount of mercury exposure may occur from the presence of dental amalgams. It is not necessary to replace amalgams just because of the mercury content; furthermore, the removal process may weaken the tooth.

Q   *Someone spilled some mercury at my child's school (or inside an occupied building). How should it be cleaned up?*

A   It is necessary to enlist a specialist's help to clean up even small mercury spills in schools and inside of buildings. Mercury should not be vacuumed or swept up because this may spread the mercury droplets and increase mercury vapor. Keep everyone out of the room where the mercury spilled. Children and pregnant women should not be allowed to help, and windows and doors in the affected rooms should be opened to the outside and closed off from other rooms. If the spilled amount is small, such as from a broken thermometer, it may be cleaned up using a damp rag or paper towels (see https://www.epa.gov/mercury/what-do-if-mercury-thermometer-breaks). If the amount of mercury appears to be more than 1 pound or 2 tablespoons (30 mL), the National Response Center (NRC) should be called for assistance. The NRC hotline operates 24 hours a day, 7 days a week. Call (800) 424-8802. The local health department may be able to assist.

Q   *I've heard that vaccines cause autism. Are they safe? Should I vaccinate my children?*

A   Thimerosal (containing ethylmercury) is added to 2 multi-dose vaccines as a preservative to prevent bacterial overgrowth. Thimerosal does not stay in the body a long time so it does not build up and reach harmful levels. When thimerosal enters the body, it breaks down to ethylmercury and thiosalicylate, which are readily eliminated. Measles, mumps, and rubella (MMR) vaccines do not and never did contain thimerosal. Varicella (chickenpox), inactivated polio (IPV), and pneumococcal conjugate vaccines also have never contained thimerosal. Influenza (flu) vaccines are currently available in both thimerosal-containing (for multi-dose vaccine vials) and thimerosal-free versions.

Vaccines do not cause autism. Many well-designed studies conducted by scientists from the Centers for Disease Control and Prevention (CDC) and by investigators outside of the CDC have not found that vaccines are associated with autism. Vaccines are rigorously tested for safety and effectiveness prior to being licensed and are continuously monitored for safety after licensure. Vaccines are among the safest medical products in use. All children should be vaccinated according to the Advisory Committee on Immunization Practices schedule so they are protected from vaccine preventable diseases that can cause illness, disability, and death.

## Resources

### Institute of Medicine
*Seafood Choices: Balancing Benefits and Risks*
Web site: https://www.nap.edu/catalog/11762/seafood-choices-balancing-benefits-and-risks

### Pediatric Environmental Health Specialty Units (PEHSUs)
Located in each of the 10 regions of the United States, PEHSUs are staffed with physicians trained in pediatrics, medical toxicology, and the Web site provides fact sheets and resources for questions about a host of environmental toxins. The Web site is: www.pehsu.net

**Poison Control Centers**

Available by telephone 24 hours daily, 7 days a week, poison control centers are staffed with health care professionals experienced in managing and advising about a wide range of poisonous and toxic substances, plants, and animals. The toll-free number is 1-800-222-1222.

**State and local public health and environmental agencies**

These agencies may be of assistance if a mercury spill occurs, if clinically significant poisoning is suspected, or to evaluate possible environmental exposure sources.

For elemental mercury spills of 1 pound (more than 2 tablespoons), the National Response Center should be contacted for assistance: 1-800-424-8802.

For questions about mercury toxicity, exposure, and clean-up of small spills, the poison control center (1-800-222-1222) and regional Pediatric Environmental Health Specialty Unit (www.pehsu.net) are good resources.

**US Environmental Protection Agency**

Web site: www.epa.gov/mercury

This Web site provides a wide array of information on mercury, including a link to state fish advisories, a list of consumer products that contain mercury, handouts about fish consumption advisories for pregnant women and children, and household hazardous waste collection centers that accept mercury-containing equipment and used fluorescent light bulbs.

**US Food and Drug Administration**

Web site: www.fda.gov/forconsumers/consumerupdates/ucm397443.htm

This Web site provides recent advice for consumers about health benefits of fish and fish to avoid because of higher mercury content.

Web site: www.fda.gov/BiologicsBloodVaccines/SafetyAvailability/VaccineSafety/UCM096228

This Web site provides details about preservatives in vaccines and lists thimerosal content in specific vaccines.

**World Health Organization**

*Children's Exposure to Mercury Compounds (2010)*

Web site: www.who.int/ceh/publications/children_exposure/en/index.html

# References

1. Food and Drug Administration. New Advice: pregnant women and young children should eat more fish. June 2014. http://www.fda.gov/forconsumers/consumerupdates/ucm397443.htm. Accessed January 19, 2018.

2. Smutna M, Kruziokova K, Marsaler P, Kopriva V, Svobodova Z. Fish oil and cod live as safe and healthy food supplements. *Neurendocrinol Lett.* 2009;30(Suppl 1):156–162

3. Maehre HK, Malde MK, Eilertsen KE, Elevoll EO. Characterization of protein, lipid and mineral contents in common Norwegian seaweeds and evaluation of their potential as food and feed. *J Sci Food Agric.* 2014;94(15):3281–3290

4. Clarkson TW, Magos L, Myers GJ. Human exposure to mercury: the three modern dilemmas. *J Trace Elem Exp Med.* 2003;16:321–343

5. Food and Drug Administration. Consumer Updates. Mercury Poisoning Linked to Skin Lightening Products. Updated July 12, 2016. https://www.fda.gov/ForConsumers/ConsumerUpdates/ucm294849.htm. Accessed January 19, 2018

6. Lynch E, Braithwaite R. A review of the clinical and toxicological aspects of 'traditional' (herbal) medicines adulterated with heavy metals. *Expert Opin Drug Saf.* 2005;4(4):769–778

7. Saper RB, Phillips RS, Sehgal A, et al. Lead, mercury, and arsenic in US- and Indian-manufactured Ayurvedic medicines sold via the Internet. *JAMA.* 2008;300(8):915–923

8. Zayas LH, Ozuah PO. Mercury use in espiritismo: a survey of botanicas. *Am J Public Health.* 1996;86(1):111–112

9. Clarkson TW. The pharmacology of mercury compounds. *Annu Rev Pharmacol.* 1972;12:375–406

10. National Research Council. *Toxicological Effects of Methylmercury.* Washington, DC: National Academies Press; 2000

11. Jaffe KM, Shurtleff DB, Robertson WO. Survival after acute mercury vapor poisoning. *Am J Dis Child.* 1983;137(8):749–751

12. Solis MT, Yuen E, Cortez PS, Goebel PJ. Family poisoned by mercury vapor inhalation. *Am J Emerg Med.* 2000;18(5):599–602

13. Taueg C, Sanfilippo DJ, Rowens B, Szejda J, Hesse JL. Acute and chronic poisoning from residential exposures to elemental mercury—Michigan, 1989–1990. *J Toxicol Clin Toxicol.* 1992;30(1):63–67

14. Fawer RF, deRibaupierre Y, Guillemin MP, Berode M, Lob M. Measurement of hand tremor induced by industrial exposure to metallic mercury. *Br J Ind Med.* 1983;40(2):204–208

15. Smith PJ, Langolf GD, Goldberg J. Effect of occupational exposure to elemental mercury on short term memory. *Br J Ind Med.* 1983;40(4):413–419

16. Forman J, Moline J, Cernichiari E, et al. A cluster of pediatric metallic mercury exposure cases treated with meso-2,3-dimercaptosuccinic acid (DMSA). *Environ Health Perspect.* 2000;108(6):575–577

17. Agner E, Jans H. Mercury poisoning and nephrotic syndrome in two young siblings. *Lancet.* 1978;2(8096):951

18. Tubbs RR, Gephardt GN, McMahon JT, et al. Membranous glomerulonephritis associated with industrial mercury exposure. Study of pathogenetic mechanisms. *Am J Clin Pathol.* 1982;77(4):409–413

19. Edlich RF, Greene JA, Cochran AA, et al. Need for informed consent for dentists who use mercury amalgam restorative material as well as technical considerations in removal of dental amalgam restorations. *J Environ Pathol Toxicol Oncol.* 2007;26(4):305–322

20. Brownawell AM, Berent S, Brent RL, et al. The potential adverse health effects of dental amalgam. *Toxicol Rev.* 2005;24(1):1–10

21. Mitchell RJ, Osborne PB, Haubenreich JE. Dental amalgam restorations: daily mercury dose and biocompatibility. *J Long Term Eff Med Implants.* 2005;15(6):709–721

22. DeRouen TA, Martin MD, Leroux BG, et al. Neurobehavioral effects of dental amalgam in children: a randomized clinical trial. *JAMA.* 2006;295(15):1784–1792

23. Bellinger DC, Trachtenberg F, Daniel D, Tavares MA, McKinlay S. A dose-effect analysis of children's exposure to dental amalgam and neuropsychological function: the New England Children's Amalgam Trial. *J Am Dent Assoc.* 2007;138(9):1210–1216

24. Bellinger DC, Caniel C, Trachtenberg F, Tavares M, McKinlay S. Dental amalgam restorations and children's neuropsychological function: the New England Children's Amalgam Trial. *Environ Health Perspect.* 2007;115(3):440–446

25. Cheek DB. Acrodynia. In: Kelley V, ed. *Brenneman's Practice of Pediatrics.* Vol I. New York, NY: Harper and Row Publishers; 1977;17D:1–12

26. Warkany J. Acrodynia—postmortem of a disease. *Am J Dis Child.* 1966;112(2):147–156

27. Gotelli CA, Astolfi E, Cox C, Cernichiari E, Clarkson TW. Early biochemical effects of an organic mercury fungicide on infants: "dose makes the poison." *Science.* 1985;227(4687):638–640

28. Agocs MM, Etzel RA, Parrish RG, et al. Mercury exposure from interior latex paint. *N Engl J Med.* 1990;323(16):1096–1101

29. van der Linde AA, Lewiszong-Rutjens CA, Verrips A, Gerrits GP. A previously healthy 11-year-old girl with behavioural disturbances, desquamation of the skin and loss of teeth. *Eur J Pediatr.* 2009;168(4):509–511

30. Weinstein M, Bernstein S. Pink ladies: mercury poisoning in twin girls. *CMAJ.* 2003;168(2):201

31. Amin-Zaki L, Majeed MA, Elhassani SB, Clarkson TW, Greenwood MR, Doherty RA. Prenatal methylmercury poisoning. Clinical observations over five years. *Am J Dis Child.* 1979;133(2):172–177

32. Debes F, Budtz-Jørgensen E, Weihe P, White RF, Grandjean P. Impact of prenatal methylmercury exposure on neurobehavioral function at age 14 years. *Neuroxicol Teratol.* 2006;28(3):363–375

33. Myers GJ, Davidson PW, Cox C, et al. Prenatal methylmercury exposure from ocean fish consumption in the Seychelles child development study. *Lancet.* 2003;361(9370):1686–1692

34. Axelrad DA, Bellinger DC, Ryan LM, Woodruff TJ. Dose-response relationship of prenatal mercury exposure and IQ; an integrative analysis of epidemiologic data. *Environ Health Perspect.* 2007;115(4):609–615

35. Debes F. Weihe P, Grandjean P. Cognitive deficits at age 22 years associated with prenatal exposure to methylmercury. *Cortex.* 2016;74:358–369

36. Strain JJ, Yeates AJ, van Wijngaarden E, et al. Prenatal exposure to methyl mercury from fish consumption and polyunsaturated fatty acids: associations with child development at 20 mo of age in an observational study in the Republic of Seychelles. *Am J Clin Nutr.* 2015;101(3): 530–537

37. Caldwell KL, Mortensen ME, Jones RL, Caudill SP, Osterloh JD. Total blood mercury concentrations in the U.S. population: 1999-2006. *Int J Hyg Environ Health.* 2009;212(6): 588–598

38. Mortensen ME, Caudill SP, Caldwell KL, Ward CD, Jones RL. Total and methyl mercury in whole blood measured for the first time in the U.S. population: NHANES 2011-2012. *Environ Res.* 2014;134:257–264

39. Axton JH. Six cases of poisoning after a parenteral organic mercurial compound (Merthiolate). *Postgrad Med J.* 1972;48(561):417–421

40. Fagan DG, Pritchard JS, Clarkson TW, Greenwood MR. Organ mercury levels in infants with omphaloceles treated with organic mercurial antiseptic. *Arch Dis Child.* 1977;52(12):962–964

41. Lowell JA, Burgess S, Shenoy S, Peters M, Howard TK. Mercury poisoning associated with hepatitis-B immunoglobulin. *Lancet.* 1996;347(8999):480

42. Matheson DS, Clarkson TW, Gelfand EW. Mercury toxicity (acrodynia) induced by long-term injection of gammaglobulin. *J Pediatr.* 1980;97(1):153–155

43. Pfab R, Muckter H, Roider G, Zilker T. Clinical course of severe poisoning with thimerosal. *J Toxicol Clin Toxicol.* 1996;34(4):453–460

44. Rohyans J, Walson PD, Wood GA, MacDonald WA. Mercury toxicity following merthiolate ear irrigations. *J Pediatr.* 1984;104(2):311–313

45. Institute of Medicine. Immunization Safety Committee. Immunization Safety Review: Vaccines and Autism. 2004. http://www.nap.edu/catalog/10997/immunization-safety-review-vaccines-and-autism. Accessed January 19, 2018

46. Thompson WW, Price C, Goodson, et al. Early thimerosal exposure and neuropsychological outcomes at 7 to 10 years. *N Engl J Med.* 2007;357(13):1281–1292

47. Parker SK, Schwartz B, Todd J, Pickering LK. Thimerosal-containing vaccines and autistic spectrum disorder: a critical review of published original data. *Pediatrics.* 2004;114(3):793–804

48. Stehr-Green P, Tull P, Stellfeld M, Mortenson PB, Simpson D. Autism and thimerosal-containing vaccines: lack of consistent evidence for an association. *Am J Prev Med.* 2003;25(2):101–106

49. Madsen KM, Lauritsen MB, Pedersen CB, et al. Thimerosal and the occurrence of autism: negative ecological evidence from Danish population-based data. *Pediatrics.* 2003;112(3 Pt 1): 604–606

50. Hviid A, Stellfeld M, Wohlfahrt J, Melbye M. Association between thimerosal-containing vaccine and autism. *JAMA.* 2003;290(13):1763–1766

51. Heron J, Golding J, ALSPAC Study Team. Thimerosal exposure in infants and developmental disorders: a prospective cohort study in the United Kingdom does not support a causal association. *Pediatrics.* 2004;114(3):577–583

52. Andrews N, Miller E, Grant A, Stowe J, Osborne V, Taylor B. Thimerosal exposure in infants and developmental disorders: a retrospective cohort study in the United Kingdom does not support a causal association. *Pediatrics.* 2004;114(3):584–591

53. Price CS, Thompson WW, Goodson B, et al. Prenatal and infant exposure to thimerosal from vaccines and immunoglobulins and risk of autism. *Pediatrics.* 2010;126(4):656–664

54. Godlee F, Smith J, Marcovitch H. Wakefield's article linking MMR vaccine and autism was fraudulent. *BMJ.* 2011;342:c7452

55. Centers for Disease Control and Prevention. *The Fourth National Report on Human Exposure to Environmental Chemicals, Updated Tables, March 2018.* http://www.cdc.gov/biomonitoring/pdf/FourthReport_UpdatedTables_Mar2018.pdf. Accessed September 1, 2018

56. Bornhorst JA, Hunt JW, Urry FM, McMillin GA. Comparison of sample preparation methods for clinical trace element analysis by inductively coupled plasma mass spectrometry. *Am J Clin Path.* 2005;123(4):578–583

57. Kershaw TB, Clarkson TW, Dharir PH. The relationship between blood levels and dose of methylmercury in man. *Arch Environ Health.* 1980;35(1):28–36

58. Nuttall KL. Interpreting hair mercury levels in individual patients. *Ann Clin Lab Sci.* 2006;36(3):248–261

59. Tominack R, Weber J, Blume C, et al. Elemental mercury as an attractive nuisance: multiple exposures from a pilfered school supply with severe consequences. *Pediatr Emerg Care.* 2002;18(2):97–100

60. Anderson O, Aaseth J. A review of pitfalls and progress in chelation treatment of metal poisonings. *J Trace Elem Med Biol.* 2016;38:74–80

61. Myers SM, Johnson CP, American Academy of Pediatrics Council on Children with Disabilities. Management of children with autism spectrum disorders. *Pediatrics.* 2007;120(5):1162–1182

# Chapter 34

# Nitrates and Nitrites in Water

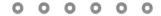

## KEY POINTS

- Nitrate and nitrite are found in some drinking water, vegetables, cured meats, fish, dairy products, beers, and cereals.
- Drinking water is the main source of nitrate for infants.
- Ingestion by infants of water containing high amounts of nitrate can cause methemoglobinemia, a condition that may result in fatality.
- To help prevent methemoglobinemia, pediatricians should recommend that families who drink well water test their water for nitrates before or shortly after a baby's birth.
- Well water with high nitrate levels should not be given to infants younger than age 1 year and should not be used to prepare infant formula or to reconstitute juice.

## INTRODUCTION

Nitrate ($NO_3^-$) and nitrite ($NO_2^-$) are natural oxidation products of nitrogen. Nitrogen is the most abundant gas in the atmosphere. The environment processes nitrogen through the nitrogen cycle. A relatively inert gas, nitrogen must be reduced to be usable by plants or animals. Nitrogen that has been reduced is also called fixed nitrogen. The nitrogen cycle describes how the environment processes nitrogen through atmospheric conditions, specific nitrogen-fixing bacteria, animal waste, and decomposition into ammonia, nitrite, and nitrate. Plants absorb and incorporate the essential nutrient nitrogen from the nitrate or ammonium in the soil. These natural sources fix between 100 to 300 teragrams (Tg, a unit of mass equal to $10^{12}$ [one trillion] grams) of nitrogen per year. The mass of reactive nitrogen passing through the nitrogen cycle has dramatically increased in the last 100 years.[1] Prior to the development of the Haber-Bosch process to convert atmospheric nitrogen into ammonia in the early 1900s, human agricultural activities produced about 15 Tg of reactive nitrogen per year.[2] Total agricultural and natural nitrogen increased from 155 to 345 Tg between 1900 and 2000.[3] Most of this reactive nitrogen is used as nitrogen fertilizers in agriculture. Other sources, such as clearing forests and grasslands for agricultural purposes, burning of biomass fuels, and increasing use of nitrogen-fixing plants contribute to this total.[1] Increased urbanization and modern agricultural activities have increased nitrate contamination of water and food supplies. Nitrogen fertilizers, intensive livestock operations, substandard septic systems, and municipal wastewater treatment discharges increase nitrate concentrations in some surface waters and ground waters.[4] These sources run off or leak into the water supply used for drinking and watering plants used for food. Surface water contamination with nitrate and nitrite often fluctuates according to the timing of precipitation. Well water, however, often demonstrates stable levels of contamination because the well typically taps into a relatively static reservoir.

Researchers and public health officials began to associate the ingestion of nitrate and nitrite with severe illness in the late 1940s and 1950s.[5,6] Physicians diagnosed children with cyanosis as "blue babies." Many of these children were found to have elevated levels of modified hemoglobin called methemoglobin. Physicians, researchers, and public health officials attributed the illness to the presence of elevated nitrate and/or nitrite in contaminated drinking water.[7] Nitrate can be reduced to nitrite, which oxidizes hemoglobin into methemoglobin. Gastrointestinal tract infections or genetic diseases can also result in methemoglobin formation in infants without exposure to high nitrate concentrations from drinking water or foods.[8] Methemoglobinemia is, therefore, often a multifactorial illness with contributions from an external exposure, genetic susceptibility, developmental stage, and inflammatory and endogenous production of nitrogen oxides.

Trends in agriculture have increased the amount of nitrate in our drinking water resources. For example, throughout the Midwestern United States, farmers have installed drainage tiling into swamplands and wetlands. Swamplands, wetlands, and other riparian (ie, relating to or situated on river banks) areas stored, filtered, and slowly released excessive rainfalls into the streams. Much of the drainage tiling was installed through support from the federal government in the early 1900s, but still continues today.[9] Drainage tile speeds the movement of water to streams and rivers and lowers the local water table. In addition to the installation of tiling, farmers have removed riparian land and often plant up to the edge of waterways. These trends have markedly decreased the land's ability to store and filter rainfall.

The combination of tiling and encroachment into riparian lands increases short-term productivity on farmland, but also increases the speed of the runoff of soil, nutrients, and chemicals applied to the land. Since the mid-1900s, modern agricultural activities, such as using nitrogen fertilizers and concentrating animal feeding operations, contribute to elevated nitrate concentrations not only in drinking water but also in local bodies of water, rivers, and streams. The nitrogen and nitrate stimulate rapid growth of algae and other plant life in these water systems. This algae and plant life dies off at the end of their growth cycle, sinks to the bottom of the water, and decomposes. The decomposition consumes large amounts of oxygen from the water and creates hypoxic areas, called "dead zones," that cannot support normal aquatic life.[10,11] These "dead zones" occur in small farm ponds and larger bodies of water, such as the Gulf of Mexico. The Mississippi River/Gulf of Mexico Watershed Nutrient (Hypoxia) Task Force tracks the area of hypoxia each year. In 2015, the area of hypoxia was 6,474 square miles (42,667 square kilometers) and had a 5-year average of more than 5,500 square miles (14,245 square kilometers).[12] This matches the size of the state of Connecticut.

Nitrate concentrations in the US water supply have generally increased.[13] The US Environmental Protection Agency (EPA) has published maximum contaminant levels (MCL) for public water supplies for nitrate (10 mg/L as nitrate-nitrogen [N] and nitrite [1 mg/L nitrite-N]).[13] Nationwide, concentrations of nitrate exceeded the MCL of 10 mg/L in approximately 7% of domestic wells tested and were more likely to occur in agricultural areas. Nitrate exceedances in the MCL in public-supply wells were less common (3%).[13] In the United States, current data suggest that groundwater nitrate concentrations greater than 5 mg/L (half of the MCL) range from 0% to 53% of the area in states across the nation.[13] A 1998 study in North Carolina sampled 1,600 wells in 15 counties where concentrated animal feeding operations were located. The samples contained nitrate concentrations above the recommended MCL in 10.2% of the wells.[14] Nitrate and nitrite in drinking water are often markers of other contamination, typically of agricultural origin, including fecal coliform bacteria and pesticides.

## ROUTES AND SOURCES OF EXPOSURE

Ingestion of nitrate- and/or nitrite-containing products is the primary route of exposure. Nitrite is oxidized into nitrate in the aerobic and bacterial conditions found in most water, making nitrate the product primarily consumed.[15] Nitrate is rapidly absorbed in the proximal small intestine. More than 70% of ingested nitrate is excreted in the urine in less than 24 hours. Approximately 25% of the ingested nitrate enters the saliva and is reduced by bacteria to nitrite. The nitrite is then rapidly absorbed into the blood in the small intestine. Nitrite exposed to acidic gastric conditions generates nitrosating agents that react with nitrosatable compounds, especially secondary amines and amides. This series of reactions may result in the generation of mutagenic N-nitroso compounds.

Nitrate and nitrite are found in some drinking water, vegetables, cured meats, fish, dairy products, beers, and cereals. Drinking water is the main source of nitrate for infants. A report from the American Academy of Pediatrics includes recommendations about drinking well water.[16] Breast feeding effectively reduces nitrate exposure.[17] Mothers do not produce breast milk with high nitrate concentrations even when ingesting nitrate-contaminated water.

Infants are at highest risk for the development of methemoglobinemia when caregivers feed infants formula made from contaminated water. The gastric pH of infants is higher than that of older children. Although this pH is likely to allow more nitrite to be oxidized to nitrate, it also may allow for a larger number of anaerobic bacteria higher in the gut. The anaerobic bacteria reduce the nitrate into nitrite. Gastrointestinal tract infection, diarrhea, and/or vomiting can lead to anaerobic conditions that increase the amount of nitrite available for absorption and are likely a major risk factor for methemoglobinemia. Infants aged younger than 6 months demonstrate lower amounts and activity of cytochrome-$b5$ reductase (also known as methemoglobin reductase), the enzyme that regenerates hemoglobin from methemoglobin. Infants, especially young infants, often still have fetal hemoglobin that is more susceptible to oxidation than other forms of hemoglobin. Infants younger than age 6 months are, therefore, at increased risk; those younger than age 1 month are at highest risk.

## SYSTEMS AFFECTED

Nitrate and nitrite are absorbed through the gastrointestinal tract and primarily affect the hematologic system in infants and children. Nitrate can be converted into nitrite by oral bacteria and gut flora. The oxidation of ferrous iron ($Fe^{+2}$) in hemoglobin to ferric iron ($Fe^{+3}$) by nitrite results in methemoglobin, which is incapable of carrying oxygen. The build-up of methemoglobin causes the majority of acute clinical effects.

## CLINICAL EFFECTS

Methemoglobinemia generally presents with few clinical signs other than cyanosis. Cyanosis and the early warning signs may be less obvious following a large ingestion of sodium or potassium nitrate salts. Methemoglobin is dark brown and causes cyanosis at concentrations as low as 3%. The symptoms increase in severity as the concentration of methemoglobin increases. The mucous membranes of infants with methemoglobinemia-induced cyanosis tend to have a brownish cast. The brown discoloration increases with the concentration of methemoglobin, as do irritability, tachypnea, altered mental status, and complaints of headache in older children. A methemoglobin concentration of greater than 25% in older children may cause headache, dyspnea, syncope, confusion, and/or palpitations. Methemoglobin concentrations of greater than 50% may result in cardiac dysrhythmias, metabolic acidosis, and/or death.

Nitrate and/or nitrite ingestion may contribute to other medical conditions that cause methemoglobinemia. Gastrointestinal tract infections, decreased enzymatic activity, inherited hemoglobin M trait, or other oxidant ingestion can cause methemoglobinemia apart from nitrate exposure. In addition, genetic variability results in various enzymatic concentrations. For example, the Blue Fugates, a small and relatively isolated community in Kentucky, and other select groups may have reduced enzymatic activity that increases their risk for the development of methemoglobinemia.[18,19] Drinking water with high concentrations of nitrate can exacerbate these conditions and result in methemoglobinemia. Research on the effects of nitrate exposure also has focused on effects of chronic exposure. The International Agency for Research on Cancer (IARC) reviewed the evidence associating the development of cancer with chronic ingestion of nitrate- or nitrite-containing substances. The IARC determined that nitrate or nitrite is "probably carcinogenic to humans" (Group 2A) when ingested under conditions that can generate $N$-nitroso compounds. Some of the $N$-nitroso compounds that could be formed are known human carcinogens.[20]

Chronic exposure to elevated concentrations of nitrate in drinking water supplies and, therefore, of $N$-nitroso compounds, has been thought to impact thyroid and steroid hormone homeostasis with adverse effects on development and reproduction.[15,21] Associations have been found between birth defects and high nitrate concentrations in water supplies.[22,23] Reports from Indiana (1991–1993) described 3 women who experienced a total of 6 spontaneous abortions; the women resided in proximity to each other and consumed drinking water from private wells containing high concentrations of nitrate.[24] Increasing concentrations of nitrate in drinking water also have been associated with an increasing risk of neural tube defects.[25–27]

## DIAGNOSTIC METHODS

The diagnostic evaluation of a child with suspected methemoglobinemia is similar to an evaluation for cyanosis.[28] In the absence of respiratory symptoms, history of cardiovascular disease, abnormal pulse, or abnormal oximetry, a diagnosis of methemoglobinemia should be considered in a child who becomes cyanotic and unresponsive to oxygen administration. Urgent supportive therapy may be necessary in cases of severe cyanosis. Arterial blood gases and pulse oximetry assist with the methemoglobin evaluation. A complete blood count with differential, peripheral blood smear, and reticulocyte count are used to evaluate the cause of the cyanosis. These tests evaluate for hemoglobinopathies, anemias, or thalassemias. Bilirubin, lactate dehydrogenase, serum haptoglobin, free serum hemoglobin, and Heinz body preparation evaluate for end organ dysfunction and/or hemolytic anemia. A chest x-ray, echocardiogram, and/or electrocardiogram may be indicated to assess cardiac and pulmonary function. The necessity of these tests is based on clinical presentation.

## TREATMENT OF CLINICAL SYMPTOMS

Health care professionals who suspect that a child has methemoglobinemia should consult with a poison control center or a toxicologist to help guide management. An asymptomatic child with cyanosis who has a methemoglobin concentration of less than 20% usually requires no treatment other than identifying and eliminating the source of exposure. For methemoglobin concentrations greater than 30%, methylene blue and 100% oxygen are therapeutic antidotes. Methylene blue acts as an electron carrier for the hexose monophosphate alternate pathway that reduces methemoglobin to hemoglobin. The cyanosis should rapidly respond to the methylene blue.

Exchange transfusions, packed red blood cells, and/or hyperbaric oxygen therapies are second-line treatments. These may be used when methylene blue is unsuccessful. Patients with erythrocyte glucose-6-phosphate dehydrogenase (G6PD) or nicotinamide adenine dinucleotide phosphate (NADPH) reductase deficiency should not receive methylene blue. Both a G6PD and a NADPH reductase deficiency can result in methemoglobinemia but through a different enzymatic pathway than the cytochrome-$b5$ reductase pathway. Methemoglobinemia caused by the ingestion of aniline dye or dapsone also may be refractory to methylene blue therapy.

## PREVENTION OF EXPOSURE

Prenatal and newborn care for families with private wells should include a recommendation for testing well water nitrate contamination and safety.[8] Water testing for nitrate, pesticides, and fecal coliforms can be performed by any reference or public health laboratory using US EPA-approved laboratory methods.

Water with elevated nitrate concentrations should not be ingested by infants aged younger than 1 year or used to prepare infant formula. Well waters with high nitrate concentrations typically have elevated concentrations of various pesticides and fecal coliform bacteria. Care must be taken when boiling water before mixing formula because this may concentrate nitrate and other chemical contaminants. Boiling water for 1 minute generally is sufficient to kill microorganisms without causing overconcentration of nitrate and other chemical contaminants. Water softeners and charcoal filters do not reduce nitrate concentration; however, reverse osmosis and ion exchange resins are able to remove nitrate from drinking water.

If methemoglobinemia has been diagnosed, the clinical team must identify and eliminate the exogenous sources of exposure because clinical treatment alone is insufficient to treat methemoglobinemia. The family residence, occupation of parents, drinking water sources, foods ingested, topical medications, and/or folk remedies may contribute to nitrate exposure. In addition, children with gastrointestinal tract infections, diarrhea, dehydration, metabolic acidosis, and some inherited conditions may be more vulnerable to nitrate exposures.

Reports of methemoglobinemia that are the result of nitrate exposure are scarce in areas that enforce appropriate drinking water regulations.

## FREQUENTLY ASKED QUESTIONS

Q  *Do commercial treatment systems sufficiently protect against nitrate contamination?*

A  Water softeners and charcoal filters do not significantly reduce nitrate concentrations. Reverse-osmosis systems and ion exchange resins do remove nitrate but are expensive.

Q  *Is low-grade nitrate contamination a risk for cancer?*

A  We do not know for sure. Published studies of exposure to nitrate in drinking water and cancer risk are not all in agreement, but the International Agency for Research on Cancer has determined that ingesting nitrate under conditions that are likely to increase formation of endogenous *N*-nitroso compounds probably increases the risk for cancer. Although health benefits have been seen in diets that include recommended intake levels of nitrate-rich vegetables, high intake of preserved meats (ie, bacon, hot dogs, ham) can lead to higher nitrate levels and increase the risk for formation of nitrosamines.

Q  *Are the current maximum contaminant levels sufficiently strict to protect the population?*

A  Most of the population is protected from methemoglobinemia or other potential adverse effects of nitrate at current maximum contaminant levels. The US EPA's drinking water standards for nitrate (10 parts per million) and nitrite (1 part per million) are designed to protect the health even of people who are considered most susceptible. These standards only apply, however, to public water supplies and not to water from private wells.

Q  *Should I have my well water tested? How often?*

A  Indications for testing a well include having a new baby, recent damage to the well, or living in a neighborhood where there is known well water nitrate contamination. Families with private wells should have them tested for nitrates and coliform bacteria on a yearly basis. Risk factors for increased nitrate contamination include shallow well depth, local cropland treated with nitrogen fertilizers, and local animal operations that contribute to regional nitrate contamination. Collect the sample during wet weather (late spring and early summer), when runoff and excess soil moisture carry contaminants into shallow groundwater sources or through defects in your well. Do not test during dry weather or when the ground is frozen.

Q  *I have a young baby and will be staying in a vacation home for a few weeks. I do not know whether the well has been tested. Can I give my baby the well water?*

A  The well water should be tested before being offered to an infant. If this is not possible, it may be safer and more convenient to use bottled water for the baby and others staying in the vacation home.

## REFERENCES

1. Zerkle AL, Mikhail S. The geobiological nitrogen cycle: from microbes to the mantle. *Geobiology*. 2017;15(3):343–352

2. Fields S. Global nitrogen: cycling out of control. *Environ Health Perspect*. 2004;112(10): A556–A563

3. Bouwman AF, Beusen AH, Griffioen J, et al. Global trends and uncertainties in terrestrial denitrification and $N_2O$ emissions. *Philos Trans R Sco Lond B Biol Sci*. 2013;386(1621):20130112

4. Wick K, Heumesser C, Schmid E. Groundwater nitrate contamination: factors and indicators. *J Environ Manage*. 2012;111:178–186

5. Bosch H, Rosenfield AB, Huston R, Shipman HR, Woodward FL. Methemoglobinemia and Minnesota well supplies. *J Am Water Works Assoc*. 1950;42(2):161–170

6. Walton G. Survey of literature relating to infant methemoglobinemia due to nitrate-contaminated water. *Am J Public Health Nations Health*. 1951;41(8 Pt 1):986–996

7. Knobeloch L, Salna B, Hogan A, Postle J, Anderson H. Blue babies and nitrate-contaminated well water. *Environ Health Perspect*. 2000;108(7):675–678

8. Greer FR, Shannon M, American Academy of Pediatrics Committee on Nutrition, American Academy of Pediatrics Committee on Environmental Health. Infant methemoglobinemia: the role of dietary nitrate in food and water. *Pediatrics*. 2005;116(3):784–786

9. Kalita PK, et al. Subsurface drainage and water quality: the Illinois experience. Transactions of the ASABE. 2007;50(5):1651–1656. http://elibrary.asabe.org/abstract.asp?aid=23963&t=2& redir=&redirType. Accessed July 3, 2018

10. Rabalais NN, Turner RE, Wiseman WJ. Hypoxia in the Gulf of Mexico. *J Environ Qual*. 2001;30(2):320–329

11. National Oceanic and Atmospheric Administration. 2015 Gulf of Mexico dead zone 'above average.' 2015. http://www.noaanews.noaa.gov/stories2015/080415-gulf-of-mexico-dead-zone-above-average.html. Accessed May 25, 2018

12. Louisiana Universities Marine Consortium. How is hypoxia mapped in the summer? 2015. http://www.gulfhypoxia.net/Research/Shelfwide%20Cruises/. Accessed May 25, 2018

13. Dubrovsky NM, Burow KR, Clark GM, et al. The quality of our Nation's waters. Nutrients in the Nation's Streams and Groundwater, 1992–2004. U.S. Geological Survey Circular 1350. https://pubs.usgs.gov/circ/1350/pdf/circ1350.pdf. Accessed May 25, 2018

14. Barros N, Rudo K, Shehee M. Importance of regular testing of private drinking water systems in North Carolina. *NC Med J.* 2014;75(6):429–434

15. U.S. Department of Health and Human Services. Agency for Toxic Substances and Disease Registry. Toxicologial profile for nitrate and nitrite. 2017. https://www.atsdr.cdc.gov/ToxProfiles/tp204.pdf. Accessed May 25, 2018

16. Rogan WJ, Brady MT, American Academy of Pediatrics Committee on Environmental Health, Committee on Infectious Diseases. Drinking water from private wells and risks to children. *Pediatrics.* 2009;123(6):e1123–e1137

17. Dusdieker LB, Stumbo PJ, Kross BC, Dungy CI. Does increased nitrate ingestion elevate nitrate levels in human milk? *Arch Pediatr Adoles Med.* 1996;150(3):311–314

18. Fermo E, Bianchi P, Vercellati C, et al. Recessive hereditary methemoglobinemia: two novel mutations in the NADH-cytochrome b5 reductase gene. *Blood Cells Mol Dis.* 2008;41(1):50–55

19. Trost C. The blue people of Troublesome Creek. *Science.* 1982;82:35–39

20. International Agency for Research on Cancer. Ingested Nitrate and Nitrite, and Cyanobacterial Peptide Toxins. IARC Monographs on Evaluation of Carcinogenic Risks to Humans, 2010. Volume 94

21. Poulsen R, Cedergreen N, Hayes T, Hansen M. Nitrate: An environmental endocrine disruptor? A review of the evidence and research needs. *Environ Sci Technol.* 2018;52(7):3869–3887

22. Croen LA, Todoroff K, Shaw GM. Maternal exposure to nitrate from drinking water and diet and risk for neural tube defects. *Am J Epidemiol.* 2001;153(4):325–331

23. Brender JD, Weyer PJ. Agricultural compounds in water and birth defects. *Curr Environ Health Rep.* 2016;3(2):144–152

24. Centers for Disease Control and Prevention. Spontaneous abortions possibly related to ingestion of nitrate-contaminated well water—LaGrange County, Indiana, 1991-1994. *MMWR Morb Mortal Wkly Rep.* 1996;45(26):569–572

25. Croen LA, Todoroff K, Shaw GM. Maternal exposure to nitrate from drinking water and diet and risk for neural tube defects. *Am J Epidemiol.* 2001;153(4):325–331

26. Brender JD, Olive JM, Felkner M, Suarez L, Marckwardt W, Hendricks KA. Dietary nitrites and nitrates, nitrosatable drugs, and neural tube defects. *Epidemiology.* 2004;15(3):330–336

27. Brender JD, Weyer PJ, Romitti PA, et al. Prenatal nitrate intake from drinking water and selected birth defects in offspring of participants in the national birth defects prevention study. *Environ Health Perspect.* 2013;121(9):1083–1089

28. Cortazzo JA, Lichtman AD. Methemoglobinemia: a review and recommendations for management. *J Cardiothoracic Vasc Anesth.* 2014;28(4):1043–1047

Chapter 35

# Noise

○ ○ ○ ○ ○ ○

## KEY POINTS

- Noise is defined as unwanted or disturbing sound.
- Excessive noise exposure often is unrecognized as an individual and public health problem.
- Noise can affect hearing, learning, result in a physiologic stress response, and cause psychological harm.
- Damage to hearing accumulates; noise exposures starting earlier in life are potentially more harmful as people age.
- Environmental modifications and behavioral interventions can mitigate noise exposure in some hospital settings.
- Pediatricians should add excessive noise, such as from headphones used with smartphones and tablets, to their list of modifiable environmental exposures to discuss with children and families.

## INTRODUCTION

Noise is usually defined as any "unwanted or disturbing sound."[1] Acoustic signals that produce a pleasant sensation are generally called "sound" whereas unpleasant sounds are called "noise."

Sound consists of waves that exert pressure on air and objects such as the tympanic membrane. Sound has frequency (pitch), intensity (loudness), periodicity, and duration.[2] The frequency of sound is measured in cycles per second and is expressed in hertz (Hz) (1 Hz = 60 cycles per second). People respond to frequencies ranging from 20 to 20,000 Hz but are most sensitive to sounds in the range of 500 to 3,000 Hz, the band of frequencies that includes human speech.

The loudness (or pressure) of sound waves is measured in pascals (Pa) or decibels (dB, a tenth of a bel). The range of sound limits in human hearing is 0.00002 Pa (the weakest sound that a keen human adult ear can detect under quiet conditions) to 200 Pa (the pressure causing pain in the adult ear). The dB scale, a logarithmic scale, is a method of compressing this range by expressing the ratio of one sound energy level to another. The unit most commonly used is dB SPL, indicating that the ratio of sound pressure levels (SPL) is being used. The loudness of human speech is approximately 50 dB SPL.

The perceived loudness of sound varies with the frequency. For example, to match the perceived loudness of a 40 dB SPL 1,000-Hz tone requires more than 80 dB SPL at 50 Hz and more than 60 dB SPL at 10,000 Hz. The 40 dB SPL equivalency curve is used to determine the measure of sound intensity, referred to as the decibel weighted by the A scale (dBA). Periodicity refers to either continuous sound or impulse sound. Duration is the total length of time of exposure to sound. Reviews of sound characteristics and hearing are available.[3,4] Noise pollution is common: vehicular traffic, railways, airplanes and airports, industrial sites, and leaf blowers contribute to widespread environmental noise exposure. Indoor sources include video games, toys, and appliances. Temporary or permanent damage to hearing can occur after exposure to loud noises. Damage to hearing can occur after exposure to less loud noises experienced over a long period of time. Some noises, such as snoring, barking, or nearby conversations, are not loud enough to damage hearing but may cause annoyance resulting in adverse health effects. Although often ignored or considered as merely a nuisance, these noises can interfere with normal activities, such as sleep and conversation, thereby disrupting or lessening quality of life.[1]

Traditionally, the main focus of preventing adverse effects of noise has been in adult occupational or military settings. Although there is a smaller research base about noise effects on children compared with the research base in adults,[5] it is increasingly evident that infants, children, and adolescents face risks from multiple sources of noise. Children may be more vulnerable to noise because of effects on developing cognition and less control over their environments.[5] Damage to hearing accumulates; noise exposures starting in earlier life are potentially more harmful as people age.[6]

## ROUTES OF EXPOSURE

Sound waves enter the external auditory canal and vibrate the eardrum. This vibration, in turn, travels through the 3 ossicles of the middle ear (the malleus, incus, and stapes), in which the stapes vibrates the oval window, vibrating the fluid of the cochlea of the inner ear. Within the cochlea, the basilar membrane covers the organ of Corti, which is composed of hair cells. Each hair cell responds to a specific frequency of the vibration and converts this signal to a nerve impulse. The impulses, transmitted by auditory nerves, are interpreted as sound or noise by the brain. Loss of hearing originating in the external auditory canal, eardrum, ossicles, or middle ear is called conductive hearing loss and is usually treatable. Loss of hearing originating in the hair cells or sites within the central nervous system is called sensorineural hearing loss and is usually irreversible. A fixed number of cochlear hair cells is present at birth. If damaged, cochlear hair cells do not regenerate.[7] Hearing develops during fetal life with the cochlea and peripheral sensory end organs completing normal development by 24 weeks' gestation. The hearing threshold (the intensity at which sound is perceived) approaches a nearly adult level of 13.5 dB by 42 weeks' gestation. Sound is transmitted well to the uterus and the fetus can therefore be exposed to excessive sound.[2] Although sound vibration also may be transmitted to the body directly through the skin, this topic is not discussed here.

## SOURCES OF EXPOSURE

Even young children can be exposed to excessive noise in their environments. Infants often are exposed in hospital well baby nurseries and Neonatal Intensive Care Unit (NICU) settings. Environmental noise is one of many stresses experienced by NICU infants from sources such as phones, ventilators, infusion pumps, monitors, incubators, alarms, and air conditioning. An infant's own crying can be a significant source of noise because loud sounds are amplified in an incubator.[8] The NICU environment is generally louder than most homes or offices and contains disturbing noises of short duration and at irregular intervals. The American Academy of Pediatrics (AAP) recommends a maximum acceptable level of 45 decibels (dBA) for NICUs,[2] but sound levels there often exceed this recommendation.[9] For example, cardiorespiratory alarms increased sound levels to 73 dB, endotracheal suctioning to 68 dB, and phone ringing to 83 dB.[10] Excessive noise also is common in Pediatric Intensive Care Units (PICUs).[11]

In the home, infant sleep machines used to produce ambient noise to help infants sleep are recommended by popular Web sites[12] that parents may consult to help with sleep issues. Infant sleep machines often exceed current standards for ambient noise in nurseries. A study examining 14 infant sleep machines played at maximum level showed that 3 machines produced output levels of 85 dBA. If played for 8 hours, these levels exceed current occupational limits for accumulated noise exposure[13] and could damage an infant's hearing.

Older children and adolescents are at risk of increased exposure to noise related to their behaviors. Children can damage hearing by playing with firecrackers and cap pistols[14] that can produce noise levels of 134 dBA (Table 35-1).[15] Teenagers may not realize that they are susceptible to the adverse effects of excessive noise and that the results of such exposure can be permanent. Approximately 60% of teenagers and young adults exposed to sounds greater than 87 dBA did not consider the noise to be too loud.[16]

Portable listening devices (PLDs), popular among youth, can cause music-induced hearing loss because of high sound levels produced by prolonged or repeated exposures. A small but substantial group of adolescents using these devices are at risk of hearing loss through their regular listening habits.[17]

| Table 35-1. Average Peak Sound Levels for Selected Toys[a] | |
|---|---|
| TOY | PEAK NOISE LEVEL (dBA) |
| Music box | 79 |
| Toy mobile phone | 85 |
| Sit-on fire truck | 87 |
| Laser pistol | 87 |
| Musical telephone | 89 |
| Robot soldier | 94 |
| Pull turtle | 95 |
| Police machine gun | 110 |
| Cap gun fired without caps | 114 |
| Cap gun fired with caps | 134 |

[a] Adapted from the National Institute of Public Health Denmark.[15]
Abbreviation: dBA, decibels weighted by the A scale.

## CLINICAL EFFECTS

### Effects on Hearing

Susceptibility to noise-induced hearing loss is highly variable; although some individuals are able to tolerate high noise levels for prolonged periods, other people in the same conditions may lose some hearing.[18]

Noise exposure that causes trauma to the hair cells of the cochlea results in hearing loss. Prolonged exposure to sounds louder than 85 dBA is potentially injurious.[19] Continuous exposure to hazardous levels of noise tends to have its maximum effect in the high-frequency regions of the cochlea. Noise-induced hearing loss usually is most severe around 4,000 Hz, with downward extension toward speech frequencies with prolonged exposure. This pattern of loss of frequency perception is true regardless of the frequency of the noise exposure. Impulse noise is more harmful than continuous noise because it bypasses the body's natural protective reaction to noise, the dampening of the ossicles mediated by the facial nerve.[20]

Noise is the most common modifiable environmental cause of hearing loss among young and middle-aged adults;[6] hearing loss is prevalent in adults with nearly 1 in 4 (24%) showing evidence of sensorineural hearing loss. Almost 1 in 4 US adults reporting excellent or good hearing had audiometric evidence of hearing loss, indicating that hearing loss often is not recognized. Hearing loss, however, is the third most common chronic physical condition in the United States today and is twice as common as diabetes mellitus or cancer.[6]

Noise affects hearing in people of all ages. The US Centers for Disease Control and Prevention (CDC) reported that during the period of 2001 to 2008, 30 million Americans aged older than 12 years were estimated to have noise-induced hearing loss in both ears; 48 million had hearing loss in at least one ear. Approximately 2.5 million youths aged 12 to 19 years had tinnitus (the sensation of ringing, buzzing, or clicking often caused by noise exposure) during the period of 2005 to 2008;[21] an estimated 12.5% of children and adolescents aged 6 to 19 years (about 5.2 million) have suffered permanent damage to their hearing from excessive exposure to noise.[22] Small children also may be at risk: pediatricians in offices now witness even very young children intently viewing noisy videos on their parents' cell phones or tablets.

Exposure to loud noise may result in tinnitus and a temporary decrease in the sensitivity of hearing. This condition, called temporary noise-induced threshold shift (NITS), sometimes occurs after a lengthy flight or following a loud concert. This situation may last for several hours, depending on the degree of exposure but may become permanent depending on the severity and duration of noise exposure. The prevalence of NITS in one or both ears found in a large national study of children aged 6 to 19 years was 12.5% (or 5.2 million children affected).[23] Most children with NITS had an early phase of NITS in only 1 ear and involving only a single frequency. However, among children with NITS, 4.9% had moderate to profound NITS. Several smaller studies also have concluded that noise-induced hearing loss in youth is concerning.[7] Farm youth may have a particularly high frequency of hearing loss and NITS.[24] The average sound level at a music festival was 95 dBA, and 36% of surveyed attendees reported tinnitus after listening to the music.[25]

The consequences of episodes of NITS may be enormous if they progress to a persistent minimal sensorineural hearing loss. In school-aged children, even minimal sensorineural hearing loss has been associated with poor school performance and social and emotional dysfunction.[26] Small amounts of hearing loss can profoundly affect speech, comprehension, communication, learning, and social development. Without intervention, children with mild to moderate hearing loss generally do not perform as well as children with no hearing loss. This gap in school performance increases as children progress through their school careers.[22]

Preterm infants may be especially sensitive to sound: hearing impairment is diagnosed in 2% to 10% of preterm infants compared with 0.1% of the general pediatric population.[9] Infants in NICUs, however, have other risk factors for the development of hearing loss including asphyxia, development of intraventricular hemorrhage, elevated bilirubin levels, and exposure to aminoglycosides. No studies have directly examined the effects of NICU noise on hearing loss in preterm infants; more research is needed.[8]

Exposure to excessive noise during fetal life can lead to high-frequency hearing loss in children.[27,28] A study of more than 1 million Swedish women showed an association between occupational noise exposure during pregnancy and hearing dysfunction in their children.[29]

## Physiologic Effects

Activation of the hypothalamus-pituitary-adrenal (HPA) axis and the subsequent release of cortisol are a major component of the physiological stress response. Noise causes a stress response as evidenced by the release of cortisol. A study among adults suggested a modification of the normal circadian cortisol rhythm in relation to aircraft noise exposure.[30] Increasing evidence links alterations in the normal circadian cortisol rhythm with cardiovascular diseases and other negative outcomes. People chronically exposed to high levels of environmental noise have increased risks of cardiovascular diseases including myocardial infarction.[31] Noise pollution affects millions of people[1] and therefore is not only an environmental nuisance but also a threat to public health.

Noise contributes to sleep deprivation.[32,33] Noise levels at 40 to 45 dBA result in a 10% to 20% increase in awakening or arousal changes on electroencephalograms (EEGs). Noise levels at 50 dBA result in a 25% probability of arousal features on EEGs.[34] One in 3 people report being annoyed during the daytime and 1 in 5 report disturbed sleep because of traffic noise.[31]

In preterm babies in NICU settings, noise may cause hypoxia, apnea, changes in oxygen saturation, and elevated heart and respiratory rates leading to increased oxygen consumption, thereby diminishing the calories available for growth.[9] Noise can affect infant sleep.[8]

## Psychologic Effects

Exposure to moderate levels of noise can cause psychological stress.[35] Annoyance, including feelings of bother, interference with activity, and symptoms such as headache, tiredness, and irritability are common psychological reactions to noise. The degree of annoyance is related to the nature of the sound and individual tolerance. Intense noise can cause personality changes and a reduced ability to cope. Sudden, unexpected noise can cause a startle reaction, which may provoke physiological stress responses.

Work performance can be affected by noise. At low levels, it can improve the performance of simple tasks. However, noise may impair intellectual function and performance of complex tasks.

Ambient noise may negatively affect understanding of speech in the classroom. Guidelines for noise standards in permanent and relocatable classrooms have been published.[36] Guidelines on classroom noise that consider child age and vulnerable conditions were also proposed.[37] Vulnerable groups—those suspected of delayed speech processing in noise—need quieter environments.

## Burden of Disease From Noise Exposure

The World Health Organization (WHO) estimated the environmental burden of disease that is the result of environmental noise. This burden is expressed as disability-adjusted life years (DALYs). Disability-adjusted life years, based on a quantitative risk assessment, "are the sum of the potential years of life lost due to premature death and the equivalent years of "healthy" life lost by virtue of being in states of poor health or disability." The WHO examined evidence linking environmental noise and health effects, such as cardiovascular disease, cognitive impairment, sleep disturbance, tinnitus, and feelings of annoyance. The WHO conservatively estimated that DALYs lost from environmental noise were "61,000 years for ischemic heart disease, 45,000 years for cognitive impairment of children, 903,000 years for sleep disturbance, 22,000 years for tinnitus, and 654,000 years for annoyance in the European Union Member States and other western European countries." Their calculations signify that "at least 1 million healthy life years are lost every year from traffic-related noise in the western part of Europe. Sleep disturbance and annoyance, mostly related to road traffic noise, comprise the main burden of environmental noise."[31]

## DIAGNOSIS OF NOISE-INDUCED HEARING LOSS

Parental concern about a child's hearing, speech, or language delay indicates a need for further evaluation.[38] A child with 1 or more risk factors on a hearing risk assessment (such as prematurity warranting a NICU stay or a history of excessive noise exposure) should have ongoing developmentally appropriate hearing screening and at least 1 diagnostic audiology assessment by age 24 to 30 months. The typical finding in noise-induced hearing loss is a dip in hearing threshold around 4,000 Hz on an audiogram. Physicians in facilities that are unable to provide pure tone audiograms should refer their patients for evaluation. An audiologic evaluation, including pure tone audiometry, should be performed to determine whether there is hearing loss (induced by noise or resulting from other causes) in children who have no evidence of acute or serous otitis media but have a history of:

- Excessive environmental noise exposure, such as prolonged exposure to cap pistols or boom boxes
- Poor school performance
- Short attention span
- Complaining of ringing in the ears, a feeling of fullness in the ears, muffling of hearing, or difficulty in understanding speech
- Speech delay

The AAP recommends hearing screening for all newborn infants and periodic screening for every child through adolescence.[39,40]

## TREATMENT OF CLINICAL SYMPTOMS

Although noise-induced threshold shifts may be temporary, there is no known treatment to reverse noise-induced hearing loss. Children with hearing loss should have appropriate referrals to otolaryngologists and audiologists to determine the severity of their hearing loss and be fitted with personal amplification devices, as necessary. Categories of hearing loss (HL) are: 20 to 40 dB HL, mild hearing loss; 41 to 60 dB HL, moderate hearing loss; 61 to 90 dB HL, severe hearing loss; greater than 90 dB HL, profound hearing loss. Pediatricians should counsel children and teenagers who have hearing loss and their parents about ways to preserve existing hearing and prevent additional hearing loss.

## PREVENTION OF EXPOSURE

Noise exposure has been underemphasized as a serious public health environmental health threat, including as a health hazard to young people. A 2016 report from the National Academies of Sciences included a call to action for government agencies to strengthen efforts to collect, analyze, and disseminate population-based data on hearing loss in adults.[41] Because hearing damage accumulates over time, noise exposure beginning earlier in life has the potential of becoming more harmful as people age. One in 5 young adults aged 20 to 29 has evidence of hearing loss, suggesting the early-life interventions must be developed.[6]

Federal standards for permissible noise exposures in work settings take into account the loudness and time of exposure.[42] Employers are required to use administrative or engineering controls when employees are subjected to sound exceeding maximum levels, and to provide personal protective equipment if those controls fail. They also are required to administer a hearing conservation program whenever employee noise exposures equal or exceed an 8-hour time-weighted average of 85 dBA. Effectively using personal protective equipment, such as earplugs and earmuffs, and avoiding loud environments have been shown to prevent hearing loss.[43]

In contrast, there are no federal regulations about exposure to nonoccupational noise. In 1972, Congress passed the Noise Control Act, giving the US Environmental Protection Agency (EPA) a mandate to regulate environmental noise. The US EPA's Office of Noise Abatement of Control was established at that time but was closed in 1982. State and local governments now have the primary responsibility of responding to many noise pollution matters. These government regulations are needed to protect infants, children, adolescents, and adults from excessive noise.

A report issued by the US EPA in 1974 identified 70 dB over 24 hours (75 dB over 8 hours) as the average exposure limit for intermittent environmental noise. Guidelines for Community Noise issued in 1999 by the WHO recommended avoiding noise exposure levels that exceed 70 dBA over a 24-hour period or 85 dBA over a 1-hour period.[6]

Pediatricians can intervene to prevent and mitigate noise exposures. Sound reduction strategies have been proposed for NICU settings with the goal of reducing the sound reaching newborns' ears to less than 45 dB. These strategies include lowering sound levels for the entire NICU unit, placing infants in more "private" rooms to reduce environmental noise, and having them wear earmuffs or earplugs. Other criteria are to maintain a 50 dBA-equivalent noise level averaged over 1 hour for infants in hospital nurseries and NICUs.[44,45] These strategies aim to help reduce the stress experienced by the infant, thereby promoting growth and reducing adverse health outcomes.[9] One small randomized controlled trial of earplugs used in the NICU setting showed a trend toward better growth and cognition.[46] A quality improvement initiative targeting environmental and behavioral modifications resulted in decreased noise levels in 1 level 4 NICU.[47] Interventions for PICU settings, such as keeping doors to patient rooms closed, also have been suggested.[48] More research is needed in this area. Pediatricians in office settings can discuss excessive noise as hazardous but preventable exposures. Small children cannot remove themselves from noisy environments and therefore must rely on parents to do so although many parents may not understand the hazard. Children and teenagers also may not understand the hazard. Concrete suggestions include:

- Avoid loud noises, especially loud impulse noise, whenever possible.
- Avoid toys that make loud noise, especially cap pistols. If a toy seems too loud for a parent, then it likely is too loud for the child. A parent may put tape over the speakers or remove the batteries of toys already owned that are too loud.[49] (Currently, there is no regulation on the amount of noise toys

can make. Voluntary noise standards are enforced by the Consumer Product Safety Commission, at their discretion.)

■ Avoid the use of firecrackers to protect hearing and to avoid other injury.

■ Reduce the volume on televisions, computers, radios, and personal music devices (iPods, etc). Turn off televisions, computers, and radios when not in use.

■ Ask parents to help children protect their hearing by teaching them to turn the volume down and take listening breaks. Parents can aim to model good listening habits.[50]

■ Protect infants and young children when they are taken to concerts and sporting events with their parents or other caregivers.

■ Use headphones and earbuds with caution. The volume level of the radio or personal digital player should be low enough so that normal conversation can still be heard.

■ When flying in a plane or riding in a train, consider using noise-cancelling headphones or earbuds that pick up ambient outside noise and emit a counter frequency that cancels out the incoming noise. Noise-cancelling headphones are useful because children will not need to turn the volume up to drown out outside noise. Parents should choose earbuds or headphones that fit well so that sound leakage is avoided, reducing the need to turn up volume.[50]

■ Use earplugs or noise-cancelling headphones or noise-cancelling earbuds if attending a loud event (such as a rock concert or dance event). If the level of noise is perceived as uncomfortable or painful, it is prudent to leave the event.

■ Create a "stimulus haven," the quietest room in the house for play and interactions.[51]

Table 35-2 lists common exposures to noise. Aircraft noise varies by position in the airplane, with high levels (90 dBA) in the back of the cabin during takeoff and average noise levels at 78 to 84 dBA over the duration of the flight.[52]

When noise reduction is not possible, hearing protectors need to be worn, such as during occupational exposures, use of power lawn mowers, recreational exposures such as loud concerts, and other situational noise exposures. Hearing protectors include earplugs, earmuffs, and noise-cancelling devices. Earplugs should fit properly; a slight tug required to remove them indicates correct fit. They are available in most drug stores or online. Earplugs should be checked while chewing because jaw motion may loosen them. Earmuffs have cups lined with sound-absorbing material that are held against the head with a spring band or oil-filled ring that provides a tight seal. Noise cancellation devices use electronic technology to cancel out ambient noise.

## Table 35-2. Decibel Ranges and Effects of Common Sounds

| EXAMPLE | SOUND PRESSURE (dBA) | COMMENTS |
|---|---|---|
| Breathing | 0–10 | Threshold of hearing |
| Whisper, rustling leaves | 20 | Very quiet |
| Quiet rural area at night | 30 | |
| Library, soft background music | 40 | |
| Quiet suburb (daytime), conversation in living room | 50 | Quiet |
| Conversation in restaurant or average office, background music, chirping bird | 60 | Intrusive |
| Freeway traffic at 15 m, vacuum cleaner, noisy office or party, TV audio | 70 | Annoying |
| Garbage disposal, clothes washer, average factory, freight train at 15 m, food blender, dishwasher, arcade games | 80 | Possible hearing damage |
| Busy urban street, diesel truck | 90 | Hearing damage |
| Power lawn mower, iPod or other MP3 player, motorcycle at 8 m, outboard motor, farm tractor, printing plant, jack hammer, garbage truck, jet takeoff (305 m away), subway | 100 | |
| Automobile horn at 1 m, boom box stereo held close to ear, steel mill, riveting | 110 | |
| Front row at live rock music concert, siren, chainsaw, stereo in cars, thunderclap, textile loom, jet takeoff (161 m away) | 120 | Human pain threshold |
| Earphones at maximum level, armored personnel carrier, jet takeoff (100 m away) | 130 | |
| Aircraft carrier deck | 140 | |
| Toy cap pistol, firecracker, jet takeoff (25 m away) | 150 | Eardrum rupture |

Abbreviations: dBA, decibels weighted by the A scale; m, meters.

## Frequently Asked Questions

Q  *Is it okay to use a white noise from a noise machine to help my new baby sleep?*

A  We now often live in noisy environments that can disturb a baby's sleep. Infant sleep machines are designed to provide noises to soothe the baby and to mask louder environmental noises that can interfere with sleep. Infant sleep machines, however, can produce dangerously loud sounds that can harm the baby's hearing, especially if the machine is placed near the baby. If you decide to use a sleep machine, locate it as far away as possible from your baby and never in the crib or on a crib rail, play it at a low volume, and use it for as short a period of time as possible.

Q. *We live in a neighborhood with a great deal of noise from leaf blowers. What steps can be taken to avoid this noise?*

A. Noise from gas-powered leaf blowers can damage hearing[53] and causes air pollution. Many communities have passed ordinances to ban leaf blowers[54] but enforcement often is an issue. Work with neighbors and local government officials to educate them about the hazard and create legislation if needed.

Q  *We live near an airport and the jets fly directly over our house as they take off and land. Will this be harmful to my newborn baby?*

A  If the noise causes discomfort to a parent, it may cause harm to the baby. The Federal Aviation Administration maintains a Web site that contains information about aircraft and airport noise and whom to contact with questions, concerns, or complaints about noise issues. (https://www.faa.gov/about/office_org/headquarters_offices/apl/noise_emissions/airport_aircraft_noise_issues). You may also want to seek help from your local government officials. Moving to a quieter setting may be an option for some families.

Q  *Are there unique hazards to the use of earbuds or headphones? How loud is too loud?*

A  There are several reports of hearing loss secondary to the use of personal audio players using either headphones or earbuds. Children and adolescents should be educated about the potential danger of loud music, whether heard at concerts, dances, and other social events or through earbuds or headphones. The personal digital audio player should be set at approximately 60% of maximum (maximum volume is about 100 to 110 dBA), and listening should be limited to 60 minutes daily. The user should be able to hear conversations going on around him or her while listening to the music. Earbuds generally have tighter seals with the ear canal than do headphones, so sound transfer may be more efficient with earbuds. Ringing or a feeling of fullness in the ear definitely means the music was too loud.

Q.  *We are thinking of moving to a rural area near a wind farm. I believe in renewable energy but I have heard that wind turbines are noisy. Will there be a problem for me or my family?*

A.  Exposure to too much noise can interfere with sleep and cause other problems. Wind turbines generate noise and a number of symptoms have been described by some people living near wind farms. Exposure to wind turbines seems to increase the risk of sleep disturbances and having feelings of annoyance.[55] The noise decreases as people get farther away from the turbines. Local governments set noise standards for communities.[56] Before you consider moving, it is a good idea to look at where your home is situated in relation to the wind turbine and investigate the regulations in your community.

Q.  *I took my family to a wedding reception where the music was so loud that I could not hear the person who was sitting at the table next to me. What can be done about this?*

A.  Many weddings and similar celebratory events have excessively loud band or DJ music. The music volume at these events often is uncomfortable or causes ear pain. It is helpful in these situations to have earplugs with you (and for family members), or to temporarily relocate while the music is playing. Asking the host to have the band or DJ lower the volume may result in some relief. You are also pointing out a larger issue: if noise was more widely understood as a major public health problem, then situations such as this would be less likely to arise. Unfortunately, many people appear to relish being in an extremely noisy music environment. A long-term approach of education and regulation is needed to avoid these situations in the future.

## Resources

### National Institute for Occupational Safety and Health
Noise and Hearing Loss Prevention
Web site: https://www.cdc.gov/niosh/topics/noise/other.html

### US Centers for Disease Control and Prevention
Hearing Loss in Children. Noise-Induced Hearing Loss
Web site: https://www.cdc.gov/ncbddd/hearingloss/noise.html

### World Health Organization
Noise
Web site: www.euro.who.int/en/health-topics/environment-and-health/noise

## References

1. US Environmental Protection Agency. Clean Air Act Title IV - Noise Pollution. https://www. epa.gov/clean-air-act-overview/clean-air-act-title-iv-noise-pollution. Accessed May 31, 2018

2. American Academy of Pediatrics Committee on Environmental Health. Noise: a hazard for the fetus and newborn. *Pediatrics*. 1997;100(4):724–727

3. Philbin MK, Graven SN, Robertson A. The influence of auditory experience on the fetus, newborn, and preterm infant: report of the sound study group of the national resource center: the physical and developmental environment of the high risk infant. *J Perinatol*. 2000;20 (8 Suppl):S1–S142

4. Nave CR. HyperPhysics: Sound and Hearing. http://hyperphysics.phy-astr.gsu.edu/hbase/ HFrame.html. Accessed May 31, 2018

5. Stansfield S, Clark C. Health effects of noise exposure in children. *Curr Environ Health Rep*. 2015;2(2):171–178

6. Carroll YI, Eichwald J, Scinicariello F, et al. Vital signs: noise-induced hearing loss among adults — United States 2011–2012. *MMWR Morb Mortal Wkly Rep*. 2017;66(5):139–144. https://www.cdc.gov/mmwr/volumes/66/wr/mm6605e3.htm?s_cid=mm6605e3_w. Accessed May 31, 2018

7. Harrison RV. The prevention of noise induced hearing loss in children. *Int J Pediatr*. Volume 2012, Article ID 473541. https://www.ncbi.nlm.nih.gov/pmc/articles/PMC3530863/pdf/ IJPED2012-473541.pdf. Accessed May 31, 2018

8. Wachman EM, Lahav A. The effects of noise on preterm infants in the NICU. *Arch Dis Child Fetal Neonatal Ed*. 2011;96(4):F305–F309

9. Almadhoob A, Ohlsson A. Sound reduction management in the neonatal intensive care unit for preterm or very low birth weight infants. Cochrane Database of Systematic Reviews. First published: 30 January 2015. http://onlinelibrary.wiley.com/doi/10.1002/14651858.CD010333. pub2/full. Accessed May 31, 2018

10. Hassanein SM, El Raggal NM, Shalaby AA. Neonatal nursery noise: practice-based learning and improvement. *J Matern Fetal Neonatal Med*. 2013;26(4):392–395

11. Kramer B, Joshi P, Heard C. Noise pollution levels in the pediatric intensive care unit. *J Crit Care*. 2016;36:111–115

12. The 5 S's for Soothing Babies. https://www.happiestbaby.com/blogs/blog/the-5-s-s-for-soothing-babies. Accessed May 31, 2018

13. Hugh SC, Wolter NE, Propst EJ, Gordon KA, Cushing SL, Papsin BC. Infant sleep machines and hazardous sound pressure levels. *Pediatrics*. 2014;133(4):677–681

14. Segal S, Eviatar E, Lapinsky J, Shlamkovitch N, Kessler A. Inner ear damage in children due to noise exposure from toy cap pistols and firecrackers: a retrospective review of 53 cases. *Noise Health*. 2003;5(18):13–18

15. National Institute of Public Health Denmark. *Health Effects of Noise on Children and Perception of the Risk of Noise*. Bistrup ML, ed. Copenhagen, Denmark: National Institute of Public Health Denmark; 2001:29

16. Mercier V, Hohmann B. Is electronically amplified music too loud? What do young people think? *Noise Health*. 2002;4(16):47–55

17. Portnuff CD. Reducing the risk of music-induced hearing loss from overuse of portable listening devices: understanding the problems and establishing strategies for improving awareness in adolescents. *Adolesc Health Med Ther*. 2016;7:27–35

18. Henderson D, Hamernik RP. Biologic bases of noise-induced hearing loss. *Occup Med*. 1995;10(3):513–534

19. Prince MM, Stayner LT, Smith RJ, Gilbert SJ. A re-examination of risk estimates from the NIOSH Occupational Noise and Hearing Survey (ONHS). *J Acoust Soc Am*. 1997;101:950–963

20. Jackler RK, Schindler DN. Occupational hearing loss. In: LaDou J, ed. *Occupational Medicine*. Norwalk, CT: Appleton and Lange; 1990:95–105

21. Centers for Disease Control and Prevention. Loud Noise Can Cause Hearing Loss. Public Health and Scientific Information. Statistics about the Public Health Burden of Noise-Induced Hearing Loss. https://www.cdc.gov/nceh/hearing_loss/public_health_scientific_info.html. Accessed May 31, 2018

22. Centers for Disease Control and Prevention. Hearing Loss in Children. Noise-Induced Hearing Loss. https://www.cdc.gov/ncbddd/hearingloss/noise.html. Accessed May 31, 2018

23. Niskar AS, Kieszak SM, Holmes AE, Esteban E, Rubin C, Brody DJ. Estimated prevalence of noise-induced hearing threshold shifts among children 6–19 years of age: the Third National Health and Nutrition Examination Survey, 1988–1994, United States. *Pediatrics*. 2001;108(1):40–43

24. Renick KM, Crawford JM, Wilkins JR. Hearing loss among Ohio farm youth: a comparison to a national sample. *Am J Ind Med*. 2009;52(3):233–239

25. Mercier V, Luy D, Hohmann BW. The sound exposure of the audience at a music festival. *Noise Health*. 2003;5(19):51–58

26. Bess FH, Dodd-Murphy J, Parker RA. Children with minimal sensorineural hearing loss: prevalence, educational performance, and functional status. *Ear Hear*. 1998;19(5):339–354

27. Lalande NM, Hetu R, Lambert J. Is occupational noise exposure during pregnancy a risk factor of damage to the auditory system of the fetus? *Am J Ind Med*. 1986;10(4):427–435

28. Lary S, Briassoulis G, de Vries L, Dubowitz LM, Dubowitz V. Hearing threshold in preterm and term infants by auditory brainstem response. *J Pediatr*. 1985;107(4):593–599

29. Selander J, Albin M, Rosenhall U, Rylander L, Lewné M, Gustavsson P. Maternal occupational exposure to noise during pregnancy and hearing dysfunction in children: a nationwide prospective cohort study in Sweden. *Environ Health Perspect*. 2016;124(6):855–860

30. Lefèvre M, Carlier MC, Champelovier P, Lambert J, Laumon B, Evrard A. Effects of aircraft noise exposure on saliva cortisol near airports in France. *Occup Environ Med*. 2017;74(8):612–618

31. World Health Organization Regional Office for Europe. Burden of disease from environmental noise. Quantification of healthy life years lost in Europe. 2011. http://www.euro.who.int/__data/assets/pdf_file/0008/136466/e94888.pdf. Accessed June 1, 2018

32. Falk SA, Woods NF. Hospital noise—levels and potential health hazards. *N Engl J Med*. 1973;289(15):774–781

33. Cureton-Lane RA, Fontaine DK. Sleep in the pediatric ICU: an empirical investigation. *Am J Crit Care*. 1997;6(1):56–63

34. Thiessen GJ. Disturbance of sleep by noise. *J Acoust Soc Am*. 1978;64(1):216–222

35. Morrison WE, Haas EC, Shaffner DH, Garrett ES, Fackler JC. Noise, stress, and annoyance in a pediatric intensive care unit. *Crit Care Med*. 2003;31(1):113–119

36. American Speech-Language-Hearing Association. American National Standard on Classroom Acoustics. http://www.asha.org/public/hearing/American-National-Standard-on-Classroom-Acoustics/. Accessed June 1, 2018

37. Picard M, Bradley JS. Revisiting speech interference in classrooms. *Audiology*. 2001;40(5):221–244

38. Harlor Jr AD, Bower C, American Academy of Pediatrics Committee on Practice And Ambulatory Medicine, Section On Otolaryngology–Head And Neck Surgery. Hearing assessment in infants and children: recommendations beyond neonatal screening. *Pediatrics*. 2009;124(4):1252–1263

39. American Academy of Pediatrics. Early Hearing Detection and Intervention. https://www.aap.org/en-us/advocacy-and-policy/aap-health-initiatives/PEHDIC/Pages/Early-Hearing-Detection-and-Intervention.aspx. Accessed June 1, 2018

40. Bright Futures/American Academy of Pediatrics. Recommendations for Preventive Pediatric Health Care. https://www.aap.org/en-us/Documents/periodicity_schedule.pdf. Accessed June 1, 2018

41. National Academies of Sciences, Engineering, and Medicine. Hearing health care for adults: priorities for improving access and affordability. Washington, DC: The National Academies Press; 2016

42. US Occupational Safety and Health Administration. Occupational Noise Exposure. https://www.osha.gov/SLTC/noisehearingconservation/standards.html. Accessed June 1, 2018

43. Themann CL, Suter AH, Stephenson MR. National research agenda for the prevention of occupational hearing loss—part 1. *Semin Hear.* 2013;34(3):145–207

44. Philbin MK, Robertson A, Hall JW III. Recommended permissible noise criteria for occupied, newly constructed or renovated hospital nurseries. The Sound Study Group of the National Resource Center. *J Perinatol.* 1999;19(8 Pt 1):559–563

45. Graven SN. Sound and the developing infant in the NICU: conclusions and recommendations for care. *J Perinatol.* 2000;20(8 Pt 2):S88–S93

46. Turk CA, Williams AL, Lasky RE. A randomized clinical trial evaluating silicone earplugs for very low birth weight newborns in intensive care. *J Perinatol.* 2009;29(5):358–363

47. Ahamed MF, Campbell D, Horan S, Rosen O. Noise reduction in the neonatal intensive care unit: a quality improvement initiative. *Am J Med Qual.* 2018;33(2):177–184

48. Kaur H, Rohlik GN, Nemergut MD, Tripathi S. Comparison of staff and family perceptions of causes of noise pollution in the Pediatric Intensive Care Unit and suggested intervention strategies. *Noise Health.* 2016;18(81):78–84

49. Hear-it AISBL. Noisy toys are not for delicate ears. http://www.hear-it.org/noisy-toys-are-not-for-delicate-ears. Accessed June 1, 2018

50. Healthychildren.org. 10 Tips to Preserve Your Child's Hearing during the Holidays. https://www.healthychildren.org/English/health-issues/conditions/ear-nose-throat/Pages/Tips-Preserve-Childs-Hearing-Holidays.aspx. Accessed June 1, 2018

51. Wachs TD. Nature of relations between the physical and social microenvironment of the two-year-old child. *Early Dev Parenting.* 1993;2(2):81–87

52. Torsten Lindgren T, Wieslander G, Nordquist T, Dammström BG, Norbäck D. Hearing status among cabin crew in a Swedish commercial airline company. *Int Arch Occup Environ Health.* 2009;82(7):887–892

53. Centers for Disease Control and Prevention. Too Loud! For Too Long! Loud noises damage hearing. https://www.cdc.gov/vitalsigns/pdf/2017-02-vitalsigns.pdf. February 2017. Accessed June 1, 2018

54. New York Times. On Banning Leaf Blowers. https://www.nytimes.com/2017/03/17/realestate/on-banning-on-leaf-blowers.html?_r=0. Accessed June 1, 2018

55. Schmidt JH, Klokker M. Health effects related to wind turbine noise exposure: a systematic review. *PLoS One.* 2014;9(12):e114183

56. New York Times. No One Satisfied With New Vermont Wind Power Sound Rules. November 12, 2017.

Chapter 36

# Perfluoroalkyl and Polyfluoroalkyl Substances (PFAS)

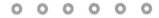

**KEY POINTS**

- PFAS are a large group of highly stable carbon-fluorine compounds with characteristics that have made them useful in consumer products and commercial processes.

- Several PFAS are environmentally persistent and have contaminated groundwater and drinking water despite US production of perfluorooctane sulfonic acid (PFOS) and perfluorooctanoic acid (PFOA) having ceased in 2002 and 2015, respectively. Serum PFOS and PFOA levels in the US general population have also declined in the past decade.

- The US Environmental Protection Agency (EPA) lifetime health advisory levels for PFOS and PFOA in drinking water were lowered in 2016, resulting in concerns about health effects at concentrations that previously were considered acceptable.

- Studies of large doses of PFAS given to laboratory animals have shown adverse effects on the liver, immune system, hormone levels, and reproduction, but the relevance of these findings to humans is uncertain.

- At the relatively low exposures that result from consuming PFAS-contaminated drinking water, no specific human health effects can be determined or predicted with certainty.

## INTRODUCTION

Perfluoroalkyl and polyfluoroalkyl substances (PFAS) is the current terminology used for chemicals that have been referred to as perfluorochemicals (PFCs). (The PFC acronym can also refer to perfluorocarbons, a different group of compounds that are greenhouse gases.) PFAS comprise a large group of human-made chemicals that contain strong carbon-fluorine bonds, a structure that makes them repellent to both water and fat, highly stable, and resistant to heat.

Produced since the 1950s, PFAS have had extensive industrial and commercial applications as surfactants, lubricants, polishes, and paper and textile coatings. Examples of common consumer products using PFAS include stain-repellent carpets and fabrics, furniture, and clothing; food packages, paper, and boxes that resist grease (eg, pizza boxes, food wrapping paper, microwave popcorn bags); floor care and cleaning products; personal care products with "perfluoro" ingredients; and foams used to fight or smother fires.[1,2] The most widely studied PFAS for human health effects are perfluorooctane sulfonic acid (PFOS) and perfluorooctanoic acid (PFOA, see Figure 36-1). Perfluorohexane sulfonic acid (PFHxS), perfluorononanoic acid (PFNA), and a few other PFAS have less frequently been measured in human studies.

PFAS are persistent in the environment, resistant to biologic and photo-chemical breakdown, and can readily migrate through soil and into groundwater and drinking water sources. As widespread exposure in humans, wildlife, and the environment became apparent in the late 20th century, major US producers voluntarily phased out production of specific PFAS: PFOS by 3M in 2002 and PFOA by DuPont in 2012.[3] Other PFOA manufacturers were encouraged to phase out production and usage entirely by 2015. Shorter chain PFAS that are less environmentally persistent and do not concentrate in wildlife, such as perfluorobutane sulfonate (PFBS) and perfluorohexanoic acid (PFHxA), have largely replaced PFOS and PFOA, both of which are still produced outside the United States.[3]

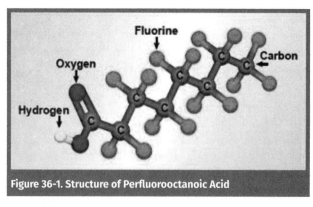

Figure 36-1. Structure of Perfluorooctanoic Acid

As concerns about environmental persistence and widespread human exposure increased during the 1990s, research and programs began to evaluate PFAS exposure in human populations. In 1999 in the United States, the Centers for Disease Control and Prevention (CDC) began measuring several PFAS in serum collected from a large sample of the US general population. The CDC has continued to make PFAS measurements in a representative sample of people aged 12 years and older who participated in the National Health and Nutritional Examination Survey (NHANES).[4] An important outcome has been the ability to monitor PFAS exposure over time, which shows that serum concentrations have declined substantially from 1999 to 2014: PFOS by 83% (Figure 36-2); PFOA by 63%; and perfluorohexane sulfonic acid (PFHxS) by 37%. The downward trend is similar across all ages and racial/ethnic groups, and in men and women. In contrast, use of PFNA seems to have led to increased exposure and higher serum concentrations in Americans since 1999.[4]

## ROUTES OF EXPOSURE

PFAS are widely disseminated in the environment, and several specific PFAS chemicals have been detected in coastal and marine waters, as well as in fresh surface waters, aquifers, and soils. These chemicals are persistent in the environment, and several PFAS bioaccumulate in the food chain. Human exposure has

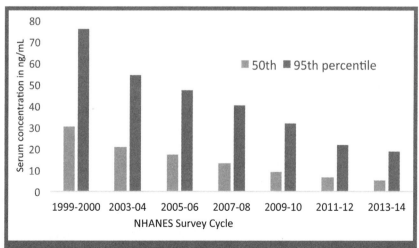

**Figure 36-2. Concentrations of perfluorooctane sulfonic acid in the blood of the US population as measured in the National Health and Nutrition Examination Survey over the period 1999-2014**

Source: Centers for Disease Control and Prevention. The National Report on Human Exposure to Environmental Chemicals, Updated Tables, March 2018. https://www.cdc.gov/exposurereport/. Accessed August 26, 2018

been demonstrated in both industrial and developing countries. The most likely exposure route for these chemicals is ingestion of food and drinking water; indoor dust may contribute to exposure in young children because of their mouthing behavior or hand-to-mouth transfer.[5] PFOS in particular has been shown to bioconcentrate in fish, and consumption of contaminated fish from contaminated fresh water can be an important dietary source.[1,6–8] Primarily PFOS and PFOA, but also other PFAS compounds, have contaminated drinking water sources in the United States and Europe as a consequence of industrial pollution, uncontrolled run-off, and soil application of contaminated bio-solids, resulting in unusually high exposures to the populations consuming the water.[9,10] PFOS and PFOA have been shown to be transferred from mother to the developing fetus, and nursing infants can be exposed through human milk.[11–15]

## SYSTEMS AFFECTED

Animal studies using high PFOS and PFOA doses have demonstrated acute and chronic toxicities, including increased liver weight, fatty liver, and lipid abnormalities; immunotoxicity; reduced thyroid hormone and testosterone concentrations; neurotoxicity; and developmental toxicity. Most animal cancer studies have examined PFOA, with results showing increases in liver, pancreatic, and testicular tumors.[16] Prenatal PFOA exposure reduced the growth and development of rat pups and reduced the litter size. It is notable that PFOS and PFOA, among the most widely studied of the PFAS chemicals, have different pharmacokinetics in animals and humans. For example, a dose of PFOS, PFOA, or PFHxS given to a rat is eliminated within days (eg, elimination half-life of days), but the elimination half-life in humans is on a scale of years: 3.5 years for PFOA; 4.8 years for PFOS; and 7.3 years for PFHxS.[17] The explanation for this difference is not entirely known, but PFAS are highly bound to serum proteins, not metabolized, and primarily eliminated in urine. Human kidneys may reabsorb PFAS from the urine, whereas rats may not, resulting in the rapid urinary elimination in rodents.[18] Further complicating the relevance of rodent data is that non-human primate studies found different effects. Studies in monkeys showed reversible and limited toxic effects on cholesterol, thyroid hormone, and body weight when large doses of PFOS were administered.[19,20] Interspecies differences in PFAS-induced activation of peroxisome proliferator–activator receptor α (PPARα) may contribute to effects in rodents that are not observed in humans. The PPAR family of receptors are important in lipid metabolism, and in rodents, PPARα activation appears to be an important pathway that leads to liver toxicity and tumors. In humans, however, PFAS do not appear to activate PPARα.[21,22]

Human epidemiologic studies have included pregnant women and children highly exposed from contaminated drinking water as well as those with "background" exposures. These health effects studies have used follow-up (cohort) as well as cross-sectional study designs and have focused on one or more of the following: birth outcomes (eg, birth weight and anthropometric data after prenatal exposure), endocrine function (eg, thyroid, metabolic, sex hormones), age at onset of puberty, liver enzymes and lipids (eg, cholesterol, lipid fractions, triglycerides), and immune response (eg, vaccine antibody titers).[12,23–37] To date, the results of these studies have been inconsistent or have uncertain clinical relevance, and no specific health effect can be attributed with certainty to PFAS exposure. Detecting health effects from PFAS is challenging in part because those persons exposed have little variability in their serum concentrations. Other limitations of PFAS studies include small sample sizes and cross-sectional study design in which serum concentrations and health effects were evaluated at the same time point so it is not possible to determine if the exposure came before or after the health effect occurred. A study of glomerular filtration rate and PFOA in children concluded that higher serum PFOA concentrations may have been a consequence of, rather than a cause of, decreased renal function.[38] Uncertainty also applies to the finding that adults or children with higher concentrations of PFOS or PFOA tend to have higher total cholesterol and LDL-C, because no relationship is apparent with HDL-C or triglycerides.[34,35] The factors described, in addition to incomplete information about confounding factors (eg, diet, genetics, medications), may be among those that contribute to inconsistent findings in human health studies and the relatively small increases in risk for health effects when they have been found (usually less than an increased risk of 2 or 3 times). Khalil et al[39] have reviewed the extensive human epidemiologic findings and their limitations.

## CLINICAL EFFECTS

The C8 Health Project was established to identify health consequences of contaminated drinking water in Ohio and West Virginia. This project included a series of epidemiologic studies conducted as part of a legal settlement between residents of the Ohio River Valley whose drinking water contamination was caused by a manufacturer of PFOA (which has an 8-carbon structure and is referred to as C8).[9] The C8 Project involved about 69,000 residents, lasted from 2005 to 2013, and evaluated PFOA exposure in relation to a number of health conditions or outcomes.[40] Serum PFOA concentrations in the affected residents were approximately 7 to 8 times higher than the general US population (geometric means of 32.9 vs. 3.92 mcg/L, respectively).[9] In this population, higher PFOA concentrations were associated with increased total cholesterol and LDL-C and older age at onset of puberty.[32,34] Several childhood conditions or those that could affect children were not associated with PFOA exposure: neurodevelopmental disorders (including attention deficit disorders and learning disabilities), infections (including influenza, colds, bronchitis, gastrointestinal infections, meningitis, and otitis media), asthma, thyroid abnormalities (specifically, TSH and total T4), birth defects, preterm birth and low birth weight, and miscarriage and stillbirth.[28,40]

Although not as extensively studied for health effects as the C8 Project, numerous episodes of drinking water contamination with PFOS, PFOA, and other PFAS chemicals have been documented. Most have shown increased serum concentrations of PFAS chemicals in people who drank the water compared with general populations exposed to "background" levels of PFAS chemicals. In West Germany, PFOA discharged into a river used for drinking water resulted in serum PFOA concentrations in adults and children that were similar to what occurred in Ohio and West Virginia.[7,41] In the United States, several communities with PFAS production facilities have experienced drinking water contamination because of run-off or discharge into rivers, streams, or lakes and from PFAS chemicals that migrated through soils and into drinking water aquifers. As expected, people who consumed contaminated drinking water had serum PFOS, PFOA, or other PFAS concentrations that were substantially higher than the general US population.[42,43]

## DIAGNOSTIC METHODS

Unlike clinical laboratory tests used to evaluate, diagnose, and manage health conditions, PFAS measurements are mostly used in research studies or community exposure assessments. The results do not predict current or future risk for health conditions or diseases. Serum PFAS measurements can determine the extent of exposure. Children tested would likely have detectable serum concentrations because PFAS exposure is widespread. Table 36-1 shows specific PFAS that the CDC's National Biomonitoring program measures to provide US population-based references ranges.[4]

Reference ranges provide useful comparisons for studies of exposed communities or groups. The CDC's reference ranges are available only for

---

**Table 36-1. Perfluoroalkyl and Polyfluoroalkyl Substances (PFAS) Measured in Serum by the CDC**

Perfluorooctanoic acid (PFOA)
Perfluorooctane Sulfonic Acid (PFOS)
Perfluorohexane Sulfonic Acid (PFHxS)
2-(N-Methyl-perfluorooctane sulfonamido) Acetic Acid (Me-PFOSA-AcOH or MeFOSAA)
Perfluorodecanoic Acid (PFDeA)
Perfluorobutane Sulfonic Acid (PFBuS)
Perfluoroheptanoic Acid (PFHpA)
Perfluorononanoic Acid (PFNA)
Perfluoroundecanoic Acid (PFUA or PFUnDA)

those persons aged 12 years and older; recently, however, the CDC measured serum PFAS in a representative sample of children aged 3 to 11 years.[44] Results in these younger children were similar to those in the adolescents and adults whose measurements were made during the same 2013 to 2014 survey period (ie, NHANES).[44] Data in younger children are severely limited although a small study of children aged birth through 12 years suggested that serum PFAS concentrations increase with age.[45]

Serum PFAS measurements are available only from specialized or research laboratories, may be costly, and may not be covered by insurance. If a physician decides to order serum PFAS measurement on a patient, it is advisable to talk with the laboratory that will do the measurement before the sample is collected. Most PFAS measured in serum have elimination half-lives on the order of several years, so measurements less than 1 year or even several years apart are unlikely to show much change, even after a known source of PFAS (eg, drinking water contamination) is eliminated.

## TREATMENT OF CLINICAL SYMPTOMS

PFAS exposure is asymptomatic, even at high exposure levels seen with drinking water contamination or in workers who were involved in production and had very high, long-term exposures.[46] No proven therapy or approved medication is available to speed up the body's natural but slow elimination of PFAS.

## PREVENTION OF EXPOSURE

In the United States, general population exposure to PFOS, PFOA, and several other PFAS have decreased over time as a result of reductions in their production and use (see Figure 36-2). PFOS and PFOA contamination of drinking water sources continue to be detected, however, perhaps largely because of the US EPA's recent testing requirements.[47] In 2016, the US EPA released lifetime health advisories for PFOS and PFOA that are intended to provide useful information to water system managers. The advisory for PFOS and for PFOA is 70 parts per trillion (ppt). The advisory for combined PFOS and PFOA in drinking water is also 70 ppt.[47] The lifetime health advisory is based on experimental and human data and is intended to protect the most sensitive groups (the developing fetus and infants). As the name suggests, the advisory assumes a concentration of PFOS or PFOA in drinking water that is continuous and is consumed over a lifetime.

In cases of drinking water contamination, using bottled water can reduce exposure. Alternative sources for showering and bathing are rarely necessary unless other chemicals or contaminants are present because PFAS chemicals are not well absorbed through the skin or inhaled from water vapor. Occasionally, high levels of PFOS and sometimes other PFAS have been found in freshwater fish taken from contaminated waters. In this situation, fish advisories were issued and people have been advised not to eat fish taken from these waters.[6]

Boiling water does not remove PFAS chemicals. Methods to remove PFOS and PFOA from water include activated charcoal filtration and reverse osmosis.[48] Removal effectiveness is determined by the extent of contamination, that is, the concentration of the PFAS chemical(s), and how well the system is maintained. Municipal water systems use PFOS and PFOA removal technology and monitor performance to ensure effectiveness. Home treatment systems can be installed if private wells become contaminated and should be certified by independent accredited third-party organizations against American National Standards Institute standards to verify their contaminant removal claims.[48]

## FREQUENTLY ASKED QUESTIONS

Q  *I've learned that my drinking water was contaminated with one or more PFAS chemicals. Should I stop or avoid breastfeeding my infant?*

A  Breastfeeding is recommended for infants. Numerous research studies have documented the broad and compelling advantages for infants, mothers, families, and society related to breastfeeding. Some of these benefits include immunologic advantages, lower obesity rates, and greater cognitive development for the infant in addition to health advantages for the lactating mother. Even though a number of environmental pollutants such as PFAS can readily pass to the infant through human milk, the advantages of breastfeeding continue to outweigh potential risks in nearly every circumstance. The American Academy of Pediatrics and other organizations recommend breastfeeding.[49] Using bottled water for drinking can reduce further exposure.

Q  *Should my child's blood be tested for PFAS?*

A  Although a number of PFAS can be measured in serum, the testing requires specialized laboratory staff and complex technology that is not available in clinical laboratories. Because the results do not guide medical therapy or predict future health effects, serum PFAS measurements are not generally available outside of research studies. In communities in which contaminated drinking water was discovered, serum PFAS measurements were part of the public health response determining the extent of exposure. However, routine measurements of serum PFAS are not recommended because few laboratories measure PFAS, the tests are costly and unlikely to be covered by insurance, and the results do not provide clinical information to guide medical management.

*Q  How can I prevent my child from being exposed to PFAS chemicals?*

A  It may not be possible to completely prevent exposure to many PFAS chemicals because they do not break down in the environment and can enter house dust, food, and drinking water. Almost all Americans who have been tested have low or "background" levels of several PFAS chemicals. However, the use of the persistent PFAS chemicals, such as PFOS, PFOA, and PFHxS, has declined in the past 30 years and Americans have less exposure now compared with the past. It is possible to reduce exposure when there are specific contamination situations involving PFAS. Large drinking water systems monitor for PFOS and PFOA and should notify residents if contamination occurs above specific levels. In this event, residents can use bottled water for drinking. Local and state public health authorities have issued fish advisories, warning people not to consume fish from lakes or rivers that were contaminated with specific PFAS chemicals, typically the result of manufacturing run-off or dumping.

*Q  What are the drinking water health advisories that the US EPA recently issued for PFOS and PFOA? If my drinking water has higher levels than the advisory, does this mean that my child will become sick?*

A  The US EPA reviews scientific studies in laboratory animals and humans and uses techniques to estimate the concentration of a chemical in drinking water that would be safe to consume over a lifetime, called a lifetime health advisory. The intent is for the advisory level to protect against adverse health effects in the most sensitive groups, the fetus and nursing infant. The current health advisory for PFOS, PFOA, or both together is 70 parts per trillion (ppt). If a system finds that the drinking water has more than 70 ppt of PFOS or PFOA, then the US EPA advises several actions, including steps to reduce the water levels of these chemicals. Consuming water with higher concentrations of these chemicals does not mean that adverse health effects will occur. The advisory assumes that drinking water with 70 ppt of PFOS, PFOA, or both will be consumed every day over a lifetime. There is no certainty that any adverse health effects will occur.

*Q  Our community had drinking water contaminated with PFOS and PFOA at levels higher than the US EPA health advisory. What kind of medical testing or monitoring should my child have?*

A  PFOA, PFOS, and other persistent PFAS chemicals have not consistently been associated with human health effects, despite a large number of epidemiologic studies. Increased total cholesterol has been found in adults and children with higher PFOS and PFOA levels, but the studies cannot prove causation because many factors that lead to higher cholesterol were not known, such as diet and family history. No PFAS-specific medical monitoring or tests exist at this time. However, infants and children who receive regular medical care and services, such as those included in the *Recommendations for Preventive Pediatric Health Care* (available at: https://www.aap.org/en-us/Documents/periodicity_schedule.pdf), effectively will have medical surveillance and early intervention for health effects, regardless of exposure to PFOS, PFOA, or other PFAS.

Q   *What can I do or give my child to help get rid of the PFAS in his or her body?*

A   In the body, PFOS, PFOA, and PFHxS are mostly bound to albumin and other serum proteins, but some of the chemicals may be stored in the liver and possibly other organs. These chemicals are not metabolized, and they are eliminated in the urine very slowly, possibly because they may be reabsorbed from urine back into the blood. There is no known medication or process to speed the body's natural mechanism for eliminating PFAS chemicals in urine or to remove them from the blood.

Q   *I've heard that the health department plans to do biomonitoring in my community because PFOA and PFOS have contaminated our drinking water. What does this mean?*

A   Biomonitoring is used to determine exposure to environmental chemicals, and it involves using blood or urine samples to measure a chemical or its metabolite(s). A serum PFOS or PFOA measurement is an example of a biomonitoring measurement. Most often, biomonitoring is used in studies or surveys to evaluate which people are exposed to a chemical and to what extent. For many environmental chemicals, biomonitoring can demonstrate that exposure has occurred, but it may not mean that any adverse health effects will result. The NHANES is an ongoing survey that samples the US general population to evaluate health and nutrition by examining and collecting blood and urine samples from the almost 5,000 participants who are interviewed each year. In addition to clinical laboratory tests, blood and urine samples are used to measure environmental chemicals, including several PFAS chemicals. Results of these measurements are used to determine reference ranges (by age group, sex, and race/ethnicity) for comparison with individual or group results, to assess effectiveness of actions to reduce exposures, and to track, over time, trends in exposure levels in the US population.

Q   *What should I do with my old nonstick ("Teflon™") cookware?*

A   You may want to dispose of cracked or chipped nonstick pots or pans. Nonstick cookware with cracks or chips will not be a good cooking surface and may allow food to stick to the exposed metal surface. Using stainless steel and iron cookware avoids this concern, but some cooks may prefer pots and pans with nonstick coatings. If used, these pans should be used at recommended temperatures (not on "high") and never be preheated to high temperatures. Above 500 degrees, the coatings may degrade and give off fumes. Do not use tools that will scratch and ruin the nonstick surface. Above all, read the instructions that come with the cookware so you can preserve its finish and use it safely.

Q    *Should I worry about my pizza box? Or microwave popcorn bag? Or fast food wrapping paper?*

A    Pizza and popcorn boxes, microwave popcorn bags, and fast food wrapping paper used to be coated with a PFOA-containing repellent to prevent food leakage and sticking. In 2016, the Food and Drug Administration (FDA) prohibited the use of several PFAS that were used as paper and cardboard coatings designed to repel oil and water in food containers such as popcorn bags, pizza boxes, as well as food take-out containers and wrappers. Health concerns and environmental persistence were the overriding reasons for the FDA ruling, but the replacement coatings are varied and have not been well studied.

## REFERENCES

1. Fromme H, Tittlemier SA, Volkel W, Wilhelm M, Twardella D. Perfluorinated compounds—exposure assessment for the general population in western countries. *Int J Hyg Environ Health.* 2009;212(3):239–270

2. Kotthoff M, Muller J, Jurling H, Schlummer M, Fiedler D. Perfluoroalkyl and polyfluoroalkyl substances in consumer products. *Environ Sci Pollut Res.* 2015;22(19):14546–14559

3. Lau C. Perfluorinated compounds: an overview. In: DeWitt JC, ed. *Toxicological Effects of Perfluoroalkyl and Polyfluoroalkyl Substances.* Switzerland: Springer International Publishing; 2015:1–21

4. Centers for Disease Control and Prevention. *The National Report on Human Exposure to Environmental Chemicals, Updated Tables, March 2018.* https://www.cdc.gov/exposurereport/. Accessed August 26, 2018

5. Karaskova P, Venier M, Melymuk L, et al. Perfluorinated alkyl substances (PFASs) in household dust in Central Europe and North America. *Environ Int.* 2016;94:315–324

6. Houde M, De Silva AO, Muir DC, Letcher RJ. Monitoring of perfluorinated compounds in aquatic biota: an updated review. *Environ Sci Technol.* 2011;45(19):7962–7973

7. Holzer J, Midasch O, Rauchfuss K, et al. Biomonitoring of perfluorinated compounds in children and adults exposed to perfluorooctanoate-contaminated drinking water. *Environ Health Perspect.* 2008;116(5):651–657

8. Stahl LL, Snyder BD, Olsen AR, Kincaid TM, Walthen JB, McCarty HB. Perfluorinated compounds in fish from U.S. urban rivers and the Great Lakes. *Sci Tot Environ.* 2014;499:185–195

9. Frisbee SJ, Brooks AP Jr, Maher A, et al. The C8 health project: design, methods, and participants. *Environ Health Perspect.* 2009;117(12):1873–1882

10. Wilhelm M, Kraft M, Rauchfuss K, Holzer J. Assessment and management of the first German case of a contamination with perfluorinated compounds (PFC) in the Region Sauerland, North Rhine-Westphalia. *J Toxicol Environ Health A.* 2008;71(11-12):725–733

11. Apelberg BJ, Goldman LR, Calafat AM, et al. Determinants of fetal exposure to perfluoroalkyl compounds in Baltimore, Maryland. *Environ Sci Technol.* 2007;41(11):3891–3897

12. Apelberg BJ, Witter FR, Herbstman JB, et al. Cord serum concentrations of perfluorooctane sulfonate (PFOS) and perfluorooctanoate (PFOA) in relation to weight and size at birth. *Environ Health Perspect.* 2007;115(11):1670–1676

13. Karman A, Ericson I, van Bavel B, et al. Exposure of perfluorinated chemicals through lactation: levels of matched human milk and serum and a temporal trend, 1996-2004, in Sweden. *Environ Health Perspect.* 2007;115(2):226–230

14. Pinney SM, Biro FM, Windham GC, et al. Serum biomarkers of polyfluoroalkyl compound exposure in young girls in greater Cincinnati and the San Francisco Bay area, USA. *Environ Pollut.* 2014;184:327–334

15. Von Ehrenstein OS, Fenton SE, Kato K, Kuklenyik Z, Calafat AM, Hines EP. Polyfluoroalkyl chemicals in the serum and milk of breastfeeding women. *Reprod Toxicol.* 2009;27(3-4): 239–245

16. Kennedy GE, Symons JM. Carcinogenicity of perfluoroalkyl compounds. In: DeWitt JC, ed. *Toxicological Effects of Perfluoroalkyl and Polyfluoroalkyl Substances.* Switzerland: Springer International Publishing; 2015:265–304

17. Olsen GW, Burris JM, Ehresman DK, et al. Half-life of serum elimination of perfluorooctanesulfonate, perfluorohexanesulfonate, and perfluorooctanoate in retired fluorochemicals production workers. *Environ Health Perspect.* 2007;115(9):1298–1305

18. Harada K, Inoue K, Moikawa A, Yoshinaga T, Saito N, Koizumi A. Renal clearance of perfluorooctane sulfonate and perfluorooctanoate in humans and their species-specific excretion. *Environ Res.* 2005;99(2):253–261

19. Chang S, Allen BC, Andres KL, et al. Evaluation of serum lipid, thyroid, and hepatic clinical chemistries in association with serum perfluorooctanesulfonate (PFOS) in Cynomolgus monkeys after oral dosing with potassium PFOS. *Toxicol Sci.* 2017;156(2):387–401

20. Seacat AM, Thomford PJ, Hansen KJ, Olsen GW, Case MT, Butenoff JL. Subchronic toxicity studies on perfluorooctanesulfonate potassium salt in Cynomolgus monkeys. *Toxicol Sci.* 2002;68(1):249–264

21. Nakamura T, Ito Y, Yangiba Y, et al. Microgram-order ammonium perfluorooctanoate may activate mouse peroxisome proliferator-activated receptor α, but not human PPARα. *Toxicology.* 2009;265(1-2):27–33

22. Ren J, Vallanat B, Nelson DM, et al. Evidence for the involvement of xenobiotic-responsive nuclear receptors in transcriptional effects upon perfluoroalkyl acid exposure in diverse species. *Reprod Toxicol.* 2009;27(3-4):266–277

23. Andersen CS, Fei C, Gamborg M, Nohr EA, Sorensen TI, Olsen J. Prenatal exposures to perfluorinated chemicals and anthropometry at 7 years of age. *Am J Epidemiol.* 2013;178(6):921–927

24. Barry V, Darrow LA, Klein M, Winquist A, Steenland K. Early life perfluorooctanoic acid (PFOA) exposure and overweight and obesity risk in adulthood in a community with elevated exposure. *Environ Res.* 2014;132:62–69

25. Braun JM, Chen A, Romano ME, et al. Prenatal perfluoroalkyl substance exposure and child adiposity at 8 years of age: the HOME study. *Obesity* (Silver Spring). 2016;24(1):231–237

26. Mora AM, Oken E, Rifas-Shiman SL, et al. Prenatal exposure to perfluoroalkyl substances and adiposity in early and mid-childhood. *Environ Health Perspect.* 2017;125(3):467–473

27. de Cock M, de Boer MR, Lamoree M, Legler J, van de Bor M. Prenatal exposure to endocrine disrupting chemicals in relation to thyroid hormone levels in infants—a Dutch prospective cohort study. *Environ Health.* 2014;13:106

28. Lopez-Espinosa MJ, Mondal D, Armstrong B, Bloom MS, Fletcher T. Thyroid function and perfluoroalkyl acids in children living near a chemical plant. *Environ Health Perspect.* 2012;120(7):1036–1041

29. Wang Y, Starling AP, Haug LS, et al. Association between perfluoroalkyl substances and thyroid stimulating hormone among pregnant women: a cross-sectional study. *Environ Health.* 2013;12(1):76

30. Fleisch AF, Rifas-Shiman SL, Mora AM, et al. Early-life exposure to perfluoroalkyl substances and childhood metabolic function. *Environ Health Perspect.* 2017;125(3):481–487

31. Lopez-Espinosa MJ, Mondal D, Armstrong BG, Eskenazi B, Fletcher T. Perfluoroalkyl substances, sex hormones, and insulin-like growth factor-1 at 6-9 years of age: a cross-sectional analysis within the C8 Health Project. *Environ Health Perspect.* 2016;124(8): 1269–1275

32. Lopez-Espinosa MJ, Fletcher T, Armstrong B, et al. Association of perfluorooctanoic acid (PFOA) and perfluorooctane sulfonate (PFOA) with age of puberty among children living near a chemical plant. *Environ Sci Technol.* 2011;45(19):8160–8166

33. Fitz-Simon N, Fletcher T, Luster MI, et al. Reductions in serum lipids with a 4-year decline in serum perfluorooctanoic acid and perfluorooctanesulfonic acid. *Epidemiology.* 2013;24(4):569–576

34. Frisbee SJ, Shankar A, Knox SS, et al. Perfluorooctanoic acid, perfluorooctanesulfonate, and serum lipids in children and adolescents. *Arch Pediatric Adolesc Med.* 2010;164(9):860–869

35. Geiger SD, Xiao J, Ducatman A, Frisbee S, Innes K, Shankar A. The association between PFOS, PFOA and serum lipid levels in adolescents. *Chemosphere.* 2014;98:78–83

36. Grandjean P, Andersen EW, Budtz-Jorgensen E, et al. Serum vaccine antibody concentrations in children exposed to perfluorinated compounds. *JAMA.* 2012;307:391–397

37. Stein CR, McGovern KJ, Pajak AM, Maglione PJ, Wolff MS. Perfluoroalkyl and polyfluoroalkyl substances and indicators of immune function in children aged 12-19 y: National Health and Nutrition Examination Survey. *Pediatr Res.* 2016;79(2):348–357

38. Watkins DJ, Josson J, Elston B, et al. Exposure to perfluoroalkyl acids and markers of kidney function among children and adolescents living near a chemical plant. *Environ Health Perspect.* 2013;121(5):625–630

39. Khalil N, Lee M, Steenland K. Epidemiological findings. In: DeWitt JC, ed. *Toxicological Effects of Perfluoroalkyl and Polyfluoroalkyl Substances.* Switzerland: Springer International Publishing; 2015:305–335

40. C8 Science Panel (C8). The C8 Science Panel. Updated January 4, 2017. http://www.c8sciencepanel.org/index.html. Accessed February 18, 2018

41. Brede E, Wilhelm M, Goen T, et al. Two-year follow-up biomonitoring pilot study of residents' and controls' PFC plasma levels after PFOA reduction in public water system in Arnsberg, Germany. *Int J Hyg Environ Health.* 2010;213(3):217–223

42. Agency for Toxic Substances and Disease Registry. Health Consultation. Exposure Investigation Report. Perfluorochemical serum sampling in the vicinity of Decatur, Alabama, Morgan, Lawrence, and Limestone counties. U. S. Department of Health and Human Services, Atlanta, GA. April 1, 2013. https://www.atsdr.cdc.gov/hac/pha/Decatur/Perfluorochemical_Serum%20Sampling.pdf. Accessed February 18, 2018

43. Minnesota Department of Health. Public Health Assessment. Perfluorochemical contamination in southern Washington county, northern Dakota county, and southeastern Ramsey county, Minnesota. U.S. Department of Health and Human Services, Agency for Toxic Substances and Disease Registry. Atlanta, GA. January 5, 2012. http://www.health.state.mn.us/divs/eh/hazardous/topics/pfcs/pha/woodbury/pha3m0112.pdf. Accessed February 18, 2018

44. Ye X, Kato K, Wong LY, et al. Per-and polyfluoroalkyl substances in the sera from children 3 to 11 years of age participating in the National Health and Nutrition Examination Survey 2013-2014. *Int J Hyg Environ Health.* 2018;221(1):9–16

45. Schecter A, Malik-Bass N, Calafat AM, et al. Polyfluoroalkyl compounds in Texas children from birth through 12 years of age. *Environ Health Perspect.* 2012;120(4):590–594

46. Olsen GW. PFAS biomonitoring in higher exposed populations. In: DeWitt JC, ed. *Toxicological Effects of Perfluoroalkyl and Polyfluoroalkyl Substances.* Switzerland: Springer International Publishing; 2015:77–125

47. U.S. Environmental Protection Agency. Drinking water health advisories for PFOS and PFOA. 2016. https://www.epa.gov/ground-water-and-drinking-water/drinking-water-health-advisories-pfoa-and-pfos. Accessed February 18, 2018

48. U.S. Environmental Protection Agency. Fact Sheet: PFOA & PFOS Drinking Water Health Advisories. May 2016. https://www.epa.gov/sites/production/files/2016-05/documents/drinkingwaterhealthadvisories_pfoa_pfos_5_19_16.final_.1.pdf. Accessed February 18, 2018

49. American Academy of Pediatrics. Section on Breastfeeding. Breastfeeding and the use of human milk. *Pediatrics.* 2012;129(3):e827–e841; and Dorea JG. Author Reply. *Pediatrics.* 2012;130(2):e462–e464

Chapter 37

# Persistent Bioaccumulative Toxic Substances (PBTs)

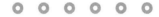

**KEY POINTS**

- Persistent bioaccumulative toxic substances (PBTs) include polybrominated diphenyl ethers (PBDEs), perchlorate, and perfluoroalkyl and polyfluoroalkyl substances (PFAS).
- PBTs degrade slowly or not at all, have the potential for long-distance transport, may bioaccumulate, and have toxic effects in wildlife and humans.
- PBTs are widely distributed across the entire earth with some of the highest levels found in the most remote areas, such as the Arctic and deep-sea trenches.
- PBTs can cause adverse health effects including cancer, reproductive disorders, immune disorders, allergies and hypersensitivity, central and peripheral nervous system effects, and alterations in normal endocrine function.
- Even after they are no longer manufactured, PBTs continue to be a human health concern because they are long-lived in the environment, particularly in marine ecosystems.
- Although PBDEs and other PBTs pass into human milk, the advantages of breastfeeding outweigh any potential risks.

## INTRODUCTION

Persistent bioaccumulative toxic substances (PBTs) include several classes of well-known environmental toxicants, the most well studied being persistent organic pollutants (POPs [see Chapter 38]). POPs were initially categorized as a group of 12 specific halogenated chemicals or mixtures (aldrin, chlordane, dichlorodiphenyltrichloroethane [DDT], dieldrin, endrin, heptachlor, hexachlorobenzene, mirex, polychlorinated biphenyls [PCBs], dioxins, dibenzofurans, and toxaphene), addressed by the 2001 Stockholm Convention on Persistent Organic Pollutants. This global treaty among over 150 member states aimed to protect human health and the environment, and later extended the listing of PBTs to many other chemicals. PBTs include toxicants with the following features: (1) they degrade slowly or not at all in the environment through exposure to sunlight, water, or other mechanisms; (2) they have the potential for long-distance transport by air or water with settling in remote regions of the globe; (3) many have long biological half-lives, leading to bioaccumulation in humans and other living creatures; and (4) they have or are strongly suspected of having toxicity in wildlife and humans. These chemicals include a broad range of substances (Table 37-1), such as organic aromatic compounds (eg, pentachlorophenol, polyaromatic hydrocarbons), metals (eg, lead, mercury), pesticides (eg, lindane), and halogenated compounds. The number of substances labeled as PBT continues to grow at an increasing rate, corresponding to their use in the manufacture of consumer products.

PBTs were released into the environment throughout the 1900s and 2000s because of human activity. As a result, PBTs are now widely distributed everywhere across the earth. Some of the highest levels are found in the most remote areas, such as the Arctic and deep-sea trenches. This extensive contamination of the environment results in chronic exposure of many species, including humans, over generations. For humans, the outcomes can include both acute and chronic toxic effects.

PBTs become more concentrated in living organisms through a process called bioaccumulation. Most PBTs are poorly soluble in water but are readily absorbed and stored in fatty tissues. Fish, predatory birds, mammals, and humans are high on the food chain and have the greatest concentrations as a result of biomagnification. Through continuous dietary exposure, concentrations can become magnified by up to 70,000 times background levels in higher trophic-level organisms.

PBTs can cause a range of adverse health effects including cancer, reproductive disorders, immune disorders, allergies and hypersensitivity, central and peripheral nervous system effects, and alterations in normal development. Some PBTs are endocrine disruptors that alter normal function of hormonal systems, leading to adverse reproductive, developmental, metabolic, and immune functioning for exposed individuals and their offspring.

## Table 37-1. Common Persistent Toxic Substances

| SUBSTANCE | COMMON SOURCES OR USES |
|---|---|
| Methyl tertiary butyl ether (MTBE) | Gasoline additive |
| Alkylphenols | Clothing treatment solutions (precursors to detergents) |
| Endosulfan | Insecticide |
| Phthalates | Plastics |
| **Metals and organometals** | |
| Lead and tetraethyl lead | Paint, gasoline additive |
| Mercury and organomercury | Air, food |
| Cadmium | Tobacco smoke |
| Organotin compounds | Marine paint, outdoor air |
| Methylcyclopentadienyl manganese tricarbonyl (MMT) | Gasoline additive |
| **Halogenated compounds** | |
| Perfluoroalkyl and polyfluoroalkyl substances (PFAS) | Teflon®, Scotchgard®, nonstick materials, GenX |
| Polybrominated diphenyl ethers (PBDEs) | Fire retardants, food, water, indoor air, dust |
| Perchlorates | Food, water |
| Lindane, DDT, organochlorines | Insecticide (lice, scabies) |
| Pentachlorophenol | Wood preservative |
| Agent Orange[a] | Herbicide |

[a] Composed of 2,4,5-trichlorophenoxyacetic acid (2,4,5-T) and 2,4-dichlorophenoxyacetic acid (2,4-D), with trace 2,3,7,8-tetrachlorodibenzodioxin (TCDD) as a contaminant of 2,4,5,-T

Among PBTs, the halogenated compounds have received the greatest attention. Halogenated chemicals have the longest history of concern, not only because of their health effects but because of their impact on diminishing stratospheric ozone (the "ozone layer"), the protective blanket that absorbs significant amounts of the sun's harmful ultraviolet radiation. This environmental damage, coupled with the suspected toxicity of halogenated compounds, led to the removal of chlorofluorocarbons (CFCs) from refrigerators, air conditioners, spray cans, and multiple-dose inhalers. Chemicals made with the halides chlorine ($Cl^-$), bromine ($Br^-$), and fluorine ($Fl^-$) remain prevalent in manufacturing and commercial goods, often because of their unique chemical properties in specific applications.

This chapter reviews 2 widely used classes of persistent toxic substances—polybrominated diphenyl ethers (PBDEs) and perchlorates. These examples illustrate issues relevant to all persistent, bioaccumulative, toxic pollutants. Perfluoroalkyl and polyfluoroalkyl substances (PFAS), another class of PBTs, are discussed in Chapter 36.

## POLYBROMINATED DIPHENYL ETHERS (PBDES)

The PBDEs are among a family of chemicals (also known as brominated flame retardants [BFRs]) used primarily as fire retardants. Structurally related to PCBs, the PBDEs have a base structure of 2 phenyl rings linked by an oxygen atom. In addition, PBDEs have attached multiple bromine atoms that vary in number ( from 1 to 10) and position to form 209 distinct chemical congeners.[1] Among the commercial PBDE flame retardants, there are 3 classes of commercial mixtures of these congeners: (1) pentabrominated diphenyl ether (pentaBDE) that contains congeners with 4 to 6 bromines; (2) octabrominated diphenyl ether (octaBDE) containing largely 5 to 9 bromines; and (3) decabrominated diphenyl ether (decaBDE), which has a full complement of 10 bromine atoms and is approximately 97% pure as a commercial product. All of these compounds are additive flame retardants, meaning that they are intercalated into products and not chemically bonded to the matrix. Therefore, they can leach out of commercial products over time.

The development and use of PBDEs were once hailed as an industrial advance and were claimed to be responsible for a marked reduction in the morbidity and mortality from fires in homes and businesses. The overall benefit of PBDEs in improving fire safety, however, particularly when compared with other means of fire prevention, lacks definitive proof in practice.[2] At the same time, their increasing use has led to increasing environmental contamination. PBDEs were once manufactured in amounts exceeding 67,000 metric tons annually, but over the last 10 years all 3 commercial mixtures have been listed as POPs under the Stockholm Convention, effectively banning their use in member states across the world. Although not a member of the Stockholm Convention, the United States has also limited or ceased use of all PBDEs through mutual agreement with chemical producers.

Although no longer used, PBDEs were ubiquitous in consumer products, and thus continue to leach out of legacy household and office products across the world. Discarded products continue to release PBDEs into the environment as the surrounding manufactured products degrade but the PBTs do not. PBDEs continue to be found in building materials, furniture, motor vehicles, paints, plastics, polyurethane foams, furniture, certain textiles, and clothing, often at concentrations as high as 5% to 30% by weight.[1]

PBDEs are similar to other persistent toxic substances because they have extensive environmental persistence and biological half-lives in humans as long as 2 to 4 years, although because of metabolism, some congeners may have short elimination half-lives of approximately 15 days.[3,4] They differ from many other PBTs because they are primarily used indoors (in consumer products) rather than outdoors and are therefore more likely to result in direct human exposure.[5] PBDE exposures also are increased when compared with exposure to other PBTs because of their disposal methods. Unlike many consumer products that must be recycled and/or managed as toxic waste because of their harmful constituents, products containing PBDEs are discarded in household trash, leading to uncontrolled discharge into the environment.[6] In many parts of the world, concentrations of PBDEs continue to rise in wildlife, including invertebrates, fish, birds, and marine mammals.[7] Concentrations in humans rose rapidly over the last few decades, particularly in the United States and China.[5,8] Women who have recently emigrated to the United States from rural Mexico have lower concentrations of PBDEs in their blood,[9] consistent with greater use of these chemicals in the United States as well as their presence in modern interior environments. Concentrations of pentaBDEs in the blood of US adults are 10 to 100 times higher than those found in Europe and Japan.[10] This finding is largely the result of the fact that the pentaBDE product was used extensively only in North America. Scientific studies have begun to investigate human exposure to PBDEs during unregulated electronic waste recycling operations that often employ children in developing countries.[11,12]

PBDEs are found extensively in fatty fish, meat, and dairy products.[13] On the basis of typical food consumption patterns, meat accounts for the highest single food source of PBDEs in children and adults. Intake from food is estimated at 2 to 5 nanograms (ng)/kg daily for children and 1 ng/kg daily in adults. PBDEs are also "recycled" back into the food chain as a result of contamination of biosolid fertilizers and amended soils (eg, compost and other soil conditioners).[14]

PBDEs are found in several gestational and reproductive tissues.[15] Because of the high lipid content in human milk, the lower brominated PBDEs (4 to 6 bromines) are present at significant concentrations.[16,17] Human milk concentrations in US women are as much as 75 times higher than concentrations in European, Asian, or other women from around the world.[6,7,15-19] As a result, the

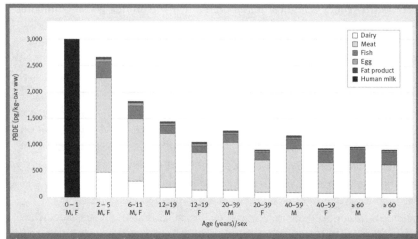

**Figure 37-1. Daily PBDE dietary intake of US population by age and food group (pg/kg body weight).**

Abbreviations: F, female; M, male; PBDE, polybrominated diphenyl ether; pg, picogram; ww, wet weight.
Reprinted with permission from Schecter et al.[5]

highest exposure in humans occurs in nursing infants, who ingest an average 307 ng/kg of body weight daily, versus 1 ng/kg daily for adults (Figure 37-1). This corresponds with average concentrations of 24 to 114 parts per billion (ppb) of PBDEs in children's blood, a concentration considerably higher than the blood concentrations in adults.

Food intake does not account entirely for the concentrations of PBDEs found in children and adults.[20] In a study of a single family, concentrations of PBDEs were higher in September than in December. They were also higher in the children than they were in the adults.[10] A primary source of PBDE exposure in the United States is house dust.[20] The lower concentration found in adults was attributed to a lower degree of exposure to dust and to the specific types of PBDEs measured because the higher brominated PBDEs have comparatively short elimination half-lives. According to current estimates, house dust accounts for up to 80% of total exposure to PBDEs in toddlers, compared with 14% for adults. Exposure to dust can also lead to as much as a 100-fold higher concentration in toddlers.[21] As surrogates for human exposure, house cats have been shown to have higher rates of hyperthyroidism when exposed to higher levels of PBDEs in home environments.[22,23] This was initially hypothesized because the behavior of cats—licking and grooming, lying on furniture and carpets—has some resemblance to that of young children.

Exposure to PBDEs is potentially toxic to the reproductive and neurologic systems. PBDEs also appear to act as primary endocrine disrupters, affecting the estrogen and thyroid axes.[24-26] According to the US Environmental

Protection Agency (EPA), PBDEs are significantly neurotoxic in experimental animals, producing hyperactivity and other changes in behavior.[27] In animal models, toxicity is similar to that of the PCBs, including endocrine disruption, reproductive and developmental toxicity, and central nervous system (CNS) effects.[1,6,7] Effects on the hypothalamic-pituitary-thyroid axis have received the most attention.[24] Exposed animals have reduced circulating thyroid hormone concentrations, which is thought to be caused by altered thyroid hormone metabolism, both glucuronidation and sulfation, and changes in transporters.[28] Altered hormone homeostasis also appears to be a CNS effect in part, attributable to disturbances of thyroid hormone signaling at multiple levels of the hypothalamic-pituitary-thyroid axis. This has led to theories that PBDEs can alter neurogenesis in the fetus and newborn infant.[7] One study reported inverse associations between PBDEs in cord blood and measures of neurodevelopment through age 6 years.[29] Lam et al[25] have since reviewed the scientific literature and concluded that there is evidence of an association between developmental PBDE exposure and reduced IQ. Further, adverse reproductive effects can be produced in laboratory animals with exposures to concentrations of less than 302 ng/g lipid weight, a concentration reached by 5% of US women.[10] The commercial PBDE mixture, DE71, was shown to be carcinogenic in rats and mice.[30]

On the basis of growing concerns, legislative and regulatory actions have been passed to reduce human exposure. In 2010, the US EPA set a reference dose for PBDEs of 7.1 mcg/kg/day.[31] A reference dose is a scientific estimate of the daily exposure level that is not expected to cause adverse health effects in adult humans. Previously in 2003, the State of California voted to ban the sale of pentaBDE and octaBDE and products containing them by January 2008. The California regulation was followed by regulations in other states including Hawaii, Maine, Massachusetts, Michigan, New York, and Washington. Internationally, the Stockholm Convention has included pentaBDE and octaBDE since 2009, and decaBDE commercial mixture since 2017. This means that countries signing the treaty must eliminate or reduce their use of these chemicals. Canada has limited the production and sale of some PBDEs since 1999.[32] The European Union eliminated the use of many PBDEs as of July 2006[33] and more recently published regulations to prohibit or restrict decaBDE in 2017.[34] Although regulatory actions and mutual agreements to phase out hazardous chemicals are designed to protect human health, they also can have the opposite effect. Typically, limitations on the production or use of a chemical are not put into place until after extensive research has been conducted including exposure studies, ecological and biological monitoring, epidemiologic studies, and studies in animals and humans demonstrating adverse health effects. Once phased out of use, regulated chemicals are often rapidly replaced by structurally similar chemicals with unknown toxicological profiles, some of which are more hazardous than the initial chemical. Thus, regulation by chemical class rather than by the individual chemical has been proposed and recently adopted by the US Consumer Product Safety Commission.[35]

Reducing exposures is possible by limiting sources in homes and when purchasing consumer products. Because many products, such as pillows and mattresses, have flame-retardant treatments, frequent dusting and vacuuming may reduce exposure. Discarding worn foam-containing furniture and bedding containing PBDEs is recommended. Risks and benefits of using alternative flame-retardant products should be weighed and compared with using PBDEs or other non-chemical fire mitigation strategies.[36]

## PERCHLORATES

Perchlorates are salts that carry the perchlorate ($ClO_4^-$) ion. Perchlorates were used until the mid-20th century as a treatment for hyperthyroidism.[37,38] Because they are potent oxidizers, perchlorates are commonly used in many industries. Ammonium perchlorate is used in the production of solid rocket fuel, propellants, explosives, automobile airbags, pyrotechnic compounds (eg, fireworks), and blasting equipment.[39] A small amount of perchlorate is formed naturally. Natural sources and use by industry have led to widespread environmental contamination.[40]

In the United States, perchlorate contamination of water wells and other drinking water sources has become more prevalent.[41-43] Analyses of urinary perchlorate concentrations in the US National Health and Nutrition Examination Survey (NHANES) showed detectable levels of perchlorate in every sample tested (detection limit = 0.05 ppb).[44] The US EPA has not established a national regulation for perchlorate in drinking water, and the permissible or recommended amounts in public water supplies differ by state or do not exist; private wells are not regulated. Consultation with the local health department about perchlorate regulations and its presence in public water or well water may be advisable in certain areas, such as the desert west, in which there is arid soil and dry conditions. Perchlorate concentrations greater than 4 mcg/L have been found in the drinking water consumed by more than 11 million people in 35 states.[37] In these water sources, concentrations of perchlorate range from 4 to 420 mcg/L.[38] People also are exposed through food. Perchlorates found in cow milk were traced back to animals grazing on crops irrigated with perchlorate-contaminated water, and in US supermarket milk samples, concentrations ranged from 1.7 to 6.34 mcg/L.[45] Perchlorates have been found in fruits, vegetables, and grains.[46,47] Human exposure is substantial as a result of this contamination of food and water. Perchlorate has been found in human milk at a mean concentration of 5.8 mcg/L[48] and readily crosses the placenta from the maternal circulation to that of the fetus.[49] Thus, adverse effects of exposures to perchlorate are of concern during critical developmental windows.

The main health concern resulting from exposure is possible inhibition of thyroid function, an effect that appears to occur predominantly by competitive inhibition of iodide transport that reduces the amount of iodide available for hormone synthesis.[43] In experimental animals, exposure to perchlorates produces abnormal CNS development; neuroanatomic disturbances in the hippocampus in the absence of overt neurotoxicity have been observed.[39] These effects may be of relevance to human neurodevelopment. In children with congenital hypothyroidism, mental retardation may develop if the hypothyroidism is not detected promptly and treated. Without treatment, children born with even mild subclinical deficiencies of thyroid function have reduced intelligence, a high incidence of attention-deficit/hyperactivity disorder, and visuospatial difficulties.[39,43,50] Most serious sequelae attributable to perchlorate exposures may be in the first trimester of pregnancy, when the fetus depends on the maternal supply of iodine and thyroid hormones, and during exclusive breastfeeding because perchlorate competes with iodine, a key component of thyroid hormone, for uptake into milk.[51] Because perchlorates accumulate in human milk, there is concern for breastfed infants because they rely completely on human milk for iodine.[43] Data also suggest that there are genetic influences on thyroid hormone synthesis, indicating that certain population subgroups are more susceptible to the effects of environmental goitrogens (substances that suppress thyroid function) such as perchlorate.[51]

Although studies in animals link perchlorate exposure prenatally and postnatally with adverse health outcomes, human epidemiologic studies associating exposure with adverse effects in children show inconsistent results. In a 2005 review, the National Academy of Sciences (NAS) noted a lack of firm evidence to show that perchlorates produced important human toxicity. On the basis of their review, however, the NAS recommended a reference dose for perchlorate in human milk of 0.0007 mg/kg/day (or 0.7 mcg/kg/day).[52] Other scientists have suggested that this dose is not low enough to protect health.[53] In 2006, scientists from the Centers for Disease Control and Prevention (CDC) described a strong association between perchlorate concentrations in US women and their circulating thyroid hormone concentrations.[54] In that study, perchlorate was a significant negative predictor of thyroxine ($T_4$) concentrations in adults. According to current theories, the goitrogenic effects of perchlorates alone may be low. In the context of exposure to other environmental goitrogens, such as thiocyanate (found in tobacco smoke) and nitrates (found in surface and well water), however, perchlorate exposure may lead to a significant effect on the thyroid axis. In this combined effect theory, the discrete effect of perchlorates might be missed in epidemiologic investigations. Among environmental goitrogens, perchlorate is estimated to be 10 times more potent than thiocyanate and 300 times more potent than nitrate at inhibiting iodide uptake by the thyroid.[51] A study in infants revealed that higher urinary concentrations of perchlorate were associated with higher urinary concentrations of thyroid-stimulating hormone (TSH) in infants who had lower urinary iodide.[55] TSH stimulates the production of $T_4$ when levels are low. In addition, mothers and children, in general, and lactating women, in particular, need adequate iodine, either through the use of iodized salt or as part of a supplement because inadequate iodine increases susceptibility to any perchlorate-induced effect on the thyroid. Some risk of thyroid axis impact can be mitigated through iodine supplementation in the diet.[56]

## FREQUENTLY ASKED QUESTIONS

Q  *Because human milk can contain PBDEs, should I stop breastfeeding my infant?*

A  Breastfeeding is recommended for infants. Numerous research studies have documented the broad and compelling advantages for infants, mothers, families, and society related to breastfeeding. Some of these benefits include immunologic advantages, lower obesity rates, and greater cognitive development for the infant in addition to health advantages for the lactating mother. Even though a number of environmental pollutants, such as PBDEs, can readily pass to the infant through human milk, the advantages of breastfeeding outweigh potential risks in nearly every circumstance. The American Academy of Pediatrics and other organizations recommend breastfeeding.

Q  *I am concerned that home dust may be contaminated with PBDE. Should I get my child's PBDE blood level measured?*

A  Although PBDEs can be measured in serum, the testing requires specialized laboratory staff and complex technology that is not available in clinical laboratories. Because the results do not guide medical therapy or predict future health effects, serum PBDE measurements are not generally available outside of research studies. Routine measurement of serum PBDEs is not recommended because few laboratories measure PBDEs, the tests are costly and unlikely to be covered by insurance, and the results do not provide clinical information to guide medical management.

Q  *I have been notified that the drinking water in my home has perchlorate contamination. Should I get my child's thyroid function tested?*

A  Use bottled water if you have concerns about the presence of perchlorates in your tap water, and you may also contact local drinking water authorities and follow their advice. Perchlorate is rapidly cleared from the body, so unless you suspect extremely high levels of exposure, thyroid function testing is likely not warranted.

Q    *Should I buy an organic mattress for my infant?*

A    If you wish to reduce PBDE exposure, several producers now offer mattresses that are free of flame retardants and will decrease childhood exposure to potentially hazardous chemicals.

## References

1. Birnbaum LS, Staskal DF. Brominated flame retardants: cause for concern? *Environ Health Perspect.* 2004;112(1):9–17

2. Betts KS. New thinking on flame retardants. *Environ Health Perspect.* 2008;116(5):A210–A213

3. Geyer HJ, Schramm KW, Darnerud PO, et al. Terminal elimination half-lives of the brominated flame retardants TBBPA, HBCD, and lower brominated PBDEs in humans. *Organohalogen Compounds.* 2004;66:3820–3825

4. Thuresson K, Höglund P, Hagmar L, Sjödin A, Bergman A, Jakobsson K. Apparent half-lives of hepta- to decabrominated diphenyl ethers in human serum as determined in occupationally exposed workers. *Environ Health Perspect.* 2006;114(2):176–181

5. Schecter A, Papke O, Harris TR, et al. Polybrominated diphenyl ether (PBDE) levels in an expanded market basket survey of U.S. food and estimated PBDE dietary intake by age and sex. *Environ Health Perspect.* 2006;114(10):1515–1520

6. Athanasiadou M, Cuadra SN, Marsh G, Bergman A, Jakobsson K. Polybrominated diphenyl ethers (PBDEs) and bioaccumulative hydroxylated PBDE metabolites in young humans from Managua, Nicaragua. *Environ Health Perspect.* 2008;116(3):400–408

7. Lema SC, Dickey JT, Schultz IR, Swanson P. Dietary exposure to 2,2',4,4'-tetrabromodiphenyl ether (PBDE-47) alters thyroid status and thyroid hormone-regulated gene transcription in the pituitary and brain. *Environ Health Perspect.* 2008;116(12):1694–1699

8. Fång J, Nyberg E, Winnberg U, Bignert A, Bergman Å. Spatial and temporal trends of the Stockholm Convention POPs in mothers' milk–a global review. *Environ Sci Pollut Res Int.* 2015;22(12):8989–9041

9. Bradman A, Fenster L, Sjodin A, Jones RS, Patterson DG Jr, Eskenazi B. Polybrominated diphenyl ether levels in the blood of pregnant women living in an agricultural community in California. *Environ Health Perspect.* 2007;115(1):71–74

10. Fischer D, Hooper K, Athanasiadou M, Athanassiadis I, Bergman A. Children show highest levels of polybrominated diphenyl ethers in a California family of four: a case study. *Environ Health Perspect.* 2006;114(10):1581–1584

11. Yu G, Bu Q, Cao Z, et al. Brominated flame retardants (BFRs): a review on environmental contamination in China. *Chemosphere.* 2016;150:479–490

12. Awasthi AK, Zeng X, Li J. Environmental pollution of electronic waste recycling in India: a critical review. *Environ Pollut.* 2016;211:259–270

13. Schecter A, Haffner D, Colacino J, et al. Polybrominated diphenyl ethers (PBDEs) and hexabromocyclododecane (HBCD) in composite U.S. food samples. *Environ Health Perspect.* 2010;118(3):357–362

14. Kim M, Li LY, Gorgy T, Grace JR. Review of contamination of sewage sludge and amended soils by polybrominated diphenyl ethers based on meta-analysis. *Environ Pollut.* 2017;220 (Pt B):753–765

15. Tang J, Zhai JX. Distribution of polybrominated diphenyl ethers in breast milk, cord blood and placentas: a systematic review. *Environ Sci Pollut Res Int.* 2017;24(27):21548–21573

16. Zhang J, Chen L, Xiao L, Ouyang F, Zhang QY, Luo ZC. Polybrominated diphenyl ether concentrations in human breast milk specimens worldwide. *Epidemiology.* 2017;28(Suppl 1): S89–S97

17. Lind Y, Darnerud PO, Atuma S, et al. Polybrominated diphenyl ethers in breast milk from Uppsala County, Sweden. *Env Res.* 2003;93(2):186–194

18. Lunder S, Jacob A. *Fire Retardants in Toddlers and Their Mothers.* Washington, DC: Environmental Working Group; 2008

19. Čechová E, Vojta Š, Kukučka P, et al. Legacy and alternative halogenated flame retardants in human milk in Europe: implications for children's health. *Environ Int.* 2017;108:137–145

20. Fromme H, Becher G, Hilger B, Völkel W. Brominated flame retardants–exposure and risk assessment for the general population. *Int J Hyg Environ Health.* 2016;219(1):1–23

21. Wu N, Webster T, Hermann T, et al. Associations of PBDE levels in breast milk with diet and indoor dust concentrations. *Organohalogen Compounds.* 2007;67:654–656

22. Walter KM, Lin YP, Kass PH, Puschner B. Association of polybrominated diphenyl ethers (PBDEs) and polychlorinated biphenyls (PCBs) with hyperthyroidism in domestic felines, sentinels for thyroid hormone disruption. *BMC Vet Res.* 2017;13(1):120

23. Dye JA, Venier M, Zhu L, Ward CR, Hites RA, Birnbaum LS. Elevated PBDE levels in pet cats: sentinels for humans? *Environ Sci Technol.* 2007;41(18):6350–6356

24. Linares V, Bellés M, Domingo JL. Human exposure to PBDE and critical evaluation of health hazards. *Arch Toxicol.* 2015;89(3):335–356

25. Lam J, Lanphear BP, Bellinger D, et al. Developmental PBDE exposure and IQ/ADHD in childhood: a systematic review and meta-analysis. *Environ Health Perspect.* 2017;125(8): 086001

26. Kuriyama SN, Talsness CE, Grote K, Chahoud I. Developmental exposure to low-dose PBDE-99: effects on male fertility and neurobehavior in rat offspring. *Environ Health Perspect.* 2005;113(2):149–154

27. US Environmental Protection Agency. Technical Fact Sheet – PBDEs and PBBs. January 2014, EPA 505-F-14-006. https://www.epa.gov/fedfac/technical-fact-sheet-polybrominated-diphenyl-ethers-pbdes-and-polybrominated-biphenyls-pbbs. Accessed June 13, 2018

28. Szabo DT, Richardson VM, Ross DG, Diliberto JJ, Kodavanti PR, Birnbaum LS. Effects of perinatal PBDE exposure on hepatic phase I, phase II, phase III, and deiodinase 1 gene expression involved in thyroid hormone metabolism in male rat pups. *Toxicol Sci.* 2009;107(1): 27–39

29. Herbstman JB, Sjodin A, Kurzon M, et al. Prenatal exposure to PBDEs and neurodevelopment. *Environ Health Perspect.* 2010;118(5):712–719

30. National Toxicology Program: NTP Technical Report on the Toxicology of a pentabromodiphenyl oxide mixture (DE71) (Cas no. 32534-81-9) in F344/N rats and B6C3F1/N mice and toxicology and carcinogenesis studies of a pentabromodi-phenyl oxide mixture (DE71) in Wistar Han [Crl:WI(Han)] rats and B6C3F1/N mice (gavage and perinatal and postnatal gavage studies) NTP TR 589; 2015. https://ntp.niehs.nih.gov/results/pubs/longterm/reports/longterm/tr500580/listedreports/tr589/index.html. Accessed June 13, 2018

31. US Environmental Protection Agency. An Exposure Assessment of Polybrominated Diphenyl Ethers. EPA/600/R-08/086F; May 2010

32. Government of Canada. Canadian Environmental Protection Act, 1999 (CEPA). https://www.canada.ca/en/environment-climate-change/services/canadian-environmental-protection-act-registry/related-documents.html. Accessed June 14, 2018

33. The European Parliament. Restriction of Hazardous Substances Directive 2002/95/EC, (RoHS 1). Directive on the restriction of the use of certain hazardous substances in electrical and electronic equipment. Official Journal of the European Union 2002/95/EC. 27 January 2002. https://eur-lex.europa.eu/legal-content/EN/TXT/?uri=CELEX%3A32002L0095. Accessed June 14, 2018

34. The European Commission. Annex XVII to Regulation (EC) No 1907/2006 of the European Parliament and of the Council concerning the Registration, Evaluation, Authorisation and Restriction of Chemicals (REACH) as regards bis(pentabromophenyl)ether. Official Journal of the European Union. 9 February 2017

35. U.S. Consumer Product Safety Commission (CPSC). Petition Requesting Rulemaking on Products Containing Organohalogen Flame Retardants (OFRs). Petition CPSC-2015-0022; September 20, 2017

36. DiGangi J, Blum A, Bergman A, et al. San Antonio statement on brominated and chlorinated flame retardants. *Environ Health Perspect.* 2010;118(12):A516–A518

37. Buffler PA, Kelsh MA, Lau EC, et al. Thyroid function and perchlorate in drinking water: an evaluation among California newborns, 1998. *Environ Health Perspect.* 2006;114(5):798–804

38. Godley AF, Stanbury JB. Preliminary experience in the treatment of hyperthyroidism with potassium perchlorate. *J Clin Endocrinol Metab.* 1954;14(1):70–78

39. Gilbert ME, Sui L. Developmental exposure to perchlorate alters synaptic transmission in hippocampus of the adult rat. *Environ Health Perspect.* 2008;116(6):752–760

40. Blount BC, Pirkle JL, Osterloh JD, Valentin-Blasini L, Caldwell KL. Urinary perchlorate and thyroid hormone levels in adolescent and adult men and women living in the United States. *Environ Health Perspect.* 2006;114(12):1865–1871

41. Kent R, Landon MK. Triennial changes in groundwater quality in aquifers used for public supply in California: utility as indicators of temporal trends. *Environ Monit Assess.* 2016;188(11):610

42. Rajagopalan S, Anderson TA, Fahlquist L, Rainwater KA, Ridley M, Jackson WA. Widespread presence of naturally occurring perchlorate in high plains of Texas and New Mexico. *Environ Sci Technol.* 2006;40(10):3156–3162

43. Steinmaus CM. Perchlorate in water supplies: sources, exposures, and health effects. *Curr Environ Health Rep.* 2016;3(2):136–143

44. Blount BC, Valentin-Blasini L, Osterloh JD, Mauldin JP, Pirkle JL. Perchlorate exposure of the US population, 2001-2002. *J Expo Sci Environ Epidemiol.* 2007;17(4):400–407

45. Kirk AB, Smith EE, Tian K, Anderson TA, Dasgupta PK. Perchlorate in milk. *Environ Sci Technol.* 2003;37(21):4979–4981

46. Lau FK, deCastro BR, Mills-Herring L, et al. Urinary perchlorate as a measure of dietary and drinking water exposure in a representative sample of the United States population 2001-2008. *J Expo Sci Environ Epidemiol.* 2013;23(2):207–214

47. Food and Drug Administration. Survey Data on Perchlorate in Food: 2005/2006 Total Diet Study Results. Center for Food Safety and Applied Nutrition; 2008. https://www.fda.gov/Food/FoodborneIllnessContaminants/ChemicalContaminants/ucm077615.htm. Accessed June 14, 2018

48. Kirk AB, Dyke JV, Martin CF, Dasgupta PK. Temporal patterns in perchlorate, thiocyanate, and iodide excretion in human milk. *Environ Health Perspect.* 2007;115(2):182–186

49. Zhang T, Ma Y, Wang D, et al. Placental transfer of and infantile exposure to perchlorate. *Chemosphere.* 2016;144:948–954

50. Haddow JE, Palomaki GE, Allan WC, et al. Maternal thyroid deficiency during pregnancy and subsequent neuropsychological development of the child. *New Engl J Med.* 1999;341(8):549–555

51. Scinicariello F, Murray HE, Smith L, Wilbur S, Fowler BA. Genetic factors that might lead to different responses in individuals exposed to perchlorate. *Environ Health Perspect.* 2005;113(11):1479–1484

52. National Research Council, Committee to Assess the Health Implications of Perchlorate Ingestion. *Health Implications of Perchlorate Ingestion.* Washington, DC: National Research Council; 2005

53. Ginsberg G, Rice D. The NAS perchlorate review: questions remain about the perchlorate RfD. *Environ Health Perspect.* 2005;113(9):1117–1119

54. Calafat AM, Wong LY, Kuklenyik Z, Reidy JA, Needham LL. Polyfluoroalkyl chemicals in the U.S. population: data from the National Health and Nutrition Examination Survey (NHANES) 2003-2004 and comparisons with NHANES 1999-2000. *Environ Health Perspect.* 2007;115(11): 1596–1602

55. Cao Y, Blount BC, Valentin-Blasini L, Bernbaum JC, Phillips TM, Rogan WJ. Goitrogenic anions, thyrotropin, and thyroid hormone in infants. *Environ Health Perspect.* 2010;118(9):1332–1337

56. American Academy of Pediatrics Council on Environmental Health, Rogan WJ, Paulson JA, et al. Iodine deficiency, pollutant chemicals, and the thyroid: new information on an old problem. *Pediatrics.* 2014;133(6):1163–1166

# Chapter 38

# Persistent Organic Pollutants — DDT, PCBs, PCDFs, and Dioxins

○ ○ ○ ○ ○ ○

## KEY POINTS

- Persistent organic pollutants (POPs) are fat-soluble compounds that persist in the body and environment for long periods.
- Food is the main source of exposure to persistent organic pollutants.
- Infants and children often are more heavily exposed than adults.
- Health effects vary by compound, exposure level, and developmental stage at exposure.
- Manufacture and use of many of these compounds are banned; amounts allowed in commercially available foods are regulated.

## INTRODUCTION

The persistent organic pollutants (POPs) are a large and diverse family of hydrocarbon compounds containing one or several aromatic rings with chlorine, bromine, or fluorine substituting for one or more of the hydrogen atoms.[1]

The POPs include polychlorinated biphenyls (PCBs), dioxins, furans, the pesticide dichlorodiphenyltrichloroethane (DDT), other chlorinated pesticides, polybrominated biphenyls (PBBs), polybrominated diphenyl ethers (PBDEs), and the perfluoroalkyl and polyfluoroalkyl substances. Because these compounds are based on highly stable carbon-halogen bonds, they resist biological degradation, break down very slowly in the environment and in living organisms, and can persist in soil and in sediments of rivers, lakes, and oceans for years or even decades.

Persistent organic pollutants are biologically persistent and fat-soluble. Because they are based on carbon-halogen bonds, they are not readily metabolized. They are not excreted in urine or via exhaled breath, but instead persist in the body for long periods of time, mainly in adipose tissue. They are also bioaccumulative. When released to the environment, POPs are ingested by bacteria and plankton that are then consumed by larger and still larger species. Because none of these organisms has the capacity to efficiently degrade carbon-halogen bonds, POPs persist and concentrate as they move up the food chain to reach very high levels in long-lived predator species at the top of the food chain, such as tuna, swordfish, seals, whales, eagles, ospreys, and humans. Biological and environmental specimens from diverse locations around the globe all contain POPs, including the bodies of humans in all countries surveyed.[2] In general, the most highly halogenated POPs are the most environmentally and biologically persistent and the most highly bioaccumulative.

The manufacture and use of POPs is highly regulated in most countries, and manufacture and use of many compounds are now banned. In the United States, the first POP to be eliminated from commerce was the pesticide DDT, which was banned following the discovery by Rachel Carson that DDT had nearly caused the extinction of top predator avian species, such as ospreys and bald eagles, by interfering with reproduction.[3-5] Polychlorinated biphenyls were the second class of POPs to be controlled in the United States, and their manufacture and use were ended by Congress under the Toxic Substances Control Act of 1977.[6]

Internationally, the manufacture, distribution, and use of POPs are controlled under the Stockholm Convention, an international treaty adopted in 2001 that aims to protect human health and the environment by eliminating and reducing worldwide production, use, and emission of POPs.[7] The Stockholm Convention initially targeted global elimination of the "dirty dozen," 12 widespread, highly toxic POPs broadly believed to have sufficient toxicity to outweigh any benefit from their continued use. In 2009, 9 additional chemicals were listed under the Stockholm Convention; these are termed living chemicals because many are still manufactured and used.[7]

## CHEMICALS BANNED OR RESTRICTED UNDER THE STOCKHOLM CONVENTION

The original list consisted of the following chemicals:

Aldrin

Chlordane

DDT

Dieldrin

Endrin

Heptachlor

Hexachlorobenzene

Mirex

Polychlorinated biphenyls (PCBs)

Polychlorinated dibenzo-*p*-dioxins (PCDDs)

Polychlorinated dibenzofurans (PCDFs)

Toxaphene

Recent additions include the following chemicals:

β-hexachlorocyclohexane

Chlordecone

Hexabromobiphenyl

Lindane

Pentachlorobenzene

Tetra- and pentabromodiphenyl ether

Perfluorooctanoic acid (PFOA) and perfluorooctane sulfonic acid (PFOS)

In this chapter, four of the "dirty dozen" POPs are discussed—DDT and its derivatives, PCBs, polychlorinated dibenzodioxins (PCDDs), especially 2,3,7,8 tetrachlorodibenzodioxin (TCDD), and dibenzofurans. Three additional organochlorine pesticides (chlordane, heptachlor, hexachlorobenzene) are discussed in Chapter 15. Other older organochlorine pesticides—aldrin, dieldrin, endrin, mirex, and toxaphene—are no longer used in the United States, and clinical questions about them seldom arise. Other persistent agents of current concern include PBBs (see Chapter 29) and PBDEs (see Chapter 37) and the perfluoroalkyl and polyfluoroalkyl substances (see Chapter 36).

## Polychlorinated Biphenyls (PCBs)

The PCBs are a class of 209 structurally similar halogenated hydrocarbons (congeners), each consisting of 2 linked phenyl rings with between 1 and 10 attached chlorine atoms (see Figure 38-1).[8] They are clear, nonvolatile,

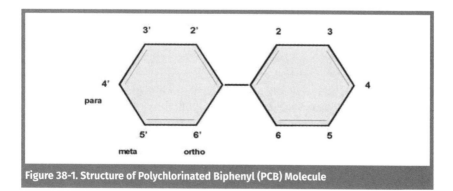

**Figure 38-1. Structure of Polychlorinated Biphenyl (PCB) Molecule**

hydrophobic oils. Approximately 1.5 million metric tons of PCBs were produced worldwide starting in 1929 until their ban in the 1970s. Because of their great stability, non-flammability, and resistance to heat and chemicals, PCBs were used widely as heat exchange fluids in electrical transformers and capacitors. PCBs were also used in consumer products, such as hydraulic fluids, immersion oil for microscopes, carbonless copy paper, electrical appliances, and fluorescent lighting ballasts.

Although PCBs have not been manufactured in the United States for more than 30 years, much of the total mass of PCBs produced is still in the environment as a consequence of their extensive past use, improper containment, and long environmental persistence.[1] Polychlorinated biphenyls cycle between air, water, and soil, and PCB vapors can be transported long distances in the atmosphere.[1] Very high concentrations are found in the circumpolar regions as a consequence of long-range atmospheric transport.[9]

Many waterways in the United States and in other countries are contaminated today with PCBs.[8] The Hudson River is heavily contaminated as the result of leakage of an estimated 1.3 million pounds of PCBs from General Electric manufacturing plants in upstate New York; PCBs have been detected in sediment, water, fish, crabs, and lobsters throughout the length of the river and as far as 200 miles downstream in New York Harbor.[10] Studies monitoring changes in PCB contamination in Hudson River sediments over time have shown that PCBs degrade very slowly and that while the river is becoming cleaner in respect to other contaminants, PCBs remain stubbornly persistent. The most heavily chlorinated PCBs are the most persistent. Parts of the Great Lakes are also contaminated with PCBs.[8]

## Dichlorodiphenyltrichloroethane (DDT)

Dichlorodiphenyltrichloroethane is the best known of the chlorinated hydrocarbon pesticides. Beginning in the 1940s until its ban in 1972, DDT was used extensively in the United States to control insect pests in agriculture and insect vectors of disease.[11] In World War II, DDT contributed importantly to malaria control.[3] DDT was banned in the United States following the report by Rachel Carson that DDT is an endocrine disruptor and reproductive toxicant.[5] Carson described this discovery and its consequences for the environment and potentially for human health in her landmark book *Silent Spring*. She observed that DDT had accumulated to reach high levels in iconic predatory bird species at the top of the food chain, most notably ospreys and bald eagles, in which it acted as an endocrine disruptor and led to the production of thin-walled, non-viable eggs that cracked prematurely leading to chick death; the DDT metabolites *o,p'*-DDT and dichlorodiphenyldichloroethylene (DDE) are weak estrogens. The result was the near extinction of ospreys and bald eagles in many areas of the United States. These species have slowly rebounded since the banning of DDT. This ban marked the beginning of the modern environmental movement and was one of the first official acts of the newly formed US Environmental Protection Agency (EPA).[4]

Dichlorodiphenyltrichloroethane continues to be manufactured and used in a number of countries around the world to control insect vectors of disease, especially the vectors that carry malaria. The World Health Organization (WHO) recommends DDT for indoor malarial vector control under certain circumstances.[12] These limited uses are permitted under the Stockholm Convention. In the environment, DDT breaks down slowly into DDE and dichlorodiphenyldichloroethane (DDD) because of the action of soil microorganisms. DDT, DDE, and DDD have long environmental half-lives and can potentially persist in soil for hundreds of years. In the United States, DDT and its breakdown products are found at many hazardous waste sites.[11]

## Dioxins and Furans

Polychlorinated dibenzofurans (PCDFs) are partially oxidized PCBs. They were never produced intentionally but are formed as contaminants in PCBs that have undergone high temperature applications or have been combusted in fires or explosions.[13,14] Polychlorinated dibenzodioxins (PCDDs), commonly referred to as dioxins, also are contaminants and are not manufactured. These are formed during the manufacture of hexachlorophene, pentachlorophenol, the phenoxy acid herbicides 2,4,5 trichlorophenoxyacetic acid (a component of Agent Orange, used as a defoliant during the Vietnam War), and silvex.

Dioxins, like PCBs, have multiple congeners with varying numbers of chlorine atoms and differing levels of toxicity. One dioxin congener, tetrachlorodibenzo-$p$-dioxin (TCDD), is among the most highly toxic of toxic synthetic chemicals. The following is the structural formula of TCDD:

Most dioxin today is formed as a by-product of industrial processes including smelting and chlorine bleaching of paper pulp. Combustion of PCBs and vinyl chloride plastics can produce dioxins. Dioxins can arise as a combustion by-product in waste incinerators when PCB-containing plastics are burned.[13]

## ROUTES AND SOURCES OF EXPOSURE

Ingestion is the principal route of exposure to POPs.[1] Because children eat more food per kilogram of body weight than do adults, they are proportionately more heavily exposed. Because POPs are not well metabolized or excreted, ingestion of even very small daily doses over many years can lead to their accumulation in tissues, and the body burdens of POPs increase with age. POPs cross the placenta from mother to fetus; therefore, maternal consumption of foods with high concentrations of POPs during or even before pregnancy can result in exposure *in utero*.

Persistent organic pollutants are fat-soluble and concentrate to reach high levels in lipid-rich human milk as described in detail in Chapter 15. Human milk is therefore a source of exposure for infants. In recent years, following restrictions in their manufacture, levels of POPs in human milk have declined, with the exception of the brominated flame retardants (see Chapter 37). Infant formula is free of POPs because the lipid in formula comes from coconuts or other sources low on the food chain. Levels of POPs are also very low in cow's milk because dairy cows do not have much exposure; in addition, a milk cow makes tons of milk during her lifetime, keeping the concentrations of pollutants low.

### Polychlorinated Biphenyls (PCBs)

The most highly concentrated food source of PCBs is sport fish taken from contaminated waters.[8] Red meat and chicken may be contaminated, and although these foods contain lower levels of POPs than fish, they are eaten in greater quantities and thus contribute significantly to population exposure.

In areas of the United States and Canada where PCB contamination has been a problem, state, provincial, and local health and environment departments have issued advisories that recommend limiting the consumption of contaminated fish.

Ballasts in older fluorescent light fixtures used PCBs as insulating fluid. When older ballasts deteriorate or break, they can release PCBs in liquid and vapor form into the indoor environment. This can be an important source of PCBs for schoolchildren, especially in US schools built prior to the ban on PCB manufacture in 1976. In New York City, the US EPA ordered that all PCB-containing ballasts be removed and replaced with PCB-free equipment. Window caulk containing PCBs is another source of exposure in older buildings, especially schools.[15]

### Dichlorodiphenyltrichloroethane (DDT)

Meat, poultry, dairy products, and fish, especially sport fish, are the principal food sources of DDT. Although environmental levels of DDT are much lower in North America today than in past decades, residual levels persist in the soil in many areas of the United States as a legacy of past use and can enter food crops. DDT can leach into waterways to contaminate fish. Food imported from countries that still use DDT is an additional exposure source.

In the human body, DDT freely crosses the placenta. Human milk is a significant source of exposure for nursing infants.[16] Levels of DDT in infant formula and cow's milk are very low to nondetectable.

People who live in countries that continue to use DDT in agriculture or vector control can be directly exposed through inhalation, skin contact, and ingestion of recently sprayed foods and contaminated drinking water. Children and adults who have grown up in countries that use DDT have higher body burdens of DDT than native-born US children.

## Dioxins and Furans

More than 90% of the daily intake of dioxins and furans comes from food, primarily meat and dairy products, and to a lesser extent fish.[13,14] To protect against dietary exposure to dioxins and furans, countries around the world have established food monitoring programs, and from time to time these programs detect excess levels of dioxins in certain foodstuffs leading to product recalls.

## Exposure to Persistent Organic Pollutants in the High Arctic

Exposure to POPs is a problem for children and families in the Arctic who eat a traditional diet of blubber from top-predator marine mammals such as seals and whales.[9] Atmospheric migration of POPs to high latitudes, coupled with bioconcentration of these compounds in predators, result in very high concentrations of POPs in these species. Dietary intakes among some aboriginal people substantially exceed established national and international guidelines.

## Occupational Exposure

Occupational exposure to POPs is rare in the United States today and most commonly occurs among workers involved in the cleanup of hazardous waste sites or repair work for electrical utilities.[8] Some heavy electrical equipment produced decades ago continues to be used, and these older transformers and capacitors may leak or become damaged during fires or explosions, thus exposing workers and the environment to PCBs or PCDFs. Substantial quantities of PCBs are still present in older industrial facilities. Women working in settings with the potential for occupational exposure are at risk of accumulating significant body burdens that can be passed to their children during pregnancy or through human milk.

DDT is still used as an indoor spray to control malaria in some countries, mostly in sub-Saharan Africa.[12] Workers who apply the pesticide and residents of sprayed houses can have high exposures. In addition, DDT is still used internationally in agriculture, and persons who handle imported food or fiber are at risk of exposure. There should be no occupational exposure to DDT in the United States today.

## SYSTEMS AFFECTED AND CLINICAL EFFECTS

Persistent organic pollutants have been associated with an array of adverse health effects that vary from compound to compound and tend to be more severe at higher exposure levels. Effects also vary with developmental stage; severe health effects can result from even very low levels of exposure in critical windows during pregnancy and early postnatal life (see Table 38-1).[16] Health effects include neurodevelopmental impairment, endocrine disruption, congenital malformations, skin lesions, and cancer.

| Table 38-1. Reported Signs and Symptoms by Age at Occurrence from PCBs, PCDFs, PCDDs, TCDD, and DDT/DDE ||
|---|---|
| **PRENATAL EXPOSURE TO LOW LEVELS OF PCBs** ||
| ■ Newborns | Decrease in birth weight[17] |
| ■ Infants | Motor delay detectable from birth to 2 years[18] |
| ■ 7-month-olds | Defects in visual recognition memory[19] |
| ■ 4-year-olds | Defects in short-term memory[20] |
| ■ 9-year-olds | Lower IQ[21] |
| ■ 11-year-olds | Delays in cognitive development[22] |
| **PRENATAL EXPOSURE TO HIGH LEVELS OF PCBs/PCDFs (ASIAN POISONINGS)** ||
| ■ Newborns | Low birth weight, conjunctivitis, natal teeth, pigmentation[23] |
| ■ Infant through school age | Delays on all cognitive domains tested; behavior disorders; growth retardation; abnormal development of hair, nails, and teeth; pigmentation; increased risk of bronchitis[24] |
| ■ Puberty | Small penis size but normal development in boys; growth delay but normal development in girls[25] |
| **DIRECT INGESTION OF HIGH DOSES OF PCBs/PCDFs** ||
| ■ Any age | Chloracne, keratoses, and pigmentation; mixed peripheral neuropathy; gastritis[26] |

| Table 38-1. Reported Signs and Symptoms by Age at Occurrence from PCBs, PCDFs, PCDDs, TCDD, and DDT/DDE (*continued*) | |
|---|---|
| **DERMAL EXPOSURE TO HIGH LEVELS OF TCDD** | |
| ▪ Children | Probably higher absorbed dose for a given exposure than adults, chloracne, liver test abnormalities[27] |
| **EXPOSURE TO LOW LEVELS OF DDT/DDE** | |
| ▪ Children | Delays in psychomotor test scores in preschool children[28] |

Abbreviations: DDT, dichlorodiphenyltrichloroethane; DDE, dichlorodiphenyldichloroethylene; PCBs, polychlorinated biphenyls; PCDDs, polychlorinated dibenzodioxins; PCDFs, polychlorinated dibenzofurans; TCDD, 2,3,7,8-tetra-chlorobenzo-*p*-dioxin.

## Polychlorinated Biphenyls (PCBs)

### Neurodevelopmental Toxicity

Prenatal exposures during vulnerable periods in early development can cause brain injury and neurodevelopmental deficits.[19–22,28–30]

Initial recognition of the developmental neurotoxicity of PCBs arose in studies of children exposed to high levels of these compounds in 2 poisoning incidents in Asia. One occurred in Japan in the late 1960s and involved approximately 1,800 infants and children.[31] The syndrome, called Yushō disease—the Japanese term for rice oil disease—resulted from PCB contamination of rice oil used in cooking. The PCBs entered the rice oil in the factory where the oil was produced as the result of a leak in a heat exchange system containing liquid PCBs. Follow-up investigation demonstrated that the PCBs were contaminated with highly toxic PCDFs formed during heating of the PCBs. In a similar incident in Taiwan, termed Yu-cheng disease (oil disease), rice oil was contaminated by a mix of PCBs and PCDFs and produced similar results.

Children's exposures to PCBs at levels commonly encountered in the North American environment today are associated with subclinical disruptions of neurobehavioral development. Prenatal exposures appear to be especially dangerous and are associated with lower developmental and IQ test scores, including lower psychomotor scores from the newborn period through age 2 years, defects in short-term memory in 7-month-old infants and 4-year-old children, and lowered IQs in 9- and 11-year-old children.[18–22] Exposure to PCBs and other POPs through human milk, though the subject of much concern, appears to be significantly less hazardous to neurobehavioral development than prenatal exposures.[18]

Epidemiologic studies of infants exposed prenatally to PCBs and followed into childhood found evidence for persistent motor problems, cognitive deficits, problems with visual recognition, deficits in executive functioning, attention-deficit/hyperactivity disorder, and autism spectrum disorders. The most serious of these deficits have generally occurred among the most heavily exposed children.[30]

### Endocrine Disruption

Research has examined the possibility that PCBs may act as endocrine disruptors. For instance, PCB exposure can lead to disruption in thyroid function, and it has been suggested that the neurobehavioral toxicity of prenatal exposure to PCBs may be mediated, at least in part, by prenatal disruption of thyroid function.[32,33] This relationship has not been definitively established in human populations at current levels of exposure.

Male fertility appears to decrease with exposure to PCBs. Inverse associations have been noted between PCB levels and sperm motility and with serum testosterone levels.[34]

Exposure to PCBs may also affect, in a complex manner, the timing of onset of male puberty. A higher total body burden of dioxin and dioxin-like PCBs appears to delay male puberty, whereas non–dioxin-like PCBs appear to accelerate the onset of puberty.[35]

### Obesity, Diabetes, and Cardiovascular Health

Emerging evidence indicates that exposures to PCBs, dioxins, and other halogenated hydrocarbons are associated with the development of obesity, metabolic syndrome, diabetes mellitus, and cardiovascular disease.[36–38] PCB-126 (a dioxin-like PCB congener) and dioxin can produce cardiovascular lesions in experimental animals, elevate serum cholesterol levels, and raise blood pressure.[39,40] Other PCB congeners, such as PCB-77, stimulate the secretion of proinflammatory adipokines that promote obesity.[41] Large-scale epidemiologic studies have shown a dose-response association between serum PCB levels at current levels of environmental exposure and cardiovascular disease mortality among US adults.[38]

### Immune Function

Data from experiments in laboratory animals indicate that exposure in early life to dioxin-like PCBs and to tetrachlorodibenzo-*p*-dioxin depresses immune function. To explore the potential immunotoxicity of PCBs in developing infants, studies of the immune response to standard childhood immunizations were conducted in a birth cohort in the Faroe Islands. Investigators found that the antibody response to diphtheria toxoid was depressed at age 18 months by 24.4% for each doubling of the cumulative PCB exposure.[42] A review of 41 studies found limited evidence for the association of prenatal exposure to DDE, PCBs, and dioxins with an increased risk of respiratory infections.[43]

## Cancer

Occupational exposure to PCBs in adult workers is associated with an increased risk of melanoma.[44] Epidemiologic studies found evidence for an association between PCB exposure and an increased risk of non-Hodgkin lymphoma (NHL), but results are variable.[45] The International Agency for Research on Cancer concluded that there is only limited evidence for an association between PCB exposure and NHL.[44]

## Dichlorodiphenyltrichloroethane (DDT)

### Toxicity

Acute high-dose exposure to DDT can cause neurotoxicity with irritability and, in extreme cases, convulsions.[3] Such exposure is not seen today except in locations where DDT is still directly applied as a pesticide.

The effects on children's health of early-life exposures to DDT, mostly in the form of the metabolic breakdown product DDE, have been studied in several cohorts of young children, with most showing some negative effects on developmental test scores. Results from a Catalan birth cohort showed that prenatal exposure to p,p'-DDE was associated with delays in mental and psychomotor development at 13 months of age.[46] A study in mostly migrant women in California showed similar developmental delays but in association with DDT, the parent compound.[47] Long-term breastfeeding was found to be beneficial to neurodevelopment in both studies, despite exposure to DDT and its breakdown products through human milk.[48]

Exposure to DDT in utero has been linked to increased risk of obesity in children.[49] The effect appears to be stronger in boys than in girls.[50]

### Breast Cancer

The possibility that DDT exposure might increase the risk of breast cancer has been the subject of intense study. Cross-sectional epidemiological studies, such as the Long Island Breast Cancer Study, examined this question by measuring serum levels of DDT and other POPs in adult women with and without breast cancer. These studies generally found very low levels of DDT and its metabolites in the serum and found little evidence for an association between DDT levels and breast cancer. Because of their cross-sectional design, the studies were limited in their ability to measure exposure during earlier periods of heavy DDT use and during critical windows of susceptibility in early development.[51]

A more recent study from California examined stored blood samples from the 1960s when DDT use was very high before it was banned. High serum levels of DDT during childhood in the 1960s were associated with a 5-fold increased risk of breast cancer among women decades later.[52] These women were younger than age 14 years in 1945, when DDT came into widespread use, and mostly still younger than age 20 years when DDT use peaked. Among women not exposed to DDT in that era, no association was observed between DDT levels and breast cancer. A second study in the same population examined the relationship between DDT exposure in utero as a consequence of maternal exposure. This study examined daughters' risk of breast cancer in relation to their mothers' serum levels of o,p'-DDT during pregnancy and found that DDT exposure in utero was linked to an increased risk of breast cancer.[53]

These findings document the potential for toxic environmental exposures during windows of developmental vulnerability in early life to influence risk of disease across the life span.

## Dioxins and Furans

Studies of persons exposed to dioxins in acute, high-dose exposure episodes, studies of workers exposed occupationally, and experimental studies in animals have produced much information on the toxicology and health effects of dioxins. Many toxic effects of dioxins and furans parallel those described previously for PCBs, but tend to be more severe and to occur at much lower levels of exposure.[13]

TCDD is a highly potent carcinogen and is categorized as a known human carcinogen by the International Agency for Research on Cancer.[54]

Two mass poisonings with furans occurred in Asia. In each case, the source of exposure was rice cooking oil inadvertently mixed with PCBs that had been heat-degraded and thus heavily contaminated with polychlorinated dibenzofurans. In 1968, in the first episode, the initial diagnostic clue was an epidemic of acne among residents of Kyushu province in Japan. It was traced to the use of contaminated cooking oil. Approximately 2,000 babies born in this time were eventually given a diagnosis of Yushō disease.[55] Among babies born to 13 women who were pregnant around the time of exposure, one was stillborn and was deeply and diffusely pigmented (a "cola-colored" baby). Some of the live-born children were small, hyperbilirubinemic, and pigmented and had conjunctival swelling with dilation of the sebaceous glands of the eyelid. Follow-up of the children up to 9 years later showed apathy, lethargy, and soft neurologic signs. The growth deficit that was apparent at birth resolved by approximately age 4 years.

An extraordinarily similar outbreak occurred in 1979 in Taiwan.[56,57] In that incident, 117 children born during or after that episode of food contamination were exposed to their mothers' body burden of PCBs and polychlorinated dibenzofurans. These children were examined in 1985 and have been followed since that time. Findings include ectodermal defects, such as excess pigmentation, carious teeth, poor nail formation, and short stature. They have persistent behavioral abnormalities and the difference in mean, full-scale IQ between exposed and unexposed children ranged from 9 to 19 points during 6 years of annual testing. Exposed boys, but not girls, showed deficits in spatial reasoning.

Developmental delays in children born to exposed mothers as long as 6 years after exposure are as severe as those seen among children born in 1979.[58]

Massive exposures to dioxins have occurred. The first was the exposure of Vietnamese civilians and US service members to 2,3,7,8-TCDD, a contaminant in the trichlorophenol herbicide known as Agent Orange, that was sprayed widely as a defoliant during the Vietnam War. The spraying left a legacy of TCDD contamination still detectable in human milk.[59] A meta-analysis found that parental exposure to Agent Orange appears to be associated with an increased risk of birth defects and that that the magnitude of association tended to increase with greater degrees of exposure.[60]

A second episode of TCDD exposure was the release of large amounts of dioxin and other chemicals in an explosion at a chemical factory in Seveso, Italy in 1975. Kilogram quantities of TCDD were discharged into the environment and exposed an estimated 37,000 people of all ages. The highest serum concentrations of TCDD recorded in humans occurred in children in the most heavily exposed areas.[61] Chloracne developed in children in the area near the explosion and it was most pronounced on areas unprotected by clothing.[62] Abnormal liver tests were found in some children.[27] Further follow-up of men exposed as infants or adolescents showed alterations in sperm production and sex hormones.[63]

Industrial workers in herbicide manufacturing plants and other industries are occupationally exposed to dioxins on an ongoing basis and thus their children are at risk of prenatal exposure, exposure via human milk, and exposure to contaminated dust carried home on their parents' shoes and clothing.[64]

## DIAGNOSTIC METHODS

Many laboratories can measure levels of DDT/DDE and PCBs in serum. No quality assurance programs or reference values are available, however, and no laboratory is licensed to measure these chemicals for diagnostic or therapeutic use. Thus, any measurement would have to be regarded as research and would be interpretable only within a research project. The polychlorinated dibenzofurans and polychlorinated dibenzodioxins are much more difficult to measure, and no clinical interpretation is available if the measurement is performed. Because any of the POPs can appear in human milk, it occasionally seems useful to measure them in a clinical setting. However, any reasonably sensitive method will detect DDE and PCBs in most samples of human milk. Thus far, all expert bodies that have considered this topic have recommended breastfeeding and do not recommend testing of human milk.[47,65,66] More information is included in Chapter 15.

## TREATMENT

No regimen is known to lower the body burden of the POPs. In Asia, treatments included cholestyramine, sauna bathing, and fasting; however, none has proven effective. Breastfeeding does lower maternal levels by approximately 20% for each 6 months of lactation. Theoretically, this would increase the risk to the child, but so far, the morbidity attributable to exposure to these compounds has come mainly from prenatal exposure to maternal body burden rather than from exposure through human milk (see Chapter 15).[18]

## REGULATION

In 1972, DDT was banned in the United States, and PCBs are banned from production throughout the world.[7] Any waste substance, such as waste oil containing more than 50 parts per million (ppm) of PCBs, must be handled as a hazardous substance and disposed of as hazardous waste.

Polychorinated biphenyls are food contaminants. Legally binding standards, termed 'tolerances' have been set to regulate permissible levels of PCBs in food.[67] If levels of PCBs in a food product exceed the tolerance, the US Food and Drug Administration (FDA) can order that the food be removed from the market. The FDA mandates tolerances of 0.2 to 3.0 ppm of PCBs for all foods, with a tolerance level in fish of 2 ppm. The FDA also limits PCBs in paper food-packaging materials to 10 ppm. There are no tolerances for polychlorinated dibenzofurans or polychlorinated dibenzodioxins.

The Food and Agriculture Organization and the WHO publish allowable daily intakes for POPs. For PCBs, the allowable daily intake is 6 mcg/kg of body weight per day, which is about the median for a 5-kg infant who is fed only human milk.[68] There are no allowable daily intakes for polychlorinated dibenzofurans or polychlorinated dibenzodioxins. There is a tolerable daily intake (reflecting greater uncertainty in the data) of 4 picograms per kilogram per day of toxic equivalents of TCDD. Similarly, there is a tolerable daily intake for total DDT of 0.01 mg/kg/day.

Although intake by breastfed children might commonly exceed this level, the WHO has explicitly advised that there be no change in the organization's policy to recommend breastfeeding despite the presence of pollutant chemicals.[65,66] The benefits of breast feeding far outweigh any possible adverse consequences from this exposure.

The concept of toxic equivalency has been devised to deal with the dilemma of regulating exposures and setting acceptable exposure levels for POPs in foods.[69] The problem is that exposure to a single compound of this class is unusual; rather, most human exposures are to mixtures of dozens or more POPs of varying toxicity, with TCDD being the most potent. Because much, if not all, of the toxicity of TCDD and other POPs is thought to relate to the strength of their binding to the aryl hydrocarbon hydroxylase (Ah) receptor in mammalian cells, assays have been developed to measure the strength of Ah receptor binding of particular compounds. Once the Ah binding affinity of a compound has been determined, it can be compared to that of TCDD to provide an index of its toxicity relative to TCDD—a toxic equivalent (TEQ) factor. The toxic equivalency of a mixture of POPs can be estimated by adding the toxic equivalents of the individual compounds in the mix.

## ALTERNATIVES

Polychlorinated biphenyls have been replaced mostly by mineral oils. Polychlorinated dibenzodioxins and polychlorinated dibenzofurans were never made deliberately, and no product is now contaminated with these compounds at the levels seen during the 1960s. In all agricultural uses, DDT has been supplanted by other pesticides or improved agricultural practice. For malaria control, DDT can most likely be replaced by bed nets and other means of controlling vectors.

## Frequently Asked Questions

Q   *How do I know whether fish or other foods contain PCBs or dioxins?*

A   Virtually all food today contains trace amounts of POPs. Commercial foods are regulated, so they should not have more than minimal amounts. Among unregulated foods, the most common source of high-level exposure to POPs is top predator sport fish. States in which exposures to POPs have been a problem, such as those surrounding the Great Lakes, have published advisories concerning the consumption of noncommercial fish, and these advisories are available from state health departments.

It is important for women to eat fish during pregnancy because the omega-3 fatty acids in fish promote fetal brain development. It is also important that pregnant women eat fish that are low in POPs and in methylmercury.[70] Authoritative guides listing the fish that are safe and unsafe to eat, especially during and before pregnancy, have been published by the Monterrey Bay Aquarium and the Natural Resources Defense Council. (See Resources at the end of the chapter)

Q   *Given that POPs are known to concentrate in human milk, is it safe for women who have eaten large quantities of game fish to breastfeed their infants?*

A   Authoritative bodies that have studied the safety of breastfeeding, including the American Academy of Pediatrics and the WHO, have concluded that the benefits of breastfeeding outweigh any risks from exposures to POPs or toxic chemicals in human milk. Breastfeeding, especially prolonged breastfeeding, conveys enormous health and psychological benefits to the child including greater resistance to infections and a reduced risk of childhood cancer.

*Q How can national governments reduce population exposure to POPs?*

A National governments can reduce exposures to POPs by curtailing and banning their manufacture and use by joining the Stockholm Convention, controlling industrial sources of their environmental release, controlling their release from landfills and hazardous waste sites, requiring incineration of PCB-contaminated waste materials at temperatures over 850°C in specially constructed incinerators in order to prevent formation of dioxins, and establishing and enforcing strict programs for monitoring of these chemicals in the food supply.

*Q How can state and local governments reduce population exposure to POPs?*

A State and local governments can reduce exposures by controlling commercial sources of release and securing landfills. Local governments can control the spread of PCBs in school environments by requiring timely removal of all PCB-containing fluorescent light ballasts. Parents can accelerate this process through citizen action.

## RESOURCES

### Fish guides

To guide families in the selection of fish species low in PCBs and other persistent pollutants, such as methylmercury, various groups have published authoritative tables listing safer and less safe fish. The following are links to those guides:

- Natural Resources Defense Council
  https://www.nrdc.org/sites/default/files/walletcard.pdf
- Environmental Working Group
  www.ewg.org/research/ewgs-good-seafood-guide?gclid=COKCjKCZtMwCF QIfhgodwOYHNQ
- Monterrey Bay Aquarium
  www.seafoodwatch.org/seafood-recommendations

### US Environmental Protection Agency (EPA)

Web site: www.epa.gov/OST/fish
This site lists EPA guidelines for states for the development of fish advisories for PCBs and other persistent contaminants.

### World Health Organization (WHO)

*Persistent Organic Pollutants: Impact on Child Health* (2010)
www.who.int/ceh/publications/persistent_organic_pollutant/en/index. html

# References

1. World Health Organization. Persistent Organic Pollutants Impact on Child Health. 2010. http://www.who.int/ceh/publications/persistent_organic_pollutant/en/. Accessed January 20, 2018

2. Centers for Disease Control and Prevention. National Biomonitoring Program. http://www.cdc.gov/biomonitoring/. Accessed January 20, 2018

3. Rogan WJ, Chen A. Health risks and benefits of bis(4-chlorophenyl)-1,1,1-trichloroethane (DDT). *Lancet*. 2005;366(9487):763–773

4. US Environmental Protection Agency. The Guardian: Origins of the EPA. https://archive.epa.gov/epa/aboutepa/guardian-origins-epa.html. Accessed March 6, 2018

5. Carson R. *Silent Spring*. Boston, MA: Houghton Mifflin; 1962

6. US Environmental Protection Agency. US Congress. Toxic Substances Control Act of 1976. https://www.epa.gov/laws-regulations/summary-toxic-substances-control-act. Accessed March 6, 2018

7. United Nations Environment Programme. Stockholm Convention on Persistent Organic Pollutants. http://chm.pops.int/TheConvention/Overview/tabid/3351/Default.aspx. Accessed March 6, 2018

8. Agency for Toxic Substances and Disease Registry. Toxicological Profile for Polychlorinated Biphenyls (PCBs). 2000. https://www.atsdr.cdc.gov/toxprofiles/tp17-p.pdf. Accessed January 20, 2018

9. Nuijten RJ, Hendriks AJ, Jenssen BM, Schipper AM. Circumpolar contaminant concentrations in polar bears (*Ursus maritimus*) and potential population-level effects *Environ Res*. 2016;151:50–57

10. US Environmental Protection Agency. Hudson River PCBs Superfund Site. https://www3.epa.gov/hudson/. Accessed January 20, 2018

11. Agency for Toxic Substances and Disease Registry. Public Health Statement for DDT, DDE, and DDD. 2002. https://www.atsdr.cdc.gov/phs/phs.asp?id=79&tid=20. Accessed January 20, 2018

12. World Health Organization. Malaria. http://www.who.int/topics/malaria/en/. Accessed January 20, 2018

13. Agency for Toxic Substances and Disease Registry. Toxicological Profile for Chlorinated Dibenzo-*p*-dioxins (CDDs). Updated September 2008. https://www.atsdr.cdc.gov/toxprofiles/tp104.pdf. Accessed January 20, 2018

14. World Health Organization. Dioxins and their effects on human health. Fact sheet No 225. 2016. http://www.who.int/mediacentre/factsheets/fs225/en/. Accessed January 20, 2018

15. Herrick RF, Stewart JH, Allen JG. Review of PCBs in US schools: a brief history, an estimate of the number of impacted schools, and an approach for evaluating indoor air samples. *Environ Sci Pollut Res Int*. 2016;23(3):1975–1985

16. Korrick SA, Sagiv SK. Polychlorinated biphenyls, organochlorine pesticides and neurodevelopment. *Curr Opin Pediatr*. 2008;20(2):198–204

17. Nieuwenhuijsen MJ, Dadvand P, Grellier J, Martinez D, Vrijheid M. Environmental risk factors of pregnancy outcomes: a summary of recent meta-analyses of epidemiological studies. *Environ Health*. 2013;12:6

18. Gladen BC, Rogan WJ, Hardy P, Thullen J, Tingelstad J, Tully M. Development after exposure to polychlorinated biphenyls and dichlorodiphenyl dichloroethene transplacentally and through human milk. *J Pediatr*. 1988;113(6):991–995

19. Jacobson JL, Jacobson SW. Evidence for PCBs as neurodevelopmental toxicants in humans. *Neurotoxicology*. 1997;18(2):415–424

20. Jacobson JL, Jacobson SW, Humphrey HE. Effects of *in utero* exposure to polychlorinated biphenyls and related contaminants on cognitive functioning in young children. *J Pediatr.* 1990;116(1):38–45

21. Stewart PW, Lonky E, Reihman J, Pagano J, Gump BB, Darvill T. The relationship between prenatal PCB exposure and intelligence (IQ) in 9-year-old children. *Environ Health Perspect.* 2008;116(10):1416–1422

22. Jacobson JL, Jacobson SW. Intellectual impairment in children exposed to polychlorinated biphenyls *in utero. N Engl J Med.* 1996;335(11):783–789

23. Miller RW. Congenital PCB poisoning: a reevaluation. *Environ Health Perspect.* 1985;60: 211–214

24. Rogan WJ, Gladen BC, Hung KL, et al. Congenital poisoning by polychlorinated biphenyls and their contaminants in Taiwan. *Science.* 1988;241(4863):334–336

25. Guo YL, Lai TJ, Ju SH, Chen YC, Hsu CC. Sexual developments and biological findings in Yucheng children. In: Fiedler H, Frank H, Hutzinger O, Parzefall W, Riss A, Safe S, eds. *Organohalogen Compounds.* 14th ed. Vienna, Austria: Federal Environmental Agency; 1993:235–238

26. Kuratsune M, Yoshimura T, Matsuzaka J, Yamaguchi A. Epidemiologic study on Yusho, a poisoning caused by ingestion of rice oil contaminated with a commercial brand of polychlorinated biphenyls. *Environ Health Perspect.* 1972;1:119–128

27. Signorini S, Gerthoux PM, Dassi C, et al. Environmental exposure to dioxin: the Seveso experience. *Andrologia.* 2000;32(4-5):263–270

28. Gaspar FW, Harley KG, Kogut K, et al. Prenatal DDT and DDE exposure and child IQ in the CHAMACOS cohort. *Environ Int.* 2015;85:206–212

29. Schantz SL, Widholm JJ, Rice DC. Effects of PCB exposure on neuropsychological function in children. *Environ Health Perspect.* 2003;111(3):357–576

30. Ribas-Fito N, Sala M, Kogevinas M, Sunyer J. Polychlorinated biphenyls (PCBs) and neurological development in children: a systematic review. *J Epidemiol Community Health.* 2001;55(8):537–546

31. Kuratsune M, Yoshimura T, Matsuzaka, Yamaguchi A. Epidemiologic study on Yusho, a poisoning caused by ingestion of rice oil contaminated with a commercial brand of polychlorinated biphenyls. *Environ Health Perspect.* 1972;1:119–128

32. Hagmar L. Polychlorinated biphenyls and thyroid status in humans: a review. *Thyroid.* 2003;13(11):1021–1028

33. Winneke G, Walkowiak J, Lilenthal H. PCB-induced neurodevelopmental toxicity in human infants and its potential mediation by endocrine dysfunction. *Toxicology.* 2002;181-182: 161–165

34. Meeker JD, Hauser R. Exposure to polychlorinated biphenyls (PCBs) and male reproduction. *Syst Biol Reprod Med.* 2010;56(2):122–131

35. Burns JS, Lee MM, Williams PL, et al. Associations of eripubertal serum dioxin and polychlorinated biphenyl concentrations with pubertal timing among Russian boys. *Environ Health Perspect.* 2016;124(11):1801–1807

36. Lee DH, Lee IK, Porta M, Steffes M, Jacobs DR Jr. Relationship between serum concentrations of persistent organic pollutants and the prevalence of metabolic syndrome among non-diabetic adults: results from the National Health and Nutrition Examination Survey 1999-2002. *Diabetologia.* 2007;50(9):1841–1851

37. Eslami B, Naddafi K, Rastkari N, Rashidi BH, Djazayeri A, Malekafzali H. Association between serum concentrations of persistent organic pollutants and gestational diabetes mellitus in primiparous women. *Environ Res.* 2016;151:706–712

38. Humblet O, Birnbaum L, Rimm E, Mittleman MA, Hauser R. Dioxins and cardiovascular disease mortality. *Environ Health Perspect.* 2008;116(11):1443–1448

39. Lind PM, Orberg J, Edlund UB, Sjoblom L, Lind L. The dioxin-like pollutant PCB 126 (3,3',4,4',5-pentachlorobiphenyl) affects risk for cardiovascular disease in female rats. *Toxicol Lett.* 2004;150(3):293–299

40. Jokinen MP, Walker NJ, Brix AE, Sells DM, Haseman JK, Nyska A. Increased cardiovascular pathology in female Sprague-Dawley rats following chronic treatment with 2,3,4,8-tetrachlorodibenzo-*p*-dioxin and 3,3',4,4',5-penatachlorobiphenyl. *Cardiovas Toxicol.* 2003;3(4):299–310

41. Arsenescu V, Arsenescu RI, King V, Swanson H, Cassis LA. Polychlorinated biphenyl-77 induces adipocyte differentiation and proinflammatory adipokines and promotes obesity and atherosclerosis. *Environ Health Perspect.* 2008;116(6):761–768

42. Heilmann C, Grandjean P, Weihe P, Nielsen F, Budtz-Jørgensen E. Reduced antibody responses to vaccinations in children exposed to polychlorinated biphenyls. *PLoS Med.* 2006;3(8):e311

43. Gascon M, Morales E, Sunyer J, Vrijheid M: Effects of persistent organic pollutants on the developing respiratory and immune systems: a systematic review. *Environ Int.* 2013;52:51–65

44. Lauby-Secretan B, Loomis D, Grosse Y, et al. Carcinogenicity of polychlorinated biphenyls and polybrominated biphenyls. *Lancet Oncol.* 2013;14(4):287–288

45. Kramer S, Hikel SM, Adams K, Hinds D, Moon K. Current status of the epidemiologic evidence linking polychlorinated biphenyls and non-hodgkin lymphoma, and the role of immune dysregulation. *Environ Health Perspect.* 2012;120(8):1067–1075

46. Eskenazi B, Marks AR, Bradman A, et al: In utero exposure to dichlorodiphenyltrichloroethane (DDT) and dichlorodiphenyldichloroethylene (DDE) and neurodevelopment among young Mexican American children. *Pediatrics.* 2006;118(1):233–241

47. Pan IJ, Daniels JL, Goldman BD, Herring AH, Siega-Riz AM, Rogan WJ: Lactational exposure to polychlorinated biphenyls, dichlorodiphenyltrichloroethane, and dichlorodiphenyldichloroethylene and infant neurodevelopment: an analysis of the pregnancy, infection, and nutrition babies study. *Environ Health Perspect.* 2009;117(3):488–494

48. Ribas-Fito N, Julvez J, Torrent M, Grimalt JO, Sunyer J. Beneficial effects of breastfeeding on cognition regardless of DDT concentrations at birth. *Am J Epidemiol.* 2007;166(10):1198–1202

49. Warner M, Wesselink A, Harley KG, Bradman A, Kogut K, Eskenazi B. Prenatal exposure to dichlorodiphenyltrichloroethane and obesity at 9 years of age in the CHAMACOS study cohort. *Am J Epidemiol.* 2014;179(11):1312–1322

50. Heggeseth B, Harley K, Warner M, Jewell N, Eskenazi B. Detecting associations between early-life DDT exposures and childhood growth patterns: a novel statistical approach. *PLoS One.* 2015;10(6):e0131443

51. National Cancer Institute. Long Island Breast Cancer Study Project (Past Initiative). https://epi.grants.cancer.gov/past-initiatives/LIBCSP/Members.html. Accessed January 20, 2018

52. Cohn BA, Wolff MS, Cirillo PM, Sholtz RI. DDT and breast cancer in young women: new data on the significance of age at exposure. *Environ Health Perspect.* 2007;115(10):1406–1414

53. Cohn BA, La Merrill M, Krigbaum NY, et al. DDT exposure in utero and breast cancer. *J Clin Endocrinol Metab.* 2015;100(8):2865–2872

54. International Agency for Research on Cancer. *Polychlorinated Dibenzo-para-dioxins and Polychlorinated dibenzofurans.* Volume 69. 1997.

55. Harada M. Intrauterine poisoning: clinical and epidemiological studies and significance of the problem. *Bull Inst Constitut Med Kumamoto Univ.* 1976;25:1–60

56. Hsu ST, Ma CI, Hsu SK, Wu SS, Hsu NH, Yeh CC. Discovery and epidemiology of PCB poisoning in Taiwan. *Am J Ind Med.* 1984;5(1-2):71–79

57. Chen YC, Yu ML, Rogan WJ, Gladen BC, Hsu CC. A six-year follow-up of behavior and activity disorders in the Taiwan Yu-Cheng children. *Am J Public Health.* 1994;84(3):415–421

58. Lai TJ, Liu X, Guo YL, et al. A cohort study of behavioral problems and intelligence in children with high prenatal polychlorinated biphenyl exposure. *Arch Gen Psychiatry.* 2002;59(11):1061–1066

59. Manh HD, Kido T, Tai PT, et al. Levels of polychlorinated dibenzodioxins and polychlorinated dibenzofurans in breast milk samples from three dioxin-contaminated hotspots of Vietnam. *Sci Total Environ.* 2015;511:416–422

60. Ngo AD, Taylor R, Roberts CL, Nguyen TV. Association between Agent Orange and birth defects: systematic review and meta-analysis. *Int J Epidemiol.* 2006;35(5):1220–1230

61. Mocarelli P, Needham LL, Morocchi A, et al. Serum concentrations of 2,3,7,8-tetrachlorodibenzo-*p*-dioxin and test results from selected residents of Seveso, Italy. *J Toxicol Environ Health.* 1991;32(4):357–366

62. Caramaschi F, del-Corno G, Favaretti C, Giambelluca SE, Montesarchio E, Fara GM. Chloracne following environmental contamination by TCDD in Seveso, Italy. *Int J Epidemiol.* 1981;10(2):135–143

63. Mocarelli P, Gerthoux PM, Patterson DG, et al. Dioxin exposure, from infancy through puberty, produces endocrine disruption and affects human semen quality. *Environ Health Perspect.* 2008;116(1):70–77

64. Chisolm JJ Jr. Fouling one's own nest. *Pediatrics.* 1978;62(4):614–617

65. Pronczuk J, Moy G, Vallenas C. Breast milk: an optimal food. *Environ Health Perspect.* 2004;112(13):A722–A723

66. Mead MN. Contaminants in human milk: weighing the risks against the benefits of breastfeeding. *Environ Health Perspect.* 2008;116(10):A426–A434

67. Agency for Toxic Substances and Disease Registry. Polychlorinated Biphenyls (PCBs) Toxicity. What Standards and Regulations Exist for PCB Exposure? http://www.atsdr.cdc.gov/csem/csem.asp?csem=30&po=8. Accessed January 21, 2018

68. Food and Agriculture Organization/World Health Organization. Acceptable Daily Intakes, Proposed MRLs and Estimated GLs. http://www.fao.org/fileadmin/templates/agphome/documents/Pests_Pesticides/JMPR/Evaluation94/annexi.pdf. Accessed January 21, 2018

69. Consultation on assessment of the health risk of dioxins; re-evaluation of the tolerable daily intake (TDI): executive summary. *Food Addit Contam.* 2000;17(4):223–240

70. Oken E, Rifas-Shiman SL, Amarasiriwardena C, et al. Maternal prenatal fish consumption and cognition in mid childhood: mercury, fatty acids, and selenium. *Neurotoxicol Teratol.* 2016;57:71–78

Chapter 39

# Personal Care Products

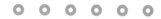

**KEY POINTS:**

- Personal care products should be kept out of the reach of young children.
- Synthetic fragrances in personal care products should be avoided.
- Regular soap is preferred over antibacterial soap.
- In addition to protective clothing, broad-spectrum sunscreen of at least SPF 15 is recommended for children.
- Chemical hair straighteners should be avoided.

**INTRODUCTION**

Personal care products are consumer products used externally to clean or care for the body. These include hygiene products (ie, cleansers, moisturizers), sunscreens, and cosmetics. Consumer products made from paper, cotton, or synthetic fiber, such as tissue and cotton swabs, may also be considered personal care products. Exposure to chemicals contained in these products is primarily through the skin, but can also occur through unintentional ingestion and inhalation. Some products are marketed for use in children, and children also may be exposed to products used by adult caregivers. Table 39-1 lists some chemicals commonly found in personal care products, health effects, and products that may contain these ingredients.

This chapter will focus on product types to which children are most commonly exposed. Specific chemicals will be discussed here; a detailed discussion of the toxicity of these and other chemicals of concern can be found in other chapters. Personal care products are regulated by the Food and

| Table 39-1. Commonly Encountered Personal Care Product Ingredients | | |
|---|---|---|
| **CHEMICAL** | **EFFECTS** | **PRODUCTS** |
| Acrylic polymers | Skin irritation | Artificial nail products |
| Ammonium thioglycolate | Foul odor, skin irritation | Hair permanent curl or straightening products |
| Antibacterial agents | Some are endocrine disruptors, may contribute to antibiotic resistance at population level | Soaps, cleansers |
| Avobenzone | In vitro estrogenic effects, not clinically significant at doses in commercially available products | Sunscreen |
| Benzocaine | Methemoglobinemia | Topical oral analgesics |
| Formaldehyde | See Chapter 20 | Multiple personal care products, most significant exposure from hair straighteners and nail polish in some settings |
| Lead | See Chapter 32 | Traditional eyeliner products manufactured outside United States, trace amounts in US cosmetics, can be higher levels in cosmetics manufactured elsewhere; lead acetate in some permanent hair dyes |
| Mercury | See Chapter 33 | Some cosmetics, especially those manufactured outside United States, some permanent hair dyes |
| Nanoparticles | No demonstrated health effects | Zinc oxide and titanium oxide in sunscreen products |
| Oxybenzone | In vitro estrogenic effects | Sunscreen |
| Parabens | In vitro estrogenic effects | Used as a preservative in multiple personal care products |
| Phthalates | Endocrine disruption | Used as color fixative or in fragrances in multiple personal care products |
| Placental protein | Endocrine effects | Specialized hair conditioning treatment |
| Sodium hydroxide (lye) | Corrosive, causes eye and respiratory irritation and burns to skin | Hair straighteners |
| Sodium lauryl sulfate | No evidence of harmful health effects | Soaps and shampoos |
| Toluene | Central nervous system effects, respiratory irritation | Solvent used in some nail care products, is being phased out in the United States |

Drug Administration (FDA) under the Federal Food, Drug, and Cosmetic Act. This law does not require "cosmetic" products or most of their ingredients to be FDA-approved before they go on the market, with the exception of color additives used in cosmetics. Under this law, "cosmetic" products are defined as products "intended to be rubbed, poured, sprinkled, or sprayed on, introduced into, or otherwise applied to the human body . . . for cleansing, beautifying, promoting attractiveness, or altering the appearance" (FD&C Act, sec. 201(i)). Products included are moisturizers, perfumes, nail polishes, facial makeup, cleansing shampoos, hair permanents, hair dyes, and deodorants, as well as any substance intended for use as an ingredient in these products. It does not include soap. Soap is regulated by the Consumer Product Safety Commission (CPSC), not the FDA. The laws and regulations enforced by the FDA and the CPSC do not contain definitions for "organic" or "natural." It should therefore not be assumed that products with these labels, or that are plant-based, are necessarily safe.

## SOAPS, LOTIONS, SHAMPOOS, AND ANTIPERSPIRANTS/DEODORANTS

Soaps may contain antibacterial agents. Some of these, such as triclosan and trilocarban, were banned by the FDA from consumer products including soaps and body washes.[1] Some soap manufacturers have replaced these chemicals with other antibacterial agents, such as benzalkonium chloride and chloroxylenol. The FDA attests that there is insufficient evidence to support the use of antibacterial soap over regular soap, and encourages consumers to choose plain soap and water.[2] Evidence has shown that triclosan and other antibacterial agents are endocrine disruptors, and there are case reports in children of the association between triclosan exposure and allergies.[3] Resistance to triclosan and other antibacterial agents may confer cross-resistance or co-resistance to other, clinically important antibiotics.[4] Consumers should therefore avoid soap marketed as "antibacterial," use plain soap and water, and employ proper handwashing techniques. In general, regular soap is less costly than antibacterial soap, providing another benefit to consumers.

Phthalates, which are esters of phthalic acid, are used in a variety of personal care products, often for their ability to fix color and fragrance. The properties and potential toxicity of phthalates are discussed in Chapters 29 and 41. Studies show increasing evidence of phthalates' endocrine disrupting properties; this is of particular concern during critical developmental windows in gestation and childhood.[5] There is insufficient evidence to identify a safe dose of phthalates. It is difficult to quantify the relative contribution of particular personal care products to a person's total phthalate exposure, partly because phthalates are found in so many products. Consumers can take steps to avoid phthalate exposure in personal care products, some of which are labeled "phthalate free." Although individual chemical components of fragrance are not required to be listed on product labels, consumers can avoid phthalates by purchasing products that are fragrance-free or labeled "no synthetic fragrance." This is true for soaps, shampoos, lotions, antiperspirants/ deodorants, and other personal care products. The word "fragrance" or "parfum" in the ingredient list means that the product is likely to contain phthalates.

Parabens are widely used as preservatives in personal care products. In vitro studies demonstrated weak estrogenic effects of these chemicals,[6] and parabens can be absorbed through the skin without breakdown.[7] Because intact paraben esters have been found in breast cancer tissue,[8] and most breast cancers are found in the upper outer quadrant, there is speculation about a possible association between paraben-containing antiperspirants and the development of breast cancer. No studies have established this association, and there is more breast tissue in the upper outer quadrant, which may explain why the upper outer quadrant is the most common location for breast tumors.[9] Parabens have also been shown to have weakly estrogenic properties, although far less potent than natural estrogens made in the body. Consumers concerned about parabens can avoid exposure by purchasing products labeled "paraben free" or by avoiding products that list any of the following ingredients: ethyl-paraben, propylparaben, butylparaben, isobutylparaben, isopropylparaben, and benzylparaben.

Formaldehyde and formaldehyde-releasing chemicals are used as preservatives in soaps, particularly liquid soaps, shampoos, and other personal care products. The toxicity of formaldehyde is discussed in detail in Chapter 20. The primary route of exposure is through inhalation, although the liquid form may be ingested. Formaldehyde exposure from most personal care products, including soaps and shampoos, is very small, especially relative to other sources in homes, such as pressed-wood building materials and cigarette smoke. Because of increasing consumer concern, there are now more formaldehyde-free soaps and shampoos in the marketplace; however, it is not clear whether there is a significant health benefit from using these products.

Sodium lauryl sulfate, an anionic surfactant found in many soaps, shampoos, and household cleaners, is often cited as a chemical of concern by the popular media. Evidence suggests, however, that sodium lauryl sulfate is safe with regard to direct health effects and downstream environmental impacts.[10] Although this chemical can be irritating to the eyes and skin in its pure formulation, this is not a significant concern in the low concentrations found in soaps, shampoos, and other cleansers. No evidence has shown that sodium lauryl sulfate has bioaccumulative properties as has been suggested by popular media, and from an environmental impact standpoint, it readily biodegrades into fatty acid byproducts that are benign to the environment.

## OTHER HAIR PRODUCTS

A small number of hair dye products contain lead or mercury. The toxicity of these chemicals is discussed in detail in Chapters 32 and 33, respectively. Although it is difficult to quantify the dose of these toxic metals attributable to hair dye, youth and caregivers should avoid these products. No safe level of lead or mercury has been identified, and unintentional ingestion is a concern if these products are in the home.

Chemical hair straighteners and home permanent kits are most commonly used by African American women and girls. Higher frequency and duration of lifetime hair relaxer use has been associated with an increased risk of uterine fibroid tumors in African American women.[11] Formaldehyde-based straighteners, which include keratin treatments, can result in significant exposure to inhaled formaldehyde. Liquid formaldehyde exposure to the scalp and neck can cause skin irritation. Straighteners and permanent kits containing ammonium thioglycolate are foul smelling, can irritate the skin through direct contact, and can cause allergic reactions.[12] To mask the smell, strong fragrances are often added that may include chemicals of concern. Alkaline hair straighteners, most commonly sodium hydroxide- (lye-) based, are corrosive. These products can burn the skin; irritate nasal, oral, and respiratory mucosa; and cause damage when in contact with the eyes. Children who unintentionally ingest these corrosive hair straighteners can sustain significant oral and gastrointestinal burns. These products should not be used in children, and adults should not use them in the presence of children. If they are used by adults, special care should be taken to keep these products out of children's reach.

Hair conditioning treatments containing placental protein contain ingredients derived from animal placentas. Although these products are not well studied, there is a potential risk of contamination from infectious agents, and a potential risk of endocrine effects of progesterone and estrogen from the animal placentas.[13]

Hairsprays commonly include alcohol-based solvents. Unintentional ingestion is a risk to children, and these products should be stored out of reach of young children. Inhalation of hairspray can produce acute respiratory irritation and coughing; contact with the eyes can cause irritation. These products should be used in a well-ventilated area. Hairspray use, along with nail polish and deodorant use, has been associated with evidence of higher phthalate exposure in women.[14]

An association has been found between the duration and frequency of use of hair products in childhood and an earlier age of menarche. This may be attributable to the presence of endocrine disrupting chemicals in these products, including placental estrogens and phthalates.[15]

## ORAL CARE PRODUCTS

Mouthwash containing alcohol and chlorhexidine gluconate can cause acute toxicity in children if ingested in large volume. Mouthwash should be stored out of the reach of young children and should not be used until children are able to swish and spit, typically at age 6 years.

Toothpastes are intended to be used in small volume, and to stay in the mouth for a short period of time (2 minutes). Toothpaste use should be followed by spitting and rinsing. Unintentional ingestion of a large volume of toothpaste could present a risk to children; therefore, toothpaste should be used in small quantities with adult supervision of young children, typically until an age of at least 6 years. Fluoride toothpaste is recommended for children by the American Dental Association[16] and the American Academy of Pediatrics.[17] Some toothpastes contain triclosan (described previously), and the use of these products is not recommended for children.

Over-the-counter topical benzocaine products marketed for teething and other oral pain are not recommended in infants and young children younger than age 2 years because of the risk for the development of methemoglobinemia.[18]

## DIAPER PRODUCTS

Perfumed diaper wipes and creams can cause skin irritation, and these products may contain phthalates. Chemicals can be avoided when cleansing the diaper area by using plain water, and if wipes are used, unscented wipes are preferred to minimize the risk of skin irritation.

## FACIAL MAKEUP AND NAIL PRODUCTS

Young children may be exposed to makeup and nail products by interacting with an adult who is using these, or by getting into an adult's products. Therefore, these products should be kept out of the reach of young children. In some cultures, facial makeup products and nail products are sometimes used in young children. In addition, adolescents may experiment with makeup and nail products.

Facial makeup may be a source of lead and other heavy metals. In particular, culturally specific makeup may be used in children. Products may be unintentionally ingested.[19,20] For example, sindoor, or vermilion powder, is used in South Asian cultures to mark the forehead during religious ceremonies, and is used on the parting of hair in women. Turmeric products may be used topically in South Asian cultures. All of these can be contaminated with lead. Traditional eyeliners used in several cultures (with names including kohl, kajal, al-kahal, surma, tiro, tozali, or kwalli) can contain especially large amounts of lead and other heavy metals. It is illegal to sell these products in the United States, but they are sometimes found in specialty markets or brought in to the country by families traveling from abroad.

Makeup sold in the United States, such as lipsticks, can have trace amounts of lead. The FDA sampled makeup products on the US market and found that 99% of those tested had lead content below 10 parts per million (ppm).[21] The FDA issued guidance to manufacturers recommending that cosmetics contain no higher lead content than 10 ppm.[22] Makeup products manufactured in other countries may have higher lead content.

Makeup and nail products may also contain phthalates for color or fragrance fixing and formaldehyde as a preservative. In particular, nail salons using formaldehyde-containing polishes and hardeners can be environments in which there is significant inhaled exposure to formaldehyde.[23] Given the other routes of exposure to phthalates and formaldehyde, makeup and nail polish likely play a relatively small role that is difficult to quantify.

Acrylic polymers used in artificial nail primers ( found in do-it-yourself home artificial nail kits and in nail salon supplies) are corrosive and can cause significant skin and nail bed irritation. These products can burn the skin, and unintentional ingestion can cause chemical burns of the gastrointestinal tract and airway.[24,25] Toluene is a solvent used in nail polishes and other nail products, but its use is being phased out.[26] Toxic effects of inhaled toluene include central nervous system and respiratory effects, and nausea. Nail products free of phthalates, formaldehyde, and toluene are available on the US market. Young children with hand-to-mouth behaviors should not use nail polish, and water-based nail polishes may be safer choices for children. Nail salon workers should use protective equipment including masks and gloves, and nail salons must be well ventilated.[21]

## FRAGRANCES

Perfumes can act as respiratory irritants or allergens and can especially provoke symptoms in children with asthma. There is no legal requirement for formulations of synthetic perfumes to be revealed publicly, nor is there a requirement for the components of those perfumes to be tested for safety. In addition, synthetic fragrances typically contain phthalates. Among personal care products, the use of perfume has been most significantly associated with higher phthalate exposure in women.[13]

## SUNSCREEN

In addition to protective clothing, a broad-spectrum sunscreen with an SPF of at least 15 is recommended to protect children against harmful UV radiation[27] whenever children are outdoors during the day.

Nanoparticles (zinc oxide and titanium dioxide) in sunscreens are commonly cited in popular media as potentially toxic. Titanium dioxide is considered a possible carcinogen based on animal studies.[28] Inhalation exposure may occur with loose powders containing titanium oxide, but there is limited evidence to show absorption of titanium dioxide particles through the skin. Zinc oxide nanoparticles are not absorbed through skin.[29] Zinc oxide provides excellent UVA and UVB protection, and no evidence suggests toxic effects.

Oxybenzone and avobenzone are sunscreen ingredients with excellent UVA and UVB protection. They have been found to have weak in vitro estrogenic properties, but at doses that far exceed those found in sunscreen products.[30] These chemicals are toxic to coral reefs and are not permitted for use on swimmers in certain protected reef areas. Toxicity of oxybenzone and avobenzone to developing coral is caused by increased susceptibility to bleaching, DNA damage, and endocrine disruption.[31]

Because sprayed sunscreens can be inhaled and may result in contact with the eyes, they can cause respiratory and eye irritation. Instead, this product may be sprayed on an adult caregiver's hands and wiped on the child's skin.

Parents can minimize chemical exposures by using zinc oxide-based sunscreen creams in addition to using protective clothing, wearing sunglasses, timing activities, and seeking shade. If zinc oxide sunscreen is not available, it is more important to use any sunscreen (to avoid the known risks of sunburn and other excessive sun exposure) rather than using no sunscreen. Sun protection advice is discussed in more detail in Chapter 44.

## Conclusion

Personal care products are used in children and by adults in households where children live. These products should always be kept out of the reach of young children, and additional steps can be taken to avoid children's exposure to chemicals of concern in these products. These steps include avoiding unnecessary use of cosmetic products in children, avoiding products containing synthetic fragrances, and, where evidence exists, avoiding the use of specific products that contain known toxic chemicals. Pediatricians can counsel parents and caregivers about the safety of personal care products and be mindful about cultural practices surrounding personal care products that may confer specific toxicity risks.

## Frequently Asked Questions

Q  *What are some online resources that have information about personal care products?*

A  Several Web sites offer information on personal care products, but many have little scientific evidence to support their recommendations. One resource that has been well received by the public and health care professionals is the

Environmental Working Group Skin Deep Database: www.ewg.org/skindeep. However, errors in interpretation of the science may still occur.

The Cosmetic Ingredient Review allows searching for specific cosmetic ingredients to yield safety information: www.cir-safety.org/

The Chemical Inspection and Regulation Service Web site includes the searchable International Nomenclature for Cosmetic Ingredients list: www.cirs-reach.com/Cosmetic_Inventory/International_Nomenclature_of_Cosmetic_Ingredients_INCI.html

Q *What are safe nipple emollients to use while breastfeeding?*

A Purified lanolin is commonly used and is safe for mother and baby. Plant-based oils can also be safe options, and human milk itself can be used to soothe and soften sore nipples.

Q *Are plant-based oils safe to use for moisturizing the skin and hair?*

A Cocoa butter, shea butter, coconut oil, and other plant-based oils are commonly used as hair and body moisturizers. No evidence exists to suggest that these products are unsafe. Like any product, they can cause irritation or allergic reaction in some persons, but if they are well tolerated they can be a safe alternative to other products that contain multiple ingredients. The methods used to harvest some of these products, especially palm oil, have raised concerns about harm to the environment. The Roundtable on Sustainable Palm Oil (RSPO) provides certification of sustainably sourced palm oil. Rainforest Alliance certification provides independent verification of environmentally sound practices for harvest of tropical plant products including many plant oils, and Fair Trade certification provides verification of fair labor practices.

Q *What are nanoparticles in sunscreen?*

A Nanoparticles in sunscreen are typically zinc oxide or titanium oxide. Titanium oxide in loose powders may be inhaled, and inhaled titanium oxide has been found to have carcinogenic effects in animal studies. In cream form, it is unclear whether titanium oxide is absorbed through the skin, and there is no evidence that it causes toxicity. Zinc oxide is not absorbed through the skin.

Q *I am concerned about the chemicals in sunscreen and the potential harm to my children. What do you recommend?*

A Using protective clothing, timing activities, and seeking shade are the most important first-line measures for sun protection. Broad-spectrum sunscreen with a minimum SPF of 15 is also recommended. Zinc-based sunscreens can be a good first choice for parents who are especially concerned about chemical ingredients in sunscreen. Inhalation of spray-on sunscreen can be avoided by spraying these into an adult's hand and wiping on the child's skin or by choosing sunscreen creams.

## References

1. Safety and Effectiveness of Consumer Antiseptics; Topical Antimicrobial Drug Products for Over-the-Counter Human Use. A Rule by the Food and Drug Administration. 09/06/2016. https://www.federalregister.gov/documents/2016/09/06/2016-21337/safety-and-effectiveness-of-consumer-antiseptics-topical-antimicrobial-drug-products-for. Accessed March 27, 2018. Docket No. FDA-1975-N-0012 Formerly Part of Docket No. 1975N-0183H. Document Number: 2016-21337

2. Antibacterial Soap? You Can Skip It, Use Plain Soap and Water. U.S. Food and Drug Administration. https://www.fda.gov/ForConsumers/ConsumerUpdates/ucm378393.htm. Accessed March 27, 2018

3. Ginsberg GL, Balk SJ. Consumer products as sources of chemical exposures to children: case study of triclosan. *Curr Opin Pediatr.* 2016;28(2):235–242

4. Yazdankhah SP, Scheie AA, Høiby EA, et al. Triclosan and antimicrobial resistance in bacteria: an overview. *Microb Drug Resist.* 2006;12(2):83–90

5. Shea KM, American Academy of Pediatrics Committee on Environmental Health. Pediatric exposure and potential toxicity of phthalate plasticizers. *Pediatrics.* 2003;111(6 Pt 1): 1467–1474

6. Golden R, Gandy J, Vollmer GA. Review of the endocrine activity of parabens and implications for potential risks to human health. *Crit Rev Toxicol.* 2005;35(5):435–458

7. Pozzo AD, Pastori N. Percutaneous absorption of parabens from cosmetic formulations. *Int J Cosmet Sci.* 1996;18(2):57–66

8. Darbre PD, Aljarrah A, Miller WR, Coldham NG, Sauer MJ, Pope GS. Concentrations of parabens in human breast tumours. *J Appl Toxicol.* 2004;24(1):5–13

9. Lee AH. Why is carcinoma of the breast more frequent in the upper outer quadrant? A case series based on needle core biopsy diagnoses. *Breast.* 2005;14(2):151–152

10. Bondi CA, Marks JL, Wroblewski LB, Raatikainen HS, Lenox SR, Gebhardt KE. Human and environmental toxicity of sodium lauryl sulfate (SLS): evidence for safe use in household cleaning products. *Environ Health Insights.* 2015;9:27–32

11. Wise LA, Palmer JR, Reich D, Cozier YC, Rosenberg L. Hair relaxer use and risk of uterine leiomyomata in African-American women. *Am J Epidemiol.* 2012;175(5):432–440

12. Burnett CL, Bergfeld WF, Belsito DV, et al. Final amended report on the safety assessment of Ammonium Thioglycolate, Butyl Thioglycolate, Calcium Thioglycolate, Ethanolamine Thioglycolate, Ethyl Thioglycolate, Glyceryl Thioglycolate, Isooctyl Thioglycolate, Isopropyl Thioglycolate, Magnesium Thioglycolate, Methyl Thioglycolate, Potassium Thioglycolate, Sodium Thioglycolate, and Thioglycolic Acid. *Int J Toxicol.* 2009;28(4 Suppl):68–133

13. Nair B, Elmore AR, Cosmetic Ingredient Review Expert panel. Final report on the safety assessment of human placental protein, hydrolyzed human placental protein, human placental enzymes, human placental lipids, human umbilical extract, placental protein, hydrolyzed placental protein, placental enzymes, placental lipids, and umbilical extract. *Int J Toxicol.* 2002;21(1):81–91

14. Parlett LE, Calafat AM, Swan SH. Women's exposure to phthalates in relation to use of personal care products. *J Expo Sci Environ Epidemiol.* 2013;23(2):197–206

15. James-Todd T, Terry MB, Rich-Edwards J, Deierlein A, Senie R. Childhood hair product use and earlier age at menarche in a racially diverse study population: a pilot study. *Ann Epidemiol.* 2011;21(6):461–465

16. American Dental Association Council on Scientific Affairs. Fluoride toothpaste use for young children. *J Am Dent Assoc.* 2014;145(2):190–191

17. Clark MB, Slayton RL, Section on Oral Health. Clinical report: fluoride use in caries prevention in the primary care setting. *Pediatrics.* 2014;134(3):626–633

18. Benzocaine and Babies: Not a Good Mix. https://www.fda.gov/ForConsumers/ ConsumerUpdates/ucm306062.htm. Accessed March 27, 2018

19. Lin CG, Schaider LA, Brabander DJ, Woolf AD. Pediatric lead exposure from imported Indian spices and cultural powders. *Pediatrics.* 2010;125(4):e828–e835

20. Centers for Disease Control and Prevention. Infant lead poisoning associated with the use of tiro, an eye cosmetic from Nigeria – Boston, Massachusetts, 2011. *MMWR Morb Mortal Wkly Rep.* 2012;61(30):574–576

21. Limiting Lead in Lipstick and Other Cosmetics. https://www.fda.gov/Cosmetics/ ProductsIngredients/Products/ucm137224.htm. Accessed March 27, 2018

22. Draft Guidance for Industry: Lead in Cosmetic Lip Products and Externally Applied Cosmetics: Recommended Maximum Level. https://www.fda.gov/Cosmetics/GuidanceRegulation/ GuidanceDocuments/ucm452623.htm. Accessed March 27, 2018

23. Health Hazards in Nail Salons. https://www.osha.gov/SLTC/nailsalons/chemicalhazards.html. Accessed March 27, 2018

24. Linden CH, Scudder DW, Dowsett RP, Liebelt EL, Woolf AD. Corrosive injury from methacrylic acid in artificial nail primers: another hazard of fingernail products. *Pediatrics.* 1998;102(4):979–983

25. Woolf A, Shaw J. Childhood injuries from artificial nail primer cosmetic products. *Arch Pediatr Adolesc Med.* 1998;152(1):41–46

26. Toluene in Nail Polishes and Other Nail Products. https://www.fda.gov/cosmetics/ productsingredients/products/ucm127068.htm#toluene. Accessed March 27, 2018

27. American Academy of Pediatrics Council on Environmental Health and Section on Dermatology. Ultraviolet radiation: a hazard to children and adolescents. *Pediatrics.* 2011;127(3):e791–e817

28. Baan R, Straif K, Grosse Y, Secretan B, Ghissassi FE, Cogliano V, on behalf of the WHO International Agency for Research on Cancer Monograph Working Group. Carcinogenicity of carbon black, titanium dioxide, and talc. *Lancet Oncol.* 2006;7(4):295–296

29. Cross SE, Innes B, Roberts MS, Tsuzuki T, Robertson TA, McCormick P. Human skin penetration of sunscreen nanoparticles: in-vitro assessment of a novel micronized zinc oxide formulation. *Skin Pharmacol Physiol.* 2007;20(3):148–154

30. Wang SQ, Burnett ME, Lim HW. Safety of oxybenzone: putting numbers into perspective. *Arch Dermatol.* 2011;147(7):865–866

31. Downs CA, Kramarsky-Winter E, Segal R, et al. Toxicopathological effects of the sunscreen UV filter, oxybenzone (Benzophenone-3), on coral planulae and cultured primary cells and its environmental contamination in Hawaii and the U.S. Virgin Islands. *Arch Environ Contam Toxicol.* 2015;70(2):265–288

Chapter 40

# Pesticides

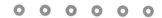

## KEY POINTS

- Pesticides are substances that are intended to reduce the impact of insects, animals, unwanted plants, fungi, or other microorganisms.
- Pesticides are widely used in homes, industry, agriculture, and as pharmaceuticals.
- When pesticides are used according to package instructions, acute poisonings should be rare.
- Because of the widespread use of pesticides, children are exposed to low levels of pesticides during critical times of development; research indicates that there may be life-long consequences as a result of exposure to certain pesticides.
- With the spread of mosquito-borne illnesses such as Zika virus, yellow fever, dengue fever, and chikungunya, careful use of appropriate pesticides can mitigate the risk of these illnesses while minimizing pesticide-related toxicity.

## INTRODUCTION

As defined by the US Environmental Protection Agency (EPA), a pesticide is a substance or mixture of substances intended for preventing, destroying, repelling, or mitigating any pest.[1] Pests include insects; mice and other animals; unwanted plants, such as weeds; fungi; or microorganisms, including bacteria and viruses. In addition to insecticides, the term "pesticide" also applies to herbicides, fungicides, and other substances used to control pests. Pesticides are ubiquitous in the environment.

The mechanism by which some pesticides kill pests includes cytotoxic or neurotoxic effects that can also harm or kill human beings. The US EPA estimates that in the year 2012, 88 million households (approximately 67%) were using 1 or more pesticides in the home or immediate environment.[2] Efforts by the US EPA to reduce residential usage of products most commonly associated with acute poisonings were associated with more than a 40% reduction in incidence of serious pesticide poisonings from 1995 to 2004.[3]

Pesticides have numerous beneficial effects. When used appropriately for control of insects and rodents, pesticides can assist in the prevention or the spread of disease. Pesticides can have a positive effect on crop yields. These compounds, however, also can be toxic to adults and children. Because pesticides are present in food, homes, schools, and parks, children are at risk for exposure from multiple sources. Children at increased risk include those whose parents are farmers or farm workers, pesticide applicators, or landscapers or children who live adjacent to agricultural areas.[4,5] Some crops require the application of multiple pesticides and each of these may contain a combination of "active" and "inactive" ingredients. The distinction between "active" and "inactive" does not refer to the human toxicity of the ingredient. Children and teenagers may work or play near their parents in the fields, where they may be exposed to pesticides. People who work with pesticides may use these agricultural-strength chemicals at home.[5] Inappropriate applications may increase exposure and cause illness and death.[6]

All pesticides sold or distributed in the United States must be registered by the US EPA. Registration is based on evaluation of scientific data and assessment of the risks and benefits of a product's use. States may have additional pesticide restrictions. The US EPA also is required by law to set tolerances for pesticide in food. A tolerance is the maximum permissible level for pesticide residues allowed in or on human food and animal feed. In response to concerns about children's exposure to pesticides via food, Congress passed the Food Quality Protection Act of 1996 (Pub L No. 104-170).[7] This law was unique in that it explicitly required that the US EPA ensure a "reasonable certainty that no harm will result in infants and children" from exposure to pesticides and that the effects of chemicals that have the same mechanism of action be considered cumulatively. Additional information regarding chronic exposure to small amounts of pesticides from food is included in Chapter 18.

This chapter focuses on acute and chronic effects of pesticides and prevention measures.

## INSECTICIDES

The major classes of insecticides are organophosphates, carbamates, pyrethrum and synthetic pyrethroids, organochlorines, biologically derived agents (toxins and live organisms), boric acid, borates, and neonicotinoids.

## Food Quality Protection Act (FQPA) of 1996

Actions generated by the Food Quality Protection Act, modifying the Federal Insecticide, Fungicide and Rodenticide Act and the Federal Food, Drug, and Cosmetic Act:

- Established a single health-based standard for all pesticides in food.

- Benefits, in general, cannot override the health-based standard.

- Prenatal and postnatal effects are to be considered.

- In the absence of data confirming the safety to infants and children, because of their special sensitivities and exposures, an additional uncertainty factor of up to 10 times is required to be added to safety values.

- Aggregate risk, the sum of all exposures to the chemical, must be considered in establishing safe levels.

- Cumulative risk, the sum of all exposures to chemicals with similar mechanisms of action, must be considered in establishing safe levels.

- Endocrine disruptors are to be included in the evaluation of safety.

- All existing pesticide registrations are to be reviewed by 2006.

- Expedited review is possible for safer pesticides.

- Risks are to be determined for 1-year and lifetime exposure.

## Organophosphates

Organophosphate pesticides are a major category of insecticides used in the United States and are a significant source of acute pesticide poisonings. Effective in 2000 and in 2003, respectively, two of the most toxic organophosphate pesticides—chlorpyrifos and diazinon—were banned for household use. A few household uses of organophosphate pesticides remain, including in flea collars (tetrachlorvinphos), in pest strips (dichlorvos), and for head lice and general use (malathion). Malathion is still widely used as a home and garden insecticide. From 2000 to 2012, organophosphate use in the United States decreased by 70%. Organophosphate pesticides make up approximately one third of all insecticides used in all market sectors in the United States.[2] When used in agriculture, there is a risk that mists of these chemicals can drift into nearby communities. Because of concerns about Zika virus in the United States, aerial spraying with an organophosphate pesticide (Naled™) has become more common. These compounds can also be detected as residues on food.

In addition, many people may still have these products stored in their homes. Therefore, clinicians should remain alert to these exposures and their risks.

## N-Methyl Carbamates

N-methyl carbamates are similar to organophosphates. The most toxic carbamate is aldicarb, which is used on food crops. Carbaryl and propoxur are available for a variety of household uses. Propoxur was used in some types of flea collars, but in 2016 companies making these flea collars agreed to stop producing them because propoxur residue on pet fur could increase children's exposure.[8] Carbaryl is a widely used garden insecticide, with 2 to 4 million pounds applied for household use in 2012.[2] These chemicals are moderately toxic, and propoxur is considered by the US EPA to be a probable human carcinogen.[9]

## Pyrethrum and Synthetic Pyrethroids

Pyrethrum, an extract of dried chrysanthemum flowers, refers to a composite of 6 insecticidal ingredients known as pyrethrins. Natural pyrethrins are used mainly for indoor bug bombs and aerosols because of their instability in light and heat. Anti-lice shampoos, such as A200™ and Rid™, contain pyrethrins. Pyrethroids, synthetic chemicals based on the structure and biological activity of pyrethrum, are modified to increase their stability. The pyrethroids are classified as type I or type II (or cyano-pyrethroids); type II pyrethroids generally are more toxic than type I. Pyrethroids are used in agriculture, gardening, and homes for control of structural pests (eg, termites), for flea control, and against lice and scabies (as permethrin [eg, Elimite™]). Permethrin (Permanone™, Duranon™) is marketed as a spray for tents and clothing and is sold in pesticide-impregnated outdoor clothing.[7,8] Pyrethrum and pyrethroids rapidly penetrate insects and paralyze them. As residential uses of organophosphate pesticides have become more restricted since 2000, pyrethrin and pyrethroids have taken their place. The incidence of calls to poison control centers and visits to health care facilities related to organophosphates steadily declined from 2000 to 2005, while those related to pyrethrum and pyrethroid pesticides correspondingly increased.[10]

## Organochlorines

Halogenated hydrocarbons were developed in the 1940s for use as insecticides, fungicides, and herbicides. Organochlorines are lipid soluble, have low molecular weight, and persist in the environment. Dichlorodiphenyltrichloroethane (DDT), chlordane, and other organochlorines were enormously successful because of their efficacy and low acute toxicity. Production of DDT and most other organochlorine compounds was banned in the United States in the 1970s because of concern about their persistence, bioaccumulation in the food chain, effects on wildlife, and possible long-term carcinogenicity. Organochlorines continue to be used in developing countries, including those exporting food to the United States. Lindane, also known as gamma benzene hexachloride or hexachlorobenzene (Kwell™), continues to be prescribed for lice and scabies, although safer preparations are available. Lindane poses a serious risk of poisoning if accidentally ingested or misused topically. According to the US Food and Drug Administration (FDA), lindane is to be used only in patients who have failed to respond to adequate doses of other approved agents and with caution in those weighing less than 110 lb (50 kilograms).[11] As of January 2002, the state of California no longer allowed the sale of pharmaceutical lindane.[12] A survey of California pediatricians indicated that the ban did not cause significant problems, and at the same time, it nearly eliminated poisonings from lindane in California.[13] The ban eliminated discharge of water contaminated with lindane into waterways by water-treatment facilities. In 2015, based on data from the Adverse Event Reporting System, the FDA added a black box warning regarding lindane, reinforcing that it should only be used as a second line drug for the treatment of lice and that repeated use of lindane is not recommended. The Centers for Disease Control and Prevention (CDC) recommends against using lindane for the treatment of children younger than 10 years.[14] The American Academy of Pediatrics (AAP) no longer recommends lindane for the treatment of head lice.[15]

## Biologically Derived Agents

One of the most widely used live biological agents is the bacterium *Bacillus thuringiensis*. This organism is cultured and then used in its spore form as an insecticide. Toxins (proteins and nucleotide-like compounds) are produced by the vegetative form that infects insects. Infections or adverse reactions in humans are very rare. Avermectin is a toxin derived from the soil bacterium *Streptomyces avermitilis* and it is used to control mites, fire ants, and other insects. Acute toxicity is rare and it is degraded rapidly by sunlight. Rotenone, derived from dried derris root, is sold as a dust, powder, or spray. It is used in gardens and on food crops. It is toxic to fish, birds, and insects, but generally is not harmful to humans. A case report describes a child who ingested a pesticide containing rotenone and eugenol who died from respiratory failure.[16] Eugenol is an oily liquid extracted from certain essential oils, especially from clove oil, nutmeg, cimmamon, basil, and bay leaf. Spinosad, a pesticide synthesized from a biologically based compound, was approved by the FDA in 2011 as a treatment for head lice. It interferes with nicotinic and gamma-aminobutyric acid (GABA) function, but has low mammalian toxicity.

## Boric Acid and Borates

Boric acid commonly is available as a pellet or powder for household insect control. Boric acid and borates generally are considered to be among the less toxic chemicals used for insect control and increasingly are used instead of organophosphate pesticides in settings where children may be present. Although less toxic, this class of compounds was used extensively in the 1950s and 1960s, with reports of significant toxicity, especially when ingested.[17,18] Poison control centers increasingly are receiving reports of ingestions of boric acid pellets or powders by children younger than 6 years, with an increase in cases from 2,445 in 1999 to 5,850 in 2015.[19]

## FLEA CONTROL PRODUCTS

Children may come into direct contact with pesticides through the use of household products. Some products readily available to consumers have significant toxicity and should be avoided when possible; others have been associated with little or no toxicity. Flea control products are widely used in the United States. Three fifths of US households contain a pet, and the market for flea control products is more than $380 million per year.[20] Because children frequently are in close contact with their pets and may sleep with them, exposure to these products is of significant concern.

Flea collars legally may contain a toxic organophosphate, such as tetra-chlorvinphos. The US EPA has reviewed human safety data and is currently working with manufacturers to address human health risks.[21] These collars are designed to slowly release pesticides onto the fur of the pet, where residues are bioavailable to children through direct contact.[22] Many pet shampoos, dips, and sprays contain permethrin. Although the toxicity of permethrin is less than that of some other insecticides, it has been identified as a likely human carcinogen by the US EPA.[23] Less toxic choices are imidacloprid (Advantage™) or fipronil (Frontline™) products, although these have some neurotoxicity and can be transferred to a child's hand when petting an animal. These newer agents are discussed later in this chapter. Selamectin (Revolution™), a botanical insecticide/antiparasitic, is a derivative of avermectin, another botanical insecticide. It is not considered to have significant health hazards, but it is a relatively new product for which fewer data are available compared with older alternatives. Neonicotinoids (discussed later) may be used for flea control.

Preferred approaches to flea control include regular flea combing and bathing of pets, regular vacuuming of carpets, and washing pets' bedding in hot water. If necessary, a systemic flea control preparation, such as lufenuron (Program™), or an insect-growth regulator, such as S-methoprene, fenoxycarb, or pyriproxyfen (Nylar™), are the least toxic alternatives.

## Fipronil

Fipronil is the most common example of another relatively newer class of insecticides known as N-phenylpyrazoles. Fipronil is also widely used on pet animals for flea control as well as lawn treatments, agricultural crops, and in bait stations for ant and roach control. These agents inhibit GABA channels, leading to hyperexcitability of nerve cells. Although this mechanism of action is similar to that of organochlorines, the N-phenylpyrazoles are selective for $GABA_A$ channels, whereas organochlorines inhibit $GABA_A$ and $GABA_C$ channels.[24]

## Neonicotinoids

Neonicotinoids may be used as flea control for pet animals. These insecticides are becoming more widely used in agricultural settings. There are several in this class, including acetamiprid, thiacloprid, and imidacloprid. The latter is the most commonly used active ingredient in this class. Neonicotinoids work as agonists to nicotinic acetylcholine receptors (nAChRs), but their uniqueness lies in their highly selective affinity for insect nAChRs, compared with those of mammals. In addition, they are water soluble, which decreases their ability to cross the mammalian blood-brain barrier; there are, however, reports of toxicity in the literature.[25,26] A study of children in an agricultural region of California demonstrated an association between exposure to neonicotinoids and tetralogy of Fallot;[27] further studies are needed to fully understand this association.

## OTHER PESTICIDES

### Herbicides

Herbicides are pesticides that kill unwanted plants in agriculture, in homes, on lawns, in gardens, in parks, on school grounds, and along roadways where children walk, play, and ride bicycles. Herbicides are used by approximately 14 million households annually, representing 21 to 33 million pounds of herbicides used for nonagricultural purposes.[2]

### Glyphosate (Roundup™, Rodeo™)

Glyphosate is a broad-spectrum herbicide used to kill unwanted plants in agriculture and landscapes. It is the second most common household pesticide in the United States, with 4 to 6 million pounds applied in 2012, according to national estimates.[2]

### Bipyridyls

The bipyridyls paraquat and diquat are nonselective herbicides. Paraquat is acutely toxic and is a restricted use pesticide unavailable to home owners. Diquat is available for household use as a general purpose weed killer.

## Chlorophenoxy Herbicides

These include 2,4-dichlorophenoxy-acetic acid (2,4-D). 2,4-D is the most common household pesticide used in the United States, with between 11 and 15 million pounds per year applied to lawns, parks, and athletic fields to kill broadleaf weeds.[2] The mixture of 2,4-D and the now-banned chlorophenoxy herbicide 2,4,5-trichlorophenoxyacetic acid was known as Agent Orange. This mixture was used heavily in South Vietnam and Cambodia for defoliation by the US Armed Forces during the Vietnam War. The mixture was contaminated with 2,3,7,8-tetrachlorodibenzo-$p$-dioxin, a known human carcinogen and developmental toxicant.

## Fungicides

Fungicides include substituted benzenes, strobilurins, organomercury compounds, thiocarbamates, ethylene bisdithiocarbamates, copper compounds, organotin compounds, cadmium compounds, thiophthalimides, triazoles, and miscellaneous compounds such as captan, benomyl, and vinclozolin. Organomercury compounds have been banned in the United States because of their extreme toxicity. Fungicides are used to protect grains and perishable produce from mold. These chemicals also are used as seed treatments, on ornamental plants, and in soil. Some fungicides are available in stores for use on garden plants. Fungicides most commonly are applied as a wettable powder or in granular form, and are generally poorly absorbed in these forms via dermal or respiratory routes.

## Wood Preservatives

Wood preservatives include pentachlorophenol and chromated copper arsenate (CCA). These preservatives were banned from materials other than wood by the US EPA in 1987. Pentachlorophenol is used as a wood preservative for utility poles, cross arms, and fence posts and is a known carcinogen. Chromated copper arsenate was used in pressure-treated wood commonly used to construct decks, porches, and playground equipment but was banned for residential use in 2004 (see Chapter 22), but other uses are still allowed, such as in wood shakes, shingles, and foundation support beams. Older outdoor wood structures may still contain arsenic, which can get on children's hands.

## Rodenticides

Rodenticides commonly used in US homes are anticoagulants or cholecalciferol. Anticoagulants interfere with the activation of vitamin K-dependent factors (II, VII, IX, X). Examples include warfarins, the 10-fold more potent indanediones, and superwarfarins (eg, brodifacoum), approximately 100 times more potent than the warfarins. Cholecalciferol (vitamin D) is poisonous to rodents at high doses. In 2008, the US EPA removed the more potent superwarfarins from products available to consumers and required retail products to be in the form of child-resistant bait stations rather than loose pellets. Yellow phosphorus, strychnine, and arsenic rodenticides no longer are registered for use but may be in use from existing stored supplies. Alumnimum and zinc phosphide are additional agents that have very high toxicity and have been associated with unintentional poisonings, particularly when misapplied.

## Insect Repellents

Insect repellents work by creating a vapor barrier that deters an arthropod from biting the skin.[28] *N,N*-diethyl-meta-toluamide (also known as *N,N*-diethyl-3-methyl-benzamide)—DEET—is the active ingredient in many insect repellent products. DEET is used to repel insects, such as mosquitoes, that may transmit viral encephalitis (eg, West Nile virus) or malaria and ticks that may carry Lyme disease. Marketed in the United States since 1956 and used by about one third of the US population each year, DEET is available in many commercial products as an aerosol, liquid, lotion, or stick and in impregnated materials, such as wristbands. Some sunscreen formulations also include DEET as a multipurpose product. Commercial products registered for direct application to human skin contain from 4% to 99.9% DEET. Concentrations less than 10% may not provide protection against ticks. The higher the concentration of DEET, the longer the protection time but concentrations above 50% provide no increase in protection time. For children, using the lowest effective dose of DEET (20% to 30%) is prudent. This concentration of DEET should provide approximately 5 hours of protection. Using separate DEET and sunscreen products at the same time is an acceptable practice. The use of combination products is not recommended because the sunscreen needs to be reapplied every 2 hours and after exertion or swimming, whereas the mosquito repellent generally does not need to be reapplied, and the risk of the repellent's toxicity increases with reapplication.

Alternatives to DEET include Picaridin (1-methylpropyl 2-[2-hydroxyethyl]-1-piperidinecarboxylate, also known as KBR 3023), oil of lemon eucalyptus or PMD, a synthesized version of oil of lemon eucalyptus, and IR3535. Picaridin and DEET have similar effectiveness at comparable concentrations. Estimated protection time varies depending on the study and type of mosquito being tested, but the range in most studies for both has been between 3 and 7 hours.[29] Oil of lemon eucalyptus (*p*-menthane-3,8-diol) is close behind DEET and Picaridin, followed by 2% soybean oil; all other substances are less effective than these.[29]

Products containing plant oils, such as cedar, cinnamon, citronella, clove, geranium, lemongrass, and others (essential oils) sold as insect repellents, are not as effective as DEET and, therefore, are not recommended when concern exists about arthropod-borne disease. In addition, some essential oils are skin irritants. Essential oils tend to be volatile and therefore have a short duration of action. For example, pure oil of eucalyptus has been found to have low activity against *Aedes aegypti*, a carrier of yellow fever, dengue fever, chikungunya, and Zika virus, and should not be used.[28,30]

## Inert Ingredients

Although there are approximately 900 pesticides registered for use in the United States, these chemicals are sold in more than 20,000 different products.[31] Each product contains one or more active ingredients (the 1 or 2 that actually kill the pest) and a mixture of other ingredients—sometimes called "inerts." A typical pesticide formulation may contain less than 2% active ingredients and more than 98% inert ingredients. These other ingredients function as dispersants, carriers, solvents, synergists, or ingredients that help the pesticide adhere to surfaces and resist rapid degradation. Despite the term "inert," these ingredients may be toxic. For example, xylene (an inert ingredient in some pyrethroid formulations) is a central nervous system depressant and reproductive toxicant. Other inert ingredients may be respiratory or dermal irritants or sensitizers or may even have potential chronic effects, such as potential carcinogenicity or reproductive toxicity. Synergists (chemicals that inhibit the detoxification process in insects), such as piperonyl butoxide and sulfoxide, generally are of low toxicity.

Inert ingredients are not subject to the same level of scrutiny as active ingredients and may be untested for toxicity. Active ingredients must be listed on the product label, whereas it is very difficult to obtain any information about the other ingredients in a pesticide product. If a patient experiences an adverse effect from exposure to a pesticide, the offending chemical may be one of the other ingredients not listed on the label. A clinician treating a patient who was exposed to a specific product can legally obtain information about other ingredients directly from the manufacturer by calling the phone number on the product label.

## SOURCES OF EXPOSURE

Children in the United States are almost universally exposed to pesticides; home and garden pesticide use may result in increased levels of exposure in both urban and rural settings.[32]

Prenatal and early childhood exposures may be especially significant because of the susceptibility of developing organ systems as well as behavioral, physiological, and dietary characteristics of children. Metabolites of organophosphate pesticides were shown to be present in the meconium of all 20 newborn infants tested in a New York City study.[33] In a study of 350 urban, suburban, and rural mother-infant dyads, at least one organophosphate metabolite was detected in all maternal urine samples during pregnancy.[34] This indicates ubiquitous exposure to these chemicals, even in utero.

The CDC conducts regular national biomonitoring surveys to test for residues of pesticides in adults and in children older than 6 years. The Fourth National Report on Human Exposure to Environmental Chemicals, published in 2009 and updated in 2017, reported on 54 pesticides and pesticide metabolites in blood or urine of the noninstitutionalized US population.[35] Six pesticides were detected in the majority of children tested. These were: 2, 4-Dichlorophenoxyacetic acid, 3-(Diethylcarbamoyl) benzoic acid (a metabolite of DEET), *p*-Nitrophenol (a metabolite of ethyl parathion, methyl parathion and nitrobenzene), 3,5,6-trichloro-2-pyridinol (a metabolite of chlorpyrifos), Dimethylthiophosphate (a metabolite of several organophosphate pesticides), and 3-Phenoxybenzoic Acid (a metabolite of Cypermethrin, Deltamethrin, and Permethrin). The CDC surveys did not provide information on whether the concentrations found in humans are toxic, but they did provide a comparison range for current exposures to certain pesticides in the general population, including children.

## ROUTES OF EXPOSURE

Children may be exposed to pesticides through inhalation, ingestion, and dermal absorption. They also may be exposed in utero from maternal exposures.

### Inhalation

Pesticides applied as dusts, mists, sprays, or gases may reach the mucous membranes or the alveoli, where they are absorbed into the bloodstream. Where suburban neighborhoods are interspersed with agricultural lands, chemicals from aerial spraying or fumigation may drift into residential areas.

Inhalation of the noninsecticide group of pesticides is usually relatively minor because their volatility is low and, with the exception of the chlorophenoxy herbicides, they are rarely distributed by aerial spraying. Fungicides may be inhaled during the process of application, but once applied they are subject to limited inhalation.

### Ingestion

Ingestion of pesticides may result in acute poisoning. Pesticides stored in food containers (eg, soft drink bottles) pose a special hazard for children. A survey conducted in California reported that 95% of households had at least one pesticide in the home (median = 4) and that 20% of pesticides were stored in the kitchen; this rate was much higher (46%) in lower income households. The survey also found that 52% of households had used a pesticide in the previous 12 months.[36]

The major problem with ingestion of pesticides is from foods that have been treated with them, especially those grown in home gardens. Infants and children may be exposed through their diets to trace amounts of pesticides applied to food crops (see Chapter 18). People also may be exposed to low levels of organochlorines by eating crops grown in contaminated soil and eating fish from contaminated waters. Pesticides are found in some water supplies; a 1999 US EPA survey found that 10.7% of community water system wells contained one or more pesticides that were not removed by standard water treatment technologies (see Chapter 17).[37]

Young children consume measurable amounts of soil, and children with pica can consume up to 100 g/day of soil that may contain persistent organic pesticides as well as heavy metals, such as arsenic or lead.

Wood treated with CCA is a potential source of children's exposure to arsenic. Arsenic is leached from the wood with aging and can accumulate on the wood surface or the soil under playground equipment and decks made with treated wood. Young children are at particular risk of exposure from hand-to-mouth activity.

Unintentional ingestion may occur with any of these compounds, especially with rodenticides. Whether by ingestion or inhalation, children—especially young children—frequently have serious exposures to pesticides, as indicated by calls to poison control centers (see Table 40-1).

### Table 40-1. Number of Calls to Poison Control Centers About Pediatric Pesticide Poisonings, 2015[19]

| PESTICIDE | AGE <6 YEARS | AGE 6–19 YEARS |
|---|---|---|
| Anticoagulant rodenticides | 6,183 | 242 |
| Pyrethroids | 5,260 | 1,939 |
| Insect repellents | 3,104 | 869 |
| Organophosphates (single agent) | 594 | 178 |
| Borates/boric acid | 5,850 | 205 |
| Glyphosate | 729 | 203 |
| Carbamates (single agent) | 430 | 118 |
| Naphthalene | 789 | 169 |
| Chlorphenoxy herbicides | 388 | 105 |

## Dermal Absorption

Many pesticides are readily absorbed through the skin. The potential for dermal exposures in children is high because of their relatively large body surface area and extensive contact with lawns, gardens, and floors by crawling and playing on the ground. Lindane (Kwell", for topical scabies and lice treatment) and DEET are absorbed through the skin. Dermal exposure to herbicides and fungicides generally results in skin irritation and rarely in systemic effects.

## SYSTEMS AFFECTED AND CLINICAL EFFECTS

### Prenatal Exposures

Effects associated with parental or prenatal pesticide exposures include intrauterine growth restriction and prematurity,[38] birth defects,[39] fetal death,[40] spontaneous abortion,[41] and childhood leukemia.[42] The evidence base supporting adverse effects on neurodevelopment as a result of prenatal exposure to organochlorine or organophosphate pesticides is growing.[43] More research is needed to further clarify whether these associations are causal. Given the concern about birth defects associated with mosquito-borne infections (ie, Zika virus), both the US EPA and the Canadian Pest Management Regulatory Agency concluded that DEET has low toxicity when applied as directed.[44]

## ACUTE EFFECTS

### Organophosphates

Organophosphates phosphorylate the active site of the enzyme acetylcholinesterase at the nerve ending, irreversibly inhibiting this enzyme. The signs and symptoms of acute organophosphate poisoning result from the accumulation of acetylcholine at cholinergic receptors (muscarinic effects) as well as at voluntary muscles (including the diaphragm) and autonomic ganglia (nicotinic effects). Accumulation of acetylcholine in the brain causes sensory and behavioral disturbances, impaired coordination, depressed cognition, and coma (see Table 40-2).

Organophosphates are rapidly distributed throughout the body after inhalation or ingestion. Symptoms usually develop within 4 hours of exposure but may be delayed up to 12 hours with dermal exposure. Initial symptoms may include headache, dizziness, miosis, nausea, abdominal pain, and diarrhea; anxiety and restlessness may be prominent. With progressive worsening, muscle twitching, weakness, bradycardia, hypersecretion (sweating, salivation, rhinorrhea, bronchorrhea), and profuse diarrhea may develop. Central nervous system effects include headache, blurred vision, anxiety, confusion, emotional lability, ataxia, toxic psychosis, vertigo, convulsions, and coma. Cranial nerve palsies have been noted.[16]

## Table 40-2. Acute Effects of Common Pesticide Classes[16]

| PESTICIDE CATEGORY | EXAMPLES | MECHANISM OF EFFECTS, ACUTE SYMPTOMS | DIAGNOSTIC TESTING AND TREATMENT |
|---|---|---|---|
| Organophosphates | Chlorpyrifos, diazinon, tetrachlorvinphos, methyl parathion, azinphos-methyl, naled, malathion, acephate | Irreversible acetylcholinesterase inhibition; nausea, vomiting, diarrhea, hypersecretion, bronchoconstriction, headache | Cholinesterase levels; supportive care, atropine, pralidoxime |
| N-methyl carbamates | Carbaryl, aldicarb, propoxur | Reversible acetylcholinesterase inhibition; nausea, vomiting, diarrhea, hypersecretion, bronchoconstriction, headache | Cholinesterase levels; supportive care, atropine |
| Pyrethrins | Pyrethrum | Allergic reactions; anaphylaxis, contact dermatitis, rhinitis, asthma, tremor, ataxia at high doses | No diagnostic test; treat allergic reactions with antihistamines and/or steroids, as needed |
| Pyrethroids | | | |
| —Type I | Allethrin, permethrin, tetramethrin | Multiple receptors in both central and peripheral nervous system affected; tremors, ataxia, irritability, enhanced startle response | No diagnostic test; decontamination, supportive care, symptomatic treatment |
| —Type II | Deltamethrin, cypermethrin, fenvalerate | Choreoathetosis, severe salivation, dizziness, fatigue, vomiting, diarrhea, paresthesias; pulmonary edema, seizures, coma in severe cases | Skin contact may cause highly unpleasant, temporary paresthesias, best treated with vitamin E oil preparations |
| Organochlorines | Lindane, endosulfan, dicofol | GABA blockade; sensory disturbances of face and extremities, dizziness, nausea, vomiting, diarrhea, uncoordination, tremors, dizziness, seizures | Detectable in blood; decontamination, supportive care, cholestyramine to clear enterohepatic recirculation |

| | | |
|---|---|---|
| Chlorophenoxy compounds | 2,4-Dichloro-phenoxyacetic acid (2,4-D) | Metabolic acidosis, neuropathy, myopathy, nausea and vomiting, myalgia, headache, myotonia, fever | Detectable in urine; decontamination, forced alkaline diuresis |
| Bipyridyl compounds | Paraquat, diquat | Free radical formation; pulmonary edema, acute tubular necrosis, hepatocellular toxicity | Urine dithionite test (colorimetric); decontamination, do NOT administer oxygen, aggressive hydration, hemoperfusion |
| Anticoagulant rodenticides | Warfarin, brodifacoum, diphencoumarin, diphacinone, pindone | Vitamin K antagonism; hemorrhage | Elevated PT; vitamin K administration |

Abbreviations: GABA, gamma-aminobutyric acid; PT, prothrombin time.

More severe intoxications result in sympathetic and nicotinic manifestations with muscle weakness and fasciculations including twitching (particularly in eyelids), tachycardia, muscle cramps, hypertension, and sweating.
Finally, paralysis of respiratory and skeletal muscles and convulsions may
develop. Children are more likely than adults to have central nervous system
signs, such as coma and seizures. Diarrhea is a relatively common symptom in
children.

### N-Methyl Carbamates

Carbamates act similarly to organophosphates in binding acetylcholinesterase,
but the bonds are more readily reversible. The clinical symptoms produced are
not easily differentiated from those of organophosphate poisoning. Although
acetylcholinesterase may be low in organophosphate poisoning, it usually is
normal in carbamate poisoning.[16] Carbamates may be highly toxic, although
the effects of exposure are more short lived, with some cases abating within 6
to 8 hours.

### Pyrethrum and Synthetic Pyrethroids

Pyrethrum and synthetic pyrethroids are absorbed systemically from the
gastrointestinal tract, but less so from the respiratory tract and skin.[16] These
agents act through delaying closure of voltage-sensitive sodium channels,
but because pyrethrins are metabolized very rapidly by the liver in mammals,
and most metabolites are promptly excreted by the kidneys, they have low
toxicity when ingested.[16] Most problematic are allergic reactions, which
have occurred in the form of contact dermatitis, anaphylaxis, or asthma.
Paresthesias (described as stinging, burning, or itching) may occur when liquid
or volatile compounds contact the skin; these rarely last more than 24 hours.[16]
Absorption of extraordinarily high doses rarely may cause incoordination,
dizziness, headaches, nausea, and diarrhea. A fatal asthma attack in a child
was described, attributed to shampooing her dog with a flea control shampoo
containing pyrethrin.[45]

### Organochlorines

The toxic action of organochlorines is primarily on the nervous system through
inhibition of $GABA_A$ and $GABA_C$ channels.[24] By interfering with the flux of
cations across nerve cell membranes, organochlorines produce abnormal
nerve function and irritability, which may result in seizures. Disturbances
of sensation, coordination, and mental function are characteristic. Lindane
poisoning presents with nausea, vomiting, and central nervous system stimulation or generalized seizures.

## Boric Acid and Borates

Boric acid dust is irritating to the skin, upper airways, and lower respiratory tract. Borates are readily absorbed by the gastrointestinal tract and can result in severe gastroenteritis, headache, lethargy, and an intensely erythematous skin rash similar in appearance to staphylococcal scalded skin syndrome in severe cases.[46] Metabolic acidosis may be observed, and shock can occur in severe cases. Chronic ingestion is more likely to cause toxicity than acute exposures.

## Neonicotinoids

Although dermal exposure has been documented, most symptomatic cases of poisoning have resulted from ingestion or inhalation. Neonicotinoids act as agonists to nicotinic acetylcholine receptors.[24] Most reports have been individual case reports, but there are now 2 series reported—one retrospective and one prospective.[25,26] Nonspecific symptoms include nausea, vomiting, dizziness, disorientation, and diaphoresis. Ulcerative lesions in the gastrointestinal tract may occur, particularly when accompanied by the solvent *N*-methyl-2-pyrrolidone (NMP). Other, more serious effects include aspiration pneumonia, respiratory failure, coma, and arrthymias.[25,26]

## Fipronil

Most reports of human poisoning to date have documented self-limiting symptoms, including nausea, vomiting, and aphthous ulcers. The mechanism of action of fipronil in the nervous system is through inhibition of $GABA_A$ channels.[24] In severe cases, mental status changes and seizures may occur. For the most part, these have not required long-term treatment beyond supportive care.[47]

## Herbicides

### *Glyphosate*

At usual exposure levels, glyphosate has a low level of acute toxicity. Ingestions of three quarters of a cup or more (usually as a suicide attempt) have been fatal.[48] Acute symptoms include mouth and throat pain, nausea, vomiting, diarrhea, and abdominal pain. In intentional ingestions, more severe symptoms have been reported: tachypnea, dysrhythmias, hypotension, pulmonary edema, kidney damage, and respiratory failure.[16] More commonly, external exposures cause skin and eye irritation. The surfactant polyethoxylated tallowamine, added to improve product application, is more toxic than the active ingredient glyphosate. The 2 mixed together (Roundup™) may show a synergistic increase in toxicity.

## Bipyridyls (Paraquat and Diquat)

Acute bipyridyl toxicity is thought to involve the production of free radical oxygen and, secondarily, interference with nicotinamide adenine dinucleotide phosphate and nicotinamide adenine dinucleotide phosphate (reduced form). Paraquat and diquat are corrosive to the tissues they contact directly. Initially, local effects of paraquat result in caustic burns to the skin or mucosa. This is followed by a period of multisystem injury with pulmonary edema and damage to the liver, kidney, myocardium, and skeletal muscle. Two to 14 days following exposure, progressive pulmonary failure occurs as a result of irreversible alveolar fibrosis. Diquat is less damaging to the skin and does not concentrate in the lungs. Intense nausea, vomiting, and diarrhea (possibly bloody) may be followed by hypertension, dehydration, renal failure, and shock. Death has occurred after ingestion of as little as 10 mL of a 20% concentration of paraquat in an adult and is common in ingestions exceeding 40 mg/kg. Sufficient amounts of paraquat may be absorbed dermally to produce systemic toxicity and death.

## Chlorophenoxy Herbicides

Chlorophenoxy herbicides primarily are irritants, causing cough, nausea, vomiting, and diarrhea. These compounds are well absorbed from the gastrointestinal tract, but few cases of large ingestions have been reported. Symptoms include gastrointestinal symptoms, headache, confusion, bizarre or aggressive behavior, peculiar odor on breath, elevated body temperature, fever, muscle weakness, and peripheral neuropathy. Renal failure and subsequent multisystem organ failure can occur in intentional ingestions.[16]

## Fungicides

Because a large variety of compounds are used in fungicides, the systems affected and clinical effects vary with each compound. Fungicides rarely are associated with acute poisonings in children because of their low toxicity, poor absorption, and use patterns (these compounds are often applied to seeds in storage). Many of these chemicals, however, are serious respiratory and skin irritants, some are associated with allergic sensitization, and some are linked to chronic effects, such as endocrine disruption.[49] Common responses to acute fungicide exposure include rashes, mucous membrane irritation, and respiratory symptoms.

# Rodenticides

## Anticoagulants

Anticoagulants may produce bleeding and are the number one cause of pesticide-related calls to poison control centers for children younger than 6 years.[19] However, data reported by the American Association of Poison Control Centers show no fatalities after anticoagulant ingestion.[19]

## Insect Repellents

Occasionally, people who use DEET experience adverse reactions, generally consisting of temporary irritation to the skin and eyes. A portion of dermally applied DEET is absorbed systemically.[50] Increased absorption of DEET has been reported in a mouse model when combined with sunscreen use.[51] In 1961, a case of encephalitis linked to DEET was reported.[52] Since that time, additional reports of adverse reactions included rashes, fevers, seizures, and death (mostly in children).[53,54] The major features of each of these cases have been reviewed.[55] Most of the cases of toxicity involved the use of DEET concentration from 10% to 50% and were related to overdose and misuse. Clinicians evaluating children with unexplained encephalopathy or seizures should consider the possibility of exposure to DEET.[56,57] Picaridin was introduced in the United States in 2005 but has been in use in Europe and Australia since 1998. Although the experience is less extensive than with DEET, no serious toxicity has been reported. No evidence of dermal, organ, or reproductive toxicity or carcinogenicity from picaridin has been demonstrated in animals.[58]

## SUBCLINICAL EFFECTS

A statistical simulation by a committee of the National Academy of Sciences suggested that for some pesticides, the reference dose (the dose of a noncancer-causing toxicant at which no health effects are likely) may be exceeded by thousands of children daily. Some children may display mild symptoms of inattention and gastrointestinal, or flulike, symptoms related to dietary pesticides.[59] Multiple exposures from a variety of sources (ie, food, yard, school) may be cumulative. Specific genetic polymorphisms may increase susceptibility to pesticide exposure.[60]

## CHRONIC SYSTEMIC EFFECTS

Although acute pesticide poisonings are relatively rare in children, low-level, chronic exposures are the focus of numerous studies. These studies have focused on interference with normal neurodevelopment, cancer risk, asthma, congenital anomalies, and endocrine-modifying effects. A technical report from the AAP Council on Environmental Health suggests that early-life and/or parental exposure to pesticides is associated with an increased risk for certain malignancies, neurodevelopmental problems, and some adverse birth outcomes.[43] An industry-sponsored systematic review of low-level, nonoccupational exposure to organophosphate pesticides indicated that there was no evidence that organophosphate pesticide exposure causes neurodevelopmental problems or birth defects in humans.[61]

## CHRONIC NEUROTOXIC EFFECTS

Many pesticides have acute neurotoxic effects. Chronic neurobehavioral or neurologic effects have been reported in a small proportion of organophosphate poisonings in adults. Symptoms reported to persist for months or years include headaches, visual difficulties, problems with memory and concentration, confusion, unusual fatigue, irritability, and depression. In serious poisonings with some organophosphates in adults, there have been reports of organophosphate-induced delayed polyneuropathy associated with paralysis in the legs, sensory disturbances, and weakness. In one well-documented case, an infant with hypertonia was diagnosed and treated for cerebral palsy prior to the discovery that she was suffering from chronic poisoning by an organophosphate pesticide. Her house had been sprayed by uncertified applicators before her birth and continued to have excessive levels of chemical 9 months later.[62]

Delayed or chronic neurotoxicity may be associated with pesticide exposure during central nervous system development. Although there is plasticity inherent in the development of the nervous system in infants and children, toxic exposures during the brain growth spurt may exert subtle, permanent effects on the structure and function of the brain. Exposure to neurotoxicants during early life may result in abnormal behavioral traits, such as hyperactivity, decreased attention span, and neurocognitive deficits. Maternal body burden of dichlordiphenyldichloroethylene (DDE, a degradation product of DDT) has been associated with impaired neurodevelopmental outcomes in children aged 6 to 24 and 42 to 60 months.[63,64] Prenatal exposure to chlorpyrifos has been associated with delays on the Psychomotor Development Index and Mental Development Index, attention problems, attention-deficit/hyperactivity disorder (ADHD), and pervasive developmental disorder at age 3 years (as identified by the Child Behavioral Checklist).[65] Other studies found similar associations between prenatal organophosphate exposure and developmental delays.[66] Pesticide exposure and children's neurodevelopment have been a major research focus for the Children's Environmental Health Centers. A pooled analysis of 4 birth cohorts (n = 936) found strong negative associations between prenatal urinary organophosphate metabolites and mental development indices in children who had a specific genetic variation in their detoxification.[67] This study also demonstrated the complexity of combining these cohorts and the influence of genetic susceptibility in determining the effects of certain pesticides.

Animal studies have demonstrated periods of vulnerability to neurotoxicants during early life. Single, relatively modest doses of organophosphate, pyrethroid, or organochlorine pesticides during the brain growth spurt in rodents led to permanent changes in muscarinic receptor levels in the brain and behavioral changes into adulthood.[68,69] These findings are supported by evidence that acetylcholinesterase may play a direct role in axonal outgrowth and neuronal differentiation.[70] The once widely used organophosphate pesticides chlorpyrifos and diazinon are suspected neuroteratogens and now have been banned by the US EPA for residential use. Chlorpyrifos is still licensed for use in agriculture.[71]

Adult rats exposed only as neonates to permethrin showed alterations in dopaminergic activity in the striatum (a part of the basal ganglia) and in behavior.[72] These findings support the hypothesis that early life exposures to pesticides increase the risk for Parkinson disease and other neurologic diseases related to aging.[73] A study of a nationally representative sample of US children aged 8 to 15 years demonstrated that boys with detectable urinary levels of 3-PBA (a metabolite of multiple pyrethroid pesticides) had a higher risk of having hyperactive-impulsive symptoms.[74]

## CARCINOGENIC EFFECTS

Some organophosphates (ie, dichlorvos, malathion) have suggestive evidence of carcinogenicity or are likely to be a human carcinogen (tetrachlorvinphos).[75] Permethrin is classified by the US EPA as a likely human carcinogen. A variety of fungicides also are suspected carcinogens. The International Agency for Research on Cancer (IARC) classified glyphosate, malathion, and diazinon as probably carcinogenic to humans.[76] Epidemiologic studies found associations between certain childhood cancers (eg, all brain cancers, non-Hodgkin lymphoma, and leukemia) and pesticide exposure.[77-79] A large review of 30 epidemiologic studies supported a possible role for pesticides in childhood leukemia.[80] Most, but not all, of the studies reported elevated risks among children whose parents were occupationally exposed to pesticides or who used pesticides in the home or garden.[81] Several studies linked home use of pesticides with childhood brain tumors.[82] Particular behaviors associated with an increased chance for the development of brain tumors included using sprays or foggers to dispense flea or tick treatments, flea collars, home pesticide bombs, fumigation for termites, pest strips, and lindane shampoo. A meta-analysis examining the association of residential exposure to pesticides during childhood with childhood cancer (excluding studies of parental occupational exposure) demonstrated a significant association between indoor insecticide use and childhood leukemia and lymphoma; herbicide exposure was also associated with increased leukemia risk.[83] The same meta-analysis observed a positive but not statistically significant association between residential pesticide or herbicide exposure and childhood brain tumors.

## ASTHMA

Occupational studies have demonstrated an increased risk of asthma excerbations in atopic farm workers who are exposed to certain pesticides, and an increased incidence of adult-onset asthma in high pesticide exposure events.[84,85] Evidence of a biological mechanism now exists to explain a pesticide-asthma association through both modification of T-helper cell activity and by alteration of airway reactivity.[43] In a case-control study of children, a report of any herbicide and/or insecticide exposure within in the first year of life was associated with an increased risk of asthma.[86] A review of epidemiological studies in which pesticide biomarkers were measured demonstrated an association between prenatal maternal or childhood DDE levels and asthma and wheezing in children.[87] This same review reported an association between permethrin in indoor air in the prenatal period and childhood wheezing, but no association between pesticide levels in breast milk or infant blood and asthma. A nationally representative cross-sectional study of children demonstrated an association between concurrent DDE levels in children and asthma in non-Hispanic Blacks, but not other ethnic/racial groups; in this study, no association between organophosphate pesticide exposure and wheezing was seen.[88] In summary, there is limited evidence to demonstrate an association between pesticide exposure and asthma in children.

## ADVERSE BIRTH OUTCOMES

Concern has been raised over exposure to a wide variety of pesticides possibly being associated with adverse birth outcomes: intrauterine growth retardation, preterm birth, congenital anomalies, and fetal death. Unfortunately, many studies rely on exposure recall, are heterogeneous in design, lack specific exposure assement, and show conflcting results. Overall, there appears to be a small increase in the risk of birth defects associated with pesticide exposure, but these findings are not strong and not characterized by specific pesticide type. Exposure to DDE during pregnancy is associated with an increased risk of preterm birth and delivering an infant who is small for gestational age. The relationship between organophosphate pesticide exposure and decreased birth weight was dependent, however, on a genetic polymorphism of organophosphate detoxification enzyme and ethnicity. In summary, the effect of pesticide exposure on birth outcomes is still not known. Although there is a link between some pesticides and adverse birth outcomes, there is a lack of data regarding pesticides currently used widely. Genetic factors appear to be important mediators of this association in some pesticides.[43]

## ENDOCRINE DISRUPTION

In the mid-1990s, evidence emerged that numerous chemicals in the environment can mimic hormones in laboratory animals, wildlife, and humans. Over the past 2 decades, much research has focused on endocrine disrupting chemicals or "endocrine disruptors." Many of the organochlorine insecticides exert some of their toxic effects through an endocrine mechanism. For example, DDT is estrogenic, and its metabolite DDE is anti-androgenic. Babies with cryptorchidism or hypospadias had a more than 2.5-fold increased risk of having detectable levels of DDT, DDE, lindane, and several other organochlorine pesticides in their blood.[89] Some pesticides, including DDE and hexachlorobenzene, suppress thyroid hormone levels in neonates.[90] The widely used herbicide atrazine is an aromatase agonist, thereby stimulating the endogenous conversion of androgens to estrogen.[91] This pesticide has been linked to intersex abnormalities in amphibian populations living near agricultural fields. Some studies have linked atrazine to mammary tumors in rats.[92] Even low-level exposures to hormonally active agents may pose a risk to infants and children because subtle alterations of hormone function during critical periods of neurologic and sexual development may have long-term effects. Endocrine disruption is discussed in greater detail in Chapter 29.

## DIAGNOSTIC METHODS

A history of exposure is of particular importance. In a review of 190 acute pesticide poisonings, laboratory tests were not often found to be diagnostically helpful.[93] In addition, symptoms of pesticide exposure are likely to be nonspecific. In the case of organophosphate or *N*-methyl carbamate poisoning, measurement of plasma pseudocholinesterase or red blood cell acetylcholinesterase concentrations are generally rapidly available and may be helpful in confirming a diagnosis. Because of population variability, however, these tests are neither sensitive nor specific and must be considered in the context of the clinical situation.

Urine metabolites of some pesticides (organophosphates, chlorophenoxy herbicides, pyrethroids) are measurable, but these tests are available only through specialty laboratories and should only be ordered in unusual circumstances. Organochlorine pesticides and their metabolites are measurable in blood. Population surveys have shown widespread low-level residues in the general population. The CDC's National Biomonitoring Study measures 54 pesticides and metabolites and has generated current reference ranges by age group, sex, and ethnicity.[35] The CDC survey includes only children older than 6 years. Testing for pesticides should be reserved for unusual circumstances, and the results interpreted with caution. The mainstay for the diagnosis of pesticide poisoning is maintaining a high index of suspicion and taking a careful exposure history.

## TREATMENT

When a poisoning has occurred, the label of the chemical should be obtained whenever possible. Many pesticides have confusingly similar names. Many different active ingredients are sold using the same trade names. Therefore, it is important to ascertain the exact ingredients for any product of concern. The US EPA-mandated label contains concise information on symptoms and signs, specific treatment guidelines, and a toll-free telephone number for manufacturer assistance. In an agricultural exposure, the county cooperative extension service agent can provide valuable knowledge of the local crops, chemical usage patterns, and modes of application.

Regional poison control centers can help with patient evaluation and management and have a medical toxicologist available for consultation. The National Pesticide Information Center can help answer questions about pesticide identification, toxicology, acute and chronic symptoms, and treatment (see Resources).

### General Concepts

Serious poisonings should be managed with guidance from a medical toxicologist and/or a regional poison control center. Immediate decontamination and attention to basic resuscitation (airway, breathing, and circulation) is important. If there is an ingestion, gastric decontamination may be indicated. If the exposure is dermal, clothing should be removed and the patient should be washed with soap and water. Caregivers should avoid exposure to the chemical. Latex examination gloves are insufficient personal protective equipment because many pesticides readily penetrate these gloves. Patients who are grossly contaminated may need to be decontaminated outside with rescuers who use chemical protective gear. Care should be taken to identify other children or adults with similar exposures and who may need evaluation and treatment. Eliminating a source of contamination may prevent future exposures.[94]

### Insecticides

#### Organophosphates

The patient should be decontaminated. Patients who are asymptomatic or have only minor symptoms should be closely observed. Individuals with muscarinic signs and symptoms of organophosphate poisoning are treated with atropine—very large doses may be required to reverse muscarinic symptoms. The most common life-threatening problem is respiratory arrest from bronchorrhea and diaphragmatic paralysis. The most reliable endpoint of adequate atropinization is control of bronchorrhea (drying of the secretions and clear lungs). Tachycardia before administration of atropine is not a contraindication to administration because early in the acute poisoning stimulation of autonomic ganglionic nicotinic receptors can activate the sympathetic pathway resulting in transient tachycardia. Eventually stimulation of cardiac muscarinic receptors predominates, resulting in bradycardia.

Pralidoxime (2-PAM, Protopam) breaks the bond in the acetylcholinesterase-phosphate complex and should be used as an antidote for most clinically significant organophosphate poisonings. Pralidoxime affects nicotinic and muscarinic effects of organophosphates. The bond in the acetylcholinesterase-phosphate complex takes up to 24 hours to become an irreversible bond that pralidoxime cannot break. Thus, it is important to administer pralidoxime early to prevent irreversible bonding and to preserve diaphragmatic function and prevent intubation. The neuromuscular junction is a nicotinic receptor and is unresponsive to atropine. If a blood sample for cholinesterase activity will be obtained, this should be done before administering pralidoxime because pralidoxime quickly reactivates the enzyme. The decision to use pralidoxime should not await blood test results but is based on the patient's clinical picture .

### N-Methyl Carbamates

Treatment with atropine for carbamate poisoning is the same as for organophosphates. Pralidoxime therapy generally is unnecessary, and in some cases, severe reactions and sudden death have occurred with its use.[95] In mixed poisonings involving organophosphates and carbamates or unidentified agents, cautious use of pralidoxime should be considered.

### Pyrethrum and Synthetic Pyrethroids

No specific antidote is available. Treatment is primarily supportive. In extremely large ingestions, intubation and lavage may be advised. Dermal paresthesias should be treated with topical application of vitamin E oil preparations. Seizures may be controlled with lorazepam. Allergic reactions should be treated as such, with follow-up intervention to prevent rechallenge with the allergen; as with any allergic reaction, allergic reactions can occur with relatively low exposures in sensitized indivduals. It is important to distinguish poisoning from pyrethrum and synthetic pyrethroids from organophosphate poisoning because some clinical features of synthetic pyrethroid poisoning can mimic organophosphate poisoning and unnecessary treatment with pralidoxime and atropine can be avoided.

### Organochlorines

No specific antidote is available. Treatment is supportive with use of anticon-vulsants for seizures and general supportive measures. Epinephrine is not advised for organolchlorine poisoning because of increased myocardial suscep-tibility to catecholamines and life-threatening dysrhythmias.

### Boric Acid and Borates

Skin, eye, and gastrointestinal tract decontamination are the principal treat-ments. Aggressive hydration, treatment of metabolic acidosis, and oxygenation can be critical to supportive care.

### Neonicotinoids

Treatment is primarily supportive. Although these agents also affect the cholin-esterase receptor, they do not require the use of oximes nor the routine use of atropine. In certain circumstances, however, some patients who presented with severe muscarinic symptoms were successfully treated with atropine.[26]

### Fipronil

No specific antidote is available. Treatment is primarily supportive. Treatment for seizures should be the same as in other insecticide poisoning.

## Herbicides

### Glyphosate

No specific antidote is available. Treatment is supportive.

### Bipyridyl Herbicides (Paraquat and Diquat)

Hemoperfusion has been shown to be ineffective in reducing mortality. In paraquat poisoning, supplemental oxygen may increase lung damage and should be avoided if possible. Renal status should be closely monitored, particularly with diquat, because dialysis may be required.

### Chlorophenoxy Herbicides

No specific antidote is available. The patient should be monitored for seizures and signs of multiple organ dysfunction (eg, gastrointestinal tract irritation or liver, kidney, and muscle damage). Alkalinization of the urine may enhance clearance.

## Fungicides

Treatment for fungicide poisoning is guided by the specific compound ingested. Generally, decontamination and supportive care are the mainstays of treatment.

## Rodenticides

### Anticoagulants

Consulting with a poison control center can assist in determining the significance of the ingestion. In general, for one-time minor ingestions of warfarin-related or superwarfarin-related rodenticides in children younger than 6 years, no hospital visits, decontamination, or prothrombin time determinations are needed. The child should be observed at home, and parents should be advised to notify a physician if bleeding or bruising occurs. More severe poisonings require monitoring of prothrombin time at 24 and 48 hours following ingestion. Vitamin $K_1$ preparations, such as phytonadione, are appropriate for treatment of poisoning with the warfarins or superwarfarins. In severe cases of poisoning with superwarfarins, treatment may need to continue for as long as 3 to 4 months.

## Insect Repellents

No specific antidote is available. Treatment for poisoning from DEET is supportive.

## PREVENTION: REDUCTION OF PESTICIDE-RELATED RISKS

With the exception of poison baits, as little as 1% of pesticides applied indoors reach the targeted pest. The rest may contaminate surfaces and air in the treated building. Outdoor pesticides may fall on nontargeted organisms, plants, animals, and outdoor furniture and play areas. Material from the outdoor environment can be tracked indoors and add to exposure from dust, floors, and carpets.[96] Pesticides applied outdoors may contaminate groundwater, rivers, or wells.

Biomagnification of long-lasting compounds may result in exposure to animals at the top of the food chain (including humans) at concentrations tens of thousands of times greater than those at the bottom of the food chain.

Exposure assessment and counseling about safe practices should be part of health maintenance visits, especially for children of farm workers, pesticide applicators, and others who work with pesticides. Safety precautions to safeguard the family's health should be stressed.

## INTEGRATED PEST MANAGEMENT

Integrated pest management (IPM) is a useful approach to minimizing pesticide use while providing long-term pest control. It integrates chemical and nonchemical methods to provide the least toxic alternative for pest control. Integrated pest management uses regular monitoring to determine if and when treatments are needed. Management tactics include physical (eg, barriers, caulking), mechanical (eg, vacuuming up white flies), agricultural (eg, choosing plants well suited to the site), biological (eg, using predators, pathogens such as *Bacillus thurigiensis*, and naturally occurring bacteria that kill insects), and educational (eg, cleaning up roach- and ant-attracting foods in the kitchen). Treatments are not based on a predetermined schedule but rather on monitoring to indicate when the pest will cause unacceptable economic, medical, or aesthetic damage. Treatments are chosen and timed to be most effective and least hazardous to nontargeted organisms and the general environment. Integrated pest management programs have been successfully adopted by personal homes, school systems, cities and counties ( for parks and roadways), gardens, and farms across the United States and often have resulted in substantial cost savings. The national PTA passed a resolution to work toward pesticide-free schools.[97,98]

Studies have demonstrated that IPM is superior to conventional pest control methods. When implemented during pregnancy, IPM was shown to reduce maternal and fetal exposure to pesticides.[99] In public housing units, IPM methods were documented to be effective as pest control and cost-effective.

## SUBCLINICAL PESTICIDE EXPOSURES

Although pesticides can cause acute toxicity, it is likely that more exposures are subclinical; these exposures are therefore not referred to poison control centers. In these cases, other resources may be able to assist. Depending on the source or nature of the exposure, consultation with the US EPA or individual state Environmental Protection Agencies may be appropriate. Local and state health departments often have some expertise with pesticide exposures. The Agency for Toxic Substances and Disease Registry (ATSDR), a part of the CDC, may be contacted for chronic or acute exposures. Pediatric Environmental Health Specialty Units are federally funded centers that provide consultation, education, and technical assistance regarding toxic exposures.[100]

## Encourage Families to Avoid the Following Unsafe Pesticide Practices[a]

- Do not enter a field that has been posted with a sign indicating pesticide treatment. Treated fields should not be entered by anyone until pesticide dust has settled, plants are dry from spray, or the worker is wearing protective clothing.

- Do not use water in drainage ditches or any irrigation system for drinking, washing food or clothing, swimming, or fishing.

- Do not carry lunch or drinks into a treated field.

- Do not put pesticides in unmarked containers or food or drink jars.

- Never take pesticide containers home for use around the house. They are unsafe.

- Do not use pesticides from work around the house.

- Do not burn pesticide bags for fuel; they can give off poisonous fumes.

## Encourage Families to Use Safe Pesticide Practices

- Wash work clothes separately from other laundry.

- Wash work clothes with detergent and hot water before wearing them again.

- Wash hands and arms after putting clothing into the washing machine.

- Change clothing and wash with soap and water before picking up or playing with your children.

- Store pesticides in an area that children cannot access.

- Cover children's skin if they are with you at work.

- Keep children and their toys and playthings indoors when there is nearby aerial spraying or spraying that may drift near the house.

- Children and teenagers should avoid work that involves mixing or spraying pesticides.

[a]Adapted from INFO Letter: Environmental and Occupational Health Briefs.[101]

## Simple Steps That May Reduce the Need for Pesticides

■ Choose plant varieties that grow well in the area. A county extension agent or nursery personnel may have advice.

■ Time the watering and fertilizing of plants according to their needs.

■ Follow recommendations given for mowing grass and pruning plants.

■ Decide what degree of damage from weeds, insects, and diseases can be tolerated, and do not take control measures unless that degree is exceeded.

■ Consider nonchemical options first when controls are needed. For example, determine whether weeds can be removed by hoeing or pulling.

## Frequently Asked Questions

Q    *I am having pest problems in my lawn and garden. Should I get regular preventive applications by a professional service?*

A    Regular lawn treatment exposes people to pesticides unnecessarily. It also may kill insects that are beneficial in controlling the pest population, thereby requiring the use of more chemicals. Weed killers, especially combination products that include a fertilizer and an herbicide, generally pose an unnecessary risk: they are used for cosmetic purposes but leave a residue on the lawn that can be tracked into the home and may pose a long-term health risk to children. If a professional lawn service is used, its personnel should (1) regularly monitor the lawn for pests and treat the lawn only when pests exist, (2) offer alternatives to the standard treatment, (3) give advance warning (including to neighbors) before applying any pesticides (this allows time to cover outdoor furniture and remove toys and pet food dishes), (4) be trained and certified, (5) give advance notification of the types of chemicals to be used and information on their health effects, and (6) avoid applications under adverse weather conditions (eg, high winds).

Q    *Is an insect repellent containing DEET safe for use on my children?*

A    Products containing DEET are the most effective mosquito repellents currently available.[29] DEET also is an effective repellent for a variety of other insect pests, including ticks. DEET should be used in areas where there is concern about illness from insect bites. It also can be used when insects are likely to be a nuisance, such as at barbecues or at the beach. Although it generally is used without any problems, there have been rare reports of adverse effects. Usually, these problems have occurred with inappropriate use; if used appropriately, DEET does not present a health risk. No definitive studies exist in the scientific literature about what concentration of DEET is safe for children. The CDC recommends using products with 20% DEET or greater on exposed skin. Use of products with the lowest effective DEET concentrations (ie, between 20% and 30%) seems most prudent for infants and young children, on whom it should be applied sparingly. Alternatives to DEET include picaridin (1-methylpropyl 2-(2-hydroxyethyl)-1-piperidinecarboxylate, also known as KBR 3023) and oil of lemon eucalyptus. Picaridin and DEET have similar effectiveness at comparable concentrations. Picaridin, derived from the pepper plant, has a favorable safety profile.

The concentration of DEET in products may range from less than 10% to 100%. The efficacy of DEET plateaus at a concentration of 30%, the maximum concentration currently recommended for infants and children. The major difference in the efficacy of products relates to their duration of action. Products with concentrations around 10% are effective for periods of approximately 2 hours. As the concentration of DEET increases, the duration of activity increases; for example, a concentration of about 24% has recently been shown to provide an average of 5 hours of protection. Concentrations greater than 50% do not provide greater protection.

The safety of DEET does not seem to relate to differences in these concentrations. Thus, products with a concentration of 30% appear to be as safe as products with a concentration of 10% when used according to the directions on the product labels. A prudent approach would be to select the lowest concentration effective for the amount of time spent outdoors. It is generally agreed that DEET should not be applied more than once a day.

Some properties of infant and toddler skin may differ from those of adult skin until children are at least age 2.[57] Because studies suggest the possibility that young skin may have greater permeability to chemicals, DEET should be applied sparingly when needed, weighing the risks of exposure to potentially life-threatening vectorborne illnesses to the possible risks of absorption. No data are available to show blood levels for infants and children following DEET application.

DEET should not be used in a product that combines the repellent with a sunscreen. Sunscreens are often applied repeatedly because they can be washed away through swimming and sweating. DEET is not water soluble and will last up to 8 hours, depending on its concentration. Repeated application may increase the potential toxic effects of DEET. Sunscreens and insect repellants may be used as individual products applied separately as indicated.

## Precautions When Using Insect Repellants

1. Read and carefully follow all directions before using the product. Do not allow children to handle the product. When using on children, apply to your own hands first and then put it on the child. Do not apply to children's hands.
2. Wear long sleeves and pants when possible and apply repellent to clothing—a long-sleeved shirt with snug collar and cuffs is best. The shirt should be tucked in at the waist. Socks should be tucked over pants, hiking shoes, or boots.
3. Use just enough repellent to cover exposed skin and/or clothing. Heavy application and saturation generally are unnecessary for effectiveness. Do not use repellents underneath clothing.
4. Do not apply to the eyes or mouth, and apply sparingly around the ears. When using sprays, do not spray directly on the face—spray on the hands first and then apply to the face.
5. Do not apply repellents over cuts, wounds, or irritated skin.
6. Wash treated skin with soap and water when returning indoors. Wash treated clothing.
7. Avoid using sprays in enclosed areas. Do not use repellents near food.
8. If a rash or other apparent allergic reaction develops in a child following use of an insect repellent, stop using the repellent, wash it off with mild soap and water, and call a pediatrician or a local poison control center for further guidance.

Q   We have rodents in and around our home. How can we safely get rid of them?

A   Most pesticides for controlling rats (rodenticides) available for home use today are the anticoagulants warfarin or superwarfarin (coumarins) or indanediones. They kill the rodents by causing internal bleeding. These anticoagulants also can cause bleeding in children if ingested and, therefore, must be used carefully. Each year, more than 7,000 children are exposed to these products, making anticoagulant baits one of the most common pesticide ingestions in children younger than 6 years. Fortunately, the amounts usually eaten by young children rarely cause serious injury. Poisoning can be avoided by following the product label and using common sense. In 2008, the US EPA took further measures aimed at decreasing the number of significant pediatric ingestions of rodenticides. "Consumer sized" products may no longer contain brodifacoum, difethialone, bromadiolone, or difenacoum (the second-generation anticoagulants). Use of tamper-resistant bait stations with solid bait will reduce children's access to these products, and therefore, sales to consumers are only allowed in this form. Because rodenticides have a long shelf-life, the older consumer products may remain in use for some time to come. If it is suspected that a child may have ingested a product containing anticoagulants, a physician or poison control center or the emergency department of the nearest hospital should be contacted immediately. In addition to rodenticides, integrated pest management techniques include careful sealing of cracks and crevices, cleaning up brush and debris from outdoor areas where rats may hide, and careful sanitation to leave no food scraps for rodents to eat. Mechanical traps can be effective for controlling a minor rodent problem. These include snap traps or glue traps. The latter are less likely to cause injuries to small children who might come into contact with the traps.

Q   *What is the best way to treat a roach problem?*

A   Hygiene measures are key. Cockroaches are found where there is water and food. Eating should be discouraged in areas other than the kitchen. All foodstuffs should be stored in closed containers. Water sources should be eliminated by caulking cracks around faucets and pipe fittings. Cracks and crevices where cockroaches can enter the home should be sealed.

A prudent approach is to minimize exposure to sprays whenever possible. Individual bait stations are recommended. If possible, baiting should be done outside the home as well. Boric acid, formulated for use as a pesticide, is comparatively less toxic than cholinesterase inhibitors and pyrethroids, and can be used in cracks and crevices in areas inaccessible to children.

If these measures are not successful, the family should consult a professional exterminator. If professional extermination is to be done, be certain that it is a licensed firm and find out what insecticide will be used and its possible toxic effects. Before using any insecticide in the home, all food, dishes, cooking utensils, children's toys, and clothing should be removed or protected from contamination. After application of the insecticide, young children and pregnant women should stay out of the area for as long as possible. The room should be aired well by cross ventilation for 4 to 8 hours before people and pets return. Crawling babies should not be allowed in the area until it has been well vacuumed or mopped and residents can be certain that the pesticide was not applied in an area that the infant can reach. For example, if the pesticide is applied to the wall, a crawling infant could hold onto the wall or wipe his hands and sustain a significant exposure.

Families should avoid using over-the-counter bug sprays and bug bombs. *The Cockroach Control Manual,* an excellent resource, is available from the University of Nebraska. It includes complete information on an integrated

## Measures That May Reduce the Danger of Exposure to Rodenticides

1. Place all rodenticides out of the reach of children and nontarget animals in tamper-proof bait boxes. Outdoors, place bait inside the entrance of a burrow and then collapse the entrance over the bait.
2. Securely lock or fasten shut the lids of all bait boxes.
3. Use a solid bait and place in the baffle-protected lockable feeding chamber, never in the runway of the box.
4. Always use sanitation measures in conjunction with pesticides to limit rodent access to food and hiding places. Work with neighbors to secure the neighborhood. If baiting alone is used without sanitation measures, the rodent population will rebound each time the baiting stops. Measures include using rat-proof garbage cans and food storage precautions (including keeping food in the refrigerator), and frequently raking up garden waste (including fallen fruit).
5. Modify the habitat by rodent-proofing buildings and changing landscaping to eliminate hiding places.
6. Continue to monitor periodically to ensure that rodents are not recolonizing.

pest management approach including "least toxic methods." It is available for purchase or free download from the Institute of Agriculture and Natural Resources, Univeristy of Nebraska Extension in Lancaster County at http://lancaster.unl.edu/pest/roachmanual.shtml.

Q  *What is the best way to control fleas on a dog or cat?*

A  There are a wide variety of flea control products. The safest approach to flea control is to avoid pesticide products altogether. This can be done by bathing the pet with a regular pet shampoo at least every other week and simultaneously washing the pet's bedding in hot water with a regular laundry detergent. Vacuuming rugs at least weekly is also very important. If your pet is scratching, then carefully comb its fur with a fine-toothed flea comb to look for "flea dirt" and adult fleas. Flea dirt is a red-brown particulate that appears rusty red if pressed onto paper. It represents the blood-filled feces from the fleas. If regular bathing, vacuuming, laundry, and flea combing are not sufficient to control fleas, then the best option is an oral agent such as lufenuron (Program™, Sentinel™). The flea products to avoid include flea collars (which generally contain tetrachlorvinphos or propoxur) and permethrin shampoos.

*Q  My house is overrun with ants. Should I get an exterminator to spray?*

A  Spraying for ants is generally ineffective. Ants are relatively easy to control using the principles of integrated pest management. First, it is important to discover how the ants are getting in to the house. Once the entry point is identified, it can be sealed off. If sealing off the entry point is not possible, ant bait can be placed in that location as long as it is out of reach of children. It is also important to discover where the ants are going and to remove all food sources by sealing food items in containers or zip lock bags. The ant trail should be wiped clean with dish soap and water to remove the scent that the ants are following. This set of actions will cause the ant problem to completely resolve within a few days. If a professional pest control company is needed, look for one that is certified by Green Shield, which maintains standards for integrated pest management pest control (www.greenshieldcertified.org).

*Q  My home has bed bugs. Is it necessary to hire a professional exterminator or can I take care of this myself with bug bombs?*

A  Bed bugs have made a big comeback in the United States over the past several years. The increase in reports of bed bug infestations appear to be the result of changes in patterns of pesticide use and increased international travel. Over-the-counter sprays and bug bombs generally are not effective against bed bugs. People may be tempted to use outdoor or expired pesticides to control bed bugs sometimes out of frustration regarding the lack of efficacy of these methods. The misuse of pesticides, ie, using pesticides not in accordance with the label, is a violation of the law and potentially hazardous. Calls to the National Pesticide Information Center regarding poisonings as a result of the misuse of pesticides to eradicate bed bugs are increasing. At least one death has been associated with this misuse. To eradicate bed bugs, consultation with a pest control professional is recommended, as well as practicing integrated pest management techniques. In the case of bed bugs, integrated pest management strategies include removing clutter, vacuuming furniture and other items that have bed bugs on them, and promptly disposing of the vacuum cleaner bag outside after placing it in a sealed plastic bag. Infested items (clothing, shoes, bedding, blankets, etc.) can be placed in a clothes dryer for at least 20 minutes to kill bed bugs and their eggs. Bed bugs are sensitive to temperature. Infested mattresses and box springs should be encased in a bed bug-proof zipped cover for 1 to 2 years because bed bugs can survive 18 months in the lab without a blood meal.

Q   *Will the US EPA ban the use of chlorpyrifos?*

A   The US EPA banned chlorpyrifos use for residential purposes in 2000, except in select cases, including when contained in ant and roach bait products. The US EPA also banned its use on some crops, such as tomatoes, and limited its use on other crops, including apples, grapes, and citrus. In 2016, the US EPA extended the timeline for its review of a total ban of chlorpyrifos. It aims to come to a clearer scientific resolution on the matter by 2022.

## Resources

### Extoxnet

Web site: ace.ace.orst.edu/info/extoxnet

A cooperative effort among the University of California at Davis, Oregon State University, Michigan State University, and Cornell University that provides updated pesticide information in understandable terms. It includes toxicology briefs and information on carcinogenicity, testing, and exposure assessment.

### National Pesticide Information Center

Phone: 800-858-7378

Web site: npic.orst.edu/index.html

A toll-free EPA and Oregon State University-sponsored information service.

### National Service Center for Environmental Publications

www.epa.gov/nscep

Use the search function to find free fact sheets on lawn care, pesticide labels, and pesticide safety.

### Organophosphate Pesticides and Child Health: A Primer for Health Care Providers

Online CME course: depts.washington.edu/opchild/

### Texas Agricultural Extension Service, Physician's Guide to Pesticide Poisoning

Web site: www.thebestcontrol.com/physicians_guide/toc.htm

### Toxnet

Web site: toxnet.nlm.nih.gov

A cluster of databases on toxicology, hazardous chemicals, and related areas.

### University of Nebraska Cooperative Extension, Signs and Symptoms of Pesticide Poisoning

Web site: extensionpubs.unl.edu/publication/9000016363839/
managing-the-risk-of-pesticide-poisoning-and-understanding-the-signs-and-symptoms/

## US Environmental Protection Agency

Web site: www.epa.gov

- Recognition and Management of Pesticide Poisonings, 6th ed.
  www.epa.gov/pesticide-worker-safety/recognition-and-management-
  pesticide-poisonings
  (available in English and Spanish)
- EPA online resources in case of suspected pesticide poisoning
  www.epa.gov/oppfead1/safety/incaseof.htm
- EPA pamphlets
  — *Citizen's Guide to Pest Control and Pesticide Safety*
  — *Pest Control in the School Environment*
  — *Healthy Lawn, Healthy Environment*
- EPA Integrated Pest Management for Schools
  www.epa.gov/managing-pests-schools

## References

1. US EPA, Office of Chemical Safety and Pollution Prevention. Basic Information about Pesticide Ingredients. *US EPA* (2013). https://www.epa.gov/ingredients-used-pesticide-products/basic-information-about-pesticide-ingredients. Accessed May 7, 2018

2. Atwood D, Paisley-Jones C. *Pesticides Industry Sales and Usage 2008 - 2012 Market Estimates.* US Environmental Protection Agency, Office of Pesticide Programs, 2015

3. Blondell JM. Decline in pesticide poisonings in the United States from 1995 to 2004. *Clin Toxicol (Phila).* 2007;45(5):589–592

4. Lu C, Fenske RA, Simcox NJ, Kalman D. Pesticide exposure of children in an agricultural community: evidence of household proximity to farmland and take home exposure pathways. *Environ Res.* 2000;84(3):290–302

5. Fenske RA, Kissel JC, Lu C, et al. Biologically based pesticide dose estimates for children in an agricultural community. *Environ Health Perspect.* 2000;108(6):515–520

6. Centers for Disease Control and Prevention. Acute illnesses associated with insecticides used to control bed bugs—seven states, 2003—2010. *MMWR Morb Mortal Wkly Rep.* 2011;60(37):1269–1274

7. Summary of the Food Quality Protection Act. US EPA. 2015. https://www.epa.gov/laws-regulations/summary-food-quality-protection-act. Accessed May 7, 2018

8. US EPA, Office of Chemical Safety and Pollution Prevention. Companies Agree to Stop Selling Pet Collars Containing Pesticide to Protect Children. 2014. https://www.epa.gov/safepestcontrol/companies-agree-stop-selling-pet-collars-containing-pesticide-protect-children. Accessed May 7, 2018

9. US EPA, Office of Chemical Safety and Pollution Prevention. Reregistration Eligibility Decision Fact Sheet: Propoxur. 1997

10. Power LE, Sudakin DL. Pyrethrin and pyrethroid exposures in the United States: a longitudinal analysis of incidents reported to poison centers. *J Med Toxicol.* 2007;3(3):94–99

11. US Food and Drug Administration. Postmarket Drug Safety Information for Patients and Providers. Lindane Shampoo and Lindane Lotion. https://www.fda.gov/Drugs/DrugSafety/PostmarketDrugSafetyInformationforPatientsandProviders/ucm110452.htm. Accessed May 7, 2018

12. Fighting lindane pollution. 2000. http://www.headlice.org/news/2000/lindaneban.htm. Accessed June 14, 2018.

13. Humphreys EH, Janssen S, Heil A, Hiatt P, Solomon G, Miller MD. Outcomes of the California ban on pharmaceutical lindane: clinical and ecologic impacts. *Environ Health Perspect.* 2008;116(3):297–302

14. Workowski KA, Bolan GA, Centers for Disease Control and Prevention. Sexually transmitted diseases treatment guidelines, 2015. *MMWR Recomm Rep.* 2015;64(RR-03):1–137

15. Devore CD, Schutze GE, American Academy of Pediatrics Council on School Health and Committee on Infectious Diseases. Head lice. *Pediatrics.* 2015;135(5):e1355–e1365

16. Roberts J, Riegart JR. *Recognition and Management of Pesticide Poisonings.* US EPA Office of Pesticide Programs, 2013

17. Goldbloom RB, Goldbloom A. Boric acid poisoning: report of four cases and a review of 109 cases from the world literature. *J Pediatr.* 1953;43(6):631–643

18. Wong LC, Heimbach MD, Truscott DR, Duncan BD. Boric acid poisoning: report of 11 cases. *Can Med Assoc J.* 1964;90:1018–1023

19. Mowry JB, Spyker DA, Brooks DE, Zimmerman A, Schauben JL. 2015 Annual Report of the American Association of Poison Control Centers' National Poison Data System (NPDS): 33rd Annual Report. *Clin Toxicol (Phila).* 2016;54(10):924–1109

20. The Neilsen Company. Nothing is Too Good for Fido: Pets That Have it All. 2015. http://www.nielsen.com/us/en/insights/news/2015/nothing-is-too-good-for-fido-pets-that-have-it-all.html. Accessed May 7, 2018

21. US EPA. Tetrachlorvinphos (TCVP). 2016. https://www.epa.gov/ingredients-used-pesticide-products/tetrachlorvinphos-tcvp. Accessed May 7, 2018

22. Davis MK, Boone JS, Moran JE, Tyler JW, Chambers JE. Assessing intermittent pesticide exposure from flea control collars containing the organophosphorus insecticide tetrachlorvinphos. *J Expo Sci Environ Epidemiol.* 2008;18(6):564–570

23. US EPA, Office of Chemical Safety and Pollution Prevention. Reregistration Eligibility Decision Fact Sheet: Permethrin. 2009

24. Ratra GS, Casida JE. GABA receptor subunit composition relative to insecticide potency and selectivity. *Toxicol Lett.* 2001;122(3):215–222

25. Mohamed F, Gawarammana I, Robertson TA, et al. Acute human self-poisoning with imidacloprid compound: a neonicotinoid insecticide. *PloS One.* 2009;4(4):e5127

26. Phua DH, Lin CC, Wu ML, Deng JF, Yang CC. Neonicotinoid insecticides: an emerging cause of acute pesticide poisoning. *Clin Toxicol (Phila).* 2009;47(4):336–341

27. Carmichael SL, Yang W, Roberts E, et al. Residential agricultural pesticide exposures and risk of selected congenital heart defects among offspring in the San Joaquin Valley of California. *Environ Res.* 2014;135:133–138

28. Nerio LS, Olivero-Verbel J, Stashenko E. Repellent activity of essential oils: a review. *Bioresour Technol.* 2010;101(1):372–378

29. Fradin MS, Day JF. Comparative efficacy of insect repellents against mosquito bites. *N Engl J Med.* 2002;347(1):13–18

30. Centers for Disease Control and Prevention. Insect Repellent Use & Safety. West Nile Virus. 2015. https://www.cdc.gov/westnile/faq/repellent.html. Accessed May 7, 2018

31. Weiss B, Amler S, Amler RW. Pesticides. *Pediatrics.* 2004;113(4 Suppl):1030–1036

32. Lu C, Knutson DE, Fisker-Andersen J, Fenske RA. Biological monitoring survey of organophosphorus pesticide exposure among pre-school children in the Seattle metropolitan area. *Environ Health Perspect.* 2001;109(3):299–303

33. Whyatt RM, Barr DB. Measurement of organophosphate metabolites in postpartum meconium as a potential biomarker of prenatal exposure: a validation study. *Environ Health Perspect.* 2001;109(4):417–420

34. Yolton K, Xu Y, Sucharew H, et al. Impact of low-level gestational exposure to organophosphate pesticides on neurobehavior in early infancy: a prospective study. *Environ Health.* 2013;12(1):79

35. Centers for Disease Control and Prevention. National Report on Human Exposure to Environmental Chemicals. 2017. https://www.cdc.gov/exposurereport/index.html. Accessed May 7, 2018

36. Guha N, Ward MH, Gunier R, et al. Characterization of residential pesticide use and chemical formulations through self-report and household inventory: the Northern California Childhood Leukemia Study. *Environ Health Perspect.* 2013;121(2):276–282

37. US EPA, Office of Water. A Review of Contaminant Occurrence in Public Water Systems. 1999

38. Longnecker MP, Klebanoff MA, Zhou H, Brock JW. Association between maternal serum concentration of the DDT metabolite DDE and preterm and small-for-gestational-age babies at birth. *Lancet.* 2001;358(9276):110–114

39. Garry VF, Schreinemacher D, Harkins ME, Griffith J. Pesticide appliers, biocides, and birth defects in rural Minnesota. *Environ Health Perspect.* 1996;104(4):394–399

40. Bell EM, Hertz-Picciotto I, Beaumont JJ. A case-control study of pesticides and fetal death due to congenital anomalies. *Epidemiology.* 2001;12(2):148–156

41. Arbuckle TE, Lin Z, Mery LS. An exploratory analysis of the effect of pesticide exposure on the risk of spontaneous abortion in an Ontario farm population. *Environ Health Perspect.* 2001;109(8):851–857

42. Metayer C, Dahl G, Wiemels J, Miller M. Childhood leukemia: a preventable disease. *Pediatrics.* 2016;138(Suppl 1):S45–S55

43. Roberts JR, Karr CJ, American Academy of Pediatrics Council on Environmental Health. Pesticide exposure in children. *Pediatrics.* 2012;130(6):e1765–e1788

44. Wylie BJ, Hauptman M, Woolf AD, Goldman RH. Insect repellants during pregnancy in the era of the Zika virus. *Obstet Gynecol.* 2016;128(5):1111–1115

45. Wagner SL. Fatal asthma in a child after use of an animal shampoo containing pyrethrin. *West J Med.* 2000;173(2):86–87

46. Tangermann RH, Etzel RA, Mortimer L, Penner GD, Paschal DC. An outbreak of a food-related illness resembling boric acid poisoning. *Arch Environ Contam Toxicol.* 1992;23(1):142–144

47. Mohamed F, Senarathna L, Percy A, et al. Acute human self-poisoning with the N-phenylpyrazole insecticide fipronil—a GABAA-gated chloride channel blocker. *J Toxicol Clin Toxicol.* 2004;42(7):955–963

48. Talbot AR, Shiaw MH, Huang JS, et al. Acute poisoning with a glyphosate-surfactant herbicide ('Roundup'): a review of 93 cases. *Hum Exp Toxicol.* 1991;10(1):1–8

49. Kelce WR, Monosson E, Gamcsik MP, Laws SC, Gray LE. Environmental hormone disruptors: evidence that vinclozolin developmental toxicity is mediated by antiandrogenic metabolites. *Toxicol Appl Pharmacol.* 1994;126(2):276–285

50. Selim S, Hartnagel RE, Osimitz TG, Gabriel KL, Schoenig GP. Absorption, metabolism, and excretion of N,N-diethyl-m-toluamide following dermal application to human volunteers. *Fundam Appl Toxicol.* 1995;25(1):95–100

51. Ross EA, Savage KA, Utley LJ, Tebbett IR. Insect repellent [correction of repellant] interactions: sunscreens enhance DEET (N,N-diethyl-m-toluamide) absorption. *Drug Metab Dispos.* 2004;32(8):783–785

52. Gryboski J, Weinstein D, Ordway NK. Toxic Encephalopathy Apparently Related to the Use of an Insect Repellent. http://dx.doi.org/10.1056/NEJM196102092640608. Accessed May 7, 2018

53. Centers for Disease Control. Seizures temporally associated with use of DEET insect repellent—New York and Connecticut. *MMWR Morb Mortal Wkly Rep.* 1989;38(39):678–680

54. Veltri JC, Osimitz TG, Bradford DC, Page BC. Retrospective analysis of calls to poison control centers resulting from exposure to the insect repellent N, N-diethyl-m-toluamide (DEET) from 1985–1989. *J Toxicol Clin Toxicol.* 1994;32(1):1–16

55. Roberts JR, Reigart JR. Does anything beat DEET? *Pediatr Ann.* 2004;33(7):444–453

56. Brown M, Hebert AA. Insect repellents: an overview. *J Am Acad Dermatol.* 1997;36(2 Pt 1): 243–249

57. Giusti F, Martella A, Bertoni L, Seidenari S. Skin barrier, hydration, and pH of the skin of infants under 2 years of age. *Pediatr Dermatol.* 2001;18(2):93–96

58. Picardin—a new insect repellent. *Med Lett Drugs Ther.* 2005;47(1210):46–47

59. National Research Council. *Pesticides in the Diets of Infants and Children.* Washington, DC: National Academies Press; 1993

60. Furlong CE, Holland N, Richter RJ, Bradman A, Ho A, Eskenazi B. PON1 status of farmworker mothers and children as a predictor of organophosphate sensitivity. *Pharmacogenet Genomics.* 2006;16(3):183–190

61. Reiss R, Chang ET, Richardson RJ, Goodman M. A review of epidemiologic studies of low-level exposures to organophosphorus insecticides in non-occupational populations. *Crit Rev Toxicol.* 2015;45(7):531–641

62. Wagner SL, Orwick DL. Chronic organophosphate exposure associated with transient hypertonia in an infant. *Pediatrics.* 1994;94(1):94–97

63. Fenster L, Eskenazi B, Anderson M, Bradman A, Hubbard A, Barr DB. In utero exposure to DDT and performance on the Brazelton neonatal behavioral assessment scale. *Neurotoxicology.* 2007;28(3):471–477

64. Torres-Sánchez L, Schnass L, Rothenberg SJ, et al. Prenatal p,p´-DDE exposure and neurodevelopment among children 3.5–5 years of age. *Environ Health Perspect.* 2013;121(2):263–268

65. Rauh VA, Garfinkel R, Perera FP, et al. Impact of prenatal chlorpyrifos exposure on neurodevelopment in the first 3 years of life among inner-city children. *Pediatrics.* 2006;118(6): e1845–e1859

66. Eskenazi B, Rosas LG, Marks AR, et al. Pesticide toxicity and the developing brain. *Basic Clin Pharmacol Toxicol.* 2008;102(2):228–236

67. Engel SM, Bradman A, Wolff MS, et al. Prenatal organophosphorus pesticide exposure and child neurodevelopment at 24 months: an analysis of four birth cohorts. *Environ Health Perspect.* 2016;124(6):822–830

68. Ahlbom J, Fredriksson A, Eriksson P. Exposure to an organophosphate (DFP) during a defined period in neonatal life induces permanent changes in brain muscarinic receptors and behaviour in adult mice. *Brain Res.* 1995;677(1):13–19

69. Ahlbom J, Fredriksson A, Eriksson P. Neonatal exposure to a type-I pyrethroid (bioallethrin) induces dose—response changes in brain muscarinic receptors and behaviour in neonatal and adult mice. *Brain Res.* 1994;645(1-2):318–324

70. Brimijoin S, Koenigsberger C. Cholinesterases in neural development: new findings and toxicologic implications. *Environ Health Perspect.* 1999;107(Suppl 1):59–64

71. US EPA. Revised Human Health Risk Assessment on Chlorpyrifos. 2017. https://www.epa.gov/ingredients-used-pesticide-products/revised-human-health-risk-assessment-chlorpyrifos. Accessed May 7, 2018

72. Nasuti C, Gabbianelli R, Falcioni ML, et al. Dopaminergic system modulation, behavioral changes, and oxidative stress after neonatal administration of pyrethroids. *Toxicology.* 2007;229(3):194–205

73. Logroscino G. The role of early life environmental risk factors in Parkinson disease: what is the evidence? *Environ Health Perspect.* 2005;113(9):1234–1238

74. Wagner-Schuman M, Richardson JR, Auinger P, et al. Association of pyrethroid pesticide exposure with attention-deficit/hyperactivity disorder in a nationally representative sample of U.S. children. *Environ Health.* 2015;14:44

75. US EPA. Office of Pesticide Programs. Chemicals Evaluated for Carcinogenic Potential. 2016

76. World Health Organization. IARC Monographs, Volume 112. Evaluation of five organophosphate insecticides and herbicides. 2015

77. Kristensen P, Andersen A, Irgens LM, Bye AS, Sundheim L. Cancer in offspring of parents engaged in agricultural activities in Norway: incidence and risk factors in the farm environment. *Int J Cancer.* 1996;65(1):39–50

78. Alexander FE, Patheal SL, Biondi A, et al. Transplacental chemical exposure and risk of infant leukemia with MLL gene fusion. *Cancer Res.* 2001;61(6):2542–2546

79. Buckley JD, Meadows AT, Kadin ME, Le Beau MM, Siegel S, Robison LL. Pesticide exposures in children with non-Hodgkin lymphoma. *Cancer.* 2000;89(11):2315–2321

80. Infante-Rivard C, Weichenthal S. Pesticides and childhood cancer: an update of Zahm and Ward's 1998 review. *J Toxicol Environ Health B Crit Rev.* 2007;10(1-2):81–99

81. Zahm SH, Ward MH. Pesticides and childhood cancer. *Environ Health Perspect.* 1998;106(Suppl 3):893–908

82. Davis JR, Brownson RC, Garcia R, Bentz BJ, Turner A. Family pesticide use and childhood brain cancer. *Arch Environ Contam Toxicol.* 1993;24(1):87–92

83. Chen M, Chang CH, Tao L, Lu C. Residential exposure to pesticide during childhood and childhood cancers: a meta-analysis. *Pediatrics.* 2015;136(4):719–729

84. Henneberger PK, Liang X, London SJ, Umbach DM, Sandler DP, Hoppin JA. Exacerbation of symptoms in agricultural pesticide applicators with asthma. *Int Arch Occup Environ Health.* 2014;87(4):423–432

85. Hoppin JA, Umbach DM, London SJ, et al. Pesticide use and adult-onset asthma among male farmers in the Agricultural Health Study. *Eur Respir J.* 2009;34(6):1296–1303

86. Salam MT, Li YF, Langholz B, Gilliland FD. Early-life environmental risk factors for asthma: findings from the Children's Health Study. *Environ Health Perspect.* 2004;112(6):760–765

87. Mamane A, Raherison C, Tessier JF, Baldi I, Bouvier G. Environmental exposure to pesticides and respiratory health. *Eur Respir Rev.* 2015;24(137):462–473

88. Perla ME, Rue T, Cheadle A, Krieger J, Karr CJ. Biomarkers of insecticide exposure and asthma in children: a National Health and Nutrition Examination Survey (NHANES) 1999–2008 analysis. *Arch Environ Occup Health.* 2015;70(6):309–322

89. Fernandez MF, Olmos B, Granada A, et al. Human exposure to endocrine-disrupting chemicals and prenatal risk factors for cryptorchidism and hypospadias: a nested case–control study. *Environ Health Perspect.* 2007;115(Suppl 1):8–14

90. Maervoet J, Vermeir G, Covaci A, et al. Association of thyroid hormone concentrations with levels of organochlorine compounds in cord blood of neonates. *Environ Health Perspect.* 2007;115(12):1780–1786

91. Fan W, Yanase T, Morinaga H, et al. Atrazine-induced aromatase expression is SF-1 dependent: implications for endocrine disruption in wildlife and reproductive cancers in humans. *Environ Health Perspect.* 2007;115(5):720–727

92. Cooper RL, Laws SC, Das PC, et al. Atrazine and reproductive function: mode and mechanism of action studies. *Birth Defects Res B Dev Reprod Toxicol.* 2007;80(2):98–112

93. Lessenger JE, Estock MD, Younglove T. An analysis of 190 cases of suspected pesticide illness. *J Am Board Fam Pract.* 1995;8(4):278–282

94. *Handbook of Common Poisonings in Children.* American Academy of Pediatrics; 1994

95. Kurtz PH. Pralidoxime in the treatment of carbamate intoxication. *Am J Emerg Med.* 1990;8(1):68–70

96. Nishioka MG, Lewis RG, Brinkman MC, Burkholder HM, Hines CE, Menkedick JR. Distribution of 2,4-D in air and on surfaces inside residences after lawn applications: comparing exposure estimates from various media for young children. *Environ Health Perspect.* 2001;109(11): 1185–1191

97. Child Proofing our Communities Campaign. Poisoned Schools: Invisible Threats, Visible Actions. 2001

98. Rose RI. Pesticides and public health: integrated methods of mosquito management. *Emerg Infect Dis.* 2001;7(1):17–23

99. Williams MK, Barr DB, Camann DE, et al. An intervention to reduce residential insecticide exposure during pregnancy among an inner-city cohort. *Environ Health Perspect.* 2006;114(11):1684–1689

100. Wilborne-Davis P, Kirkland KH, Mulloy KB. A model for physician education and consultation in pediatric environmental health—The Pediatric Environmental Health Specialty Units (PEHSU) program. *Pediatr Clin North Am.* 2007;54(1):1–13

101. Environmental and Health Risk Communications Division. INFO Letter: Environmental and Occupational Health Briefs. Piscataway NJ. 9, 1996

Chapter 41

# Plasticizers

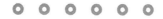

## KEY POINTS

- Plastics are composed of polymers or resins, and additives.
- The term "plasticizer" refers to a chemical added to polymers or resins. Plasticizers impart useful properties, such as flexibility or rigidity, to a product.
- Common plasticizers include phthalates and bisphenol A (BPA).
- Plasticizers may leach from products. Exposure to plasticizers may have adverse effects on human health.
- Consumers can take steps to decrease their exposures to plasticizers.

## INTRODUCTION

Plastics are made up of 2 types of components. The main components are polymers or resins that make up the bulk of the plastic material. Examples include polyvinyl chloride (PVC), polycarbonate (PC), high-density polyethylene (HDPE), and polypropylene (PP). The second components are additives. Additives are small but important parts of the overall plastic composition. Additives give plastics useful properties, such as color, fire resistance, strength, or flexibility. To a large extent, it is additives that give plastics most of their functions.

"Plasticizer" is a term used to describe some of the additives added to polymers or resins to give them more flexibility (eg, phthalates), or to make them more rigid (eg, bisphenol A [BPA]). This chapter focuses on some of the most commonly used and well-studied additives that have known or potential links to human health, particularly in children.

## PHTHALATES

Phthalates are a class of commonly used plasticizers.[1] In particular, dioctyl phthalate (DOP) is extensively used as a plasticizer for polyvinyl chloride. Factors such as flexibility and wide availability make phthalates optimal chemicals for industrial use. Phthalates migrate to the surface of plastics and can then evaporate or leach into the surrounding environment. Because of their widespread use, phthalates have become some of the most abundant industrial pollutants in the environment.[2] Many phthalates, including DOP, are classified as toxic chemicals by the US Environmental Protection Agency's (EPA) Toxic Release Inventory. Low-molecular weight phthalates, such as diethyl phthalate (DEP) and dibutyl phthalate (DBP), are commonly used as components of fragrance and color stabilizers in cosmetics and personal care products. They are found in lotions, aftershave, perfumes, nail polish, and other products used on a daily basis. High-molecular weight phthalates include di(2-ethylhexyl) phthalate (DEHP) and benzyl butyl phthalate (BBP). DEHP is used in polyvinyl chloride products, flexible plastics, and intravenous (IV) tubing.

## ROUTES OF EXPOSURE

Phthalates leach out of products easily and can, therefore, be inhaled, ingested, or dermally absorbed or enter the bloodstream directly through the IV route. Children are exposed to phthalates through multiple sources and routes of exposure (Table 41-1). Phthalates leach from products at higher concentrations when they are heated.

## SYSTEMS AFFECTED AND CLINICAL EFFECTS

Phthalates are known as "endocrine disrupting chemicals" or "endocrine disruptors" that affect the endocrine system through multiple mechanisms of action (see Chapter 29). DEHP and DBP are the most toxic to the reproductive system. Studies in animals have found anti-androgenic effects in fetal and early postnatal development leading to male reproductive tract abnormalities, including undescended testes, hypospadias, and decreased fertility. These studies are difficult to assess however, given the ubiquity of phthalates in animal feed, cages, and other products (Table 41-1). The most sensitive time period for phthalate exposure and effects in humans is thought to be during weeks 10 to 13 of gestation, a period of extensive reproductive system development. In male infants, increased maternal urinary concentrations of DEHP metabolite during the mother's third trimester of pregnancy (which may or may not be a surrogate for first trimester exposure) were associated with decreased anogenital distance (a sensitive measure of fetal anti-androgen exposure).[3] In a recent review,[4] these anti-androgenic effects were shown

## Table 41-1. Sources of Phthalate Exposure

| PHTHALATE PARENT COMPOUND | POTENTIAL SOURCES OF EXPOSURE |
| --- | --- |
| Di(2-ethylhexyl) phthalate (DEHP) | Polyvinyl chloride-containing medical tubing, blood storage bags, medical devices, food contamination, food packaging, indoor air, plastic toys, wall coverings, tablecloths, floor tiles, furniture upholstery, shower curtains, garden hoses, swimming pool liners, rainwear, baby pants, dolls, some toys, shoes, automobile upholstery and tops, packaging film and sheets, sheathing for wire and cable |
| Diethyl phthalate (DEP) | Cosmetics, nail polish, deodorant, perfumes/cologne, lotions, aftershave, pharmaceuticals/herbal products, insecticide |
| Di-isononyl phthalate (DINP) | Children's toys |
| Dibutyl phthalate (DBP) | Nail polish, makeup, aftershave, perfumes, coatings on pharmaceuticals/herbal products, chemiluminescent glow sticks |
| Di-*n*-octyl phthalate (DnOP) | Children's toys |
| Di-*n*-butyl phthalate (DnBP) | Medicines, cosmetics, cellulose acetate plastics, latex adhesives, nail polish and other cosmetic products, plasticizers in cellulose plastics, solvent for certain dyes |
| Benzyl butyl phthalate (BBP) | Vinyl flooring, adhesives, sealants, food packaging, furniture upholstery, vinyl tile, carpet tiles, artificial leather, adhesives |
| Dimethyl phthalate (DMP) | Insecticides, indoor air, adhesives, hairstyling products, shampoo, aftershave |

through exposure to mono (2-ethylhexyl) phthalate (MEHP), the hydrolytic metabolite of DEHP. A significant correlation between urinary and environmental concentrations of phthalates (DEHP, DBP, DEP) and sperm motility, sperm concentration, and DNA damage also were demonstrated. The review suggested that phthalates might contribute to reproductive damage through a decline in reproductive semen quality, reductions in gestation, preterm delivery, and spontaneous abortion. These results were confirmed with reduced sperm motility from exposure to DEHP.[5] Increased phthalate exposure through human milk has been associated with changes in luteinizing hormone, free testosterone, and sex-hormone binding globulin in male infants.[6]

In addition to male reproductive effects, there are significant threats to female reproductive health. Recent studies suggest disruptions to estrous cycles and ovarian cysts,[7] and direct damage to the ovaries.[8] Some studies suggest if pregnancy is possible, there are effects on placental formation after phthalate exposure,[9] and lead to preeclampsia, intrauterine growth retardation, and adverse birth outcomes.[10]

Exposures to DEHP and BBP have been associated with changes in inflammatory and immunologic function. In a cross-sectional study, BBP in indoor dust was associated with an increased risk of allergic rhinitis and eczema among school-aged children, and DEHP in dust was associated with an increased risk of asthmatic symptoms.[11] It is hypothesized that MEHP induces proinflammatory prostaglandins and thromboxanes in the lungs, leading to increased respiratory symptoms. Laboratory studies in mice show that phthalate exposure exerts an adjuvant effect with a co-allergen (ovalbumin), leading to increased atopic-like skin lesions.[12]

Exposure to phthalates was implicated in potential nervous system inflammation in a study in which prenatal phthalate exposure was associated with changes in Brazelton scores in newborn infants.[13] Epidemiologic studies found that prenatal phthalate exposure was associated with both an increase[14] and decrease in gestational age.[15-18] One proposed mechanism is via perturbation of prostaglandin or other inflammatory mechanisms, leading to uterine contractions.

Neurologic effects from phthalate exposure appear to be toxic even after the prenatal period. Recent studies suggest that exposure to phthalates in household dust in children aged 2 to 5 years is associated with developmental delay, and with attention deficit/hyperactivity disorder (ADHD) among male children.[19]

Scientific panels, advocacy groups, and industry groups have analyzed literature on DEHP and di-isononyl phthalate (DINP) and have come to different conclusions about safety. The controversy exists because risk to humans must be extrapolated from animal data that demonstrate differences in toxicity depending on the species, route of exposure, and age at exposure, and because of persistent uncertainties in the data on human exposure. It is important to note that effects in animals are usually demonstrated at high doses, well above exposures encountered in the general human population.

## PREVENTION

Phthalates are ubiquitous in the environment and childhood exposures are widespread. Pediatricians can inform families about how to avoid exposure and identify alternatives to phthalate-containing products. It is important to know sources of exposure (see Table 41-1), and how to avoid phthalate exposures, including avoiding heating up plastics and using safer alternatives (Table 41-2). Pediatricians may suggest that parents avoid plastics with

| Table 41-2. Tips on How to Avoid Exposures to Phthalates and Bisphenol A |
|---|
| ■ Look at the recycling code on the bottom of products to find the plastic type. |
| ■ Avoid plastics with recycling codes No. 3 (phthalates), No. 6 (styrenes), and No. 7 (bisphenol A) unless plastics labeled No. 7 are labeled as "biobased" or "greenware," meaning that they are made from corn and do not use bisphenol A. |
| ■ Plastic codes No. 1, 2, 4, and 5 are considered safer alternatives. |
| ■ Do not microwave food or beverages (including infant formula) in plastic. |
| ■ Do not microwave or heat plastic cling wraps. If you must use plastic wrap in the microwave, ensure it does not touch the food. |
| ■ Avoid placing plastics in the dishwasher. |
| ■ Use alternatives, such as glass, when possible. |
| ■ Buy phthalate-free toys or those approved by the European Union. |
| ■ Make sure that pacifiers and bottle nipples you buy are phthalate- and BPA-free. |

recycling codes No. 3 (polyvinyl chloride or vinyl may contain phthalates), No. 6, and No. 7. It is difficult to know whether a specific product contains phthalates because labeling is not required by federal law. In August 2008, the federal government enacted the Consumer Product Safety Act that created a permanent ban on DEHP, DBP, and BBP in toys for children younger than 12 years and all child-care items for children aged 3 years and younger. It also created an interim ban on 3 additional phthalates (DINP, di-isodecyl phthalate [DIDP], and di-*n*-octyl phthalate [DnOP]) until more research is conducted about potential adverse health outcomes. Several state-based policies are being developed. In general, it may be prudent to avoid exposure to phthalates when possible until the scientific basis of safety or harm from low-level exposure is more clearly established.

## BISPHENOL A

Bisphenol A (BPA) is a chemical produced in large quantities, primarily to impart rigidity in the production of polycarbonate plastics and epoxy resins. Polycarbonate plastics have applications including use in some food and drink packaging (eg, water and infant bottles), compact discs, impact-resistant safety equipment, and medical devices. Epoxy resins are used as lacquers to coat metal products, such as food cans, bottle tops, and water supply pipes. Some dental sealants and composites may also contribute to BPA exposure.

Human exposure to BPA is widespread. Since 1999, more than a dozen studies using different analytical techniques have measured free, unconjugated BPA in human serum at concentrations ranging from 0.2 to 20 ng/mL.[20] The relatively high concentrations of BPA in the sera of pregnant women, umbilical cord blood, and fetal plasma indicate that BPA crosses the placenta. The 2003-2004 Third National Health and Nutrition Examination Survey (NHANES III) conducted by the Centers for Disease Control and Prevention (CDC) found detectable concentrations of BPA in 93% of 2,517 urine samples from a representative sample of people in the United States aged 6 years and older.[21]

## SYSTEMS AFFECTED AND CLINICAL EFFECTS

Assays are available to measure the *in vitro* estrogenic activity of possible endocrine disruptors, including BPA.[22] Assays to determine the *in vivo* estrogenicity of BPA demonstrated that estrogen receptor binding is very weak, compared with the natural estrogen 17 β-estradiol. When prepubescent CD-1 mice were treated with doses of BPA ranging from 0.1 to 100 mg/kg of body weight, estrogenic responses, including increased uterine wet weight, luminal epithelial height, and increased expression of the estrogen-inducible protein lactoferrin, were observed.[23] Evidence also shows that BPA binds to thyroid hormone receptor, acting as a thyroid hormone antagonist by preventing the binding of $T_3$. One study found that the affinity of BPA for this receptor was lower than its affinity for the estrogen receptors.[24]

Some studies demonstrate effects in laboratory animals exposed to BPA[25] including multigenerational effects of BPA. Prenatal BPA exposure in mice has negative effects on development of the reproductive system, even for multiple generations. After pregnant mice were exposed to BPA, reproductive effects were seen in the first (equivalent to children), second (equivalent to grandchildren) and third (equivalent to great-grandchildren) generations.[26]

Few human epidemiologic data exist to connect BPA exposure in children to health effects. Limited cross-sectional data from studies among adults link exposure to BPA with reduced sexual function,[27] including ovarian dysfunction;[28] higher rates of diabetes mellitus[29] and heart disease;[30] and other potential consequences.[31] One small study in pregnant women[32] linked prenatal exposure to BPA with behavioral changes in children. Newer studies associated exposure to BPA with body mass index (BMI),[33] with some studies showing an association with lower BMI at younger ages, but a more rapid increase in BMI in later years.[33–36]

## PREVENTION

Guidance is available about reducing exposures to BPA in infants and children (see Table 41-2).

### Frequently Asked Questions

*Q   Why is there controversy over bisphenol A?*

A   Studies have shown effects on endocrine functions in animals exposed to bisphenol A (BPA). The controversy arises because there are few studies showing harmful effects in infants or children. There is concern, however, that children are rapidly growing and developing and may, therefore, be especially susceptible to chemicals such as BPA. Additional research studies and reviews by the US Food and Drug Administration may determine what level of exposure to BPA might cause similar effects in humans.

Q   *What precautionary measures can parents take to reduce babies' exposure to BPA?*

A   Avoid clear plastic bottles or containers with the recycling No. 7 and the letters "PC" (indicating "polycarbonate") imprinted on them—many of these contain BPA. Alternatives include polyethylene or polypropylene that should not contain BPA. Glass is also an alternative but can be hazardous if dropped or broken. Because heat may cause the release of BPA from plastic, it is prudent to consider the following:
— Do not boil polycarbonate bottles;
— Do not microwave polycarbonate bottles; and
— Do not wash polycarbonate bottles in the dishwasher.
— If pacifiers are used to reduce the risk of sudden infant death syndrome (SIDS), consistent with AAP recommendations, use pacifiers certified by the European Union to be free of BPA and phthalates.

Q   *Should I stop using canned liquid formula?*

A   The lining of cans may contain BPA, so avoiding canned formula is one way to reduce exposure. If you are considering switching from liquid to powdered formula, note that the mixing procedures may differ, so pay special attention when preparing formula from powder.
— If your baby is on a special formula to address a medical condition, you should not switch to another formula because the known risks would outweigh any potential risks posed by BPA. Speak to your pediatrician before you consider changing your baby's formula.
— Risks associated with giving your baby homemade condensed milk formulas or soy or goat milk are far greater than the potential effects of BPA.

Q   *Will breastfeeding reduce my baby's exposure to BPA?*

A   Although low concentrations of BPA have been detected in human milk, breastfeeding a baby is one way to reduce exposure to BPA that leaches from plastic bottles or formula can linings. The American Academy of Pediatrics recommends exclusive breastfeeding for a minimum of 4 months but preferably for 6 months. Breastfeeding should be continued, with the addition of complementary foods, at least through the first 12 months of age and thereafter as long as mutually desired by the mother and infant.

Q   *Is anything being done to advocate for safety testing of chemicals before they are put on the market? It appears that we are always finding possible and actual hazards of new chemicals, but not until after they have been released into the environment.*

A   The American Academy of Pediatrics and other organizations strongly advocate for protecting children, pregnant women, and the general population from the hazards of chemicals before the chemicals are marketed.[37]

## Resources For Providers And Patients

### BPA Fact Sheet
Web site: https://www.niehs.nih.gov/health/topics/agents/sya-bpa/index.cfm

### Children's Environmental Health and Disease Prevention Research Centers
Web site: https://www.niehs.nih.gov/research/supported/centers/prevention/index.cfm

### Environmental Protection Agency
Web site: https://www.epa.gov/assessing-and-managing-chemicals-under-tsca/frank-r-lautenberg-chemical-safety-21st-century-act

### National Institute of Environmental Health Sciences (NIEHS) fact sheet
Web site: www.niehs.nih.gov/health/docs/bpa-factsheet.pdf

### Pediatric Environmental Health Specialty Units (PEHSUs)
Web site: www.pehsu.net

### Phthalates Fact Sheet
Web site: https://www.cdc.gov/biomonitoring/phthalates_factsheet.html

### US Food and Drug Administration
Subcommittee Report on Bisphenol A (17-page summary)
Web site: www.fda.gov/ohrms/dockets/ac/08/briefing/2008-4386b1-05.pdf

## References

1. Shea KM; American Academy of Pediatrics, Committee on Environmental Health. Pediatric exposure and potential toxicity of phthalate plasticizers. *Pediatrics*. 2003;111(6 Pt 1): 1467–1474
2. Phthalates activate estrogen receptors. *Sci News*. 1995;148(3):47
3. Swan SH, Main KM, Liu F, et al. Decrease in anogenital distance among male infants with prenatal phthalate exposure. *Environ Health Perspect*. 2005;113(8):1056–1061
4. Giulivo M, Lopez de Alda M, Capri E, Barcelo D. Human exposure to endocrine disrupting compounds: their role in reproductive systems, metabolic syndrome and breast cancer. A review. *Environ Res*. 2016;151:251–264

5. Barakat R, Lin PP, Rattan S, et al. Prenatal exposure to DEHP induces premature reproductive senescence in male mice. *Toxicol Sci.* 2017;156(1):96–108

6. Main KM, Mortensen GK, Kaleva MM, et al. Human breast milk contamination with phthalates and alterations of endogenous reproductive hormones in infants three months of age. *Environ Health Perspect.* 2006;114(2):270–276

7. Zhou C, Gao L, Flaws JA. Prenatal exposure to an environmentally relevant phthalate mixture disrupts reproduction in F1 female mice. *Toxicol Appl Pharmacol.* 2017;318:49–57

8. Zhou C, Flaws JA. Effects of an environmentally relevant phthalate mixture on cultured mouse antral follicles. *Toxicol Sci.* 2017;156(1):217–229

9. Ferguson KK, McElrath TF, Cantonwine DE, Mukherjee B, Meeke JD. Phthalate metabolites and bisphenol-A in association with circulating angiogenic biomarkers across pregnancy. *Placenta.* 2015;36(6):699–703

10. Ferguson KK, McElrath TF, Chen YH, Mukherjee B, Meeker JD. Urinary phthalate metabolites and biomarkers of oxidative stress in pregnant women: a repeated measures analysis. *Environ Health Perspect.* 2015;123(3):210–216

11. Bornehag CG, Sundell J, Weschler CJ, et al. The association between asthma and allergic symptoms in children and phthalates in house dust: a nested case-control study. *Environ Health Perspect.* 2004;112(14):1393–1397

12. Hill SS, Shaw BR, Wu AH. Plasticizers, antioxidants, and other contaminants found in air delivered by PVC tubing used in respiratory therapy. *Biomed Chromatogr.* 2003;17(4):250–262

13. Engel SM, Zhu C, Berkowitz GS, et al. Prenatal phthalate exposure and performance on the Neonatal Behavioral Assessment Scale in a multiethnic birth cohort. *Neurotoxicology.* 2009;30(4):522–528

14. Wolff MS, Engel SM, Berkowitz GS, et al. Prenatal phenol and phthalate exposures and birth outcomes. *Environ Health Perspect.* 2008;116(8):1092–1097

15. Whyatt RM, Adibi JJ, Calafat AM, et al. Prenatal di(2-ethylhexyl)phthalate exposure and length of gestation among an inner-city cohort. *Pediatrics.* 2009;124(6):e1213–e1220

16. Rais-Bahrami K, Nunez S, Revenis ME, Luban NL, Short BL. Follow-up study of adolescents exposed to di(2-ethylhexyl) phthalate (DEHP) as neonates on extracorporeal membrane oxygenation (ECMO) support. *Environ Health Perspect.* 2004;112(13):1339–1340

17. Latini G, De Felice C, Presta G, et al. In utero exposure to di-(2-ethylhexyl)phthalate and duration of human pregnancy. *Environ Health Perspect.* 2003;111(14):1783–1785

18. Adibi JJ, Hauser R, Williams PL, et al. Maternal urinary metabolites of di-(2-Ethylhexyl) phthalate in relation to the timing of labor in a US multicenter pregnancy cohort study. *Am J Epidemiol.* 2009;169(8):1015–1024

19. Philippat C, Bennett DH, Krakowiak P, Rose M, Hwang HM, Hertz-Picciotto I. Phthalate concentrations in house dust in relation to autism spectrum disorder and developmental delay in the Childhood Autism Risks from Genetics and the Environment (CHARGE) study. *Environ Health.* 2015;14:56

20. Vandenberg LN, Hauser R, Marcus M, Olea N, Welshons WV. Human exposure to bisphenol A (BPA). *Reprod Toxicol.* 2007;24(2):139–177

21. Calafat AM, Ye X, Wong LY, Reidy JA, Needham JL. Exposure of the U.S. population to bisphenol A and 4-tertiary-octylphenol: 2003–2004. *Environ Health Perspect.* 2008;116(1):39–44

22. Soto AM, Maffini MV, Schaeberle CM, Sonnenschein C. Strengths and weaknesses of in vitro assays for estrogenic and androgenic activity. *Best Pract Res Clin Endocrinol Metab.* 2006;20(1):15–33

23. Markey CM, Michaelson CL, Veson EC, Sonnenschein C, Soto AM. The mouse uterotrophic assay: a re-evaluation of its validity in assessing the estrogenicity of bisphenol A. *Environ Health Perspect.* 2001;109(1):55–60

24. Moriyama K, Tagami T, Akamizu T, et al. Thyroid hormone action is disrupted by bisphenol A as an antagonist. *J Clin Endocrinol Metab.* 2002;87(11):5185–5190

25. National Toxicology Program. NTP-CERHR Monograph on the Potential Human Reproductive and Development Effects of Bisphenol A. https://ntp.niehs.nih.gov/ntp/ohat/bisphenol/bisphenol.pdf. Accessed April 4, 2018

26. Ziv-Gal A, Wang W, Zhou C, Flaws JA. The effects of in utero bisphenol A exposure on reproductive capacity in several generations of mice. *Toxicol Appl Pharmacol.* 2015;284(3):354–362

27. Vandenberg LN, Maffini MV, Sonnenschein C, Rubin BS, Soto AM. Bisphenol-A and the great divide: a review of controversies in the field of endocrine disruption. *Endocr Rev.* 2009;30(1):75–95

28. Takeuchi T, Tsutsumi O, Ikezuki Y, Takai Y, Taketani Y. Positive relationship between androgen and the endocrine disruptor, bisphenol A, in normal women and women with ovarian dysfunction *Endocr J.* 2004;51(2):165–169

29. Lang IA, Galloway TS, Scarlett A, et al. Association of urinary bisphenol A concentration with medical disorders and laboratory abnormalities in adults. *JAMA.* 2008;300(11):1303–1310

30. Melzer D, Rice NE, Lewis C, Henley WE, Galloway TS. Association of urinary bisphenol A concentration with heart disease: evidence from NHANES 2003/06. *PLoS One.* 2010;5(1):e8673

31. Lakind JS, Naiman DQ. Daily intake of bisphenol A and potential sources of exposure: 2005–2006 National Health and Nutrition Examination Survey. *J Exp Sci Environ Epidemiol.* 2011;21(3):272–279

32. Braun JM, Yolton K, Dietrich KN, et al. Prenatal bisphenol A exposure and early childhood behavior. *Environ Health Perspect.* 2009;117(12):1945–1952

33. Yang TC, Peterson KE, Meeker JD, et al. Bisphenol A and phthalates in utero and in childhood: association with childhood BMI z-score and adiposity. *Environ Res.* 2017;156:326–333

34. Braun J, Lanphear BP, Calafat A, et al. Early life bisphenol A exposure and child body mass index: a prospective cohort study. *Environ Health Perspect.* 2014;122(11):1239–1245

35. Volberg V, Harley K, Calafat AM, et al. Maternal bisphenol a exposure during pregnancy and its association with adipokines in Mexican-American children. *Environ Mol Mutagen.* 2013;54(8):621–628

36. Harley KG, Schall RA, Chevrier J, et al. Prenatal and postnatal bisphenol A exposure and body mass index in childhood in the CHAMACOS cohort. *Environ Health Perspect.* 2013;121:514–520

37. American Academy of Pediatrics, Council on Environmental Health. Policy statement: chemical management policy: prioritizing children's health. *Pediatrics.* 2011;127(5):983–990

Chapter 42

# Radon

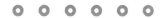

## KEY POINTS

- Radon is a gas released from certain rocks and soil.
- Radon is a carcinogen, causing about 21,000 lung cancer deaths yearly from inhaling radon.
- Smoking further increases a radon-exposed person's risk for the development of lung cancer.
- Radon exposure is a significant and preventable cause of lung cancer.
- The US Environmental Protection Agency advises testing homes and schools for radon and taking remediation steps if levels are elevated.

## INTRODUCTION

Radon is a colorless, odorless, inert radioactive gas released during the natural decay of thorium and uranium, which are common, naturally occurring elements found in varying amounts in rock and soil.[1-3] Radon-222 decays into radioactive elements, including polonium, bismuth, and lead. These decay products are often termed daughters or progeny. Some of these radioactive progeny, such as polonium-218 and polonium-214, emit alpha particles that can cause tissue damage. Radon is classified as a Class A human carcinogen by the US Environmental Protection Agency (EPA), meaning that it is known to cause cancer in humans.[2] Radon in air is measured in picocuries per liter (pCi/L); a picocurie is 1 trillionth of a curie. The curie is a standard measure for the intensity of radioactivity contained in a sample of radioactive material.

## SOURCES AND ROUTES OF EXPOSURE

Radon accounts for approximately 55% of total background radiation.[4] Outdoors, radon is diluted and poses minimal risk. Higher levels may be found indoors or in areas with poor ventilation. Radon gas in the soil can enter homes and other buildings through cracks in concrete floors and walls, floor drains, construction joints, and tiny cracks or pores in hollow-block walls.[2] A study of predictors of indoor radon concentrations in Pennsylvania found a positive trend in home radon levels related to increases in the number of unconventional natural gas wells (hydraulic fracturing, or fracking, wells).[5] Other predictors included the geology of the home location and the presence of a private well.

Inhalation of radon gas is the major route of exposure. The US EPA estimates that nearly 1 in 15 homes has elevated radon levels.[2] Different parts of the country have varying levels of radon in the ground. The US EPA or state radon offices can provide information on which areas have higher levels. The amount of radon within an individual home and between neighboring homes can be variable because of differences in ventilation, construction, and design. The most important component of radon dose comes from its short-lived decay products.[6,7] Radon itself is an inert gas with a half-life of about 4 days, and almost all the gas that is inhaled will be exhaled. Because the decay products are isotopes of solid elements, however, they may attach to molecules of water and other atmospheric gases. These decay products are then deposited on the surface of the respiratory tract and, because of their short half-lives (less than 30 minutes), will decay there. This may result in local tissue damage.

Radon is soluble in water but it is also highly volatile and, thus, mostly removed from public water supplies.[4] Its concentration in water can vary widely, however, depending on geographic location and water source. Ingestion as a route of exposure may be important if high radon concentrations are present in drinking water.[6,7] Estimates of the length of time that ingested radon may stay in the stomach are based on studies of water and food gastrointestinal tract transit times. The most significant organ to receive a radon dose through ingestion appears to be the stomach wall.[4] After passing from the stomach to the small intestine, any remaining radon is transferred to the blood and rapidly removed from the body. It is possible for radon gas to be released from water during showering. In most instances, radon entering the home through water is a small source of risk.

## SYSTEMS AFFECTED AND CLINICAL EFFECTS

### Lung Cancer

Underground miners were noted to have increased rates of lung cancer nearly a century ago.[1] A large number of independent epidemiological studies of thousands of miners around the world carried out over more than 50 years have shown increased lung cancer rates in underground miners, even after controlling for other exposures, such as smoking, asbestos, silica, diesel fumes, arsenic, chromium, nickel, and ore dust.[8-11] Laboratory studies of animals support this finding. Mice exposed to radon have increased rates of lung cancer, pulmonary fibrosis, emphysema, and a shortened lifespan.[8]

Several challenges exist in converting cancer risk estimates in individuals occupationally exposed to radon to individuals with only residential exposures. Underground miners are exposed to radon at much higher levels than are nonminers, and may have other risk factors for cancer or lung disease. Several epidemiological studies have found, however, that there is an increased risk of lung cancer from residential radon exposure.[12-16] Consensus meetings of the US EPA, the National Research Council, and the World Health Organization (WHO) have concluded that radon is a human carcinogen that contributes to a large number of lung cancer deaths each year.[1-3] Radon is estimated to cause approximately 21,000 lung cancer deaths in the United States each year.[2] Smoking greatly increases the risk of lung cancer at a given level of radon exposure. For instance, with lifetime exposure at a radon level of 4 pCi/L of air, the percentage of people estimated to develop lung cancer is 6.2% for smokers, a rate nearly 9 times higher than the percentage of 0.7% for nonsmokers.[17] Table 42-1 illustrates risks for smokers and nonsmokers at different levels of lifetime radon exposure.

| Table 42-1. Lifetime Risk of Lung Cancer Death (per Person) from Radon Exposure in Homes[17,a] | | | |
|---|---|---|---|
| **RADON LEVEL (pCi/L)[b]** | **NEVER SMOKERS** | **CURRENT SMOKERS** | **GENERAL POPULATION[c]** |
| 20 | 36 out of 1,000 | 260 out of 1,000 | 110 out of 1,000 |
| 10 | 18 out of 1,000 | 150 out of 1,000 | 56 out of 1,000 |
| 8 | 15 out of 1,000 | 120 out of 1,000 | 45 out of 1,000 |
| 4 | 7.3 out of 1,000 | 62 out of 1,000 | 23 out of 1,000 |
| 2 | 3.7 out of 1,000 | 32 out of 1,000 | 12 out of 1,000 |
| 1.25 | 23 out of 10,000 | 200 out of 10,000 | 73 out of 10,000 |
| 0.4 | 7.3 out of 10,000 | 64 out of 10,000 | 23 out of 10,000 |

[a] Estimates are subject to uncertainties as discussed in Chapter VII of EPA's *Assessment of Risks from Radon in Homes.*[17]
[b] Assumes constant lifetime exposure in homes at these levels.
[c] Includes smokers and nonsmokers.
Abbreviation: pCi/L, picocuries per liter.

Radon represents a significant and preventable cause of lung cancer. The public health impact of the 21,000 US deaths attributable to radon in 2003 can be compared with deaths in 2001 from drunk driving (17,400), falls in the home (8,000), drowning (3,900), and home fires (2,800).[2] The National Radon Action Plan is a national effort led by the American Lung Association to mitigate 5 million homes with high radon levels by 2020, which should prevent an estimated 3,200 lung cancer deaths by 2020.[18] This effort builds on an earlier federal effort to increase measurement and remediation of radon in homes, schools, and child care settings.

## Stomach Cancer

Higher rates of stomach cancer were noted in atomic bomb survivors[19] and in miners exposed to radon.[20,21] However, the studies of miners did not find trends in mortality related to dose. Few studies of cancer and ingestion of water containing radon are available. A case-cohort study of radon, radium-226, and natural uranium in Finland found no association with stomach cancer.[22] One ecological study reported a positive correlation between stomach cancer and radon levels reported by county in Pennsylvania.[23] Ecological studies look at groups and area-wide exposure data but cannot make links at an individual level.

## Leukemia

The effects of radon exposure in childhood are not well understood. It is possible that radon exposure could increase the risk of leukemia because bone marrow is vulnerable to the effects of ionizing radiation. Most studies to date have focused on residential radon exposure and childhood leukemia. Eleven of 12 descriptive (ecological) studies suggest that there could be increased risk of childhood cancer associated with radon exposure (reviewed in Evrard et al[24] and Raaschou-Nielsen[25]). In some of these studies, the effect of radon exposure was higher for acute myelogenous leukemia than for acute lymphocytic leukemia. The 7 case-control studies conducted to date, however, have shown inconsistent results; some found an association between residential radon and childhood leukemia, but others did not (reviewed in Evrard et al[24] and Raaschou-Nielsen[25]). A recent cohort study in Norway found no association with childhood leukemia and a nonsignificant, elevated risk of central nervous system tumors.[26]

Overall, the literature suggests that there may be an association between leukemia and residential radon exposure. Larger, prospective studies are required to more thoroughly understand these risks.

## DIAGNOSTIC METHODS AND MEASUREMENT OF EXPOSURE

The US EPA recommends that all homes below the third floor be tested for radon; additional details can be found on the US EPA's Web site and in the publication *A Citizen's Guide to Radon*.[2] Two general methods are used to test homes for radon: short-term testing and long-term testing. Testing should usually be performed in the basement or on the first floor because radon levels are usually higher than on upper floors. Short-term testing is generally carried out for between 2 and 90 days. Several types of detectors used for short-term testing can give good results, but because radon levels can vary daily, they do not give a good year-round estimate. The most common form of detector is charcoal-based. In a blinded study that tested commercially available short-term radon detectors, it was noted that increased humidity and temporal fluctuations in radon concentrations could have a negative influence on the accuracy and precision of some short-term detectors.[27] Long-term tests remain in the home for more than 90 days and are more likely to give a better estimate of year-round average of radon levels in the home. Anyone can perform these tests without professional help. Test kits are generally reliable, inexpensive, and readily available through state radon offices or directly from commercial vendors. The test kit is sent back to the company in a prepaid mailer for analysis, and processing time is measured in days.

## PREVENTION OF EXPOSURE

The US EPA, the WHO, and other groups have strongly recommended initiatives to reduce indoor exposure to radon.[2,3] Some municipalities require new homes to be constructed in a radon-resistant manner, that radon testing be conducted whenever a home is sold, and that radon testing be performed in all schools. When levels of radon higher than 4 pCi/L are found, repairs should be made to reduce the level. Remediation should be considered at levels between 2 and 4 pCi/L. It is often difficult to reduce radon levels that are below 2 pCi/L. The average indoor air radon level is estimated at about 1.3 pCi/L.

In general, radon exposure can be reduced by increasing ventilation and by reducing the influx of radon in the home. These repairs are not expensive and can usually be completed for about the same cost as other common home repairs. Key components of radon remediation include:

- Adjusting existing central ventilation systems
- Sealing cracks in the foundation
- Creating negative pressure under the basement floor with the installation of a radon sub-slab soil suction system
- Prohibiting the use of building materials containing excessive radium

More detailed information about home radon abatement measures is available from the US EPA (www.epa.gov/radon).

Most importantly, pediatricians should advise families about the hazards of radon exposure and that testing and remediation are easy and affordable. They should also point out that cigarette smoking dramatically magnifies the radon-induced risk of lung cancer.

## Frequently Asked Questions

*Q*  *Should I test for radon in my home?*

A  The US EPA recommends that all home floors below the third floor be checked for radon. An inexpensive home-testing kit can be obtained from home improvement stores and from some local or state radon programs. The sample obtained should be sent to a certified laboratory for analysis. Mitigation measures should be taken if the level of radon exceeds 4 pCi/L and considered for levels between 2 and 4 pCi/L. Further information can be obtained from the Resources section at the end of this chapter.

*Q*  *What are the health effects from exposure to radon?*

A  There are no immediate medical problems related to radon exposure. However, radon in indoor air is estimated to cause about 21,000 lung cancer deaths in the United States each year. Some studies suggest an increased risk of childhood leukemia with radon exposure. There is no evidence that respiratory diseases such as asthma are caused by radon exposure.

*Q*  *What about radon in schools?*

A  Children spend a third or more of their weekdays in schools, making radon in schools a potential concern. The US EPA recommends that all schools be tested for radon. Radon problems in schools are often remedied by adjusting settings of central ventilation systems. The other approaches listed previously in the chapter can also be applied. More detailed information is available at https://www.epa.gov/iaq-schools/managing-radon-schools.

## Resources

**Kansas State University National Radon Program Services (order discounted test kits)**
> Web site: http://sosradon.org/test-kits

**State and regional indoor environments contact information**
> Web site: www.epa.gov/iaq/whereyoulive.html

**The International Radon Project**
> Web site: www.who.int/ionizing_radiation/env/radon/en/index.html
> A World Health Organization initiative to reduce lung cancer risk around the world.

**US Environmental Protection Agency (EPA)**
> Web site: www.epa.gov/radon/pubs
> This Web site has links to several publications, information on home testing and remediation, and geographical maps of radon exposure.
> US EPA Radon Hotline: 800-767-7236

# References

1. National Research Council, Committee on Health Risks of Exposure to Radon. *The Health Effects of Exposure to Radon: BEIR VI*. 1999. http://www.nap.edu/read/5499/chapter/1. Accessed January 18, 2018

2. US Environmental Protection Agency. *A Citizen's Guide to Radon: The Guide to Protecting Yourself and Your Family From Radon*. 2009. Publication No. US EPA 402-K-07-009. https://www.epa.gov/sites/production/files/2016-02/documents/2012_a_citizens_guide_to_radon.pdf. Accessed January 18, 2018

3. World Health Organization. *WHO Handbook on Indoor Radon: A Public Health Perspective*. Geneva, Switzerland: World Health Organization; 2009. http://www.who.int/ionizing_radiation/env/radon/en/index1.html. Accessed January 18, 2018

4. National Research Council, Committee to Assess Health Risks from Exposure to Low Levels of Ionizing Radiation. *Health Risks from Exposure to Low Levels of Ionizing Radiation: BEIR VII Phase 2*. Washington, DC: National Academies Press; 2006. http://www.nap.edu/download/11340. Accessed July 10, 2018

5. Casey JA, Ogburn EL, Rasmussen SG, et al. Predictors of indoor radon concentrations in Pennsylvania, 1989-2013. *Environ Health Perspect*. 2015;123(11):1130–1137

6. Kendall GM, Smith TJ. Doses to organs and tissues from radon and its decay products. *J Radiol Prot*. 2002;22(4):389–406

7. Kendall GM, Smith TJ. Doses from radon and its decay products to children. *J Radiol Prot*. 2005;25(3):241–256

8. US Environmental Protection Agency. *A Physician's Guide – Radon*. 1999. Publication No. US EPA 402-K-93-008. https://www.epa.gov/radon/physicians-guide-radon. Accessed January 18, 2018

9. Lubin JH, Boice JD Jr, Edling C, et al. Lung cancer in radon-exposed miners and estimation of risk from indoor exposure. *J Natl Cancer Inst*. 1995;87(11):817–827

10. Vacquier B, Caer S, Rogel A, et al. Mortality risk in the French cohort of uranium miners: extended follow-up 1946-1999. *Occup Environ Med*. 2008;65(9):597–604

11. Samet JM, Eradze GR. Radon and lung cancer risk: taking stock at the millenium. *Environ Health Perspect*. 2000;108(Suppl 4):635–641

12. Darby S, Hill D, Deo H, et al. Residential radon and lung cancer—detailed results of a collaborative analysis of individual data on 7148 persons with lung cancer and 14,208 persons without lung cancer from 13 epidemiologic studies in Europe. *Scand J Work Environ Health*. 2006;32(Suppl 1):1–83

13. Field RW. Environmental factors in cancer: radon. *Rev Environ Health*. 2010;25(1):23–31

14. Lubin JH, Boice JD Jr. Lung cancer risk from residential radon: meta-analysis of eight epidemiologic studies. *J Natl Cancer Inst*. 1997;89(1):49–57

15. Noh J, Sohn J, Cho J, Kang DR, Joo S, Kim C, Shin DC. Residential radon and environmental burden of disease among non-smokers. *Ann Occup Environ Med*. 2016;28:12

16. Pavia M, Bianco A, Pileggi C, Angelillo IF. Meta-analysis of residential exposure to radon gas and lung cancer. *Bull World Health Organ*. 2003;81(10):732–738

17. US Environmental Protection Agency. *Report: EPA's Assessment of Risks from Radon in Homes*. 2003. Publication No. US EPA 402-R-03-003. https://www.epa.gov/sites/production/files/2014-11/documents/402-r-03-003.pdf. Accessed January 18, 2018

18. US Environmental Protection Agency. The National Radon Action Plan - A Strategy for Saving Lives. https://www.epa.gov/radon/national-radon-action-plan-strategy-saving-lives. Accessed January 18, 2018

19. Preston DL, Shimizu Y, Pierce DA, Suyama A, Mabuchi K. Studies of mortality of atomic bomb survivors. Report 13: Solid cancer and noncancer disease mortality: 1950-1997. *Radiat Res.* 2003;160(4):381–407

20. Darby SC, Radford EP, Whitley E. Radon exposure and cancers other than lung cancer in Swedish iron miners. *Environ Health Perspect.* 1995;103(Suppl 2):45–47

21. Walsh L, Grosche B, Schnelzer M, Tschense A, Sogl M, Kreuzer M. A review of the results from the German Wismut uranium miners cohort. *Radiat Prot Dosimetry.* 2015;164(1-2):147–153.

22. Auvinen A, Salonen L, Pekkanen J, Pukkala E, Ilus T, Kurttio P. Radon and other natural radionuclides in drinking water and risk of stomach cancer: a case-cohort study in Finland. *Int J Cancer.* 2005;114(1):109–113

23. Kjellberg S, Wiseman JS. The relationship of radon to gastrointestinal malignancies. *Am Surg.* 1995;61(9):822–825

24. Evrard AS, Hemon D, Billon S, et al. Ecological association between indoor radon concentration and childhood leukaemia incidence in France, 1990-1998. *Eur J Cancer Prev.* 2005;14(2):147–157

25. Raaschou-Nielsen O. Indoor radon and childhood leukaemia. *Radiat Prot Dosimetry.* 2008;132(2):175–181

26. Del Risco Kollerud R, Blaasaas KG, Claussen B. Risk of leukaemia or cancer in the central nervous system among children living in an area with high indoor radon concentrations: results from a cohort study in Norway. *Br J Cancer.* 2014;111(7):1413–1420

27. Sun S, Budd G, McLemore S, Field RW. Blind testing of commercially available short-term radon detectors. *Health Phys.* 2008;94(6):548–557

# Chapter 43

# Tobacco Use and Tobacco Smoke Exposure

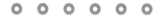

## KEY POINTS

- Secondhand and thirdhand smoke exposure cause significant pediatric morbidity and mortality with 41% of children aged 3 to 11 years in the United States exposed to tobacco smoke; African-American children are disproportionately exposed.
- Most smokers begin smoking before the age of 18 years, influenced in part by marketing and advertising by tobacco companies.
- Pediatric health care providers can provide brief but effective tobacco dependence treatment to parents and caretakers to improve child health.

## INTRODUCTION

Tobacco use and tobacco smoke exposure are uniquely linked in the pediatric setting. The most significant source of child tobacco smoke exposure is combustible cigarette use by an adult living with the child.[1] Other tobacco products, including cigars and hookah, also are sources of tobacco smoke exposure, and electronic cigarettes (e-cigarettes) are sources of exposure to nicotine and other chemicals.[2] Most tobacco use begins before age 18 years, influenced by exposure to tobacco use by parents or peers, glamorous depictions in movies and other media, advertising that targets children and adolescents, and other environmental, social, and cultural factors.[3,4] The connection between children and tobacco use is so strong that the Commissioner of the US Food and Drug Administration (FDA) declared smoking to be a "pediatric disease" in 1995.[5]

Tobacco smoke exposure is a combination of secondhand smoke (SHS) and thirdhand smoke. The 2006 Surgeon General's Report, *The Health Consequences of Involuntary Exposure to Tobacco Smoke,* determined that there is no safe level of exposure to tobacco smoke.[6] Cigarette smoking is the most important factor determining the level of particulate matter in the indoor air, and concentrations of particulates less than 2.5 micrometers (a size that reaches the lower airways) can be 2 to 3 times higher in homes with smokers than in homes without smokers.[7]

Secondhand smoke is a dynamic mixture of exhaled smoke and smoke released from the smoldering end of cigarettes, cigars, and pipes. Secondhand smoke contains more than 4,000 chemical compounds, many of which are poisons, and some carcinogens.[8] Thirdhand smoke refers to the residual smoke contamination that remains after the cigarette is extinguished.[9] This residual comprises particulate matter that settles on surfaces (including walls, furniture, carpeting, and other hard surfaces) and in loose household dust; these particles are re-emitted into the gas phase, or react with oxidants in the environment to yield secondary pollutants.[10,11]

The prevalence of cigarette use and tobacco smoke exposure continues to slowly decline; in 2015, however, 15.1% of US adults (36.5 million people) continued to be current cigarette smokers.[12] Among the Americans who continue to smoke, adults who are male, younger, multiracial or American Indian/Alaska Native, less educated, live below the federal poverty level, live in the South or Midwest, have disabilities or limitations, or who are lesbian, gay, or bisexual are disproportionately affected.[12] Although the prevalence of SHS exposure among nonsmokers has declined (52.5% during 1999 to 2000 compared with 25.3% in 2011 to 2012), significant disparities still exist. For example, 67.9% of African-American children aged 3 to 11 years in the United States are exposed to SHS compared with 37.2% of white children.[13] These numbers are much higher outside the United States in countries in which tobacco use is more prevalent and people may be less aware of the dangers of exposure.[14] Using data from 192 countries, the World Health Organization estimated that the burden of disease worldwide from exposure to SHS was approximately 1% of total mortality, and 0.7% of total worldwide burden of disease in disability-adjusted life years (DALYs).[15]

## ROUTES AND SOURCES OF EXPOSURE

The primary route of tobacco smoke exposure is through active smoking and inhalation of SHS and thirdhand smoke, although some exposure may occur through contact with particles that settle on surfaces and then are ingested through the gastrointestinal tract.[16] Because thirdhand smoke can remain long after the source of smoke is extinguished, exposure can occur after the smoker has left.[17]

Most children exposed to tobacco smoke are exposed in their own homes, and because many young children spend a large proportion of their time indoors with their families, exposure may be significant.[1] Even when parents smoke only outdoors, children can be exposed at levels that are associated with harm.[16] Children also can be exposed in the homes of relatives and friends, motor vehicles, child care settings, schools, health care facilities, dormitories, entertainment venues, parks and athletic facilities, shopping centers, restaurants, and leisure facilities. Adolescents may be exposed in their workplaces.[18]

Another source that is increasingly being recognized is tobacco smoke exposure among children living in multi-unit housing in which SHS drifts from other apartments (tobacco smoke incursion).[19] Children living in apartments have demonstrated higher levels of tobacco smoke exposure, as measured by serum cotinine, than those living in detached houses.[19]

## MECHANISMS OF EFFECT

Secondhand smoke contains more than 50 carcinogens, including polycyclic aromatic hydrocarbons, $N$-nitrosamines, aromatic amines, aldehydes, and other organic (eg, benzene) and inorganic (eg, metals, polonium$^{210}$) compounds.[6] Although the mechanisms of carcinogenesis have not been determined for all of these chemicals, tobacco-specific carcinogens have been measured in the urine of nonsmokers, including children, exposed to SHS.[20] Constituents of thirdhand smoke include nicotine, tobacco-specific carcinogens, and nitrosamines.[11]

Mechanisms by which SHS exposure causes injury to the respiratory tract have been described.[6] Prenatal exposure to nicotine causes changes in synthesis in airway tissues. These changes may be attributed to effects on nicotinic acetylcholine receptors that are abundant in the developing lung.[6] Postnatal exposure induces bronchial hyperreactivity, possibly attributable to increases in the lung's neuroendocrine cells that synthesize and release bronchoconstrictors.[6] Other mechanisms include altered neural control of the airway that results in bronchoconstriction, mucus secretion, and microvascular leakage. Increased concentrations of serum immunoglobulin E and poor immune cell function have been described in exposed children.[6] These altered immune responses may contribute to the increased prevalence of wheezing, asthma, impaired macrophage function, altered mucociliary clearance, enhanced bacterial adherence, and disruption of the respiratory epithelium.[6] Changes in nitric oxide production contribute to bronchial hyperreactivity.[6]

Infants exposed to SHS have an increased risk of Sudden Infant Death Syndrome (SIDS).[6] Although the mechanism explaining increased risk is not completely understood, studies have demonstrated deficient cardiorespiratory control, probably resulting from nicotine's effects on nicotinic receptors in the peripheral and central nervous systems during fetal development.[6]

Changes in the cardiovascular system associated with exposure to SHS include inflammatory responses, vasodilation, platelet activation, lower high-density lipoprotein levels, impaired oxygen delivery, formation of free radicals, and changes in heart rate.[6]

## Effects of Nicotine on the Developing Brain

Nicotine has neurotoxic effects on the developing brain, including the fetal brain.[21] Nicotine is the primary psychoactive component that causes addiction to tobacco products.[22] Evidence has shown that teenagers become addicted more quickly than adults. Nicotine's effect on the adolescent brain is more likely to result in the use of other substances; therefore, nicotine can be considered to be a "gateway" drug, especially in adolescents.[23]

## CLINICAL EFFECTS

The enormous burden of mortality and morbidity caused by tobacco use and tobacco smoke exposure is irrefutable; smoking is still the leading cause of preventable death and disease in the United States.[24] The 2014 Surgeon General Report, *The Health Consequences of Smoking: 50 Years of Progress*, extensively details the diseases linked to cigarette smoking, affecting almost every organ of the body.[24]

Tobacco smoke exposure causes significant disease and disability in nonsmokers.[6] Each year, SHS kills 41,000 nonsmokers including an estimated 430 deaths from SIDS.[8] In adult nonsmokers, the effects of SHS exposure include increased risk of some cancers, stroke, and cardiovascular, reproductive, and respiratory effects.[6,8,24]

The adverse health effects of exposing fetuses, infants, and children to SHS are well established. Research suggests that children are more susceptible to these health effects than are adults.[6] Short-term effects are primarily respiratory and include increased incidence and severity of upper and lower respiratory infections, otitis media with effusion, and asthma exacerbations.[8] Each year in the United States, SHS exposure causes 24,500 infants to be born with low birth weight; 71,900 preterm births; 202,300 episodes of asthma; and 790,000 health care visits for otitis media.[8]

A growing body of evidence indicates that childhood tobacco smoke exposure results in decreased lung function, increased prevalence and severity of asthma (including asthma in adulthood), and increased incidence of cancers.[6,21,25] Several authors have demonstrated a gene-environment association for these and other illnesses associated with SHS exposure.[8,26,27] Children exposed to SHS are more likely to develop dental caries and have respiratory complications when undergoing general anesthesia.[28,29] Among children aged 4 to 16 years, exposure is significantly associated with 6 or more days of school absence in the past year, and children with even low levels of exposure have decreased performance on reading, math, and block design tests.[30,31] Children living in households with smokers are at greater risk of injury and death from fires.[32] For children younger than 10 years, playing with cigarette lighters or matches causes approximately 100,000 fires and 300 to 400 child deaths each year.[33]

The effects on the fetus from maternal smoking have been well characterized, including reduction in birth weight and increased risk for preterm delivery, premature rupture of membranes, placenta previa, and placental abruption.[6] Maternal smoking during pregnancy reduces infant lung function and increases the risk for SIDS.[6] *In utero* exposure to tobacco smoke is linked to an increase in cleft lip and palate and the risk of being overweight in childhood.[25] Although the biologic basis of the effects of *in utero* tobacco smoke exposure are not known, maternal inflammatory oxidative stress is postulated as a mechanism.[34] Maternal smoking also increases the risk of learning and neurobehavioral problems and findings of preclinical atherosclerosis.[21]

## SCREENING METHODS

The American Academy of Pediatrics (AAP) recommends that pediatricians screen children and adolescents for tobacco use and tobacco smoke exposure at health supervision visits and health care visits resulting from diseases that may be caused or worsened by tobacco smoke exposure.[18] Screening for children's exposure to SHS in the clinical setting is typically done by questioning the child or accompanying adult. Groner et al[35] used hair nicotine levels to validate a series of 3 questions: (1) Does the mother smoke?; (2) Do others smoke?; and (3) Do others smoke inside? The authors then developed a decision tree with probabilities for use in the clinical setting.[35]

Sample questions to identify tobacco smoke exposure for parents/caregivers include[18]

1. Does your child live with anyone who uses tobacco?
2. Does anyone who provides care for your child smoke?
3. Does your child visit places where people smoke?
4. Does anyone ever smoke in your home?
5. Does anyone ever smoke in your car?
6. Do you ever smell smoke from your neighbors in or near your home or apartment?

Sample questions to screen for adolescent tobacco use include[18]

1. Do any of your friends use tobacco?
2. Have you ever tried a tobacco product?
3. How many times have you tried (name of tobacco product)?
4. How often do you use (name of tobacco product)?
5. Do your friends use e-cigarettes, e-hookah, or vape?
6. Have you tried e-cigarettes, e-hookah, or vape?

## PREVENTION OF EXPOSURE

The only way to completely protect children from household exposure to tobacco smoke is for parents and caretakers to stop using tobacco products.[21] In addition, comprehensive smoke-free policies are crucial to protect children and youth in the environments in which they learn, play, and work.[21]

If a parent or caretaker is not able or not willing to quit smoking, smoke-free bans in the car and home should be instituted.[18] Smoking should not be allowed within any structure attached to the home or within range of open windows or doors or in any vehicle used to transport children. Because components of SHS persist in the environment for days after the source of smoke is gone, smoke-free rules should be enforced even when children are absent.[16] This may reduce (but does not eliminate) exposure to tobacco smoke.[18]

### Counseling Parents to Quit Smoking

Pediatricians are in a unique position to provide tobacco dependence treatment to parents and caretakers. Because many parents lack health insurance and access to primary health care for themselves, pediatricians may be the only physicians some parents visit on a regular basis, serving as the primary source of health information for the family.[36,37] Pediatricians counsel parents about diet and safety and provide chemoprophylaxis in certain circumstances (ie, exposure to meningococcemia, pertussis, influenza). To decrease the harm to children from tobacco smoke exposure, it is appropriate for pediatricians to counsel parents about quitting, and to discuss and consider prescribing quit-smoking pharmacotherapies to parents who smoke. Both the AAP and the US Public Health Service Guideline, *Treating Tobacco Use and Dependence*, recommend that clinicians offer parents smoking cessation advice and assistance.[18,38] When a child has a medical condition exacerbated by SHS, such as asthma or recurrent otitis media, it is often a teachable moment for parents and caretakers.[39]

Counseling parents to eliminate children's SHS exposure is effective in increasing parents' showing interest in stopping tobacco use, making attempts at quitting, and succeeding at those attempts.[40,41] A meta-analysis of parental smoking cessation interventions found that interventions did increase parental cessation rates from 23% in the intervention group compared with 18% in the control group.[42]

Parents who use electronic devices should be encouraged to quit tobacco and nicotine use completely, utilizing the same resources recommended to tobacco smokers, including FDA-approved pharmacotherapy and referral to Quitline services.

## The Process of Quitting

At baseline, without counseling or any other intervention, approximately 4% to 8% of tobacco users quit each year.[38] Success increases with each quit attempt, and interventions such as advice to quit, counseling, and pharmacotherapies increase the likelihood of success for each attempt.[38] Approximately 10% of smokers who receive counseling from a physician stop smoking.[38] Although this rate may not seem significant within the context of an individual practice, it reflects a tremendous public health impact at a population level. If there were a 10% rate of cessation in patients in all physician practices in the United States, 2 million smokers would quit each year.[38] Over time, advice from physicians also may influence family members to quit using tobacco entirely, reduce the numbers of cigarettes they smoke, or change the venue of smoking (ie, from indoors to outdoors).

## Treating Adult Tobacco Use and Dependence

The US Public Health Service updated its Clinical Practice Guideline on tobacco dependence treatment in 2008.[38] In addition to comprehensively reviewing the efficacy of therapies, the guideline strongly recommends that all health care professionals routinely assess tobacco use status at every medical visit, regardless of the reason for the visit.[38] Health care professionals are urged to provide counseling at each visit and assess the eligibility of their patients for pharmacotherapies.[38] Table 43-1 gives further information on evidence-based tobacco dependence treatment.

Despite barriers, counseling parents in the context of a busy practice is possible because the intervention can be brief. The simple statement, "you should quit smoking," when delivered by a member of the health care team, increases quit attempts and the success of quit attempts.[38] Following up on the advice with further assistance and referral to the tobacco quit smoking telephone line (1-800-QUIT-NOW) or other community-based tobacco dependence treatment are important next steps.

## Table 43-1. Strategies for Counseling Parents and Caregivers in Tobacco Cessation[18,25,38,43–45]

The **"Five A's"** tobacco use cessation approach includes the following components:

1. **Ask** about tobacco use at every opportunity and assess status with specific attention to the user's motivation and barriers to change.
2. **Advise** the tobacco user to quit.
3. **Assess** by determining the tobacco user's readiness to quit within the next 2 to 4 weeks.
4. **Assist** the tobacco user with the change.
5. **Arrange** follow-up.

Although these steps are fairly brief, concern is frequently expressed about the limited time available for cessation counseling during a child's visit. Even brief advice from pediatricians, however, may have a positive impact on reducing parental tobacco use and relapse rates.

The Clinical Effort Against Secondhand Smoke Exposure (CEASE) program (www.ceasetobacco.org) is a practical alternative that uses **2 A's and an R** to address parental tobacco dependence treatment.[43]

*Ask* about tobacco use at every opportunity ("Does your child live with anyone who uses tobacco?")

*Assist* the tobacco user to quit using evidence-based tobacco dependence treatment that includes both counseling and first-line nicotine replacement pharmacotherapy. Consider recommending or prescribing nicotine replacement pharmacotherapies whenever appropriate. ("As your child's pediatrician, I can help you quit tobacco and help you have a tobacco-free home and car.")

*Refer* the tobacco user to 1-800-QUIT-NOW or other cessation resource as well as to their health care provider.

**Pharmacotherapies**

Nicotine is highly addictive, and nicotine replacement therapy (NRT) plays an important role in tobacco dependence treatment. Unfortunately, many people do not use NRT correctly, including using medications for too short a period of time. Pediatricians should understand the correct use of NRT and barriers to use, even if they do not prescribe them for parents or family members of patients. Many resources are available, including:

— American Academy of Pediatrics Julius B. Richmond Center of Excellence at www2.aap.org/richmondcenter/CounselingAboutSmokingCessation.html[18]
— US Department of Health and Human Services Clinical Practice Guideline Treating Tobacco Use and Dependence: 2008 Update[38]
— MD Anderson Cancer Center QuitMedKit apps at https://www.mdanderson.org/education-training/professional-education/tobacco-outreach-program.html[45]
— American College of Chest Physicians' Tobacco Dependence Treatment Toolkit at http://tobaccodependence.chestnet.org[44]

## *Billing for Counseling Parents About Smoking Cessation*

Unfortunately, there is currently no reimbursement or *Current Procedural Terminology* (CPT) code for counseling parents of pediatric patients about tobacco use cessation. Documentation and using appropriate coding for diagnosis and treatment of tobacco smoke exposure are important steps, however, to develop the evidence supporting the benefits of tobacco dependence treatment in the pediatric setting. International Classification of Diseases, 10th Revision, Clinical Modification (ICD-10-CM) Code examples are as follows[46]:

Z77.22 Contact with and (suspected) exposure to environmental tobacco smoke

Z81.2 Family history of tobacco abuse and dependence

Z71.89 Counseling, other specified

Because the consequences of SHS exposure are so great, and the time needed to deliver a brief "don't start using tobacco" or "stop using tobacco" is short, many pediatricians find the time to provide this important service.

## Adolescent Tobacco Use Prevention

Most smokers begin smoking by age 18 years.[3] Preventing initiation of and experimentation with tobacco use is an important goal for pediatricians. It is important to discuss the role of the media in tobacco use initiation and maintenance. Advertisements for tobacco products, including chewing tobacco, cigars, and snuff, are pervasive in the United States despite the 1998 ban on youth-targeted tobacco advertisements.[38,47] More subtle advertising aimed at youth is delivered by depicting tobacco use in movies, on television, the Internet, and other media. Multiple studies demonstrate that when children and adolescents view smoking in movies, they are more likely to accept and initiate tobacco use.[4] The popularity of e-cigarettes, an example of Electronic Nicotine Delivery Systems (ENDS), has been fueled by unregulated marketing and promotion in the media, including television, movies, video games, social media, among celebrity role models, on the Internet, in radio and print media, on billboards, and through point-of-sale advertising.[2]

It is important to identify adolescents at risk of tobacco use. The US Surgeon General identified 4 categories of risk factors for adolescent tobacco use.[48]

- *Personal*—belief that use of tobacco will make the teenager fit better into the social scene

- *Behavioral*—lack of strong educational goals, lack of attachment to school and social clubs
- *Socioeconomic*—low socioeconomic status
- *Environmental*—tobacco use by peers and/or parents, exposure to tobacco products and advertisements

Once adolescents initiate tobacco use, the transition from intermittent to daily smoking and nicotine dependence can progress quickly.[18] Research on the effectiveness of adolescent tobacco dependence is limited.[18] Behaviorally based programs have shown benefit for adolescents with minimal to mild tobacco dependence.[38] A list of adolescent behaviorally based tobacco dependence treatment resources is available from the AAP.[18] The US Public Health Service guideline recommends using the same counseling strategies with teenagers that are effective with adults but with advice tailored to teenagers.[38] Messages can focus on short-term effects of smoking, such as cost, bad breath, smelly clothes, decreased physical performance, and social unacceptability. It may be useful to raise teenagers' awareness of attempts by tobacco companies to "hook" them through seductive advertising campaigns. Discussing the effects of SHS exposure with children and teenagers also may be useful in reducing their exposure and increasing the rate at which their parents quit.[38] Clinicians should also ask adolescents whether they use e-cigarettes; e-cigarette use is more prevalent in teens and data suggest that their use leads teens to using combustible tobacco products (see Chapter 28).

Few studies have evaluated the effectiveness of pharmacotherapy for adolescent tobacco dependence treatment; these studies have been limited by short courses of treatment with high rates of nonadherence.[18] The AAP recommends considering tobacco dependence pharmacotherapy for moderately to severely tobacco-dependent adolescents.[18] Prior to behavioral or pharmacotherapy treatment, clinicians should determine how many cigarettes are smoked on a typical day, the degree of dependence, any contraindications to or concerns about using pharmacotherapy, body weight, and the teenager's intent to quit. Confidentiality can be an issue, especially when pharmacotherapies are prescribed for teenagers. Clinicians should be aware that prescribing pharmacotherapies such as NRT to teenagers is not approved by the FDA and therefore is considered off-label use.[18] Table 43-2 identifies steps to help teenagers stop using tobacco.

### Strategies for Preadolescents

It is important for pediatricians to begin disseminating a "don't start smoking" message as early as possible and to engage parents, even those who smoke, during this stage. One powerful message that can be delivered by a parent who uses tobacco is that "quitting is hard, and I wish I had never started." Teenagers

## Table 43-2. Steps to Help Teenagers Stop Using Tobacco

1. Ask teenagers to consider that most adults who smoke started when they were teenagers and wish that they had quit as teenagers. Mention that tobacco companies actively solicit teenagers to try smoking.

2. Ask teenagers to make a list of reasons why someone might want to quit. Then talk about any that might apply to them.

3. Point out that the longer a person smokes, the harder it is to quit.

4. Ask teenagers who are not willing to discontinue use to promise that they will not increase the amount that they smoke.

5. Ask teenagers who say that tobacco is not a problem for them, "At what point would tobacco become a problem for you?"

6. Ask teenagers who say that they are not addicted to enter into a verbal contract with you to avoid tobacco for a month. Follow up by telephone.

7. Once the teenager has made a commitment to stop, the pediatrician's task is to encourage and educate. Suggest that teenagers who are determined to give up tobacco do the following:

   — Consider the logical arguments in favor of cessation, including decreasing their risk of associated health hazards.

   — Learn about ways to quit.

   — Think about how and why they use tobacco.

   — Develop a plan to cope with (or avoid) situations where the urge to use is great, such as at parties, restaurants, clubs, etc.

   — Get the help they need (eg, schedule a follow-up appointment, use national, state, and local resources).

   — Consider prescribing first-line pharmacotherapy such as Nicotine Replacement Therapy (NRT) if there is no contraindication. Clinicians should be aware that NRT is not FDA-approved for use in persons younger than age 18 years.

   — Decide on a cessation plan and stay with it.

   — Anticipate and prepare for occasional urges to smoke long after discontinuing use.

   — Refer the teen to Teen.Smokefree.gov, a NIH-supported Web site that is tailored for the teen smoker (https://teen.smokefree.gov).

whose parents use tobacco are more likely to use tobacco themselves. The process of initiation is rapid and can occur within moments of the first inhalation.[48]

## REDUCING TOBACCO USE INITIATION

To achieve the *Healthy People 2020* objective to reduce cigarette smoking among adults to 12% or less by the year 2020, there must be a comprehensive strategy to decrease youth tobacco initiation. The Institute of Medicine (IOM) proposed a strategy in which each state should fund a comprehensive tobacco control program at the level recommended by the Centers for Disease Control and Prevention (CDC). The IOM's strategy includes: (1) strengthening and fully implementing currently proven tobacco control measures; and (2) changing the regulatory landscape to permit policy innovations.[49]

The CDC's *Best Practices for Comprehensive Tobacco Control Programs-2014* describes an integrated structure for implementing effective interventions and is an evidence-based guide to help states plan and establish tobacco control programs.[50] The major strategies proposed include

1. State and community interventions that support, implement, and unite organizations, systems, and networks that encourage and support tobacco-free behavior choices.

2. Mass-reach health communication interventions that deliver strategic, culturally appropriate and high-impact messages supporting tobacco-free behavior choices through many venues and groups.

3. Cessation interventions that focus on promoting health systems change, expanding coverage of evidence-based tobacco dependence therapies, and supporting state quitline efforts.

4. Surveillance and evaluation of tobacco-related attitudes, behaviors, and health outcomes at regular intervals.

5. Infrastructure that is adequately funded to support comprehensive sustainable tobacco control programs with skilled staff and strong leadership to implement these programs.

Tobacco 21 is an initiative that aims to raise the tobacco purchase age to 21. Tobacco 21 has gained traction in states and localities over the last several years. The AAP Julius B. Richmond Center has information about Tobacco 21 (https://www.aap.org/en-us/advocacy-and-policy/aap-health-initiatives/Richmond-Center/Pages/Tobacco-21.aspx).

The ASPIRE Program of the MD Anderson Cancer Center helps middle and high school students learn about being tobacco free using a free, bilingual online program (https://www.mdanderson.org/about-md-anderson/community-services/aspire.html).

## ALTERNATIVE TOBACCO PRODUCTS

Although there has been a decrease in cigarette use over the past few decades, the use of alternative tobacco products, including other combustible tobacco products such as hookah (waterpipes), cigarillos, cigars, bidis, kreteks, and smokeless tobacco (snuff, dip, snus, and chewing tobacco) has increased significantly over recent years.[51] A listing and description of tobacco products is found in Chapter 28. The growing popularity of e-cigarettes poses health risks for youth users and nonusers.[2] E-cigarettes are hand-held devices that deliver an aerosolized solution typically containing nicotine, propylene glycol or glycerol, and flavorings. They were initially patented in the United States (without scientific evidence) as smoking cessation devices.[52] Between 2011 and 2014, there was an 890% increase in youth use with 13.4% of high school students reporting current use.[2] In 2014, more youth used e-cigarettes than any other tobacco product. Data suggest that youth and young adults who use e-cigarettes progress to conventional cigarette use.[53,54] Secondhand waterpipe and e-cigarette aerosol exposure have implications for smoke-free air laws and occupational safety.[55]

## THE PEDIATRICIAN'S ROLE IN ELIMINATING TOBACCO USE AND TOBACCO SMOKE EXPOSURE

Pediatricians and other pediatric clinicians play important roles in delivering messages about eliminating tobacco use and tobacco smoke exposure (Table 43-3).[38] One of the most important steps is screening all patients and families for tobacco use and exposure to SHS. A systematic screening procedure can be as simple as adding "tobacco use or exposure to secondhand smoke" to the vital signs collected at every visit. The information should be recorded in a standard place on the patient's chart. When developing or updating electronic health records (EHRs), pediatricians should make sure the EHR section on vital signs has the capability to reflect active smoking and/or SHS exposure. Making cessation materials and resources readily available, including the 1-800-QUIT-NOW telephone number, is another important step (see Table 43-3).

## Table 43-3. Office Interventions[a]

1. **Set an example.**
   As role models, pediatricians should not use tobacco. Clinical buildings and associated grounds should be tobacco free, have signs stating so, and have enforcement plans. Subscribe to magazines that do not carry tobacco advertisements or advertisements written by tobacco manufacturers.
2. **Systematically assess parents' tobacco use status and children's exposure to secondhand smoke.**
   Systematic strategies for identifying tobacco users, such as stickers on the medical chart or a vital sign form in the paper record or EHR that includes tobacco use status, should be implemented. The goal is to prompt any staff member who has contact with patients or parents who use tobacco to provide information about cessation and smoke-free homes. It is important to ask about the tobacco use status of parents and household members in the context of a child's health assessment. The issue of tobacco use by parents or household members should be entered into the problem list and addressed at each visit. Patients and parents should be educated about the adverse health effects of active smoking and of secondhand and thirdhand smoke exposure.
3. **Consider incorporating tobacco use and exposure into Safe Sleep or Social Determinants of Health screening tools.**
4. **Involve several staff members in providing information about smoking cessation.**
   Educating additional office staff (eg, a nurse or health educator) in tobacco use cessation counseling can extend the physician's efforts and provide effective support.
5. **Serve as an "agenda setter."**
   The pediatrician may serve as a catalyst for a parent to quit using tobacco. The pediatrician may initiate the process and then provide referrals to resources for cessation and maintenance of a tobacco-free lifestyle.
6. **Provide patient education materials.**
   Materials can be obtained free or at low cost from many organizations (see Resources) and on the Internet.
7. **Use local resources. Local resources are available in most areas.**
   Physician referrals should include a specific agency or program, telephone number, and description of what to expect. Self-help materials are available from many agencies. The makers of tobacco use cessation pharmacotherapies offer self-help programs as adjuncts to their products.

[a] Adapted from Fiore et al[38]

## Frequently Asked Questions

Q *If I smoke, can I breastfeed?*

A Breastfeeding is best for infants, whether or not you use tobacco. However, nicotine and other toxicants are transferred to the infant through a mother's milk. Thus, for the same reasons that pregnant women should not use tobacco, breastfeeding mothers should not use tobacco. Another reason is that infants of women who smoke are weaned at an earlier age. If you do continue to use tobacco, never breastfeed while smoking because a high concentration of smoke will be near your infant. In addition, smoking or vaping any tobacco product, including vaping e-cigarettes, should be banned inside the home or vehicle.

Q   *When visitors come to my home, they ask if they can smoke in another room. What should I tell them?*

A   Children's homes and vehicles should be completely smoke-free. Even if smokers smoke in a separate room, smoke-filled air is spread throughout the home, exposing everyone in the house to secondhand smoke. Visitors to your home should honor your request not to smoke during their visit. If they cannot do this, insist that they smoke outside, away from open doors and windows. Keep in mind that thirdhand smoke remains on their hair, clothing, and skin even after the cigarette is extinguished and is another source of exposure to toxicants.

Q   *I can't stop smoking right now. How can I reduce my child's exposure to secondhand smoke?*

A   Because your child will be exposed to secondhand and thirdhand smoke if you smoke in any part of your home or vehicle, be sure that you only smoke outside the house, and never smoke in your car or any vehicle in which a child rides. Choose a smoke-free child care setting, and avoid taking your child to places where smoking is permitted, such as bars or restaurants (even if there is a separate smoking area), airport smoking lounges, etc.

Q   *Is there good evidence that exposure to secondhand smoke is linked to the development of asthma in young children?*

A   Yes, there is sufficient evidence showing a strong association between exposure to secondhand smoke and the development of asthma or wheezing in young children.

Q   *We live in my parent's home. They smoke in their bedroom. How can I ask them to smoke outside of their own home?*

A   There are a couple of things you can do. If you feel comfortable (and safe) telling them about how harmful secondhand and thirdhand smoke is to your child, you can say that the pediatrician asked if they would make their home smoke-free. Or, if you prefer, your pediatrician can write a note to them asking them to make their home smoke-free. Making their home smoke-free may have the added benefits of reducing the number of cigarettes they smoke and encouraging them to take the next step toward quitting.

Q   *I've tried to quit using the gum and the patch before. They didn't work. Why should I try them now?*

A   Nicotine-containing gum and the patch can be used together. The patch controls your baseline urge to smoke. Adding a piece of gum in place of a cigarette is used to control any cravings for a cigarette, even if you already are using a patch. Make sure you are using the gum correctly by first chewing it, then "parking" it between the gums and cheek. Some people think that the gum should be chewed like regular gum–but then it will not work. Also, each time you make a quit attempt, you learn more about the quitting process and what works (or does not work) to help you quit. Most people make several attempts at quitting before they succeed. I recommend you call 1-800-QUIT-NOW and talk to a counselor who will help you plan your next quit attempt. The service is free, and it works.

Q   *I've heard that the medicine varenicline is very helpful. What do you know about it?*

A   Varenicline has been effective in helping many smokers quit, but there also are concerns about its safety in some users. It is a good idea to discuss the benefits and risks of using this medication with your doctor or nurse practitioner. Another good source for information is 1-800-QUIT-NOW.

Q   *We do not smoke but we live in a large apartment building and we smell smoke through the walls. Is this a problem, and if so, what can we do about it?*

A   This is a problem. Children in apartments, on average, have higher cotinine levels than do children in detached houses.[19] Potential causes for this result could be seepage through walls or shared ventilation systems. You should consider working for a smoking ban in your apartment building. Smoking bans in multi-unit housing may reduce children's exposure to tobacco smoke.[56] A ruling about smoke-free multi-unit public housing issued by the US Department of Housing and Urban Development took effect on February 3, 2017 with full compliance due by July 31, 2018. This ruling states that public housing agencies "must design and implement a policy prohibiting the use of prohibited tobacco products in all public housing living units and interior areas (including but not limited to hallways, rental and administrative offices, community centers, daycare centers, laundry centers, and similar structures), as well as at outdoor areas within 25 feet of public housing and administrative office buildings (collectively, referred to as "restricted areas") in which public housing is located."[57] Monitoring the implementation of this rule will be important.

Q   *I've heard that e-cigarettes are safer for teens to use compared with regular cigarettes. Is this true?*

A   This is not true. Scientific studies are showing that teens who previously never smoked are more likely to use regular cigarettes after they start using e-cigarettes. Teens' brains are still developing so they are prone to become addicted to the nicotine contained in e-cigarettes. They then often go on to use traditional cigarettes and become addicted to them. Using e-cigarettes is hazardous for teens and is not recommended.[58–60]

## Resources

### Agency for Healthcare Research and Quality (AHRQ)
Phone: 800-358-9295
Web site: www.ahrq.gov

### American Academy of Pediatrics (AAP), Julius B. Richmond Center of Excellence
Phone: 847-434-4264
Web site: www.aap.org/richmondcenter

### American Cancer Society (ACS)
Phone: 800-ACS-2345
Web site: www.cancer.org

### American Lung Association (ALA), Environmental Health
Phone: 800-LUNG-USA or 800-548-8252 or 202-785-3355
Web site: www.lungusa.org
Freedom From Smoking: www.ffsonline.org

### Asthma and Allergy Foundation of America
Phone: 800-7-ASTHMA or 800-727-8462 or 202-466-7643
Web site: www.aafa.org

### Centers for Disease Control and Prevention (CDC), Office on Smoking and Health
Phone: 800-CDC-INFO or 800-232-4636 or 770-488-5701
Web site: www.cdc.gov/tobacco

### Clinical Effort Against Secondhand Smoke Exposure (CEASE)
Web site: www.ceasetobacco.org

### National Cancer Institute
Phone: 800-4-CANCER or 800-422-6237
Web site: www.nci.nih.gov

### Nicotine Anonymous
Phone: 415-750-0328
Web site: www.nicotine-anonymous.org

### Smoke Free Homes
Phone: 202-476-4746
Web site: www.kidslivesmokefree.org

## United States Environmental Protection Agency (EPA), Indoor Air Quality Publications
Phone: 800-490-9198
Web site: www.epa.gov/iaq/pubs

## United States Environmental Protection Agency (EPA), Smoke-free Homes and Cars Program
Phone: 866-SMOKE-FREE or 866-766-5337
Web site: www.epa.gov/smokefree

## References

1. Schwab M, McDermott A, Spengler J. Using longitudinal data to understand children's activity patterns in an exposure context: data from the Kanawha County Health Study. *Environ Int.* 1992;18:173–189
2. Walley SC, Jenssen BP. Electronic nicotine delivery systems. *Pediatrics.* 2015;136(5):1018–1026
3. US Department of Health and Human Services. *Preventing Tobacco Use Among Youth and Young Adults: A Report of the Surgeon General.* Centers for Disease Control and Prevention, National Center for Chronic Disease Prevention and Health Promotion, Office on Smoking and Health, 2012
4. Wellman RJ, Sugarman DB, DiFranza JR, Winickoff JP. The extent to which tobacco marketing and tobacco use in films contribute to children's use of tobacco: a meta-analysis. *Arch Pediatr Adolesc Med.* 2006;160(12):1285–1296
5. FDA head calls smoking a "pediatric disease." *Columbia University Record.* March 24, 1995
6. US Department of Health and Human Services. *The Health Consequences of Involuntary Exposure to Tobacco Smoke: A Report of the Surgeon General.* Centers for Disease Control and Prevention, Coordinating Center for Health Promotion, National Center for Chronic Disease Prevention and Health Promotion, Office on Smoking and Health, 2006
7. Spengler JD, Dockery DW, Turner WA, Wolfson JM, Ferris BG Jr. Long-term measurements of respirable sulfates and particles inside and outside homes. *Atmosph Environ.* 1981;15(1):23–30
8. California Environmental Protection Agency. *Proposed Identification of Environmental Tobacco Smoke as a Toxic Air Contaminant.* Air Resources Board, Office of Environmental Health Hazard Assessment; 2005
9. Winickoff JP. Beliefs about the health effects of "thirdhand smoke." *Pediatrics* 2009;123:e74
10. Martins-Green M, Adhami N, Frankos M, et al. Cigarette smoke toxins deposited on surfaces: implications for human health. *PLoS ONE.* 2014;9(1):e86391
11. Matt GE, Quintana PJ, Destaillats H, et al. Thirdhand tobacco smoke: emerging evidence and arguments for a multidisciplinary research agenda. *Environ Health Perspect.* 2011;119(9):1218–1226
12. Centers for Disease Control and Prevention. Cigarette Smoking Among Adults–United States, 2005–2015. *MMWR Morb Mortal Wkly Rep.* 2016;65(44):1205–1211. https://www.cdc.gov/mmwr/volumes/65/wr/mm6544a2.htm?s_cid=mm6544a2_w. Accessed February 19, 2018.
13. Homa DM, Neff LJ, King BA, et al. Vital signs: disparities in nonsmokers' exposure to secondhand smoke—United States, 1999-2012. *MMWR Morb Mortal Wkly Rep.* 2015;64(4):103–108. https://www.cdc.gov/mmwr/preview/mmwrhtml/mm6404a7.htm?s_cid=mm6404a7_w. Accessed February 19, 2018
14. The GTSS Collaborative Group. A cross country comparison of exposure to secondhand smoke among youth. *Tob Control.* 2006;15(Suppl 2):ii4–ii19

15. Oberg M, Jaakkola MS, Woodward A, Peruga A, Pruss-Usten A. Worldwide burden of disease from exposure to second-hand smoke: a retrospective analysis of data from 192 countries. *Lancet.* 2011;377(9760):139–146

16. Matt GE, Quintana PJ, Hovell MF, et al. Households contaminated by environmental tobacco smoke: sources of infant exposures. *Tob Control.* 2004;13(1):29–37

17. Sleiman M, Logue JM, Luo W, Pankow JF, Gundel LA, Destaillats H. Inhalable constituents of thirdhand tobacco smoke: chemical characterization and health impact considerations. *Environ Sci Technol.* 2014;48(22):13093–13101

18. Farber HJ, Walley SC, Groner JA, Nelson KE. Clinical practice policy to protect children from tobacco, nicotine, and tobacco smoke. *Pediatrics.* 2015;136(5):1008–1017

19. Wilson KM, Klein JD, Blumkin AK, Gottlieb M, Winickoff JP. Tobacco-smoke exposure in children who live in multiunit housing. *Pediatrics.* 2011;127(1):85–92

20. Hecht SS, Ye M, Carmella SG, et al. Metabolites of a tobacco-specific lung carcinogen in the urine of elementary school-aged children. *Cancer Epidemiol Biomarkers Prev.* 2001;10(11):1109–1116

21. Farber HJ, Groner J, Walley S, Nelson K. Protecting children from tobacco, nicotine, and tobacco smoke. *Pediatrics.* 2015;136(5):e1439–e1467

22. US Department of Health and Human Services. *How Tobacco Smoke Causes Disease: The Biology and Behavioral Basis for Smoking-Attributable Disease: A Report of the Surgeon General.* Centers for Disease Control and Prevention, National Center for Chronic Disease Prevention and Health Promotion, Office on Smoking and Health, 2010

23. Kandel ER, Kandel DB. Shattuck lecture. A molecular basis for nicotine as a gateway drug. *N Engl J Med.* 2014;371(10):932–943

24. The Health Consequences of Smoking—50 Years of Progress: A Report of the Surgeon General. National Center for Chronic Disease Prevention and Health Promotion (US) Office on Smoking and Health. Atlanta (GA): Centers for Disease Control and Prevention, 2014

25. Chuang SC, Gallo V, Michaud D, et al. Exposure to environmental tobacco smoke in childhood and incidence of cancer in adulthood in never smokers in the European Prospective Investigation into Cancer and Nutrition. *Cancer Causes Control.* 2011;22(3):487–494

26. Palmer CN, Doney AS, Lee SP, et al. Glutathione S-transferase M1 and P1 genotype, passive smoking, and peak expiratory flow in asthma. *Pediatrics.* 2006;118(2):710–716

27. Wang C, Salam MT, Islam T, Wenten M, Gauderman WJ, Gilliland FD. Effects of in utero and childhood tobacco smoke exposure and β2-adrenergic receptor genotype on childhood asthma and wheezing. *Pediatrics.* 2008;122(1):e107–e114

28. Aligne CA, Moss ME, Auinger P, Weitzman M. Association of pediatric dental caries with passive smoking. *JAMA.* 2003;289(10):1258–1264

29. Drongowski RA, Lee D, Reynolds PI, et al. Increased respiratory symptoms following surgery in children exposed to environmental tobacco smoke. *Paediatr Anaesth.* 2003;13(4):304–310

30. Mannino DM, Moorman JE, Kingsley B, Rose D, Repace J. Health effects related to environmental tobacco smoke exposure in children in the United States: data from the Third National Health and Nutrition Examination Survey. *Arch Pediatr Adolesc Med.* 2001;155(1):36–41

31. Yolton K, Dietrich K, Auinger P, Lanphear BP, Hornung R. Exposure to environmental tobacco smoke and cognitive abilities among U.S. children and adolescents. *Environ Health Perspect.* 2005;113(1):98–103

32. Leistikow BN, Martin DC, Milano CE. Fire injuries, disasters, and costs from cigarettes and cigarette lights: a global overview. *Prev Med.* 2000;31(2 Pt 1):91–99

33. Leistikow BN, Martin DC, Jacobs J, Rocke DM, Noderer K. Smoking as a risk factor for accident death: a meta-analysis of cohort studies. *Accid Anal Prev.* 2000;32(3):397–405

34. Møller SE, Ajslev TA, Andersen CS, Dalgård C, Sørensen TI. Risk of childhood overweight after exposure to tobacco smoking in prenatal and early postnatal life. *PLoS One.* 2014;9(10):e109184

35. Groner JA, Hoshaw-Woodard S, Koren G, Klein J, Castile R. Screening for children's exposure to environmental tobacco smoke in a pediatric primary care setting. *Arch Pediatr Adolesc Med.* 2005;159(5):450–455

36. Devoe JE, Baez A, Angier H, Krois L, Edlund C, Carney PA. Insurance + access not equal to health care: typology of barriers to health care access for low-income families. *Ann Fam Med.* 2007;5(6):511–518

37. Weissman JS, Zaslavsky AM, Wolf RE, Ayanian JZ. State Medicaid coverage and access to care for low-income adults. *J Health Care Poor Underserved.* 2008;19(1):307–319

38. Fiore M, Jaen C, Baker T, et al. *Treating Tobacco Use and Dependence: 2008 Update. Clinical Practice Guideline.* Rockville, MD: US Department of Health and Human Services, Public Health Service; 2008

39. McBride CM, Emmons KM, Lipkus IM. Understanding the potential of teachable moments: the case of smoking cessation. *Health Educ Res.* 2003;18(2):156–170

40. Winickoff JP, Buckley VJ, Palfrey JS, Perrin JM, Rigotti NA. Intervention with parental smokers in an outpatient pediatric clinic using counseling and nicotine replacement. *Pediatrics.* 2003;112(5):1127–1133

41. Winickoff JP, Hillis VJ, Palfrey JS, Perrin JM, Rigotti NA. A smoking cessation intervention for parents of children who are hospitalized for respiratory illness: the stop tobacco outreach program. *Pediatrics.* 2003;111(1):140–145

42. Rosen LJ, Noach MB, Winickoff JP, Hovell MF. Parental smoking cessation to protect young children: a systematic review and meta-analysis. *Pediatrics.* 2012;129(1):141–152

43. Winickoff JP. Implementation of a parental tobacco control intervention in pediatric practice. *Pediatrics.* 2013;132(1):109–117

44. American College of Chest Physicians' Tobacco Dependence Treatment Toolkit. http://tobaccodependence.chestnet.org. Accessed February 19, 2018

45. MD Anderson Cancer Center QuitMedKit apps. https://www.mdanderson.org/education-training/professional-education/tobacco-outreach-program.html. Accessed February 19, 2018

46. American Academy of Pediatrics. Julius B. Richmond Center Web site. http://www2.aap.org/richmondcenter/CodingPayment.html. Accessed February 19, 2018

47. National Association of Attorneys General. Master Settlement Agreement. *Settlement Documents.* http://www.naag.org/settlement_docs.php. Accessed February 19, 2018

48. Sims TH, American Academy of Pediatrics Committee on Substance Abuse. Technical report—tobacco as a substance of abuse. *Pediatrics.* 2009;124:e1045–e1053

49. Ending the Tobacco Problem: A Blueprint for the Nation. https://iom.nationalacademies.org/Reports/2007/Ending-the-Tobacco-Problem-A-Blueprint-for-the-Nation.aspx. Accessed February 19, 2018

50. Centers for Disease Control and Prevention. Best Practices for Comprehensive Tobacco Control Programs — 2014. Atlanta: US Department of Health and Human Services, National Center for Chronic Disease Prevention and Health Promotion, Office on Smoking and Health, 2014

51. Centers for Disease Control and Prevention. Consumption of cigarettes and combustible tobacco—United States, 2000–2011. *MMWR Morb Mortal Wkly Rep.* 2012;61(3):565–569

52. Grana R, Benowitz N, Glantz SA. E-cigarettes: a scientific review. *Circulation.* 2014;129(19):1972–1986

53. Arrazola RA, Singh T, Corey CG, et al. Tobacco use among middle and high school students—United States, 2011-2014. *MMWR Morb Mortal Wkly Rep.* 2015;64(14):381–385

54. Primack BA, Soneji S, Stoolmiller M, Fine MJ, Sargent JD. Progression to traditional cigarette smoking after electronic cigarette use among US adolescents and young adults. *JAMA Pediatr.* 2015;169(11):1018–1023

55. Kumar SR, Davies S, Weitzman M, Sherman S. A review of air quality, biological indicators and health effects of second-hand waterpipe smoke exposure. *Tob Control.* 2015;24(Suppl 1): i54–i59

56. Kline RL. Smoke knows no boundaries: legal strategies for environmental tobacco smoke incursions into the home within multi-unit residential dwellings. *Tob Control.* 2000;9(2):201–205

57. US Department of Housing and Urban Development. Smoke-Free Public Housing and Multifamily Properties. https://www.hud.gov/program_offices/healthy_homes/smokefree. Accessed February 19, 2018

58. Dutra LM, Glantz SA. Electronic cigarettes and conventional cigarette use among U.S. adolescents: a cross-sectional study. *JAMA Pediatr.* 2014;168(7):610–617

59. US Department of Health and Human Services. E-Cigarette Use Among Youth and Young Adults: A Report of the Surgeon General. Atlanta, GA: US Department of Health and Human Services, Centers for Disease Control and Prevention, National Center for Chronic Disease Prevention and Health Promotion, Office on Smoking and Health; 2016

60. McCabe SE, West BT, McCabe VV. Associations between early onset of E-cigarette use and cigarette smoking and other substance use among US adolescents: a national study. *Nicotine Tob Res.* 2018;20(8):923–930

Chapter 44

# Ultraviolet Radiation

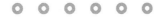

## KEY POINTS

- Overexposure to ultraviolet radiation from the sun and from artificial sources, such as tanning beds, raises skin cancer risk.
- Skin cancer is the most common cancer in the United States.
- Although cancer is not common in young people, melanoma (the skin cancer most likely to result in fatality) is one of the most common cancers in teens and young adults.
- The 2014 "Surgeon General's Call to Action to Prevent Skin Cancer" aims to raise awareness about skin cancer and calls for actions to reduce risk.
- Pediatricians can play key roles in counseling about skin cancer prevention. Skin cancer prevention steps include avoiding deliberate suntanning and artificial tanning, wearing clothing and hats, timing activities, and using sunscreen.

## INTRODUCTION

The sun sustains life on earth: it is needed for photosynthesis, provides warmth, drives biological rhythms, and promotes feelings of well-being. Sunlight is needed for vitamin D production in skin. Despite beneficial effects, overexposure to the ultraviolet (UV) component of the sunlight spectrum, and to other sources of ultraviolet radiation (UVR), can result in adverse effects on human health.

The sun emits electromagnetic radiation ranging from short-wavelength high-energy x-rays to long-wavelength lower energy radio waves. Ultraviolet radiation (UVR, "above violet") waves range from 200 to 400 nanometers (nm). UVR waves are longer than x-rays and shorter than visible light (400 to 700 nm) and infrared radiation (greater than 700 nm, "below red" or "heat"). UVR is divided into UVA (320 to 400 nm, further subdivided into UVA2 [320 to 340] and UVA1 [340 to 400]), also called black (invisible) light; UVB (290 to 320 nm); and UVC (less than 290 nm). UVC rays possess the highest energy but are completely absorbed by stratospheric ozone; no UVC reaches the earth's surface. Thus, UVB, UVA, visible light, and infrared waves have the greatest biological significance.

Solar radiation that reaches the earth's surface comprises about 95% UVA and 5% UVB.[1] Most UVB is absorbed by stratospheric ozone, and about one half of UVA is absorbed.[2] The ozone layer functions as a "natural sunscreen," protecting the earth and its inhabitants from UVR. In the 1970s, scientists discovered that chlorofluorocarbons (CFCs), chemicals commonly used as refrigerants and propellants, were drifting into the upper atmosphere, resulting in thinning of the ozone layer. Information about this enlarging "ozone hole" eventually led to the Montreal Protocol, a multinational treaty designed to protect the ozone layer in the upper atmosphere.[3,4]

UVB is more intense during the summer than during the winter, at midday compared with early morning or late afternoon, in places closer to the equator than in temperate zones, and at high altitudes compared with sea level. Sand, snow, concrete, and water can reflect up to 85% of sunlight, resulting in greater exposure.[5] Water is not a good photoprotectant because UVR can penetrate to a depth of 60 cm, resulting in significant exposure. In contrast to the variability of UVB, UVA is relatively constant throughout the day and the year.

UVR can be produced by manmade lamps (eg, sunlamps used in tanning beds) and tools (eg, welding tools), but the sun is the primary source of UVR for most people. UVR has been used for decades to treat skin diseases, especially psoriasis.[1]

## ROUTE OF EXPOSURE

Individuals are exposed to UVR through direct contact to the skin and eyes while they are outdoors in the sunlight or when they are exposed to artificial sources of UVR emitted by sunlamps and sunbeds.

## SYSTEMS AFFECTED

The skin, eyes, and immune system are affected.

## CLINICAL EFFECTS

### Effects on Skin

The skin is the organ most exposed to environmental UVR. The epidermis (the top layer of skin) is composed of basal cells, squamous cells (together called keratinocytes), and melanocytes (cells that produce melanin). The topmost layer is the stratum corneum ("horny layer"), composed of dead, keratin-filled cells that have migrated upward from the basal layer.

#### *Erythema and Sunburn*

Erythema and sunburn are acute reactions to excessive amounts of UVR. Exposure to UVR causes vasodilation and an increase in the volume of blood in the dermis, resulting in erythema. The minimal erythema (or erythemal) dose depends on factors such as skin type and thickness, the amount of melanin in the epidermis and the capacity of the epidermis to produce melanin after sun exposure, and the intensity of the radiation. The Fitzpatrick classification of 6 sun-reactive skin types takes into account an individual's expected sunburn and tanning tendency (Table 44-1).[6]

The ability of UVR to produce erythema depends on the radiation wavelength expressed as the erythema "action spectrum." For erythema and sunburn, the action spectrum is mainly in the UVB range.[7]

#### *Tanning*

Tanning is a protective response to sun exposure.[8] Immediate tanning (or immediate pigment darkening) is the result of oxidation of existing melanin after exposure to visible light and UVA. Immediate pigment darkening

### Table 44-1. Fitzpatrick Classification of Sun-reactive Skin Types

| SKIN TYPE | HISTORY OF SUNBURNING OR TANNING |
|---|---|
| I | Always burns easily, never tans |
| II | Always burns easily, tans minimally |
| III | Burns moderately, tans gradually and uniformly (light brown) |
| IV | Burns minimally, always tans well (moderate brown) |
| V | Rarely burns, tans profusely (dark brown) |
| VI | Never burns, deeply pigmented (black) |

becomes visible within several minutes and usually fades within 1 to 2 hours. Delayed tanning occurs when new melanin is formed as a result of UVB exposure. Delayed tanning becomes apparent 2 to 3 days after exposure, peaks at 7 to 10 days, and may persist for weeks or months. The tanning response means that DNA damage has occurred in the skin.[9]

### Phototoxicity and Photoallergy

Chemical photosensitivity refers to an adverse cutaneous reaction that occurs when certain chemicals or drugs are applied topically or taken systemically at the same time that a person is exposed to UVR or visible radiation. Phototoxicity is a form of chemical photosensitivity that can occur in any individual and essentially is an exaggerated sunburn response that occurs hours after exposure to the offending agent and UVR.[10] Most phototoxic agents are activated in the UVA range (320 to 400 nm). Agents associated with phototoxic reactions include those used by adolescents, such as nonsteroidal anti-inflammatory drugs (NSAIDs), tetracyclines, antipsychotic drugs, psoralens, anti-arrhythmic medications, diuretics, and St John's Wort.[10] Photoallergy is a delayed hypersensitivity response that occurs in reactive individuals after sensitization, an incubation period (7 to 10 days), and then reexposure to the agent plus UVR.[10] Photoallergy develops in a small percentage of people exposed to these agents. Sunscreen agents, antibacterial products, and fragrances are responsible for most photoallergic reactions.[10]

People who take medications or use topical agents that are sensitizing should avoid all sun exposure, if possible, and completely avoid all UVA from artificial sources. The consequences of exposure can be uncomfortable, serious, or life threatening.

Phytophotodermatitis is a skin eruption resulting from the interaction of sunlight and photosensitizing compounds. The most common phototoxic compounds are the furocoumarins (psoralens) contained in a wide variety of plants, such as limes, lemons, and celery.

Up to 80% of patients with systemic lupus erythematosus have photosensitivity. The threshold UV dose triggering cutaneous or systemic reactions is much lower than that for sunburn. Many patients are not aware of the association of flares with UVR exposure because the latency period between exposure and skin eruptions can range from several days to 3 weeks.[11]

### Skin Aging (Photoaging)

Chronic unprotected exposure to UVR weakens the skin's elasticity, resulting in sagging, deeper facial wrinkles, and skin discoloration later in life. Photo-aged skin is characterized by alterations of cellular components and of the extracellular matrix.

## Wound Healing

UVB exposure interferes with wound healing.[12]

## Nonmelanoma Skin Cancer

Nonmelanoma skin cancer includes basal cell carcinoma and squamous cell carcinoma. In the US adult population, nonmelanoma skin cancer is by far the most common cancer, with approximately 5.4 million cases occurring in 3.3 million Americans every year.[13] Most are basal cell carcinomas. The number of nonmelanoma skin cancers in the United States is not precisely known because physicians are not required to report these to cancer registries. Nonmelanoma skin cancer is rarely fatal unless left untreated; nevertheless, the American Cancer Society estimated that 2,000 people die of nonmelanoma skin cancer each year, mostly from squamous cell carcinoma.[13] The Nevoid Basal Cell Carcinoma Syndrome (Gorlin syndrome) is a rare genetic condition. People with this syndrome have a high risk for the development of many basal cell carcinomas and may have abnormalities of the jaw, eyes, and nervous tissue. For children with this syndrome, the development of basal cell carcinoma begins early in life.[14]

In general, nonmelanoma skin cancer occurs in maximally sun-exposed areas of fair-skinned people and is uncommon in people with increased natural pigmentation. Nonmelanoma skin cancer is more common in people older than 50 years, with the incidence in this age group rapidly increasing.[15] The incidence of nonmelanoma skin cancer also is increasing in young adults, especially in young women.[16] Sun exposure is the main environmental cause of nonmelanoma skin cancer. Cumulative exposure over long periods, resulting in photodamage, is considered important in the pathogenesis of squamous cell carcinoma. In general, there is an inverse relationship between skin cancer incidence and skin pigmentation of people in various countries in the world. Superficial epidermal melanin decreases the transmission of UVR. This may protect keratinocytes and melanocytes from sunlight-induced changes that lead to their malignant transformation.[8] Nonmelanoma skin cancer is extremely rare in children in the absence of predisposing conditions.

## Melanoma

Melanoma is primarily a disease of the skin. Primary extracutaneous sites include the eye, mucous membranes, gastrointestinal tract, genitourinary tract, leptomeninges, and lymph nodes. Ninety-five percent of melanomas occur in the skin.[17]

Although much less common than nonmelanoma skin cancer, cutaneous melanoma (hereafter referred to as "melanoma") is a serious public health issue. In the United States, melanoma is the fifth most common cause of new cancers in men and the sixth most common cause of new cancers in women.[18] The incidence of melanoma continues to rise in the United States[19] and melanoma is one of the most common cancers in teens and young adults.[18] Melanoma accounts for about 1% of skin cancer cases but causes most skin cancer deaths. The American Cancer Society estimated that 91,270 melanomas would be diagnosed in 2018; approximately 9,320 people were estimated to die of the disease.[20] Melanoma has an excellent prognosis if detected in its early stages. Survival is strongly associated with stage at diagnosis; individuals diagnosed at a later stage have poorer survival rates.[21] Thus, efforts have been directed toward prevention and early detection.

The reason for the increase in the incidence of melanoma is complex and incompletely understood but likely is related to changing patterns of dress favoring more skin exposure, a decrease in the earth's protective stratospheric ozone layer, more opportunities for leisure activities, and increased exposure to artificial sources of UVR through indoor tanning at salons and other venues.

**Evidence That Solar UVR Causes Skin Cancer**

In 1992, the International Agency for Research on Cancer (IARC, a part of the World Health Organization) reviewed the evidence for the carcinogenicity of solar radiation. The IARC concluded that "There is sufficient evidence in humans for the carcinogenicity of solar radiation. Solar radiation causes cutaneous malignant melanoma and non-melanocytic skin cancer."[1] Both UVB and UVA cause DNA damage that can result in skin cancer. UVB produces cyclobutane pyrimidine dimers that cause mutations (UVB "fingerprint" mutations) that may lead to skin cancer; UVA also triggers DNA damage via the production of cyclobutane pyrimidine dimers. DNA damage by UVA occurs mainly through generation of reactive oxygen species resulting in the formation of oxidative products, which are mutagenic. In addition, one of the most important defense mechanisms protecting skin against UV radiation involves the p53 tumor suppressor gene. Normally, sunlight exposure leads to upregulation of the p53 tumor suppressor gene, resulting in increased repair of DNA, cell cycle arrest, and apoptosis of damaged keratinocytes. However, p53 is also susceptible to mutagenesis, making cancerous cells resistant to apoptosis.[22]

**Risk Factors for the Development of Melanoma**

- **Age**

  Increasing age is a risk factor; most melanomas occur in people older than age 50. The average age at diagnosis is 63 years.[20] Melanoma incidence also is increasing in men and women aged 15 to 39 years but more so in young women.[23]

  Although rare, melanoma occurs in children. Ferrari et al[24] reviewed a 25-year experience with 33 Italian children who were aged 14 years or younger at presentation. The children's lesions were not typical of melanoma lesions in adults. Melanoma lesions in adults generally follow the "ABCDEs": they are **A**symmetric; with irregular **B**orders; variegated **C**olor; **D**iameter larger than 6 mm, the size of a pencil eraser; and changing or **E**volving. In the Ferrari series, many lesions were amelanotic (pink, pink-white, or red), tended to be raised, and had regular borders.[24] The key to diagnosis was recognizing that the melanoma lesions were unlike any other lesions on the child.[24] In another retrospective study of 70 patients younger than age 20 (19 patients age 10 years and younger; 51 patients aged 11 to 19 years), 60% of the younger group and 40% of the older group also did not present with conventional ABCDE criteria.[25] The authors proposed that alternative "ABCD" criteria (**A**melanotic; **B**leeding, **B**ump; **C**olor uniformity; **D**e novo, any **D**iameter) be used in conjunction with conventional ABCDE criteria to facilitate earlier recognition and treatment of melanoma in children.[25]

- **Gender**
Melanoma is more likely to occur in males. Among individuals younger than age 50, however, melanoma is more common among females.[26]

- **Skin type**
Melanoma is most common in non-Hispanic whites. People at highest risk have light skin and eyes and sunburn easily. Overall, the lifetime risk for the development of melanoma is approximately 1 in 38 for white people, 1 in 172 for Hispanic people, and 1 in 1,000 for black people.[20]

- **Nevi**
Nevi (moles) are benign pigmented tumors. Acute sun exposure is implicated in the development of nevi in children. The number of nevi increases with age,[27] nevi occur with more frequency on sun-exposed areas, and the number of nevi on exposed areas increases with the total cumulative sun exposure during childhood and adolescence.[28] Children with light skin who tend to burn rather than tan have more nevi at all ages, and children who have more severe sunburns have more nevi. Although the chance of any one nevus becoming cancerous is very low, any person with many irregular or large nevi is at increased risk for the development of melanoma. Congenital melanocytic nevi (CMN) are pigment cell malformations formed during gestation and visible at or shortly after birth. Small nevi are usually inconsequential, but large nevi increase the risk of melanoma (and may have a devastating psychologic effect). The risk of malignant transformation varies; larger CMN carry a significantly higher risk of malignant transformation. However, melanoma will not develop in most people with CMN.[29]

- **Family history**
A greater risk of melanoma exists for anyone with 1 or more first-degree relatives (parent, brother, sister, child) who has had melanoma. Approximately

10% of people with melanoma have a positive family history. The increased risk may be the result of a family's tendency toward fair skin, their patterns of sun exposure, mutations that occur in a family, or a combination of factors.[26] Certain families with germline mutations in CDKN2A and other genes are at increased risk for the development of dysplastic nevi and melanoma.[30]

- **Xeroderma pigmentosum**

  Xeroderma pigmentosum is a rare, inherited condition that affects skin cells' ability to repair UV radiation-induced damage to DNA. People with xeroderma pigmentosum have an extremely high risk for the development of melanoma and other skin cancers beginning in childhood, especially on sun-exposed areas.

- **Immune suppression**

  People who have had organ transplants, and are thus taking immune suppressive agents, have a higher risk for the development of all forms of skin cancer. Individuals with AIDS and other illnesses that suppress the immune response also are at higher risk.

- **Exposure to UV radiation from the sun**

  Most skin cancers are caused by exposure to UV radiation from the sun and artificial tanning devices.[31,32] The pattern of sun exposure is important in the etiology of basal cell carcinoma, squamous cell carcinoma, and melanoma. Personal sun exposure is usually characterized by (1) total sun exposure over time; (2) occupational exposure (signifying a more chronic exposure); and (3) nonoccupational or recreational exposure (signifying intermittent exposure).[33] Squamous cell carcinoma is significantly associated with estimated total sun exposure and with occupational exposure. Chronic exposure to UVB is now considered as the main environmental cause of squamous cell carcinoma. Squamous cell carcinoma appears to be most straightforwardly related to the total sun exposure: these tumors occur on skin areas that are most regularly exposed ( face, neck, and hands), and the risk rises with the lifelong accumulated dose of UVR.[34] Basal cell carcinoma and melanoma are significantly associated with intermittent sun exposure (ie, sunburning), but squamous cell carcinoma does not show this relationship. Melanoma is more strongly associated with intermittent sun exposure than is basal cell carcinoma.[32] Although some research shows that sunburns, especially in childhood and adolescence, raise the risk of melanoma, other studies show that sunburns at any age are harmful.[35,36]

- **Exposure to artificial sources of UVR**

  Exposure to sunbeds and sunlamps also is associated with increased risk for the development of basal cell carcinoma, squamous cell carcinoma, and melanoma.

## Effects on the Eye

In adults, more than 99% of UVR is absorbed by the anterior structure of the eye, although some of it reaches the retina.[37] Acute exposure to UVR can result in photokeratitis.[38] Gazing directly into the sun (as can occur during an eclipse) can cause focal burns to the retina (solar retinopathy).[39] Sunlight exposure is a risk factor for cataract development in adults.[40] Melanoma of the uveal tract, the most common primary intraocular malignant neoplasm in adults, is associated with light skin color, blond hair, and blue eyes.

## Effects on the Immune System

UVR exposure is thought to have 2 effects: skin cancer induction and immune suppression, which is increasingly recognized as important in the development of skin cancer.[41] Experiments in mice chronically exposed to UVR show that tumors induced by UVR are highly antigenic and are recognized and rejected by animals with normal immune systems. The tumors grow progressively, however, when transplanted into mice whose immune systems are compromised.[41] UVR exposure induces "systemic" immune suppression so that exposure on one body site suppresses the immune response when the antigen is introduced at a distant site that was not irradiated.[41] In humans, chronic exposure to UVR results in decreased function of all immune cells in the skin, including lymphocytes, mast cells, macrophages, and dendritic cells. Immune suppressive changes include increased production of the anti-inflammatory cytokine interleukin-10 (IL-10) and an increase in CD25+ regulatory T cells ($T_{reg}$).[42]

Skin cancers are common in people exposed to immunosuppressive agents. In people with renal transplants, lifelong immunosuppressive treatment needed for adequate graft function leads to a reduction of immunosurveillance and an increased risk of various cancers, including nonmelanoma skin cancer. People who have had renal transplants also have an increased incidence of melanoma and other skin cancers.[43] Because ongoing immunosurveillance is lacking, skin cancers in people who have received organ transplants are likely to behave aggressively with higher rates of local recurrence and a greater tendency to be invasive and metastatic.[44]

## Artificial Sources of UVR

Sunlamps and sunbeds are the main sources of artificial UVR used for deliberate purposes. The tanning industry has been very popular, especially with teen girls and young women. By 2009, more than one third (37%) of non-Hispanic white high school girls reported tanning indoors in the past 12 months; about half (49%) of all non-Hispanic white females who tanned indoors reported frequent use (10 times or more in the same period).[45] Prevalence has begun to decline but artificial tanning in salons is a still common among teenage girls and young women.[46]

Tanning beds primarily emit UVA radiation, although a small amount (less than 5%) is in the UVB range.[47] In terms of biological activity, the intensity of UVA radiation produced by large, powerful tanning units may be 10 to 15 times higher than that of the midday sun. Frequent indoor tanners may receive an annual UVA dose that is 1.2 to 4.7 times more than that received from sun exposure, in addition to doses received from the sun.[48] The intensity of tanning bed exposure is a phenomenon not found in nature.

Even though UVB is much more potent than UVA in causing sunburn, high fluxes of UVA can cause erythema in individuals sensitive to sunlight. In people who tan easily, exposure to tanning appliances will lead first to immediate pigment darkening. A more permanent tan will occur with accumulated exposure, depending on individual tanning ability and the amount of UVB present in the light spectrum of the tanning lamps. Immediate pigment darkening has no photoprotective effect against UVR-induced erythema or sunburn.

Artificial UVR exposure has been repeatedly shown to induce erythema and sunburn. Erythema or burning effects were reported by 18% to 55% of users of indoor tanning equipment in Europe and North America.[47] Almost 2,000 indoor tanning-related injuries were treated in emergency departments in 2012; most of these injuries were skin burns.[49] More than 15,000 tanning bed burns, including burns to the eyes or eyelids, were reported on Twitter in 2013.[50] Other frequently reported effects of artificial tanning include skin dryness, pruritus, nausea, photodrug reactions, disease exacerbation (eg, systemic lupus erythematosus), and disease induction (eg, polymorphous light eruption).

Long-term health effects include skin aging, effects on the eyes (eg, cataract formation), and carcinogenesis. A case-control study demonstrated a significant association between using any tanning device and the incidence of squamous cell carcinoma and basal cell carcinoma.[51] In 2006, the IARC published an updated analysis of studies of the carcinogenicity of artificial UVR with regard to melanoma, squamous cell carcinoma, and basal cell carcinoma.[47] Based on those data, in 2009, the IARC elevated UVR from tanning beds to a group 1 carcinogen, meaning "carcinogenic to humans." The group 1 designation places tanning beds in the same category as plutonium, tobacco, and asbestos.[52] More recent evidence shows that tanning bed use occurring earlier in life and with greater frequency increases melanoma risk. Indoor tanning prevalence, although decreasing, remains common among adolescent girls and young women. In a 2015 national US survey, 7.3% of high school students reported tanning device use (excluding getting a spray-on tan) at least once over the past year. Use was greater among females (10.6%) than males (4.0%) and increased with age. Even though indoor tanning decreased significantly among all high school students (15.6% to 7.3%) from 2009 to 2015, more than 15% of non-Hispanic white high school girls reported this practice in 2015.[46]

Because of mounting evidence about the carcinogenicity of artificial UVR, support for regulations to limit teenagers' access to tanning facilities has been widespread.[47] As of October 2017, at least 44 states regulated minors' use of tanning facilities. Indoor tanning laws include age limits and parental consent requirements. Seventeen states and the District of Columbia ban the use by minors younger than age 18. Eleven other states introduced legislation to ban minors from using tanning beds in 2017.[53] State laws may be effective in reducing teen tanning rates, especially if laws mandate age restrictions.[54] Tanning legislation, however, is often not enforced.[55,56]

In May 2014, the Food and Drug Administration (FDA) issued an order (or "Black Box Warning") requiring that sunlamp products used in tanning salons carry a visible boxed warning stating: "Attention: This sunlamp product should not be used on persons under the age of 18 years". The Black Box warning, usually applied to drugs, means that "There is an adverse reaction so serious in proportion to the potential benefit that it is essential that it be considered in assessing the risks and benefits of using the drug."[57] Despite advocacy efforts by skin cancer prevention experts, federal regulation that would ban minors younger than age 18 from tanning in salons has not been passed (as of August 2018). There is evidence that indoor tanning may be addictive in certain individuals.[58]

## TREATMENT

Pediatricians will rarely encounter patients with nonmelanoma skin cancer or melanoma. Patients at high risk, including children with xeroderma pigmentosum and related disorders, and those with a large number of nevi and a family history of melanoma, should be followed in collaboration with a dermatologist. Sunburns should be treated with cool compresses and analgesics. Instruction about preventing future sunburns should be given at the time of the burn.

## PREVENTION OF EXPOSURE

In 2014, "The Surgeon General's Call to Action to Prevent Skin Cancer" report called on partners in prevention from different sectors—including the health care sector—to address skin cancer as a major public health issue. The report emphasized that skin cancer, the most common cancer in the United States, is mainly preventable. It listed 5 strategic prevention goals: "increase opportunities for sun protection in outdoor settings; provide individuals with the information they need to make informed, healthy choices about UV radiation exposure; promote policies that advance the national goal of preventing skin cancer; reduce harms from indoor tanning; and strengthen research, surveillance, monitoring, and evaluation related to skin cancer prevention."[59] Pediatricians can help to accomplish some of these goals by providing information to patients and families. Pediatricians' counseling on skin cancer prevention has improved over the last decade but more counseling efforts still are needed.[60]

Prevention advice begins in infancy and continues when developmental stages result in new patterns of sun exposure (eg, when the child begins to walk, before starting school, before entering adolescence). In March 2018, the United States Preventive Services Task Force (USPSTF), an organization of experts who evaluate and make recommendations regarding the effectiveness of clinical preventive health services, updated its recommendations on skin cancer prevention counseling based on evidence showing the effectiveness of counseling starting at very young ages. The new recommendation calls for clinicians to counsel "young adults, adolescents, children, and parents of young children about minimizing exposure to UV radiation for persons aged 6 months to 24 years with fair skin types to reduce their risk of skin cancer."[61] The previous USPSTF recommendation applied only to fair skinned individuals aged 10 to 24 years. The new recommendation has clear relevance to pediatricians. This recommendation received the USPSTF "B" rating, meaning "that there is high certainty that the net benefit is moderate or there is moderate certainty that the net benefit is moderate to substantial."[62]

All parents and children should receive advice about protection from UVR. Not all children sunburn easily, but people of all skin types can experience skin cancer, skin aging, and sun-related damage to the immune system. Children who should receive special attention include those with xeroderma pigmentosum (who must avoid all UVR) and those with excessive numbers of nevi and/or freckles, or with first-degree family members with melanoma. Preteens and teenagers need special reinforcement because they often are susceptible to societal notions of beauty and health. Teen counseling should include a recommendation not to patronize tanning salons (or other venues that have tanning beds) for any reason, including the desire for a "prevacation" or "preprom" tan. Performing a careful skin examination as part of a complete physical examination seems prudent and affords an opportunity to provide counseling especially if there is a burn, tan, freckling, or nevi.

The American Cancer Society,[63] the Centers for Disease Control and Prevention (CDC),[64] Healthy People 2020,[65] and the National Council on Skin Cancer Prevention[66] recommend UVR-protective behaviors that include:

1. Do not burn. Avoid sun tanning and tanning beds.
2. Wear protective clothing and hats.
3. Seek shade.
4. Use extra caution near water, snow, and sand.
5. Apply sunscreen.
6. Wear sunglasses.

## Avoiding Exposure

Sunburning still is common. Among young adults, 50% reported at least 1 sunburn in the past 12 months,[67] and children and adolescents also continue to experience high rates of sunburning.[68] Advice about avoiding sunburning may be given during routine visits and at other times, such as when the child or teen is noted to have a tan or presents with a sunburn.

Infants younger than 6 months should be kept out of direct sunlight. They should be dressed in cool, comfortable clothing and wear hats with brims. Whenever feasible, children's activities may be planned to limit peak-intensity midday sun (10 AM to 4 PM). Advice should be framed in the context of promoting outdoor play, other physical activity, and visiting parks, zoos, and other natural environments.

## Clothing and Hats

Clothing has been used for sun protection for thousands of years. Clothing offers the simplest and often most practical means of sun protection. Protective factors include style, weave, and chemical enhancement. Clothes that cover more of the body provide more protection; sun-protective styles cover to the neck, elbows or wrists, and knees. A tighter weave lets in less sunlight than a looser weave. Darker and heavier clothing generally offers more protection. Treating fabrics with certain dyes or chemical additives can help to increase UVR protectiveness.[69]

Standards for quantifying the sun protection offered by clothing were first developed in Australia and New Zealand in 1996. Two standard-setting organizations (ASTM International [formerly known as the American Society for Testing and Materials] and the American Association of Textile Chemists and Colorists) were involved in setting the US standard.[70] The ultraviolet protection factor (UPF) measures a fabric's ability to block UVR from passing through the fabric and reaching the skin. The UPF is classified from 15 to 50+; 15 to 24 is rated as "Good," 25 to 39 is rated "Very Good," and 40 to 50+ is rated "Excellent" UV protection. The UPF of fabrics can be altered by shrinking, stretching, and wetness. Shrinking increases the UPF; stretching decreases the UPF. If cotton fabrics get wet, the UPF decreases. The UPF rating is available for only a small proportion of clothing in the marketplace.

Hats provide variable protection for the head and neck, depending on the brim width, material, and weave. A wide-brimmed hat (3 inches) provides an SPF of 7 for the nose, 3 for the cheek, 5 for the neck, and 2 for the chin. Medium-brimmed hats (1 to 3 inches) provide an SPF of 3 for nose, 2 for the cheek and neck, and none for the chin. A narrow-brimmed hat provides an SPF of 1.5 for the nose but little protection for the chin and neck.[5]

## Shade

Seeking shade is somewhat useful, but people can still sunburn because light is scattered and reflected. A fair-skinned person sitting under a tree can burn in less than an hour. Shade provides relief from heat, possibly providing a false sense of security about UVR protection. Clouds decrease UVR intensity but not to the same extent that they decrease heat intensity, which also may result in overexposure.[5]

## Window Glass

Americans spend most of their time indoors; thus, UVR transmission through window glass can be an important source of exposure. Standard clear window glass absorbs wavelengths below 320 nm (UVB). UVA, visible light, and infrared radiation are transmitted through standard clear window glass.[71] Tests of UVA protection provided by front windshields in 29 automobiles from different manufacturers showed consistently high UVA protection; side window UVA protection was lower and highly variable. Researchers suggested that results could partially explain the reported increased rates of cataracts in left eyes and left-sided facial skin cancers[72] (in nations where the driver side is the left).

## Sunscreen

Sunscreen is the most commonly used sun protection method. Sunscreens reduce the intensity of UVR affecting the epidermis, thus preventing erythema and sunburn. Formulating, testing, and labeling of sunscreen products are regulated as over-the-counter drugs by the FDA. FDA-approved sunscreen agents ("filters") comprise organic or inorganic chemicals, each of which is effective at certain wavelengths. Fifteen organic filters are approved in the United States. Organic filters absorb UV energy and dissipate the energy as heat. The inorganic ("physical") filters, zinc oxide and titanium dioxide, primarily absorb but also reflect and scatter UV photons. Historically, zinc oxide and titanium dioxide gave skin a white appearance and were thus not widely accepted as sunscreens. Since the early 1990s, inorganic agents have been micronized and nanosized, thus making them more cosmetically acceptable. Combinations of chemicals are needed to provide broad-spectrum protection and increase photostability.[73]

The sun protection factor (SPF) is a grading system developed to quantify the degree of protection from erythema provided by using a sunscreen. SPF pertains only to UVB; the higher the SPF, the greater the protection. For example, a person who would normally experience a sunburn in 10 minutes can be protected up to about 150 minutes (10 × 15) with an SPF-15 sunscreen. Sunscreens with an SPF of 15 or more theoretically filter more than 93% of the UVB responsible for erythema; sunscreens with an SPF of 30 filter out approximately 97% of the UVB. In actual use, the SPF often is substantially lower than expected because the amount used is less than half the recommended amount.[74] For most users, proper application and reapplication are more important factors than using a product with a higher SPF. The Skin Cancer Foundation[75] recommends using sunscreen with an SPF of at least 15; the American Academy of Dermatology[74] advises using a sunscreen with an SPF of at least 30.

The FDA approved 17 sunscreen chemicals for use in the United States. Several more are available in the European Union. Four chemicals effective in the UVA range are approved for use in the United States. In May 1999, the FDA published its final rule for over-the-counter sunscreen products that protect against UVB. Regulations concerning UVA were delayed until reliable testing methods could be developed. In June 2011, the FDA issued new rules regarding labeling of sunscreen products. Previous rules dealt almost exclusively with protection against UVB only. The 2011 FDA rule established a standard broad-spectrum test procedure to measure UVA radiation protection in relation to UVB radiation protection. Sunscreen products that pass the broad-spectrum test are allowed to be labeled as "broad spectrum," indicating protection against UVB and UVA. For "broad-spectrum" sunscreens, the SPF also indicates the overall amount of protection provided. For broad-spectrum sunscreens with SPF values of 15 or higher, the FDA allows manufacturers to claim that these formulations help protect against not only sunburn but also skin cancer and early skin aging when used as directed with other sun-protection measures. These sun-protection measures include limiting time in the sun and wearing protective clothing. For sunscreen products labeled with SPF values but not as "broad spectrum," the FDA states that the SPF value indicates the amount of protection against sunburn only. The rule also states that manufacturers cannot label sunscreens as "waterproof" or "sweatproof" or identify their products as "sunblock" because these claims overstate effectiveness. Sunscreens cannot claim to provide sun protection for more than 2 hours without reapplication or to provide protection immediately after application (eg, "instant protection") without submitting data to support these claims and obtaining FDA approval. Water resistance claims on the front label must indicate whether the product remains effective for 40 minutes or 80 minutes while swimming or sweating, based on standard testing. Sunscreens that are not water resistant must include a direction instructing consumers to use a water-resistant sunscreen if swimming or sweating. All sunscreens must include standard "Drug Facts" information on the back and/or side of the container.[76] Another FDA rule proposed in 2011 would limit the maximum SPF value on sunscreen labels to "50+" because the FDA states that data are not sufficient to show that products with SPF values higher than 50 provide greater protection for users than products with SPF values of 50.[77] This rule has not been finalized.

Regular use of a broad-spectrum sunscreen preparation has been shown to prevent solar (actinic) keratoses, lesions that may evolve to become squamous cell carcinoma.[78,79] One randomized clinical trial showed that regular sunscreen use compared with no regular sunscreen use decreased the incidence of squamous cell carcinoma.[80] Results of a randomized trial of regular sunscreen use for a 5-year period showed a 50% reduction in the incidence of new primary melanomas for up to 10 years after trial cessation. The statistical significance of this finding was borderline, however, because of the development of melanoma in only a small number of individuals.[81] Sunscreen use—especially sunscreen with good UVA protection—has been demonstrated to protect individuals from UV-induced immunosuppression.[82] The American Cancer Society, the American Academy of Dermatology, the Skin Cancer Foundation, and many other organizations recommend sunscreen use as part of an overall program of reducing UVR exposure.

Sunscreens may be systemically absorbed. In 1 study, sunscreen products were studied in vitro to assess the extent of absorption following application to excised human skin. Half of the products were marketed specifically for children. Of the 5 chemical sunscreen ingredients present in the products, only oxybenzone (benzophenone-3 or BP-3) penetrated the skin.[83] In another report, CDC researchers examined more than 2,500 urine samples collected during 2003 to 2004 for oxybenzone. The samples selected were representative of the US population aged 6 years and older as part of the National Health and Nutrition Examination Survey (NHANES), an ongoing survey that assesses the health and nutritional status of the US civilian population. The analysis found oxybenzone in 97% of the samples,[84] suggesting widespread exposure of the population. Females and non-Hispanic white people had the highest concentrations regardless of age. Higher benzophenone-3 levels were also found in non-Hispanic whites and females in the CDC's NHANES 2005-2010.[85] NHANES data are not available for children younger than age 6 years. Sunscreen ingredients have been found in human milk.[86]

Studies have shown alterations in liver, kidney, and reproductive organs in rats given oral or transepidermal doses of oxybenzone.[87] A study of 6 commonly used UVB and UVA sunscreens was conducted to determine estrogenicity in vivo and in vitro. Five of the 6 sunscreen ingredients (BP-3, homosalate, 4-methyl-benzylidene camphor [4-MBC], octyl methoxycinnamate [OMC], and octyl-dimethly-PABA) increased cell proliferation in breast cancer cells, and the sixth ingredient, butyl-methoxydibenzoylmethane (avobenzone), was inactive. In the in vivo analysis, rats fed large doses of the sunscreen ingredients OMC, 4-MBC, and BP-3 showed dose-dependent increases in uterine weight. Epidermal application of one of the products (4-MBC) also increased uterine weight.[88] Researchers investigating human prenatal exposures to phthalate and phenol metabolites and their relationship to birth weight found that higher maternal concentrations of BP-3 were associated with a decrease in birth weight in girls but a greater birth weight in boys.[89]

Sunscreen products containing zinc and titanium oxides are increasingly manufactured using nanotechnology—the design and manipulation of materials on atomic and molecular scales. Nanoscale particles are measured in nanometers (nm), or billionths of a meter. Using nanoscale particles renders products containing zinc and titanium oxides nearly transparent, increasing cosmetic acceptability. Concerns have been raised, however, about the dearth of safety information available about nanoscale ingredients, including to skin that is damaged by sunburn. No data are available about the effects of these products on infants and children. Advocacy groups have called on the FDA to require more testing and increased regulatory oversight.

Sunscreens should be used when a child might sunburn. Burning has no benefits, and it should be avoided. Using sunscreen is recommended to decrease the known risks of sun exposure and sunburning, both of which increase the risk for the development of skin cancer.

Recommendations vary about using sunscreen on infants younger than age 6 months. Increased absorption of sunscreen by immature skin is a potential concern. No scientific consensus exists, however, about when in development the characteristics of newborn and infant skin become similar to those of adult skin. Some researchers conclude that the skin continues to develop throughout the first year of life.[90] Other researchers state that infant skin is in a developmental stage structurally and functionally up to age 3 months.[91] Others conclude that skin barrier function of a full-term infant is similar to an adult's skin barrier function at birth or within 2 to 4 weeks; in contrast, the skin of a premature infant has a poor epidermal barrier with few cornified layers, leading to a higher risk of increased permeability to exogenous materials.[92] Even when skin becomes functionally mature and resembles adult skin during later infancy, young children have a higher surface area relative to body weight compared with adults. Therefore, greater relative percutaneous absorption of any topically applied agent is likely.

Toxicity in infants and children from absorption of sunscreen ingredients has not been reported. On the basis of available evidence, it is reasonable to tell parents what is known about the safety of sunscreens in infants aged younger than 6 months and to emphasize the importance of avoiding high-risk exposure to UVR. In situations in which the infant's skin is not protected adequately by clothing, it may be reasonable to apply sunscreen to small areas, such as the face and the backs of the hands, as long as the infant will not ingest the sunscreen from the hands and feet.

Preparations that contain a combination of sunscreen with the insecticide N-N-diethyl-m-toluamide (DEET) should not be used because they may result in overexposure to DEET (see Chapter 37).

## The Ultraviolet (UV) Index

The UV index was developed in 1994 by the National Weather Service in consultation with the US Environmental Protection Agency (EPA) and the CDC. The UV index predicts the intensity of UV light for the following day on the basis of the sun's position, cloud movements, altitude, ozone data, and other factors. It is conservatively calculated on the basis of effects on skin types that burn easily. Higher numbers predict more intense UV light during midday of the following day: 0 to 2 = minimal; 3 to 4 = low; 5 to 6 = moderate; 7 to 9 = high; and 10+ = very high, with greater recommended avoidance behaviors as the UV index increases (eg, avoiding outdoor exposures from 10 AM to 4 PM if the UV index is 7 or higher). The index is available online for thousands of cities at www.weather.com. It is printed in the weather section of many daily newspapers and reported through weather reports of local radio, television, and weather stations.

## Sunglasses

Sunglasses protect against sun glare and harmful radiation. The first sunglass standard was published in Australia in 1971; standards were subsequently adopted in Europe and the United States. In the United States, nonprescription sunglasses are regulated as medical devices by the Center for Devices and Radiological Health of the FDA. Standards for nonprescription sunglasses are set by the American National Standards Institute.[93] This standard is voluntary and is not followed by all manufacturers.[94]

Major US visual health organizations recommend that sunglasses absorb 99% to 100%[38,94] of the full UV spectrum (up to 400 nm). Expensive sunglasses do not necessarily provide better UVR protection. Purchasing sunglasses that meet standards for a safe level of UVR should be the goal. Wearing a hat with a brim can greatly reduce the UVR exposure to the eyes and surrounding skin. It is recommended that people wear sunglasses outdoors when working, driving, participating in sports, taking a walk, or running errands.[38] Sunglasses for infants and children are available.

## Avoiding Indoor Tanning

Teens should be discouraged from engaging in indoor tanning. Reducing the harms of indoor tanning is 1 of 5 goals outlined in the 2014 US Surgeon General's report. A mother's attitudes and own tanning practices may influence whether or not her child tans; discussions with a mother may reduce her tanning behavior and lead to reduced tanning initiation and frequency of her child's tanning.[95] It is prudent to discuss avoiding indoor tanning with preteens and their mothers, and with teens themselves. Overexposure to UVR from sunlight and exposure to UVR from artificial sources increase the risk of skin cancer, photoaging, and other adverse effects and should be avoided.

## VITAMIN D

Sun exposure and vitamin D concentrations are intricately intertwined. Humans get vitamin D from exposure to sun, from dietary sources (such as fortified milk and oily fish), and from vitamin supplements. Vitamin D synthesis in skin depends on skin type. An individual who burns easily after a first moderate UVR exposure will rapidly achieve maximal vitamin D synthesis. In contrast, dark-skinned individuals will have relatively limited vitamin D synthesis because UVR will be absorbed by melanin rather than other cellular targets.[96] Because excess previtamin $D_3$ or vitamin $D_3$ is destroyed by sunlight, exposure to sunlight does not cause vitamin D intoxication.[97] The action spectrum that induces cutaneous vitamin $D_3$ synthesis is in the UVB range.[98]

Vitamin D is essential for normal growth and skeletal development. The actions of vitamin D that extend beyond bone mineral metabolism are increasingly becoming understood.[99] Many children, adolescents, and adults have insufficient or deficient levels of vitamin D.[99] Vitamin D is available through foods, supplements, and incidental sun exposure. Because current intake levels of vitamin D by children and adolescents may not prevent vitamin D deficiency, the AAP recommends that breastfed infants (as well as infants who consume less than 1,000 mL of infant formula per day) should receive daily supplementation with 400 International Units (IU) of vitamin D. The recommended daily allowance for vitamin D allowance for children aged older than 1 year, including adolescents, is 600 IU per day.[100] Additional vitamin D supplementation and laboratory evaluations of vitamin D status may be needed for some children in some areas.

## CHALLENGES

Pediatricians alone cannot change social concepts in which a suntan is equated with health and beauty. School programs and public education campaigns must continue to address this issue.

Several challenges to successful skin cancer prevention efforts have been identified.[101] Sun protection messages that talk about avoiding or limiting time during peak sun hours may conflict with messages that promote physical activity. This potential conflict may be resolved by following the example of Australia, the country with the world's highest incidence of melanoma, to "Slip, Slop, Slap"—slip on a shirt, slop on some sunscreen, and slap on a hat. This message is consistent with conducting outdoor physical activity in a sun-protective manner. Next, controversy exists about how much sun exposure is needed for vitamin D synthesis, possibly resulting in excessive exposure to the sun and deliberate exposure to artificial UVR. Third, it has been reported that skin cancer risk behaviors cluster with other risky behaviors, such as smoking and risky drinking. A greater understanding of these behaviors may help with interventions in high-risk groups. It is possible that intentional outdoor tanning will increase as the prevalence of indoor tanning decreases among teens and young adults.[102] Pediatricians increasingly face time constraints that can limit counseling time. These challenges suggest that it is uncertain whether primary prevention efforts to reduce skin cancer through UVR protection will be successful.

## Frequently Asked Questions

Q   *Why is a baby at special risk from sunburn?*

A   Babies cannot tell you if they are too hot or beginning to burn and cannot get out of the sun without an adult's help. Even dark-skinned babies may be sunburned. Babies also need an adult to keep them away from direct sunlight, dress them properly, and apply sunscreen.

Q   *What can I do to protect my child?*

A   Babies younger than age 6 months should be kept out of direct sunlight to reduce their exposure to damaging UV rays. They should be moved under a tree, umbrella, or stroller canopy, although on reflective surfaces, an umbrella or canopy may reduce UVR exposure by only 50%.

To avoid sunburn, infants and children may be dressed in cool, comfortable clothing, such as shirts and pants made of cotton, and should wear hats. Swimwear and other garments made of materials with high UPF ratings are available online and in brick and mortar stores. Sunscreen should be applied to the parts of the skin that will be exposed to the sun. Parents should apply sunscreen liberally and rub it in well before going outdoors, covering all exposed areas, especially the child's face, nose, ears, feet, and hands, and the backs of the knees. Sunscreen should be used even on cloudy days because the sun's rays can penetrate through clouds. When choosing a sunscreen, parents should look for the words "broad spectrum" on the label, meaning that the sunscreen will screen out most of the UVB and UVA rays. An SPF of 15 should be adequate in most cases. It is important to reapply after sweating or swimming. It is also important to remember that using sunscreen is only one part of a total program of sun protection. Sunscreens should be used to prevent burning and not as a reason to stay in the sun longer. Sunscreen may be applied to infants who are younger than age 6 months to small areas of skin uncovered by clothing and hats.

Q   *I left my bottle of sunscreen in the car for a day. Is it still ok to use?*

A   Temperature extremes (such as can occur in a hot car) may make sunscreen ingredients degrade so they are no longer effective. Avoid keeping your sunscreen in a hot car and try to keep the sunscreen bottle covered or in the shade when you are outside.[73]

Q   *I bought sunscreen with an SPF of 30. Does that mean that it is twice as effective as a sunscreen with an SPF of 15?*

A   Although some people believe that a sunscreen with an SPF of 30 offers twice as much protection as one with an SPF of 15, this is not the case. When properly applied, SPF 15 sunscreen blocks about 93% of burning rays and SPF 30 blocks about 97%. More important than SPF is making sure that the sunscreen is labeled as "broad spectrum," that you use enough (about 1 ounce for an adult or teen per sitting), and reapply every 2 hours and also reapply after swimming or sweating. A sunscreen with an SPF of 15 or 30 should be adequate for most people. Also wear protective clothing and hats whenever possible, and use properly labelled sunglasses to protect your eyes.

Q   *Can I use a sunscreen spray on my child?*

A   Many sunscreen spray products (like certain other spray products) contain flammable ingredients, such as alcohol. If you choose to use a spray product, make sure to keep yourself and your child away from any open flame because burns have been reported in people using sunscreen sprays. To avoid inhaling any sunscreen, it is best to spray the product on your hands first, then apply it to your child.

Q   *What factors in clothing can offer protection against sunburn?*

A   Some fabrics have a UPF rating showing how much sun protection they offer. Even if a fabric does not have a UPF rating, it may offer excellent sun protection. Some fabrics, such as polyester crepe, bleached cotton, and viscose, are quite transparent to UVR and should be avoided in the sun. Other fibers, such as unbleached cotton, can absorb UVR. High-luster polyesters and even thin, satiny silk can be highly protective because they reflect radiation. A fabric's weave also is important; in general, the tighter the weave or knit, the higher the protection offered. To assess protection, parents can hold the material up to a window or lamp and see how much light gets through. Darker clothes also generally offer more protection. Virtually all garments lose about a third of their sun-protective ability when wet.

Q  *I am concerned that using sunscreen on my child when she goes outside will
lead to a low vitamin D level. Is this true?*

A  Vitamin D helps the body to absorb calcium and so is needed for bone
health in infants, children, teens, and adults. The other actions of vitamin
D are being studied by researchers. Although vitamin D is generated when
the skin is exposed to direct sunlight, exposing the skin to the sun's ultraviolet rays raises the risk for the development of skin cancer. Fortunately,
vitamin D is available from certain foods (such as dairy products, salmon,
and sardines) and vitamin supplements. Infants and children should, therefore, be protected from sun exposure with clothing, hats, and sunscreen.
To ensure that infants and young children are protected from rickets (a
bone disease that occurs when vitamin D levels are very low), the American
Academy of Pediatrics recommends that all breastfed infants (as well as
infants consuming less than 1,000 mL of infant formula per day) receive
daily supplementation with 400 IU of vitamin D.[100] The American Academy
of Pediatrics recommends that children older than age 1 and teenagers
receive 600 IU of vitamin D per day.[100] Deliberate sun exposure or using
tanning salons as a way to increase vitamin D levels, or for other reasons,
raises skin cancer risk and should be avoided.

Q  *I have heard that some sunscreen ingredients are absorbed into the body and
are not safe. What should I do?*

A  Scientific research shows that some sunscreen chemicals are absorbed by
people. Studies in laboratory animals show that some chemical sunscreen
ingredients have hormone-like effects. Concern has been raised that
the vitamin A derivatives retinol and retinyl palmitate, added to many
sunscreens, may raise cancer risk. The physical sunscreens titanium
dioxide and zinc oxide are increasingly manufactured through nanotechnology, a method that uses tiny particles. It is possible that these particles
may be absorbed into the body; there are no research studies in children
about this technology.

These concerns must be weighed against the known risks of sun exposure
and sunburning. Keeping these pros and cons in mind, it is reasonable
to use sunscreen with the goals of preventing sunburning and possibly
decreasing the risk of certain skin cancers. Sunscreen use should be part of
a total program of limiting sun exposure. It may be prudent to avoid using
products containing oxybenzone, a chemical with known hormone-like
effects, especially on children.[99,103]

Q  *Are tanning salons safe?*

A  People who use sunlamps or go to tanning salons are exposed primarily to
UVA. The tan that occurs represents a protective response to the harmful
ultraviolet rays. Skin damage occurs whether a tan comes from the sun

itself or from artificial light from a tanning salon. Tanning in a tanning salon (or other venues such as gyms) raises the risk for the development of skin cancer. Tanning salons are not safe and should not be used by teenagers or others. The American Academy of Pediatrics, the World Health Organization, the American Academy of Dermatology, and the American Medical Association have urged states to pass legislation that prohibits minors younger than age 18 years from accessing tanning salons.[99,103]

Q   *Is using a spray tan safe?*

A   "Spray tans," also known as "sunless" or "self-tanning" products, are sometimes used by people to substitute for going outside or visiting a tanning salon. Sunless tanners use dihydroxyacetone (DHA), a chemical that reacts with amino acids in the stratum corneum (the top layer of skin) to form brown-black compounds, melanoidins, which deposit in the skin. DHA is a mutagen that induces DNA strand breaks in certain strains of bacteria; it has not been shown to be carcinogenic in animal studies.[104] DHA is the only color additive approved by the US FDA for use as a tanning agent. DHA-containing tanning preparations may be applied to the consumer's bare skin by misters at sunless tanning booths. Bronzers are water-soluble dyes that temporarily stain the skin. Bronzers are easily removed with soap and water.

DHA-induced tans become apparent within 1 hour; maximal darkening occurs within 8 to 24 hours. Most users report that color disappears over 5 to 7 days. Because neither DHA nor melanoidins afford any significant UVR protection, consumers must be advised that sunburn and sun damage may occur unless they use sunscreen and other sun protection methods. Consumers must also be warned that any sunless products containing added sunscreen provide UVR protection during a few hours after application and that additional sun protection must be used during the duration of the artificial tan. Potential spray tan users may also be advised that it is probably healthier to "love the skin you're in" rather than seeking a darker look.

Q   *How do I choose sunglasses for my child?*

A   There are no government regulations on the amount of UVR that sunglasses must block. Sunglasses are regulated as medical devices by the FDA and may be labeled as UV protective if they meet certain standards. Parents should look for a label that states that the lenses block at least 99% of UVA and 99% of UVB rays.

Protection is provided by a chemical coating applied to the lenses. Lens color has nothing to do with UV protection. Ski goggles and contact lenses with UV protection also are recommended.

It is never too early for a child, even an infant, to wear sunglasses. Larger lenses, well-fitted and close to the surface of the eye, provide the best protection.

Q   *I am concerned about the environment and have read that some sunscreen ingredients are washed off from the skin into ocean water and may contribute to bleaching of coral reefs. Is this true?*

A   Some researchers contend that certain sunscreen ingredients, such as oxybenzone, contribute significantly to coral reef bleaching and are therefore hazardous to coral reefs.[105] Other reports suggest that climate change is the main hazard to coral reefs.[106] More research is needed in this area. We strongly recommend that you continue to take steps needed to prevent sunburning and other overexposure to the sun.

## Resources

**American Academy of Pediatrics**
Web site: www.aap.org
The AAP provides a patient education brochure titled "Fun in the Sun."

**American Cancer Society**
Web site: https://www.cancer.org/cancer/skin-cancer.html

**Centers for Disease Control and Prevention**
Web site: https://www.cdc.gov/cancer/skin/index.htm

**National Council on Skin Cancer Prevention**
Web site: www.skincancerprevention.org
The National Council comprises organizations (including the AAP) whose staffs have experience, expertise, and knowledge in skin cancer prevention and education.

**Skin Cancer Foundation**
Web site: www.skincancer.org
The foundation is dedicated to nationwide public and professional education programs aimed at increasing public awareness, sun protection and sun safety, skin self-examination, children's education, melanoma understanding, and continuing medical education.

**US Environmental Protection Agency**
Web site: https://www.epa.gov/sunsafety

**World Health Organization (WHO)**
What are simple action steps for sun protection?
Web site: www.who.int/features/qa/40/en/

# References

1. International Agency for Research on Cancer. *IARC Monographs on the Evaluation of Carcinogenic Risks to Humans. Volume 55. Solar and Ultraviolet Radiation. Summary of Data Reported and Evaluation.* Lyon, France: World Health Organization; 1997. http://monographs.iarc.fr/ENG/Monographs/vol55/mono55.pdf. Accessed June 4, 2018

2. National Aeronautics and Space Administration. Ozone Hole Watch. http://ozonewatch.gsfc.nasa.gov/facts/SH.html. Accessed June 4, 2018

3. Gillis J. The Montreal Protocol, a Little Treaty That Could. New York Times, December 9, 2013. http://www.nytimes.com/2013/12/10/science/the-montreal-protocol-a-little-treaty-that-could.html?_r=0. Accessed June 4, 2018

4. United Nations Environment Programme Ozone Secretariat. The Montreal Protocol on Substances that Deplete the Ozone Layer. http://ozone.unep.org/en/treaties-and-decisions/montreal-protocol-substances-deplete-ozone-layer. Accessed June 4, 2018

5. Gilchrest BA. Actinic injury. *Annu Rev Med.* 1990;41:199–210

6. Fitzpatrick TB. The validity and practicality of sun-reactive skin types I through VI. *Arch Dermatol.* 1988;124(6):869–871

7. Diffey BL. Ultraviolet radiation and human health. *Clin Dermatol.* 1998;16(1):83–89

8. Gilchrest BA, Eller MS, Geller AC, Yaar M. The pathogenesis of melanoma induced by ultraviolet radiation. *N Engl J Med.* 1999;340(17):1341–1348

9. Fisher DE, James WD. Indoor tanning—science, behavior, and policy. *N Engl J Med.* 2010;363(10):901–903

10. Kane KS, Nambudiri VE, Stratigos AJ. Drug-induced photosensitivity. In: *Color Atlas & Synopsis of Pediatric Dermatology.* 3rd ed, 2016. http://accesspediatrics.mhmedical.com.elibrary.einstein.yu.edu/content.aspx?bookid=1870&sectionid=136754879. Accessed June 4, 2018

11. Obermoser G, Zelger B. Triple need for photoprotection in lupus erythematosus. *Lupus.* 2008;17(6):525–527

12. Liu H, Yue J, Lei Q, et al. Ultraviolet B inhibits skin wound healing by affecting focal adhesion dynamics. *Photochem Photobiol.* 2015;91(4):909–916

13. American Cancer Society. Key Statistics for Basal and Squamous Cell Skin Cancers. http://www.cancer.org/cancer/skincancer-basalandsquamouscell/detailedguide/skin-cancer-basal-and-squamous-cell-key-statistics. Accessed June 4, 2018

14. American Cancer Society. Basal and Squamous Cell Skin Cancer Causes, Risk Factors, and Prevention. https://www.cancer.org/content/dam/CRC/PDF/Public/8819.00.pdf. Accessed June 4, 2018

15. Rogers HW, Weinstock MA, Feldman SR, Coldiron BM. Incidence estimate of nonmelanoma skin cancer (keratinocyte carcinomas) in the US population, 2012. *JAMA Dermatol.* 2015;151(10):1081–1086

16. Christenson LJ, Borrowman TA, Vachon CM, et al. Incidence of basal cell and squamous cell carcinomas in a population younger than 40 years. *JAMA.* 2005;294(6):681–690

17. Markovic SN, Erickson LA, Rao RD, et al. Malignant melanoma in the 21st century, part 1: epidemiology, risk factors, screening, prevention, and diagnosis. *Mayo Clin Proc.* 2007;82(3):364–380

18. Siegel RL, Miller KD, Jemal A. Cancer statistics, 2017. *CA Cancer J Clin.* 2017;67(1):7–30. http://onlinelibrary.wiley.com/doi/10.3322/caac.21387/epdf. Accessed June 4, 2018

19. Weir HK, Marrett LD, Cokkinides V, et al. Melanoma in adolescents and young adults (ages 15-39 years): United States, 1999-2006. *J Am Acad Dermatol.* 2011;65(5 Suppl 1):S38–S49

20. American Cancer Society. Key Statistics for Melanoma Skin Cancer. https://www.cancer.org/cancer/melanoma-skin-cancer/about/key-statistics.html. Accessed June 4, 2018

21. Balch CM, Gershenwald JE, Soong SJ, et al. Final version of 2009 AJCC melanoma staging and classification. *J Clin Oncol.* 2009;27(36):6199–6206

22. Woo DK, Eide MJ. Tanning beds, skin cancer, and vitamin D: an examination of the scientific evidence and public health implications. *Dermatol Ther.* 2010;23(1):61–71

23. Purdue MP, Beane Freeman LE, Anderson WF, Tucker MA. Recent trends in incidence of cutaneous melanoma among US Caucasian young adults. *J Invest Dermatol.* 2008;128(12):2906–2908

24. Ferrari A, Bono A, Baldi M, et al. Does melanoma behave differently in younger children than in adults? A retrospective study of 33 cases of childhood melanoma from a single institution. *Pediatrics.* 2005;115(3):649–654

25. Cordoro KM, Gupta D, Frieden IJ, McCalmont T, Kashani-Sabet M. Pediatric melanoma: results of a large cohort study and proposal for modified ABCD detection criteria for children. *J Am Acad Dermatol.* 2013;68(6):913–925

26. American Cancer Society. Risk Factors for Melanoma Skin Cancer. https://www.cancer.org/cancer/melanoma-skin-cancer/causes-risks-prevention/risk-factors.html. Accessed June 4, 2018

27. Gallagher RP, McLean DI, Yang CP, et al. Suntan, sunburn, and pigmentation factors and the frequency of acquired melanocytic nevi in children. Similarities to melanoma: the Vancouver Mole Study. *Arch Dermatol.* 1990;126(6):770–776

28. Holman CD, Armstrong BK. Pigmentary traits, ethnic origin, benign nevi, and family history as risk factors for cutaneous malignant melanoma. *J Natl Cancer Inst.* 1984;72(2):257–266

29. Alikhan A, Ibrahimi OA, Eisen DB. Congenital melanocytic nevi: Where are we now? Part I. Clinical presentation, epidemiology, pathogenesis, histology, malignant transformation, and neurocutaneous melanosis. *J Am Acad Dermatol.* 2012;67(4):495.e1–17

30. Tsao H, Rodgers L, Patel D. Inherited susceptibility to melanoma. UpToDate. http://www.uptodate.com/contents/inherited-susceptibility-to-melanoma?source=search_result&search=familial=melanoma&selectedTitle=1%7E11. Accessed June 4, 2018

31. Armstrong BK, Kricker A. How much melanoma is caused by sun exposure? *Melanoma Res.* 1993;3(6):395–401

32. Lucas RM, McMichael AJ, Armstrong BK, Smith WT. Estimating the global disease burden due to ultraviolet radiation exposure. *Int J Epidemiol.* 2008;37(3):654–667

33. Armstrong BK, Kricker A. The epidemiology of UV induced skin cancer. *J Photochem Photobiol B.* 2001;63(1-3):8–18

34. de Gruijl FR, van Kranen HJ, Mullenders LH. UV-induced DNA damage, repair, mutations and oncogenic pathways in skin cancer. *J Photochem Photobiol B.* 2001;63(1-3):19–27

35. Dennis LK, Vanbeek MJ, Beane Freeman LE, Smith BJ, Dawson DV, Coughlin JA. Sunburns and risk of cutaneous melanoma: does age matter? A comprehensive meta-analysis. *Ann Epidemiol.* 2008;18(8):614–627

36. Wu S, Han J, Laden F, Qureshi AA. Long-term ultraviolet flux, other potential risk factors, and skin cancer risk: a cohort study. *Cancer Epidemiol Biomarkers Prev.* 2014;23(6):1080–1089

37. American Optometric Association. Statement on Ocular Ultraviolet Radiation Hazards in Sunlight. St Louis, MO: American Optometric Association; 1993. https://www.aoa.org/Documents/optometrists/ocular-ultraviolet.pdf. Accessed June 4, 2018

38. American Optometric Association. UV Protection. Protecting Your Eyes from Solar Radiation. https://www.aoa.org/patients-and-public/caring-for-your-vision/uv-protection. Accessed June 4, 2018

39. Wong SC, Eke T, Ziakas NG. Eclipse burns: a prospective study of solar retinopathy following the 1999 solar eclipse. *Lancet.* 2001;357(9251):199–200

40. Jacobs DS. Cataract in adults. UpToDate. Last updated August 30, 2017. http://www.uptodate. com/contents/cataract-in-adults?source=preview&search=cataracts&language=en-US&an chor=H2&selectedTitle=1,150#H2. Accessed June 4, 2018

41. Ullrich SE. Sunlight and skin cancer: lessons from the immune system. *Mol Carcinog.* 2007;46(8):629–633

42. Bonilla FA. Secondary immunodeficiency due to underlying disease states, environmental exposures, and miscellaneous causes. UpToDate. https://www.uptodate.com/contents/ secondary-immunodeficiency-due-to-underlying-disease-states-environmental-exposures- and-miscellaneous-causes?source=search_result&search=sun%20exposure%20immune%20 suppression&selectedTitle=1,150#H32. Accessed June 4, 2018

43. Fattouh K, Ducroux E, Decullier E, et al. Increasing incidence of melanoma after solid organ transplantation: a retrospective epidemiological study. *Transpl Int.* 2017;30(11):1172–1180

44. Ho WL, Murphy GM. Update on the pathogenesis of post-transplant skin cancer in renal transplant recipients. *Br J Dermatol.* 2008;158(2):217–224

45. Guy GP Jr, Berkowitz Z, Tai E, Holman DM, Everett Jones S, Richardson LC. Indoor tanning among high school students in the United States, 2009 and 2011. *JAMA Dermatol.* 2014;150(5):501–511

46. Guy GP Jr, Berkowitz Z, Everett Jones S, Watson M, Richardson LC. Prevalence of indoor tanning and association with sunburn among youth in the United States. *JAMA Dermatol.* 2017;153(5):387–390

47. International Agency for Research on Cancer Working Group on artificial ultraviolet (UV) light and skin cancer. The association of use of sunbeds with cutaneous malignant melanoma and other skin cancers: a systematic review. *Int J Cancer.* 2006;120(5):1116–1122

48. Miller SA, Hamilton SL, Wester UG, Cyr WH. An analysis of UVA emissions from sunlamps and the potential importance for melanoma. *Photochem Photobiol.* 1998;68(1): 63–70

49. Guy GP, Jr, Watson M, Haileyesus T, Annest JL. Indoor tanning-related injuries treated in a national sample of U.S. hospital emergency departments. *JAMA Intern Med.* 2015;175(2): 309–311

50. Seidenberg AB, Pagoto SL, Vickey TA, et al. Tanning bed burns reported on Twitter: over 15,000 in 2013. *Transl Behav Med.* 2016;6(2):271–276

51. Karagas M, Stannard VA, Mott LA, Slattery MJ, Spencer SK, Weinstock MA. Use of tanning devices and risk of basal cell and squamous cell skin cancers. *J Natl Cancer Inst.* 2002;94(3):224–226

52. International Agency for Research on Cancer. Sunbeds and UV Radiation. http://www.iarc.fr/ en/media-centre/iarcnews/2009/sunbeds_uvradiation.php. Accessed June 4, 2018

53. National Conference of State Legislatures. Tanning restrictions for minors. A state-by-state comparison. http://www.ncsl.org/research/health/indoor-tanning-restrictions.aspx. Accessed June 4, 2018

54. Guy GP Jr, Berkowitz Z, Jones SE, et al. State indoor tanning laws and adolescent indoor tanning. *Am J Public Health.* 2014;104(4):e69–e74

55. Mayer JA, Hoerster KD, Pichon LC, Rubio DA, Woodruff SI, Forster JL. Enforcement of state indoor tanning laws in the United States. *Prev Chronic Dis.* 2008;5(4). http://www.cdc.gov/ pcd/issues/2008/oct/07_0194.htm. Accessed June 4, 2018

56. Bulger AL, Mayer, JE, Gershenwald JE, Guild SB, Gottlief MA, Geller AC. Enforcement provisions of indoor tanning bans for minors: an analysis of the first 6 US states. *Am J Public Health.* 2015;105(8):e10–e12

57. Gottleib M, Balk SJ, Geller AC, Gershenwald JE. Teens and indoor tanning: time to act on the US Food and Drug Administration's Black-box warning. *Ann Surg Oncol.* 2015;22(3):701–703

58. Balk SJ, Fisher DE, Geller AC. Indoor tanning: a cancer prevention opportunity for pediatricians. *Pediatrics*. 2013;131(4):772–785

59. US Department of Health and Human Services. US Surgeon General's Call to Action to Prevent Skin Cancer. Washington, DC: U.S. Department of Health and Human Services; 2014

60. Balk SJ, Gottschlich LA, Holman DM, Watson M. Counseling on sun protection and indoor tanning. *Pediatrics*. 2017;140(6):1680–1686

61. US Preventive Services Task Force. Skin Cancer Prevention: Behavioral Counseling. https://www.uspreventiveservicestaskforce.org/Page/Document/UpdateSummaryFinal/skin-cancer-counseling2?ds=1&s=skin. Accessed June 4, 2018

62. United States Preventive Services Task Force. Grade Definitions. https://www.uspreventiveservicestaskforce.org/Page/Name/grade-definitions#brec2. Accessed June 4, 2018

63. American Cancer Society. How Do I Protect Myself from UV Rays? https://www.cancer.org/cancer/skin-cancer/prevention-and-early-detection/uv-protection.html. Accessed June 4, 2018

64. Centers for Disease Control and Prevention. What Can I Do to Reduce My Risk of Skin Cancer? https://www.cdc.gov/cancer/skin/basic_info/prevention.htm. Accessed June 4, 2018

65. US Department of Health and Human Services. Healthy People 2020. https://www.healthypeople.gov/2020/topics-objectives/topic/cancer/objectives. Accessed June 4, 2018

66. National Council on Skin Cancer Prevention. Skin Cancer Prevention Tips. https://www.skincancerprevention.org/skin-cancer/prevention-tips. Accessed June 4, 2018

67. Centers for Disease Control and Prevention. Sunburn and sun protective behaviors among adults aged 18–29 years–United States, 2000–2010. *MMWR Morb Mortal Wkly Rep*. 2012;61(18):317–322

68. Centers for Disease Control and Prevention. QuickStats: Percentage of Teens Aged 14—17 Years Who Had a Sunburn* During the Preceding 12 Months,† by Race/Ethnicity§—National Health Interview Survey, United States, 2010. https://www.cdc.gov/mmwr/preview/mmwrhtml/mm6030a6.htm. Accessed June 4, 2018

69. The Skin Cancer Foundation. Everyday and High-UPF Sun-Protective Clothing. http://www.skincancer.org/publications/the-melanoma-letter/summer-2012-vol-30-no-2/clothing. Accessed June 4, 2018

70. American Society for Testing and Materials. UV-Protective Textile Standards. January 2001. https://www.astm.org/SNEWS/JANUARY_2001/insight_jan01.html. Accessed June 4, 2018

71. Almutawa F, Vandal R, Wang, SQ, Lim HW. Current status of photoprotection by window glass, automobile glass, window films, and sunglasses. *Photodermatol Photoimmunol Photomed*. 2013;29(2):65–72

72. Boxer Wachler BS. Assessment of levels of ultraviolet A light protection in automobile windshields and side windows. *JAMA Ophthalmol*. 2016;134(7):772–775

73. Mancuso JB, Maruthi R, Wang SQ, Lim HW. Sunscreens: an update. *Am J Clin Dermatol*. 2017;18(5):643–650

74. American Academy of Dermatology. Sunscreen FAQs. https://www.aad.org/media/stats/prevention-and-care/sunscreen-faqs. Accessed June 4, 2018

75. The Skin Cancer Foundation. Prevention Guidelines. http://www.skincancer.org/prevention/sun-protection/prevention-guidelines. Accessed June 4, 2018

76. US Food and Drug Administration. Questions and Answers: FDA announces new requirements for over-the-counter (OTC) sunscreen products marketed in the U.S. http://www.fda.gov/Drugs/ResourcesForYou/Consumers/BuyingUsingMedicineSafely/UnderstandingOver-the-CounterMedicines/ucm258468.htm. Accessed June 4, 2018

77. US Food and Drug Administration. Revised Effectiveness Determination; Sunscreen Drug Products for Over-the-Counter Human Use. Proposed Rule. https://www.gpo.gov/fdsys/pkg/FR-2011-06-17/pdf/2011-14769.pdf. Accessed June 4, 2018

78. Thompson SC, Jolley D, Marks R. Reduction of solar keratoses by regular sunscreen use. *N Engl J Med.* 1993;329(16):1147–1151

79. Naylor MF, Boyd A, Smith DW, Cameron GS, Hubbard D, Nelder KH. High sun protection factor sunscreens in the suppression of actinic neoplasia. *Arch Dermatol.* 1995;131(2):170–175

80. Green A, Williams G, Neale R, et al. Daily sunscreen application and betacarotene supplementation in prevention of basal-cell and squamous-cell carcinomas of the skin: a randomised controlled trial. *Lancet.* 1999;354(9180):723–729

81. Green AC, Williams GM, Logan V, Strutton GM. Reduced melanoma after regular sunscreen use: randomized trial follow-up. *J Clin Oncol.* 2011;29(3):257–263

82. Moyal DD, Fourtanier AM. Broad-spectrum sunscreens provide better protection from solar ultraviolet-simulated radiation and natural sunlight-induced immunosuppression in human beings. *J Am Acad Dermatol.* 2008;58(5 Suppl 2):S149–S154

83. Jiang R, Roberts MS, Collins DM, Benson HAE. Absorption of sunscreens across human skin: an evaluation of commercial products for children and adults. *Br J Clin Pharmacol.* 1999;48(4):635–637

84. Calafat AM, Wong LY, Ye X, Reidy JA, Needham JL. Concentrations of the sunscreen agent benzophenone-3 in residents of the United States: National Health and Nutrition Examination Survey 2003–2004. *Environ Health Perspect.* 2008;116(7):893–897

85. US Centers for Disease Control and Prevention. National Biomonitoring Program. Benzophenone-3. https://www.cdc.gov/biomonitoring/Benzophenone-3_Biomonitoring Summary.html. Accessed June 3, 2018

86. Schlumpf M, Kypke K, Vökt CC, et al. Endocrine active UV filters: developmental toxicity and exposure through breast milk. *Chimie.* 2008;62:345–351

87. National Toxicology Program. NTP Technical Report on Toxicity Studies of 2-5 Hydroxy-4-methoxybenzophenone (CAS Number: 131-57-7) Administered Topically and in Dosed Feed to F344/N Rats and B6C3F1 Mice. Research Triangle Park, NC: National Toxicology Program, National Institute of Environmental Health Sciences, US Department of Health and Human Services; 1992. https://ntp.niehs.nih.gov/ntp/htdocs/st_rpts/tox021.pdf. Accessed June 4, 2018

88. Schlumpf M, Cotton B, Conscience M, Haller V, Steinmann B, Lichtensteiger W. In vitro and in vivo estrogenicity of UV screens. *Environ Health Perspect.* 2001;109(3):239–244

89. Wolff MS, Engel SM, Berkowitz GS, et al. Prenatal phenol and phthalate exposures and birth outcomes. *Environ Health Perspect.* 2008;116(8):1092–1097

90. Telofski LS, Morello III P, Correa MCM, Stamatas GM. The infant skin barrier: can we preserve, protect, and enhance the barrier? *Dermatol Res Pract.* 2012;2012:198789

91. Miyauchi Y, Shimaoka Y, Fujimura T, et al. Developmental changes in neonatal and infant skin structures during the first 6 months: in vivo observation. *Pediatr Dermatol.* 2016;33(3):289–295

92. Visscher MO, Adam R, Brink S, Odio M. Newborn infant skin: physiology, development, and care. *Clin Dermatol.* 2015;33(3):271–280

93. American National Standards Institute. ANSI Z80.3 - Sunglasses Requirements. https://ansidotorg.blogspot.com/2016/05/ansi-z803-sunglasses-requirements.html. Accessed June 4, 2018

94. American Academy of Ophthalmology. Recommended Types of Sunglasses. https://www.aao.org/eye-health/glasses-contacts/sunglasses-recommended-types. Accessed June 4, 2018

95. Baker MK, Hillhouse JJ, Liu X. The effect of initial indoor tanning with mother on current tanning patterns. *Arch Dermatol.* 2010;146(12):1427–1428

96. Gilchrest BA. Sun protection and vitamin D: three dimensions of obfuscation. *J Steroid Biochem Mol Biol*. 2007;103(3-5):655–663

97. Holick MF. Vitamin D deficiency. *N Engl J Med*. 2007;357(3):266–281

98. Lim HW, Carucci JA, Spencer JM, Rigel DS. Commentary: a responsible approach to maintaining adequate serum vitamin D levels. *J Am Acad Dermatol*. 2007;57(4):594–595

99. Balk SJ; American Academy of Pediatrics Council on Environmental Health and Section on Dermatology. Ultraviolet radiation: a hazard to children and adolescents. *Pediatrics*. 2011;127 (3):e791–e817

100. Golden NH, Abrams SA, American Academy of Pediatrics Committee on Nutrition. Optimizing bone health in children and adolescents. *Pediatrics*. 2014;134(4):e1229–e1243

101. Weinstock MA. The struggle for primary prevention of skin cancer. *Am J Prev Med*. 2008;34(2):171–172

102. Hay JL, Riley KE, Geller AC. Tanning and teens: is indoor exposure the tip of the iceberg? *Cancer Epidemiol Biomarkers Prev*. 2017;26(8):1170–1174

103. American Academy of Pediatrics Council on Environmental Health and Section on Dermatology, Balk SJ. Ultraviolet radiation: a hazard to children and adolescents. *Pediatrics*. 2011;127(3):588–597

104. National Toxicology Program. Nomination Summary for Dihydroxyacetone (N98013). https://ntp.niehs.nih.gov/testing/noms/search/summary/nm-n98013.html. Accessed June 4, 2018

105. Downs CA, Kramarsky-Winter E, Segal R, et al. Toxicopathological effects of the sunscreen UV filter, oxybenzone (Benzophenone-3), on coral planulae and cultured primary cells and its environmental contamination in Hawaii and the U.S. Virgin Islands. *Arch Environ Contam Toxicol*. 2016;70(2):265–288

106. Great Barrier Reef Marine Park Authority 2016, Interim report: 2016 coral bleaching event on the Great Barrier Reef, GBRMPA, Townsville. http://elibrary.gbrmpa.gov.au/jspui/ bitstream/11017/3044/5/Interim%20report%20on%202016%20coral%20bleaching%20 event%20in%20GBRMP.pdf. Accessed August 12, 2018

Chapter 45

# Antimicrobial Use and Resistance in Animal Agriculture

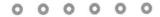

## KEY POINTS

- Antibiotic use drives the emergence and spread of antibiotic resistance.
- Approximately three quarters of antibiotics of medical importance sold in the United States are for use in livestock or poultry production, many of them for healthy animals.
- Because overuse of medically important antibiotics in food animal production contributes to worsening resistance, the World Health Organization (WHO) now recommends an end to the routine practice of feeding these drugs to flocks or herds of healthy animals.
- Advocating for policies consistent with WHO recommendations to restrict unnecessary antibiotic use in healthy food-producing animals is good for public health and complements other measures to maintain antibiotic efficacy and delay antibiotic resistance.

## INTRODUCTION

Antimicrobial resistance is "one of the most serious threats to public health globally and threatens our ability to treat infectious diseases."[1] The crisis is worsening.

Antibiotic resistance already is widespread in pathogens commonly affecting children, including community-acquired infections caused by *Campylobacter* and *Salmonella* species, and hospital-acquired (eg, *Enterococcus* species,

*Staphylococcus aureus*) infections. Among gram-negative pathogens, resistance has emerged to "last-resort" antibiotics, such as carbapenems and colistin, that are more commonly used in adults but also are given to very ill children.

Any use of antibiotics can eliminate susceptible bacteria, allowing resistant bacteria to survive. By adding to the pressure on bacterial populations that selects for resistant strains, antibiotic overuse hastens the emergence and spread of bacterial resistance.[2] Overuse and misuse in human medicine are significant drivers of the problem. Overuse and misuse in the production of food animals (cattle, pigs, poultry, etc.) also are important, although the significance of use in animals has not been well-appreciated by medical practitioners until more recently.[1]

## ANTIMICROBIAL USE IN FOOD ANIMAL PRODUCTION

### Scope of Use

According to data collected by the US Food and Drug Administration (FDA) since 2009, antimicrobial sales (by active ingredient) for use in food animals are extensive.[3] This widespread use creates environmental reservoirs in which bacteria are routinely exposed to antibiotics, contributing significantly to the development and dissemination of resistance. Heightened risks to infants and children derive from their exposure to antibiotic-resistant bacterial pathogens on meat and poultry products, as well as from exposure to bacteria acquiring resistance indirectly from environmental reservoirs.

At their recent peak in 2015, sales of medically important antibiotics for use in food animals totaled more than 21.4 million pounds of antibiotic active ingredients. (Sales decreased for the first time in 2016, but remain 9% above 2009 levels.)[3] Sales of antibiotics for use in human medicine in 2015—the last year for which data are available—totaled 7,025,863 pounds (E. Kline; Center for Disease Dynamics, Economics, & Policy; personal communication; December 7, 2017). Comparing same-year sales, around 75% of medically important antibiotics are sold in the United States for use in animals, not humans. Medically important antibiotics used in food animal production include critically important classes such as fluoroquinolones, cephalosporins, macrolides, tetracyclines, penicillins, sulfonamides, streptogramins, and aminoglycosides.

In the United States, there also is significant food animal use of antibiotics that are not medically important, chiefly ionophores, but their use does not carry the same threat of cross resistance. Cross resistance describes how the use of one antibiotic in animals can trigger the development of resistance not only to that drug, but also to other antibiotics from that same class used in human medicine.

Only recently have efforts been made to compare use of antimicrobials (medically and nonmedically important) in food animals from one country to the next, using common metrics. An independent, multi-year review, commissioned by the United Kingdom's (UK) Prime Minister's Office, recently compared antimicrobial use in food animal production in European Union (EU) countries with that in select, non-EU countries including the United States. Estimated usage in the United States (approximately 180 mg of antimicrobial active ingredient/kilogram of food animal biomass produced) is lower than that for Italy or Spain (at or above 300 mg/kg), but several times higher than use in major meat-producing countries such as Australia, Denmark, or the Netherlands.[4] The same review now recommends that individual countries, beginning with high income countries, set a target for reducing food animal use of antibiotics to no more than 50 mg/kg of animal biomass within a decade.

## Indications for Use

Antibiotics that are medically important have been FDA-approved in food animals for uses including disease treatment, disease control, and disease prevention, and for production uses such as feed efficiency and growth promotion.[5] As in human medicine, treatment use of antibiotics that are medically important refers to curative doses given for a relatively short duration to diseased animals. Diseased larger animals, including cows or pigs, may be individually treated via injection. For disease detected in a poultry flock, however, administering antibiotics *en masse*, via medicated feed or water, is the only feasible means of treatment.[6] Metaphylaxis, or disease control, refers to mass-dosing of a herd or flock to treat some diseased animals while controlling the spread of disease to other, healthy creatures. Like antibiotics for disease treatment, metaphylaxis typically involves antibiotics administered at higher dosage levels for short periods of time.

Among those antibiotics considered medically important and consumed in US food animal production through 2016, those used for disease prevention (prophylaxis) and growth promotion/feed efficiency likely accounted for the vast majority. Antibiotics for either purpose typically have been delivered to flocks or herds as additives to animal feed or drinking water; 2016 data indicate that 95% of these antibiotics for food animal use were sold as additives to animal feed (72%) or drinking water (23%).[7]

Production uses of antibiotics, including growth promotion and feed efficiency, are unrelated to animal health or disease management. Feeding antibiotics to animals for these purposes began a half century ago, but without rigorous testing as to efficacy. Today, there still is no consensus to explain how antibiotics promote growth, and few published studies demonstrate a growth promotion effect that is significant.[8] In January 2017, the FDA ended legal use of medically important antibiotics in animal feed for production purposes. The pharmaceutical industry, however, has consistently claimed that antibiotics for growth promotion accounted for no more than 10% to 15% of total use.[9] Disease prevention, meanwhile, also consists of giving antibiotics in feed or water to flocks or herds of healthy animals when they may be at risk, such as during transportation, or when confined in a crowded facility as is typical of livestock or poultry raised today under industrial conditions.[1]

In November 2017, the WHO issued new guidelines recommending against the use of medically important antibiotics in animals in whom disease is absent (ie, no use for growth promotion and prevention without diagnosis). Only under exceptional circumstances should antibiotics be used to prevent disease if it has been diagnosed in other animals in the same flock, herd, or fish population.[10] The guidelines aim to help preserve the effectiveness of antibiotics important in human medicine by reducing their unnecessary use in animals. Concurrently, the Lancet published a WHO-commissioned systematic review of 179 published studies constituting the scientific support for the recommendations.[11] In the previous year, the European Medicines Agency (the FDA equivalent for the EU) also issued guidance recommending against the marketing of EU-approved antibiotics for routine disease prevention in food-producing animals.[12]

In contrast, the FDA's recent action to end growth promotion allows many of the same antibiotics that are medically important to continue being administered at similar dosages to groups of healthy animals in the name of disease prevention, as long as it is under a veterinarian's direction. In 1973, the FDA considered antibiotics added to animal feeds both for disease prevention and for growth promotion to be "subtherapeutic" uses.[13] Currently, however, the FDA defines antibiotics used for disease prevention explicitly as "therapeutic" use, along with disease treatment or metaphylaxis.[14]

Some public interest groups worry that this loophole in the FDA's approach, in addition to being contrary to the WHO's recommendations, also carries the risk that excess sales and uses of these antibiotics in US food animal production will continue.[15,16] In 2016, those sales decreased for the first time since reporting began in 2009, but continue to outpace sales of the same drugs for human medicine.

No matter how the FDA refers to them, antibiotics used for growth promotion or disease prevention share important similarities from a human risk standpoint. First, they are delivered to animals at what physicians would consider subtherapeutic (lower than disease treatment) levels, via feed or drinking water. Second, antibiotics are given to basically healthy flocks or herds that show no signs of clinical illness; no diagnosis is made, no target organism is identified, and susceptibility testing is not done. Third, individual animals in the flock or herd receive variable dosages, depending on their intake of feed or water, resulting in no control of the dose received. Finally, because there is no specific diagnosis (and in the case of disease prevention, the perceived risk is fairly open-ended), the duration of antibiotic use is often prolonged rather than finite. Taken together, these factors add to the pressure that selects for resistant bacterial strains, thereby hastening the emergence and spread of resistance.

## ANTIBIOTIC RESISTANCE AND ANTIBIOTIC USE IN FOOD ANIMALS

Overuse or misuse of antibiotics places pressure on bacteria, selecting for resistant strains.[1]

With approximately 75% of medically important antibiotics in the United States sold for use in animals, the selection pressure being exerted by this volume of drugs is significant. In addition, 95% of these animal antibiotics are formulated as products to be added at sublethal levels to feed or drinking water, and therefore with poor dose control and often without duration limits. Given the basics of selection pressure, these are ideal conditions for the formation and spread of bacterial resistance.

Food animal production sites are now reservoirs for plasmids that carry antibiotic resistance genes; plasmids are extra-chromosomal strands of DNA that can transfer between bacteria in the same species, or among different species. "Co-resistance" describes the presence of more than one resistance gene on a plasmid; in fact, plasmids can carry physically linked genes conferring resistance to up to 10 (or even more) different antibiotics. When co-resistance exists, "co-selection" describes how the exposure of bacteria to one antibiotic can supply the selection for them to acquire resistance to all antibiotics represented on that plasmid. Long-term exposure of food animals to even a single antibiotic can foster resistance to multiple agents, not simply that one, as an experiment by Levy et al[17] clearly demonstrated 4 decades ago.

### Resistance is Ecological

Under optimal conditions, resistance can develop from a new mutation and begin to spread within hours or days.[18] Bacteria acquire most resistance genes, however, from other bacteria, via horizontal transfer.[19] Increasing numbers of studies document resistance gene movement between commensal bacteria and pathogens, and transfer of these genes among animal species, including humans.[20] The diverse mechanisms by which bacteria share genetic material have caused experts to go beyond considering movement of resistant bacterial cells to studies of the ecology and movement of resistance genes in reservoirs in which bacteria and antibiotics coexist.[21]

Environmental and animal reservoirs are important contributors to the movement of resistance genes. Important reservoirs include the rumen and/ or gut of food animals eating antibiotic-containing feed, and the gut of humans exposed to antibiotics.[22] Antibiotics also have been measured in water near animal waste lagoons,[23] surface waters, and river sediments.[24] Investigators have found resistance genes identical to those found in swine waste lagoons in groundwater and soil microbes hundreds of meters downstream.[25]

## TRANSMISSION OF ANTIBIOTIC RESISTANCE TO HUMANS

Increasingly, food animals in the United States are raised in large numbers under close confinement, transported in large groups to slaughter, and processed very rapidly.[14] These stressful conditions cause increased bacterial shedding and inevitable contamination of hide, carcass,[26] and meat[27] with fecal bacteria.

It is common for food animals under these industrialized conditions to be exposed to multiple antibiotics over the course of their lives. When food animals are colonized by bacteria carrying resistance genes, that resistance can be transferred via multiple pathways to the human population: through the food chain; via direct contact with the animals; or through contamination of food crops, drinking water, or swimming areas by excreta.[17] Dissemination of resistant bacteria via the food chain is facilitated by centralized food processing and packaging, particularly of ground meat products, and broad distribution through food wholesalers and retail chains.[28] Farmers, farm workers, farm families,[13] and casual visitors[29] are at documented increased risk of infection with resistant organisms.

Studies that date back decades—including studies in children—directly link use of antibiotics in livestock with antibiotic-resistant bacteria, and with infections traceable back to farm animals or contaminated food. In 2013, according to the Centers for Disease Control and Prevention (CDC)'s Foodborne Disease Active Surveillance Network, which covers only 15% of the US population, there were 19,056 foodborne infections in infants and children and 80 deaths, including those that were the result of infection with *Campylobacter, Salmonella,* and *E. coli.*[30]

### Salmonella

Of 1.2 million annual infections caused by non-typhoidal *Salmonella*, an estimated 100,000 are the result of drug-resistant strains, with 3% of these infections resistant to ceftriaxone, the first-line therapy for children. Over the past 15 years, ceftriaxone resistance among *Salmonella* serotype Dublin bacteria collected by the National Antimicrobial Resistance Monitoring System (NARMS) increased from 0% to 86% in cattle isolates and from 0% to 92% in human isolates.[31] In 1983, 18 people in 4 Midwestern states became ill with a *S.* Newport resistant to ampicillin, carbenicillin, and tetracycline, carried on a transmissible plasmid. An investigation concluded that the patients, including

3 children, had eaten hamburger from South Dakota beef cattle fed subtherapeutic levels of chlortetracycline given for growth promotion.[32]

## Campylobacter

In 2013, Consumer Reports tested 316 packages of raw chicken breasts sold at
American supermarkets and found that 43% harbored *Campylobacter*.[33] Almost
a quarter of 1.3 million annual cases of *Campylobacter* infection are thought
to be drug–resistant; the prevalence of resistance to macrolide antibiotics, the
treatment class of choice for children with severe infections, was 2% in 2013.[34]
As of 2014, ciprofloxacin resistance in *C. jejuni* (which accounts for 90% of
human *Campylobacter* infections) was 27%, up from 22% the previous year.[35]

## Methicillin-resistant *Staphylococcus aureus* (MRSA)

An expanding reservoir of "livestock-associated" MRSA strains exists in food
animals worldwide.[36] Livestock-associated MRSA, especially the CC 398
clone, is transmitted to the human population via retail poultry[36] and meat.[37]
*Staphylococcus* bacteria, including MRSA, are not considered foodborne pathogens, and NARMS does not conduct surveillance on MRSA. MRSA is, however,
a common meat contaminant transmitted via the food supply, in addition to
being transmitted via direct contact with animals.

## Extraintestinal *E. coli*

*E. coli* bacteria, mostly harmless, live in the guts of people and animals. Some
*E. coli* are enteric pathogens, causing diarrhea. Others, known as extra-
intestinal pathogenic *E. coli*, or ExPEC strains, cause millions of nonenteric
infections each year, including sepsis and urinary tract infections; they are
the most common cause of hospital- and community-acquired nonenteric
infections.[38]

Some strains of ExPEC *E. coli* may carry resistance to extended-spectrum
cephalosporins, making the infections caused by them increasingly hard to
manage. Cephalosporin resistance among ExPEC strains is mostly conferred
by the spread and acquisition of genes that encode extended-spectrum
beta-lactamases (ESBLs), and/or plasmid-mediated AmpC-beta-lactamases
(pAmpC).[39] The global spread of ExPEC bacteria in humans and food animals,
especially the spread of the *E. coli* sequence type 131 (ST131) clone, is problematic. Of equal concern is that ESBL and pAmpC resistance genes usually reside
on plasmids that have great potential to spread horizontally through the bacterial population.[39] One hypothesis is that animals and food contaminated with
ESBL/pAmpC-producing *E. coli* may serve as reservoirs for transfer of these
pathogens to people. An increasing number of studies support this hypothesis,
including those finding shared gene sequences and other similarities among
ExPEC *E. coli* isolated from humans and from food animals and/or meat.

## Colistin-resistant *Enterobacteriaceae*

Polymyxin antibiotics, such as colistin, have been widely used in food animal production in China, Europe, and many other places; two polymyxins are FDA-approved for use in poultry,[40] sheep, and cattle in the United States,[41] but they are not being actively marketed. Until recently, their toxicity prevented common use in human medicine; now, however, colistin is considered an important human antibiotic of last resort. For example, colistin has been used in patients infected with carbapenem-resistant *Enterobacteriaceae* (CRE). The CDC identifies CRE, which causes 600 deaths in the United States annually, as one of its top three most urgent threats from the resistance epidemic.[1]

In late 2015, starting in China and then in the United States, strains of highly drug-resistant *E. coli* were identified in pigs and humans. The strains had colistin resistance (conferred by the mcr-1 gene) carried on an easily transmissible plasmid.[42] Widespread concern exists about the global spread of plasmids carrying the mcr-1 gene because it is likely that plasmid-mediated colistin resistance will eventually be acquired by gram negative pathogens that are already pan-resistant to carbapenem and other antibiotics. The result would be infections rendered virtually untreatable in children and adults. For now, mcr-1–mediated colistin resistance has been identified only in 2 pigs in the United States, and not from any retail meats. There are clear signs that reservoirs for transmissible colistin resistance exist in human and food animal settings, making future foodborne transmission more than a hypothetical threat.

## CONCLUSION

Antibiotic resistance is a serious and worsening problem. Strong evidence shows that overuse of medically important antibiotics in food animal production contributes significantly to the crisis. Our understanding of the scope of that impact is growing.

In food animal settings, antibiotic stewardship entails not only using antibiotics judiciously when animals are sick, but also doing everything possible to avoid using antibiotics in the first place. New WHO guidelines recommend that medically important antibiotics no longer be used as preventive tools in livestock production in the absence of disease. Ending the routine use of medically important antibiotics for disease prevention was one of 11 core recommendations in the report issued recently by the independent *Expert Commission on Addressing the Contribution of Livestock to the Antibiotic Resistance Crisis.*[43] The complete recommendations are endorsed by the Academic Pediatric Association, the American Pediatric Society, the Pediatric Infectious Diseases Society, and the Infectious Diseases Society of America, among other medical groups.

The WHO sees these recommendations for reducing antibiotic use in food animals as clearly within its public health mandate because the most effective way to prevent transmission of antibiotic-resistant bacteria from food-producing animals to humans is by preventing emergence and spread of this resistance in these animals in the first place. The American Academy of Pediatrics also is committed to preserving the effectiveness of antibiotics for treating disease in children by reducing unnecessary antibiotic use. Consumers, pediatricians, and public officials should support the WHO recommendations among other antibiotic stewardship measures, to preserve their future efficacy and delay the emergence of antibiotic resistance in animal and medical settings.

The Expert Commission report carries an appendix titled, "*Tools for Health Professionals To Improve Use of Medically Important Antibiotics in Livestock.*"[43] The toolkit includes steps for practicing clinicians that include advising families to buy and serve meat and poultry produced without routine or unnecessary antibiotics. The toolkit also details steps to take in hospitals, clinics, or professional organizations.

Through advocacy for meat produced without these antibiotics, pediatricians may help leverage the purchasing power of hospitals, schools, and supermarkets to reduce the overall consumption of antibiotics, and decrease the selection pressure that contributes significantly to the worsening crisis in antibiotic resistance.

## Frequently Asked Questions

Q   *Do the antibiotics added to animal feed stay in the animals and eventually reach humans who consume meat and poultry?*

A   The greater health concern is not for antibiotic residues in food, but rather for the creation of agricultural reservoirs of resistance that may reach humans. A good illustration of the problem is how an mcr-1 gene conferring resistance to the last-resort antibiotic, colistin, after first being detected in pigs, on meat, and in human patients in China,[40] was quickly identified in over 30 different countries, as well. Because the resistance was detected more often in animals than in people, authors of the original study concluded that colistin resistance most likely originated in food animals and then spread from that reservoir to the human population.[44]

With respect to residues, there are regulations requiring specific "washout" periods. Antibiotics must be stopped for a prescribed number of days or weeks, depending on the drug, prior to slaughter of animals or collection of dairy products. These restrictions are designed to prevent animal proteins from containing unsafe residue levels of antibiotics at the time of slaughter or harvest. The success of these regulations depends on the compliance of food animal producers and the adequacy of enforcement and inspection programs.

Q *Can animals be successfully raised and brought to slaughter without the use of antibiotics to prevent illness?*

A Yes. The European Union now restricts marketing of antibiotics for disease prevention in flocks or herds. In addition, some major livestock-producing member nations, including Denmark and the Netherlands, specifically prohibit use of any medically important antibiotics for growth promotion or disease prevention. Europe also promotes the use of vaccines, better nutrition and breeding, and improvements to animal husbandry and hygiene to promote animal health and prevent unnecessary antibiotic use in the first place. In the United States, organic producers certified by the US Department of Agriculture (USDA) cannot use any antibiotics as a condition of their certification. Use of medically important antibiotics is also prohibited in US poultry production that is verified to conform to criteria under the Certified Responsible Antibiotic Use (CRAU) program.

Q *Is meat and poultry from animals raised without routine antibiotics prohibitively expensive?*

A Not necessarily. It depends on the kind of meat, and where it is purchased. In many parts of the United States, parents can buy meat or poultry produced with no antibiotics or reduced antibiotics directly from farmers, at only small price increases compared with retail supermarket prices. It is possible to identify these producers online, or via state and federal programs highlighting community-supported agriculture. Many school districts with limited food budgets are now buying poultry produced under the CRAU label at little to no price increase over other poultry products. The number of fast food and casual restaurant chains offering chicken products produced with no medically important antibiotics is rapidly increasing. Retail or restaurant products containing pork or beef raised without medically important antibiotics generally are less available, or available only at a price premium. Recent announcements by major American meat companies may indicate that situation also is changing in response to consumer demand.

## References

1. Paulson JA, Zaoutis TE. American Academy of Pediatrics Council on Environmental Health and Committee on Infectious Diseases. Nontherapeutic use of antimicrobial agents in animal agriculture: implications for pediatrics. *Pediatrics*. 2015;136(6):e1670–e1677

2. American Academy of Pediatrics Committee on Infectious Diseases. Antimicrobial stewardship: appropriate and judicious uses of antimicrobial agents. In: Kimberlin DW, Brady MT, Jackson MA, Long SS. eds. *Red Book: 2018 Report of the Committee on Infectious Diseases*. Itasca, IL: American Academy of Pediatrics; 2018:802–806

3. Food and Drug Administration (2017). 2016 Summary Report on Antimicrobials Sold or Distributed for Use in Food-Producing Animals (Table 10, p. 51). https://www.fda.gov/ForIndustry/UserFees/AnimalDrugUserFeeActADUFA/ucm042896.htm. Accessed April 27, 2018

4. Global Review on Antimicrobial Resistance. Antimicrobials in agriculture and the environment: reducing unnecessary use and waste (8 December 2015). http://amr-review.org/. Accessed April 27, 2018. Note that in October 2016, the European Medicines Agency (EMA) provided updated 2014 sales data for agricultural antimicrobials across 29 EU/EEA nations. http://www.ema.europa.eu/ema/index.jsp?curl=pages/regulation/document_listing/document_listing_000302.jsp. Accessed April 27, 2018

5. Alliance for Prudent Use of Antibiotics. The need to improve antimicrobial use in agriculture: ecological and human health consequences. *Clin Infect Dis.* 2002;34(Suppl 3):S71–S144. https://academic.oup.com/cid/issue/34/Supplement_3. Accessed June 14, 2018

6. McEwen SA, Fedorka-Cray PJ. Antimicrobial use and resistance in animals. *Clin Infect Dis.* 2002;34(Suppl 3):S93–S106. https://academic.oup.com/cid/issue/34/Supplement_3. Accessed August 31, 2018

7. Food and Drug Administration. *2016 Summary Report on Antimicrobials Sold or Distributed for Use in Food-Producing Animals.* 2017. https://www.fda.gov/downloads/ForIndustry/UserFees/AnimalDrugUserFeeActADUFA/UCM588085.pdf. Table 7, page 45. Accessed June 14, 2018

8. Graham JP, Boland JJ, Silbergeld E. Growth promoting antibiotics in food animal production: an economic analysis. *Public Health Rep.* 2007;122(1):79–87

9. Hoffman B. "New FDA 'Rules' Not Likely To Reduce Antibiotic Use On Farm," Forbes (2013). https://www.forbes.com/sites/bethhoffman/2013/12/13/new-fda-rules-will-not-reduce-antibiotic-use-on-farm/#47e284e278fe. Accessed April 27, 2018

10. World Health Organization. Press release and WHO guidelines on use of medically important antimicrobials in food-producing animals. November 7, 2017. http://www.who.int/mediacentre/news/releases/2017/antibiotics-animals-effectiveness/en/. Accessed April 27, 2018

11. Tang KL, Caffrey NP, Nobrega DB, et al. Restricting the use of antibiotics in food-producing animals and its associations with antibiotic resistance in food-producing animals and human beings: a systematic review and meta-analysis. *Lancet Planet Health.* 2017;1(8):e316–e327

12. European Medicines Agency, Veterinary Medicines Division (2016). Question and answer on the CVMP guideline on the SPC for antimicrobial products (EMEA/CVMP/SAGAM/383441/2005), February 18, 2016. EMA/CVMP/414812/2011-Rev.2. http://www.ema.europa.eu/docs/en_GB/document_library/Other/2011/07/WC500109155.pdf. Accessed April 27, 2018

13. Food and Drug Administration. Antibiotic and sulfonamide drugs in the feed of animals. National Archives and Records Administration. *Fed Regist.* 1973;(38):9811–9813. https://www.loc.gov/item/fr038076/. Accessed April 27, 2018

14. Food and Drug Administration. Guidance for Industry #213: New Animal Drugs and New Animal Drug Combination Products Administered in or on Medicated Feed or Drinking Water of Food-Producing Animals Recommendations for Drug Sponsors for Voluntarily Aligning Product Use Conditions with GFI #209 (2013). https://www.fda.gov/downloads/AnimalVeterinary/GuidanceComplianceEnforcement/GuidanceforIndustry/UCM299624.pdf. Accessed June 14, 2018

15. Pew Charitable Trusts. Gaps in FDA's Antibiotics Policy. November 30, 2014. http://www.pewtrusts.org/en/research-and-analysis/issue-briefs/2014/11/gaps-in-fdas-antibiotics-policy. Accessed April 27, 2018

16. Natural Resources Defense Council fact sheet. FDA's efforts fail to end misuse of livestock antibiotics. December 2015. https://www.nrdc.org/sites/default/files/fda-guidance-213.pdf. Accessed April 27, 2018

17. Levy SB, FitzGerald GB, Macone AB. Changes in intestinal flora of farm personnel after introduction of a tetracycline-supplemented feed on the farm. *N Engl J Med*. 1976;295(11): 583–588

18. Pray L. Antibiotic resistance, mutation rates and MRSA. *Nature Education*. 2008;1(1):30. American Society of Microbiology. *Antimicrobial Resistance: An Ecological Perspective*. https://www.nature.com/scitable/topicpage/antibiotic-resistance-mutation-rates-and-mrsa-28360. Accessed June 14, 2018

19. Levy SB, Marshal BM. Genetic transfer in the natural environment. In: Sussman M, Collins GH, Skinner FA, Stewart-Tall DE, eds. *Release of Genetically-engineered Micro-organisms*. London, England: Academic Press; 1988:61–76

20. Hummel R, Tschape H, Witte W. Spread of plasmid-mediated nourseothricin resistance due to antibiotic use in animal husbandry. *J Basic Microbiol*. 1986;26(8):461–466

21. Mazel D, Davies J. Antibiotic resistance in microbes. *Cell Mol Life Sci*. 1999;56(9-10):742–754

22. Shoemaker NB, Wang GR, Salyers AA. Evidence of natural transfer of a tetracycline resistance gene between bacteria from the human colon and bacteria from the bovine rumen. *Appl Environ Microbiol*. 1992;58(4):1313–1320

23. Campagnolo ER, Johnson KR, Karpati A, et al. Antimicrobial residues in animal waste and water resources proximal to large-scale swine and poultry feeding operations. *Sci Total Environ*. 2002;299(1-3):89–95

24. Halling-Sorensen B, Nors Nielsen S, Lanzky PF, et al. Occurrence, fate and effects of pharmaceutical substances in the environment—a review. *Chemosphere*. 1998;36(2):357–393

25. Chee-Sanford JC, Aminov RI, Krapac IJ, Garrigues-Jeanjean N, Mackie RI. Occurrence and diversity of tetracycline resistance genes in lagoons and groundwater underlying two swine production facilities. *Appl Environ Microbiol*. 2001;67(4):1494–1502

26. Barkocy-Gallagher GA, Arthur TM, Siragusa GR, et al. Genotypic analyses of Escherichia coli O157:H7 and O157 nonmotile isolate recovered from beef cattle and carcasses at processing plants in the Midwestern states of the United States. *Appl Environ Microbiol*. 2001;67(9): 3810–3818

27. Millemann Y, Gaubert S, Remy D, Colmin C. Evaluation of IS200-PCR and comparison with other molecular markers to trace Salmonella enterica subsp enterica serotype typhimurium bovine isolates from farm to meat. *J Clin Microbiol*. 2000;38(6):2204–2209

28. Center for Science in the Public Interest, Environmental Defense Fund, Food Animal Concerns Trust, Public Citizen's Health Research Group, Union of Concerned Citizens. *Petition to Rescind Approvals for the Subtherapeutic Use of Antibiotics in Livestock Used in (or Related to Those Used in) Human Medicine*. http://www.cspinet.org/ar/petition_3_99.html. Accessed April 27, 2018

29. Centers for Disease Control and Prevention. Outbreaks of *Escherichia coli* O157:H7 infections among children associated with farm visits—Pennsylvania and Washington, 2000. *MMWR Morb Mortal Wkly Rep*. 2001;50(15):293–297

30. Crim SM, Iwamoto M, Huang JY, et al. Incidence and trends of infection with pathogens transmitted commonly through food: Foodborne Diseases Active Surveillance Network, 10 US sites, 2006–2013. *MMWR Morb Mortal Wkly Rep*. 2014;63(15):328–332

31. Food and Drug Administration. NARMS Integrated Report: 2012-2013. http://www.fda.gov/AnimalVeterinary/SafetyHealth/AntimicrobialResistance/NationalAntimicrobialResistanceMonitoringSystem/ucm059103.htm. Accessed April 27, 2018

32. Holmberg SD, Osterholm MT, Senger KA, Cohen ML. Drug-resistant *Salmonella* from animals fed antimicrobials. *N Engl J Med*. 1984;311(10):617–622

33. Consumer Reports. The High Cost of Cheap Chicken (2014). http://www.consumerreports.org/cro/magazine/2014/02/the-high-cost-of-cheap-chicken/index.htm. Accessed April 27, 2018

34. Centers for Disease Control and Prevention. Antibiotic Resistance. Threat Report 2013. Atlanta, GA: Centers for Disease Control and Prevention; 2013. https://www.cdc.gov/drugresistance/pdf/ar-threats-2013-508.pdf. Accessed June 14, 2018

35. Centers for Disease Control and Prevention. NARMS 2014 Human Isolates Surveillance Report. Atlanta, GA: Centers for Disease Control and Prevention; 2014. https://www.cdc.gov/narms/pdf/2014-annual-report-narms-508c.pdf. Accessed June 14, 2018

36. Larsen J, Stegger M, Andersen PS, et al. Evidence for human adaptation and foodborne transmission of livestock-associated methicillin-resistant *Staphylococcus aureus*. *Clin Infect Dis*. 2016;63(10):1349–1352

37. Verkade E, Kluytmans J. Livestock-associated *Staphylococcus aureus* CC398: animal reservoirs and human infections. *Infect Genet Evol*. 2014;21:523–530

38. Manges AR. *Escherichia coli* and urinary tract infections: the role of poultry-meat. *Clin Microbiol Infect*. 2016;22(2):122–129

39. Mo SS, Slettemeås JS, Berg ES, Norström M, Sunde M. Plasmid and host strain characteristics of *Escherichia coli* resistant to extended-spectrum cephalosporins in the Norwegian Broiler Production. *PloS One*. 2016;11(4):e0154019

40. Food and Drug Administration. Approved Animal Drug Products. NADA 141-069, NADA 031-944. https://animaldrugsatfda.fda.gov/adafda/views/#/search. Accessed April 27, 2018

41. Food and Drug Administration. Approved Animal Drug Products. NADA 008-763. https://animaldrugsatfda.fda.gov/adafda/views/#/search. Accessed April 27, 2018

42. Liu Y, Wang Y, Walsh TR, et al. Emergence of plasmid-mediated colistin resistance mechanism MCR-1 in animals and human beings in China: a microbiological and molecular biological study. *Lancet Infect Dis*. 2016;16(2):161–168

43. Expert Commission on Addressing the Contribution of Livestock to the Antibiotic Resistance Crisis. Combating Antibiotic Resistance: A Policy Roadmap to Reduce Use of Medically Important Antibiotics in Livestock. http://battlesuperbugs.com/PolicyRoadmap. Accessed April 27, 2018. The list of endorsing organizations is at the same Web site

44. American Society of Microbiology online journal, *Cultures*. The Antibiotic Resistance Issue – Interview with Boudewijn Catry. 2016;3:1. http://asmcultures.org/3-1/. Accessed April 27, 2018

# Chapter 46

# Arts and Crafts

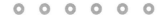

## KEY POINTS

- Play activity and creative projects have many benefits, are critical to child development, and should be encouraged and facilitated in a safe manner.
- Because some art materials contain hazardous ingredients, parents and teachers should read labels carefully and select materials with appropriate safety designations.
- Taking preventive measures such as hand washing after use, ventilation of rooms during art activities, supervising young children while using art supplies, and storing art supplies securely and in original containers may greatly reduce exposure to arts and crafts hazards.
- Children with special vulnerabilities such as asthma or developmental delays should be identified, and appropriate measures should be taken to protect their health while using art supplies.
- Caregivers who engage in art activities at home professionally or as a hobby may have contaminated workspaces. Therefore, steps should be taken to reduce the risk of harmful exposures to the artist and family members.

## INTRODUCTION

Play activity and creative projects have many benefits and are critical to child development. This chapter discusses potential hazards from arts and crafts materials and ways to limit exposures that may be toxic. Simple interventions (eg, hand washing, not eating while using art supplies, storing materials only in original labeled containers, ensuring ventilation) will often prevent potentially toxic exposures.

Arts and crafts materials abound in homes, child care settings, schools, churches, and park and recreation facilities. Although there are some published case reports and reviews of occupationally related hazards for adult artists,[1-4] there is little peer-reviewed literature about toxic exposures from children's use of arts and crafts materials. Toxicity from specific arts and crafts materials typically becomes apparent only after reports are made public. Many arts and crafts products contain ingredients known to be hazardous. Parents, teachers, and adults and teenagers working with children may not be aware of the potential health hazards associated with these common materials. Dangerous chemicals found in art materials include metals, solvents, and dusts or fibers.[5]

Lead, mercury, cadmium, and cobalt are metals found in paints, pastels, pigments, inks, glazes, enamels, and solder.[6] Legal bans on lead and other metals in paint do not apply to artists' paint, which is used in painting, drawing, ceramics, silk-screening, making stained glass, and other art activities that may involve children or adolescents.[2] Some papier-mâché products contain heavy metals from inks found in magazines. Hazardous organic solvents, such as turpentine, kerosene, mineral spirits, xylene, benzene, methyl alcohol, and formaldehyde, are used in painting, silk-screening, and shellacking as well as in cleaning tools and preparing work surfaces.[7] Rubber cement, spray-on enamels, and spray-on fixatives are common products that also contain organic solvents.[8] Materials containing dust and fibers, such as asbestos, silica, and talc, may be present in some clays, sculpture materials, and powdered pigments.

Physical hazards result from exposure to noise, dangerous mechanical and power tools, machinery and materials storage, and waste disposal practices. These are most likely to occur in industrial arts settings and often are regulated under federal Occupational Safety and Health Administration (OSHA) regulations, US Environmental Protection Agency (EPA) rules, state workers' compensation laws, or local fire prevention laws.[9]

## ROUTES OF EXPOSURE

The wide variety of arts and crafts materials used by children and adolescents permits the full spectrum of routes of exposure. The types of exposures depend on the activity, materials used, the age of the child, and environmental conditions, such as ventilation. Inhalation is a major route of exposure for volatile organic solvents, dusts, and fibers. Exposure can occur during normal use, especially if ventilation is inadequate or the necessary personal protective equipment is not available or properly used. Inhalational exposure can also occur through inappropriate exploring of new materials by sniff testing.

Intentional inhalation, such as glue sniffing, can result in high-level exposure. Heating art work (eg, during pottery glazing) can volatilize metals.

Unintentional ingestion is the route of exposure for many art hazards and may occur when common art materials are improperly stored in unlabeled or empty food containers. Even properly labeled art materials may be ingested by young or developmentally delayed children. Using homemade art as food or beverage containers can cause exposure if these products are contaminated. Ingestion also may occur through nail biting, thumb sucking, or other hand-to-mouth behaviors common in children. A potential source of toxicants in paint is licking the brush prior to dabbing it into paints. Cleaned used paint brushes may contain residual paint, and toxicity has been reported with this as an exposure source.[7]

Dermal absorption may occur from improper handling of hazardous art materials, accidental spills, or contact with cuts or abrasions. Exposure through the conjunctivae may occur from spills, splashes, and eye rubbing.

Arc welding used in sculpting potentially has the hazards of occupational welding, including ocular keratitis, respiratory tract irritation, inhalational exposure of metals, and metal fume fever (flulike symptoms and a metallic taste that commence approximately 12 hours after inhaling metals).[10]

## Nonchemical Exposures

Physical hazards cause injury in several ways. Standards developed to protect adult workers from noise may be exceeded in secondary school industrial arts workshops, exposing children to noise levels that may cause hearing loss. Use of potentially dangerous equipment may result in cuts, crush injuries, fractures, punctures, or amputations. Power equipment may cause electrical injury or fires and can release carbon monoxide. Techniques requiring repetitive motion may cause tendinitis, carpal tunnel syndrome, or other injuries. Most of these hazards can be minimized through evaluations performed by industrial hygienists, engineering measures, and use of personal protective equipment.

## SYSTEMS AFFECTED AND CLINICAL EFFECTS

Although relatively little is known about the effects on children of chronic low-level exposures to hazardous art materials, health problems among adult artists have been described.[1,2,4,7] These experiences in adults raise the possibility that chronic low-level exposures to hazardous art materials could exacerbate or cause allergies, asthma, central and peripheral nerve damage, psychological and behavioral changes, respiratory damage, skin changes, or cancer. Women of childbearing age and pregnant women who are exposed to certain components of hazardous art materials (eg, solvents, heavy metals) may be at increased risk of reproductive or fetal health impacts. For example, prenatal exposure to lead has been linked to neurodevelopmental and growth problems in children.[11] Emerging evidence suggests that maternal occupational exposure to organic solvents is linked to problems such as fetal growth restriction and neural tube defects.[12,13]

## Diagnostic Methods and Treatment

In general, if an art-related exposure is thought to be the cause of symptoms, the source should be identified and removed from the child's environment. Diagnosis and treatment are specific to each type of exposure and illness.

## Prevention of Exposure

Taking preventive measures may greatly reduce exposure to arts and crafts hazards. Subacute toxicity from long-term, low-level childhood exposure has not been studied or documented. Nonetheless, it is prudent to implement measures designed to prevent exposures that could be harmful. Some measures apply to all environments in which children use arts and crafts materials; others apply specifically to institutions.

Prevention begins with selection of the safest materials. At district or state levels in public schools and other large institutions, central ordering can facilitate the selection of safe art materials. The California Office of Environmental Health Hazard Assessment (OEHHA) has developed guidelines on the safe purchasing and use of arts and crafts materials for children that includes a list of products that should not be purchased for use by school-aged children (see Resources at the end of the chapter). For children, only materials certified to be safe should be selected (see Table 46-1 for art selection recommendations and a summary of the key labels that indicate safer products for children). The US Consumer Product Safety Commission (CPSC) considers a child to be anyone younger than 13 years or attending grade school or below. Adolescents are

### Table 46-1. Recommendations for Selecting Art Materials for Children Younger Than 13 Years

- Read the label and instructions on all arts and craft materials.
- Buy only products labeled "Conforms to ASTM D4236" and that bear the AP (Approved Product) label. Products bearing the Cautionary Label should not be used by children.
- Do not use materials labeled "Keep out of Reach of Children" or "Not for Use by Children."
- Do not use materials marked with the words "Poison," "Danger," "Warning," or "Caution," or that contain hazard warnings on the label.
- Do not use donated or found materials unless they are in the original containers with full labeling.

usually better able to follow directions, use precautions, and understand risks and are generally more able to use adult art materials and techniques.

Arts and crafts materials are labeled in a variety of ways. The familiar AP (Approved Product), CP (Certified Product), and HL Health Label (Non-Toxic) seals of the Art & Creative Materials Institute (ACMI) certify that an art material can be used by everyone, even children and adults who have impairments, without risk of acute or chronic health hazards. A new AP seal, with or without performance certification, is currently being phased in to replace the previous non-toxic ACMI seals (CP, AP, and HL). The ACMI labeling program covers approximately 80% of all children's art materials and approximately 95% of all fine art materials sold in the United States. Although these labels cannot guarantee complete safety of a product, they are preferable to products that do not carry this label. The ACMI also has a CL (Cautionary Label) designation, which indicates that the product contains hazardous ingredients, but can be used safely by certain people (adults) if used according to directions. Products with CL labels should not be used by children or by anyone with a physical or mental handicap who is not able to read and understand safety labeling on product packages.

Another common designation for art supplies created by the American Society for Testing and Materials (ASTM) is ASTM D4236 - Labeling of Art Materials for Chronic Health Hazards. This standard requires that art materials be evaluated by a toxicologist and, if labeling is required, that they conform to stringent labeling that includes identifying hazardous ingredients, risks associated with use, precautions to prevent harm, first aid measures, and sources of further information. All products certified by the ACMI (discussed previously) have conformed to this standard since its inception. Initially voluntary, the ASTM D4236 standard is now mandatory for all art materials imported or sold in the United States. This standard was made mandatory by the Hazardous Art Materials Act, which is administered by the CPSC. The standard also requires that hazardous consumer products, including art materials, have warnings to "keep out of reach of children" (for acute health hazards) or that they "should not be used by children" (for chronic health hazards).

Some art supplies may carry a generic non-toxic label; this should be interpreted with caution. Federal law does not have a specific definition for non-toxic art supplies and does not prohibit use of the non-toxic label on products that do not require cautionary (hazardous) labeling. Some of the products labeled "non-toxic" may be harmful, especially if used in an unintended manner.[14]

Occasionally, art materials available for purchase are improperly labeled. Crayons containing high levels of lead have been labeled non-toxic. To make sure that an art material has been evaluated by a toxicologist, parents should look for the statement, "conforms to ASTM D4236" covering chronic health hazards and an ACMI seal for acute and chronic health hazards.[15]

In addition to labeling guidelines, the following recommendations highlight specific materials of concern for school children that can result in higher exposures. Children should not be exposed to the following: solvent or solvent-based supplies (eg, certain glues, inks, permanent markers), processes that produce airborne dust that can be inhaled, materials with heavy metals, materials in self-pressurized containers, aerosols/sprays, and high-temperature hot glue guns.[14,16]

Aside from safe purchasing practices, a key component of prevention involves the safe use of art products and the creation of a safe classroom environment (Table 46-2). Simple behavioral interventions and careful selection of art materials may eliminate much of the risk. Behavior interventions include hand washing after use of materials, not eating or drinking while using art supplies, wearing proper protective gear when appropriate, and closely supervising students to ensure safe and correct use of materials (eg, no licking of paint brushes). Close supervision of children during arts and crafts activities can prevent injuries and poisonings, ensure proper use of materials, and allow observation of adverse reactions. Special attention should be paid to students with physical or mental disabilities, which may affect safe use of the supplies. Surplus materials should be stored away from children. Cuts and abrasions should be covered if they may come into contact with materials.

It is also important to ensure good ventilation in rooms used for arts and crafts activities by introducing clean air and circulating vapors away from students (see Chapter 20). Air disturbance should be minimized when using powders to avoid suspension and potential inhalation.[14] Materials should be properly labeled, purchased new or sealed in original containers with full instructions, and used with adult supervision according to manufacturers'

## Table 46-2. Recommendations for Safe Use of Art Materials[14,16]

- Wash hands with soap and water after using materials.
- Do not eat or drink while using art supplies.
- Wear proper protective gear when appropriate.
- Supervise students closely to ensure they are using materials correctly and safely.
- Store surplus materials out of the reach of children.
- Cover exposed cuts and abrasions with bandages when using art materials.
- Ventilate rooms used for arts and crafts activities.
- Store materials in original containers, fully labeled, sealed, and out of reach of children.
- After use, instructors should properly clean all tools, wipe down surfaces with a wet cloth/mop, and properly store art materials.
- Emergency protocols should be in place in case of an injury, poisoning, or allergic reaction.

instructions. After use, proper storage and cleanup are essential, storing materials in original, fully labeled containers. Appropriate cleanup at the end of an art session includes closing and storing containers, cleaning all tools, wiping down surfaces with a wet cloth or wet mop, and washing hands thoroughly. Adult art and hobby materials should be similarly labeled and stored out of children's reach. Half of all artists work in home studios, many of which are in living areas where children also live and may be exposed.

Emergency protocols should be in place in case of an injury, poisoning, or allergic reaction. The local poison control center number should be prominently posted. Adequate flushing facilities should be provided in the event of spills or eye splashes. Safety Data Sheets should be available on-site for all hazardous materials that may be used in high school industrial arts classes. Adult supervisors should have proper first aid and emergency response skills and training.

Art safety education for all supervising adults and teenagers is desirable. Art activities are common in church schools, child care settings, preschools, elementary and secondary schools, hospitals, chronic care institutions, therapeutic facilities, and at art festivals. Art teachers should be thoroughly trained in safety for all techniques used in the classroom. Children with special vulnerabilities should be identified and appropriate measures taken to protect their health. Children at higher risk include those with asthma and allergies who may be especially sensitive to exposures tolerated by children without these conditions. Children with physical, psychological, or learning disabilities may need special assistance in the use of some equipment or in understanding instructions and following safety techniques.[17]

Industrial arts programs should follow OSHA, US EPA, and state guidelines for ventilation, physical plant, fire safety systems, and personal protective equipment. These programs for older children and young adults should have a formal health and safety component.

## Frequently Asked Questions

Q   Are water-based art supplies always safe?

A   In general, water-based supplies are preferable because they avoid organic solvents. Accidental ingestion of even small amounts of organic solvents can be fatal. Coloring agents used in paints and inks can contain toxic substances, such as metals. Some water-based, cold-water dyes are sensitizers. Long-term health effects have not been thoroughly studied, and therefore, safer alternatives are preferred. Because some water-based paints may contain formaldehyde preservative, choose formaldehyde-free products. Water-based, unscented markers are preferable over permanent or dry erase markers. It is best to wash hands after using any art product. Make sure to avoid ingestion (such as licking paint brushes).

Q    *Can I use glazed ceramic art to store food or beverages?*

A    Glazes may contain metals. Although the lead content of glaze has been limited in dishes made in the United States for commercial sale, some glaze colors used for art projects may contain lead or other metals. These glazes may have labels recommending that they should not be used by children. Pottery made in foreign countries, particularly low- or middle-income countries, may contain lead or other metals. Metal contamination has been reported from products made in Mexico and China. Hot foods or acidic foods or drinks stored in such glazed containers may result in leaching of metals found in glaze, resulting in exposure. Glazed ceramic art and pottery from outside the United States should only be used for decoration, not for holding food or drinks.

Q    *I heard on the news that some crayons may contain asbestos fibers. How can I make sure the crayons I buy do not have asbestos?*

A    The Environmental Working Group (EWG) released a report in 2015 revealing that four crayon brands tested in independent laboratories contained detectable levels of asbestos fibers. All four crayon types were made in China. The source of the asbestos contamination is from the use of talc, which is used as a binding agent in crayons. The risk of significant exposure to asbestos fibers from typical use of these crayons is low. Given the health effects associated with asbestos exposure (see Chapter 23), it is prudent to avoid possible sources of asbestos exposure. When purchasing crayons, ensure that the company does not include talc in the ingredients, and that the product complies with ASTM D4236 and has the seal of the ACMI. The EWG report was the third study in 15 years to document the presence of asbestos in children's products, highlighting the ongoing nature of the issue and need for reform on a federal level. To view the EWG report: www.asbestosnation.org/facts/tests-find-asbestos-in-kids-crayons-crime-scene-kits/

Q    *I am a painter and work out of an art studio in my home. How can I protect my children from potentially harmful exposures from the paint and other materials I use?*

A    The occupational health and safety of artists, such as painters, is a unique concern because of potential exposures to a variety of toxic chemicals in art supplies and the unregulated setting in which they frequently perform their work (ie, the home). Artists may work in small and intensely contaminated home workspaces, leading to exposures for themselves and their families.[7] Potential hazards in paints and related product include heavy metals (eg, lead, mercury, cadmium), solvents (eg, xylene, toluene, benzene), and others (eg, methylene chloride, acids, alkalis).[7,16] Children and family members should be kept out of home art studios and other locations where potentially hazardous materials are used, stored, or discarded. Home art studios should follow basic principles of hygiene and safety that include selection of less toxic materials when possible, appropriate ventilation, use of proper protective gear, implementation of proper clean-up methods, and appropriate storage and disposal of materials. Before re-entering other areas of the home, painters should wash hands thoroughly and change work clothing and shoes. Details on these principles can be found through agencies such as the OSHA and the US CPSC (see Resources at the end of the chapter). In addition, the OSHA provides free consultations on health and safety practices for small businesses with high-risk exposures (some home studios may qualify): https://www.osha.gov/dcsp/smallbusiness/consult.html. An organization called Arts, Crafts & Theatre Safety has a hotline that provides advice about health and safety issues in the arts field: www.artscraftstheater-safety.org/hotlines.html. Some unions, such as United Scenic Artists, provide health and safety information to their members: https://www.usa829.org/HealthSafety.aspx.

Q   *What are safe art materials to purchase for my children?*

A   To ensure that an art material has been evaluated by a toxicologist for safety, parents should look for materials with the statement "conforms to ASTM D4236" and has an ACMI Approved Product seal. Although this label cannot guarantee complete safety of a product, products bearing this label are preferable to products that carry the Cautionary Label. Do not purchase art materials labeled "Keep out of Reach of Children" or "Not for Use by Children," or have the words Poison, Danger, Warning, or Caution, or that contain hazard warnings on the label. Do not use donated or found materials unless they are in the original containers with full labeling. Children should be supervised when using art materials. Materials should be kept properly labeled and stored. Safe clean up, including hand washing (with soap and water) is important.

## Resources

### American Industrial Hygiene Association (AIHA)

Phone: 703-849-8888; fax: 703-207-3561

Web site: www.aiha.org

e-mail: infonet@aiha.org

This organization gives guidance to institutions about designing and managing industrial arts facilities and programs.

## Art & Creative Materials Institute (ACMI)

Phone: 781-556-1044; fax: 781-207-5550

Web site: www.acminet.org

The ACMI, an organization of art and craft manufacturers, develops standards for the safety and quality of art materials. The ACMI manages a certification program to ensure the safety of children's art and craft materials and the accuracy of labels of adult art materials that are potentially hazardous. The organization also develops and distributes information on the safe use of art and craft materials and provides lists of certified products (those that are safe for children and adult art materials that may have a hazard potential) to individuals, to the US CPSC, state health agencies, and school authorities; and provides consultations for concerned individuals. The ACMI has access to toxicologists to answer questions about health concerns.

## California Office of Environmental Health Hazard Assessment (OEHHA)

The OEHHA has developed information to assist school personnel in selecting and using safe art and craft products in the classroom in a publication titled "Art and Craft Materials in Schools: Guidelines for Purchasing and Safe Use" (updated September 2016). https://oehha.ca.gov/risk-assessment/document-general-info/art-and-craft-materials-schools-guidelines-purchasing-and-safe

## Public Interest Research Group (PIRG)

Phone: 202-546-9707 (Federal Advocacy Office); 617-747-4370 (Main Office)

Web site: www.uspirg.org

e-mail: uspirg@pirg.org

Several state PIRGs have conducted surveys of art hazards in schools. Similar methodology was employed by all. Reports may be obtained from individual state groups. The PIRG also releases annual reports on toy safety.

## US Consumer Product Safety Commission (CPSC)

Phone: 800-638-2772

Web site: www.cpsc.gov

The CPSC is responsible for developing and managing regulations to support the Labeling for Hazardous Art Materials Act and the Federal Hazardous Substances Act. The CPSC instigates actions on mislabeled products and/or misbranded hazardous substances (products whose labels do not conform to these acts). Actions may involve confiscations, product recalls, or other legal actions. The CPSC's Web site contains general product safety information and recent press releases and an "Art and Craft Safety Guide." To report a dangerous product or product-related injury or illness, call the CPSC's hotline at 800-638-2772 or online at www. cpsc.gov. This CPSC Web site explains art material testing and certifications: www.cpsc.gov/Business--Manufacturing/Business-Education/ Business-Guidance/Art-Materials/

### US Occupational Safety and Health Administration (OSHA)

The OSHA sets and enforces occupational health standards and provides training, outreach, education, and assistance to employers and employees. Web site: www.osha.gov

## References

1. Dorevitch S, Babin A. Health hazards of ceramic artists. *Occup Med.* 2001;16(4):563–575

2. McCann MF. Occupational and environmental hazards in art. *Environ Res.* 1992;59(1):139–144

3. Ryan TJ, Hart EM, Kappler LL. VOC exposures in a mixed-use university art building. *AIHA J (Fairfax, Va).* 2002;63(6):703–708

4. Zuskin E, Schachter EN, Mustaibegović J, Pucarin-Cvetković J, Lipozencić J. Occupational health hazards of artists. *Acta Dermatovenerol Croat.* 2007;15(3):167–177

5. Klaassen CD, ed. *Casarett and Doull's Toxicology: The Basic Science of Poisons.* 8th ed. New York, NY: McGraw Hill; 2013

6. Babin A, Peltz PA, Rossol M. *Children's Art Supplies Can Be Toxic.* New York, NY: Center for Safety in the Arts; 1992

7. Lesser SH, Weiss SJ. Art hazards. *Am J Emerg Med.* 1995;13(4):451–458

8. McCann M. *Artist Beware.* New York, NY: Lyons and Burford Publishers; 1992

9. McCann M. *School Safety Procedures for Art and Industrial Art Programs.* New York, NY: Center for Safety in the Arts; 1994

10. LaDou J, Harrison RJ. *Current Diagnosis & Treatment: Occupational & Environmental Medicine.* 5th ed. McGraw-Hill Education; 2014

11. Ettinger AS, Wengrovitz AG, eds. National Center for Environmental Health/Centers for Disease Control and Prevention. Guidelines for the Identification and Management of Lead Exposure in Pregnant and Lactating Women. Published November 2010. https://www.cdc.gov/nceh/lead/publications/leadandpregnancy2010.pdf. Accessed January 18, 2018

12. Desrosiers TA, Lawson CC, Meyer RE, et al. National Birth Defects Prevention Study. Assessed occupational exposure to chlorinated, aromatic and Stoddard solvents during pregnancy and risk of fetal growth restriction. *Occup Environ Med.* 2015;72(8):587–593

13. Desrosiers TA, Lawson CC, Meyer RE, et al. National Birth Defects Prevention Study. Maternal occupational exposure to organic solvents during early pregnancy and risks of neural tube defects and orofacial clefts. *Occup Environ Med.* 2012;69(7):493–499

14. California Environmental Protection Agency-Office of Environmental Health Hazard Assessment. Art and Craft Materials in Schools: Guidelines for Purchasing and Safe Use. October 2014. http://www.oehha.ca.gov/education/art/guidelinesforart.html. Accessed January 18, 2018

15. Lu PC. A health hazard assessment in school arts and crafts. *J Environ Pathol Toxicol Oncol.* 1992;11(1):12–17

16. U.S. Consumer Product Safety Commission. Art and Craft Safety Guide. Publication No. 5015. https://www.cpsc.gov/s3fs-public/5015.pdf. Accessed January 23, 2018

17. Rossol M. The first art hazards course. *J Environ Pathol Toxicol Oncol.* 1992;11(1):28–32

Chapter 47

# Asthma

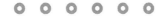

## KEY POINTS

- The development of asthma likely involves a complex interaction of genes, physical environment, and social environment.
- Asthma is a complex disease representing more than one phenotype, so it is likely that different risk factors exist for each individual and for different susceptible populations.
- Mitigating environmental risks for asthma exacerbations is increasingly recognized as a key part of asthma management.
- Additional research is needed to clearly elucidate risk factors and protective factors for asthma development.

## INTRODUCTION

Asthma is a chronic respiratory disease characterized by bronchial hyperresponsiveness, intermittent reversible airway obstruction, and airway inflammation.[1] This chapter will briefly review environmental factors that influence the development of asthma and then focus on environmental triggers in children with asthma.

## ASTHMA DEVELOPMENT

Asthma is a complex disease representing more than one phenotype. It is likely that many combinations of genetic and environmental factors contribute to the development of asthma, and prenatal and/or early life exposures appear to play an important role. Poverty and other social determinants may potentiate these environmental and genetic risks by affecting risk of and response to environmental exposures. Rates of asthma have risen over recent decades to a current plateau, and given that human genes change over generations, it is likely that recent changes in children's environments have contributed to the increasing prevalence of asthma. It is also possible that epigenetic factors play a role in the development of asthma.[2-4]

A commonly supported hypothesis involves a shift in T helper cell response influencing the development of allergic reactivity and asthma. Studies suggest that the neonatal immune system tends to favor an allergic (immunoglobulin E [IgE]-promoting) response to any potential allergens. This response is mediated in part through infant T helper cells that tend to release a series of cytokines that promote the development of an "allergic" B cell response—the generation of specific IgE—to certain environmental allergens. The end result of the T cell cytokine profile that favors an IgE response is termed a Th2 response. In contrast, as the immune system matures, naïve T cells develop along a different path, releasing a mix of cytokines in response to exposure to environmental allergens that favor a Th1 (pro-inflammatory) response. Recent work has expanded the paradigm to include a role for regulatory T cells and other immune cells, but a detailed discussion of this paradigm is beyond the scope of this chapter.

It is postulated that differences in exposures to environmental stimuli during early childhood could either perpetuate Th2 responses and the pathway toward asthma or shift the balance toward the expected Th1 response, depending on the types of stimuli and/or an individual's genetic predisposition.[1,5] Proposed hypotheses on environmental factors that may favor the Th2 response include improved hygiene, changes in diet, changes in intestinal flora because of increased use of antibiotics and/or dietary changes (leading to alterations in the microbiome), increased exposure to allergens because of changes in housing and lifestyle, obesity and reduced physical activity, and changes in the prenatal environment.[6] The "hygiene hypothesis" postulates that early childhood infections (which promote a Th1 response) are becoming less frequent, favoring a persistent Th2 imbalance.[1,7] Supporting this hypothesis are observations that the presence of an older sibling and early child care attendance are associated with a reduced incidence of asthma. The development of a Th2 (IgE) response to common environmental contaminants (eg, house-dust mite, cockroach, mouse, cat, and dog allergens) is strongly correlated with the development of childhood asthma.[5,8] Some studies have suggested that exposure to pet allergens during infancy may be protective, although the data show mixed results.[7,9-11] Associations between early exposure to airborne particulates or pollutant gases and childhood asthma development also have been suggested.[12] Emerging evidence supports the role of chemicals found in plastics (such as phthalates and bisphenol A) in the development of asthma.[13–17] Investigators are evaluating the potential role of microbiome and modifications of the microbiome in asthma risk and risk reduction.[18] Data about the protective role of breastfeeding and early diet in the development of asthma show conflicting results.[19] In summary, despite several proposed risk and protective factors, the relationship between prenatal and early life exposures and asthma development is not completely understood.

## ENVIRONMENTAL TRIGGERS OF ASTHMA EXACERBATIONS

The most recently revised guidelines for asthma management promulgated by the National Asthma Education and Prevention Program (NAEPP) presented 4 components of managing asthma exacerbations and prevention of exacerbations.[6] One of the 4 components was control of environmental factors that affect asthma, recognizing the important role of environment in triggering asthma exacerbations. The guidance recommends, "measures to control exposures to allergens and pollutants or irritants that make asthma worse."[6] Indoor triggers of asthma[20] include secondhand tobacco smoke (SHS); respiratory irritants such as volatile organic compounds (VOCs) and fragrances (see Chapter 20); animal and insect allergens (eg, pet dander, rodent and cockroach antigens), and fungi, commonly known as molds.

Outdoor triggers include pollens, outdoor air pollutants, and molds (see Chapter 21).[21,22] Table 47-1 lists common asthma triggers.

## Indoor Environmental Asthma Triggers

### Secondhand Tobacco Smoke

The prevalence of tobacco use and exposure to SHS has declined significantly, but more than 15% of US adults still used tobacco in 2015.[23] Children are among the most heavily exposed to SHS (see Chapter 43). Children whose mothers smoke have more wheezing symptoms and a higher incidence of lower respiratory tract illnesses compared with those whose mothers do not smoke.[24] The greatest effect seems to be related to maternal smoking during pregnancy and/or early infancy.[25–28] A meta-analysis of 79 prospective epidemiologic studies published between 1997 and 2011 assessing the association between tobacco smoke exposure and the incidence of wheeze or asthma in childhood concluded that prenatal maternal smoking and household SHS exposure were associated with an increased risk of asthma.[29] Exposure to SHS is associated with an increase in asthma attacks, earlier asthma symptom onset, increased medication use, and a more prolonged recovery from acute attacks.[24] Acute short-term exposure to SHS increases bronchial hyperreactivity, requiring as

## Table 47-1. Common Indoor and Outdoor Asthma Triggers

| AGENT | MAJOR SOURCES |
| --- | --- |
| **INDOOR** | |
| Secondhand tobacco smoke | Cigarettes, cigars, other tobacco products |
| Wood smoke | Fireplaces and wood-burning stoves |
| Fungi (molds) | Floods, roof leaks, plumbing leaks, wet basements, air-conditioning units |
| Nitrogen oxides | Space heaters, gas-fueled cooking stoves |
| Odors or fragrances | Sprays, deodorizers, cosmetics, household cleaning products, pesticides |
| Volatile organic compounds (VOCs) | Building and insulation materials, cleaning agents, solvents, pesticides, sealants, adhesives, combustion products, molds |
| Dust mites | Bedding (pillows, mattresses, box springs, bed linens), carpets, soft upholstered furniture, draperies, stuffed toys |
| Animals | Cat and dog dander and saliva, rodent urine |
| Cockroaches | Cockroach feces and regurgitated digestive matter |
| **OUTDOOR** | |
| Pollens | Seasonal release from pollen-generating plants |
| Molds | Ubiquitous in soil, increased in wet environments and decaying organic matter (eg, wood chips) |
| Ozone ($O_3$) | Combustion sources (eg, motor vehicle exhaust, power plants) |
| Particulate matter ($PM_{10}$, $PM_{2.5}$, $PM_{1.0}$) | Combustion sources (eg, diesel engines, industry, wood burning) |
| Sulfur dioxide ($SO_2$) | Burning of coal (coal-fired power plants, other industrial sources) |

Abbreviations: $PM_{10}$, indicates particulate matter less than 10 mcm in aerodynamic diameter; $PM_{2.5}$, particulate matter less than 2.5 mcm in aerodynamic diameter; $PM_{1.0}$, particulate matter less than 1 mcm in aerodynamic diameter.

long as 3 weeks to recover baseline pulmonary function following exposure.[24] A systematic review and meta-analysis found that exposure to SHS after birth promoted the expression of immunological markers of allergic sensitization and increased the risk of atopic disease among children, especially those younger than age 7 years.[30]

### Other Airborne Irritants

Other common sources of air pollutants that may be respiratory irritants include gas stoves and wood stoves, space heaters (gas or kerosene) and fireplaces, and furnishings and construction materials that release organic gases and vapors.[31,32] Epidemiologic evidence for the role of these pollutants in exacerbating asthma is limited but suggests associations between exposures and asthma exacerbations.[31-33]

Gas stoves or ovens can generate high levels of nitrogen dioxide indoors, especially when there is inadequate ventilation or the gas stove is used as an ancillary heat source.[34] Poorly ventilated fireplaces can produce substantial levels of wood smoke indoors.

Volatile organic compounds and fragrances may induce acute asthma episodes in sensitive individuals.[35] The mechanism of action is unknown but presumed to be nonspecific irritation. Formaldehyde is emitted from many consumer products, including new carpets, paper products (eg, tissues, towels, bags), urea-formaldehyde foam insulation, and glues used in plywood and pressed-board products. Formaldehyde is a known respiratory irritant in the occupational setting and a common air pollutant in the home (see Chapter 20).[31,32,36]

## Allergenic Triggers

### Animal Allergens

Animal allergens are glycoproteins that often induce an IgE response in humans. These allergens usually are found in saliva, sebaceous glands (dog and cat), or sometimes in urine (rodents). Allergies to cow hair or horsehair and dander also have been reported, often through occupational or hobby exposures.[31,32] The spread of allergens in the environment has been studied primarily for cats; however, the pathway of spread is likely to be similar for other domestic furry animals.[31,32] Cat allergen-containing material dries and adheres to many surfaces (eg, animal fur or hair, bedding, clothing) and can be transported to other environments via these sources. Once an animal enters the room, small airborne allergen-containing particles (diameter <5 mcm) can be detected, but an animal does not need to enter a room for airborne allergen to be detected. These small particles remain suspended in the air for hours. Once allergen-containing particles are inhaled, they are easily deposited in distal airways. Clinical manifestations of animal allergy range from mild cutaneous symptoms, such as urticaria, to rhinoconjunctivitis to life-threatening bronchospasm and anaphylaxis.

## Cats

More than 6 million US residents have allergies to cats, and up to 40% of atopic patients demonstrate skin test sensitivity.[37] The major allergen *Fel d I* is present in high concentration in the saliva and sebaceous and anal glands of cats. The grooming habits of cats result in a large amount of saliva on the fur, and cat allergen can be spread via small airborne particles.[38] Children with cats can transmit cat allergens to schoolrooms, which may create an environment that can precipitate asthma in sensitized children.[39] Once a cat is removed from an indoor environment, the allergen may persist for many months in reservoirs, such as bedding. Analysis of data from a birth cohort in the United Kingdom documented that pet ownership during pregnancy and childhood was associated with a reduced risk of aeroallergen sensitization and atopic asthma at age 7 years, but was associated with an increased risk of nonatopic asthma.[40] No clear evidence exists for a protective or harmful effect of cat ownership on sensitization to animal dander.[41,42]

## Dogs

Dogs are the most common domesticated animal species found in US homes. Five percent to 30% of atopic patients have a positive skin test to the major allergen *Can f I*, although many do not demonstrate clinical symptoms or have positive bronchoprovocation tests.[43] There appears to be variation in clinical sensitivity to different dog breeds, and breed-specific allergens have been suggested.[44] Nevertheless, no dog breed is considered nonallergenic. As with cat allergen, the highest concentrations of *Can f I* are found in canine fur and dander.[44]

## Rodents

People may be exposed to rodents if they are present as pests or pets in the home. Rat and mouse allergens are present primarily in their urine.[44,45] Through transfer, the fur and dander often contain high amounts of allergen. The prevalence of mouse and rat allergens can be widespread in inner-city homes.[44,45] Among children with asthma living in inner cities, there is an association between mouse allergen in house-dust samples and sensitization to mouse allergen, especially among children with asthma who exhibit atopy to multiple allergens on skin testing. Similar results have been found regarding rat allergen; sensitization and exposure are associated with increased asthma morbidity in inner-city children. Early mouse exposure has been associated with early wheeze and atopy later in life.[45–47]

## Birds

In the occupational setting, hypersensitivity pneumonitis can be associated with antigens from bird excreta and proteinaceous materials found in dust dispersed from birds; however, it is unclear whether birds cause allergy and asthma.[31,32] Large quantities of dust mites have been documented in feathers, and dust-mite allergen is the likely source of the allergic stimulus from feather-containing items in the home, including pillows, comforters, bedding, and down-filled clothes.[31,32]

### Insect Allergens

#### Cockroaches

Cross-sectional studies suggest the prevalence of cockroach hypersensitivity is related to the degree of infestation in the living environment, although nonresidential exposures (eg, schools) may cause sensitization in persons whose homes are not infested. Cockroach infestations are more common in warm, moist environments with readily accessible food sources. Although the highest allergen levels typically are found in the kitchen, significantly elevated concentrations of cockroach allergen also are found in bedrooms or television-watching areas, particularly if food is consumed in these places.

Numerous species of cockroaches have been described in the United States, and 3 predominant species have been associated with IgE antibody production. The German cockroach, *Blattella germanica,* is the source of 2 primary antigens, *Bla g 1* and *Bla g 2*; however, significant cross-reactivity exists between cockroach allergens. Cockroach allergens have been described as principal triggers of allergic rhinitis and asthma. Positive skin tests to cockroach antigens can be found in up to 60% of urban residents with asthma. Cockroach fecal material and regurgitated material ("frass") is the source of common allergens. Cockroach allergens may behave like the dust-mite antigen; that is, they are carried on large particles that are only airborne for short periods of time during active disturbance. Levels of allergen in places where children spend a significant amount of time may be most important. Children with asthma, cockroach allergen sensitization, and exposure to elevated levels of cockroach allergen in bedroom dust had more days of wheezing, more missed school days, and more emergency department visits and hospitalizations than did nonsensitized and/or nonexposed asthmatic children.[31,32,48] In addition, hospitalization rates for children who were sensitized and exposed to higher levels of cockroach allergen were nearly 3 times as high as for those with low exposure and sensitivity.

#### House-dust Mites (*Dermatophagoides*)

House-dust mites most likely play a major role in inducing asthma and triggering asthma exacerbations in sensitized children. Mite antigen commonly is found where human dander is found, and the principal allergens—*Der p I* and *Der p II*—are found in the outer membrane of mite fecal particles. Indoor environments that provide optimal growth conditions for *Dermatophagoides* species have a relative humidity greater than 55% and temperatures between

22°C and 26°C (71°F and 79°F), but dust mites can survive laundering at moderate temperatures. Under optimal conditions, mites proliferate on mattress surfaces, carpeting, and upholstered furniture, each of which contains a large amount of human dander, its primary food source. A gram of dust may contain 1,000 mites and 250,000 fecal pellets. Pellet diameters range in size from 10 to 40 mcm and, therefore, are not easily transported into the lower airway passages. Exposure occurs either by proximity of the nasopharyngeal mucosa to mite reservoirs (especially mattresses, pillows, carpets, bed linens, clothes, and soft toys) or to airborne antigen that is resuspended during house-cleaning activities.

### Fungi (Molds)

Molds are most prominent in climates with increased ambient humidity, although some can grow in relatively dry areas. Species of common indoor molds (eg, *Aspergillus, Penicillium,* and *Cladosporium* species) require sufficient moisture for growth, and places where indoor mold growth is commonly found include household areas with high humidity (eg, basements, crawl spaces, ground floors, bathrooms, and areas with standing water, such as air-conditioner condensers) and areas with recent moisture damage. Carpeting, ceilings, and paneled or hollow walls also are common reservoirs.

Dampness and the presence of mold should be suspected when there is visible mold or mildew in the home, a moldy or musty smell, evidence of water condensation on windowsills (except immediately after showers or cooking in the kitchen), or the use of a humidifier. Many epidemiologic studies have documented an association between dampness and mold in the home and asthma and allergy symptoms.[31,32,49–56] Because dampness and visible mold growth could be indicators for dust-mite allergen exposure, the relative contribution of molds versus other allergens (eg, house-dust mite) is not entirely clear. Several studies have documented, however, that the association between mold and asthma persists even after adjusting for levels of dust-mite allergen.[57,58] A systematic review of 16 studies concluded that exposure to visible mold was associated with increased risk for asthma.[59] A birth cohort study demonstrated that exposure during infancy to 3 mold species common to water-damaged buildings (*Aspergillus ochraceus, Aspergillus unguis*, and *Penicillium variable*) was associated with childhood asthma at age 7 years.[60]

### Miscellaneous Allergens

#### Latex

Latex may cause an allergic response either by direct contact or by inhalation of latex particles. Symptoms range from cutaneous eruption, sneezing, and bronchospasm to anaphylaxis.[61] Widespread use of latex gloves and revised processing procedures, making the allergen more potent, may have contributed to the increase in reported cases. Most sensitivities occur in medical personnel, food service workers, or environmental service workers, although household exposures to balloons, gloves, condoms, and certain sporting equipment also may trigger allergic and asthmatic responses. Children with increased exposure to latex (eg, those with urogenital abnormalities, cerebral palsy, and preterm infants) are at increased risk for the development of latex allergy. Up to one third of children with spina bifida have been reported to have positive skin tests to latex.[61] Recently, latex allergy has become rarer than in the past.

### Food

Many foods contain allergenic proteins that can trigger asthma or anaphylactic reactions in sensitized persons. Peanuts, tree nuts, fish, shellfish, eggs, and milk are the most commonly associated foods.[62] Although oral ingestion typically is needed to elicit symptoms, contact with aerosolized particulates and oils that contain the offending antigens can induce symptoms in highly allergic persons. In rare individuals, food additives, including sulfites and food coloring—especially tartrazine (a synthetic yellow dye) or cochineal (a red dye made of the dried and pulverized bodies of female cochineal insects)—also can be highly allergenic. Asthma symptoms are frequent among children experiencing anaphylaxis but are rarely the sole manifestations of food allergy.

## Outdoor Environmental Triggers

### Outdoor Air Pollution

Millions of Americans live in areas that fail to meet the National Ambient Air Quality Standards. These are standards set by the US Environmental Protection Agency (EPA) for widespread air pollutants considered harmful to the public and environment (see Chapter 21). Pollutants are generally considered to be particulate or gaseous and certain criteria particulates are regulated by the US EPA. Ozone and particulate matter are of special concern. Levels of these air pollutants are high enough in many parts of the United States to present respiratory hazards to children with asthma. During 2007 to 2009, an estimated 36.2% of the US population lived in nonattainment counties for the 2008 8-hour ozone standard. During 2006 to 2008, 13.6% of the US population lived in nonattainment counties for the 2006 24-hour $PM_{2.5}$ standard.[63] This is concerning because improvements in air quality can be associated with improved lung-function growth in children.[64]

### Ozone

Ambient (outdoor) ozone is formed by the action of sunlight on nitrogen oxides and reactive hydrocarbons (both of which are emitted by motor vehicles and industrial sources) under stable weather conditions. The levels tend to be highest on warm, sunny, windless days and often peak in the mid-afternoon.

During the warm season, ozone concentrations often exceed the National Ambient Air Quality Standards in many urban and rural areas of the United States, with the highest levels often being reached in suburban regions of major metropolitan areas.

Ozone is a powerful oxidant and respiratory irritant. Increased rates of hospitalization and acute visits for asthma exacerbations have been associated with high ozone days.[65,66] One study found an increased incidence of asthma associated with heavy exercise among children living in communities with high levels of ozone air pollution.[67]

### Particulate Matter

Particulate matter is a heterogeneous mixture of airborne particles. In urban areas, motor vehicle exhaust (especially diesel), industry, and wood smoke are important sources of particulate pollution. Particulate pollution has been associated with asthma exacerbations and bronchitis symptoms in children with asthma. In addition to their irritant properties, diesel particulates may enhance the allergic response.

### Sulfur Dioxide

Sulfur dioxide ($SO_2$) is a potent respiratory irritant that can cause asthma exacerbations. Principal sources of $SO_2$ include coal-fired power plants, paper and pulp mills, refineries, and other industries. Although ambient levels of $SO_2$ are below the national air quality standard in most areas of the United States, $SO_2$ levels can be increased in areas near these sources.

For additional information on health effects of outdoor air pollution, see Chapter 21.

### Outdoor Allergens

Outdoor air contains a variety of allergens, most of which arise from plant pollens and mold spores. Exposures to high concentrations of tree, grass, and ragweed pollens that occur in the spring, summer, and early fall can induce respiratory symptoms, such as sneezing, rhinitis, and bronchospasm in sensitized children. Spores from mold, such as *Alternaria* and *Aspergillus* species, commonly are found in damp, wooded areas, including the wood chips often used as ground cover in playgrounds. These allergens also can cause acute and recurrent asthma exacerbations.[68,69] Outdoor exposure to mold spores has been implicated in fatal exacerbations of asthma.[69,70] Asthma attacks that occur during thunderstorms also have been linked to increased mold spores and grass pollen in the outdoor air.[71,72]

## DIAGNOSIS

To establish a diagnosis of asthma, clinicians should take a detailed medical history. They should determine that the patient has a history of episodic symptoms of airflow obstruction or airway hyperresponsiveness. A physical examination should be performed, focusing on the upper respiratory tract, chest, and skin. Alternative diagnoses should be excluded.[6] Atopy and a family history of asthma and/or atopy are strong predictors of persistent asthma. Pulmonary function testing in children younger than 5 years is difficult to conduct and poorly reproducible. A response to a therapeutic trial of bronchodilator and/or anti-inflammatory medications frequently is helpful in confirming the diagnosis. Chest radiographs should not routinely be used to diagnose asthma, but they may reveal the presence of peribronchial thickening and hyperinflation, which may help to evaluate other diagnostic possibilities such as a congenital anomaly or foreign body. Baseline pulmonary function testing may demonstrate a decreased forced expiratory volume in 1 second ($FEV_1$), and a decreased mid-expiratory phase ($FEV_{25-75}$) compared with predicted norms, but most children with asthma have normal lung function. Prebronchodilator and postbronchodilator spirometry ($>12\%$ $FEV_1$ improvement), methacholine, exercise, or cold air bronchoprovocation ($\geq20\%$ $FEV_1$ decrease) may help support a diagnosis of asthma in the patient with mild symptoms. Daily or diurnal variability in peak flow measurements also may help.

## TREATMENT

As noted previously, the National Institutes of Health, through the NAEPP, provides evidence-based guidelines discussing all aspects of asthma treatment.[6] Goals of treatment include preventing chronic and troublesome symptoms, maintaining normal pulmonary function, maintaining a normal quality of life, reducing the number of exacerbations, and minimizing emergency department visits and hospitalizations. Medications are categorized into 2 general classes: (1) long-term preventive medications that achieve and maintain control of persistent asthma; and (2) quick-relief medications that treat acute symptoms and exacerbations. The "step care" approach to asthma therapy emphasizes initiating higher-level therapy at the onset of treatment to control symptoms, and then "stepping down" the use of quick-relief medications followed by control medications. Preventive medications include inhaled corticosteroids and nonsteroidal medications, such as leukotriene receptor antagonists and long-acting beta-adrenergic agonists; newer biologic treatments (anti IgE) are available for more severe asthma. Relief medications are largely inhaled rapid-acting adrenergic agonists.[6]

Uncontrolled asthma is a risk factor for severe anaphylaxis to food allergens. Management of asthma symptoms that occur as part of an anaphylactic reaction requires the use of intramuscular epinephrine, rather than use of an inhaled adrenergic agonist.[73]

Allergen immunotherapy is available for many allergens and has had some success.[74] Immunotherapy should not take the place of efforts to control exposure to allergens, irritants, and other triggers.

## MANAGEMENT OF ENVIRONMENTAL TRIGGERS OF ASTHMA

Reducing exposure to inhalant indoor allergens and irritants can improve asthma control.[6] Several exposure reduction strategies are summarized in Table 47-2. Focusing on one allergen reduction strategy may be ineffective and generally, a multifaceted approach is required.[6] Multifaceted home environmental intervention strategies in combination with community health worker-based assessments and parent education can be cost-effective and represent an effective public health strategy, especially in inner-city communities.[6,75,76] These environmental interventions can be as effective as the use of inhaled corticosteroids in treating asthma symptoms.[6]

### Control Measures for Allergens and Irritants

Avoiding environmental allergens and irritants is one of the primary goals of good asthma management. Skin testing or in vitro testing and counseling about appropriate environmental control strategies are recommended for all children with persistent asthma who are exposed to perennial indoor allergens.[6]

Most control measures have been directed at the control of chronic asthma symptoms and the prevention of asthma exacerbations.[75,77,78] Possible interventions to decrease the risk for the development of asthma currently are being investigated.[6] To date, food allergen avoidance diets prenatally or postnatally have not been successful in decreasing the incidence of asthma. A randomized controlled trial to evaluate the use of house-dust mite-impermeable bedding on severe asthma exacerbations in children found that the bedding reduced the number of children coming to the hospital with asthma attacks but not the number requiring oral prednisolone.[79] Primary prevention of asthma should include efforts to reduce exposure to SHS in children and adolescents. Pregnant women should not smoke and should avoid exposure to SHS.

Complete control of many of the environmental allergens is difficult, and multiple intervention strategies are recommended. Several reviews outline priorities for allergen avoidance.[6,31,32,80–83] Recommendations follow the basic principles of control of sources. Recommendations for aggressive and continual attention to multiple reservoirs are especially relevant for children who require multiple medications to control their symptoms. Barriers to implementation of indoor environmental control strategies for low-income children with asthma have been evaluated.[76] Models are emerging in which insurance companies pay for environmental interventions that are being evaluated, and there is some early evidence evaluating home visitation programs to reduce exposures.[84]

In 1999, Congress directed the US Department of Housing and Urban Development (HUD) to address children's environmental health. In response, HUD launched its Healthy Homes Initiative (HHI) aimed at protecting children and families from housing-related health and safety hazards. One focus of the HHI is improving the home environment for children with asthma. In many locations, HHI programs support home interventions to control allergens for children with asthma.

### Secondhand Tobacco Smoke and Other Indoor Irritants

Pediatricians should ask about children's exposure to SHS. They should counsel parents and caregivers who smoke to quit smoking and to eliminate sources of smoke in the child's environment (see Chapter 43). There is no evidence to show that ventilation can decrease a child's exposure to SHS.[31,32] High-efficiency particulate air (HEPA) filters used in homes of children with asthma where there are smokers may result in a 25% to 50% decrease in indoor PM (SHS is the major contributor to indoor PM). The HEPA filter groups showed improvements in measures of asthma control and/or morbidity.[85,86] Adequate ventilation is imperative for indoor combustion appliances (eg, gas or kerosene space heaters, gas stoves, wood-burning fireplaces, wood stoves). Gas or kerosene space heaters, often used in cold climates in which they may be on for prolonged periods,[31,32] should not be used in unvented spaces because of the risk of carbon monoxide poisoning. Sealant coatings or coverings are sometimes applied over formaldehyde-containing materials to decrease emissions. Furniture, carpets, and building materials emit the highest levels of VOCs during the first months after manufacturing, and adequate ventilation should be supplied during and immediately after installation. Low-emission carpets, adhesives, and building materials are commercially available, but there are no clinical studies comparing asthma exacerbations among children in homes with traditional versus low-emission carpets. Using alternative products that contain few or no VOCs or fragrances, such as paint and finishes with low levels of VOCs, non-aerosol and unscented cleaners, and cosmetics, should be encouraged.

### Indoor Allergens

#### Animal Allergens

The preferred treatment for animal allergy is to avoid animals that provoke the reaction. Removing the animal from the home or keeping it outdoors (eg, in the garage) are strongly recommended. Other measures, such as restricting the pet to an area of the home, keeping the child's bedroom as a "safe zone," and using air purifiers, have not been effective because animal allergens are airborne, travel throughout a home, and stick to surfaces throughout the home. If removal is not possible or acceptable, efforts should be made to control all sites where pet allergens accumulate as well as the source, but the child is likely to continue to have significant exposure to the allergen. Other than service dogs, animals should be avoided or limited in schools and child care settings.[83]

Control of the major cat allergen *Fel d I* is difficult. Removing the cat results in marked reduction in allergen levels, but this will likely take months. A weekend at home without the cat is not a sufficient test to determine whether the child's asthma will improve if the cat is removed from the home. Aggressive cleaning (eg, removing carpets, washing walls and furniture) may accelerate the process of allergen removal once the pet is removed. Many cat-sensitive patients are exposed to cat allergens outside their home and should receive advice about avoiding these other settings. If the cat remains in the home, measures should include restricting pets to one area and creating a "safe room" in the child's bedroom by not allowing pets into the room and keeping the door closed, but this will not remove exposure—it will only reduce it. Dense filter material may be placed over forced air outlets to trap airborne dander particles. Washing cats may temporarily decrease the amount of cat dander and dried saliva in the environment, but this is impractical because the allergen quickly reaccumulates.[6,81] Other methods include removing carpeting and heavily contaminated items, using HEPA filter vacuums and filters, regular damp mopping, weekly cat bathing, and washing cat-contaminated items. Many of these methods have been found to temporarily reduce airborne cat allergen levels by about 90%, but emphasis should be placed on the word temporary.[87,88] HEPA filters are effective for cat allergen only when used with the other measures.[30] Although these efforts focus on reduction of exposure for children with asthma, limited studies suggest that in some children, early contact with cats and dogs may, in fact, prevent allergy more effectively than avoiding these animals.[9,10,40–42,89,90]

Dog allergens provoke significant bronchial hyperresponsiveness in people less often than do cat allergens because dog allergy is less prevalent. Guidelines recommended for minimizing cat allergen exposure should also be followed for minimizing dog allergen exposure.

Levels of airborne rodent urinary allergens have been reduced in most laboratory environments by regulations that mandate rapid room air exchanges and high-efficiency filters. Intervention strategies for pest control have been studied for people exposed to infestations in housing and have demonstrated reduction in allergen levels but mixed results on asthma symptom outcomes.[91-93] These pest control strategies employed Integrated Pest Management (IPM), a method of pest control that aims to minimize pesticide applications. IPM practitioners seek to block pests' entry points, remove their food sources, and aim for using pesticide gels and baits rather than sprays.

### Cockroaches

Cockroaches may be found wherever water, heat, and organic material are present.[82] It is essential to minimize organic material on open surfaces to reduce infestation. Other control measures include storing all foodstuffs in sealed containers, eliminating water sources, eating only in the kitchen, taking trash out daily, caulking all cracks around faucets and pipe fittings, and placing roach gel baits and bait stations in kitchens and bathrooms.[6,94,95] Boric acid can be used in areas not accessible to children. Gel baits have been demonstrated to reduce allergen levels in homes and decrease asthma morbidity in children.[95] When considering using other pesticides, families must balance the risks of cockroaches, the severity of asthma, and the risks of pesticide use. IPM for pest control should be employed (see Table 47-2 and Chapter 40). Families should avoid using over-the-counter "bug sprays," because they may cause toxic reactions and may also exacerbate asthma. Cockroach allergens are carried on particles similar in size to dust-mite allergens. Therefore, exposure to cockroach allergens may be related to brief resuspension of settled dust. Concentrations of cockroach allergen are higher in kitchens but often are found in bedrooms. The same physical barrier and cleaning interventions recommended for dust-mite allergen may reduce exposure to cockroach allergen. Reducing cockroach allergen in infested homes decreases asthma symptoms and complications in children.[95,96]

### Dust Mites

Eliminating dust-mite exposure reduces symptoms and the degree of nonspecific bronchial hyperreactivity.[97] Because dust-mite allergen is carried on relatively large particles, exposure is likely mostly related to breathing allergen that is resuspended during activity. Encasing mattresses, pillows, and box springs in allergen-impermeable covers and washing bedding regularly in hot water are the most important avoidance measures to reduce dust-mite exposure. Plastic or vinyl covers are an economical choice for box springs but may be uncomfortable for use on mattresses and pillows.[98] Vapor- or air-permeable covers that prevent the passage of allergens are available for a comparable price.[78,79-98] Clinical intervention trials have shown substantial allergen reduction and improvement in asthma symptoms with dust-mite allergen reduction methods (impervious pillow and mattress covers and weekly hot water washing of bed linens). Normal laundering (adequate room, moderately

## Table 47-2. Reducing Exposures in the Home, School, and Child Care Setting[a]

| ENVIRONMENTAL TRIGGERS | STRATEGIES TO REDUCE EXPOSURES |
|---|---|
| **Animal dander** | Remove animal from indoor environment; at a minimum, keep animal out of the child's room |
| **House-dust mites** | **Recommended:**<br>■ Encase mattress in an allergen-impermeable cover<br>■ Encase pillow in an allergen-impermeable cover or wash it weekly<br>■ Wash sheets and blankets on the child's bed in hot water weekly<br>■ Prolonged exposure to dry heat or freezing can kill mites but does not remove the allergen<br><br>**Desirable:**<br>■ Reduce indoor humidity to or below 60%, ideally 30%–50%<br>■ Remove carpets from the bedroom<br>■ Avoid sleeping or lying on upholstered furniture<br>■ Remove carpets that are laid on concrete<br>■ Select floor coverings at schools and child care settings on the basis of functional use |
| **Cockroaches** | ■ Use poison bait or traps to control insects; intensive cleaning is necessary to reduce reservoirs<br>■ Do not leave food or garbage exposed<br>■ Use integrated pest management (IPM) methods |
| **Rodents** | ■ Use IPM methods<br>■ Do not leave food or garbage exposed |

| Pollens (from trees, grass, or weeds) and outdoor molds | ▪ If possible, stay indoors with windows closed during periods of peak pollen exposure, usually during midday and afternoon<br>▪ Run air conditioning on recirculation setting if possible<br>▪ At school and child care settings, schedule physical activities indoors when pollen or pollutant levels are excessive |
|---|---|
| **Indoor molds** | ▪ Fix all leaks and eliminate other sources of water intrusion<br>▪ Clean moldy surfaces and remove reservoirs of indoor and relevant outdoor mold<br>▪ Reduce indoor humidity to or below 60%, ideally 30%–50%<br>▪ Dehumidify basements if possible<br>▪ Ensure that exhaust fans or other sources of ventilation are used in areas of increased humidity (eg, bathrooms, kitchens) and that they are functioning effectively |
| **Secondhand tobacco smoke** | ▪ Advise parents and others in the home who smoke to stop smoking. Smoking outside the home will reduce but will not eliminate the child's exposure<br>▪ Advise the adolescent smoker to stop smoking<br>▪ Promote tobacco-free schools and child care centers |
| **Indoor/Outdoor pollutants and irritants** | ▪ Discuss ways to reduce exposures to:<br>▪ Wood-burning stoves or fireplaces<br>▪ Unvented gas stoves or heaters<br>▪ Other irritants (eg, perfumes, cleaning agents, sprays)<br>▪ Sources of volatile organic compounds (VOCs), such as new carpeting, particle board, paint |

[a] Adapted from National Institutes of Health Asthma Practice Guidelines, 2007.[6]

warm water, and a variety of commercial laundry detergents) is sufficient to extract most dust mite and cat allergens from bedding.[99] Further studies are needed to determine whether there are differences in clinical outcomes after different laundering conditions.

Alternatives to hot water washing that kill mites include drying bedding outside in the sun (dust mites are sensitive to sunlight), drying in a tumble dryer at 130°F (54°C) for at least 20 minutes, and placing soft toys in the freezer for 24 hours.[6,96] Dry cleaning of blankets kills mites but is less effective in removing allergens.

Carpeting, a major source of mite antigen and proliferation, should be removed when possible, especially in bedrooms. A single vacuuming may decrease the dust-mite burden by only 35% for a carpeted surface but by 80% for a solid surface. If possible, upholstered furniture should be replaced with washable vinyl, leather, or wood. Window shades are preferable to curtains or venetian blinds. If curtains are used, they should be made of washable fabric. Blinds should be made of vinyl. Although acaricides (chemicals that kill mites) containing benzyl benzoate or tannic acid may reduce antigen levels on carpeting and upholstery, they must be reapplied every 3 months. Using acaricides is far less effective than removing carpet followed by regular damp mopping of hardwood or vinyl flooring. Therefore, many experts no longer recommend the use of acaricides in routine management of allergen avoidance.[6]

Because dust-mite allergen becomes airborne only during disturbances and falls rapidly, there is little opportunity for air cleaners to have an effect. Vacuum cleaners that incorporate a HEPA filter or double-thickness bag to prevent leakage of allergen may be helpful.

Strategies to control humidity to limit growth of dust mites vary according to climate.[31,32,89] In humid climates (ie, at least 8 months per year with relative outdoor humidity 50%), controlling reservoirs for dust mites is key. Successful dehumidification of homes is very difficult in truly humid climates (eg, the southeastern United States). Air conditioning to maintain indoor relative humidity below 50% requires tight housing and may be expensive to achieve. Air conditioning in the bedroom may be considered. In areas of moderate or seasonal humidity, mite growth may be strongly seasonal and growth can be substantially higher in areas of the house that maintain humidity (eg, carpets laid on a concrete slab). During dry seasons, opening windows for an hour per day will ensure removal of humidity from the house.[31,32] In dry climates (eg, the upper Midwest, the mountain states [altitude 5,000 feet]) and the southwestern United States, growth of dust mites in homes is minimal unless the house is humidified.

## Fungi (Molds)

Home remediation to reduce moisture sources is effective in decreasing asthma morbidity.[100,101] Because mold growth requires water, the water source must be eliminated to prevent and control mold growth. Sources of water include leaking roofs or pipes, prior flooding or rainwater, and condensation on pipes and ductwork within interior or exterior structure walls. To keep a home dry, exhaust fans in the kitchen and bathrooms should be in working order and used. Dehumidifiers can be considered for areas with consistently elevated humidity levels, with a target of <50% relative humidity. Dehumidifiers reduce ambient humidity but do not significantly reduce mold growth on surfaces in contact with groundwater.

### Outdoor Air Pollution and Allergens

In communities with recognized periods of increased ozone levels, pediatricians should counsel patients with asthma and their families about the health effects of ozone. Parents, physical education teachers, and coaches should consider modifying sports practice schedules on days with high ozone levels (see Chapter 21).

It is important to identify seasonal allergens that trigger a patient's asthma. The physician can then initiate prophylactic antihistamine and/or anti-inflammatory therapies and/or recommend using air conditioning, if available. Staying indoors during the afternoon hours may help symptoms. Molds, especially *Alternaria* species, may be present outdoors year-round in moderate climates but are greatly reduced following the onset of frost or recurrent freezing temperatures. Affected persons should be instructed to follow pollution alerts for high pollen counts, especially during the summer months.

### Frequently Asked Questions

Q   *Do you recommend any special air filtration system for patients with asthma?*

A   Avoid room humidifiers and keep central furnace system humidification below 50% during winter months. Filters on central forced-air systems and furnaces should be changed regularly, according to manufacturers' recommendations. The MERV rating (Minimum Efficiency Reporting Value) is the standard method for comparing the efficiency of air filters. The higher the MERV rating, the better the filter is at removing particles from the air. Upgrading to a medium-efficiency filter (rated at 20%–50% efficiency at removing particles between 0.3 and 10 mcm [MERV 8–12]) will improve air quality and is economical. Electrostatic filters/precipitators in central furnace and air-conditioning systems may be beneficial for airborne particles (eg, cat allergen). Avoid the use of air cleaners (usually labeled as electrostatic) that generate ozone.

Room HEPA filters also may be beneficial. However, they only work in a single room, and the noise generated may not be acceptable. Preferably, they should be used in the child's bedroom.

Q   *Do you recommend a special vacuum cleaner for patients with asthma?*

A   Other strategies to reduce allergen exposure are more beneficial. However, an efficient vacuum cleaner that avoids resuspension of allergens may be useful for removing allergens, especially from hard surfaces. Leakage of allergen is minimized in vacuum cleaners that incorporate a double-thickness bag and have tight-fitting junctions within the cleaner; a HEPA filter is not always necessary, depending on vacuum design. Unfortunately, there is no certification process to guide consumers.

Q   *How can we better prepare the house to prevent asthma attacks from occurring?*

A   Quit smoking if you smoke and eliminate exposures to SHS by making sure your home and car are kept smoke-free. Reduce dust mites, cockroaches, and home dampness or molds. Consider removing carpeting. Remove pets to which the child demonstrates specific allergy. If removing the pet is not possible, keep pets out of the bedroom and routinely perform allergen reduction measures (vacuuming, minimizing reservoirs of dander—eg, pillows). If the pet is not removed, it will be nearly impossible to avoid exposure. Consider using a vacuum cleaner that is efficient at cleaning and avoids resuspension of allergens (such as one equipped with a HEPA filter).

Q   *Can odors of cooking foods cause an allergic reaction (eg, asthma) in susceptible patients?*

A   Allergenic proteins aerosolized from foods during the cooking process may cause reactions in some patients. For example, frying an egg or fish in a pan in a closed area without sufficient ventilation can lead to airway symptoms in children with an egg or fish allergy. The presence of a positive skin-prick test or the presence of an elevated IgE to a given food should not necessarily lead to an elimination diet, however, because positive tests are not necessarily highly predictive of clinical food allergy. Children with a suspected reaction or a positive IgE test should be evaluated by an allergist.

Q   *Should I use a humidifier?*

A   Humidifiers should be avoided. A relative humidity of greater than 50% promotes the growth of dust mites and mold. If used, the humidifier must be cleaned frequently to prevent the growth of mold.

Q   *Are foam pillows safe for children or can they also be allergenic?*

A   All pillows, regardless of content, may serve as reservoirs for dust mites and other allergens. An allergen-impermeable pillow cover should be used as a physical barrier between dust-mite reservoirs in pillows and the child.

Q   *My family lives in a multi-unit building where there is pest infestation and cigarette smoking in common areas. What can I do about this?*

A   If other families share your concerns about issues such as pest control, mold problems, and cigarette smoking, you may want to organize as a group to alert management to your concerns for your children's health. Many health departments have regulations regarding pest infestation and cigarette smoking in multifamily housing, so consult your local health department.

Q   *Should I worry about my young child swimming in a chlorinated pool?*

A   Some studies have demonstrated that repeated exposure to chlorine byproducts among recreational swimmers may lead to lung harm.[102] In addition, some studies have been published on the issue of the possible harmful effects of swimming on a baby's respiratory health. Concerns are primarily with indoor chlorinated pools. Long-term studies are needed to clarify this issue.

Q   *I have heard that antioxidants can prevent asthma in my child. Should I give her a supplement?*

A   Studies of vitamins and antioxidants have not shown consistent results regarding preventing the development of asthma or improving asthma control.[103,104]

Q   *I have mold in my home. Should I worry that my daughter is allergic to it?*

A   Testing for sensitivity to mold in children without allergy symptoms is not recommended. Performing these tests in patients who do not have symptoms may lead to an incorrect diagnosis. Positive skin tests or serologic tests do not necessarily translate into clinical disease. The interpretation of IgE-specific results must be done in the context of the patient's clinical presentation. Moldy surfaces should, however, be cleaned, and it is important to fix leaks and other sources of water intrusion to prevent further mold growth.

Q   *My child has asthma, but I don't have any mold, animals, or insects in my home that I can see. Could she have an allergy to dust mites?*

A   If your child has asthma and allergy symptoms, allergy testing will typically be done. Dust mites are common indoor allergens and will be part of the allergy test panel. They are a known trigger of asthma and there is evidence that avoidance improves asthma outcomes. Allergy shots may help patients with asthma who are sensitized to dust mites. Allergy testing may include a skin test or a blood test.

## Resources

**Allergy & Asthma Network – Mothers of Asthmatics, Inc**
Phone: 800-878-4403
Web site: www.aanma.org

**American Lung Association**
Phone: 800-LUNG-USA
Web site: www.lungusa.org

**Asthma and Allergy Foundation of America**
Phone: 202-466-7643
Web site: www.aafa.org

**California Indoor Air Quality Program**
Air cleaners: www.arb.ca.gov/research/indoor/aircleaners.htm

**National Environmental Education Foundation**
Phone: 202-833-2933
Web site: www.neefusa.org

**National Heart Lung and Blood Health Information Center**
Phone: 301-592-8573 (Public) or 1-800 877-8339 (Federal Relay Service)
Web site: www.nhlbi.nih.gov/health/infoctr/index.htm

**National Institutes of Health, National Heart Lung and Blood Institute**
Web site: www.nhlbi.nih.gov

**University of California**
Residential, Industrial, and Institutional Pest Control. 2nd ed. Pesticide
Application Compendium,
Vol 2. Davis, CA: University of California; 2006.
Web site: www.ipm.ucdavis.edu/IPMPROJECT/ADS/manual_
riipestcontrol.html

**US Environmental Protection Agency, Indoor Environments Division**
IAQ Tools for Schools Program: www.epa.gov/iaq/schools
Asthma: www.epa.gov/asthma

**US Environmental Protection Agency, Transportation and Air Quality
Division**
National Clean Diesel Campaign – Clean School Bus USA: www.epa.gov/
cleanschoolbus

# References

1. Busse WW, Lemanske RF Jr. Asthma. *N Engl J Med.* 2001;344(5):350–362
2. DeVries A, Vercelli D. Early predictors of asthma and allergy in children: the role of epigenetics. *Curr Opin Allergy Clin Immunol.* 2015;15(5):435–439
3. Murphy TM, Wong CC, Arseneault L, et al. Methylomic markers of persistent childhood asthma: a longitudinal study of asthma-discordant monozygotic twins. *Clin Epigenetics.* 2015;7:130
4. Yang IV, Pedersen BS, Liu A, et al. DNA methylation and childhood asthma in the inner city. *J Allergy Clin Immunol.* 2015;136(1):69–80
5. Holgate ST. Pathogenesis of asthma. *Clin Exp Allergy.* 2008;38(6):872–897
6. National Institutes of Health, National Asthma Education Program. *Expert Panel Report 3 (EPR-3): Guidelines for the Diagnosis and Management of Asthma.* Bethesda, MD: National Institutes of Health, National Heart, Lung, and Blood Institute; 2007. Publication NIH 08-4051. Updated April 2012. https://www.nhlbi.nih.gov/files/docs/guidelines/asthsumm.pdf. Accessed March 6, 2018
7. Bufford JD, Gern JE. The hygiene hypothesis revisited. *Immunol Allergy Clin North Am.* 2005; 25(2):247–262
8. Platts-Mills TA, Blumenthal K, Perzanowski M, Woodfolk JA. Determinants of clinical allergic disease. The relevance of indoor allergens to the increase in asthma. *Am J Respir Crit Care Med.* 2000;162(3 Pt 2):S128–S133
9. Platts-Mills TA. Paradoxical effect of domestic animals on asthma and allergic sensitization. *JAMA.* 2002;288(8):1012–1014
10. Celedon JC, Litonjua AA, Ryan L, Platts-Mills T, Weiss ST, Gold DR. Exposure to cat allergen, maternal history of asthma, and wheezing in first 5 years of life. *Lancet.* 2002;360(9335):781–782
11. O'Connor GT, Lynch SV, Bloomberg GR, et al. Early-life home environment and risk of asthma among inner-city children. *J Allergy Clin Immunol.* 2017;Sep 12. pii: S0091-6749(17)31204-6 (Epub ahead of print)
12. Gehring U, Wijga AH, Brauer M, et al. Traffic-related air pollution and the development of asthma and allergies during the first 8 years of life. *Am J Respir Crit Care Med.* 2010;181(6): 596–603
13. Donohue KM, Miller RL, Perzanowski MS, et al. Prenatal and postnatal bisphenol A exposure and asthma development among inner-city children. *J Allergy Clin Immunol.* 2013;131(3):736–742
14. North ML, Takaro TK, Diamond ML, Ellis AK. Effects of phthalates on the development and expression of allergic disease and asthma. *Ann Allergy Asthma Immunol.* 2014;112(6):496–502
15. Robinson L, Miller R. The impact of bisphenol A and phthalates on allergy, asthma, and immune function: a review of latest findings. *Curr Environ Health Rep.* 2015;2(4):379–387
16. Shu H, Jonsson BA, Larsson M, Nanberg E, Bornehag CG. PVC flooring at home and development of asthma among young children in Sweden, a 10-year follow-up. *Indoor Air.* 2014;24(3):227–235
17. Spanier AJ, Kahn RS, Kunselman AR, et al. Prenatal exposure to bisphenol A and child wheeze from birth to 3 years of age. *Environ Health Perspect.* 2012;120(6):916–920
18. Johnson CC, Ownby DR. The infant gut bacterial microbiota and risk of pediatric asthma and allergic diseases. *Transl Res.* 2017;179:60–70
19. Dick S, Friend A, Dynes K, et al. A systematic review of associations between environmental exposures and development of asthma in children aged up to 9 years. *BMJ Open.* 2014;4(11): e006554
20. Gaffin JM, Phipatanakul W. The role of indoor allergens in the development of asthma. *Curr Opin Allergy Clin Immunol.* 2009;9(2):128–135

21. Etzel RA. How environmental exposures influence the development and exacerbation of asthma. *Pediatrics*. 2003;112(1 Pt 2):233–239

22. Yu O, Sheppard L, Lumley T, Koenig JQ, Shapiro GG. Effects of ambient air pollution on symptoms of asthma in Seattle-area children enrolled in the CAMP study. *Environ Health Perspect*. 2000;108(12):1209–1214

23. Jamal A, King BA, Neff LJ, Whitmill J, Babb SD, Graffunder CM. Cigarette smoking among adults—United States, 2005-2015. *MMWR Morb Mortal Wkly Rep*. 2016;65(44):1205–1211

24. US Department of Health and Human Services. *The Health Consequences of Involuntary Exposure to Tobacco Smoke: A Report of the Surgeon General*. Centers for Disease Control and Prevention, Coordinating Center for Health Promotion, National Center for Chronic Disease Prevention and Health Promotion, Office on Smoking and Health; 2006

25. Duijts L, Jaddoe VWV, van der Valk RJP, et al. Fetal exposure to maternal and paternal smoking and the risks of wheezing in preschool children: the Generation R Study. *Chest*. 2012;141(4):876–885

26. Cohen RT, Raby BA, Van Steen K, et al. In utero smoke exposure and impaired response to inhaled corticosteroids in children with asthma. *J Allergy Clin Immunol*. 2010;126(3):491–497

27. Oh SS, Tcheurekdjian H, Roth LA, et al. Effect of secondhand smoke on asthma control among black and Latino children. *J Allergy Clin Immunol*. 2012;129(6):1478–1483.e7

28. Hollams EM, de Klerk NH, Holt PG, Sly PD. Persistent effects of maternal smoking during pregnancy on lung function and asthma in adolescents. *Am J Respir Crit Care Med*. 2014;189(4):401–407

29. Burke H, Leonardi-Bee J, Hashim A, et al. Prenatal and passive smoke exposure and incidence of asthma and wheeze: systematic review and meta-analysis. *Pediatrics*. 2012;129(4):735–744

30. Feleszko W, Ruszczynski M, Jaworska J, Strzelak A, Zalewsli BM, Kulus M. Environmental tobacco smoke exposure and risk of allergic sensitization in children: a systematic review and meta-analysis. *Arch Dis Child*. 2014;99(11):985–992

31. Institute of Medicine. *Clearing the Air: Asthma and Indoor Air Exposures*. Washington, DC: National Academies Press; 2000

32. Kanchongkittiphon W, Mendell MJ, Gaffin JM, Wang G, Phipatanakul W. Indoor environmental exposures and exacerbation of asthma: an update to the 2000 review by the Institute of Medicine. *Environ Health Perspect*. 2015;123(1):6–20

33. Delfino RJ. Epidemiologic evidence for asthma and exposure to air toxics: linkages between occupational, indoor, and community air pollution research. *Environ Health Perspect*. 2002;110(Suppl 4):573–589

34. Hansel NN, Breysse PN, McCormack MC, et al. A longitudinal study of indoor nitrogen dioxide levels and respiratory symptoms in inner-city children with asthma. *Environ Health Perspect*. 2008;116(10):1428–1432

35. Shim C, Williams MH Jr. Effect of odors in asthma. *Am J Med*. 1986;80(1):18–22

36. McGwin G, Lienert J, Kennedy JI. Formaldehyde exposure and asthma in children: a systematic review. *Environ Health Perspect*. 2009;118(3):313–317

37. Wood RA, Eggleston PA. Management of allergy to animal danders. *Pediatr Asthma Allergy Immunol*. 1993;7(1):13–22

38. Luczynska CM, Li Y, Chapman MD, Platts-Mills TA. Airborne concentrations and particle size distribution of allergen derived from domestic cats *(Felis domesticus)*. Measurements using cascade impactor, liquid impinger, and a two-site monoclonal antibody assay for *Fel d I*. *Am Rev Respir Dis*. 1990;141(2):361–367

39. Almquist C, Wickman M, Perfetti L, et al. Worsening of asthma in children allergic to cats, after indirect exposure to cat at school. *Am J Respir Crit Care Med*. 2001;163(3 Pt 1):694–698

40. Collin SM, Granell R, Westgarth C, et al. Pet ownership is associated with increased risk of non-atopic asthma and reduced risk of atopy in childhood: findings from a UK birth cohort. *Clin Exp Allergy.* 2015;45(1):200–210

41. Lodrup Carlsen KC, Roll S, Carlsen KH, et al. Does pet ownership in infancy lead to asthma or allergy at school age? Pooled analysis of individual participant data from 11 European birth cohorts. *PLoS One.* 2012;7(8):e43214

42. Konradsen JR, Fujisawa T, van Hage M, et al. Allergy to furry animals: new insights, diagnostic approaches, and challenges. *J Allergy Clin Immunol.* 2015;135(3):616–625

43. de Groot H, Goei KG, van Swieten P, Aalberse RC. Affinity purification of a major and a minor allergen from dog extract: serologic activity of affinity-purified *Can f I* and of *Can f I*-depleted extract. *J Allergy Clin Immunol.* 1991;87(6):1056–1065

44. Lindgren S, Belin L, Dreborg S, Einarsson R, Pahlman I. Breed-specific dog-dandruff allergens. *J Allergy Clin Immunol.* 1988;82(2):196–204

45. Phipatanakul W, Eggleston PA, Wright EC, Wood RA. Mouse allergen. I. The prevalence of mouse allergen in inner-city homes. The National Cooperative Inner-City Asthma Study. *J Allergy Clin Immunol.* 2000;106(6):1070–1074

46. Perry T, Matsui E, Merriman B, Duong T, Eggleston P. The prevalence of rat allergen in inner-city homes and its relationship to sensitization and asthma morbidity. *J Allergy Clin Immunol.* 2003;112(2):346–352

47. Phipatanakul W, Celedon JC, Hoffman EB, Abdulkerim H, Ryan LM, Gold DR. Mouse allergen exposure, wheeze and atopy in the first seven years of life. *Allergy.* 2008;63(11):1512–1518

48. Rosensteich DL, Eggleston P, Kattan M, et al. The role of cockroach allergy and exposure to cockroach allergen in causing morbidity among inner-city children with asthma. *N Engl J Med.* 1997;336(19):1356–1363

49. Peat JK, Dickerson J, Li J. Effects of damp and mould in the home on respiratory health: a review of the literature. *Allergy.* 1998;53(2):120–128

50. Thacher JD, Gruzieva O, Pershagen G, et al. Mold and dampness exposure and allergic outcomes from birth to adolescence: data from the BAMSE cohort. *Allergy.* 2017;72(6):967–974

51. Institute of Medicine. *Damp Indoor Spaces and Health.* Washington, DC: National Academies Press; 2004

52. American Academy of Pediatrics Committee on Environmental Health. Policy statement: spectrum of noninfectious health effects from molds. *Pediatrics.* 2006;118(6):2582–2586

53. Mazur LJ, Kim J, American Academy of Pediatrics Committee on Environmental Health. Technical report: spectrum of noninfectious health effects from molds. *Pediatrics.* 2006;118(6):e1909–e1926

54. Pongracic JA, O'Connor GT, Muilenberg ML, et al. Differential effects of outdoor vs indoor fungal spores on asthma morbidity in inner-city children. *J Allergy Clin Immunol.* 2010;125(3):593–599

55. Iossifova YY, Reponen T, Ryan PH, et al. Mold exposure during infancy as a predictor of potential asthma development. *Ann Allergy Asthma Immunol.* 2009;102(2):131–137

56. World Health Organization. *WHO Guidelines for Indoor Air Quality: Dampness and Mold.* Copenhagen, Denmark: World Health Organization; 2009

57. Nafstad P, Oie L, Mehl R, et al. Residential dampness problems and symptoms and signs of bronchial obstruction in young Norwegian children. *Am J Respir Crit Care Med.* 1998;157(2):410–414

58. Dales RE, Miller D. Residential fungal contamination and health: microbial cohabitants as covariates. *Environ Health Perspect.* 1999;107(Suppl 3):481–483

59. Tischer C, Chen CM, Heinrich J. Association between domestic mould and mould components, and asthma and allergy in children: a systematic review. *Eur Respir J.* 2011;38(4):812–814

60. Reponen T, Lockey J, Bernstein DI, et al. Infant origins of childhood asthma associated with specific molds. *J Allergy Clin Immunol.* 2012;130(3):639–644

61. Landwehr LP, Boguniewicz M. Current perspectives on latex allergy. *J Pediatr.* 1996;128(3): 305–312

62. Sicherer SH, Sampson HA. Food allergy. *J Allergy Clin Immunol.* 2010;125(2 Suppl 2):S116–S125

63. Yip FY, Pearcy JN, Garbe PL, Truman BI, Centers for Disease Control and Prevention. Unhealthy air quality – United States, 2006 – 2009. *MMWR Suppl.* 2011;60(1):28–32

64. Gauderman WJ, Urman R, Avol E, et al. Association of improved air quality with lung development in children. *N Engl J Med.* 2015;372(10):905–913

65. White MC, Etzel RA, Wilcox WD, Lloyd C. Exacerbations of childhood asthma and ozone pollution in Atlanta. *Environ Res.* 1994;65(1):56–68

66. American Academy of Pediatrics Committee on Environmental Health. Ambient air pollution: respiratory hazards to children. *Pediatrics.* 1993;91(6):1210–1213

67. McConnell R, Berhane K, Gilliland F, et al. Asthma in exercising children exposed to ozone: a cohort study. *Lancet.* 2002;359(9304):386–391

68. Licorish K, Novey HS, Kozak P, Fairshter RD, Wilson AF. Role of *Alternaria* and *Penicillium* spores in the pathogenesis of asthma. *J Allergy Clin Immunol.* 1985;76(6):819–825

69. O'Hollaren MT, Yunginger JW, Offord KP, et al. Exposure to an aeroallergen as a possible precipitating factor in respiratory arrest in young patients with asthma. *N Engl J Med.* 1991;324(6):359–363

70. Targonski PV, Perskey VW, Ramekrishnan V. Effect of environmental molds on risk of death from asthma during the pollen season. *J Allergy Clin Immunol.* 1995;95(5 Pt 1):955–961

71. Dales RA, Cakmak S, Judek S, et al. The role of fungal spores in thunderstorm asthma. *Chest.* 2003;123(3):745–750

72. Rangamuwa KB, Young AC, Thien F. An epidemic of thunderstorm asthma in Melbourne 2016: asthma, rhinitis, and other previous allergies. *Asia Pac Allergy.* 2017;7(4):193–198

73. Simmons FE. Anaphylaxis: recent advances in assessment and treatment. *J Allergy Clin Immunol.* 2009;124(4):625–636

74. Denning DW, O'Driscoll BR, Powell G, et al. Randomized controlled trial of oral antifungal treatment for severe asthma with fungal sensitization: the Fungal Asthma Sensitization Trial (FAST) Study. *Am J Respir Crit Care Med.* 2009;179(1):11–18

75. Wu F, Takaro TK. Childhood asthma and environmental interventions. *Environ Health Perspect.* 2007;115(6):971–975

76. Krieger JK, Takaro TK, Allen C, et al. The Seattle-King County healthy homes project: implementation of a comprehensive approach to improving indoor environmental quality for low-income children with asthma. *Environ Health Perspect.* 2002;110(Suppl 2):311–322

77. Etzel RA. Indoor air pollution and childhood asthma: effective environmental interventions. *Environ Health Perspect.* 1995;103(Suppl 6):55–58

78. Tovey E, Marks G. Methods and effectiveness of environmental control. *J Allergy Clin Immunol.* 1999;103(2 Pt 1):179–191

79. Murray CS, Foden P, Sumner H, Shepley E, Custovic A, Simpson A. Preventing severe asthma exacerbations in children. A randomized trial of mite-impermeable bedcovers. *Am J Respir Crit Care Med.* 2017;196(2):150–158

80. Portnoy J, Chew GL, Phipatanakul W, et al. Environmental assessment and exposure reduction of cockroaches: a practice parameter. *J Allergy Clin Immunol.* 2013;132(4):802–808.e1–25

81. Portnoy J, Miller JD, Williams PB, et al. Environmental assessment and exposure control of dust mites: a practice parameter. *Ann Allergy Asthma Immunol.* 2013;111(6):465–507

82. Gold Dr, Adamkiewicz G, Arshad SH, et al. NIAID, NIEHS, NHLBI and MCAN Workshop report: the indoor environment and childhood asthma-implications for home environmental intervention in asthma prevention and management. *J Allergy Clin Immunol*. 2017;140(4): 933–949

83. American Academy of Pediatrics Committee on School Health, National Association of School Nurses. *Health, Mental Health, and Safety Guidelines for Schools*. Taras H, Duncan P, Luckenbill D, et al, eds. Elk Grove Village, IL: American Academy of Pediatrics; 2004

84. Tschudy MM, Sharfstein J, Matsui E, et al. Something new in the air: paying for community-based environmental approaches to asthma prevention and control. *J Allergy Clin Immunol*. 2017;140(5):1244–1249

85. Lanphear BP, Hornung RW, Khoury J, Yolton K, Lierl M, Kalkbrenner A. Effects of HEPA air cleaners on unscheduled asthma visits and asthma symptoms for children exposed to secondhand tobacco smoke. *Pediatrics*. 2011;127(1):93–101

86. Butz AM, Matsui EC, Breysse P, et al. A randomized trial of air cleaners and a health coach to improve indoor air quality for inner-city children with asthma and secondhand smoke exposure. *Arch Pediatr Adolesc Med*. 2011;165(8):741–748

87. Sulser C, Schulz G, Wagner P, et al. Can the use of HEPA cleaners in homes of asthmatic children and adolescents sensitized to cat and dog allergens decrease bronchial hyperresponsiveness and allergen contents in solid dust? *Int Arch Allergy Immunol*. 2009;148(1):23–30

88. Kerkhof M, Wijga AH, Brunekreef B, et al. Effects of pets on asthma development up to 8 years of age: the PIAMA study. *Allergy*. 2009;64(8):1202–1208

89. Call RS, Smith TF, Morris E, Chapman MD, Platts-Mills TA. Risk factors for asthma in inner city children. *J Pediatr*. 1992;121(6):862–866

90. House JS, Wyss AB, Hoppin JA, et al. Early-life farm exposures and adult asthma and atopy in the Agricultural Lung Health Study. *J Allergy Clin Immunol*. 2017;140(1):249–256

91. Phipatanakul W, Cronin B, Wood RA, et al. Effect of environmental intervention on mouse allergen levels in homes of inner-city Boston children with asthma. *Ann Allergy Asthma Immunol*. 2004;92(4):420–425

92. Pongracic JA, Visness CM, Gruchalla RS, Evans R 3rd, Mitchell HE. Effect of mouse allergen and rodent environmental intervention on asthma in inner-city children. *Ann Allergy Asthma Immunol*. 2008;101(1):35–41

93. Matsui EC, Perzanowski M, Peng RD, et al. Effect of an integrated pest management intervention on asthma symptoms among mouse-sensitized children and adolescents with asthma: a randomized clinical trial. *JAMA*. 2017;317(10):1027–1036

94. O'Connor GT, Gold DR. Cockroach allergy and asthma in a 30-year-old man. *Environ Health Perspect*. 1999;107(3):243–247

95. Rabito FA, Carlson JC, He H, Werthmann D, Schal C. A single intervention for cockroach control reduces cockroach exposure and asthma morbidity in children. *J Allergy Clin Immunol*. 2017;140(2):565–570

96. Morgan WJ, Crain EF, Gruchalla RS, et al. Results of a home-based environmental intervention among urban children with asthma. *N Engl J Med*. 2004;351(11):1068–1080

97. von Mutius E. Towards prevention. *Lancet*. 1997;350(Suppl 2):SII14–SII17

98. Murray CS, Foden P, Sumner H, Shepley E, Custovic A, Simpson A. Preventing severe asthma exacerbations in children: a randomized trial of mite-impermeable bedcovers. *Am J Respir Crit Care Med*. 2017;196(2):150–158

99. Tovey ER, Taylor DJ, Mitakakis TZ, De Lucca SD. Effectiveness of laundry washing agents and conditions in the removal of cat and dust mite allergen from bedding dust. *J Allergy Clin Immunol*. 2001;108(3):369–374

100. Kercsmar CM, Dearborn DG, Schluchter M, et al. Reduction in asthma morbidity in children as a result of home remediation aimed at moisture sources. *Environ Health Perspect.* 2006;114(10):1574–1580

101. Burr ML, Matthews IP, Arthur RA, et al. Effects on patients with asthma of eradicating visible indoor mould: a randomised controlled trial. *Thorax.* 2007;62(9):767–772

102. Uyan ZS, Carraro S, Piacentini G, Baraldi E. Swimming pool, respiratory health, and childhood asthma: should we change our beliefs? *Pediatr Pulmonol.* 2009;44(1):31–37

103. Strait RT, Camargo CA. Vitamin E and the risk of childhood asthma. *Expert Rev Respir Med.* 2016;10(8):881–890

104. Riccioni G, Barbara M, Bucciarelli T, di Ilio C, D'Orazio N. Antioxidant vitamin supplementation in asthma. *Ann Clin Lab Sci.* 2007;37(1):96–101

Chapter 48

# Birth Defects and Other Adverse Developmental Outcomes

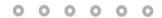

## KEY POINTS

- Although much of embryonic and fetal development is determined by genetics, environmental factors also may impact fetal growth and development either directly when a toxicant interferes with organ system development, or indirectly through epigenetic mechanisms.
- Clinicians should inform women of childbearing age to take appropriate precautions to avoid potentially toxic substances, such as tobacco; eat nutritious foods; exercise; see their clinician regularly; and take at least 400 mcg of folic acid daily.
- Economic, social, and emotional factors may have significant impacts that can be mitigated by good nutrition, emotional and social supports, and close monitoring of mother and baby.

## INTRODUCTION

Birth defects are structural or functional abnormalities present at birth that can cause physical disability, intellectual and developmental disability, and/or other adverse health outcomes. Their etiologies include genetic conditions, such as chromosome anomalies, environmental factors, or a combination of both. Serious birth defects are the leading cause of death for infants during the first year of life.[1,2]

Prenatal exposure to environmental chemicals can produce adverse pregnancy outcomes, including fetal or neonatal death, structural alterations (birth defects), and functional impairments as a result of alterations in brain structure or function (see Chapter 52), often accompanied by growth restriction.[3-9] These outcomes may be caused by maternal or paternal exposures related to infections, medications, occupational or environmental chemical pollutants,[10-13] and natural or man-made disasters (such as Hurricanes Rita, Katrina, Sandy, and Maria, as well as the World Trade Center collapse). Outcomes occur either through the direct exposure to toxicants or to indirect effects of stress associated with the consequences of dislocation and disruption of daily life and family and community cohesion.[14]

Birth defects and other developmental disorders are recognized in approximately 3% of infants at birth, 6% of children at age 1 year, and 12% of children at age 7 years. The understanding of the etiology of adverse developmental outcomes has changed because appreciation of the increasing number of environmental factors as possible causes has grown, insight into developmental neurobiology has increased, and the roles of genetics and epigenetics are coming to light (Table 48-1) (see Chapter 52).

Most adverse developmental outcomes are of unknown etiology and reported to be between 30% to 70% of all causes. Environmental factors are

**Table 48-1. Estimates of the Etiology of Birth Defects and Other Developmental Disorders[15]**

| CAUSE OF DEVELOPMENTAL DISORDER | PERCENTAGE OF CHILDREN WITH DEVELOPMENTAL DISORDER AT BIRTH |
|---|---|
| *Genetic* | |
| Monogenic conditions | 8–20 |
| Chromosomal disorders | 3–10 |
| *Environmental* | |
| Known Environmental factors | 2–9 |
| Maternal diabetes | 0.1–1.4 |
| Medicinal products | 0.2–1.3 |
| Maternal infection | 1.1–2.0 |
| *Multifactorial and Unknown* | |
| Multifactorial | 20–49 |
| Unknown | 34–70 |

thought to represent less than 10% of known causes. The "multifactorial" category—referring to a model in which risk is a consequence of the interaction among environmental, social, and biological factors—represents about 20% to 50% (Table 48-2). Thus, the effect of environmental factors on adverse developmental outcomes may be significantly under-recognized. It can be inferred from these estimates that various reports find different percentages. Knowledge in this field is evolving.

| ENVIRONMENTAL | SOCIAL | BIOLOGICAL | DEVELOPMENTAL OUTCOME | REFERENCES |
|---|---|---|---|---|
| Active smoking | Community reinforcement and peer pressure | Specific genes interact with tobacco smoke to increase risk of orofacial clefts | Learning disabilities, ADHD, orofacial clefting | 16–18 |
| Air pollution | Exposure is influenced by location of residence and socioeconomic status | Nutritional factors, which vary with socio-economic status, are important in affecting birth weight | Birth weight, preterm birth, with consequent long-term cognitive, learning, or behavioral disorders; low birth weight and preterm birth contribute to increased perinatal mortality | 8,19,20 |
| Exposures to environmental toxins, such as fumonisin, folic acid deficiency | Dietary preferences (corn contaminated with fumonisin), preconception awareness, and household socioeconomic status | Exposures to mycotoxins such as fumonisin that block folate transport, or the use of medications that have anti-folate properties, specific genes, obesity | Neural tube defects | 21–33 |

**Table 48-2. Multifactorial Etiologies of Birth Defects and Other Developmental Disorders**

Abbreviations: ADHD, attention-deficit/hyperactivity disorder

## ADVERSE PREGNANCY OUTCOMES

### Death

If the consequences of chromosomal or genetic abnormalities are significantly disruptive, they may result in embryonic, fetal, or neonatal death. Death attributable to a congenital malformation has been associated with certain paternal occupations.[11–13,34] There are data linking a variety of environmental exposures with fetal and neonatal mortality;[35] for example, increased fetal death rates (thought to be a consequence of reduction in renal blood flow) have been reported when pregnant women were treated with angiotensin-converting enzyme (ACE) inhibitors to control blood pressure.[36]

### Malformation

Malformations are birth defects that occur because of disorders in the development of structural organs, often as a result of genetic and/or chromosomal anomalies (Table 48-3). For certain malformations, environmental exposures can either increase or decrease risk. Neural tube defects (NTDs) result as a consequence of the interaction between genetic and environmental factors (ie, exposure to certain medications, chemicals, and environmental toxicants). NTDs are more likely to occur if a pregnant woman is deficient in folic acid. The U.S. Centers for Disease Control and Prevention (CDC) therefore recommends that women of childbearing age take a daily folic acid supplement of 400 to 800 mcg.[21] Maternal supplementation with folic acid also reduces the risk of congenital heart disease.[37] NTDs are more likely to occur if a pregnant woman is exposed to fumonisin, a mycotoxin found on corn that blocks folate transport,[22–26,38–41] and with other exposures not related to deficiencies in folic acid.[27]

Prenatal exposure to other chemicals and infectious agents have resulted in human structural malformations.[4,6–9] This topic is covered extensively in traditional reviews.[4–7,16,42–44]

| Table 48-3. Outcomes of a Variety of Environmental Exposures During Pregnancy | | | | |
|---|---|---|---|---|
| SITUATION OR TOXIC SUBSTANCE | BIRTH WEIGHT | LENGTH OF GESTATION | STRUCTURAL OR FUNCTIONAL DEFECT | DEATH |
| Agricultural work[45–50] | X | | Total anomalous pulmonary venous return, anencephaly (both maternal and paternal exposures), ocular malformations, orofacial clefts | X (spontaneous abortion) |
| Benzene[51] | X | | Neural tube defects, major cardiac defects | |
| Carbon monoxide[52–54] | X | | | X |

## Table 48-3. (continued)

| SITUATION OR TOXIC SUBSTANCE | BIRTH WEIGHT | LENGTH OF GESTATION | STRUCTURAL OR FUNCTIONAL DEFECT | DEATH |
|---|---|---|---|---|
| Chloroform and other trihalomethanes[55] | X | | Central nervous system defects, orofacial clefts, major cardiac defects | |
| Electronics assembly[34] | X | | | X (paternal exposure) |
| Fumonisins (mycotoxins on corn)[22–26] | | | Neural tube defects | X |
| Hair dye[56] | | | Cardiac defects | |
| Hazardous waste[57] | X | X | Cardiac and circulatory defects, neural tube defects, hypospadias, gastroschisis | |
| Lead[58,59] | X | X | Total anomalous pulmonary venous return, neurodevelopmental impairment | X |
| Methylmercury[60,61] | | | Central nervous system defects, cerebral palsy, orofacial clefts | |
| Paint/paint stripping[56] | | | Total anomalous pulmonary venous return, anencephaly | |
| Particulate matter[62,63] | X | X | | |
| Pesticides[64,65] | | | Neurodevelopmental impairment, childhood cancer | |
| Polychlorinated biphenyls[59,66] | X | | "Yusho" syndrome, orofacial clefts, neurodevelopmental impairment, thyroid function disturbance, motor deficits | |
| Solvents[67,68] | X | | Anencephaly, gastroschisis, cardiac malformations | |
| Tetrachloroethylene[69] | X | | Orofacial clefts | X |
| Trichloroethylene[55,68] | | | Central nervous system defects, neural tube defects, orofacial clefts | |

Table adapted from Table 11.7 in Mattison DR. Developmental toxicology. In: Yaffe SJ, Aranda JV, eds. *Neonatal and Pediatric Pharmacology.* 4th ed. Philadelphia, PA: Lippincott Williams and Wilkins; 2010:130–143. (X indicates that exposure to the toxic substance or occupation is associated with this outcome.)

## Functional Disorders

Functional disorders differ from structural malformations in that there is an impact on function—most significantly affecting the brain with consequent impacts on child development. These disorders may result from adverse prenatal exposures (see Chapter 52). For example, lead is one of the most common neurotoxicants in children; in utero lead exposure may also result in lasting neurodevelopmental abnormalities.[58] Paternal or maternal lead exposure may increase the risk of spontaneous abortion as well as impair fetal growth and neurodevelopment. Because lead in maternal bone can be mobilized during pregnancy, exposures producing abnormal fetal development may have occurred many years prior to the pregnancy (see Chapter 32).[58] Many adult conditions and diseases are thought to have origins in fetal life;[70] this is particularly relevant for families with few resources where stress is an aggravating factor in perpetuating a life cycle of health disparities (see Chapter 52).

## Developmental Outcomes

Examples of environmental exposures associated with birth defects and other developmental outcomes are listed in Table 48-3. Much still remains to be understood about these sometimes controversial associations.[8] Length of gestation is included in Table 48-3 because preterm birth is a significant public health problem. Evidence exists showing that gestational length is altered by some exposures as well as by social determinants of health (see Chapter 52).

## Growth

Body size, birth weight, and rate of growth after birth are influenced by factors including genetics, metabolism, and nutrition; growth is also influenced by certain environmental stressors, including chemical exposures. For example, prenatal exposure to tobacco smoke and alcohol increase fetal growth retardation and the incidence of low birth weight.[3,71-73]

## PRENATAL EXPOSURE TO SELECTED AGENTS AND THEIR STRUCTURAL AND DEVELOPMENTAL CONSEQUENCES

Pregnancy represents a unique situation because a mother's environmental exposures often reach the fetus. Consequently, understanding fetal dose and timing of exposure during pregnancy is important for characterizing potential risks (Figure 48-1). Concern about fetal exposures to environmental hazards comes from an understanding that the fetus is sensitive during certain critical windows of development. Differing windows of vulnerability exist for many systems, including respiratory, immune, reproductive, nervous, cardiovascular, and endocrine systems. Exposures may affect general growth and may also result in later adverse outcomes, such as childhood- and adult-onset cancers and other effects such as adult-onset diseases (see Figure 48-1).[61,62,74-76] Drugs and chemicals often result in adverse effects only during "critical periods" of development. Exposures outside of those critical periods may pose minimal or no risk of developmental disorders.[4,7,9,43,44]

## Thalidomide

Thalidomide[77] is perhaps the most emblematic and dramatic example of a specific agent that causes birth defects. Thalidomide first entered the German market in 1957 as a sedative, tranquilizer, and antiemetic. It was also proclaimed a "wonder drug" for insomnia, coughs, colds, and headaches. It was advertised as "completely safe" for everyone, including mother and child, "even during pregnancy," because its developers "could not find a dose high enough to kill a rat." By 1960, thalidomide was marketed in 46 countries, with sales nearly matching those of aspirin. In 1961, reports began to emerge associating the drug with severe birth defects of the limbs called phocomelia. An estimated 10,000 to 20,000 infants were born with phocomelia. By March of 1962, the drug was banned in most countries in which it was previously sold.

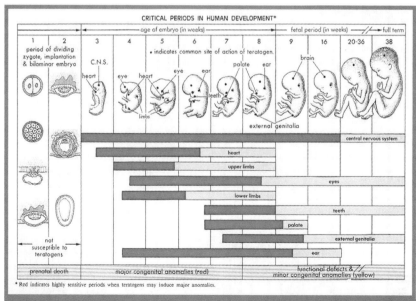

**Figure 48-1. Schema of Embryogenesis and Fetal Development – the timing of an insult during pregnancy will have an impact depending on which organ or organ system is in active development. (Source: Free Google Images)**

In the United States, Dr. Frances O. Kelsey, a recent appointee in the US Food and Drug Administration in the thalidomide era, was concerned that the drug might have adverse side effects and held up its approval, much to the frustration of the drug company. In so doing, she limited the use of the drug in the United States, thus preventing many cases of phocomelia. For this action, she received the President's Award for Distinguished Federal Civilian Service from President John Kennedy in 1962.[78] She then wrote the rules that govern most clinical drug trials today.

## Anticonvulsants

Seizure disorders occur in approximately 800,000 US women of childbearing age (0.3% to 0.5% of pregnant women), with 95% of women with epilepsy continuing anticonvulsant drug use during pregnancy. The use of anticonvulsants by women of childbearing age illustrates the utility of preconception counseling as well as the risk-benefit analysis needed to determine any potential consequences of exposures during pregnancy.[79] Much attention has focused on the developmental effects produced by prenatal anticonvulsant use. During a seizure, however, changes in the mother can also produce adverse developmental consequences.[80,81] Gene-environment interactions may play significant roles in developmental disorders observed in children whose mothers have seizure disorders. It appears that the risk of developmental disorders is not increased in children of women with epilepsy who do not require medications for seizure control during pregnancy.

Most women with epilepsy need to continue anticonvulsant use during pregnancy to control seizures, which can be life threatening. Exposure to various anticonvulsants during pregnancy increases the risk of developmental disorders two- to three-fold. The risk of malformation varies substantially among the medications used to treat different disorders. Valproic acid used during the first 3 months of pregnancy is associated with an increased risk of major congenital malformations.[82] Disagreement exists about the effects of seizure disorders on development.[79,83] Women with epilepsy who are of reproductive age should consume at least 0.4 mg/day of folic acid.[84] Some recommendations for women with epilepsy suggest increasing the dose to 5 mg/day for at least 3 months prior to conception.[85,86]

## Anticoagulants

The warfarin derivatives (coumadin, warfarin sodium) include anticoagulants that interrupt vitamin K-dependent clotting factors. They are used to treat coagulation disorders that occur among women of reproductive age.[87,88] Treatment is necessary because untreated coagulation disorders can be life threatening. Use of warfarin derivatives results in an increased risk of developmental abnormalities, including underdevelopment of the nose, growth retardation, and vertebral abnormalities. Heparin use does not result in the same adverse fetal consequences of warfarin derivatives. Women with coagulation disorders who are attempting to become pregnant often switch to heparin before conception and continue using it during pregnancy. Clinicians who treat women with coagulation disorders should discuss the risks of warfarin use with women of childbearing age. This is an example of the importance of preconception counseling.

## Cancer in Pregnancy

Treatment of cancer during reproductive ages in men and women raises concerns about possible impact on fertility, genetic effects increasing the risk of developmental disease in subsequent offspring, and risks of any treatment during pregnancy. Radiotherapy and chemotherapy are associated with early menopause. The risk of having a child with a developmental disorder is increased when conception occurs during or shortly after treatment. If fertility has been preserved and as distance of time from the treatment increases, there is good evidence that the risk of developmental disorder is no greater than in the general population.[9,89]

## Diethylstilbestrol (DES)

Although diethylstilbestrol (DES) is no longer in use, it causes birth defects of the female genital tract, and more significantly results in increased risks of breast cancer and of clear cell adenocarcinoma of the vagina in female offspring[90] years after fetal exposure. This effect is one example of endocrine disruption that can have effects even after long latency periods (see Chapter 29).

## Environmental Exposures

Environmental exposures arise from pollutants in air, water, food, soil, consumer products, and other substances. Examples include secondhand smoke (SHS), air pollutants from motor vehicles and industrial facilities, pesticides, heavy metals, plasticizers, flame retardants, chemical byproducts of drinking water disinfection, and pharmaceuticals or other chemicals that are incompletely removed during drinking water processing.

Although fetal exposures to environmental hazards are often assumed to result from maternal exposures during pregnancy, fetal exposures to certain chemicals can also be nonconcurrent with the maternal exposure (see Chapter 8). For certain persistent chemicals, such as dioxins, lead, and organochlorine and organophosphate pesticides, fetal exposure can occur from maternal body burdens resulting from exposures before conception. Paternal exposures may also contribute to fetal risk through mutagenic and epigenetic mechanisms involving sperm; in some instances, the chemical can be carried in semen, with fetal exposure following conception (see Chapter 8).[11,12]

Although there are few data to determine the potentially toxic developmental effects of exposure to most environmental chemicals, current epidemiological techniques may be used to assess whether the exposure is likely to represent a developmental risk. Data about selected chemicals and exposures are summarized in Table 48-4.

| Table 48-4. Select Environmental Exposures Associated With Adverse Developmental Outcomes | | |
|---|---|---|
| **ENVIRONMENTAL EXPOSURE** | **DEVELOPMENTAL OUTCOME(S) OBSERVED** | **ESTIMATED RISK** |
| Tobacco smoke[35, 91] | Spontaneous abortion, stillbirth, birth weight, gestational length, orofacial clefts, Sudden Infant Death Syndrome (SIDS), certain birth defects | Clear evidence demonstrates that maternal smoking independently decreases birth weight by about 200 grams and reduces gestational length. Evidence also supports an association between maternal smoking and SIDS. Maternal secondhand smoke exposure reduces birth weight by about 20 grams. Limited evidence supports an association between maternal active smoking and orofacial clefts, cardiac defects, spontaneous abortion, and stillbirth. |
| Particulate matter[8,63] | Birth weight, gestational length, cardiac defects, orofacial clefts | Evidence suggests there may be an association between particulate matter and birth weight and gestational length. Limited evidence supports an association between particulate matter and cardiac defects and orofacial clefts. |
| Pesticides[11, 35, 71,92] | Birth weight, gestational length, neurodevelopmental impact, spontaneous abortion | There is inadequate evidence linking maternal or paternal exposures to most pesticides and increased risk of spontaneous abortion, stillbirth, preterm birth, or growth restriction. Some data suggest an association between paternal exposure and spontaneous abortion. Limited evidence supports a relationship between maternal levels of DDT/DDE and preterm birth and growth restriction. |
| Fumonisin (a mycotoxin found on corn and in corn flour)[22–25] | Neural tube defects | Neural tube defects along the US-Mexico border linked to consumption of corn contaminated with fumonisin. Fumonisin can produce neural tube defects in experimental animals (diminished by folic acid). |
| Methylmercury [60,61] | Brain damage | Six percent of infants in a Japanese fishing village in which seafood was contaminated demonstrated delayed developmental milestones and had cognitive, motor, visual, and auditory deficits. |

## Table 48-4. Select Environmental Exposures Associated With Adverse Developmental Outcomes (*continued*)

| ENVIRONMENTAL EXPOSURE | DEVELOPMENTAL OUTCOME(S) OBSERVED | ESTIMATED RISK |
|---|---|---|
| Hypoxia[93] | Growth restriction, persistent ductus arteriosus | Functional closure of the patent ductus arteriosus is delayed in children living at altitudes ≥4 km. Asymptomatic pulmonary hypertension and other alterations of pulmonary hemodynamics also are increasingly found in these children. |
| Ethyl alcohol[94] | Brain damage, growth retardation, cardiac and joint defects | Clear evidence: 30% occurrence in infants of women who manifest chronic alcoholism. |

Abbreviations: DDE, dichlorodiphenyldichloroethylene; DDT, dichlorodiphenyltrichloroethane.
Table adapted from: Table 11.6 in Mattison DR. Developmental toxicology. In: Yaffe SJ, Aranda JV, eds. *Neonatal and Pediatric Pharmacology*. 4th ed. Philadelphia, PA: Lippincott Williams and Wilkins; 2010:130–143

## Tobacco

Many studies demonstrate that infants born to women who smoke weigh less than infants born to nonsmokers. Maternal exposure to SHS is also considered a causal factor for reduction in birth weight;[91] the evidence also suggests that SHS causes preterm birth. Accumulating evidence shows that prenatal tobacco exposure causes likely permanent brain changes, thus increasing the likelihood of early and addictive nicotine use later in life.[95,96] Sensitization of the fetal brain to nicotine results in increased likelihood of addiction when the brain is exposed to nicotine at a later stage, such as adolescence. Studies of rodents[97] and primates[98] exposed prenatally to tobacco demonstrate subtle brain changes that persist into adolescence and are associated with tobacco use and nicotine addiction.[99,100] Population-based studies demonstrate associations between prenatal tobacco exposure and early tobacco experimentation[101] as well as an increased likelihood of tobacco use during adolescence and adulthood.[102,103]

## Particulate Matter

Particulate matter is the mixture of solid particles and liquid droplets found in the air. Some particles are emitted directly from a source, such as construction sites, unpaved roads, fields, smokestacks, or fires. Others form from reactions in the atmosphere of chemicals such as sulfur dioxides and nitrogen oxides emitted from power plants, industrial sources, and automobiles. See Chapter 21 for additional information about particulate matter.

Epidemiologic studies conducted in countries with relatively high levels of particulate matter found evidence of an association with growth retardation.[35] Studies of preterm birth in the Czech Republic, China, southern California, Pennsylvania, and California found associations between preterm birth and particulate matter. The associations tend to be relatively small, although they typically are statistically significant.[35]

## Pesticides

The agricultural sector accounts for more than 75% of the nation's total conventional pesticide use, suggesting that persons engaged in agricultural work and/or who reside in or near agricultural areas may be at greatest risk of exposure.[71,92] Exposure to various pesticides has been correlated with preterm birth and reduced fetal growth.[35] A study about the effect of agricultural organophosphate pesticides found a significant positive association between maternal exposure and the occurrence of growth retardation. This finding is supported by studies of inner-city and minority populations, who are more likely to be exposed to indoor pesticides. In the first study, exposure of the fetus to chlorpyrifos was inversely associated with birth weight.[104] The second study found that the inverse association between chlorpyrifos and birth weight was highly significant when limited to the newborn infants born before the US Environmental Protection Agency (EPA) banned residential use of this pesticide in 2000. Newborn infants born later had much lower exposure levels, and the significant correlation between chlorpyrifos and birth weight was not found.[105] Other studies of organophosphate metabolite concentrations and fetal growth have been less conclusive.[106-108] Exposure to triazine and other herbicides, common contaminants of rural drinking water sources, also may be associated with decreased fetal growth.[109,110]

## Methylmercury

When inorganic mercury is dumped into water, aquatic organisms metabolize it to methylmercury. Methylmercury, an organic form of mercury, concentrates in the muscle of fish and other sea animals. When consumed by humans, it is concentrated in fat-rich tissues, including the brain. Two disastrous events provided information about the developmental effects of human exposures to methylmercury.[35] In 1971, Iraqis were exposed to methylmercury when they inadvertently consumed seed grain that had been treated with methylmercury to repel rodents. In the mid 1950s, Japanese villagers were exposed to methylmercury when they consumed fish and other aquatic species living in Minamata Bay. Since the 1930s, the bay had become polluted with industrial releases of mercury that was converted to methylmercury, which subsequently concentrated in fish. Children exposed in utero displayed marked neurodevelopmental effects.[61,62] See Chapter 33 for additional information about mercury.

## Hypoxia

Several types of hypoxia may occur during pregnancy. In communities at high altitude, the partial pressure of oxygen in the air is less than that at sea level. Pregnancy complications related to oxygen deprivation are observed in these communities, particularly relating to birth weight.[93] Complications depend on the level, duration, and timing of the deprivation. Lack of oxygen also results from carbon monoxide exposure, frequently a consequence of a faulty combustion device, such as an unventilated space heater. Carbon monoxide exposure, depending on the level and duration, may produce headache, nausea, and ultimately unconsciousness and death. At the level producing unconsciousness, carbon monoxide can damage the fetus and affect the developing nervous system (see Chapter 25).

## Ethyl Alcohol

Ethyl alcohol has been used socially for thousands of years. Its adverse effect on embryonic and fetal development had been suggested but it was not until the early 1970s that the impact on fetal development was explicitly defined.[94] Exposure to ethyl alcohol occurs primarily as a consequence of ingestion in social settings, but in the broadest sense is considered to be an environmental exposure. In some settings, occupational exposure can occur during the production of ethyl alcohol-containing products. Ethyl alcohol produces abnormal development of the face and central nervous system in a dose-dependent fashion across multiple species, including humans. A safe dose during pregnancy or during development is not known.[94] Prenatal ethyl alcohol exposure is the most common known and preventable cause of significant developmental disorders (see Chapter 52).

## Congenital Infections

A dramatic example of the impact of an intrauterine infection on fetal growth and development occurred during the rubella epidemic of 1963 to 1965.[111] Prenatal rubella infection caused 30,000 miscarriages, and 20,000 pregnant women who contracted the disease gave birth to infants with congenital anomalies and major neurodevelopmental consequences including seizure disorders, blindness, deafness, intellectual disabilities, and autism spectrum disorder.[112] Intrauterine infections with potentially teratogenic effects include toxoplasmosis, rubella, cytomegalovirus, herpes (collectively known as the acronym TORCH) and the Zika virus.[113] Zika virus outbreaks and their association with microcephaly and other congenital malformations have raised great concern across the world, particularly in the Americas. The virus interferes with the duplication of neural stem cells, resulting in a depletion of the number of eventual cells in the brain, and hence smaller brains and microcephaly.[114] Other viral, bacterial, and parasitic infections can occur during pregnancy and may have potentially adverse outcomes, particularly in low-income countries.[115]

## Social and Economic Factors

Social and economic factors are responsible for approximately 40% to 50% of premature births. Adverse social factors are associated with lower education level, limited employment, lower income, poorer nutrition, single parent status, depression, and an increased risk for substance abuse and domestic violence. The common denominator may be related to increased stress and stress hormones.[116] Children who experience persistent and unremitting stress in the absence of a supportive parental figure, resulting in the chronic elevation of stress hormones (particularly cortisol), are prone to the development of the "toxic stress" syndrome.[117] Toxic stress often results in adverse long-term effects on brain function with resulting developmental and behavioral disorders. The neuroendocrine system may be affected with an increased likelihood for hypertension, obesity, diabetes mellitus, and autoimmune disorders. Children who experienced toxic stress may experience added stress when they become pregnant, thereby increasing the risk of prematurity in their offspring (see Chapter 52).[118,119]

## CONCLUSIONS

Our understanding of birth defects and adverse developmental outcomes is changing; we are beginning to recognize that the impact of exposures during fetal development may manifest across the life of the individual into adulthood.[73] Structural birth defects are only one manifestation of developmental toxicity; others include disorders of function and of growth. In addition, we now know that paternal exposures can result in adverse developmental outcomes in offspring.[11–13]

Testing systems are available to identify toxicants that are likely to cause human developmental disease. Clearly, the highest degree of certainty that a chemical, physical, or a biological agent is a human developmental toxicant derives from studies in which the agent is shown to produce developmental disorders in human populations. Human data are available, however, only when exposure has already occurred and adverse developmental consequences have been discovered. Clinicians and public health practitioners cannot wait until data in humans are available before evaluating the potential toxicity of a chemical and acting to limit or prevent exposure.

In all but a few cases, human epidemiological research data are too sparse to support chemical risk assessments for developmental toxicity. Experimental data from research in animals, in vitro experimental data, and theoretical data can be used effectively to identify potential developmental hazards. Thus, preliminary conclusions can be drawn about the likelihood that developmental disorders are attributable to specific drugs, environmental chemicals, or biological agents.

To address the rising concern about environmental toxicants that can cause birth defects and other adverse neurodevelopmental outcomes, a group of scientists, advocates, and clinicians formed an alliance called TENDR: *Targeting Environmental Neurodevelopmental Risks to Protect Children.* The alliance published a consensus statement about the links between exposures to toxic chemicals and children's resulting risks for neurodevelopmental disorders. With greater awareness about potential adverse effects of environmental toxicants, and knowledge about how to avoid them, each woman can experience a healthier pregnancy and the greater likelihood that a healthy baby will grow and develop into a healthy adult.[120,121]

Given the number of known developmental toxicants relative to the number of agents that have been tested for developmental toxicity, and the number of agents for which there are no developmental toxicity data, it is likely that additional developmental hazards will be identified; therefore, it is wise to adopt the Precautionary Principle (see Chapter 64).

NOTE: Portions of this chapter were adapted in part from: (1) Mattison DR. Developmental toxicology. In: Yaffe SJ, Aranda JV, eds. *Neonatal and Pediatric Pharmacology.* 4th ed. Philadelphia, PA: Lippincott Williams and Wilkins; 2010:130–143; (2) Stillerman KP, Mattison DR, Giudice LC, Woodruff TJ. Environmental exposures and adverse pregnancy outcomes: a review of the science. *Reprod Sci.* 2008;15(7):631–650; and (3) Giacoia G, Mattison D. Obstetric and fetal pharmacology. In: The Global Library of Women's Medicine. *Fetal Physiology.* London, England: Sapiens Global Library Ltd; 2008. Available at: http://www.glowm.com/index.html?p=glowm.cml/section_view&articleid=196. Accessed April 5, 2018.

## Frequently Asked Questions

Q  *What can I do to ensure the healthiest possible pregnancy and to reduce the chance that my baby will have a birth defect?*

A  Schedule a preconception visit with your doctor (or other clinician). Preconception health care is care that a woman of childbearing age receives before pregnancy; interconception care is care between pregnancies. A preconception visit can help you and your doctor to identify and treat health conditions that may adversely affect your pregnancy. These conditions include high blood pressure, diabetes mellitus, seizure disorders, and certain infections. The visit gives your clinician the opportunity to discuss important subjects such as nutrition, weight, exercise, stress reduction, smoking cessation, and secondhand smoke exposure, avoiding alcohol, avoiding fish high in mercury, and avoiding recreational and occupational exposures that may pose risks. This is also an opportunity for your clinician to administer any missing vaccines and to make adjustments to any medications you are taking to ensure that they are the safest possible.

In addition to asking about your health history, your clinician will also ask about your partner's and family's health. If you or your partner have a history of birth defects or preterm births, or if either of you has a high risk for a genetic disorder on the basis of family history, ethnic background, or age, your clinician may suggest that you see a genetic counselor.

Your clinician will suggest that you take 0.4 mg of folic acid daily to prevent certain types of birth defects. A higher dose of folic acid may be recommended in some situations, especially if you have already had a child with a certain kind of birth defect or if you are taking certain medications.

Q  *I am pregnant and live in a building that is old; I am worried about lead. Will it affect my baby?*

A  If you have an elevated lead level, it could have an adverse effect on your baby. It would be a good idea to get your blood lead level checked. If it is high, then you should find out whether there is lead in the paint or some other source, such as tap water. Once the source is identified, you should either have the lead removed or find a way to move out of harm's way. If you are worried, you should contact the local Poison Control Center, the Regional Environmental Protection Agency office, or the regional Pediatric Environmental Health Specialty Unit (pehsu.net)

Q  *I did not know I was pregnant and went to a wedding in Florida where I had champagne and where people were smoking. I am worried that the champagne, the smoke, and the risk of having contracted Zika will harm my baby. What should I do?*

A  It is appropriate that you are concerned about these potential risks to your baby. Although we cannot clearly and accurately evaluate the risks of each of those exposures in the abstract, it is most important that you see an obstetrician as soon as possible to discuss your concerns and avail yourself of good prenatal care and close monitoring of your pregnancy. These actions go a long way toward reducing risks and ensuring a promising positive outcome.

## References

1. NIH Birth Defects. https://www.nichd.nih.gov/health/topics/birthdefects/Pages/default.aspx. Accessed August 4, 2018
2. Mathews TJ, MacDorman MF, Thoma ME. Division of Vital Statistics. Infant Mortality Statistics From the 2013 Period Linked Birth/Infant Death Data Set. National Vital Statistics Reports. Volume 64, Number 9. August 6, 2015. https://www.cdc.gov/nchs/data/nvsr/nvsr64/nvsr64_09.pdf. Accessed April 5, 2018

3. Mattison DR. Environmental exposures and development. *Curr Opin Pediatr.* 2010;22(2): 208–218

4. Shepard TH, Lemire RJ. *Catalog of Teratogenic Agents.* 13th ed. Baltimore, MD: The Johns Hopkins University Press; 2010

5. Kolb VM. Teratogens: Chemicals Which Cause Birth Defects. 2nd ed. University of Wisconsin-Parkside; 2013

6. Friedman JM, Polifka J. *Teratogenic Effects of Drugs. A Resource for Clinicians (TERIS).* 2nd ed. Baltimore, MD: The Johns Hopkins University Press; 2000

7. Kalter H. Teratology in the 20th century: environmental causes of congenital malformations in humans and how they were established. *Neurotoxicol Teratol.* 2003;25(2):131–282

8. Woodruff TJ, Parker JD, Darrow LA, et al. Methodological issues in studies of air pollution and reproductive health. *Environ Res.* 2009;109(3):311–320

9. Schaefer C, Peters P, Miller RK, eds. *Drugs During Pregnancy and Lactation. Treatment options and risk assessment.* 2nd ed. Amsterdam, The Netherlands: Elsevier; 2007

10. Winchester PD, Huskins J, Ying J. Agrichemicals in surface water and birth defects in the United States. *Acta Paediatr.* 2009;98(4):664–669

11. Cordier S. Evidence for a role of paternal exposures in developmental toxicity. *Basic Clin Pharmacol Toxicol.* 2008;102(2):176–181

12. Anderson D, Brinkworth M, eds. *International Conference on Male-Mediated Developmental Toxicity.* Cambridge, UK: RSC Publishing; 2007

13. Olshan AF, Mattison DR, eds. *Male-Mediated Developmental Toxicity.* Springer Science & Business Media; 2012

14. Xiong X, Harville EW, Mattison DR, Elkind-Hirsch K, Pridjian G, Buekens P. Exposure to Hurricane Katrina, post-traumatic stress disorder and birth outcomes. *Am J Med Sci.* 2008;336(2):111–115

15. Feldkamp ML, Carey JC, Byrne JLB, Krikov S, Botto LD. Etiology and clinical presentation of birth defects: population based study. *BMJ.* 2017;357:j2249

16. Shepard TH, Brent RL, Friedman JM, et al. Update on new developments in the study of human teratogens. *Teratology.* 2002;65(4):153–161

17. Shi M, Wehby GL, Murray JC. Review on genetic variants and maternal smoking in the etiology of oral clefts and other birth defects. *Birth Defects Res C Embryo Today.* 2008;84(1):16–29

18. MacLehose RF, Olshan AF, Herring AH, Honein MA, Shaw GM, Romitti PA; National Birth Defects Prevention Study. Bayesian methods for correcting misclassification: an example from birth defects epidemiology. *Epidemiology.* 2009;20(1):27–35

19. Maantay J. Mapping environmental injustices: pitfalls and potential of geographic information systems in assessing environmental health and equity. *Environ Health Perspect.* 2002;110(Suppl 2):161–171

20. de Medeiros AP, Gouveia N, Machado RP, et al. Traffic-related air pollution and perinatal mortality: a case-control study. *Environ Health Perspect.* 2009;117(1):127–132

21. Rasmussen SA, Erickson JD, Reef SE, Ross DS. Teratology: from science to birth defects prevention. *Birth Defects Res A Clin Mol Teratol.* 2009;85(1):82–92

22. Greene ND, Copp AJ. Mouse models of neural tube defects: investigating preventive mechanisms. *Am J Med Genet C Semin Med Genet.* 2005;135C(1):31–41

23. Marasas WF, Riley RT, Hendricks KA, et al. Fumonisins disrupt sphingolipid metabolism, folate transport, and neural tube development in embryo culture and in vivo: a potential risk factor for human neural tube defects among populations consuming fumonisin-contaminated maize. *J Nutr.* 2004;134(4):711–716

24. Gelineau-van Waes J, Starr L, Maddox J, et al. Maternal fumonisin exposure and risk for neural tube defects: mechanisms in an in vivo mouse model. *Birth Defects Res A Clin Mol Teratol.* 2005;73:487–497

25. Missmer SA, Suarez L, Felkner M, et al. Exposure to fumonisins and the occurrence of neural tube defects along the Texas-Mexico border. *Environ Health Perspect.* 2006;114(2):237–241

26. Kimanya ME, De Meulenaer B, Roberfroid D, Lachat C, Kolsteren P. Fumonisin exposure through maize in complementary foods is inversely associated with linear growth of infants in Tanzania. *Molecular Nutrition and Food Research.* 2010;54(11):1659–1667

27. Heseker HB, Mason JB, Selhub J, Rosenberg IH, Jacques PF. Not all cases of neural-tube defect can be prevented by increasing the intake of folic acid. *Br J Nutr.* 2009;102(2):173–180

28. Suarez L, Brender JD, Langlois PH, Zhan FB, Moody K. Maternal exposures to hazardous waste sites and industrial facilities and risk of neural tube defects in offspring. *Ann Epidemiol.* 2007;17(10):772–777

29. Schwarz EB, Sobota M, Gonzales R, Gerbert B. Computerized counseling for folate knowledge and use: a randomized controlled trial. *Am J Prev Med.* 2008;35(6):568–571

30. Yang J, Carmichael SL, Canfield M, Song J, Shaw GM; National Birth Defects Prevention Study. Socioeconomic status in relation to selected birth defects in a large multicentered US case-control study. *Am J Epidemiol.* 2008;167(2):145–154

31. Brouns R, Ursem N, Lindemans J, et al. Polymorphisms in genes related to folate and cobalamin metabolism and the associations with complex birth defects. *Prenat Diagn.* 2008;28(6):485–493

32. Stothard KJ, Tennant PW, Bell R, Rankin J. Maternal overweight and obesity and the risk of congenital anomalies: a systematic review and meta-analysis. *JAMA.* 2009;301(6):636–650

33. Emes RD, Clifford H, Haworth KE, et al. Antiepileptic drugs and the fetal epigenome. *Epilepsia.* 2013;54(1):e16–e19

34. Sung TI, Wang JD, Chen PC. Increased risks of infant mortality and of deaths due to congenital malformation in the offspring of male electronics workers. *Birth Defects Res A Clin Mol Teratol.* 2009;85(2):119–124

35. Wigle DT, Arbuckle TE, Turner MC, et al. Epidemiologic evidence of relationships between reproductive and child health outcomes and environmental chemical contaminants. *J Toxicol Environ Health B Crit Rev.* 2008;11(5-6):373–517

36. Quan A. Fetopathy associated with exposure to angiotensin converting enzyme inhibitors and angiotensin receptor antagonists. *Early Hum Dev.* 2006;82(1):23–28

37. Feng Y, Wang S, Chen R, Tong X, Wu Z, Mo X. Maternal folic acid supplementation and the risk of congenital heart defects in offspring: a meta-analysis of epidemiological observational studies. *Sci Rep.* 2015;5:8506

38. Jurenka J. Folic acid antagonists during pregnancy and the risk of birth defects. *Altern Med Rev.* 2001;6(1):109

39. Hernandez-Diaz S, Werler MM, Walker AM, Mitchell AA. Neural tube defects in relation to use of folic acid antagonists during pregnancy. *Am J Epidemiol.* 2001;153(10):961–968

40. Sayed AR, Bourne D, Pattinson R, Nixon J, Henderson B. Decline in the prevalence of neural tube defects following folic acid fortification and its cost-benefit in South Africa. *Birth Defects Res A Clin Mol Teratol.* 2008;82(4):211–216

41. Mosley BS, Cleves MA, Siega-Riz AM, et al. Neural tube defects and maternal folate intake among pregnancies conceived after folic acid fortification in the United States. *Am J Epidemiol.* 2009;169(1):9–17

42. Toepoel M, Steegers-Theunissen RP, Ouborg NJ, et al. Interaction of PDGFRA promoter haplotypes and maternal environmental exposures in the risk of spina bifida. *Birth Defects Res A Clin Mol Teratol.* 2009;85(7):629–636

43. Brent RL. How does a physician avoid prescribing drugs and medical procedures that have reproductive and developmental risks? *Clin Perinatol.* 2007;34(2):233–262

44. Brent RL. Environmental causes of human congenital malformations: the pediatrician's role in dealing with these complex clinical problems caused by a multiplicity of environmental and genetic factors. *Pediatrics.* 2004;113(4 Suppl):957–968

45. Weselak M, Arbuckle TE, Wigle DT, Walker MC, Krewski D. Pre- and post-conception pesticide exposure and the risk of birth defects in an Ontario farm population. *Reprod Toxicol.* 2008;25(4):472–480

46. Gonzalez BS, Lopez ML, Rico MA, Garduno F. Oral clefts: a retrospective study of prevalence and predisposal factors in the State of Mexico. *J Oral Sci.* 2008;50(2):123–129

47. Bretveld RW, Hooiveld M, Zielhuis GA, Pellegrino A, van Rooij IA, Roeleveld N. Reproductive disorders among male and female greenhouse workers. *Reprod Toxicol.* 2008;25(1):107–114

48. Batra M, Heike CL, Phillips RC, Weiss NS. Geographic and occupational risk factors for ventricular septal defects: Washington State, 1987-2003. *Arch Pediatr Adolesc Med.* 2007;161(1):89–95

49. Rull RP, Ritz B, Shaw GM. Validation of self-reported proximity to agricultural crops in a case-control study of neural tube defects. *J Expo Sci Environ Epidemiol.* 2006;16(2):147–155

50. Brender JD, Felkner M, Suarez L, Canfield MA, Henry JP. Maternal pesticide exposure and neural tube defects in Mexican Americans. *Ann Epidemiol.* 2010;20(1):16–22

51. Wennborg H, Magnusson LL, Bonde JP, Olsen J. Congenital malformations related to maternal exposure to specific agents in biomedical research laboratories. *J Occup Environ Med.* 2005;47(1):11–19

52. Woodruff TJ, Darrow LA, Parker JD. Air pollution and postneonatal infant mortality in the United States, 1999-2002. *Environ Health Perspect.* 2008;116(1):110–115

53. Son JY, Cho YS, Lee JT. Effects of air pollution on postneonatal infant mortality among firstborn infants in Seoul, Korea: case-crossover and time-series analyses. *Arch Environ Occup Health.* 2008;63(3):108–113

54. Wang L, Pinkerton KE. Air pollutant effects on fetal and early postnatal development. *Birth Defects Res C Embryo Today.* 2007;81(3):144–154

55. Bove FJ, Fulcomer MC, Klotz JB, Esmart J, Dufficy EM, Savrin JE. Public drinking water contamination and birth outcomes. *Am J Epidemiol.* 1995;141(9):850–862

56. Wilson PD, Loffredo CA, Correa-Villaseñor A, Ferencz C. Attributable fraction for cardiac malformations. *Am J Epidemiol.* 1998;148(5):414–423

57. Fielder HM, Poon-King CM, Palmer SR, Moss N, Coleman G. Assessment of impact on health of residents living near the Nant-y-Gwyddon landfill site: retrospective analysis. *BMJ.* 2000;320(7226):19–22

58. Jelliffe-Pawlowski LL, Miles SQ, Courtney JG, Materna B, Charlton V. Effect of magnitude and timing of maternal pregnancy blood lead (Pb) levels on birth outcomes. *J Perinatol.* 2006;26(3):154–162

59. Mendola P, Selevan SG, Gutter S, Rice D. Environmental factors associated with a spectrum of neurodevelopmental deficits. *Ment Retard Dev Disabil Res Rev.* 2002;8(3):188–197

60. Rice DC. Overview of modifiers of methylmercury neurotoxicity: chemicals, nutrients, and the social environment. *Neurotoxicology.* 2008;29(5):761–766

61. Grandjean P. Methylmercury toxicity and functional programming. *Reprod Toxicol.* 2007;23(3):414–420

62. Wigle DT, Arbuckle TE, Walker M, Wade MG, Liu S, Krewski D. Environmental hazards: evidence for effects on child health. *J Toxicol Environ Health B Crit Rev.* 2007;10(1-2):3–39

63. Huynh M, Woodruff TJ, Parker JD, Schoendorf KC. Relationships between air pollution and preterm birth in California. *Paediatr Perinat Epidemiol.* 2006;20(6):454–461

64. Colborn T. A case for revisiting the safety of pesticides: a closer look at neurodevelopment. *Environ Health Perspect*. 2006;114(1):10–17

65. Weselak M, Arbuckle TE, Foster W. Pesticide exposures and developmental outcomes: the epidemiological evidence. *J Toxicol Environ Health B Crit Rev*. 2007;10(1-2):41–80

66. Yoshizawa K, Heatherly A, Malarkey DE, Walker NJ, Nyska A. A critical comparison of murine pathology and epidemiological data of TCDD, PCB126, and PeCDF. *Toxicol Pathol*. 2007;35(7):865–879

67. Thulstrup AM, Bonde JP. Maternal occupational exposure and risk of specific birth defects. *Occup Med (Lond)*. 2006;56(8):532–543

68. Watson RE, Jacobson CF, Williams AL, Howard WB, DeSesso JM. Trichloroethylene-contaminated drinking water and congenital heart defects: a critical analysis of the literature. *Reprod Toxicol*. 2006;21(2):117–147

69. Beliles RP. Concordance across species in the reproductive and developmental toxicity of tetrachloroethylene. *Toxicol Ind Health*. 2002;18(2):91–106

70. Grandjean P. Late insights into early origins of disease. *Basic Clin Pharmacol Toxicol*. 2008;102(2):94–99

71. Hanson MA, Gluckman PD. Developmental origins of health and disease: new insights. *Basic Clin Pharmacol Toxicol*. 2008;102(2):90–93

72. Shea AK, Steiner M. Cigarette smoking during pregnancy. *Nicotine Tob Res*. 2008;10(2):267–278

73. Grandjean P, Barouki R, Bellinger D, et al. Life-long implications of developmental exposure to environmental stressors: new perspectives. *Endocrinology*. 2015;156(10):3408–3415

74. Rasmussen SA, Erickson JD, Reef SE, Ross DS. Teratology: from science to birth defects prevention. *Birth Defects Res A Clin Mol Teratol*. 2009;85(1):82–92

75. Selevan SG, Kimmel CA, Mendola P. Windows of susceptibility to environmental exposures in children. *Children's Health and the Environment*. 2004:17:725–735

76. Euling SY, Selevan SG, Pescovitz OH, Skakkebaek NE. Role of environmental factors in the timing of puberty. *Pediatrics*. 2008;121(Suppl 3):S167–S171

77. Kim JH, Scialli AR. Thalidomide: the tragedy of birth defects and the effective treatment of disease. *Toxicol Sci*. 2011;122 (1):1–6

78. McFadden RD. Frances Oldham Kelsey, who saved U.S. babies from thalidomide, dies at 101. *Science*. August 7, 2015

79. Battino D, Tomson T. Management of epilepsy during pregnancy. *Drugs*. 2007;67(18):2727–2746

80. Uziel D, Rozental R. Neurologic birth defects after prenatal exposure to antiepileptic drugs. *Epilepsia*. 2008;49(Suppl 9):35–42

81. Holmes LB, Harvey EA, Coull BA, et al. The teratogenicity of anticonvulsant drugs. *N Engl J Med*. 2001;344(15):1132–1138

82. Jentink J, Loane MA, Dolk H, et al. Valproic acid monotherapy in pregnancy and major congenital malformations. EUROCAT Antiepileptic Study Working Group. *N Engl J Med*. 2010;362(23):2185–2193

83. Bromfield EB, Dworetzky BA, Wyszynski DF, Smith CR, Baldwin EJ, Holmes LB. Valproate teratogenicity and epilepsy syndrome. *Epilepsia*. 2008;49(12):2122–2124

84. Harden CL, Hopp J, Ting TY, et al. Practice parameter update: management issues for women with epilepsy—focus on pregnancy (an evidence-based review): obstetrical complications and change in seizure frequency: report of the Quality Standards Subcommittee and Therapeutics and Technology Assessment Subcommittee of the American Academy of Neurology and American Epilepsy Society. *Neurology*. 2009;73(2):126–132

85. Tomson T, Hiilesmaa V. Epilepsy in pregnancy. *BMJ*. 2007;335(7623):769–773

86. Walker SP, Permezel M, Berkovic SF. The management of epilepsy in pregnancy. *BJOG*. 2009;116(6):758–767

87. Cho FN. Management of pregnant women with cardiac diseases at potential risk of thromboembolism—experience and review. *Int J Cardiol.* 2009;136(2):229–232

88. Shannon MS, Edwards MB, Long F, Taylor KM, Bagger JP, De Swiet M. Anticoagulant management of pregnancy following heart valve replacement in the United Kingdom, 1986-2002. *J Heart Valve Dis.* 2008;17(5):526–532

89. Meirow D, Schiff E. Appraisal of chemotherapy effects on reproductive outcome according to animal studies and clinical data. *J Natl Cancer Inst Monogr.* 2005;(34):21–25

90. Herbst AL, Anderson D. Diethylstilbestrol (DES) pregnancy treatment: a promising widely used therapy with unintended adverse consequences. *AMA J Ethics.* 2015;17(9):865–870

91. Office of the Surgeon General. The health consequences of smoking: a report of the Surgeon General. Washington, DC: US Department of Health and Human Services, Public Health Service; 2004

92. Eskenazi B, Rosas LG, Marks AR, et al. Pesticide toxicity and the developing brain. *Basic Clin Pharmacol Toxicol.* 2008;102(2):228–236

93. Waldhoer T, Klebermass-Schrehof K. The impact of altitude on birth weight depends on further mother- and infant-related factors: a population-based study in an altitude range up to 1600 m in Austria between 1984 and 2013. *J Perinatol.* 2015;35(9):689–694

94. Henderson J, Gray R, Brocklehurst P. Systematic review of effects of low-moderate prenatal alcohol exposure on pregnancy outcome. *BJOG.* 2007;114(3):243–252

95. Abreu-Villaça Y, Seidler FJ, Tate CA, Cousins MM, Slotkin TA. Prenatal nicotine exposure alters the response to nicotine administration in adolescence: effects on cholinergic systems during exposure and withdrawal. *Neuropsychopharmacology.* 2004;29(5):879–890

96. Abreu-Villaça Y, Seidler FJ, Slotkin TA. Does prenatal nicotine exposure sensitize the brain to nicotine-induced neurotoxicity in adolescence? *Neuropsychopharmacology.* 2004;29(8):1440–1450

97. Nordberg A, Zhang XA, Fredriksson A, Eriksson P. Neonatal nicotine exposure induces permanent changes in brain nicotinic receptors and behaviour in adult mice. *Brain Res Dev Brain Res.* 1991;63(1-2):201–207

98. Slotkin TA, Seidler FJ, Qiao D, et al. Effects of prenatal nicotine exposure on primate brain development and attempted amelioration with supplemental choline or vitamin C: neurotransmitter receptors, cell signaling and cell development biomarkers in fetal brain regions of rhesus monkeys. *Neuropsychopharmacology.* 2005;30(1):129–144

99. Ernst M, Moolchan ET, Robinson ML. Behavioral and neural consequences of prenatal exposure to nicotine. *J Am Acad Child Adolesc Psychiatry.* 2001;40(6):630–641

100. Slotkin TA, Tate CA, Cousins MM, Seidler FJ. Prenatal nicotine exposure alters the responses to subsequent nicotine administration and withdrawal in adolescence: serotonin receptors and cell signaling. *Neuropsychopharmacology.* 2006;31(11):2462–2475

101. Niaura R, Bock B, Lloyd EE, Brown R, Lipsitt LP, Buka S. Maternal transmission of nicotine dependence: psychiatric, neurocognitive and prenatal factors. *Am J Addict.* 2001;10(1):16–29

102. Al Mamun A, O'Callaghan FV, Alati R, et al. Does maternal smoking during pregnancy predict the smoking patterns of young adult offspring? A birth cohort study. *Tob Control.* 2006;15(6):452–457

103. Roberts KH, Munafo MR, Rodriguez D, et al. Longitudinal analysis of the effect of prenatal nicotine exposure on subsequent smoking behavior of offspring. *Nicotine Tob Res.* 2005;7(5):801–808

104. Perera FP, Rauh V, Tsai WY, et al. Effects of transplacental exposure to environmental pollutants on birth outcomes in a multiethnic population. *Environ Health Perspect.* 2003;111(2):201–205

105. Whyatt RM, Rauh V, Barr DB, et al. Prenatal insecticide exposures and birth weight and length among an urban minority cohort. *Environ Health Perspect*. 2004;112(10):1125–1132

106. Berkowitz GS, Wetmur JG, Birman-Deych E, et al. In utero pesticide exposure, maternal paraoxonase activity, and head circumference. *Environ Health Perspect*. 2004;112(3):388–391

107. Eskenazi B, Harley K, Bradman A, et al. Association of in utero organophosphate pesticide exposure and fetal growth and length of gestation in an agricultural population. *Environ Health Perspect*. 2004;112(10):1116–1124

108. Bjorling-Poulsen M, Andersen HR, Grandjean P. Potential developmental neurotoxicity of pesticides used in Europe. *Environ Health*. 2008;7:50

109. Dabrowski S, Hanke W, Polanska K, Makowiec-Dabrowska T, Sobala W. Pesticide exposure and birthweight: an epidemiological study in Central Poland. *Int J Occup Med Environ Health*. 2003;16(1):31–39

110. Villanueva CM, Durand G, Coutté MB, Chevrier C, Cordier S. Atrazine in municipal drinking water and risk of low birth weight, preterm delivery, and small-for-gestational-age status. *Occup Environ Med*. 2005;62(6):400–405

111. Maldonado YA. Rubella virus. In: Long SS, Pickering LK, Prober CG, eds. *Principles and Practice of Pediatric Infectious Diseases*. 3rd ed. (rev reprint). New York, NY: Churchill Livingstone; 2009

112. Chess S. Autism in children with congenital rubella. *J Autism Child Schizophr*. 1971;1(1):33-47. http://www.neurodiversity.com/library_chess_1971.pdf. Accessed April 5, 2018

113. Centers for Disease Control and Prevention. Zika Virus. https://www.cdc.gov/zika/index.html. Accessed April 5, 2018

114. Onorati M, Li Z, Liu F, et al. Zika virus disrupts Phospho-TBK1 localization and mitosis in human neuroepithelial stem cells and radial glia. *Cell Rep*. 2016;16(10):2576–2592

115. Waldorf KM, McAdams RM. Influence of infection during pregnancy on fetal development. *Reproduction*. 2013;146(5):R151–R162

116. Dole N, Savitz DA, Hertz-Picciotto I, Siega-Riz SM, McMahon MJ, Buekens P. Maternal stress and preterm birth. *Am J Epidemiol*. 2003;157(1):14–24

117. Shonkoff JP, Garner AS. The lifelong effects of early childhood adversity and toxic stress. *Pediatrics*. 2012;129(1):e232–e246

118. Hogue CJ, Bremner JD. Stress model for research into preterm delivery among black women. *Am J Obstet Gynecol*. 2005;192(5 Suppl):S47–S55

119. Jo H, Schieve LA, Sharma AJ, Hinkle SN, Li R, Lind JN. Maternal prepregnancy body mass index and child psychosocial development at 6 years of age. *Pediatrics*. 2015;135(5):e1198–e1209

120. Hirtz D, Campbell C, Lanphear B. Targeting environmental neurodevelopmental risks to protect children. *Pediatrics*. 2017;139(2):e20162245

121. Bennett D, Bellinger DC, Birnbaum LS, et al. Project TENDR: targeting environmental neuro-developmental risks the TENDR consensus statement. *Environ Health Perspect*. 2016;124(7):A118–A122

Chapter 49

# Cancer

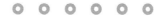

## KEY POINTS

- The incidence of childhood cancers has increased in the United States and other developed countries over the past 40 years.
- Leukemia, the most common childhood cancer, has been linked to exposures to radiation, secondhand smoke, pesticides, and solvents.
- Pediatricians and obstetricians can play important roles in educating parents to reduce exposures to these environmental risk factors.
- Additional research is needed to determine risk factors and protective factors for most childhood cancers.

## INTRODUCTION

Cancer in children is relatively rare, accounting for only about 1% of all cancers, but in industrialized nations, cancer is the most common cause of death from disease and the second most common cause of death (after injuries) in children aged 5 to 14. An estimated 10,270 new cancer cases were expected in 2017 in US children younger than age 15.[1] From 2010 to 2014, in the 18 areas covered by the National Cancer Institute-Surveillance Epidemiology and End Results (NCI-SEER) registries (approximately 30% of the US population), the average annual incidence rate for childhood cancer was 16.2 cases per 100,000, while the cancer incidence rate for all cancers among adults was about 443 per 100,000.[2] The most common types of pediatric cancers (children aged 0 to 14) are acute lymphoblastic leukemia (ALL) (26%) and brain and central nervous system (CNS) malignancies (21%). The other childhood tumors consist of a heterogeneous group of malignancies, including neuroblastoma (7%), non-Hodgkin lymphoma (6%), Wilms tumor (5%), acute myeloid leukemia (AML) (5%), bone tumors (4%), and Hodgkin lymphoma (4%).[1] Because the distribution and the histology of cancer among children are different than in adults, childhood cancer has its own classification system, the International Classification of Childhood Cancer. Updated in 2005, it includes 12 major histologically based subtypes and 47 subgroups.[3]

The major categories and subtypes of childhood cancers differ in the age of onset, ethnicity, race, and gender-related characteristics (Table 49-1).[1] For example, ALL, the most common childhood cancer, has a peak incidence at age 2 to 3 years; it is more common in boys and Caucasians in the United States. In contrast, osteosarcoma, a primary bone cancer, peaks during adolescence and is slightly more common in blacks in the United States.[4] Ewing sarcoma, which also peaks during adolescence and young adulthood, is extremely rare in blacks.[1] Genetically determined variations in carcinogen metabolism, immune function, growth, and other functional processes appear to account for some of the observed differences in cancer incidence. Gender differences have been noted in several types of childhood malignancies, including higher male-to-female ratios for Hodgkin disease, ependymomas, and primitive neuroectodermal tumors in contrast with other forms of CNS tumors. A notable female predominance is apparent for thyroid carcinoma and for melanoma in children and adolescents.

## TIME TRENDS IN INCIDENCE AND MORTALITY

Childhood cancer rates (younger than age 15) increased 38% between 1975 and 2014 in the United States based on data from 9 US population-based registries. The average annual percent change was 0.6%, which was a statistically significant increase.[2] The incidence of leukemia, the most common childhood cancer, increased significantly by 0.7% over the entire period resulting in a 42% change; the increases were greatest for Hispanic children.[5] For brain and other nervous system cancers, incidence increased from 2.3 to 3.3 per 100,000, with a higher average annual percent change from 1975 to 1990 (2.1%) than from 1990 to 2014 (0.3%).[2] The large increase in incidence occurred after improvements in diagnosis and changes in classification in the mid 1980s. The average annual percent change in incidence of non-Hodgkin lymphoma in children and adolescents aged 0 to 19 increased significantly by 1.2% from 1975 to 2014, whereas a significant decline in Hodgkin lymphoma rates occurred over the same period. Among adolescents and young adults aged 15 to 19, the largest increases in cancer incidence occurred for testicular cancer among boys and thyroid cancer, which occurred mostly among girls.[2]

## Table 49-1. Incidence and Major Risk Factors for Childhood Cancers (ages 0–19)[a]

| CANCER TYPE | AGE PEAK | MALE: FEMALE RATIO | WHITE: BLACK RATIO | INCIDENCE (PER MILLION) | KNOWN RISK FACTORS | SUGGESTED RISK FACTORS |
|---|---|---|---|---|---|---|
| **All cancer** | | 1.1 | 1.4 | 178 | | |
| **Leukemias** | | 1.2 | 1.6 | 49.4 | Birth weight >4,000 g, ionizing radiation, sibling with leukemia, Down syndrome, inherited disorders (ataxia-telangiectasia, inherited bone marrow failure syndromes, Bloom syndrome, neurofibromatosis), treatment with chemotherapy for another cancer | |
| – Acute lymphoblastic leukemia | 2–4 y | 1.3 | 1.9 | 35.5 | | Parental pesticide exposures and paternal smoking; inverse association with proxies of early life exposure to common infections (daycare attendance, birth order); inverse association with breastfeeding and maternal folic acid intake |
| – Acute myeloid leukemia | Infancy | 1.0 | 1.1 | 8.9 | Benzene 1,3- butadiene | Parental occupational exposures such as benzene and pesticides; traffic-related benzene exposure |
| **Hodgkin lymphoma** | Adolescence | 1.1 | 1.3 | 12.0 | Affected sibling, Epstein-Barr virus linked with some forms | |

[a]Ratios and rates from references 1 and 2

(*continued*)

## Table 49-1. Incidence and Major Risk Factors for Childhood Cancers (ages 0-19)[a] (*continued*)

| CANCER TYPE | AGE PEAK | MALE: FEMALE RATIO | WHITE: BLACK RATIO | INCIDENCE (PER MILLION) | KNOWN RISK FACTORS | SUGGESTED RISK FACTORS |
|---|---|---|---|---|---|---|
| **Non-Hodgkin lymphoma (except Burkitt)** | Adolescence | 2.0 | 1.0 | 9.5 | Immunosuppressive therapy, congenital immunodeficiency syndromes, HIV infection | |
| **Central Nervous System** | | | | | | |
| – All CNS tumors (includes benign brain/CNS tumors) | Infancy | 1.2 | 1.4 | 47.2 | Ionizing radiation, inherited disorders (neurofibromatosis, tuberous sclerosis, nevoid basal cell syndrome, Turcot syndrome, Li-Fraumeni syndrome) | Maternal diet during pregnancy (positive association with cured meats; inverse association with fruits/vegetables), sibling or parent with brain tumor; parental occupation in agriculture |
| – Ependymoma | | 1.3 | 1.4 | 3.7 | | |
| – Astrocytoma | | 1.1 | 1.5 | 16.5 | | |
| – Medulloblastoma | | 1.5 | 1.8 | 5.9 | | |
| **Neuroblastoma and ganglioneuro-blastoma** | Infancy | 1.1 | 1.2 | 7.9 | | Pesticide exposures; maternal sex hormone use |
| **Bone Tumors** | | | | | | |
| – Osteosarcoma | Adolescence | 1.2 | 0.9 | 5.2 | Radiation therapy for cancer, inherited disorders (Li-Fraumeni syndrome, retinoblastoma, Rothmund-Thomson syndrome) | High birth weight; taller than peers |
| – Ewing sarcoma | Adolescence | 1.4 | 9.7 | 2.8 | | Pesticide exposures |

**Soft-tissue Sarcomas**

| Cancer | Peak age | | | | Genetic risk factors | Environmental risk factors |
|---|---|---|---|---|---|---|
| – Rhabdomyosarcoma | Infancy | 1.3 | 0.8 | 4.7 | At least one congenital abnormality (up to one third of patients), inherited disorders (Li-Fraumeni syndrome, neurofibromatosis) | |
| **Wilms tumor** | Infancy | 0.8 | 0.9 | 5.9 | Inherited disorders (WAGR syndrome, Beckwith-Wiedemann syndrome, Perlman syndrome, Denys-Drash syndrome) | Father employed as a welder or mechanic; pesticide exposures |
| **Hepatic tumors** | Infancy | 1.6 | 2.3 | 2.5 | Inherited disorders (Beckwith Wiedemann syndrome, hemihypertrophy, familial adenomatous polyposis, Gardner syndrome) | |
| **Testicular germ cell tumors** | Adolescence–young adult | | 7.8 | 9.0 | Cryptorchidism | Organochlorine insecticides |
| **Thyroid carcinoma** | Adolescence | 0.2 | 3.2 | 9.4 | Ionizing radiation, inherited cancer predisposition syndromes (multiple endocrine neoplasia, familial polyposis) | |
| **Melanoma** | Adolescence | 0.6 | 14.2 | 3.9 | Ultraviolet radiation from sun, artificial sources (tanning salons), sunburns in childhood/adolescence, number of nevi and dysplastic nevi, inherited disorders (xeroderma pigmentosum) | |
| **Retinoblastoma** | Infancy | 0.9 | 1.0 | 3.3 | Inherited disorders (mutations in retinoblastoma [RB] gene) | 13q deletion syndrome |

[a]Ratios and rates from references 1 and 2

Significant advancements in treatment of childhood cancers have led to significant decreases in childhood cancer mortality over this same period. From 1975 to 2014, childhood leukemia mortality (ages 0 to 19) decreased from 2.0 to 0.6 deaths per 100,000 children (average annual percent change was −3.6% from 1975 to 1998 and −3.2% from 2001 to 2014). As a result, there was an overall decrease in mortality from all childhood cancers (ages 0 to 19) from slightly more than 5 per 100,000 in 1975 to about 2.1 per 100,000 from 2010 to 2014.[1] The American Cancer Society estimated that approximately 1,190 children younger than age 15 years would die of malignancy in 2017.[6] The increasing incidence rates and decreases in mortality for many childhood cancers has resulted in increasing numbers of cancer survivors who may experience adverse health effects related to their treatment, including an increased risk of adult cancer. As of 2010, in the United States, there were approximately 380,000 survivors of cancer diagnosed in childhood or adolescence (younger than age 20).[2]

## INTERPRETING EPIDEMIOLOGIC STUDIES OF CHILDHOOD CANCER RISK

Designing and interpreting studies that attempt to evaluate environmental exposures and cancer risk are challenging, even for common adult-onset cancers.[7] The rarity of childhood cancer further adds to these challenges. Childhood cancers comprise a biologically and clinically heterogeneous group of disorders in which different environmental exposures and genetic risk factors may play a role. Careful definition of the specific disease types is very important when designing and interpreting studies of childhood cancer risk factors. For example, ALL and AML are leukemias with very different ages of onset and clinical outcomes. Even within ALL, there are subtypes with differences in age of onset, outcomes, chromosomal abnormalities, and molecular aberrations in the leukemic cells. In epidemiologic studies of childhood leukemia, there has been an emphasis to consider subgroups defined by genetics or immunophenotype. Ongoing research suggests that these different disease subtypes could have different etiologic factors.[8]

To date, most etiologic studies of childhood cancer have been case-control studies. These studies can be limited by selection of controls and recall bias (differential recall of exposures among cases and controls). Longitudinal cohort studies that enroll healthy participants, follow them for years or even decades, and study disease outcomes are powerful studies that can elucidate risk factors with less potential for biases than case-control studies. This approach has usually not been feasible in rare disorders, including childhood cancer. For example, even in a cohort of 1 million children, with a disease incidence of 1 in 2,000 (similar to ALL), only approximately 500 cases would occur. Clinical and biological heterogeneity would further reduce the power to find statistically meaningful associations. Investigators from around the world have formed the International Childhood Cancer Cohort Consortium, which seeks to study childhood cancer etiology through combining data from existing birth cohorts.[9] In 2000, the NCI pediatric cooperative clinical trials groups merged to form the Children's Oncology Group (COG); over 220 hospitals and institutions in the United States and Canada are affiliated with COG, which has enabled epidemiologic research on the causes of childhood cancer. In 2007, through an informed consent process, all COG institutions began registration of childhood cancer cases in the Childhood Cancer Research Network, which will enable researchers to follow the health of patients into adulthood and streamline etiologic studies.[10]

The method and quality of the exposure assessment should also be considered when etiologic studies are interpreted. For example, assessments are generally made of self-reported exposure to any type of pesticide versus studying specific pesticides. Many chemicals are rapidly metabolized, making the evaluation of clinical specimens challenging. The timing of the exposure (preconception, prenatal, or postnatal) and the latency period between exposure and cancer development also are considerations. In the absence of environmental or biological measurements, it often is difficult to interpret a child's exposure because exposure levels or use may change over time as a result of growth, development, and behavioral changes. Finally, epidemiologic studies looking at many potential risk factors for childhood cancer might by chance alone find at least one factor meeting the traditional definition of "statistically significant" ($P < 0.05$).

## KEY FEATURES OF CARCINOGENESIS IN CHILDHOOD CANCERS

Although many chemical and physical agents are known to be associated with cancer risk in humans,[11,12] the etiology of most childhood malignancies is not known. The latency period between a potential carcinogenic exposure and the onset of childhood cancer, however, is relatively short in comparison with cancers in older adults. A relatively short latency period could exist for a carcinogenic exposure occurring during the prenatal period (such as the pregnant mother exposed to diagnostic x-rays) or postnatally (such as chemotherapy with DNA-damaging drugs, eg, epipodophyllotoxin). The latency period may be longer for carcinogenic exposures occurring before conception (such as paternal cigarette smoking) that may increase the risk of childhood cancer in offspring. The carcinogenicity of environmental agents may be enhanced or diminished by interaction with one another or by genetic influences. Studies of familial cancer clusters have led to the identification of rare inherited disorders that increase the risk of childhood cancers (Table 49-1). These studies continue to result in the discovery of cancer susceptibility genes. Most childhood cancers, however, likely develop from a combination of host susceptibility factors, immune factors, and chemical or other exposures.[13]

## ROUTES OF EXPOSURE

Routes of exposures to carcinogens include absorption through the skin, ingestion, and inhalation. Children are exposed to carcinogens that occur as air and water pollutants, in tobacco products, in medications, in the diet, in household products, and through parental occupational exposures brought into the home. Occasionally, what is at first considered a therapeutic advance has eventually proved to have deleterious effects, including cancer, so practitioners must remain vigilant to the potential hazards of therapeutic innovations. In addition, endogenous reactions, such as oxidation after ingestion, or other types of metabolic change may result in cancer in children and adults. Several forms of exogenous chemical agents do not cause cancer until they undergo one or more endogenous chemical reactions.

Children are potentially exposed to environmental contaminants at higher levels than are adults (see Chapter 3). Young children spend more time on the floor or ground and put more things in their mouths. They have a higher intake of food, water, and air per body unit of weight. Children also have a higher surface-to-volume ratio than adults and, therefore, can absorb proportionally greater amounts of a contaminant. Developmentally disabled older children may be exposed to higher levels of environmental contaminants. These children may continue to put more things in their mouths for longer periods of time, may spend more time on the floor because of an inability to walk or because they engage in age-inappropriate behaviors, and may fail to understand that some substances are dangerous.

## BIOLOGICAL PROCESSES AND CLINICAL EFFECTS

Environmental carcinogens may act through several different mechanisms. Many carcinogens, such as ionizing radiation and certain chemotherapeutic medications, induce DNA damage.[14] Cellular processes usually repair the DNA damage, but occasionally, abnormal cellular proliferation and malignant transformation may result. Two major categories of cancer genes have been described. Oncogenes are a class of latent cancer genes that, when activated, transform normal cells to cancer cells. Tumor suppressor genes, the other main class of cancer genes, normally regulate development (eg, of the eye or kidney). When these genes are inactivated (mutated), they no longer regulate growth of the organ, and cancer develops (eg, retinoblastoma or Wilms tumor).

Carcinogens also may act by disrupting normal cellular proliferation in tissues of the fetus, developing child, or adult. Endocrine disruptors are exogenous agents that interfere with the mechanisms of natural hormones and may result in abnormal gene regulation or activation.[15,16] Disordered immune regulation, attributable to immunosuppressive agents or infection, also is associated with cancer risk. In this instance, immunosurveillance, which is responsible for the destruction of the earliest neoplastic cells, is reduced. The carcinogenic effect of a chemical is detectable when the dose is high or chronic, as in medicinal, occupational, or large accidental exposures. For physical and chemical exposures, it is hypothesized that parental exposure (before conception, prenatally, or postnatally) may play an important role in the development of childhood cancer. It is also hypothesized that there are critical windows of exposure during childhood and adolescence during which exposures to contaminants may result in an increased cancer risk later in life.

## RISK FACTORS

Some characteristic features of the major childhood cancer categories (and a limited number of subtypes) are shown in Table 49-1. More details about childhood cancer types and incidence can be found in the National Cancer Institute monograph.[17] Although epidemiologic studies of childhood cancers have evaluated many postulated risk factors, there are few established risk factors.[13,18] Familial and genetic factors seem to occur in no more than 5% to 15% of different categories of childhood cancer.[19] Some risk factors, such as exposure to ionizing radiation, have been established as causal. In moderate to high doses, ionizing radiation has been linked with increased risks of several types of pediatric cancers (ALL, AML, CNS tumors, malignant bone tumors, and thyroid carcinoma). Other risk factors have been linked with specific forms of childhood cancer. For example, treatment with alkylating agents has been linked to an increased risk of AML in some children. An increased incidence of several types of childhood cancers occurs among children with certain genetic syndromes or congenital disorders. Suggestive or limited data link certain maternal reproductive factors, parental occupational exposures, air pollution, residential pesticides, cured meats, paternal smoking, and other exposures with increased risk of some types of childhood cancers.

## Physical Agents

### Solar and Artificial Ultraviolet Radiation

A substantial proportion of all cancers in humans involve the skin. Skin cancers may be induced by ultraviolet radiation (UVR) from sun exposure.[20] Exposure to artificial sources of UVR, as occurs when teenagers and young adults visit tanning salons, also increases the risk of melanoma and other skin cancers. Because of the long latent period, skin cancers rarely occur in childhood, except among children with conditions in which there is markedly heightened sensitivity (eg, xeroderma pigmentosum, which has an inherent DNA repair defect, or albinism, which has a lack of skin pigment to protect against UVR damage). In the general population, persons with darker pigmentation have a lower risk of skin cancer. Maps of cancer mortality show that mortality attributable to melanoma is significantly higher in the southern United States than in the northern United States. The incidence of melanoma has increased more rapidly than that of most cancers, and children and adolescents who experience repeated sunburns are at greater risk (see Chapter 44).[21]

### Ionizing Radiation

Ionizing radiation (IR) is high-energy radiation that is strong enough to cause displacement of electrons and break chemical bonds. Exposure causes genotoxicity (DNA damage resulting from strand breaks and/or mutations) that can result in abnormal cell division and/or cell death. Ionizing radiation is a well-described carcinogen. Types of ionizing radiation exposure range from diagnostic radiation, such as x-rays, to radioactive materials emitted from nuclear power plant accidents. See Chapter 31 for more details.

Studies that began more than 50 years ago suggested a 1.6-fold excess of almost every type of cancer in children younger than 10 years after maternal exposure to diagnostic abdominal x-rays during pregnancy.[22] Most subsequent epidemiologic studies confirmed these findings, but some did not.[23,24] The potential carcinogenic effects of postnatal diagnostic radiation exposure have been much less studied.[24] Large-scale data collection on pediatric exposure to diagnostic medical radiation began in the mid 1990s. Adolescents who underwent repeated exposure to diagnostic radiation examinations for scoliosis were documented to have an increased risk of breast cancer later in life.[25,26]

Computed tomography (CT) scans have been increasingly used in pediatric patients to aid in the diagnosis of illnesses and injuries. CT scanning[24,27] and pediatric interventional and fluoroscopic imaging modalities expose patients to much higher levels of ionizing radiation than do x-rays. A large study of CT scans in children in Great Britain found positive associations between the radiation dose from CT scans and both leukemia and brain tumors.[28] Although the absolute risks are small because of the rarity of these cancers, it is prudent to reduce exposure to diagnostic radiation whenever possible.[28,29]

In the Childhood Cancer Survivor Study cohort, radiotherapy is associated with an increased risk of second primary cancers, including cancers of the breast, thyroid, CNS, gastrointestinal tract, and sarcomas.[30] Among children with some genetic disorders, such as hereditary retinoblastoma, nevoid basal cell carcinoma syndrome, and ataxia telangiectasia, an increased susceptibility to radiogenic cancers has been found.

Numerous studies have been conducted among Japanese survivors of the atomic bombs. High rates of leukemia were initially noted among survivors, and approximately 30 years after the detonation, the rates of leukemia returned to baseline.[31] Long-term studies found an increased risk of breast cancer at younger ages among people younger than 20 years at the time of the bomb detonations.[32,33] Subsequent studies of solid cancer incidence among adolescents and adults who were exposed in utero or before age 6 years found excess risks of solid tumors in persons aged 12 to 55 years.[34]

In 1986, a partial meltdown at a nuclear reactor in Chernobyl, Ukraine, resulted in fallout of substantial amounts of radioactive isotopes, primarily in Ukraine and Belarus, in neighboring countries, and to a lesser extent, throughout the world. In addition to the acute exposure, individuals were further exposed through food, milk, and water supplies. Increased rates of thyroid cancer in children, which is typically very rare, and in adults were found in several studies.[35,36] The incidence of leukemia following the accident did not increase in children or power plant workers involved in the cleanup.[37,38]

### Nonionizing Radiation

Nonionizing radiation refers to electromagnetic radiation that does not carry enough energy to cause displacement of electrons and break chemical bonds in living tissue. Nonionizing radiation includes static electric and magnetic fields, low-frequency electric and magnetic fields, radiofrequency electromagnetic fields (see Chapter 27), and microwaves. Radiofrequency waves are generated as part of global telecommunications networks or as part of industrial processes using this energy for heating. A recent pooled analysis of studies of childhood leukemia among children living in the vicinity of radio and television broadcast towers found an approximately two-fold increased risk at exposures 0.4 or greater microtesla ($\mu$T); whereas a pooled analyses of childhood brain tumors found no associations at these exposure levels.[39] On the basis of these studies, electromagnetic fields were classified as a possible carcinogen to humans.[40] Selection bias is a concern in case-control studies because participants with low socioeconomic status have a higher likelihood of being exposed to electromagnetic fields and may be underrepresented among controls, which may have led to an overestimation of the association. However, even if it is assumed that the observed association is causal, the fraction of childhood leukemias attributable to magnetic field exposure is small—only approximately 2% to 4% in North America. Experimental data from animal studies in support of the associations observed in the epidemiologic studies are limited. The NIH National Toxicology Program (NTP) is currently conducting studies in rats and mice on cellular phone radiofrequency radiation using frequencies and modulations currently used in the United States. The NTP found low incidences of tumors in the brains and hearts of male rats, but not in female rats, and studies in mice are continuing.[41]

## Asbestos

Exposure to asbestos fibers increases the frequency of lung cancer, especially in smokers; asbestos exposure causes mesothelioma after a latent period as long as 40 years.[42] The precise mechanism of asbestos-related carcinogenesis is still under investigation; postulated mechanisms include DNA damage attributable to free radicals generated by the fibers, alteration of proto-oncogene/tumor suppressor genes, and viral-host interactions. During the 1950s, schoolroom ceilings were routinely sprayed with asbestos, which deteriorated with time. As a result of public health initiatives, asbestos has been removed or walled off, but it is conceivable that mesothelioma may develop in adults exposed as school children, and those who smoke will have an increased risk of lung cancer (see Chapter 23).

## Environmental Chemical Exposures

Children are exposed to a wide range of chemical agents in residences, schools, child care settings, and other environments. Environmental chemical exposures of particular concern include secondhand smoke (SHS); air pollutants; pesticides; endocrine disruptors; contaminants of drinking water; N-nitroso compounds; mycotoxins, such as aflatoxin in peanuts; and hydrocarbons and solvents used in residences and other settings.

### Tobacco

Active smoking is a well-established cause of cancer and tobacco smoke contains the leukemogen, benzene. Many studies have evaluated parental smoking prior or during pregnancy and SHS exposure to the child in relation to the risk of childhood leukemia.[43] Most studies have generally shown no association with maternal smoking; however, a review and meta-analysis of 18 studies of paternal smoking found positive associations for an increased risk of leukemia with paternal smoking before conception and during the pregnancy.[43] The association between parental smoking during pregnancy and the risk of childhood brain tumors is inconsistent. A meta-analysis of 17 studies of parental smoking[44] found no association; however, a large cohort study in Sweden found positive associations between maternal smoking and astrocytomas diagnosed in children aged 5 to 9.[45] Another study found that children who were exposed to tobacco smoke during pregnancy and who had genes that more rapidly activated polycyclic aromatic hydrocarbons (PAHs) were at increased risk.[46] The risk of lung cancer is increased after exposure in childhood to SHS from parents who smoke (see Chapter 43). Smokeless tobacco causes oral cancer in young adults.[47] The practice of chewing tobacco has grown among high school students, who may view professional athletes as role models. The American Medical Association has advocated for a ban on advertising and promotion of all tobacco products.[48] Pediatricians have an opportunity and responsibility to prevent tobacco-related cancers and other tobacco-related conditions.[49]

## Air Pollution

Air pollution is composed of a variable mixture of compounds that includes particulate pollutants, benzene, PAHs, nitrogen and sulfur oxides, carbon monoxide, and ozone (see Chapter 21). Levels of exposure vary on the basis of location, time of day, and season. In 2013, the International Agency for Research on Cancer (IARC) reviewed the evidence for air pollution and cancer and concluded that air pollution and particulate matter (PM) in particular are carcinogenic to humans.[50] In 2012, an IARC review concluded that diesel engine exhaust, an important component of transportation-related air pollution from diesel cars, trucks, trains, and ships, was carcinogenic to humans.[51] More than 20 analytic epidemiologic studies of childhood cancer and air pollution with individual-level estimates of exposure have been published.[50,52] The IARC working group concluded that outdoor air pollution was a possible cause of childhood leukemia, especially ALL, based on positive associations in large studies with validated exposure assessment and limited potential for selection and recall biases. A meta-analysis of traffic-related air pollution and other sources of benzene exposure in children (parental occupational exposure, household use of benzene and other aromatic-containing products) and childhood ALL and AML that included studies from 1999 to 2014,[53] found significantly increased summary relative risks for traffic-related air pollution and ALL and AML, with stronger associations for AML and in studies with detailed models of traffic pollution. Maternal occupational exposure and use of aromatic-containing household products were also associated with increased risk in most studies, with consistent associations for AML. Other childhood cancers have not been as well-studied in relation to air pollution, and associations with lymphoma, childhood brain tumors, and neuroblastoma are inconsistent.[50] A recent registry-based study in Texas found a relationship between roadway density near birth homes and a higher incidence of CNS tumors, particularly ependymona.[54] Large prospective studies are needed and should include improved exposure assessment and characterization of cancer subtypes.

## Endocrine Disruptors

Endocrine disrupting compounds (also known as endocrine disruptors or disrupters) are defined as exogenous agents that change endocrine function and cause adverse effects at the level of the organism, its progeny, and/or subpopulations of organisms (see Chapter 29).[55] Diethylstilbestrol (DES) is an endocrine disrupting compound that is also the only definitively established human transplacental chemical carcinogen.[56] DES is a synthetic estrogen that was used to prevent miscarriage from the late 1940s through the 1970s. It is now known to be associated with an increased risk of vaginal clear cell carcinoma in young women whose mothers took DES during pregnancy. DES also is associated with increased rates of reproductive organ malformation and dysfunction in both male and female offspring.

The dioxin 2,3,7,8-tetrachlorodibenzo-*p*-dioxin (TCDD) is a highly toxic manmade compound with endocrine disrupting properties. It is a known human carcinogen, causing an increase in total cancer.[57] Rodent models suggest that altered mammary gland development and/or abnormal maternal estrogen or prolactin levels may contribute to its carcinogenic mechanism. Other endocrine disrupting compounds have been evaluated as potential cancer risk factors. For example, di(2-ethylhexyl) phthalate, used in medical devices such as medical tubing, was evaluated by the IARC and deemed to be "possibly carcinogenic to humans" (IARC cancer classification Group 2B).[58] The US EPA's endocrine disruptor screening program has evaluated over 50 pesticide active ingredients and 9 other chemicals, including phthalates used as inactive ingredients in pesticides, to determine their potential for disrupting estrogen, androgen, and thyroid hormone pathways,[59] with another list of more than 100 chemicals planned for evaluation.

## *Pesticides*

Pesticides are a heterogeneous group of chemicals with diverse mechanisms of action. The IARC classified the organochlorine insecticide lindane as a human carcinogen and 7 other pesticides as probable human carcinogens. Several of the latter are still registered for use in the United States and more are still in use in other countries, most notably the organochlorine insecticide dichlorodiphenyltrichloroethane (DDT). For endocrine disrupting chemicals, such as DDT, it is hypothesized that there are critical windows of exposure during childhood and adolescence during which exposures can increase cancer risk later in life. Findings from a study of breast cancer among a cohort of women and their daughters support this hypothesis. Among women exposed to DDT before age 14, serum DDT concentrations were associated with an increased breast cancer risk; there was no increased risk in women who were first exposed at older ages.[60] In a later study of breast cancer risk among the daughters,[61] an increased risk was found among women with higher in utero exposure to DDT.

Exposures to pesticides come from sources such as farming, manufacturing, and home and garden uses (see Chapter 40). Most studies of childhood cancer and pesticide exposures have been case-control studies of leukemia and brain tumors.[62-70] Although many of these case-control studies were limited by sample size, exposure assessment, and disease heterogeneity, the results from these studies and some cohort studies suggest that there is a small increase in the risk of leukemia and brain tumors with pesticide exposures from residential use and parental occupational exposure. More recent meta-analyses of leukemia and brain tumors and pooled analyses of childhood leukemia have attempted to evaluate the magnitude of risk by maternal and paternal exposures, general type of pesticide (insecticides, herbicides), and by timing of use (during the pregnancy, child's early life). In the most recent meta-analysis,[64] the associations for childhood leukemia were stronger for maternal exposure (residential use and occupational exposures) than for paternal exposures; whereas paternal exposures appear to be more important for childhood brain cancer. A meta-analysis of 15 studies of childhood leukemia and residential pesticide exposures[66] concluded that residential exposure to insecticides and herbicides during pregnancy and to insecticides during early childhood resulted in increased risks. A meta-analysis of parental occupational exposure to pesticides and childhood leukemia[68] found that maternal exposure during the prenatal period was associated with an increased risk of childhood leukemia; whereas weaker associations were observed for exposures during the child's postnatal life. No consistent associations were found with paternal exposures. Farm-related pesticide exposures were associated with somewhat stronger risks than other occupational pesticide exposures.[68] A meta-analysis of 9 studies of paternal pesticide exposure and neuroblastoma found no increased risk.[71] Future large, cohort studies of parental occupational and childhood exposures to pesticides and childhood cancers are needed to further assess the risks that pesticide exposures may confer. Until then, it appears prudent to reduce and, if possible, eliminate pesticide exposure of children.

### Hydrocarbons and Solvents

Hydrocarbons are organic compounds that include gasoline, paint thinner, solvents, trichloroethylene, and others. Benzene, a known human carcinogen, is used as an additive in motor fuels (see Chapter 30) and hobby glues and in the manufacture of plastics and is also formed by the incomplete combustion of fossil fuels. The dose-response relationship between benzene exposure and adult leukemia (especially AML) risk is well established among adults with occupational exposures.[11,12]

Studies of parental occupations, parental hobbies, and home projects that involve hydrocarbons and solvents in paints and plastics have mostly focused on childhood leukemia.[72,73] A meta-analysis of 13 case-control studies of ALL and AML participating in the Childhood Leukemia International Consortium (CLIC)[72] found no association between paternal or maternal occupational exposure to paints and the risk of either cancer. There was, however, an increased risk of ALL with residential paint exposures shortly before conception, during the pregnancy, and/or after birth, with greater risk for specific cytogenetic subtypes of ALL.

### Arsenic

Arsenic is a well-documented human carcinogen that is associated with the development of adult-onset cancer of the skin, lungs, bladder, and possibly liver (see Chapter 22).[74,75] It induces oxidative damage to DNA and has been shown to be an endocrine disrupting compound. Arsenic crosses the placenta and has been associated with growth retardation and fetal loss. The long-term effects of arsenic exposure and childhood cancer risk are not well established.

### Infection

Exposure to infectious agents during childhood may contribute to cancer risk in adults and children.[8,76] Unless an infant is immunized shortly after birth, vertical transmission from infected mother to infant of hepatitis B virus (HBV) is common. Chronic hepatitis B virus infection will develop in more than 90% of infants infected perinatally with hepatitis B virus, and hepatitis B virus-related hepatocellular carcinoma or cirrhosis will eventually develop in up to 25% of infants and older children who have acquired hepatitis B virus infection. Immunization shortly after birth with hepatitis B vaccine and hepatitis B immune globulin, followed by routine administration of 2 additional doses of hepatitis B vaccine, will prevent chronic hepatitis B virus infection and consequences in most infants.[77]

In childhood, Burkitt lymphoma results from Epstein-Barr virus infection and is endemic in parts of Africa. It is rarely seen in North America and Europe, suggesting possible gene-environment interactions in susceptibility. Epstein-Barr virus is also associated with childhood Hodgkin lymphoma, nasopharyngeal carcinoma, and the majority of cases of post-transplant lymphoproliferative disorder. Infection with other agents raises risks of certain cancers in adults. They include Kaposi sarcoma in individuals infected with HIV, hepatitis C-associated liver cancer, and *Helicobacter pylori*-associated gastric cancer. Young women are at risk of cervical cancer and other cancers caused by human papillomavirus (HPV); young men are at risk of penile cancer and other cancers caused by HPV. Human papillomavirus vaccine can be given to girls and boys as early as age 9 years and is universally recommended for girls and boys as young as age 9 years, adolescents, and young adults.[77]

Several studies found that children who have fewer recorded common infections (eg, upper respiratory tract infections) in the first year of life and less social contact (ie, through child care settings) are at increased risk of childhood leukemia.[8,76,78] Investigators hypothesize that early exposure to common childhood illnesses leads to a more "mature" immune system and that immune dysregulation may contribute to childhood leukemia risk. Further data are needed to fully understand these findings.

## Diet

A number of natural chemicals in food are animal carcinogens and possible human carcinogens. These include aflatoxins, sassafras, cycasin, and bracken (their natural constituents are carcinogens). Preliminary studies have associated maternal consumption of DNA topoisomerase II inhibitor-containing foods (including specific fruits and vegetables, soy, coffee, wine, tea, and cocoa) with an increased risk of infant leukemia.[79] Some food constituents protect against cancer in experimental animals. Among these anti-carcinogens are carotenoids, flavonoids, vitamin C, and other antioxidants.[80] A review of 11 studies of maternal diet and childhood ALL found that a diet composed largely of vegetables, fruits, and protein sources before and during pregnancy reduced ALL risk in offspring.[81] Maternal consumption of cured meats during pregnancy has been associated with an increased risk of childhood brain tumors in most studies.[82] In a recent IARC review of the evidence for human carcinogenicity of red and processed meat,[83] red meat was classified as a probable human carcinogen and processed meat was classified as a human carcinogen, based on epidemiologic studies showing consistent increased risk of colorectal cancer with higher intakes. Meat processing by curing and smoking can result in the formation of carcinogenic chemicals, including N-nitroso-compounds (NOC) and PAHs. High-temperature cooking, (eg, by pan frying, grilling, barbecuing) produces known or suspected carcinogens, including heterocyclic amines and PAHs. Previously, the IARC also determined that ingested nitrate or nitrite under conditions that result in endogenous nitrosation (formation of NOC in the body) is "probably carcinogenic to humans" (IARC cancer classification Group 2A)[84] based on limited evidence from epidemiologic studies of dietary nitrite intake (mostly derived from processed meats) and stomach cancer as well as strong animal and mechanistic studies.

Although data from epidemiologic studies, clinical observations, and animal experiments are insufficient to allow for strong recommendations to be made about specific dietary nutrients, adhering to established cancer prevention guidelines about nutrition and physical activity was shown to significantly decrease overall cancer incidence and mortality.[85] Reductions in risk were seen for breast cancer incidence (19% to 60%), endometrial cancer (23% to 60%), and colorectal cancer in men and women. Other dietary guidelines are recommended to decrease cancer risk. These include reducing fat consumption from 40% to 30% of calories; including whole-grain cereals, citrus fruits, and green and yellow vegetables in the daily diet; limiting consumption of cured foods and alcoholic beverages; and maintaining optimal body weight.[80]

## Parental Occupation

Since the mid 1970s, parental occupational exposures to potential carcinogens have been implicated in the etiology of many types of childhood cancers.[13,18,86] Exposures have been studied before conception, prenatally, and postnatally. Agents such as ionizing radiation, asbestos, benzene, pesticides, and many others have been implicated in the etiology of childhood cancers. The strategy used to assess such exposures in most studies, however, has been limited to identifying exposures from job titles on birth or death certificates or a job history obtained from one or both parents. The most consistent associations have been with parental occupational pesticide exposure and childhood leukemias.[67-69] For other occupational exposures, the strongest evidence is for childhood leukemia and paternal exposure to solvents, paints, and employment in motor vehicle-related occupations; and for childhood nervous system cancers and paternal exposure to paints.[73,86] The relationship between other parental occupational exposures and specific childhood cancers has often been inconsistent. The application of more accurate methods to ascertain exposure is more likely to clarify the relationship of specific occupational exposures with specific forms of childhood cancer.[87]

## WHAT TO DO IF CLUSTERS ARE OBSERVED

Clusters of cancers occasionally occur within a neighborhood or school district, often by chance. It is possible that cancers may be environmentally induced (ie, the histories of the affected people reveal a common exposure, usually to a drug or occupational chemical).[88,89] In office practice, pediatricians can make novel observations about environmental or other causes of specific types of childhood cancers. If a cluster is suspected, the pediatrician should report this observation to the state health department. It is important to determine whether the cancers are of the same or related types. Cancers of the same type are more likely than diverse types to be induced by an environmental carcinogen. Cases should be excluded if the latent period is too short or if the neoplasm was present before the child resided, attended school, or was otherwise exposed in the area. If the exclusions do not dispel the clusters, an environmental epidemiologist from the state health department should be consulted.

An association between two events need not be causal. Establishing causality is enhanced by showing (1) a logical time sequence (ie, the presumed causal event preceded the effect); (2) specificity of the effect (ie, one type rather than multiple types of cancer caused by a given exposure); (3) a dose-response relationship; (4) biologic plausibility (ie, the new information is consistent with previous knowledge); (5) consistency with other observations about cause and effect (eg, determining whether the relationship of processed meat consumption to colon cancer rates is demonstrated in other countries); (6) the exclusion of concomitant variables (alternative explanations) in the analysis; and (7) disappearance of the effect when the cause is removed. Not all of these elements can be evaluated or will hold true for even the most fully studied effects of an environmental exposure. It is not the pediatrician's job to establish causality but to work with epidemiologists and health departments to evaluate the situation.[90]

## SEARCHING FOR CLUES TO CANCER CAUSES

In searching for clues to cancer causes, a careful history can provide important information. A detailed family history should be taken. The medical history for a child with cancer should include a recent pedigree showing illnesses and age of onset in each first-degree relative (parents, siblings, and children of the index case), as well as information about other relatives with cancer or other potentially related diseases, such as immunologic disorders, blood dyscrasias, or congenital malformations. Second, pediatricians should inquire about parents' occupations and the parents' and child's environmental exposures (including smoking) before, during, and after the pregnancy. Despite the extensive studies of environmental exposures and childhood cancers, this knowledge has not been routinely integrated into clinical practice as demonstrated by a recent survey on environmental history-taking and perceptions among pediatric hematologists and oncologists.[91] Exposures of particular relevance to childhood cancer include SHS, pesticides, solvents, radiation, and unusual infections. When asking these questions, it is important to frame queries sensitively so as not to have parents feel guilt or blame. Other findings that may be important in determining the causes of childhood cancers are coexistent disease (such as multiple congenital malformations), multifocal or bilateral cancer in paired organs (a possible clue to hereditary transmission), cancer of an unusual histologic type, cancer at an unusual age (eg, adult-type cancers in childhood), cancer at an unusual site, or marked overreaction to conventional cancer therapy (eg, acute reaction to radiotherapy for lymphoma in ataxia telangiectasia). This information, especially regarding family history, may be relevant to the risk of malignancy in the child's siblings or other relatives. Epidemiologists also can use this information to gain new understandings of the origins of childhood cancer.

Pediatricians and obstetricians can also play important roles in educating parents to reduce exposures to environmental risk factors. Information about prenatal folic acid supplementation, preventing tobacco use and SHS exposure, and a healthy diet for mother and child can be a part of education on childhood cancer prevention.[92]

## Frequently Asked Questions

Q  *What steps can I take to prevent cancer in my child?*

A  Although the causes of many childhood cancers are unknown, there is consistent evidence for an increased risk of childhood leukemia with exposures to pesticides, solvents, traffic-related air pollution, and paternal smoking.[92] Therefore, limiting these exposures during pregnancy and throughout the child's life is prudent. Breastfeeding, folic acid supplementation during pregnancy, and a healthy diet, which includes limited or no consumption of cured/smoked meats and fish, and frequent intake of fruits and vegetables has been shown to reduce childhood leukemia risk.[92] Children should be encouraged not to smoke, use electronic cigarettes or similar devices, or use smokeless tobacco products. Adults should be encouraged to quit smoking; if they choose to keep smoking, they should never smoke indoors or in the car to prevent family members from being exposed to secondhand smoke. Children should be encouraged to wear clothing and hats and to use sunscreen when outdoors so that they do not become sunburned. Teenagers should not be allowed to tan in tanning salons or other venues, such as health clubs, that may have tanning beds. Other important preventive measures include testing the home for radon and making sure no friable asbestos exists in the home.

Q  *Why did neuroblastoma develop in my 3-month-old child?*

A  We know that damage to DNA (a mutation) occurs at a specific location in one chromosome in neuroblastoma, but we do not know what causes the mutation. Mutations may occur during normal reshuffling of genetic material. Usually, the damage is repaired and cancer does not develop, but unfortunately, this defense is sometimes breached.

Q  *The cat has been sick. Could the cat have caused my child's leukemia?*

A  There is no evidence that pets transmit cancer to humans. Cats develop a similar disease caused by a virus, which they can transmit to other cats but not to humans. The same is true of chickens and cattle, in which a leukemia-like disease is virally induced.

Q  *Several children in our neighborhood have cancer. Could it be caused by the same thing?*

A  Although most environmental causes of cancer in humans have been first recognized by the occurrence of a cluster of cases, such discoveries are infrequent and generally involve rare cancers attributable to heavy exposures to a carcinogen. The many types of cancer (more than 80) give rise to thousands of random clusters each year in the United States in neighborhoods, schools, social clubs, sports teams, and other groups of people. By focusing on the location of cases, an otherwise random clustering of cases may seem to be unusual. To establish a cause, however, more evidence than a cluster is needed, including a dose-response effect (the bigger the dose, the more frequent the effect) and biologic plausibility considering other knowledge about cancer. In most clusters, there are many different types of cancers and many different causes, rather than a single cause.

Q   *Will my child with cancer give my other children cancer?*

A   Cancer is not transmitted from one person to another. Occasionally, a genetic predisposition to specific cancers is transmitted from parents to children, which may have implications for other children in the family.

For example, retinoblastoma (a rare cancer of the eye) runs in families. Usually, signs of predisposition to hereditary cancer can be detected in the histories of families with genetic disorders. For children at risk, early detection and treatment can improve survival and well-being. Thus, few children die of retinoblastoma today.

Q   *A member of our household smokes. Could that be the cause of my child's cancer?*

A   There is increasing evidence that paternal smoking (but not maternal smoking) before and during the pregnancy increases the risk of childhood leukemia in offspring. Cancers in children younger than 15 years generally are of a different microscopic category from adult cigarette-induced cancers, and no evidence currently exists that the childhood cancers are inducible by secondhand smoke. On the other hand, adult cancers, such as lung cancer, leukemia, and lymphoma, have been associated with exposure to maternal smoking that occurs before the child reaches age 10 years.

Q   *Is it possible that the drugs I took during pregnancy started my child's cancer?*

A   Diethylstilbestrol (DES) is the only known medication given to pregnant mothers that is associated with increased cancer risk in their children. It has not been used since the 1970s and was associated primarily with vaginal clear cell adenocarcinoma in young women whose mothers took DES during pregnancy. Other drugs commonly used during pregnancy have not been shown to be carcinogenic in the offspring. Drugs that have been shown to present a risk of either malformations or a theoretical risk of cancer are generally avoided during pregnancy.

Q   *I have heard that peanut butter may cause cancer. Is this true?*

A   Peanuts can be contaminated with molds that produce aflatoxins, which are toxic chemicals and known carcinogens. The US Food and Drug Administration allows aflatoxins at low levels in nuts, seeds, and legumes because they are considered "unavoidable contaminants." If a particular batch of peanut butter is tested and the concentration of aflatoxin is over the action level, it will be subject to a recall. Aflatoxins have been shown to increase the risk of liver cancer in adults; however, there is no evidence of a link with childhood cancers.

Q   *Is childhood cancer increasing?*

A   Yes. Rates of childhood cancer (age younger than 15) increased 38% between 1975 to 2014 in the United States.[2] For leukemia, the most common childhood cancer, there was a 42% increase in incidence rates; increases were greatest for Hispanic children.[2,5] For brain cancer and other nervous system cancers, incidence increased in the 1980s because of improvements in diagnostic procedures and changes in classification. Rates were stable from 1987 to 2014. Among children and adolescents (age younger than 20), non-Hodgkin lymphoma increased; whereas, Hodgkin lymphoma rates decreased over the same period.

Q   *Does living near a nuclear power plant increase my child's risk of cancer?*

A   One study in Germany showed that children younger than age 5 with leukemia were more than twice as likely as a comparison group of children to live within 5 km of a nuclear power plant.[93] It is not clear whether this association is causal. Additional studies are needed to clarify the risk of living near a nuclear power plant.

## Resources

**Center for Integrative Research on Childhood Leukemia and the Environment (at University of California, Berkeley).** Includes a multimedia eBook dedicated to children's environmental health research translation for clinicians and parents:

http://circle.berkeley.edu/translation-and-outreach/for-clinicians/
http://circle.berkeley.edu/translation-and-outreach/for-parents/

**Children's Oncology Group and Cure Search**
Web sites: www.childrensoncologygroup.org
www.curesearch.org

**National Cancer Institute**
Phone: 800-4-CANCER
Web site: www.cancer.gov

## Reference List

1.  National Cancer Institute. Cancer in Children and Adolescents. http://www.cancer.gov/types/childhood-cancers/child-adolescent-cancers-fact-sheet. Accessed August 29, 2018

2.  Howlader N, Noone AM, Krapcho M, et al, eds. SEER Cancer Statistics Review, 1975-2014. National Cancer Institute. Bethesda, MD. https://seer.cancer.gov/csr/1975_2014/. Accessed May 9, 2018

3. Steliarova-Foucher E, Stiller C, Lacour B, Kaatsch P. International Classification of Childhood Cancer, third edition. *Cancer*. 2005;103(7):1457–1467

4. Mirabello L, Troisi R, Savage SA. Osteosarcoma incidence and survival rates from 1973 to 2004: data from the surveillance, epidemiology, and end results program. *Cancer*. 2009;115(7): 1531–1543

5. Barrington-Trimis JL, Cockburn M, Metayer C, Gauderman WJ, Wiemels J, McKean-Cowdin R. Rising rates of acute lymphoblastic leukemia in Hispanic children: trends in incidence from 1992 to 2011. *Blood*. 2015;125(19):3033–3034

6. American Cancer Society. Cancer Facts & Figures 2014. Special Section: Cancer in Children & Adolescents. https://www.cancer.org/content/dam/cancer-org/research/cancer-facts-and-statistics/annual-cancer-facts-and-figures/2014/special-section-cancer-in-children-and-adolescents-cancer-facts-and-figures-2014.pdf. Accessed May 9, 2018

7. Linet MS, Wacholder S, Zahm SH. Interpreting epidemiologic research: lessons from studies of childhood cancer. *Pediatrics*. 2003;112(1 Pt 2):218–232

8. Wiemels J. Perspectives on the causes of childhood leukemia. *Chem Biol Interact*. 2012;196(3):59–67

9. Brown RC, Dwyer T, Kasten C, et al. Cohort profile: the International Childhood Cancer Cohort Consortium (I4C). *Int J Epidemiol*. 2007;36(4):724–730

10. Children's Oncology Group. Childhood Cancer Research Network (CCRN). https://childrensoncologygroup.org/index.php/childhood-cancer-research-network-ccrn. Accessed May 9, 2018

11. Belpomme D, Irigaray P, Hardell L, et al. The multitude and diversity of environmental carcinogens. *Environ Res*. 2007;105(3):414–429

12. Clapp RW, Jacobs MM, Loechler EL. Environmental and occupational causes of cancer: new evidence 2005-2007. *Rev Environ Health*. 2008; 23(1):1-37

13. Ross JA, Spector L. Cancers in children. In: Schottenfeld D, Fraumeni JF Jr, eds. *Cancer Epidemiology and Prevention*. 3rd ed. Oxford University Press; 2006

14. Anderson LM. Environmental genotoxicants/carcinogens and childhood cancer: bridgeable gaps in scientific knowledge. *Mutat Res*. 2006;608(2):136–156

15. Birnbaum LS, Fenton SE. Cancer and developmental exposure to endocrine disruptors. *Environ Health Perspect*. 2003;111(4):389–394

16. Fenton SE, Birnbaum LS. Timing of environmental exposures as a critical element in breast cancer. *J Clin Endocrinol Metab*. 2015;100(9):3245–3250

17. Linet MS, Ries LA, Smith MA, Tarone RE, Devesa SS. Cancer surveillance series: recent trends in childhood cancer incidence and mortality in the United States. *J Natl Cancer Inst*. 1999;91(12):1051–1058

18. Bunin GR. Nongenetic causes of childhood cancers: evidence from international variation, time trends, and risk factor studies. *Toxicol Appl Pharmacol*. 2004;199(2):91–103

19. Stiller CA. Epidemiology and genetics of childhood cancer. *Oncogene*. 2004;23(38):6429–6444

20. Leiter U, Eigentler T, Garbe C. Epidemiology of skin cancer. *Adv Exp Med Biol*. 2014;810: 120–140

21. American Academy of Pediatrics Council on Environmental Health, Section on Dermatology, Balk SJ. Ultraviolet radiation: a hazard to children and adolescents. *Pediatrics*. 2011;127(3):588–597

22. Bithell JF, Stewart AM. Pre-natal irradiation and childhood malignancy: a review of British data from the Oxford Survey. *Br J Cancer*. 1975;31(3):271–287

23. Schulze-Rath R, Hammer GP, Blettner M. Are pre- or postnatal diagnostic X-rays a risk factor for childhood cancer? A systematic review. *Radiat Environ Biophys*. 2008;47(3):301–312

24. Linet MS, Kim KP, Rajaraman P. Children's exposure to diagnostic medical radiation and cancer risk: epidemiologic and dosimetric considerations. *Pediatr Radiol*. 2009;39(Suppl 1):S4–S26

25. Hoffman DA, Lonstein JE, Morin MM, Visscher W, Harris BS III, Boice JD Jr. Breast cancer in women with scoliosis exposed to multiple diagnostic x rays. *J Natl Cancer Inst*. 1989;81(17): 1307–1312

26. Ronckers CM, Doody MM, Lonstein JE, Stovall M, Land CE. Multiple diagnostic X-rays for spine deformities and risk of breast cancer. *Cancer Epidemiol Biomarkers Prev*. 2008;17(3): 605–613

27. Brody AS, Frush DP, Huda W, Brent RL. Radiation risk to children from computed tomography. *Pediatrics*. 2007;120(3):677–682

28. Pearce MS, Salotti JA, Little MP, et al. Radiation exposure from CT scans in childhood and subsequent risk of leukaemia and brain tumours: a retrospective cohort study. *Lancet*. 2012;380(9840):499–505

29. Goske MJ, Applegate KE, Boylan J, et al. The 'Image Gently' campaign: increasing CT radiation dose awareness through a national education and awareness program. *Pediatr Radiol*. 2008;38(3):265–269

30. Morton LM, Onel K, Curtis RE, Hungate EA, Armstrong GT. The rising incidence of second cancers: patterns of occurrence and identification of risk factors for children and adults. *Am Soc Clin Oncol Educ Book*. 2014:e57–e67

31. Ichimaru M, Ishimaru T. Review of thirty years study of Hiroshima and Nagasaki atomic bomb survivors. II. Biological effects. D. Leukemia and related disorders. *J Radiat Res*. 1975;16(Suppl):89–96

32. Land CE, Tokunaga M, Koyama K, et al. Incidence of female breast cancer among atomic bomb survivors, Hiroshima and Nagasaki, 1950-1990. *Radiat Res*. 2003;160(6):707–717

33. Miller RW. Delayed effects of external radiation exposure: a brief history. *Radiat Res*. 1995;144(2):160–169

34. Preston DL, Cullings H, Suyama A, et al. Solid cancer incidence in atomic bomb survivors exposed in utero or as young children. *J Natl Cancer Inst*. 2008;100(6):428–436

35. Ron E. Thyroid cancer incidence among people living in areas contaminated by radiation from the Chernobyl accident. *Health Phys*. 2007;93(5):502–511

36. Brenner AV, Tronko MD, Hatch M, et al. I-131 dose response for incident thyroid cancers in Ukraine related to the Chornobyl accident. *Environ Health Perspect*. 2011;119(7):933–993

37. Ostroumova E, Hatch M, Brenner A, et al. Non-thyroid cancer incidence in Belarusian residents exposed to Chernobyl fallout in childhood and adolescence: Standardized Incidence Ratio analysis, 1997-2011. *Environ Res*. 2016;147:44–49

38. Hatch M, Ostroumova E, Brenner A, et al. Non-thyroid cancer in Norther Ukraine in the post-Chernobyl period: short report. *Cancer Epidemiol*. 2015;39(3):279–283

39. Schüz J. Exposure to extremely low-frequency magnetic fields and the risk of childhood cancer: update of the epidemiological evidence. *Prog Biophys Mol Biol*. 2011;107(3):339–342

40. International Agency for Research on Cancer. IARC Monographs on the evaluation of carcinogenic risks to humans, Vol 80. Non-ionizing Radiation, Part 1: Static and Extremely Low-Frequency (ELF) Electric and Magnetic Fields. Lyon, France: International Agency for Research on Cancer; 2002

41. Wyde M, Cesta M, Blystone C, et al. Report of Partial findings from the National Toxicology Program Carcinogenesis Studies of Cell Phone Radiofrequency Radiation in Hsd: Sprague Dawley® SD rats (Whole Body Exposure). BioRxiv. http://dx.doi.org/10.1101/055699. Accessed May 9, 2018

42. Cugell DW, Kamp DW. Asbestos and the pleura: a review. *Chest*. 2004;125(3):1103–1117

43. Chang JS. Parental smoking and childhood leukemia. *Methods Mol Biol*. 2008;472:103–137

44. Huang Y, Huang J, Lan H, Zhao G, Huang C. A meta-analysis of parental smoking and the risk of childhood brain tumors. *PLoS One*. 2014;9(7):e102910

45. Tettamanti G, Ljung R, Mathiesen T, Schwartzbaum J, Feychting M. Maternal smoking during pregnancy and the risk of childhood brain tumors: results from a Swedish cohort study. *Cancer Epidemiol*. 2016;40:67–72

46. Barrington-Trimis JL, Searles Nielsen S, Preston-Martin S, et al. Parental smoking and risk of childhood brain tumors by functional polymorphisms in polycyclic aromatic hydrocarbon metabolism genes. *PLoS One*. 2013;8(11):e79110

47. National Institutes of Health State-of-the-Science Conference Statement on Tobacco Use: Prevention, Cessation, and Control. *NIH Consens State Sci Statements*. 2006;23(3):1–26

48. American Medical Association. Tobacco Advertising and Media H-495.984. https://policysearch.ama-assn.org/policyfinder/detail/tobacco?uri=%2FAMADoc%2FHOD.xml-0-4516.xml. Accessed May 9, 2018

49. Farber HJ, Nelson KE, Groner JA, Walley SC. Public policy to protect children from tobacco, nicotine, and tobacco smoke. *Pediatrics*. 2015;136(5):998–1007

50. International Agency for Research on Cancer. IARC Monographs on the Evaluation of Carcinogenic Risks to Humans Vol. 109. Outdoor air pollution. Lyon, France: International Agency for Research on Cancer; 2016

51. Benbrahim-Tallas L, Baan RA, Grosse Y, et al. Carcinogenicity of diesel-engine and gasoline-engine exhausts and some nitroarenes. *Lancet Oncol*. 2012;13(7):663–664

52. Raaschou-Nielsen O, Reynolds P. Air pollution and childhood cancer: a review of the epidemiological literature. *Int J Cancer*. 2006;118(12):2920–2929

53. Carlos Wallace FM, Zhang L, Smith MT, Rader G, Steinmaus C. Parental, in utero, and early-life exposure to benzene and the risk of childhood leukemia: a meta-analysis. *Am J Epidemiol*. 2015;183(1):1–14

54. Danysh HE, Zhang K, Mitchell LE, Scheurer ME, Lupo PJ. Maternal residential proximity to major roadways at delivery and childhood central nervous system tumors. *Environ Res*. 2016;146:315–322

55. US Environmental Protection Agency. Endocrine Disruptor Screening Program. http://www.epa.gov/endo/index.htm. Accessed May 9, 2018

56. Newbold RR. Prenatal exposure to diethylstilbestrol and long-term impact on the breast and reproductive tract in humans and mice. *J Dev Orig Health Dis*. 2012;3(2):73–82

57. International Agency for Research on Cancer. IARC Monographs on the Evaluation of Carcinogenic Risks to Humans Vol. 100F. Chemical Agents and Related Occupations. Lyon, France: International Agency for Research on Cancer; 2012

58. International Agency for Research on Cancer. IARC Monographs on the Evaluation of Carcinogenic Risks to Humans. Volume 101: Some Chemicals in Industrial and Consumer Products, Some Food Contaminants and Flavourings, and Water Chlorination By-Products. Lyon, France: International Agency for Research on Cancer; 2011

59. US Environmental Protection Agency. Endocrine Disruptor Screening Program (EDSP) Overview. https://www.epa.gov/endocrine-disruption/endocrine-disruptor-screening-program-edsp-overview. Accessed May 9, 2018

60. Cohn BA, Wolff MS, Cirillo PM, Sholtz RI. DDT and breast cancer in young women: new data on the significance of age at exposure. *Environ Health Perspect*. 2007;115(10):1406–1414

61. Cohn BA, La Merrill M, Krigbaum NY, et al. DDT Exposure in utero and breast cancer. *J Clin Endocrinol Metab*. 2015;100(8):2865–2872

62. Zahm SH, Ward MH. Pesticides and childhood cancer. *Environ Health Perspect*. 1998;106(Suppl 3):893–908

63. Infante-Rivard C, Weichenthal S. Pesticides and childhood cancer: an update of Zahm and Ward's 1998 review. *J Toxicol Environ Health B Crit Rev.* 2007;10(1-2):81–99

64. Chen M, Chang CH, Tao L, Lu C. Residential exposure to pesticide during childhood and childhood cancers: a meta-analysis. *Pediatrics.* 2015;136(4):719–729

65. Vinson F, Merhi M, Baldi I, Raynal H, Gamet-Payrastre L. Exposure to pesticides and risk of childhood cancer: a meta-analysis of recent epidemiological studies. *Occup Environ Med.* 2011;68(9):694–702

66. Turner MC, Wigle DT, Krewski D. Residential pesticides and childhood leukemia: a systematic review and meta-analysis. *Environ Health Perspect.* 2010;118(1):33–41

67. Van Maele-Fabry G, Hoet P, Lison D. Parental occupational exposure to pesticides as risk factor for brain tumors in children and young adults: a systematic review and meta-analysis. *Environ Int.* 2013;56:19–31

68. Wigle DT, Turner MC, Krewski D. A systematic review and meta-analysis of childhood leukemia and parental occupational pesticide exposure. *Environ Health Perspect.* 2009;117(10):1505–1513

69. Bailey HD, Fritschi L, Infante-Rivard C, et al. Parental occupational pesticide exposure and the risk of childhood leukemia in the offspring: findings from the childhood leukemia international consortium. *Int J Cancer.* 2014;135(9):2157–2172

70. Bailey HD, Infante-Rivard C, Metayer C, et al. Home pesticide exposures and risk of childhood leukemia: findings from the childhood leukemia international consortium. *Int J Cancer.* 2015;137(11):2644–2663

71. Moore A, Enquobahrie DA. Paternal occupational exposure to pesticides and risk of neuroblastoma among children: a meta-analysis. *Cancer Causes Control.* 2011;22(11): 1529–1536

72. Bailey HD, Metayer C, Milne E, et al. Home paint exposures and risk of childhood acute lymphoblastic leukemia: findings from the Childhood Leukemia International Consortium. *Cancer Causes Control.* 2015;26(9):1257–1270

73. Schüz J, Kaletsch U, Meinert R, Kaatsch P, Michaelis J. Risk of childhood leukemia and parental self-reported occupational exposure to chemicals, dusts, and fumes: results from pooled analyses of German population-based case-control studies. *Cancer Epidemiol Biomarkers Prev.* 2000;9(8):835–838

74. Vahter M. Health effects of early life exposure to arsenic. *Basic Clin Pharmacol Toxicol.* 2008;102(2):204–211

75. Karagas MR, Gossal A, Pierce B, Ahsan H. Drinking water arsenic contamination, skin lesions, and malignancies: a systematic review of the global evidence. *Curr Environ Health Rep.* 2015;2(1):52–68

76. Greaves M. Infection, immune responses and the aetiology of childhood leukaemia. *Nat Rev Cancer.* 2006;6(3):193–203

77. American Academy of Pediatrics Committee on Infectious Diseases. Kimberlin DW, Brady MT, Jackson MA, Long SS, eds. *Red Book*: 2018 Report of the Committee on Infectious Diseases. 31st ed. Itasca, IL: American Academy of Pediatrics; 2018

78. Urayama KY, Buffler PA, Gallagher ER, Ayoob JM, Ma X. A meta-analysis of the association between day-care attendance and childhood acute lymphoblastic leukaemia. *Int J Epidemiol.* 2010;39(3):718–732

79. Ross JA. Maternal diet and infant leukemia: a role for DNA topoisomerase II inhibitors? *Int J Cancer Suppl.* 1998;11:26–28

80. Key TJ, Schatzkin A, Willett WC, Allen NE, Spencer EA, Travis RC. Diet, nutrition and the prevention of cancer. *Public Health Nutr.* 2004;7(1A):187–200

81. Abiri B, Kelishadi R, Sadeqhi H, Azizi-Soleiman F. Effects of maternal diet during pregnancy on the risk of childhood acute lymphoblastic leukemia: a systematic review. *Nutr Cancer.* 2016;68(7):1065–1072

82. Dietrich M, Block G, Pogoda JM, Buffler P, Hecht S, Preston-Martin S. A review: dietary and endogenously formed N-nitroso compounds and risk of childhood brain tumors. *Cancer Causes Control.* 2005;16(6):619–635

83. Bouvard V, Loomis D, Guyton KZ, et al. Carcinogenicity of consumption of red and processed meat. *Lancet Oncol.* 2015;16(16):1599–1600

84. IARC Monograph Working Group on the Evaluation of the Carcinogenic Risk to Humans. Ingested Nitrate and Nitrite, and Cyanobacterial Peptide Toxins. Vol 94; 2010. http://monographs.iarc.fr/ENG/Monographs/vol94/mono94.pdf. Accessed May 9, 2018

85. Kohler LN, Garcia DO, Harris RB, Oren E, Roe DJ, Jacobs ET. Adherence to diet and physical activity cancer prevention guidelines and cancer outcomes: a systematic review. *Cancer Epidemiol Biomarkers Prev.* 2016;25(7):1018–1028

86. Colt JS, Blair A. Parental occupational exposures and risk of childhood cancer. *Environ Health Perspect.* 1998;106(Suppl 3):909–925

87. Schüz J, Spector LG, Ross JA. Bias in studies of parental self-reported occupational exposure and childhood cancer. *Am J Epidemiol.* 2003;158(7):710–716

88. Kingsley BS, Schmeichel KL, Rubin CH. An update on cancer cluster activities at the Centers for Disease Control and Prevention. *Environ Health Perspect.* 2007;115(1):165–171

89. Benowitz S. Busting cancer clusters: realities often differ from perceptions. *J Natl Cancer Inst.* 2008;100(9):614–615

90. Hill AB. The environment and disease: association or causation? *Proc R Soc Med.* 1965;58:295–300

91. Metayer C, Dahl G, Wiemels J, Miller M. Childhood leukemia: a preventable disease. *Pediatrics.* 2016;138(Suppl 1):S45–S55

92. Zachek CM, Miller MD, Hsu C, et al. Children's cancer and environmental exposures: professional attitudes and practices. *J Pediatr Hematol Oncol.* 2015;37(7):491–497

93. Kaatsch P, Spix C, Schulze-Rath R, Schmiedel S, Blettner M. Leukaemia in young children living in the vicinity of German nuclear power plants. *Int J Cancer.* 2008;122(4):721–726

Chapter 50

# Chelation (Non-Approved Use for Environmental Toxicants)

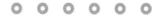

## KEY POINTS

- Chelation therapy is indicated for the treatment of severe cases of childhood poisoning caused by selected metals (eg, lead, arsenic, iron). Chelation also is associated with a significant risk of adverse reactions that must be weighed in assessing its possible therapeutic benefit.
- No scientific evidence is available to suggest that pharmaceutical chelation is an effective intervention for autism spectrum disorder, except in those cases in which the child with autism spectrum disorder also suffers from moderate to severe lead poisoning.
- Clinicians who are caring for a child with significant poisoning from metals who might benefit from chelation are advised to consult first with an expert in medical toxicology or pediatric environmental health, or an agency such as a poison control center (PCC) or a Pediatric Environmental Health Specialty Unit (PEHSU).

## INTRODUCTION

This chapter focuses on the non-approved use by some clinicians of chelation to treat environmental toxicants, usually in patients who have chronic health conditions, where there is no accepted scientific evidence of efficacy. This chapter is not about chelation of patients who have inherited or have iatrogenic toxicity from iron-overload or aluminum-loading. It is not about children with moderate to severe lead poisoning who are symptomatic and/or have high concentrations of lead in their blood. In these situations, chelation is approved and indicated.

The most frequently encountered non-approved uses of chelation agents in the pediatric setting are for treatment of neurodevelopmental disabilities, including attention-deficit/hyperactivity disorder (ADHD), autism spectrum disorder (ASD), and others. Although chelation therapy does not treat these conditions, these conditions can be effectively managed with evidence-based behavioral therapies for ASD and medications for ADHD.[1,2] Families may seek treatment outside of the usual medical system or ask their child's pediatrician for chelation therapy for heavy metal toxicity. It is important to understand and acknowledge the basis for these requests.

"Heavy metal" is a loosely defined term referring to metals with specific gravity of 5 or higher (although metalloids are sometimes called "heavy" as well), including copper, lead, zinc, cadmium, chromium, arsenic, mercury, and nickel.[3] The term may be used to mean that the metal is toxic when ingested or absorbed. Chelation is the treatment of heavy metal poisoning using agents that bind with a metal ion to form a complex with different chemical, biological, and/or physical properties. The resulting complexes are more easily removed or excreted from the body than the non-complexed metal.[4] Ideal chelation agents are water soluble to enter the bloodstream, are stable, are able to reach physiological compartments in which metals accumulate, form nontoxic complexes with the metal, and can be excreted without causing harm. Most chelation agents have some affinity for all metals; it is important to select the agent that is best suited to form complexes with the metal of concern without depleting other essential minerals, such as calcium and zinc.[5]

Chelation agents are classified mainly by their affinity for organic states. Hydrophilic chelators enhance renal excretion of metals and do not readily cross cellular walls; as a result, they have limited effects on intracellular metal concentrations. Lipophilic chelators decrease intracellular storage sites but may redistribute toxic metals to other lipophilic compartments such as the brain. Excretion rates may differ as well.[4]

This chapter describes the on-label (approved uses of chelation therapy) and the associated adverse effects with indicated use. The chapter also describes the historical context spurring off-label practices and the ongoing non-approved uses of chelation therapy especially in vulnerable pediatric populations, such as those with neurodevelopmental disabilities.

## ON-LABEL (APPROVED) USES OF CHELATION THERAPY

Chelation therapy is indicated for treatment of childhood lead poisoning ( for example, children with blood lead levels ≥45 mcg/dL) (see Chapter

32). In addition, chelation therapy during pregnancy or early infancy may be warranted in certain circumstances, especially where the maternal or neonatal blood lead exceeds ≥45 mcg/dL.[6] Although it is approved by the Food and Drug Administration (FDA) for hemochromatosis, the treatment of choice for hemochromatosis is blood donation.

The frequency of chelation therapy for elevated blood lead levels has decreased significantly as a result of a multi-pronged approach to widespread testing of children, enforcement of the housing code, facilitated residential inspection and mitigation and abatement efforts, and educational outreach to both the lay public and health care providers. Because of these efforts, a pediatrician in primary care practice rarely encounters a child with an elevated blood lead level for which chelation therapy is indicated. Children are at higher risk of lead exposure if they are members of racial-ethnic minority groups, live in poverty, live in substandard housing, are recent immigrants, and have parents who are exposed to occupational sources of lead.[7]

The use of chelants in the management of childhood lead poisoning has been reviewed elsewhere.[8] Pediatricians and other health care professionals are strongly advised to consult experts in pediatric environmental health and to weigh benefits and harms of the disease and the treatment before initiating chelation therapy.[9] For specific exposures and treatments, a pediatrician experienced in managing children with lead poisoning should be consulted—these physicians can be found through the American Academy of Pediatrics (AAP) Council on Environmental Health or through lead poisoning prevention programs at state health departments (www.cdc.gov/nceh/lead/programs/default.htm). Physicians with expertise in pediatric environmental health as well as guidelines for medical management of childhood lead poisoning can also be found by contacting a regional PEHSU at: www.pehsu.net.[9]

## ADVERSE EFFECTS OF CHELATION AGENTS

Chelation therapy is associated with significant risks of morbidity and mortality,[10–12] and there is increasing evidence of a lack of beneficial outcomes associated with its use for the treatment of ASD.[13] Table 50-1 lists many of the adverse effects of general classes of agents used for chelation. It is critical that a harm-benefit analysis be performed prior to initiating treatment with chelation agents, whether "off-" or "on-label."

Although chelation can promote excretion of heavy metals, most chelation agents do not uniformly decrease the body burden of heavy metals.[11,17] Some agents do not cross the blood-brain barrier efficiently; others do not enter the intracellular space. Most are effective in binding with metals in the vascular system, which can cause release of metals from other compartments, resulting in an increase in blood levels of the target metal. Such an increase in blood

## Table 50-1. Toxicities of Chelation Agents[4]

| AGENT | APPROVED USE | TOXICITY |
|---|---|---|
| British anti-lewisite[14] (BAL [2,3-dimercatopropanol]), dimercaprol, and related agents, such as 2,3-dimercapto-1-propanesulfonic acid (DMPS) | ▪ Only given parenterally (deep intramuscular)<br>▪ Arsenic, gold, mercury, acute lead poisoning (when used concomitantly with CaNa$_2$EDTA)[14] | ▪ Dosage exceeding 5 mg/kg will usually be followed by vomiting, convulsions, and stupor, beginning within 30 minutes and subsiding within 6 hours following injection.[14]<br>▪ Toxicities are dose-dependent and doses require small fractional dosages in the pediatric population.<br>▪ Contraindicated in children allergic to nuts (medication is dissolved in peanut oil)<br>▪ Contraindicated in children with glucose-6-phosphatase deficiency because it can lead to hemolysis in this patient population<br>▪ Can cause nausea, emesis, fever, rashes, significant hypertension/tachycardia; headache; burning sensation in lips, mouth, throat; feeling of throat, chest, or hand constriction; transient decline in percent polymorphonuclear leukocyte count<br>▪ Can cause liver and kidney dysfunction or zinc deficiency<br>▪ Can cause pain or sterile abscesses at the injection site<br>▪ Children often are at risk for the development of fever, which abates with cessation of treatment |
| Edetate calcium disodium[15] (CaNa$_2$EDTA; calcium disodium ethylenediamine tetraacetate; Brand name: calcium disodium Versenate) | ▪ Only given parenterally<br>▪ Indicated for the reduction of blood levels and depot stores of lead in lead poisoning (acute and chronic) and lead encephalopathy[15]<br>▪ Chelation therapy should not replace effective measures to eliminate or reduce further exposure to lead.[15] | ▪ Renal toxicities; malaise and fatigue; chills, fever; headache; anorexia, nausea, and vomiting; transitory hypotension; prolonged prothrombin time; T-wave inversion on electrocardiogram<br>▪ Depletion of essential trace metals<br>▪ Thrombophlebitis |

| | | |
|---|---|---|
| Deferoxamine | ▪ Not recommended for treatment of primary hemochromatosis (treat with phlebotomy)<br>▪ Iron<br>▪ Aluminum (dialysis patients) | ▪ Pruritus, wheals, rash, anaphylaxis, dysuria, abdominal discomfort, diarrhea, fever, leg cramps, tachycardia, cataract formation, neurotoxicity associated with long-term, high-dose use (typically for treatment of thalassemia major), including visual and auditory changes<br>▪ May cause renal failure, especially if patient is volume-depleted (hydrate first)<br>▪ Contraindicated if renal insufficiency, anuria, pregnancy |
| 2,3-dimercaptosuccinic acid (DMSA)[16] | ▪ Indicated for the treatment of lead poisoning in pediatric patients with blood lead levels ≥45 mcg/dL[16]<br>▪ It is not indicated for prophylaxis of lead poisoning in a lead-containing environment; chelation therapy should always be accompanied by identification and removal of the source of the lead exposure.[16] | ▪ Mild elevation in hepatic transaminase is the most common adverse effect of DMSA therapy<br>▪ Adverse dermatological reactions and fixed drug eruptions; the pathogeneses are poorly understood<br>▪ Reported hemolysis in patients with glucose-6-phosphate dehydrogenase deficiency<br>▪ Gastrointestinal distress including nausea, vomiting, diarrhea<br>▪ Depletion of essential trace metals |
| Disodium EDTA (Na$_2$EDTA) | ▪ Not approved for use in children | ▪ Hypocalcemic tetany can occur with too-rapid infusion<br>▪ Has caused death in children |
| Pentetic acid (diethylenetriaminepentaacetic acid [DTPA]) | ▪ Investigational | ▪ Limited use because of poor access to intracellular sites of metal stores |

level can theoretically promote additional dispersion of the metal. Early studies of mice treated with British anti-lewisite (BAL, 2,3-dimercatopropanol) showed increased distribution of mercury to the brain following treatment.[18–22] In some instances, chelation may actually cause more harm than no treatment. For example, lead stored in bone is relatively inert if calcium intake is sufficient and bone stores of calcium are not resorbed to supply calcium.

Little evidence exists to show that chelation reverses neurologic damage from lead poisoning. In a multisite, randomized, controlled trial, investigators studied the effect of chelation with 2,3-dimercaptosuccinic acid (DMSA or succimer) on neurodevelopmental outcomes of children aged 12 to 33 months whose blood lead levels were 20 to 44 mcg/dL.[23] The blood lead levels of the children who had undergone chelation decreased, but 1 year following the start of chelation the study found no differences between the blood lead levels of children who received chelation and those who received a placebo; and there were no differences between treated and untreated groups in neurodevelopmental outcomes at age 7 years.[23,24]

Chelation agents are not selective for specific metals. This lack of selectivity is the cause of one of the most important adverse effects of chelation therapy—concomitant loss of essential metals and minerals, especially calcium and zinc, during treatment.[25] Calcium and zinc are essential metals that can be depleted below critical limits, posing serious health threats to patients. Thus, the potential secondary targets of chelation agents must be identified prior to chelation. The agent most frequently implicated in deaths associated with chelation is edentate disodium ($Na_2EDTA$).[10,12,26] The on-label indications for this agent are hypercalcemia and ventricular arrhythmias attributable to digitalis toxicity. $Na_2EDTA$ use in children is contraindicated because of the high risk of hypocalcemia and fatal tetany. The chelation agent edetate disodium calcium ($CaNa_2EDTA$), which can be used for chelation, has a similar name. Despite the risks associated with $Na_2EDTA$, some pharmacies stock both types; confusion of the two has resulted in case-reportable pediatric deaths. A child with ASD died after the "off-label" use of chelation with $Na_2EDTA$; death was caused by acute cerebral hypoxic-ischemic injury, with secondary necrosis resulting from profound hypocalcemia.[10,12,26]

## Autism Spectrum Disorder and Mercury

Thimerosal (sodium ethylmercury thiosalicylate, also known as merthiolate), an organic compound of ethylmercury, has been used in multidose vaccine vials to prevent bacterial and fungal contamination since it was patented in 1928.[27] As the number of childhood vaccinations increased, concerns arose that the amount of mercury to which infants were exposed as a result of delivery of multiple thimerosal-containing vaccines might reach toxic levels. As a result, the FDA and Institute of Medicine reviewed the use of thimerosal in childhood vaccines and found that the body of epidemiological evidence reviewed "favors a rejection of a causal relationship" between thimerosal-containing vaccines and ASD.[27,28] Despite the absence of evidence of harm attributable to thimerosal-containing vaccines, the US Public Health Service and the AAP recommended minimizing exposure to thimerosal-containing vaccines and eventual removal of thimerosal from vaccines.[29] Since 2001, all vaccines recommended for children 6 years and younger have contained no thimerosal or only "trace" or insignificant amounts (defined as a concentration of less than 0.0002%), with the exception of multidose vials of inactivated influenza vaccine.[27] Single-dose units of influenza vaccine formulated for pediatric use are thimerosal-free. For more information, see www.fda.gov/cber/vaccine/thimerosal.htm and www.nap.edu/catalog/10997.html.

In 2001, a group of parents of children with ASD published an article posing the idea that ASDs are a "novel form of mercury poisoning" in *Medical Hypotheses*, a journal that states it " . . . will publish radical ideas, so long as they are coherent and clearly expressed . . ."[30,31] Authors cited evidence such as a similarity between the clinical signs of mercury toxicity and manifestations of ASD, temporal association between the increase in the prevalence of ASD and the increased number of immunizations administered in early childhood, and higher levels of mercury in people with ASD than in people without. Each of these claims has been addressed and refuted in the peer-reviewed literature.[32-34] In 2001, the Institute of Medicine published the findings of an extensive review concluding that no proof could be found linking thimerosal-containing vaccines and ASD, ADHD, speech or language delays, or other neurodevelopment disabilities.[28,35] One of the arguments against the link is the unfortunate persistence of the increase in prevalence of ASD after the removal of thimerosal from childhood vaccines.[36] In addition, several epidemiologic studies have found no association between receiving thimerosal-containing vaccines and later neurodevelopmental disabilities or ASD.[37,38]

## Autism Spectrum Disorders and Lead

Children with developmental disorders and neurological syndromes who have persistent pica (ingestion of non-food items) behaviors and/or poor cognitive discriminatory recognition of acceptable food from non-food, may have increased risk of lead contamination.[39,40] Their increased risk may persist into school age and adolescence. Prenatal and early childhood exposure to heavy metals has been associated with adverse effects on neurodevelopment and cognition. Exposure to heavy metals prenatally or during early childhood can disrupt normal patterns of development, although no direct associations between lead exposure and ASD have been published. Evidence from case studies of children with ASD and lead is inadequate to draw any conclusions regarding causation. One report described the development of ASD or autism-like symptoms in 2 children following exposure to lead; both children received chelation therapy.[41] Both were reevaluated several years after treatment and found to have intellectual and functional impairments that did not fulfill the diagnostic criteria for ASD. Another case report of a child with symptoms of ASD, ADHD, and a blood lead level of 42 mcg/dL showed decreased repetitive behaviors during chelation, but the behaviors returned once treatment was discontinued.[42] Other cases have been reported.[39,43]

## OFF-LABEL USES OF CHELATION AGENTS

In the United States, the FDA allows physicians to prescribe approved medications for purposes other than their intended indications—called "off-label" use. A growing number of clinicians who practice complementary and alternative medicine are using chelation agents to treat neurologic diseases, such as ASD. Reports suggest that 6% to 11% of families of children with ASD in a number of English-speaking countries, including the United States, Canada, and Australia, have sought out and tried chelation therapy.[13,44–46] Notably, the AAP's Committee on Children with Disabilities has issued a report on the management of children with ASD that does not endorse use of chelation or other 'detoxification' measures.[47]

Exposure to high concentrations of heavy metals, such as lead and mercury, is associated with considerable toxicity (see Chapters 32 and 33). Studies of lead-exposed children document adverse neurocognitive effects at blood levels below 5 mcg/dL—the CDC's current reference level.[48–51] Comparable studies of the effects of mercury concentrations below the US Environmental Protection Agency "reference dose" have not been performed, although retrospective studies of children from populations with high fish intake suggest an inverse association of prenatal exposure to mercury and IQ.[52] One randomized trial found that administration of a course of the chelant, dimercaptosuccinic acid (DMSA), did not significantly reduce blood mercury concentrations in young children.[53]

Similarly, our understanding of the benefits and harms of chelation therapy is incomplete. The evidence supporting chelation as an effective treatment for ASD and other neurodevelopmental disabilities does not exist at present. A recent Cochrane review on chelation for ASD found that there was no clinical trial evidence to suggest that pharmaceutical chelation is an effective intervention for ASD.[13] Given prior reports of serious adverse events, such as hypocalcemia, renal impairment, and reported death, the risks of using chelation for ASD currently outweigh proven benefits.[13] This review excluded 9 studies because they were nonrandomized trials or were withdrawn before enrollment, and included data from only one study, which had limitations in its methodology.[13] Although chelation can lower the body's burden of heavy metals and slow or eliminate further decline associated with ongoing exposures, it has not been shown to reverse effects that have already occurred.[23,24,52,53] Evidence of harm from chelation is robust, no causal link between heavy metals and ASD exists, and as such, there is a potentially serious health risk of using chelation for ASD without any proven benefits.[13,54] Because of ethical and logistical challenges of research in this field, most studies are limited to animal subjects or case reports in people. Because of ethical concerns, in 2008, the National Institutes of Health withdrew support for a study of chelation among children with ASD after preliminary results linked chelation to brain damage in rats.[55,56]

## 'Detoxification' Products

Some clinicians inappropriately promote the chelation of children with ASD or other chronic health conditions to "detoxify" them of mercury and other metals. These clinicians are using a variety of chelation agents and routes of administration for neurodevelopmental disabilities. Several of these agents are not approved for use or are given through unlicensed and unstudied routes of administration, such as rectal and transdermal.[57] Bentonite clay, a naturally occurring clay, is marketed as a chelation agent for ASD and other childhood neurologic and behavioral diseases. According to a Web site on which the clay is sold, when mixed with water, the clay creates a negatively charged bath. The positive metals are purportedly drawn electrostatically through the pores and absorbed by the clay.[58] Many clinicians who treat children with ASD using chelation cite case studies reporting improved cognitive function as evidence of therapeutic effect. One case series of 11 children (10 boys, 1 girl) with ASD treated for 2 to 7 months with leuprolide acetate (an antiandrogen) and *meso*-1,3,-dimercaptosuccinic acid was published in 2006.[59] The work was seriously flawed by the absence of a control group, the combination of two unproven therapies, and the lack of use of a validated evaluation tool. For these reasons, it was 1 of 9 studies excluded from the Cochrane review.[13] Behaviors of children, including children with neurodevelopment disabilities, such as ASD, are expected to improve over time and with behavioral therapy; without a control group, controlling for age and other concurrent behavioral and educational therapies, confounding factors may better account for symptom improvement.

## Chelant Provocative Testing

One technique used to demonstrate increased concentrations of heavy metals is "provocation" testing.[60] Provocation analysis has been used to measure urinary excretion of metals after administration of a chelation agent, such as $CaNa_2EDTA$ or DMSA; however, there are no validated "provoked" urine metal references ranges in children. The theory behind provocation testing is circuitous: excretion of heavy metals following chelation is cited as evidence that the subject had an elevated body burden of heavy metals. Despite this reasoning, one study that used this technique reported significantly higher concentrations of mercury in the urine of 221 children with ASD following chelation, compared with urine collected from a group of 18 normal children who were tested for exposure to heavy metals but did not receive chelation.[61] A more recent study did not find increased heavy metal excretion after provocation in children with ASD.[62] A study of 65 children aged 3 to 8 years with ASD by Adams et al[63,64] found 49 children to be high excreters of heavy metals. These children continued on to receive a 3-day regimen of oral DMSA or placebo with the cycle repeated up to 6 times. No significant differences were found with regard to symptoms.[63,64] The selective reporting bias in this study causes concern because the level of urinary excretion of toxic metals in the control group and the potential differences in excretion levels between the two study phases were not reported during the second phase of the study.[13,64]

A position statement by the American College of Medical Toxicology and the 2012 joint statement by the American Academy of Clinical Toxicology and the PEHSU do not recommend the use of provoked urine samples for the assessment of metal toxicity or body burden for the previously listed reasons.[60,65]

## RECOMMENDATIONS

Pediatricians should understand that appropriate uses of chelation are limited; Chapter 32 describes indications for chelation of children with lead poisoning. Families may ask pediatricians about the efficacy of off-label use of chelation agents to treat chronic neurodevelopmental disabilities, such as ASD.[66] The evidence base for the use of chelation to treat neurodevelopmental disabilities is poor; many studies cited by clinicians who recommend chelation are poorly designed, have small sample sizes, and have conflicting results. It is important for pediatricians to be aware of the quality and quantity of the evidence cited in support of off-label uses of chelation. A fact sheet on chelation at the PEHSU Web site, with information designed for use by the general public, is a resource for pediatric clinicians.[60]

*Recommendations for Pediatricians and Other Health Care Providers*
1. Be ready to address chelation and heavy metal toxicities if parents of children with chronic health problems wish to learn more.
2. It is important not to be dismissive of parents' questions about chelation because they may be considering it for their child. By keeping avenues for communication open and respectful, pediatricians can review the safety concerns and lack of efficacy of chelation therapy. In this way, the family may be more open to a dialogue that reviews lack of efficacy and potential

harm of chelation therapy and may inform the clinician of future questions about other treatments.[67]

3. It is important for pediatricians to be informed about evidence-based behavioral therapies for ASD and other developmental disabilities so that these can be shared with parents.[68]

4. Ask families about use of chelation therapy—as well as herbal products, dietary supplements, vitamins, and other nonprescription drugs and treatments.[69]

5. Learn about the misuses of chelation therapy: the potential harms and its limited benefits.[69]

## Frequently Asked Question

Q   *The parents of a 3-year-old child recently diagnosed with ASD asked about chelation for heavy metal poisoning. They have information from a parent support group that suggests that chelation could help their child. What do I tell them?*

A   Thank them for bringing the subject up with you. Emphasize the importance of open discussion of treatments they are considering for their child. Be supportive of the family's desire to find effective treatments. Acknowledge that medicine does not yet offer curative treatments for this condition.

Explore issues such as parental guilt and worries about prenatal exposures that may have contributed to development of ASD. In particular, ask about environmental exposures about which parents may be concerned, including vaccines, anti-Rho D immunoglobin, diet, and stress.[70] Address specific concerns about heavy metals, and emphasize possible exposures in your history taking.[67] Does the child have a history of exposure to heavy metals? Can local sources of heavy metals, such as incinerators or power plants, be identified? Does the child have a history of pica? Does the child have a history of lead exposure? Does the family eat a lot of fish and, if so, what kinds? Have the parents (or other household members) ever had jobs in which they were exposed to heavy metals? Describe the strength of the evidence showing no association between exposure to heavy metals and ASD. Discuss the pitfalls of provocation testing. If appropriate, discuss the risks of chelation, such as hypocalcemia, toxicities of the drugs, potential harm from intravenous catheter placement, and others. Point out that children, including children with ASD, continue to develop, and that uncontrolled studies may conclude that improvements in behaviors are attributable to treatment, when the improvements may actually be attributable to development. Inform parents of evidence-based behavioral therapies that they can safely pursue and that have been associated with improved outcomes in young children with ASD.

# References

1. Myers SM, Johnson CP, American Academy of Pediatrics Council on Children With Disabilities. Management of children with autism spectrum disorders. *Pediatrics.* 2007;120(5):1162–1182

2. Subcommittee on Attention-Deficit/Hyperactivity Disorder, Steering Committee on Quality Improvement and Management, Wolraich M, et al. ADHD: clinical practice guideline for the diagnosis, evaluation, and treatment of attention-deficit/hyperactivity disorder in children and adolescents. *Pediatrics.* 2011;128(5):1007–1022

3. Duffus JH. "Heavy metals"—a meaningless term? *Pure Appl Chem.* 2002;74(5):793–807

4. Goyer R. Toxic effects of metals. In: Klaassen C, ed. *Casarett and Doull's Toxicology: The Basic Science of Poisons.* 5th ed. New York, NY: McGraw-Hill; 1995:694–696

5. Klaassen C. Heavy metal and heavy-metal antagonists. In: Gilman A, Rall T, Nies A, Taylor P, eds. *Goodman and Gilman's The Pharmacological Basis of Therapeutics.* New York, NY: Pergamon Press; 1990:1592–1614

6. Work Group on Lead and Pregnancy, CDC Advisory Committee on Childhood Lead Poisoning Prevention. Guidelines for the identification and management of lead exposure in pregnant and lactating women. 2010. http://www.cdc.gov/nceh/lead/publications/leadandpregnancy2010.pdf. Accessed February 20, 2018

7. Centers for Disease Control and Prevention. At-risk populations. http://www.cdc.gov/nceh/lead/tips/populations.htm. Updated 2015. Accessed February 20, 2018

8. Woolf AD, Goldman R, Bellinger DC. Clinical approach to childhood lead poisoning. *Pediatr Clin North Am.* 2007;54(2):271–294

9. Newman N, Binns HJ, Karwowski M, Lowry J, PEHSU Lead Working Group. Medical management of childhood lead exposure and poisoning. 2013. http://www.pehsu.net/_Childhood_Lead_Exposure.html. Accessed February 20, 2018

10. Brown MJ, Willis T, Omalu B, Leiker R. Deaths resulting from hypocalcemia after administration of edetate disodium: 2003-2005. *Pediatrics.* 2006;118(2):e534–e536

11. Risher JF, Amler SN. Mercury exposure: evaluation and intervention the inappropriate use of chelating agents in the diagnosis and treatment of putative mercury poisoning. *Neurotoxicology.* 2005;26(4):691–699

12. Centers for Disease Control and Prevention. Deaths associated with hypocalcemia from chelation therapy—Texas, Pennsylvania, and Oregon, 2003-2005. *MMWR Morb Mortal Wkly Rep.* 2006;55(8):204–207

13. James S, Stevenson SW, Silove N, Williams K. Chelation for autism spectrum disorder (ASD). *Cochrane Database Syst Rev.* 2015;5:CD010766

14. Taylor Pharmaceuticals. BAL in oil ampules (dimercaprol injection, USP). https://www.accessdata.fda.gov/drugsatfda_docs/label/2007/005939s007lbl.pdf. Updated 2006. Accessed February 20, 2018

15. Graceway Pharmaceuticals. I. Calcium disodium versenate (edetate calcium disodium injection, USP). https://www.accessdata.fda.gov/drugsatfda_docs/label/2009/008922s016lbl.pdf. Accessed February 20, 2018

16. Schwarz Pharma Mfg. I. Chemet (succimer). http://www.accessdata.fda.gov/drugsatfda_docs/label/2007/019998s013lbl.pdf. Updated July, 2007. Accessed February 20, 2018

17. Stangle DE, Strawderman MS, Smith D, Kuypers M, Strupp BJ. Reductions in blood lead overestimate reductions in brain lead following repeated succimer regimens in a rodent model of childhood lead exposure. *Environ Health Perspect.* 2004;112(3):302–308

18. Agency for Toxic Substances and Disease Registry. Toxicological profile for mercury. Atlanta, GA: U.S. Department of Health and Human Services; 1999

19. Agency for Toxic Substances and Disease Registry. Addendum to the Toxicological Profile for Mercury (Alkyl and Dialkyl Compounds). Atlanta, GA: Division of Toxicology and Human Health Science; 2013. http://www.atsdr.cdc.gov/toxprofiles/mercury_organic_addendum.pdf. Accessed February 20, 2018

20. Berlin M, Lewander T. Increased brain uptake of mercury caused by 2,3-dimercaptopropanol (bal) in mice given mercuric chloride. *Acta Pharmacol Toxicol (Copenh)*. 1965;22:1–7

21. Berlin M, Ullrebg S. Increased uptake of mercury in mouse brain caused by 2,3-dimercaptopropanol. *Nature*. 1963;197:84–85

22. Berlin M, Rylander R. Increased brain uptake of mercury induced by 2,3-dimercaptopropanol (bal) in mice exposed to phenylmercuric acetate. *J Pharmacol Exp Ther*. 1964;146:236–240

23. Rogan WJ, Dietrich KN, Ware JH, et al. The effect of chelation therapy with succimer on neuropsychological development in children exposed to lead. *N Engl J Med*. 2001;344(19):1421–1426

24. Dietrich KN, Ware JH, Salganik M, et al. Effect of chelation therapy on the neuropsychological and behavioral development of lead-exposed children after school entry. *Pediatrics*. 2004;114(1):19–26

25. Bradberry S, Vale A. A comparison of sodium calcium edetate (edetate calcium disodium) and succimer (DMSA) in the treatment of inorganic lead poisoning. *Clin Toxicol (Phila)*. 2009;47(9):841–858

26. Baxter AJ, Krenzelok EP. Pediatric fatality secondary to EDTA chelation. *Clin Toxicol (Phila)*. 2008;46(10):1083–1084

27. Center for Biologics Evaluation and Research. Thimerosal in vaccines questions and answers. http://www.fda.gov/cber/vaccine/thimfaq.htm. Updated 2015. Accessed February 20, 2018

28. Institute of Medicine. Immunizations Safety Review: Vaccines and Autism. Washington DC: The National Academies Press; 2004. http://www.nap.edu/catalog/10997/immunization-safety-review-vaccines-and-autism. Accessed February 20, 2018

29. Centers for Disease Control and Prevention. Thimerosal in vaccines: a joint statement of the American Academy of Pediatrics and the public health service. *MMWR Morb Mortal Wkly Rep*. 1999;48(26):563–565

30. Bernard S, Enayati A, Redwood L, Roger H, Binstock T. Autism: a novel form of mercury poisoning. *Med Hypotheses*. 2001;56(4):462–471

31. The Aims and Scope of the Journal *Medical Hypotheses*. http://www.journals.elsevier.com/medical-hypotheses/. Updated 2015. Accessed February 20, 2018

32. Nelson KB, Bauman ML. Thimerosal and autism? *Pediatrics*. 2003;111(3):674–679

33. Andrews N, Miller E, Grant A, Stowe J, Osborne V, Taylor B. Thimerosal exposure in infants and developmental disorders: a retrospective cohort study in the United Kingdom does not support a causal association. *Pediatrics*. 2004;114(3):584–591

34. Verstraeten T, Davis RL, DeStefano F, et al. Safety of thimerosal-containing vaccines: a two-phased study of computerized health maintenance organization databases. *Pediatrics*. 2003;112(5):1039–1048

35. Institute of Medicine (US) Immunization Safety Review Committee. Thimerosal-Containing Vaccines and Neurodevelopmental Disorders. Washington DC: The National Academies Press; 2001. http://www.nap.edu/catalog/10208/immunization-safety-review-thimerosal-containing-vaccines-and-neurodevelopmental-disorders. Accessed February 20, 2018

36. Schechter R, Grether JK. Continuing increases in autism reported to California's developmental services system: mercury in retrograde. *Arch Gen Psychiatry*. 2008;65(1):19–24

37. Price CS, Thompson WW, Goodson B, et al. Prenatal and infant exposure to thimerosal from vaccines and immunoglobulins and risk of autism. *Pediatrics*. 2010;126(4):656–664

38. Thompson WW, Price C, Goodson B, et al. Early thimerosal exposure and neuropsychological outcomes at 7 to 10 years. *N Engl J Med*. 2007;357(13):1281–1292

39. George M, Heeney MM, Woolf AD. Encephalopathy from lead poisoning masquerading as a flu-like syndrome in an autistic child. *Pediatr Emerg Care*. 2010;26(5):370–373

40. Zeager M, Heard T, Woolf AD. Lead poisoning in two children with Landau-Kleffner syndrome. *Clin Toxicol (Phila)*. 2012;50(5):448

41. Lidsky TI, Schneider JS. Autism and autistic symptoms associated with childhood lead poisoning. *J Applied Res*. 2005;5(1):80–87

42. Eppright TD, Sanfacon JA, Horwitz EA. Attention deficit hyperactivity disorder, infantile autism, and elevated blood-lead: a possible relationship. *Mo Med*. 1996;93(3):136–138

43. Accardo P, Whitman B, Caul J, Rolfe U. Autism and plumbism: a possible association. *Clin Pediatr (Phila)*. 1988;27(1):41–44

44. Green VA, Pituch KA, Itchon J, Choi A, O'Reilly M, Sigafoos J. Internet survey of treatments used by parents of children with autism. *Res Dev Disabil*. 2006;27(1):70–84

45. Brent J. Commentary on the abuse of metal chelation therapy in patients with autism spectrum disorders. *J Med Toxicol*. 2013;9(4):370–372

46. Harrington JW, Allen K. The clinician's guide to autism. *Pediatr Rev*. 2014;35(2):62–78

47. American Academy of Pediatrics Committee on Children With Disabilities. Technical report: the pediatrician's role in the diagnosis and management of autistic spectrum disorder in children. *Pediatrics*. 2001;107(5):E85

48. Lanphear BP, Hornung R, Khoury J, et al. Low-level environmental lead exposure and children's intellectual function: an international pooled analysis. *Environ Health Perspect*. 2005;113(7):894–899

49. Canfield RL, Kreher DA, Cornwell C, Henderson CR, Jr. Low-level lead exposure, executive functioning, and learning in early childhood. *Child Neuropsychol*. 2003;9(1):35–53

50. Canfield RL, Henderson CR, Jr, Cory-Slechta DA, Cox C, Jusko TA, Lanphear BP. Intellectual impairment in children with blood lead concentrations below 10 microg per deciliter. *N Engl J Med*. 2003;348(16):1517–1526

51. Centers for Disease Control and Prevention. CDC response to advisory committee on childhood lead poisoning prevention recommendations in "low level lead exposure harms children: A renewed call of primary prevention." Atlanta, GA: National Center for Environmental Health, CDC; 2012. http://www.cdc.gov/nceh/lead/acclpp/cdc_response_lead_exposure_recs.pdf. Accessed February 20, 2018

52. Axelrad DA, Bellinger DC, Ryan LM, Woodruff TJ. Dose-response relationship of prenatal mercury exposure and IQ: an integrative analysis of epidemiologic data. *Environ Health Perspect*. 2007;115(4):609–615

53. Cao Y, Chen A, Jones RL, et al. Efficacy of succimer chelation of mercury at background exposures in toddlers: a randomized trial. *J Pediatr*. 2011;158(3):480–485

54. McKay CA, Jr. Role of chelation in the treatment of lead poisoning: discussion of the treatment of lead-exposed children trial (TLC). *J Med Toxicol*. 2013;9(4):339–343

55. Boyles S. Chelation study for autism called off. *WebMD Health News*. September 18, 2008. http://www.webmd.com/brain/autism/news/20080918/chelation-study-autism-called-off. Accessed February 20, 2018

56. Mitka M. Chelation therapy trials halted. *JAMA*. 2008;300(19):2236

57. Sinha Y, Silove N, Williams K. Chelation therapy and autism. *BMJ*. 2006;333(7571):756

58. McCoy C. Battle autism with bentonite clay. *NaturalNews.com*. June 26, 2009. http://www.naturalnews.com/026508_clay_autism_environment.html. Accessed February 20, 2018

59. Geier DA, Geier MR. A clinical trial of combined anti-androgen and anti-heavy metal therapy in autistic disorders. *Neuro Endocrinol Lett*. 2006;27(6):833–838

60. Goldman RH, Woolf AD. Chelation therapy - guidance for parents and families. July 2012. http://www.pehsu.net/Public_Chelation_Therapy.html . Accessed February 20, 2018

61. Bradstreet J, Geier DA, Kartzinel JJ, Adams JB, Geier MR. A case-control study of mercury burden in children with autistic spectrum disorders. *J Am Phys Surg.* 2003;8(3):76–79

62. Soden SE, Lowry JA, Garrison CB, Wasserman GS. 24-hour provoked urine excretion test for heavy metals in children with autism and typically developing controls, a pilot study. *Clin Toxicol (Phila).* 2007;45(5):476–481

63. Adams JB, Baral M, Geis E, et al. Safety and efficacy of oral DMSA therapy for children with autism spectrum disorders: part A—medical results. *BMC Clin Pharmacol.* 2009;9:16

64. Adams JB, Baral M, Geis E, et al. Safety and efficacy of oral DMSA therapy for children with autism spectrum disorders: part B—behavioral results. *BMC Clin Pharmacol.* 2009;9:17

65. Charlton N, Wallace KL. American College of Medical Toxicology position statement on post-chelator challenge urinary metal testing. *J Med Toxicol.* 2010;6(1):74–75

66. Myers SM, Johnson CP, American Academy of Pediatrics Council on Children With Disabilities. Management of children with autism spectrum disorders. *Pediatrics.* 2007;120(5):1162–1182

67. McClafferty H, Vohra S, Bailey M, et al. Pediatric integrative medicine. *Pediatrics.* 2017;140(3):e20171961

68. Dawson G, Rogers S, Munson J, et al. Randomized, controlled trial of an intervention for toddlers with autism: the early start Denver model. *Pediatrics.* 2010;125(1):e17–e23

69. Woolf AD, Gardiner P. Use of complementary and alternative therapies in children. *Clin Pharmacol Ther.* 2010;87(2):155–157

70. Hussain J, Woolf AD, Sandel M, Shannon MW. Environmental evaluation of a child with developmental disability. *Pediatr Clin North Am.* 2007;54(1):47–62

# Chapter 51

# Chemical and Biological Terrorism

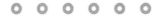

## KEY POINTS

- Children may be among the victims of chemical and biological terrorism, and their physiology and anatomy may render them more susceptible to certain chemical and biological agents.
- Recognition of these agents can be difficult—particularly for the delayed symptoms associated with biological agents—and may depend on syndromic surveillance.
- Public health agencies and pediatricians can play important roles in preparedness for chemical and biological terrorism.
- Decontamination and treatment protocols can mitigate illness and injury and can limit mortality.
- Behavioral and mental health consequences of terrorist attacks must be considered.

## INTRODUCTION

Terrorism of all forms has the goal of producing injury, fear, or chaos in an effort to disable or intimidate a population. Recent terrorist acts have included, and at times targeted, child victims. In 2004, more than 750 children were among the 1,100 hostages in the 3-day siege of a school in Beslan, North Ossetia, of the Russian Federation. Children have been among the victims in other well-known acts of terrorism, including the release of the nerve agent sarin in the Tokyo subway system, and the bombing of the Oklahoma City federal building, both in 1995; the distribution of anthrax-containing letters through the US Postal Service in 2001; and the Syrian sarin attacks in 2013 and 2017.[1,2]

The release of chemical or biological agents can have tremendous impacts on children, adolescents, and their environments including physiological, psychological, and developmental impacts.[1,3] If children are the victims of a terrorist attack, any vulnerabilities within pediatric emergency medical systems and hospitals and lack of surge capacity will create great challenges to medical management and care capabilities for ill and injured children.[4,5] Pediatricians should be prepared to consider the clinical issues that arise after exposure to these agents, as well as the safety of water and food supplies, and the potential contamination of soil and air. The principles of consequence management, designed to minimize morbidity and mortality after a chemical or biological agent release, must involve multiple pediatric disciplines including environmental health, emergency medicine, critical care, behavioral medicine and mental health, primary care, and infectious diseases. Response plans must address recognition, triage, diagnosis, and management. Moreover, an effective partnership between government agencies and pediatricians must be forged in advance of any terrorist attack to promote preparedness and minimize the effects on children. In the aftermath of a chemical or biological attack, pediatric emergency departments need to be prepared to see many frightened patients who are concerned that they are ill, but in fact are not physically affected.

Potential "weapons of mass destruction" may be formed from chemical, biological, radiological, nuclear, or explosive agents.[6] Chemical and explosive agents may be misused as "weapons of opportunity," requiring limited planning or financial resources.[1,7] For example, an intentional detonation involving a railcar carrying hazardous chemicals could result in contamination of a nearby community, causing major hardship and emotional distress.

Community planning, hospital staff training, medication stockpiling, and preparation for chemical, biological, radiological, nuclear, or explosive events, especially for incidents that might involve numerous children, all present daunting logistical challenges. As part of the network of health responders, pediatricians need to be able to answer questions, recognize signs of possible exposure to a chemical or biological weapon, understand first-line response, and participate in disaster planning to ensure that the needs of children are addressed.[6] This chapter does not attempt to serve as a stand-alone reference on chemical or biological terrorism, but instead provides an introduction to the topic, especially with regard to pediatric environmental health concerns; more information is available (see Resources). Radiological emergencies are the focus of the American Academy of Pediatrics's (AAP's) 2003 policy statement on Radiation Disasters and Children;[8] a revision is in press.[9,10]

## AGENTS OF CONCERN

### Chemical

A large number of toxic chemicals have the potential to be used as terrorist weapons. They include nerve agents, cyanide, vesicants (chemicals that cause blistering), and pulmonary agents (Table 51-1).[11–15] The release of the nerve agent sarin in the Tokyo subway attack in Japan demonstrated the ease with which a chemical agent can be dispersed and the resulting effects.[15] Relatively easy to manufacture, sarin, like all nerve agents, acts like an organophosphate pesticide, inhibiting the enzyme acetylcholinesterase. Victims of sarin exposure, therefore, present with a picture of cholinergic excess. Most common symptoms are miosis, nausea, and vomiting. More significant exposures produce lacrimation, salivation, and diarrhea. Moderate exposures to nerve agents stimulate nicotinic receptors, leading to muscle fasciculation and generalized weakness. Severe exposures produce central nervous system toxicity, manifested as seizures and coma. Death from sarin exposure results

## Table 51-1. Potential Chemical Agents for Use in Terrorism[a]

| CLASS | EXAMPLES |
|---|---|
| Nerve agents | Tabun<br>Sarin<br>Soman<br>VX |
| Vesicants | Mustard gas<br>Nitrogen mustard |
| Irritants/corrosives | Chlorine<br>Bromine<br>Ammonia |
| Choking agents | Phosgene |
| Cyanogens | Hydrogen cyanide |
| Incapacitating agents: central nervous system depressants, anticholinergics, lacrimators | 3-quinuclidinyl benzilate (BZ), capsaicin, cannabinoids, barbiturates |

[a] From the American Academy of Pediatrics[1,3]

from respiratory failure or complications of central nervous system toxicity. Sarin also has unique chemical properties that enhance its toxicity. It is denser than air and settles close to the ground, in the breathing zones of children. Sarin is viscous and oily, leading to deposition on clothing and skin. It is readily absorbed through intact skin and through standard barriers (such as surgical gloves) used by health care personnel. Finally, because it can remain on clothing or skin until it is removed, sarin can secondarily affect anyone not wearing personal protective equipment while handling a contaminated victim. Sarin vapors can enter the ventilation system of a building or hospital, thereby affecting individuals throughout the structure.[16-18] Information on management of exposure to specific chemical weapons can be found in several reviews.[6,7,10,19-22]

## Biological

Infectious agents and their toxins have been used as weapons. Unlike chemical agents, in which the release is usually obvious and casualties appear promptly, biological agents can be released covertly, with casualties appearing over a period of days, potentially leading to a significant delay in recognition and diagnosis.[23-25] Because of this time delay, victims typically become ill away from the site of exposure, and the epicenter of the release can be very difficult to identify. Victims of certain bioterror infections can, themselves, subsequently spread agents to diverse additional locations, analogous to the spread of severe acute respiratory syndrome.

According to the National Academy of Sciences, several dozen biological agents or toxins are potential candidates for use as bioweapons.[9] Included among these are agents that the Centers for Disease Control and Prevention (CDC) identifies as "category A agents." These agents have the following characteristics:

- Can be easily disseminated or transmitted person-to-person;
- Cause high mortality, with potential for major public health impact;
- Have the potential for causing public panic and social disruption; and
- Require special attention for public health preparedness.

The 6 biological agents designated as category A are *Bacillus anthracis* (anthrax), *Yersinia pestis* (plague), *Variola major* (smallpox), *Francisella tularensis* (tularemia), *Clostridium botulinum* toxin, and filoviruses and arenaviruses (viral hemorrhagic fevers). Public health efforts have focused primarily on the category A agents; hospitals, pediatricians, and government agencies have been called on to improve preparedness (eg, by stockpiling and developing a distribution plan for antibiotics, vaccines, and antidotes).[9,26] Preparedness efforts should also address the potential risks posed by the many other agents, including those in categories B and C, but these are beyond the scope of this chapter (Table 51-2).

| Table 51-2. Biological Weapons of Concern[a] |
|---|
| **CATEGORY A** |
| Anthrax *(Bacillus anthracis)*<br>Smallpox *(Variola major)*<br>Tularemia *(Francisella tularensis)*<br>Plague *(Yersinia pestis)*<br>Botulinum (*Clostridium botulinum* toxin)<br>Viral hemorrhagic fevers (filoviruses [eg, Ebola, Marburg] and arenaviruses [eg, Lassa]) |
| **CATEGORY B** |
| Q fever *(Coxiella burnetii)*<br>Brucellosis (*Brucella* species)<br>*Clostridium perfringens* (*C. perfringens*)<br>Glanders *(Burkholderia mallei)*<br>Melioidosis *(Burkholderia pseudomallei)*<br>Viral encephalitis (alphaviruses, Venezuelan equine encephalomyelitis, eastern equine encephalomyelitis, western equine encephalomyelitis)<br>Typhus *(Rickettsia prowazekii)*<br>Biotoxins (ricin, staphylococcal enterotoxin B)<br>Psittacosis *(Chlamydia psittaci)*<br>Food-safety threats (eg, *Salmonella* species, *Escherichia coli* O157:H7)<br>Water-safety threats (eg, *Vibrio cholerae, Cryptosporidium parvum*) |
| **CATEGORY C** |
| Emerging threat agents (eg, Nipah virus, hantavirus) |

[a] From American Academy of Pediatrics and Centers for Disease Control and Prevention[1,27]

## PEDIATRIC IMPLICATIONS

Children may be especially susceptible to the effects of chemical and biological agents because of their anatomic and physiologic differences and unique behavioral characteristics (Table 51-3).[28,29] Infants and children have an increased surface area-to-volume ratio compared with adults, higher minute ventilation, and breathing zones that are closer to the ground (where some agents may settle), and therefore are often at higher risk of exposure to and absorption of many agents. With regard to skin permeability, there is no scientific consensus about precisely when newborn and infant skin attain the same barrier function and other functions that adult skin has.[30,31] The skin of premature infants, however, has a poorly developed epidermal barrier; this results in a risk of increased permeability to topical agents.

Children often require different medical countermeasures than do adults, including different dosages, antibiotics, or antidotes. They have greater susceptibility to dehydration and shock from biological and chemical agents. Children

| Table 51-3. Factors Enhancing Children's Vulnerability to Biological Agents[29] | |
| --- | --- |
| FACTOR | RELEVANT AGENTS |
| **Anatomic and physiologic differences**<br>■ Increased ratio of surface area-to-volume<br>■ Higher minute ventilation<br>■ Breathing air closer to ground | ■ T-2 mycotoxins<br>■ All aerosolized agents<br>■ Denser aerosolized agents |
| **Unique susceptibility/severity** | ■ Smallpox, T-2 mycotoxins, VEE |
| **Developmental considerations**<br>■ Dependent on others for care, more likely to lack knowledge or independent means to seek care or identify and avoid danger | ■ All agents |

Abbreviation: VEE, Venezuelan equine encephalitis

often depend on others for care, and their developmental abilities and cognitive levels may impede their ability to escape danger. In addition, they cannot be easily or rapidly decontaminated in adult decontamination units. Children have unique psychological needs and vulnerabilities, and special management plans are needed in the event of mass casualties and evacuation. For all these reasons, emergency responders, medical professionals, and health care institutions require special expertise and training to ensure that children receive optimal medical and psychological care.

Certain groups of children may be especially vulnerable to bioterror agents. Neonates and young infants are relatively immunocompromised compared with older children and adults. Preschool children have high hand-to-mouth activity and are also less likely than older children and adults to maintain personal hygiene (eg, cough etiquette and hand washing), thereby facilitating the spread of certain agents, particularly among similarly aged children; older children and adolescents are more likely to engage in risk-taking behavior that may place them at higher risk.

## Identification of Sentinel Events

Nuclear, incendiary, chemical, and explosive disasters are typically recognized immediately. By contrast, identification of a biological terror event can be very difficult and requires a high index of suspicion. After the covert release of a biological agent, victims may present for medical care over several days; in the early phases of their illness, children and adults may seek medical attention with nonspecific complaints. Easily misdiagnosed, victims may then infect others (if the illness is communicable) before clinical manifestations become more characteristic.

Education of clinicians about agents used as biological weapons and the illnesses they produce is a cornerstone of effective planning.[32,33] An important component of a physician's role in protecting populations against biological terror is biosurveillance or syndromic surveillance; the CDC has created a National Biosurveillance Strategy for Human Health that may be useful to pediatricians (http://sites.google.com/site/nbshh10).

A key principle of consequence management for biological terrorism is recognizing that pediatricians, whether in emergency departments, inpatient settings, or primary care settings, may be the first to encounter victims. Because early diagnosis and treatment substantially reduce the number of affected individuals, pediatricians and others who provide care to children must develop sufficient knowledge to recognize the first signal of a bioterrorist event. For example, skin lesions seen in initial cases of cutaneous anthrax in October 2001 (including the sole pediatric patient) were mistaken for spider bites. All physicians must acquaint themselves with the manifestations of diseases caused by the most common biological agents, including anthrax, plague, smallpox, botulism, and ricin.[7] Detailed descriptions of many biological agents are available in the AAP *Red Book* (http://aapredbook.aappublications. org). A physician who suspects a biological outbreak should immediately notify the local health department and ask for further assistance.

## MANAGEMENT OF MASS CASUALTIES

In addition to producing large numbers of casualties, terrorist events typically produce an even larger number of patients with minor physical problems and well individuals with psychological distress. The latter groups may exceed the seriously injured or infected patients by ratios as high as 10:1. This ratio may be magnified in a pediatric population because young children are unable to communicate effectively. Because they are concerned about possible exposure, parents are then likely to consult health care providers about symptoms, or to request a thorough assessment even in the absence of symptoms or signs. Depending on the number of victims in each group (psychologically distressed, wounded, and severely injured), pediatric offices and emergency departments may become overwhelmed. After the release of the nerve agent sarin in Japan, patients came to emergency departments at a rate as high as 500 per hour, rapidly overwhelming hospital resources.[17] Moreover, because most patients came by foot, car, or taxi, there was no opportunity to perform out-of-hospital ("field") triage to separate healthy from contaminated patients. The principal lesson learned after that event was that office- and hospital-based emergency planning must include contingency plans for managing large numbers of victims ("surge-capacity" planning), with special attention to pediatric needs. An additional challenge arises when creating algorithms to facilitate assessment of young, preverbal children.

## DECONTAMINATION, TREATMENT, AND PROPHYLAXIS

Protocols for treatment and postexposure prophylaxis of children exposed to chemical and biological weapons remain poorly developed. For example, some decontamination protocols for chemical agents have recommended a 10-minute shower with soap or diluted bleach.[14] In children, such a regimen risks hypothermia and serious skin or eye irritation. This risk can be minimized by using warmed water and with attention paid to timely drying, warming, and reclothing. It may be particularly difficult to decontaminate an exposed child or to interact with the child when a rescuer is wearing personal protective gear. The process may be made smoother and the child's anxiety and fear may be alleviated if a parent is present during the decontamination. It is important to incorporate these principles to develop appropriate pediatric decontamination protocols.[34,35]

Treatment of nerve-agent exposures includes supportive care and prompt administration of the antidotes atropine and, when organophosphates are implicated, pralidoxime. A review of pharmacokinetic data considered the benefit of timely atropine dosing following a nerve agent exposure versus the risk of overdose; on balance, it appears that relatively large initial doses of atropine are well tolerated and can mitigate excessive bronchorrhea and prevent respiratory failure.[36] Auto-injectors that deliver premeasured doses of both medications can be lifesaving. This is especially true when large numbers of victims are exposed and first responders are in personal protective gear that limits their fine motor skills. In these situations, it is difficult to prepare timely and accurate medication doses based on weight using multidose vials; intravenous dosing in such situations also is impractical. The Food and Drug Administration (FDA) recently established pediatric dosing recommendations and labeling for pralidoxime. As of 2017, however, auto-injectors that allow for rapid administration of both medications (atropine and pralidoxime) were not approved by the FDA for use in younger children.[37] The FDA has taken steps to encourage production and approval of these devices in the future to address this pressing need. In the interim, consensus recommendations are available to guide the use of currently available auto-injectors for symptomatic children.[38]

In the case of biological weapons, recommendations for pediatric patients have been rudimentary, although some recommendations specific to children and pregnant women have been released. The CDC Web site (www.cdc.gov/anthrax) contains recommendations for prophylaxis and treatment of children and pregnant women who have been exposed to or are suffering from anthrax.

Local supplies of antibiotics, antidotes, and other medical supplies may be quickly depleted. The CDC, under its Strategic National Stockpile (SNS) program, oversees a national stockpile of materials for rapid delivery to local communities. Should a terror event occur, public health and government entities in states and cities have developed plans to rapidly request deployment of pharmaceuticals and equipment from the SNS for distribution to a point of care in the relevant jurisdiction. Unfortunately, because many medical counter-measures have not been evaluated or approved for use in children, the SNS does not include these pediatric formulations or dosages.

Hospital administrators must consider how to protect hospitalized patients from an airborne release of chemical and biological weapons. Guidance has been prepared for protecting building environments from airborne chemical, biological, or radiological attacks.[39]

Radioactive iodine may be released after a nuclear power plant accident, nuclear weapon detonation, or terrorist event. Expeditious treatment with KI can be effective in protecting the thyroid gland, but not other organs. Guidance about treatment with KI is available (see Chapter 31).

## BEHAVIORAL AND MENTAL HEALTH CONSEQUENCES

All forms of terrorism, including hoaxes, can produce significant psychological distress that may persist long after any risk of adverse health effects has passed. However, the greatest potential for long-term or permanent emotional distur-bances is found in mass casualty incidents that produce injury or death. As the events of September 11, 2001, proved, children are at high risk for the devel-opment of significant and persistent adjustment difficulties, including acute stress reactions and posttraumatic stress disorder, anxiety, depression, and other mental health problems. In situations in which deaths have occurred, bereavement may be the predominant or concurrent challenge. Manifestations of adjustment difficulties after a terrorist event may include somatic complaints (eg, change in appetite, headache, abdominal pain, malaise); fear, anxiety, or school avoidance; sadness or depression; difficulty concentrat-ing and learning; regression; acting out or risk-taking, including onset of or increase in alcohol or other substance use; and emotional withdrawal or avoid-ance of previously enjoyed activities. Sleep problems include trouble falling or staying asleep, as well as nightmares (which are common in children).[26,38–43] After a terrorist event, pediatricians can educate parents about how to commu-nicate with and support their children, limit their exposure to media reports, and recognize and seek treatment for adjustment reactions. Community-level disaster preparedness includes developing a network of mental health services to address psychological needs and developing ways to deliver psychologi-cal first aid, bereavement counseling, and other supportive services to large numbers of children, often in community sites such as schools.[5,44,45]

## Planning by Government

Rapid, effective response to terrorist acts relies on the actions of a number of government agencies at all levels. State and local government agencies are essential collaborators in the process of disaster planning, especially as it relates to first responders. State and local agencies must realize that they will be largely unsupported by federal resources in the initial hours after an attack and must prepare accordingly. Planning for disasters at all levels must consider the unique needs of children and families and should include input from pediatricians.

Depending on the type and impact of an event, responding federal agencies will likely include the US Department of Homeland Security/Federal Emergency Management Agency (FEMA), the US Department of Health and Human Services (DHHS), the CDC, the US Environmental Protection Agency, the US Department of Agriculture, and potentially a number of others. The US DHHS oversees the National Disaster Medical System, which coordinates the rapid deployment of Disaster Medical Assistance Teams (DMATs) of professional and para-professional medical personnel to disaster sites. The DMATs supplement local medical care and assist with triage and evacuation as needed.[46] Acts of terrorism require not only the involvement of public health systems but also, as criminal acts, they involve many branches of law enforcement, including the Federal Bureau of Investigation and state and local police. In contrast to natural disasters such as earthquakes, acts of terrorism require that these systems work together. By necessity, law enforcement agencies will need to work with public health agencies and health care providers to facilitate investigations (eg, collecting clothing and specimens as evidence, embargoing sensitive or classified information, interviewing victims). This process poses challenges for pediatricians, emergency physicians, nurses, and other health care providers.

Following the anthrax attacks of 2001, Congress passed the Project BioShield Act of 2003, a comprehensive effort of the US DHHS and its partners to stockpile medical countermeasures, such as anthrax vaccine and immune globulin, botulinum antitoxin, pediatric formulation of potassium iodide, and diethylenetriaminepentaacetate (DTPA), a chelating agent for certain radiological particles.[47]

## COMMUNITY PLANNING

Disaster planning also takes place at the community level. Planning should be based on a thorough hazard vulnerability analysis that takes into account unique characteristics and vulnerabilities of a community. An assessment of natural disaster and terrorism-based threats must consider the locations (eg, schools, child care settings) and needs of children, including those with special health care needs. Hazard vulnerability analysis and disaster planning should include input from pediatricians.

Important activities include identifying shelter facilities appropriate for children and families. These facilities must be large enough to care for large numbers of victims if a local area becomes uninhabitable. Alternate sites should be prepared to provide at least a 2- to 3-day supply of age-appropriate nutrition, water, toiletries, clothing, and other basic needs. Plans should ensure that mass care shelter environments are safe and secure for children, and have appropriate access to essential services and supplies, such as infant formula and food for toddlers.[5]

Schools and child care facilities must be included in community-level planning because children spend much of their time in these settings.[1,40,42] Schools may also be targets for such attacks, as exemplified by the Beslan school hostage crisis in the Russian Federation in 2004. Issues for planning in schools include establishing protocols for sheltering in place, lockdown, and/ or rapid evacuation of children; identifying safe sites should a facility require immediate evacuation; developing mechanisms for notifying parents and reuniting them with their children as quickly as possible; arranging care for children whose parents are incapacitated or out of contact; providing first aid; arranging for *in loco parentis* treatment of children when their parents cannot be reached; addressing how medical countermeasures can be administered to children as appropriate; and planning support strategies for children's adjustment to, and recovery from, disasters.[48]

## PEDIATRIC PLANNING FOR TERRORIST EVENTS

Children or adolescents may appear in pediatricians' offices or health centers after exposure. Pediatricians in these settings must

(1) become knowledgeable about agents and their clinical manifestations and contribute to biosurveillance efforts;

(2) become effective educators and communicators about chemical and biological agents, as well as blast injuries,[49] and how these agents affect children;

(3) become involved in local disaster planning to advocate for pediatric preparedness including administering KI to infants, children and lactating women after an event that potentially releases radioactive iodine;

(4) ensure that offices have emergency care plans and protocols that permit evaluation of victims, protect unaffected patients, and review the need for personal protective equipment;

(5) develop surge-capacity protocols;

(6) develop skills in providing psychological first aid and brief interventions for children who experience loss and crisis; and

(7) develop and test office/practice plans for disasters to limit disruption of essential services provided to patients and families.

For many of these tasks, pediatricians can adopt algorithms being developed by federal agencies or seek guidance from the AAP Children & Disasters Web site (http://www.aap.org/disasters). This site reviews or provides links to resources concerning evaluation and management of crisis events, provides guidance to prepare pediatricians and practices for disasters, and provides materials appropriate for families. Materials are available to help practices develop written disaster plans (http://www.aap.org/disasters/practice.cfm).

Because pediatric residents generally are not adequately knowledgeable about this topic, their education and training may be improved by including a curriculum in medical schools and pediatric residencies.[50] An educational intervention in pediatric disaster medicine was conducted for pediatric and pediatric emergency medicine residents at a tertiary care teaching hospital. Participants increased their short-term knowledge and showed moderate retention of information.[51]

## Frequently Asked Questions

Q  *What is a weapon of opportunity?*

A  Examples are explosives or chemicals intended for a legitimate purpose that are misused as weapons.

Q  *Why is the nerve agent sarin particularly toxic for children?*

A  Sarin is viscous and lipophilic, with a tendency to remain on clothing and exposed skin, and to be absorbed through gloves and intact skin. Children have a relatively higher surface area-to-volume ratio; therefore, compared with adults, they are likely to absorb more of any substance that contacts skin. In addition, sarin is denser than air, so it accumulates close to the ground in the breathing zone of children.

Q  *Why are biological weapons generally more difficult to detect than chemical ones?*

A  Biological agents may be released covertly, and symptoms may not appear for several days. Victims, particularly younger children, may present with nonspecific complaints. A high index of clinical suspicion, as well as syndromic surveillance, are often necessary to detect the effects of biological agents.

Q  *How can pediatricians prepare for chemical and biological terrorism?*

A  In addition to understanding the classes of agents and their effects, pediatricians must be prepared to triage behavioral and mental health consequences of terrorism that may persist long after medical effects have resolved.

# Resources

### American Academy of Pediatrics
Children, Terrorism & Disasters Web site: www.aap.org/disasters; www.aap.org/disasters/terrorism-biological.cfm; and www.aap.org/disasters/terrorism-chemical.cfm

### Centers for Disease Control and Prevention
Emergency Preparedness and Response Web site: http://emergency.cdc.gov

### Markenson D, Reynolds S, American Academy of Pediatrics Committee on Pediatric Emergency Medicine and Task Force on Terrorism.
Technical report: the pediatrician and disaster preparedness. *Pediatrics.* 2006;117(2):e340–e362

# References

1. American Academy of Pediatrics Committee on Environmental Health, Committee on Infectious Diseases. Chemical-biological terrorism and its impact on children. *Pediatrics.* 2006;118(3):1267–1278

2. Rosman Y, Eisenkraft A, Milk N, et al. Lessons learned from the Syrian sarin attack: evaluation of a clinical syndrome through social media. *Ann Intern Med* 2014;160(9):644–648

3. American Academy of Pediatrics Committee on Environmental Health, Committee on Infectious Diseases. Chemical-biological terrorism and its impact on children: a subject review. *Pediatrics.* 2000;105(3 Pt 1):662–670

4. Institute of Medicine, Committee on the Future of Emergency Care in the United States Health System. *Emergency Care for Children: Growing Pains.* Washington, DC: National Academies Press; 2006

5. National Commission on Children and Disasters. *2010 Report to the President and Congress.* Rockville, MD: Agency for Healthcare Research and Quality 2010. AHRQ Publication No. 10-M037. http://www.ahrq.gov/prep/nccdreport. Accessed February 21, 2018

6. American Academy of Pediatrics. *Pediatric Terrorism and Disaster Preparedness: A Resource for Pediatricians.* Foltin GL, Schonfeld DJ, Shannon MW, eds. Rockville, MD: Agency for Healthcare Research and Quality; 2006. AHRQ Publication No. 06(07)-0056

7. Macintyre AG, Christopher GW, Eitzen E Jr, et al. Weapons of mass destruction events with contaminated casualties: effective planning for health care facilities. *JAMA.* 2000;283(2):242–249

8. American Academy of Pediatrics Committee on Environmental Health. Radiation disasters and children. *Pediatrics.* 2003;111(6 Pt 1):1455–1466

9. Paulson JA, American Academy of Pediatrics Council on Environmental Health. Pediatric considerations before, during and after radiological/nuclear emergencies. Policy Statement. *Pediatrics,* in press

10. Linet MS, Kazzi Z, Paulson JA, American Academy of Pediatrics Council on Environmental Health. Pediatric considerations before, during and after radiological /nuclear emergencies. Technical Report. *Pediatrics,* in press

11. National Research Council. *Chemical and Biological Terrorism: Research and Development to Improve Civilian Medical Response*. Washington, DC: National Academies Press; 1999

12. US Army Medical Research Institute of Chemical Defense. *Field Management of Chemical Casualties Handbook*. Aberdeen Proving Ground, MD: US Army Medical Research Institute of Chemical Defense; 1996

13. Dunn MA, Sidell FR. Progress in medical defense against nerve agents. *JAMA*. 1989;262(5):649–652

14. Holstege CP, Kirk M, Sidell FR. Chemical warfare: nerve agent poisoning. *Crit Care Clin*. 1997;13(4):923–942

15. Okumura T, Takasu N, Ishimatsu S, et al. Report on 640 victims of the Tokyo subway sarin attack. *Ann Emerg Med*. 1996;28(2):129–135

16. Okumura T, Suzuki K, Fukuda A, et al. The Tokyo subway sarin attack: disaster management, part 1: community emergency response. *Acad Emerg Med*. 1998;5(6):613–617

17. Okumura T, Suzuki K, Fukuda A, et al. The Tokyo subway sarin attack: disaster management part 2: hospital response. *Acad Emerg Med*. 1998;5(6):618–624

18. Okumura T, Suzuki K, Fukuda A, et al. The Tokyo subway sarin attack: disaster management, part 3: national and international responses. *Acad Emerg Med*. 1998;5(6):625–628

19. *Pediatric Emergency Preparedness for Natural Disasters, Terrorism and Public Health Emergencies: A National Consensus Conference*. Markenson D, Redlener M, eds. New York, NY: National Center for Disaster Preparedness, Mailman School of Public Health, Columbia University; 2007. https://academiccommons.columbia.edu/catalog/ac:126146. Accessed September 3, 2018

20. Shenoi R. Chemical warfare agents. *Clin Pediatr Emerg Med*. 2002;3:239–247. https://www.sciencedirect.com/science/article/pii/S1522840102900364. Accessed September 3, 2018

21. Rodgers GC Jr, Condurache CT. Antidotes and treatments for chemical warfare/terrorism agents: an evidence-based review. *Clin Pharmacol Ther*. 2010;88(3):318–327

22. Craig JB, Culley JM, Tavakoli AS, Svendsen ER. Gleaning data from disaster: a hospital-based data mining method to study all-hazard triage from a chemical disaster. *Am J Disaster Med*. 2013;8(2):97–111

23. Christopher GW, Cieslak TJ, Pavlin JA, Eitzen EM Jr. Biological warfare. A historical perspective. *JAMA*. 1997;278(5):412–417

24. Danzig R, Berkowsky PB. Why should we be concerned about biological warfare? *JAMA*. 1997;278(5):431–432

25. Holloway HC, Norwood AE, Fullerton CS, Engel CC Jr, Ursano RJ. The threat of biological weapons. Prophylaxis and mitigation of psychologic and social consequences. *JAMA*. 1997;278(5)425–427

26. Chung S, Shannon M. Hospital planning for acts of terrorism and other public health emergencies involving children. *Arch Dis Child*. 2005;90(12):1300–1307

27. Centers for Disease Control and Prevention. Emergency Preparedness and Response. Bioterrorism Agents/Diseases. http://emergency.cdc.gov/agent/agentlist-category.asp. Accessed February 21, 2018

28. Schonfeld D. Supporting children after terrorist events: potential roles for pediatricians. *Pediatr Ann*. 2003;32(3):182–187

29. Cieslak TJ, Henretig FM. Bioterrorism. *Pediatr Ann*. 2003;32(3):154–165

30. Telofski LS, Morello AP, Mack Correa MC, Stamatas GN. The infant skin barrier: can we preserve, protect, and enhance the barrier? *Dermatol Res Pract*. 2012;2012:198789

31. Miyauchi Y, Shimaoka Y, Fujimura T, et al. Developmental changes in neonatal and infant skin structures during the first 6 months: in vivo observation. *Pediatr Dermatol*. 2016;33(3):289–295

32. Henretig FM, Cieslak TJ, Eitzen EM Jr. Biological and chemical terrorism. *J Pediatr.* 2002;141(3):311–326

33. Henretig FM, Cieslak TJ, Kortepeter MG, Fleisher GR. Medical management of the suspected victim of bioterrorism: an algorithmic approach to the undifferentiated patient. *Emerg Med Clin North Am.* 2002;20(2):351–364

34. Heon D, Foltin GL. Principles of pediatric decontamination. *Clin Pediatr Emerg Med.* 2009;10(3):186–194

35. New York City Department of Health and Mental Hygiene. *Pediatric Disaster Toolkit: Hospital Guidelines for Pediatrics During Disasters. Section 8 – Decontamination of the pediatric patient. 2006.* https://www.omh.ny.gov/omhweb/disaster_resources/pandemic_influenza/hospitals/bhpp_focus_ped_toolkit.html. Accessed September 3, 2018

36. Sandilands EA, Good AM, Bateman DN. The use of atropine in a nerve agent response with specific reference to children: are current guidelines too cautious? *Emerg Med J.* 2009;26(10):690–694

37. Food and Drug Administration. *Approved Drug Products With Therapeutic Equivalence Evaluations.* 37th ed. 2017. https://www.fda.gov/downloads/drugs/developmentapprovalprocess/ucm071436.pdf. Accessed February 21, 2018

38. *Pediatric Emergency Preparedness for Natural Disasters, Terrorism and Public Health Emergencies: A National Consensus Conference.* Garrett A, Redlener M, eds. New York, NY: National Center for Disaster Preparedness, Mailman School of Public Health, Columbia University; 2009. https://academiccommons.columbia.edu/catalog/ac:126143. Accessed September 3, 2018

39. Centers for Disease Control and Prevention. *Guidance for Protecting Building Environments from Chemical, Biological, or Radiological Attacks.* Washington, DC: National Institute for Occupational Safety and Health; 2002

40. Hagan JF Jr; American Academy of Pediatrics Committee on Psychosocial Aspects of Child and Family Health, Task Force on Terrorism. Clinical report: psychosocial implications of disaster or terrorism on children: a guide for the pediatrician. *Pediatrics.* 2005;116(3):787–795

41. Burkle FM Jr. Acute-phase mental health consequences of disasters; implications for triage and emergency medical services. *Ann Emerg Med.* 1996;28(2):119–128

42. American Academy of Pediatrics Committee on Pediatric Emergency Medicine, Committee on Medical Liability, Task Force on Terrorism. The pediatrician and disaster preparedness. *Pediatrics.* 2006;117(2):560–565

43. Pynoos RS, Goenjian AK, Steinberg AM. A public mental health approach to the postdisaster treatment of children and adolescents. *Child Adolesc Psychiatry Clin North Am.* 1998;7(1):195–210

44. Schonfeld D, Gurwitch R. Addressing disaster mental health needs of children: practical guidance for pediatric emergency healthcare providers. *Clin Pediatr Emerg Med.* 2009;10(3):208–215

45. Schonfeld D. Helping children deal with terrorism. In: Osborn L, DeWitt T, First L, Zenel J, eds. *Pediatrics.* Philadelphia, PA: Elsevier Mosby; 2005:1600–1602

46. National Disaster Medical System: Disaster Medical Assistance Team (DMAT). US Department of Health and Human Services. https://www.phe.gov/Preparedness/responders/ndms/Pages/default.aspx. Accessed September 3, 2018

47. Russell PK. Project BioShield: what it is, why it is needed, and its accomplishments so far. *Clin Infect Dis.* 2007;45(Suppl 1):568–572

48. Chung S, Shannon M. Reuniting children with their families during disasters: a proposed plan for greater success. *Am J Disaster Med.* 2007;2(3):113–117

49. Hamele M, Poss WB, Sweney J. Disaster preparedness, pediatric considerations in primary blast injury, chemical, and biological terrorism. *World J Crit Care Med.* 2014;3(1):15–23

50. Schobitz EP, Schmidt JM, Poirier MP. Biologic and chemical terrorism in children: an assessment of residents' knowledge. *Clin Pediatr (Phila).* 2008;47(3):267–270

51. Cicero MX, Blake E, Gallant N, et al. Impact of an educational intervention on residents' knowledge of pediatric disaster medicine. *Pediatr Emerg Care.* 2009;25(7):447–451

Chapter 52

# Developmental Disabilities

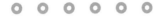

## KEY POINTS

- Many environmental toxicants can impact central nervous system development, leading to disturbances in cognitive, motor, sensory, behavioral, and/or social functioning.
- The developing central nervous system is exquisitely sensitive to environmental factors at all stages of development from the early embryonic period through childhood and adolescence.
- In general, the earlier the stage of brain development, the more vulnerable it is to environmental toxicants and the more likely it is that there will be neurodevelopmental consequences.
- Adverse social and economic factors can directly affect brain development and indirectly increase exposure to neurodevelopmental toxicants.
- Pediatricians, obstetricians, and other clinicians who care for pregnant women, children, and families should advise them about potentially hazardous exposures to environmental toxicants.

## INTRODUCTION

Developmental disabilities represent a diverse and complex set of neurologic conditions with origins in early life. Developmental disabilities are characterized by significant delays or differences in early childhood development resulting from an insult (or insults) to the developing brain that manifest in one or more functional domains. Developmental disabilities require timely identification, appropriate intervention, and medical, therapeutic, and psychosocial support to ensure optimal functioning of the child and family. This conceptualization addresses etiology, neurologic nature, manifestations, and the dynamic approach to recognition, diagnosis, and management.[1]

## INCREASING PREVALENCE OF DEVELOPMENTAL DISABILITIES

Learning and behavioral problems are increasing in children. Parents report that 1 in 6 children in the United States, 17% more than a decade ago, have a developmental disability, including learning disabilities (also known as "learning differences"), attention-deficit/hyperactivity disorder (ADHD), autism spectrum disorder (ASD), and other developmental disorders.[2] As of 2012, 1 in 10 (or more than 5.9 million) children in the United States were estimated to have ADHD.[3] As of 2014, 1 in 68 children in the United States had ASD.[4] The prevalence of prematurity, which contributes to a greater risk for developmental disabilities, also increased substantially over the decades to about 10% in the United States.[5] The US Centers for Disease Control and Prevention (CDC) recognizes that behavioral, socioeconomic, and environmental factors play substantial roles in causing prematurity.[6]

## CENTRAL NERVOUS SYSTEM DEVELOPMENT AND VULNERABILITIES

The central nervous system (CNS) begins forming shortly after conception and continues developing into early adulthood. It therefore remains vulnerable to environmental influences over a considerable period. In general, the earlier and more severe the insult to the developing brain, the more dramatic the outcome will be. The type of insult and the stage during which it occurs are important determinants of the extent and nature of the resulting developmental disability.[7]

On approximately day 18 of gestation, the neural plate invaginates and, over approximately 8 to 10 days, fuses to form the neural tube. At this point, neural crest cells begin to migrate. This is a critical period of neuronal migration in which neuronal connections develop, laying the network of connections for more complex aspects of brain function. Disturbances in the developing nervous system during these times can alter neuronal microarchitecture and neurotransmitter production, release, and reuptake. These disturbances can affect how the brain processes stimuli and coordinates tasks. Significant insults early in gestation are likely to result in more obvious anatomical malformations with a greater impact on development. For example, failure of brain septation can result in syndromes of agenesis of the corpus callosum with resulting motor and cognitive deficits; failure to close the neural tube results in spina bifida. Insults later in pregnancy tend to cause microanatomical and microarchitectural changes that manifest in more subtle functional disturbances in motor coordination, or have impacts on cognition. Early childhood is a particularly vulnerable time when environmental toxicants, as well as psychological, social, and cultural factors, can have a significant impact on brain function for a lifetime.

## SPECIFIC DEVELOPMENTAL DISABILITIES

Developmental disabilities may be broadly categorized as motor, sensory, cognitive, or behavioral/psychological, although many involve multiple elements (Figure 52-1).

The underlying principle is that any insult to the developing brain has a consequence on brain function depending on the nature, intensity, and timing of the insult. Insults that often have relatively milder consequences include learning disabilities, speech delays, sensory impairment and sensory integration disorders, motor coordination difficulties, and ADHD. More severe insults, often with major consequences, include intellectual disabilities, visual or hearing impairment, ASD, and cerebral palsy (CP).

### Learning Disabilities

Learning disabilities are characterized by difficulties with reading, mathematics, or written expression that significantly interfere with academic achievement or negatively affect activities of daily living.[8] They often are associated with cognitive processing deficits involving visual perception, language, attention, and memory. Approximately 4.6 million children aged 3 to 17 years (7.5%) have been diagnosed with at least one learning disability. Although underlying neurological mechanisms involved in learning disabilities are present at a very young age, they are usually not recognized until the child reaches school age and experiences academic difficulties.

### Speech Development and Delay

Speech development is critical to social interaction. It is important to be aware of normal milestones of speech development to respond in a timely and appropriate manner to parental concerns.[9] Delays or disorders in speech development can be a result of hearing impairment, a general developmental delay that may be associated with cognitive and motor delays as well, or, commonly, as part of the symptomatology of ASD.

### Sensory Impairment and Sensory Integration Disorder

Sensory integration disorder is a relatively new concept in pediatrics presenting with unusual reactions to sensory stimuli, such as difficulty with perceptual processing; heightened or reduced emotional reactivity; and difficulties with physiological functions, such as sleep, eating, and toileting as well as with language acquisition and development. Because sensory processing is a fundamental aspect of brain functioning, these disorders may be expressed as inattention and hyperactivity associated with ADHD, and/or behaviors associated with ASD.[10]

## Motor Delays and Coordination Disorders

Developmental delays in infancy are often identified in the first year of life because of delays in the typical dramatic progress in attaining motor skills. Delays may be mild with the attainment of milestones shortly after their expected appearance or milestones may be delayed by many months or longer. The long-term outcome is variable and related to the cause and severity of the disorder resulting in the delay.

## Attention-deficit/Hyperactivity Disorder (ADHD)

Attention-deficit/hyperactivity disorder is the most common neurobehavioral developmental disorder in childhood. It is characterized by an ongoing pattern of inattention and/or hyperactivity-impulsivity that can interfere with learning, development, and function. The CDC estimates that more than 1 in 10 (11%) US school-aged children, 1 in 5 high school boys and 1 in 11 high school girls, received an ADHD diagnosis by a health care provider by 2011, as reported by parents. The CDC reports that for children aged 4 to 17 years there was an increase in diagnosis from 7.8% prevalence in 2003 to 11% in 2011.[11] Children with ADHD may have co-existing conditions, such as learning disabilities.[12,13] Although children with ADHD or learning disabilities often face challenges, many also go on to be highly successful in life.

## Intellectual Disability

Intellectual disability is characterized by significant limitations in intellectual functioning with an IQ of 70 or below, and in difficulties with adaptive behavior, that manifest before age 18 years. Intellectual disability has been estimated to occur in 1.2% to 1.6% of the US population.[14] Although IQ scores are helpful in understanding and identifying areas of difficulty for a child, the current understanding and diagnosis of intellectual disability also involves impairments of general mental abilities that determine how well a person copes with everyday tasks.[15]

## Visual or Hearing Impairment

Sensory impairments can exist in isolation or be part of other conditions. Approximately 12 children in 10,000 have a hearing impairment originating congenitally or during early childhood. Childhood hearing impairment may be genetic or be caused by infections, hyperbilirubinemia, head trauma, noise, and exposure to aminoglycosides or other neurotoxicants. Childhood visual impairment also occurs in about 12 children per 10,000.[16] Preterm infants are at especially high risk for the development of vision impairment secondary to retinopathy following exposure to high concentrations of oxygen and high ventilator pressure. Sensory impairments should be detected as early as possible to institute early interventions designed to ensure optimal functional outcome.

## Autism Spectrum Disorder (ASD)

The understanding of ASD has changed over the past 7 to 8 decades since the term "autism" was originally used by Kanner in the 1940s to describe the child's focus on the self rather than the social world.[17] As of the 2013 publication of the *Diagnostic and Statistical Manual of Mental Disorders, Fifth Edition* (DSM-V), the diagnosis of autism is officially termed "Autism Spectrum Disorder" (ASD). This diagnosis is classified into different levels depending on the severity of expression and need for therapies, interventions, education, and behavior management.[18,19] ASD is formally characterized primarily by significant, qualitative difficulties in communication and reciprocal social interaction skills, an insistence on adhering to routines, and/or restrictive, repetitive, and stereotyped or repetitive behavior, interests, and activities.[20,21] Persons with ASD also may have characteristic speech patterns including echolalia, sensory processing difficulties, emotional reactions including anxiety, and unusual repetitive motor patterns.

ASD is indeed a spectrum with a high variability in presentation and characteristics. This may be confusing to parents and clinicians. It is important to make a diagnosis as early as possible and to promptly institute the necessary therapeutic and educational interventions to ensure an optimal outcome. Some children on the autism spectrum, particularly those in the high-functioning or "Asperger's" range, go on to become successful in society. Because of different or unusual ways of looking at the world, some people with ASD are able to make positive, innovative changes to society. It is suspected that some very famous and successful people are on the autism spectrum.

### Prevalence of ASD

The CDC estimates that the prevalence of ASD in children is 1 in 68,[22] with a prevalence in boys of 1 in 42 and in girls of 1 in 189. Variation exists from state to state with 1 in 45 children in New Jersey diagnosed with ASD, while in Wisconsin, Arkansas, and South Carolina the prevalence was approximately 1 in 80 to 100. This variation likely reflects many factors unique to the social, economic, and cultural character of each state that impact the availability and quality of diagnostic and therapeutic services.

It is unclear whether the dramatic increase in prevalence of ASD in past decades is the result of a true increase in ASD, whether this instead reflects an expansion of the diagnostic umbrella, or whether there is an increase in awareness and hence increase in diagnosis. In addition, questions remain about the extent to which environmental exposures play a part in the increase of ASD.

## Cerebral Palsy

Cerebral palsy (CP) describes a group of disorders affecting movement and posture as a result of insults to the developing fetal or infant brain.[23] The prevalence of cerebral palsy in the United States is approximately 3.6 cases per 1,000 births.[24] Although motor impairment and associated orthopedic consequences are hallmarks of cerebral palsy, there are often also seizure disorders, sensory disorders, and disturbances of cognition, communication, perception, and behavior. Etiology, timing of insult, parts of the brain affected, and the severity of the injury determine the nature and severity of the clinical manifestation in each child. The clinical picture varies from mild to severe and takes into consideration muscle tone, unusual movements, patterns of limb and trunk involvement, and the degree of cognitive ability. The Gross Motor Functional Classification Scale (GMFCS)[25] ranges from 1 to 5 from the mildest to the most impaired clinical picture. Medical complications include orthopedic problems such as contractures and scoliosis, neurological problems including spasticity and seizures, gastrointestinal problems such as constipation and gastroesophageal reflux, feeding difficulties with aspiration pneumonia and reactive airway disease, and impairments of vision and/or hearing. Children with cerebral palsy often require many therapies, hospitalizations, surgeries, subspecialty care, and adaptive equipment. This condition is best managed by an interdisciplinary team and is the prototype for conditions requiring a medical home.[26]

## ETIOLOGY OF DEVELOPMENTAL DISABILITIES

The etiology of the CNS insult often determines the pattern and severity of symptoms, which, in turn, determine the impact on health and well-being.[26]

The etiology of developmental disabilities can be viewed from the temporal perspective—prenatal, perinatal, or postnatal. The temporal paradigm is helpful because it is often possible to identify and recognize the timing of events in relation to vulnerabilities of the fetus, the newborn infant, and the growing child. Figure 52-1 provides an overview of etiologies in specific time periods and how outcomes of the CNS dysfunction manifest in the variety of developmental disabilities.[27]

Many environmental factors operate in the prenatal and postnatal periods. Some of these may operate across the lifespan, particularly with respect to social determinants. Although the distinction between the genetic and environmental etiologies of developmental disabilities represent the "nature versus nurture" question, there is a dynamic interaction between genetics and

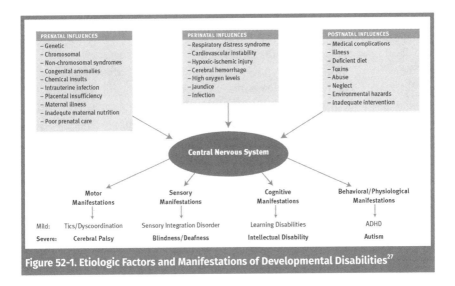

**Figure 52-1. Etiologic Factors and Manifestations of Developmental Disabilities[27]**

the environment through epigenetic mechanisms. The genetic code confers definitive physical, behavioral, and health-related characteristics on a person, while environmental factors operate epigenetically to alter the expressions of specific genetic codes, thereby modifying physical, physiological, and psychological functions.[28] The epigenetic process and its consequences provide an initial understanding of a mechanism whereby the environment can alter the growth, health, and development of children toward their ultimate future as functioning adults.

Most causes of developmental disabilities (50% to 70%) take place during the prenatal period, with 10% to 20% attributed to perinatal and 10% to 20% to postnatal causes.[29,30] Most perinatal causes in the United States are related to prematurity, which, in many cases, also has prenatal etiologies.[31]

## GENETIC INFLUENCES

Many developmental disabilities stem from specific genetic or chromosomal abnormalities. Autosomal-recessive disorders, including inborn errors of metabolism (ie, aminoacidopathies, lipoidoses, mucopolysaccharidoses), are among the most serious because they usually involve progressive neurodegeneration. Some genetic conditions are sex-linked, such as Fragile X syndrome and Rett syndrome. Disorders of chromosome number include Down syndrome, associated with an extra chromosome 21. Microdeletion anomalies such as DiGeorge syndrome, velocardiofacial syndrome, and various other malformations have been described in association with deletions and translocations involving human chromosome 22q11, or the Smith-Magenis syndrome, with a microdeletion on chromosome 17. An excellent reference for this set of conditions is *Smith's Recognizable Patterns of Human Malformation*, now in its seventh edition.[32] Disorders of mitochondrial DNA, which are primarily maternally transmitted via mitochondria in the fertilized ovum, also result in neurologic disorders that may manifest in other family members to varying degrees.[33] Other developmental disabilities appear to involve a strong genetic predisposition, although the actual mechanism of inheritance is unclear. Spina bifida likely has a genetic predisposition but can be prevented by ingesting adequate folic acid. The US Preventive Services Task Force (USPSTF) recommends that all women of child-bearing age, especially those planning a pregnancy, take a daily supplement containing 0.4 to 0.8 mg (400 to 800 mcg) of folic acid to prevent the likelihood of spina bifida in any future pregnancy.[34] ADHD and ASD also fall into this category because of genetic predisposition that very likely involves complex interactions between 1 or more genes with 1 or more environmental factors.[35,36]

Although studies of families have revealed a genetic pattern in how ADHD manifests,[37] there are multiple environmental factors associated with ADHD, such as maternal smoking during pregnancy, preterm birth, alcohol exposure, viral infections, endocrine disorders,[38] and exposures to lead, particularly among children living in older, poorer neighborhoods, with other associated psychosocial and other environmental factors.[39] Similarly, although ASD has some genetic basis,[40–42] ASD more likely results from gene-environment interactions than from a single genetic factor or etiologic agent.[43]

Because of coding of the human genome, advances in technology, and progress toward genetic diagnosis, we now see many more variations in gene sequences, some of which explain known conditions. Genetic causes of other conditions, many of which are associated with developmental disabilities, have yet to be elucidated. Epigenetics explores and serves to explain how environmental factors can modify gene expression to influence growth, development, and health.[44]

## ENVIRONMENTAL INFLUENCES

Environmental factors play major roles in brain development and brain function that can result in the manifestation of developmental disabilities. Stages of development, dose and duration of exposure, and resilience are a few of many variables that can determine the nature and extent of disability. It is helpful to examine these factors in a temporal context, ie, before, during, or after birth (see Figure 52-1).

## Prenatal Environment

### Exposure to Metals During Pregnancy

Awareness of the effect of mercury on the developing brain came in the 1950s from the disaster near Minamata, Japan in which a chemical company discharged tons of mercury waste into Minamata Bay. The mercury then entered the food chain and resulted in major neurological disorders in children, especially in newborn infants who had intrauterine exposures.[45] Although exposures to large amounts of mercury result in major neurological disturbances, exposures to smaller doses of mercury have more subtle but nonetheless significant adverse outcomes. Because oceans and lakes have been polluted with mercury, the US government has issued advisories about fish and seafood consumption during pregnancy (see Chapter 33).[46]

Lead can cause damage to the fetal brain because lead easily crosses the placenta. Pregnancy also is associated with a marked increase in maternal bone turnover, so that prenatal lead exposure can occur not only through current maternal environmental exposures but also through mobilization of the mother's accumulated stores of bone lead. Prenatal lead exposure can affect fetal DNA, which, in turn, may influence long-term epigenetic programming and disease susceptibility.[47] To address this issue, the US Department of Health and Human Services (DHHS) published *Guidelines for the Identification and Management of Lead Exposure in Pregnant and Lactating Women* (see Chapter 32).[48]

### Pesticides, Polychlorinated Biphenyls, Polycyclic Aromatic Hydrocarbons, and Other Chemicals

Exposure to several commonly used chemicals during pregnancy may result in developmental disabilities either by directly causing CNS damage or epigenetically by modifying DNA, thereby predisposing a child to greater vulnerability to environmental toxicants. Prenatal exposure to organophosphate pesticides increases the risk of memory deficits, poorer motor performance, and other conditions.[49] Prenatal exposure to pesticides may increase the likelihood of having a child with ASD.[50] Polychlorinated biphenyls (PCBs) are mixtures of chlorinated compounds once used as cooling and insulating fluids in electronic components. Prenatal exposure to PCBs can adversely affect neurologic functions, such as planning efficiency, executive working memory, speed of information processing, verbal abilities, and visual recognition memory.[51] Polycyclic aromatic hydrocarbons (PAHs) are widely distributed air pollutants generated by motor fuel combustion, coal-fired power plants, tobacco smoking, and residential heating and cooking. Exposure to high levels of these well-recognized human mutagens and carcinogens is associated with adverse effects on birth weight and cognitive development.[52]

A study conducted by the CDC through the National Health and Nutrition Examination Survey (NHANES) in 2003-2004 found that certain PCBs, organochlorine pesticides, perfluoroalkyl and polyfluoroalkyl substances, phenols, polybrominated diphenyl ethers (PBDEs), phthalates, PAHs, and perchlorate were detected in 99% to 100% of pregnant women.[53]

## Alcohol

A range of neurologic and other problems collectively referred to as fetal alcohol spectrum disorders (FASD) result from prenatal exposure to alcohol.[54] Although chronic consumption of alcohol and binge drinking are especially likely to have adverse consequences on the CNS in utero, any prenatal alcohol exposure may result in harm.[55] In the United States, approximately 4 million infants are born with prenatal alcohol exposure each year, and 1,000 to 6,000 infants are diagnosed with fetal alcohol syndrome (FAS) and more with the broadened spectrum of partial FAS and alcohol-related neurodevelopmental disorder. The classic and more severe form of FAS is characterized by certain physical features, developmental disabilities, and significant behavioral problems. The behavior problems may be exacerbated by the same environmental factors that initially may have contributed to the mother's substance abuse (eg, toxic stress, neglect and abuse, domestic violence, homelessness, family discord). Milder forms of FASD may manifest with learning disabilities, ADHD, and behavior difficulties.

Fetal exposure to alcohol is preventable. Warning labels on bottles of alcohol integrated with other educational, policy, and programmatic initiatives can help shift social norms and reduce risks of alcohol consumption during pregnancy.[56]

## Smoking

Maternal smoking during pregnancy is associated with low birth weight, prematurity, birth defects, and sudden infant death syndrome (SIDS), as well as developmental delays, cognitive problems, learning disorders, and behavioral difficulties that may be aggravated by the prematurity and low birth weight status. Pregnant mothers' exposure to secondhand tobacco smoke (SHS) also is associated with adverse pregnancy outcomes.[57] The severity may vary depending on the dose, timing, other associated exposures, and epigenetic susceptibility. The impact of fetal exposure to tobacco smoke not only affects the offspring but also subsequent generations.[58] Tobacco use is more prevalent among lower income, minority, and stressed individuals and communities.[59]

## Maternal Substance Abuse

Prenatal use of drugs, such as opioids, cocaine, methamphetamines, and cannabis, can potentially cause neurologic symptoms in children, including inattention, impulsivity, and cognitive impairment.[60] Strong evidence shows the negative effects of these prenatal exposures on infant behavior, long-term behavior, cognition, language, and achievement.[61] The long-term effects of these exposures depend on the specific drug, and the timing, dose, and duration of exposure.

### Maternal Medications

Prescription medications, including the anticonvulsants phenytoin and valproic acid, may cause neurologic syndromes with recognizable physical characteristics and neurodevelopmental consequences.[32,62] The safety of medications that may be used during pregnancy and lactation is regulated by the FDA and information is available about all FDA-approved medications.

### Maternal Infections

A dramatic example of the impact of an intrauterine infection on fetal growth and development occurred during the rubella epidemic of 1963 to 1965.[63] Babies born to mothers who contracted rubella during pregnancy had significant brain damage with consequent functional complications such as intellectual disabilities, visual impairment, and autistic behaviors.[64] The degree and nature of the impact was related to the timing of the infection—the earlier in pregnancy that a mother was infected, the greater the degree of brain damage and neurological complications. Congenital defects occurred in more than 80% of infants infected in the first trimester; virtually no defects were found in infants infected after the first 16 weeks of gestation. The gestational age at the time of fetal infection also affects the distribution of congenital defects: infection in the first trimester is more likely to result in multiple congenital defects, whereas infection after 11 to 12 weeks' gestation is more likely to result in isolated deafness or retinopathy as clinical manifestations.[65]

Other prenatal infections, including toxoplasmosis, cytomegalovirus, syphilis, herpes, and HIV, may have adverse effects.[66] The Zika virus was recently recognized as a cause of significant microcephaly and brain damage in offspring exposed prenatally. Efforts are underway to study the virus and its transmission via the *Aedes Egypti* mosquito, and to develop prevention and management strategies.[67]

### Maternal Illness and Chronic Conditions

Other maternal illnesses during pregnancy may affect fetal growth and development. Chronic conditions, such as diabetes mellitus, may be particularly problematic, especially if blood glucose is not well controlled. Maternal stress, malnutrition, physical trauma secondary to domestic abuse, and illness may adversely affect the fetus. High maternal body mass index (BMI) can be associated with adverse outcomes in offspring, such as emotional symptoms, peer problems, psychosocial difficulties, ADHD, ASD, or developmental delays, and receipt of speech language therapy, psychological services, or any special needs service.[68]

Maternal stress and depression during pregnancy is an independent risk factor for low fetal birth weight and premature delivery. Other illnesses, such as anxiety disorders, eating disorders, psychotic illness, and maternal infection, may also be associated with adverse birth outcomes and the later risk for developmental, learning, and behavioral challenges.[69-71]

## THE PERINATAL ENVIRONMENT

The two most common perinatal events associated with developmental disabilities are seen in (1) full-term infants who experience a difficult birth and sustain birth trauma or hypoxic ischemic insults, and (2) infants born prematurely (at a gestational age of less than 37 weeks) and with a birth weight of less than 2,500 grams. In the United States, most perinatal causes of developmental disabilities are related to prematurity and the degree of prematurity.[72,73] For example, the prevalence of cerebral palsy was approximately 20% at 24 to 26 weeks' gestation, compared with 4% at 32 weeks.[74]

It is increasingly recognized that the prevalence of ADHD and ASD are associated with prematurity,[75,76] as well as other cognitive, motor, learning, and behavior challenges.[77-79] Preterm birth is often associated with teenage pregnancy and lack of prenatal care, as well as maternal alcohol use, tobacco use, and drug use and other maternal and social factors.

### Postnatal Environments

A range of postnatal insults may contribute to developmental disabilities. Central nervous system damage may be caused by infection (eg, meningitis, encephalitis); injury associated with falls, motor vehicle crashes, near-drowning, and child abuse; and chemical and physical agents found in soil, water, and air. Although prenatal exposure of the developing fetus to neurotoxicants generally has a greater impact on the development of the brain and hence adverse neurodevelopmental outcomes, postnatal exposures also present serious risks to the growing and developing child. The toxicants with the greatest impact on brain function are the metals, but other chemicals also can have adverse outcomes that are more subtle and may result in lower IQ scores, learning disabilities, and ADHD.[80,81]

#### Metals

Exposure to metals may be associated with brain damage in early life. For more than 100 years, lead has been recognized as a neurotoxicant in children. High blood lead levels can result in significant brain damage; even blood lead levels of 5 mcg/dL and below may have adverse effects on IQ, learning, and behavior. Lead exposure in early childhood is associated with diminished school performance and with delinquent behavior later in life (see Chapter 32).[82]

Methylmercury's adverse effects on the developing brain are seen most dramatically with prenatal exposure but postnatal exposure also is neurotoxic (see Chapter 33). Although trace amounts of manganese are necessary for health and normal development, high levels of manganese can damage the developing nervous system. Arsenic exposure, mainly through drinking water, but also from some rice products (see Chapter 22), has been linked to adverse cognitive effects.[81]

In their review of environmental chemicals responsible for developmental neurotoxicity in children, Grandjean and Landrigan[83] recognized the greater adverse impact on the fetus but also listed the following as having adverse impact after postnatal exposure:

PCBs are associated with reduced cognitive function in infancy and childhood. PCBs are often present in foods, particularly fish, and can be passed along in breast milk (see Chapter 38). Organic pesticides, including chlorpyrifos and DDT, are linked to structural abnormalities of the brain and neurodevelopmental problems (see Chapter 40). Tetrachloroethylene solvents are linked to hyperactivity and aggressive behavior and an increased risk of psychiatric diagnosis. The PBDEs are linked to neurodevelopmental disorders in children (see Chapter 37). Bisphenol A (BPA) (see Chapter 41) is recognized as an endocrine disruptor and is strongly suspected to affect neurodevelopment in children. Phthalates have been linked to shortened attention span and impaired social interactions in children (see Chapter 41). Exposure to SHS during childhood is associated with behavioral problems and learning disabilities (see Chapter 43).[84]

Research about the neurologic effects of many chemicals is quite limited so safe levels of exposure are often unknown. Few regulations have been implemented to reduce the potential effects of numerous chemicals on the developing brain.

## THE SOCIAL AND ECONOMIC ENVIRONMENT

An impoverished social and economic environment is associated with developmental disabilities. Poverty, racism, low socioeconomic status, mental illness, and substance abuse may coexist with residence in communities in which exposures to environmental hazards are prevalent and resources are limited. Preterm birth, low birth weight, CNS abnormalities, and prolonged hospitalizations can drain family resources and interfere with parent-infant bonding.[85,86]

Nutritional and psychosocial environments have significant influence on health and development. Children with poor nutrition and those who receive inadequate sensory stimulation and nurturing in their early years are at higher risk of having developmental delays and disabilities.[87] Child maltreatment and other traumatic events may cause permanent physical damage to the brain and changes to CNS structure and functioning that can manifest as developmental disabilities.[88] The collective adverse effects on a child who lives in poverty result in a measurable reduction in brain growth, smaller white and cortical gray matter, and hippocampal and amygdala volumes, with changes in brain function.[89]

For many children, the social and economic risks are compounded during their early years. Poverty remains one of the most complex and far-reaching risk factors because it affects so many aspects of a child's life.[90] In 2015, 20% of all US children aged 0 to 17 lived in poverty.[91] The rate for children of all ages living in single female-headed families was 42%. During that same year, approximately 23% of children (16.9 million) lived in households with food insecurity (defined as a condition existing when people lack sustainable access to enough safe, nutritious, and socially acceptable food for a healthy and productive life). Children who were impoverished were also more likely to have a blood lead level of 5 mcg/dL or greater. The risk of teen pregnancy is 10 times higher among the most poor compared with the more affluent with an increased risk of premature births and the risk of remaining a single parent and in poverty in the future.[90] Moreover, living in low-income areas decreases children's access to appropriate educational, health care, and habilitative services. As an example, ADHD is less likely to be properly diagnosed and treated in disadvantaged children; as a consequence, they are more likely to experience long-term, negative psychological and social consequences and adverse educational outcomes (eg, high grade retention and dropout rates).[92] They are therefore less likely to have gainful employment or a steady and solid income, and more likely to become trapped in a cycle of poverty and environmental health disparities. It often is difficult to escape these situations unless they are interrupted by outside social forces or by the resilience and extraordinary efforts of individuals and families (Figure 52-2).[86,93,94]

Children from low income communities are more likely to experience a cumulative set of insecurities, insults, and stress termed "toxic stress."[95] Toxic stress refers to a pattern of multiple, repeated, and relentless psychological, emotional, and physiological insults with limited, inadequate, or unpredictable nurturing, support, and guidance of a parent or other caring adult. This results in persistently elevated levels of stress hormones, particularly cortisol, that can disrupt developing brain architecture. Toxic stress may lead to adverse effects on learning, executive functioning, decision-making, working memory, behavioral self-regulation, and mood and impulse control. When these children become adolescents and then adults, those

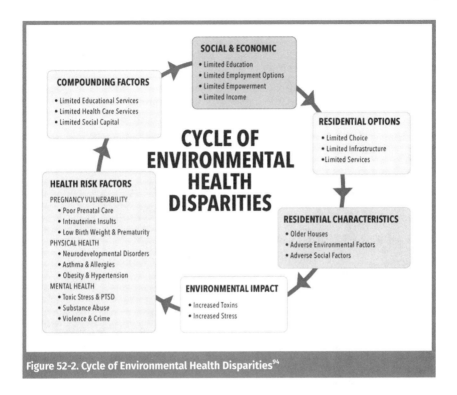

**Figure 52-2. Cycle of Environmental Health Disparities**[94]

who experienced toxic stress manifest higher rates of school failure, risk-taking behaviors, gang membership, unemployment, poverty, homelessness, violent crime, incarceration, and becoming single parents. The inflammatory impact of chronically elevated cortisol levels can result in metabolic disorders such as obesity and diabetes mellitus, and cardiovascular effects such as hypertension and stroke in adults, adversely affecting adult health and potentially resulting in early death.[95]

Just as the developing brain is vulnerable to adverse environmental influences, it is likewise susceptible to positive influences, which offers a reason for optimism about the promise of early intervention. Even in the most extreme cases of adversity, well-timed changes to children's environments can improve outcomes. Pediatricians are uniquely positioned to develop and improve strategies for preventing toxic stress in each family and in a larger public health context.[96,97] Advocacy can occur in individual clinical settings, through chapters of the American Academy of Pediatrics, and its committees, councils, and sections, and through programs such as Community Access to Child Health (CATCH).

## INTERNATIONAL CONSIDERATIONS

Children living in low- and middle-income nations may be at especially high risk of developmental disabilities (see Chapter 14). Major risk factors include specific genetic diseases, a higher frequency of births to older mothers, consanguinity, micronutrient deficiencies, and infections.[98] Toxic exposures to lead have been documented after informal mining activities in Nigeria[99] and among the Roma people of Kosovo displaced by war.[100] Displacement by natural and man-made disasters (eg, war) can result in physical, chemical, and psychological effects on a child's brain development and functional outcome. Data on epidemiology, etiology, screening, and intervention services are often lacking.[101,102]

## ROLE OF THE PEDIATRICIAN

Because pediatricians see children frequently in the first and second years of life, they are well positioned to identify delays and unusual patterns of a child's development and behavior. It is important to ask questions about family history, occupations of parents, and environmental risk factors, especially the age of the home and about smoking. When indicated, referrals should be made for neurologic, genetic, metabolic, or toxicological workups and for developmental evaluations and therapies. Developmental screening and early detection of developmental issues and subsequent referral to early intervention and other specialty services can positively affect the child's development and the family's stability and well-being.[103,104] Children, especially those from low resource communities, who participate in an early intervention program have positive benefits with enhanced developmental outcomes.[97] The complex developmental, educational, psychological, medical, and social considerations for a child with a developmental disability are best addressed in the context of a medical home.[26] Pediatricians should be aware of local, state, and federal programs for children with disabilities. Programs include birth-to-3 early intervention programs; therapeutic services; special needs preschool programs and special education services through the public school systems; transition planning for adolescents to prepare for graduation and independence; special programs such as the State Title V programs for Children with Special Health Care Needs; and parent support groups.

The following questions should be considered in an environmental history:

What are the occupations of the parents? Are they from or have they been in a foreign country? Where do they live? Is the setting rural or urban? What is the age and condition of the house in which they live? Do the parents smoke, drink alcohol, or take drugs or medication, and did the mother do so during pregnancy? Do they use alternative or natural medications or remedies?

Answers may lead to exploring possible environmental exposures that occurred before or during pregnancy. This may lead to focused testing and identifying a cause and, if possible, removing the causative agent with potential improvement of outcome or preventing further harm.

Women who are pregnant should be asked about exposure to pesticides, lead, other metals and SHS, mold, and other forms of air pollution. Pregnant women should be encouraged to receive regular prenatal care and given information about sleep, stress reduction, and exercise. They should be counseled about nutrition and dietary recommendations related to fish consumption and the benefits of breastfeeding. Clinicians should stress the importance of daily intake of folic acid during the childbearing years.[105] It is recommended that all women of child-bearing age, especially those who are planning a pregnancy, take a daily supplement containing 0.4 to 0.8 mg (400 to 800 mcg) of folic acid.[34]

When asking about potential environmental etiologies for a developmental disability, it also is important to keep in mind that parents may experience guilt and sadness about their possible role in contributing to the child's problems. Pediatricians may offer help to parents whose child has a developmental disability by offering an understanding that the cause of any developmental disability likely is multifactorial rather than related to one exposure, and that early identification and early intervention often yield excellent results.

## CONCLUSION

Developmental disabilities are common in pediatric practice. It behooves pediatricians to be aware of the conditions and perform timely screening, make referrals for further diagnostic evaluation as necessary, and refer for early intervention, necessary therapies, and appropriate education.

The causes of developmental disabilities can be genetic or environmental and, more likely, a combination of both through epigenetic mechanisms. Pediatricians should become familiar with common environmental causes and include relevant environmental questions when taking a history and exploring a diagnostic etiology.

Pediatricians should promote health literacy about known environmental causes and incorporate advice about prevention of environmental exposures into anticipatory guidance for families.

Parents often need and appreciate reassurance, support, and encouragement. When appropriate, pediatricians can inform parents that many children with developmental disabilities make excellent progress and lead productive lives. It is the clinician's role to guide the parents to the most appropriate services that will help the child reach his or her full potential.

## Frequently Asked Questions

Q  *I read on the Internet about vaccines causing autism. Should I have my child vaccinated?*

A  I certainly understand your concern about your child's well-being; however, findings from many research studies show no connection between vaccines and autism. Vaccines are safe and effective. Vaccines prevent your child from contracting diseases that can cause great harm, even death. I have seen children harmed from these illnesses and do not want harm to come to your child. Let me give you the Vaccine Information Statements from the CDC so you can read more about the vaccines I would like to administer today. Please let me know if you have other questions.

## References

1. Rubin IL, Merrick J, Greydanus DE, Patel DR, eds. *Health Care for People With Intellectual and Developmental Disabilities Across the Lifespan.* Switzerland: Springer; 2016

2. Boyle CA, Boulet S, Schieve LA, et al. Trends in the prevalence of developmental disabilities in US children, 1997–2008. *Pediatrics.* 2011;127(6):1034–1042

3. Bloom B, Jones LI, Freeman G. Summary health statistics for U.S. Children: National health interview survey, 2012. Vital and health statistics Series 10. Data from the National Health Survey; 2013:1–81

4. Centers for Disease Control and Prevention. Prevalence of autism spectrum disorder among children aged 8 years - autism and developmental disabilities monitoring network, 11 sites, United States, 2010. *MMWR.* 2014;63(2):1–21

5. Hamilton BE, Martin JA, Osterman MJK, Curtin SC, Mathews TJ. Births: final data for 2014. *Nat Vital Stat Rep.* 2015;64(12):1–64

6. Centers for Disease Control and Prevention Health Disparities and Inequalities Report — United States, 2011. *Morbidity and Mortality Weekly Report.* Supplement Vol. 60. January 14, 2011. https://www.cdc.gov/mmwr/pdf/other/su6001.pdf. Accessed April 6, 2018

7. Rice D, Barone S. Critical periods of vulnerability for the developing nervous system: evidence from humans and animal models. *Environ Health Perspect.* 2000;108(Suppl 3):511–533

8. Centers for Disease Control and Prevention. Learning Disorders. http://www.cdc.gov/ncbddd/childdevelopment/learning-disorder.html. Accessed April 6, 2018

9. University of Michigan. Speech and Language Development. http://www.med.umich.edu/yourchild/topics/speech.htm. Accessed April 6, 2018

10. Grapel JN, Cicchetti DV, Volkmar FR. Sensory features as diagnostic criteria for autism: sensory features in autism. *Yale J Biol Med.* 2015;88(1):69–71

11. Visser S, Danielson M, Bitsko R, et al. Trends in the parent-report of health care provider-diagnosis and medication treatment for ADHD disorder: United States, 2003–2011. *J Am Acad Child Adolesc Psychiatry.* 2014;53(1):34–46.e2

12. American Academy of Pediatrics Subcommittee on Attention-Deficit/Hyperactivity Disorder, Steering Committee on Quality Improvement and Management, Wolraich M, et al. ADHD: clinical practice guideline for the diagnosis, evaluation, and treatment of attention-deficit/hyperactivity disorder in children and adolescents. *Pediatrics.* 2011;128(5):1007–1022

13. Tarver J, Daley D, Sayal K. Attention-deficit hyperactivity disorder (ADHD): an updated review of the essential facts. *Child Care Health Dev.* 2014;40(6):762–774

14. Bhasin TK, Brocksen S, Avchen RN, Braun KVN. Prevalence of four developmental disabilities among children aged 8 years—Metropolitan Atlanta Developmental Disabilities Surveillance Program, 1996 and 2000. *MMWR Surveill Summ.* 2006;55(1):1–9

15. American Psychiatric Association Diagnostic and Statistical Manual Fifth Edition. DSM-5 2013. http://dsm.psychiatryonline.org/pb-assets/dsm/update/DSM5Update2016.pdf. Accessed April 6, 2018

16. Centers for Disease Control and Prevention. Metropolitan Atlanta Developmental Disabilities Surveillance Program (MADDSP). Atlanta, GA: Centers for Disease Control and Prevention; 2000. https://www.cdc.gov/ncbddd/developmentaldisabilities/MADDSP.html. Accessed April 6, 2018

17. Kanner L. Autistic disturbances of affective contact. *Nervous Child.* 1943;2:217–250

18. American Psychiatric Association. Autism Spectrum Disorder. American Psychiatric Publishing; 2013. https://www.psychiatry.org/psychiatrists/practice/dsm. Accessed April 6, 2018

19. Autism Speaks. Diagnostic Criteria of the Autism Spectrum Disorders. https://www.autismspeaks.org/what-autism/diagnosis/dsm-5-diagnostic-criteria. Accessed April 6, 2018

20. Autism Speaks. Answers to Frequently Asked Questions about DSM-5. https://www.autismspeaks.org/dsm-5/faq. Accessed April 6, 2018

21. Johnson CP, Myers SM, American Academy of Pediatrics Council on Children With Disabilities. Identification and evaluation of children with autism spectrum disorders. *Pediatrics.* 2007;120(5):1183–1215

22. Christensen DL, Baio J, Braun KV, et al. Prevalence and characteristics of autism spectrum disorder among children aged 8 Years — Autism and Developmental Disabilities Monitoring Network, 11 Sites, United States, 2012. *MMWR Surveill Summ.* 2016;65(3):1–23

23. Bax M, Goldstein M, Rosenbaum P, et al. Proposed definition and classification of cerebral palsy, April 2005. *Dev Med Child Neurol.* 2005;47(8):571–576

24. Yeargin-Allsopp M, Braun KV, Doernberg NS, Benedict RE, Kirby RS, Durkin MS. Prevalence of cerebral palsy in 8-year-old children in three areas of the United States in 2002: a multisite collaboration. *Pediatrics.* 2008;121(3):547–554

25. Palisano R, Rosenbaum P, Walter S, Russell D, Wood E, Galuppi B. Development and reliability of a system to classify gross motor function in children with cerebral palsy. *Dev Med Child Neurol.* 1997;39(4):214–223

26. Medical Home Initiatives for Children With Special Needs Project Advisory Committee, American Academy of Pediatrics. The medical home. *Pediatrics.* 2002;110(1 Pt 1):184–186

27. Rubin IL, Crocker AC. *Medical Care for Children and Adults with Developmental Disabilities.* 2nd ed. Baltimore, MD: Paul Brookes; 2006

28. Rivera RM, Bennett LB. Epigenetics in humans: an overview. *Curr Opin Endocrinol Diabetes Obes.* 2010;17(6):493–499

29. Wellesley D, Hockey A, Stanley F. The aetiology of intellectual disability in Western Australia: a community-based study. *Dev Med Child Neurol.* 1991;33(11):963–973

30. Centers for Disease Control and Prevention. Postnatal causes of developmental disabilities in children aged 3- 10 years — Atlanta, Georgia, 1991. *MMWR Morb Mortal Wkly Rep.* 1996;45(6):130–134

31. Huang J, Zhu T, Qu Y, Mu D. Prenatal, perinatal and neonatal risk factors for intellectual disability: a systemic review and meta-analysis. *PLoS One.* 2016;11(4):e0153655

32. Jones KL, Jones MC, del Campo M. *Smith's Recognizable Patterns of Human Malformation.* 7th ed. Elsevier; 2013

33. Chinnery PF. *Mitochondrial Disorders Overview.* http://www.ncbi.nlm.nih.gov/books/NBK1224/. Accessed April 6, 2018

34. Bibbins-Domingo K, Grossman DC, Curry SJ, et al. Folic acid supplementation for the prevention of neural tube defects: US Preventive Services Task Force Recommendation Statement. *JAMA*. 2017;317(2):183–189

35. Rossignol DA, Genuis SJ, Frye RE. Environmental toxicants and autism spectrum disorders: a systematic review. *Transl Psychiatry*. 2014;4:e360

36. Lai MC, Lombardo MV, Baron-Cohen S. Autism. *Lancet*. 2014;383(9920):896–910

37. Goos LM, Crosbie J, Payne S, Schachar R. Validation and extension of the endophenotype model in ADHD patterns of inheritance in a family study of inhibitory control. *Am J Psychiatry*. 2009;166(6):711–717

38. Millichap JG. Etiologic classification of attention-deficit/hyperactivity disorder. *Pediatrics*. 2008;121(2):e358–e365

39. Froehlich TE, Lanphear BP, Epstein JN, Barbaresi WJ, Katusic SK, Kahn RS. Prevalence, recognition, and treatment of attention-deficit/hyperactivity disorder in a national sample of US children. *Arch Pediatr Adolesc Med*. 2007;161(9):857–864

40. Moss J, Howlin P. Autism spectrum disorders in genetic syndromes: implications for diagnosis, intervention and understanding the wider autism spectrum population. *J Intellect Disabil Res*. 2009;53(10):852–873

41. Frazier TW, Thompson L, Youngstrom EA, et al. A twin study of heritable and shared environmental contributions to autism. *J Autism Dev Disord*. 2014;44(8):2013–2025

42. Grønborg T, Schendel DE, Parner ET. Recurrence of autism spectrum disorders in full- and half-siblings and trends over time: a population-based cohort study. *JAMA Pediatr*. 2013;167(10):947–953

43. Centers for Disease Control and Prevention Community Report from the Autism and Developmental Disabilities Monitoring (ADDM) Network. A Snapshot of Autism Spectrum Disorder among 8-year-old Children in Multiple Communities across the United States in 2012. United States Department of Health and Human Services 2016. http://www.cdc.gov/ncbddd/autism/documents/community_report_autism.pdf. Accessed April 6, 2018

44. Perera F, Herbstman J. Prenatal environmental exposures, epigenetics, and disease. *Reprod Toxicol*. 2011;31(3):363–373

45. Environmental Health and Safety Division Environmental Health Department. Lessons from Minamata Disease and Mercury Management in Japan. Ministry of the Environment, Japan 2011

46. US Environmental Protection Agency. Fish and Shellfish Advisories and Safe Eating Guidelines. https://www.epa.gov/choose-fish-and-shellfish-wisely/fish-and-shellfish-advisories-and-safe-eating-guidelines. Accessed April 6, 2018

47. Pilsner RJ, Hu H, Ettinger A, et al. Influence of prenatal lead exposure on genomic methylation of cord blood DNA. *Environ Health Perspect*. 2009;117(9):1466–1471

48. Ettinger AS, Wengrovitz AG. Guidelines for the Identification and Management of Lead Exposure in Pregnant and Lactating Women. U.S. Department of Health and Human Services; 2010

49. Rauh V, Arunajadai S, Horton M, et al. Seven-year neurodevelopmental scores and prenatal exposure to chlorpyrifos, a common agricultural pesticide. *Environ Health Perspect*. 2011;119(8):1196–1201

50. Shelton JF, Geraghty EM, Tancredi DJ, et al. Neurodevelopmental disorders and prenatal residential proximity to agricultural pesticides: the CHARGE study. *Environ Health Perspect*. 2014;122(10):1103–1109

51. Boucher O, Muckle G, Bastien CH. Prenatal exposure to polychlorinated biphenyls: a neuropsychologic analysis. *Environ Health Perspect*. 2009;117(1):7–16

52. Perera FP, Rauh V, Whyatt RM, et al. Effect of prenatal exposure to airborne polycyclic aromatic hydrocarbons on neurodevelopment in the first 3 years of life among inner-city children. *Environ Health Perspect.* 2006;114(8):1287–1292

53. Woodruff TJ, Zota AR, Schwartz JM. Environmental chemicals in pregnant women in the United States: NHANES 2003-2004. *Environ Health Perspect.* 2011;119(6):878–885

54. Centers for Disease Control and Prevention. Fetal Alcohol Spectrum Disorders. https://www.cdc.gov/ncbddd/fasd/facts.html. Accessed April 6, 2018

55. Bertrand J, Floyd RL, Weber MK, et al. Guidelines for identifying and referring persons with fetal alcohol syndrome. *MMWR Recomm Rep.* 2005;54(RR-11):1–14

56. Thomas G, Gonneau G, Poole N, Cook J. The effectiveness of alcohol warning labels in the prevention of Fetal Alcohol Spectrum Disorder: A brief review. *Int J Alcohol And Drug Research.* 2014;3(1):91–103

57. Chen R, Clifford A, Lang L, Anstey KJ. Is exposure to secondhand smoke associated with cognitive parameters of children and adolescents? A systematic literature review. *Ann Epidemiol.* 2013;23(10):652–661

58. Bruin JE, Gerstein HC, Holloway AC. Long-term consequences of fetal and neonatal nicotine exposure: a critical review. *Toxicol Sci.* 2010;116(2):364–374

59. Jamal A, King BA, Neff LJ, Whitmill J, Babb SD, Graffunder CM. Current cigarette smoking among adults – United States, 2005-2015. *MMWR Morb Mortal Wkly Rep.* 2016;65(44): 1205–1211

60. Minnes S, Lang A, Singer L. Prenatal tobacco, marijuana, stimulant, and opiate exposure: outcomes and practice implications. *Addict Sci Clin Pract.* 2011;6(1):57–70

61. Behnke M, Smith VC, American Academy of Pediatrics Committee on Substance Abuse, Committee on Fetus and Newborn. Prenatal substance abuse: short- and long-term effects on the exposed fetus. *Pediatrics.* 2013;131(3):e1009–e1024

62. Wlodarczyk BJ, Palacios AM, George TM, Finnell RH. Antiepileptic drugs and pregnancy outcomes. *Am J Med Genet A.* 2012;158A(8):2071–2090

63. Webster WS. Teratogen update: congenital rubella. *Teratology.* 1998;58(1):13–23

64. Chess S. Autism in children with congenital rubella. *J Autism Child Schizophr.* 1971;1(1):33–47

65. Maldonado YA. Rubella virus. In: Long SS, Pickering LK, Prober CG, eds. *Principles and Practice of Pediatric Infectious Diseases.* 3rd ed. (rev reprint). New York, NY: Churchill Livingstone; 2009

66. Adams Waldorf KM, McAdams RM. Influence of infection during pregnancy on fetal development. *Reproduction.* 2013;146(5):R151–R162

67. Centers for Disease Control and Prevention. Zika Virus. http://www.cdc.gov/zika/. Accessed April 6, 2018

68. Jo H, Schieve LA, Sharma AJ, Hinkle SN, Li R, Lind JN. Maternal prepregnancy body mass index and child psychosocial development at 6 years of age. *Pediatrics.* 2015;135(5):e1198–e1209

69. Karam F, Sheehy O, Huneau MC, et al. Impact of maternal prenatal and parental postnatal stress on 1-year-old child development: results from the OTIS antidepressants in pregnancy study. *Arch Womens Ment Health.* 2016;19(5):835–843

70. Kinsella MT, Monk C. Impact of maternal stress, depression & anxiety on fetal neurobehavioral development. *Clin Obstet Gynecol.* 2009;52(3):425–440

71. Simanek AM, Meier HCS. Association between prenatal exposure to maternal infection and offspring mood disorders: A review of the literature. *Curr Probl Pediatr Adolesc Health Care.* 2015;45(11):325–364

72. Winter S, Autry A, Boyle C, Yeargin-Allsopp M. Trends in the prevalence of cerebral palsy in a population-based study. *Pediatrics.* 2002;110(6):1220–1225

73. Pakula AT, Van Naarden Braun K, Yeargin-Allsopp M. Cerebral palsy: classification and epidemiology. In: Michaud LJ, ed. *Cerebral Palsy.* Philadelphia, PA: W.B. Saunders Company; 2009;437

74. Ancel PY, Livinec F, Larroque B, et al. Cerebral palsy among very preterm children in relation to gestational age and neonatal ultrasound abnormalities: the EPIPAGE study group. *Pediatrics.* 2006;117(3):828–835

75. Sucksdorff M, Lehtonen L, Chudal R, et al. Preterm birth and poor fetal growth as risk factors of attention-deficit/hyperactivity disorder. *Pediatrics.* 2015;136(3):e599–e608

76. Padilla N, Eklöf E, Mårtensson GE, Bölte S, Lagercrantz H, Ådén U. Poor brain growth in extremely preterm neonates long before the onset of autism spectrum disorder symptoms. *Cereb Cortex.* 2017;27(2):1245–1252

77. Msall ME, Park JJ. The spectrum of behavioral outcomes after extreme prematurity: regulatory, attention, social, and adaptive dimensions. *Semin Perinatol.* 2008;32(1):42–50

78. Hack M, Taylor HG, Schluchter M, Andreias L, Drotar D, Klein N. Behavioral outcomes of extremely low birth weight children at age 8 years. *J Dev Behav Pediatr.* 2009;30(2):122–130

79. McCormick MC, Litt JS. The outcomes of very preterm infants: is it time to ask different questions? *Pediatrics.* 2017;139(1):e20161694

80. Vrijheid M, Casas M, Gascon M, Valvi D, Nieuwenhuijsen M. Environmental pollutants and child health: a review of recent concerns. *Int J Hyg Environ Health.* 2016;219(4-5):331–342

81. Wright RO, Amarasiriwardena C, Woolf AD, Jim R, Bellinger DC. Neuropsychological correlates of hair arsenic, manganese, and cadmium levels in school-age children residing near a hazardous waste site. *Neurotoxicology.* 2006;27(2):210–216

82. American Academy of Pediatrics Council on Environmental Health. Prevention of childhood lead toxicity. *Pediatrics.* 2016;38(1):e20161493

83. Grandjean P, Landrigan PJ. Neurobehavioural effects of developmental toxicity. *Lancet Neurol.* 2014;13(3):330–338

84. Farber HJ, Groner J, Walley S, Nelson K. Protecting children from tobacco, nicotine, and tobacco smoke. *Pediatrics.* 2015;136(5):e1439–e1467

85. Rubin IL, Nodvin JT, Geller RJ, Teague WG, Holzclaw BL, Felner EI. Environmental health disparities and social impact of industrial pollution in a community – the model of Anniston, AL. *Pediatr Clin North Am.* 2007;54(2):375–398

86. Rubin IL, Geller RJ, Martinuzzi K, et al. The costs and benefits of breaking the cycle of environmental health disparities in environmental health disparities: costs and benefits of breaking the cycle. In: Rubin IL, Merrick J, eds. *Public Health: Practices, Methods and Policies Series.* New York, NY: Nova Publishers; 2016

87. Institute of Medicine. *From Neurons to Neighborhoods: The Science of Early Childhood Development.* Shonkoff JP, Phillips DA, eds. Washington, DC: National Academies Press; 2000

88. McGowan PO, Sasaki A, D'Alessio AC, et al. Epigenetic regulation of the glucocorticoid receptor in human brain associates with childhood abuse. *Nature Neuroscience.* 2009;12(3):342–348

89. Hair NL, Hanson JL, Wolfe BL, Pollak SD. Association of child poverty, brain development, and academic achievement. *JAMA Pediatr.* 2015;169(9):822–829

90. Pascoe JM, Wood DL, Duffee JH, Kuo A, American Academy of Pediatrics Committee on Psychosocial Aspects of Child and Family Health, Council on Community Pediatrics. Mediators and adverse effects of child poverty in the United States. *Pediatrics.* 2016;137(4):e20160340

91. Federal Interagency Forum on Child and Family Statistics. America's Children in Brief: Key National Indicators of Well-Being. Washington, DC: US Government Printing Office; 2017. https://www.childstats.gov/pdf/ac2016/ac_16.pdf. Accessed April 6, 2018

92. Coker TR, Elliott MN, Toomey SL, et al. Racial and ethnic disparities in ADHD diagnosis and treatment. *Pediatrics*. 2016;138(3):e20160407

93. Wu G, Feder A, Cohen H, et al. Understanding resilience. *Front Behav Neurosci*. 15 February 2013. http://dx.doi.org/10.3389/fnbeh.2013.00010. Accessed April 6, 2018

94. Rubin IL, Geller RJ, Martinuzzi K, et al. Break the cycle of environmental health disparities: an ecological framework. *Int Public Health J*. 2017;9(2):115–127

95. Shonkoff JP, Garner AS, American Academy of Pediatrics Committee on Psychological Aspects of Child and Family Health, Committee on Early Childhood, Adoption, and Dependent Care, and Section on Developmental and Behavioral Pediatrics. The lifelong effects of early childhood adversity and toxic stress. *Pediatrics*. 2012;129(1):e232–e246

96. Johnson SB, Riley AW, Granger DA, Riis J. The science of early life toxic stress for pediatric practice and advocacy. *Pediatrics*. 2013;131(2):319–327

97. Bann CM, Wallander JL, Do B, et al. Home-based early intervention and the influence of family resources on cognitive development. *Pediatrics*. 2016;137(4):e20153766

98. Rubin IL. Africa. In: Rubin IL, Merrick J, Greydanus DE, Patel DR, eds. *Health Care for People With Intellectual and Developmental Disabilities Across the Lifespan*. Dordrecht: Springer; 2016:581–590

99. Dooyema CA, Neri A, Lo YC, et al. Outbreak of fatal childhood lead poisoning related to artisanal gold mining in northwestern Nigeria, 2010. *Environ Health Perspect*. 2012;120(4): 601–607

100. Brown MJ, McWeeney G, Kim R, et al. Lead poisoning among internally displaced Roma, Ashkali and Egyptian children in the United Nations-Administered Province of Kosovo. *Eur J Public Health*. 2010;20(3):288–292

101. Maulik PK, Darmstadt GL. Childhood disability in low- and middle-income countries: overview of screening, prevention, services, legislation, and epidemiology. *Pediatrics*. 2007;120(Suppl 1):S1–S55

102. Simkiss DE, Blackburn CM, Mukoro FO, Read JM, Spencer NJ. Childhood disability and socio-economic circumstances in low and middle income countries: systematic review. *BMC Pediatr*. 2011;11:119

103. Guevara JP, Gerdes M, Localio R, et al. Effectiveness of developmental screening in an urban setting. *Pediatrics*. 2013;131(1):30–37

104. Bann CM, Wallander JL, Do B, et al. Home-based early intervention and the influence of family resources on cognitive development. *Pediatrics*. 2016;137(4):e20153766

105. Johnson K, Posner SF, Biermann J, et al. Recommendations to improve preconception health and health care—United States. A report of the CDC/ATSDR Preconception Care Work Group and the Select Panel on Preconception Care. *MMWR Recomm Rep*. 2006;55(RR-6):1–23. http:// www.cdc.gov/mmwr/preview/mmwrhtml/rr5506a1.htm. Accessed April 6, 2018

Chapter 53

# Emerging Technologies and Materials

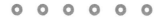

## KEY POINTS

- Many new technologies and chemicals have profoundly benefited health.
- Other new technologies and new chemicals have caused repeated episodes of disease, death, and environmental degradation.
- A root cause of these tragedies has been failure to systematically examine the safety of new technologies and to assess the toxicity of new chemicals prior to commercial introduction. New technologies and chemicals have been presumed harmless until proven to cause disease.
- Legally mandated premarket assessment of the safety and toxicity of new technologies and chemicals is essential for disease prevention. The current presumption of innocence needs to be replaced by a more skeptical and precautionary approach.
- Nanotechnology and genetically modified (GM) foods are presented as examples of new technologies that have been widely adopted in recent years with little assessment of their potential hazards.

## INTRODUCTION

The pace of scientific discovery has been more rapid in the past 50 years than at any previous time in human history and continues to accelerate. This age of discovery has seen the development of hundreds of new technologies, the synthesis of tens of thousands of new chemicals, and the release of millions of new products.

These scientific discoveries, emerging technologies, and new products have shaped and reshaped our lives. Discoveries create new industries and new ways of thinking. Automobiles and commercial aviation revolutionized transport. Refrigeration brought fresh fruits in winter. New building materials have made possible modern cities. Breakthroughs in microelectronics and physics produced desktop computing and the Internet. Continuing advances in information and communication technology, biotechnology, and nanotechnology are rapidly changing methods of social interaction, medical treatments, and data evaluation strategies.

Some new technologies and chemicals have profoundly benefited children's health. Drinking water disinfectants, vaccines, and antibiotics have helped control the major communicable diseases. Chemotherapy agents have made possible the cure of many childhood cancers. Cellular telephones and electronic data platforms are bringing modern medical technology to the farthest corners of the earth.

Emerging technologies and new chemicals have, however, too often been responsible for disease, death, and environmental degradation. Many of these tragic episodes have resulted in severe injury to children. A two-step sequence has typically marked these events. First has been the enthusiastic introduction of the new technology or new chemical with its incorporation into consumer products and subsequent dissemination into the environment. These actions have then been followed years or decades later by the belated realization that some of the materials that initially appeared to be so beneficial actually posed serious threats to children's health or to the environment, threats that were neither imagined nor in any way sought before their introduction.

Classic examples of chemicals and medications that were initially thought to be beneficial but later found to cause great harm include lead added to paint and later to gasoline (see Chapter 32), asbestos (see Chapter 23), dichlorodiphenyltrichloroethane (DDT) (see Chapter 38), thalidomide, polychlorinated biphenyls (PCBs) (see Chapter 38), diethylstilbestrol (DES) (see Chapter 48), and the ozone-destroying chlorofluorocarbons (CFCs). A recurrent theme has been that commercial introduction and wide dissemination of each of these new technologies preceded any systematic effort to assess its potential safety or toxicity.

More recent examples of chemicals that became widespread before any assessment of their potential hazards and that are now of concern include the organophosphate pesticides, the herbicide glyphosate, bisphenol A (see Chapter 41), phthalates (see Chapter 41), brominated flame retardants, and perfluoroalkyl and polyfluoroalkyl substances. These chemicals are produced in quantities of millions of tons per year, and many are used in myriad consumer products. All have become widespread in children's environments.

Only now, decades after their introduction, are their possible hazards to children's health beginning to be recognized and assessed.

## NEW TECHNOLOGIES AND CHILDREN'S HEALTH

Early warnings that emerging technologies might pose hazards to children's health and the environment have frequently been ignored. As a result, efforts to control exposures and to prevent injury to children have often been delayed, sometimes for decades.[1] In some instances, industries with deeply vested commercial interests in protecting markets for hazardous technologies have actively opposed efforts to understand and control children's exposures to hazardous materials. These industries have used highly sophisticated disinformation campaigns similar to those deployed by the tobacco industry to confuse the public and delay regulation.[2] They have attacked the credibility of heroic pediatricians such as Herbert Needleman, who discovered widespread, low-level toxicity among American children exposed to lead from paint and gasoline, and of pioneering environmental scientists, such as Irving Selikoff, who established the links between asbestos and human cancer.[3,4]

Chemical production has increased drastically (Figure 53-1). Today, there are more than 85,000 chemicals registered for commercial use with the US Environmental Protection Agency (EPA). Most of these chemicals are new synthetics. Nearly all have been invented in the past 50 years. Most did not exist previously in nature.[5]

Children are at greatest risk of exposure to the 3,000 synthetic chemicals that are produced in quantities of more than 1 million pounds per year.[5] The

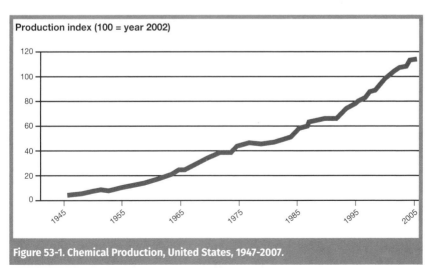

**Figure 53-1. Chemical Production, United States, 1947-2007.**

Source: Center for American Progress

US EPA classifies these as high production volume (HPV) chemicals. High production volume chemicals are used in an enormous array of consumer goods, such as cosmetics, medications, motor fuels, building materials, toys, and baby bottles. These chemicals escape from these products, become widely disseminated in the environment, and are detectable today in air, food, and drinking water in even the most remote regions of the earth. Persons of all ages, including children, are exposed to them, and in national surveys conducted by the Centers for Disease Control and Prevention, measurable quantities of nearly 200 HPV chemicals are routinely detected in the blood and urine of virtually all Americans, including pregnant women.[6,7]

Children's widespread exposure to synthetic chemicals is cause for concern because only about half of the 3,000 most widely used chemicals have undergone any safety or toxicity testing. Moreover, information on developmental toxicity or capacity to harm infants and children is available for fewer than 20% of these most widely used chemicals.[5] Little is understood about the effects on children's health of simultaneous exposures to multiple synthetic chemicals or how these chemicals may interact with one another in children's bodies.

Children are put at risk when we do not understand the possible hazards associated with their exposures to untested chemicals. Epidemiological studies are needed to specifically seek out what adverse effects are occurring in children and developing fetuses from these exposures; otherwise, subtle effects may not be recognized. The epidemic of childhood lead poisoning is an excellent example.[8,9] During the 1940s to the 1970s, lead was added to gasoline as an anti-knock agent. Millions of American children breathed in the lead in the air and had elevated levels of lead in their blood, which may have resulted in loss of IQ points, disruptive behavior, and shortened attention span. Sufficient evidence could be marshaled to mandate the removal of lead from gasoline, household paint, and consumer products.[8] The lead industry fought these interventions at every step.

Failure to test chemicals for toxicity reflects failure of the chemical industry to take responsibility for the safety of its products coupled with failure of the US federal government to exercise its responsibility to protect the environment and the health of the public. Failure of the government in this instance reflects failure of the Toxic Substances Control Act of 1976 (see Chapter 66).[10] Reflecting on the sorry state of chemical safety testing in the United States, the late Dr. David P. Rall, former Director of the National Institute of Environmental Health Sciences observed, "If thalidomide, instead of causing the birth of children with missing limbs, had instead reduced their intellectual potential by 10%, it is not likely that we would be aware even today of its toxic potency."[11]

The likelihood is high that beyond the chemicals already known to be toxic to children's early development, additional chemicals are present in commerce whose toxicity to infants and children has not yet been recognized

(Figure 53-2).[5] These currently undiscovered toxicants will most likely be found among the thousands of new synthetic chemicals that have been invented in the past half century and are in wide use today.[9]

## EMERGING TECHNOLOGIES OF CURRENT INTEREST: TWO CASE STUDIES

Two relatively new technologies that were introduced to markets with great fanfare are nanotechnology and GM food crops. They are currently in wide use but were never subjected to systemic premarket assessment of safety or toxicity. Unanticipated health hazards are now beginning to be recognized for these technologies, thus illustrating the continuing weakness of current efforts to address the risks of new technologies.[12]

### Nanotechnology

Nanotechnology is a technology based on the precisely engineered assembly of atoms and molecules to produce nanoparticles, nanotubules, and a wide array of molecular-scale nanodevices, such as pumps and switches.[13] A nanometer (nm) is one-billionth of a meter. By definition, a nanomaterial must have at least one dimension measuring 100 nm or less. Nanomaterials are of the same size range as viruses, DNA, and protein molecules.[13]

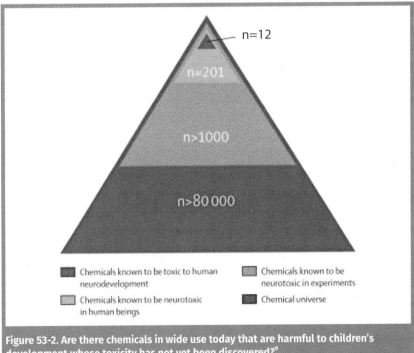

**Figure 53-2. Are there chemicals in wide use today that are harmful to children's development whose toxicity has not yet been discovered?**[9]

Source: Grandjean and Landrigan[9]

Strong, lightweight products made from nanomaterials have the potential to reduce energy consumption, pollution, and greenhouse gas emissions. Other applications could make possible the development of new medical devices.[14] Hundreds of nanotechnology-based products, such as cosmetics, inorganic sunscreens (zinc oxide and titanium dioxide), pharmaceuticals, electronics, cerium oxide fuel additives, and fuel cells, are already in commerce.

Worldwide investment in nanotechnology is exploding and is strongly supported in the United States through the National Nanotechnology Initiative.[15] The global market in nanotechnology was reported to total $200 billion in 2008 and is projected to grow to more than $3 trillion by 2020, an annual growth rate of 25% to 30%.[15]

Nanomaterials have extraordinarily high surface-to-volume ratios and unique chemical and physical properties.[13,14] These characteristics raise the possibility that nanomaterials may interact with cells and organisms in novel ways quite different from those of their parent materials. Carbon nanotubules, for example, appear to be far more hazardous than the graphite from which they are manufactured.[13,16]

Knowledge of the toxicity of nanomaterials is scant, and knowledge of their possible toxicity to early human development is virtually nil. However, hints of potential toxicity are beginning to emerge and are cause for concern. Emerging data suggest, for example, that nanoparticles may be able to produce toxic and carcinogenic effects because of their ability to enter cells. The small size of nanoparticles enhances cell entry and appears to be a major determinant of toxicity. Once within cells, nanoparticles appear to cause injury through several mechanisms, among them oxidative stress, lipid peroxidation, and protein misfolding. Protein misfolding is of concern because it is associated with neuronal degeneration and degeneration of insulin-producing beta cells in the pancreas. Nanotubules, by contrast, because they are predominantly fibrous, do not enter cells, but instead remain in the extracellular spaces where they can induce chronic inflammation. In a recent study in rodents, carbon nanotubules introduced into the lung were found to produce pathologic and carcinogenic effects (ie, lung cancer and malignant mesothelioma) similar to those caused by asbestos.[17]

This information suggests the need to exercise considerable caution in adopting nanotechnology and in introducing nanomaterials into the environment. Expert advisory groups have called for prudent assessment of the potential hazards of nanotechnology before further dissemination.[18]

## Genetically Modified Foods

Genetically modified food crops are grown from seeds whose DNA has been modified using the technology of genetic engineering to introduce new traits.[19,20] The application of biotechnology to agriculture builds on the ancient practice of selective breeding. Unlike traditional breeding, genetic engineering vastly expands the range and speed with which novel characteristics can be moved into plants. Depending on the traits selected, genetically engineered crops could be designed with a range of beneficial phenotypes, such as increased yields, the ability to thrive when irrigated with salty water, or the ability to produce fruits and vegetables resistant to mold and rot.

Herbicide resistance, especially resistance to the broad-spectrum herbicide glyphosate (Roundup®), is the principal characteristic that the biotechnology industry has chosen to introduce into food crops.[19] Corn and soybeans with genetically engineered tolerance to glyphosate were first introduced in the mid-1990s. These "Roundup Ready" crops now account for more than 90% of the corn and soybeans planted in the United States, and glyphosate has become the most widely used herbicide in the world.[20]

The great advantage of herbicide-resistant crops, especially in the first years after introduction, is that they greatly simplify weed management. Farmers can spray herbicide both before and during the growing season, leaving their crops unharmed. Widespread adoption of herbicide-resistant crops has led to overreliance on herbicides and, in particular, on glyphosate.[21] In the United States, glyphosate use has increased by a factor of more than 250, rising from 0.4 million kg in 1974 to 113 million kg in 2014. Global use has increased by a factor of more than 10. Glyphosate-resistant weeds have emerged and are found today on nearly 100 million acres of cropland in 36 states. To control these resistant weeds, fields must now be treated with ever-increasing doses of glyphosate and with multiple additional herbicides, including 2,4-D, a component of the Agent Orange herbicide mixture used in the Vietnam War.[19] The increasing application of herbicides to food crops later in the growing season increases the likelihood that measurable levels of herbicides, termed residues, will be present in food crops at harvest.

Two reviews by the National Academy of Sciences (NAS) of the safety of GM food crops in the 2000s concluded that GM crops pose no hazards to human health.[22,23] The NAS noted that genetic transformation could produce unanticipated allergens or toxins; therefore, they recommended postmarketing surveillance. The NAS concluded that there were no unique hazards associated with genetic engineering *per se*. However, both NAS reviews focused almost exclusively on the genetic aspects of plant biotechnology and did not consider the possible health hazards of the herbicides applied to GM food crops.

In 2015, the International Agency for Research on Cancer (IARC), an agency of the World Health Organization, determined glyphosate to be a probable human carcinogen.[24] The IARC found that glyphosate is linked to dose-related increases in malignant tumors at multiple anatomical sites in experimental animals and to an increased incidence of non-Hodgkin lymphoma in exposed humans.[24]

The IARC finding on the probable carcinogenicity of glyphosate suggests that GM foods and the herbicides applied to them were never properly examined and may pose hazards to the health of children. In July 2017, the State of California added glyphosate to the list of chemicals known to the state to cause cancer.[25] The manufacturer of glyphosate has stated that it disagrees with the IARC's determination that glyphosate is a probable human carcinogen.[2,26]

Labeling of foods as GM has been proposed as a strategy for assisting families in their purchasing decisions.[19] GM labeling is legally required in 64 countries outside of the United States. Labeling is essential for tracking emergence of any novel food allergies that may be associated with GM food crops and is needed for epidemiologic assessment of health effects of herbicides applied to GM crops.

Families who choose to avoid the possible hazards of GM foods can do so by purchasing fruits and vegetables that are certified as organic by the US Department of Agriculture. Organic certification requires that foods be grown without fertilizer, chemical pesticides, antibiotics, or irradiation, and that no genetically modified seed be used to produce the crops.[27] Epidemiologic studies of children who eat an organic diet have found that these children have significantly lower levels of pesticide residues in their urine than do people who eat a conventionally produced diet.[28,29]

## CONCLUSION

The introduction of new technologies and chemicals raises many questions with important implications for children's health. To protect children against emerging technologies and new synthetic chemicals, a paradigm shift is needed in public policy to a scenario in which new chemicals and technologies must be demonstrated to be safe before they are allowed to enter markets rather than presumed to be harmless until after they have caused great harm.[1,30] In such a scenario, industry would bear the responsibility for determining that a new chemical or material is safe before bringing it to market.[31] This anticipatory strategy is termed the "Precautionary Principle" (see Chapter 64). The Precautionary Principle has recently been introduced into national and international law.[32]

## References

1. Gee D. Late lessons from early warnings: toward realism and precaution with endocrine-disrupting substances. *Environ Health Perspect.* 2006;114(Suppl 1):152–160
2. Michaels D. *Doubt Is Their Product: How Industry's Assault on Science Threatens Your Health.* London, England: Oxford University Press; 2008
3. Needleman HL, Gunnoe C, Leviton A, et al. Deficits in psychologic and classroom performance of children with elevated dentine lead levels. *N Engl J Med.* 1979;300(13):689–695

4. Selikoff IJ, Seidman H. Asbestos-associated deaths among insulation workers in the United States and Canada, 1967-1987. *Ann N Y Acad Sci.* 1991;643:1–14

5. Landrigan PJ, Goldman L. Children's vulnerability to toxic chemicals: a challenge and opportunity to strengthen health and environmental policy. *Health Affairs.* 2011;30(5):842–850

6. Centers for Disease Control and Prevention. National Report on Human Exposure to Environmental Chemicals. 2015. http://www.cdc.gov/exposurereport/. Accessed January 19, 2018

7. Woodruff TJ, Zota AR, Schwartz JM. Environmental chemicals in pregnant women in the United States: NHANES 2003-2004. *Environ Health Perspect.* 2011;119(6):878–885

8. Grosse SD, Matte TD, Schwartz J, Jackson RJ. Economic gains resulting from the reduction in children's exposure to lead in the United States. *Environ Health Perspect.* 2002;110(6):563–569

9. Grandjean P, Landrigan PJ. Developmental neurotoxicity of industrial chemicals: a silent pandemic. *Lancet.* 2006;368(9553):2167–2178

10. Environmental Protection Agency. Summary of the Toxic Substances Control Act. http://www.epa.gov/regulations/laws/tsca.html. Accessed January 19, 2018

11. Weiss B. Food additives and environmental chemicals as sources of childhood behavior disorders. *J Am Acad Child Psychiatry.* 1982;21(2):144–152

12. Goldman LR. Preventing pollution? US toxic chemicals and pesticides policies and sustainable development. *Environ Law Report News Analysis.* 2002;32:11018–11041

13. Balbus JM, Maynard AD, Colvin VL, et al. Meeting report: hazard assessment for nanoparticles—report from an interdisciplinary workshop. *Environ Health Perspect.* 2007;115(11):1654–1659

14. Sargent JF. Nanotechnology: A Policy Primer. Washington, DC: Congressional Research Service. December 16, 2013.

15. Roco MC. The long view of nanotechnology development: The National Nanotechnology Initiative at 10 years. *J Nanopart Res.* 2011;13(2):427–445

16. Manke A, Luanpitpong S, Rojanasakul Y. Potential occupational risks associated with pulmonary toxicity of carbon nanotubes. *Occup Med Health Aff.* 2014;2. pii: 1000165

17. Suzui M, Futakuchi M, Fukamachi K, et al. Multiwalled carbon nanotubes intratracheally instilled into the rat lung induce development of pleural malignant mesothelioma and lung tumors. *Cancer Sci.* 2016;107(7):924–935

18. Nyland JF, Silbergeld EK. A nanobiological approach to nanotoxicology. *Hum Exp Toxicol.* 2009;28(6-7):393–400

19. Landrigan PJ, Benbrook C. GMOs, herbicides, and public health. *New Engl J Med.* 2015;373(8):693–695

20. US Department of Agriculture, Economic Research Service. Adoption of genetically engineered crops in the U.S. http://www.ers.usda.gov/data-products/adoption-of-genetically-engineered-crops-in-the-us.aspx. Accessed January 19, 2018

21. Duke SO. Perspectives on transgenic, herbicide-resistant crops in the United States almost 20 years after introduction. *Pest Manag Sci.* 2015;71(5):652–657

22. National Research Council, Committee on Identifying and Assessing Unintended Effects of Genetically Engineered Foods on Human Health. Safety of genetically engineered foods: approaches to assessing unintended health effects. Washington, DC: National Academies Press; 2004

23. National Academies of Sciences, Engineering, and Medicine. *Genetically Engineered Crops: Experiences and Prospects.* Washington, DC: The National Academies Press; 2016. https://doi.org/10.17226/23395. Accessed January 19, 2018

24. Guyton KZ, Loomis D, Grosse Y, et al. Carcinogenicity of tetrachlorvinphos, parathion, malathion, diazinon, and glyphosate. *Lancet Oncol.* 2015;16(5):490–491

25. State of California. Office of Environmental Health Hazard Assessment. Glyphosate Listed Effective July 7, 2017, as Known to the State of California to Cause Cancer. https://oehha.ca.gov/proposition-65/crnr/glyphosate-listed-effective-july-7-2017-known-state-california-cause-cancer. Accessed January 19, 2018

26. Cressey D. Widely used herbicide linked to cancer. *Scientific American.* https://www.scientific american.com/article/widely-used-herbicide-linked-to-cancer/. Accessed January 19, 2018

27. US Department of Agriculture, Agricultural Marketing Service. Organic Certification and Accreditation. https://www.ams.usda.gov/services/organic-certification. Accessed January 19, 2018

28. Lu C, Toepel K, Irish R, Fenske RA, Barr DB, Bravo R. Organic diets significantly lower children's dietary exposure to organophosphorus pesticides. *Environ Health Perspect.* 2006;114(2):260–263

29. Curl CL, Fenske RA, Elgethun K. Organophosphorus pesticide exposure of urban and suburban preschool children with organic and conventional diets. *Environ Health Perspect.* 2003;111(3):377–382

30. American Academy of Pediatrics, Council on Environmental Health. Chemical-management policy: prioritizing children's health. *Pediatrics.* 2011;127(5):983–990

31. US Environmental Protection Agency. Essential Principles for Reform of Chemicals Management Legislation. 2009. https://www.epa.gov/assessing-and-managing-chemicals-under-tsca/essential-principles-reform-chemicals-management-0. Accessed January 23, 2018

32. Grandjean P. Toxicology research for precautionary decision-making and the role of human & experimental toxicology. *Hum Exp Toxicol.* 2015;34(12):1231–1237

Chapter 54

# Environmental Disasters

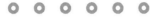

## KEY POINTS

- Children are among the most vulnerable to environmental disasters because of their size, physiology, and developmental immaturity.
- Climate change appears to be associated with an increase in the number and intensity of natural disasters. Therefore, individuals, communities, states, and the federal government must be ready to respond.
- Pediatricians have pivotal roles in helping families and communities prepare for disasters, including ensuring that families develop plans. This is especially important for families with children who have medically complex problems and for families living in underserved areas.
- Pediatricians can support families after disasters by assessing children for adjustment reactions and helping to provide other needed support.

## INTRODUCTION

Environmental health problems can accrue after many types of catastrophic events. Events can range from natural disasters such as earthquakes, floods, hurricanes, tornadoes, and wildfires, to human-made disasters such as the release of 2,3,7,8-tetrachlorodibenzodioxin in Seveso, Italy in 1976; the release of methyl isocyanate in Bophal, India in 1984; radiologic and nuclear disasters such as in Chernobyl (1986) and Fukushima (2011); and the release of millions of gallons of crude oil into the Gulf of Mexico in 2010. The terrorist events leading to the destruction of the World Trade Center buildings in September

2001 released a large cloud of toxic materials, resulting in respiratory illnesses in many first responders and people living in proximity to the disaster. Follow-up investigations of victims, including first responders and children, revealed evidence of long-term illness resulting from this unprecedented event. Whether intentional or natural, environmental disasters can result in significant morbidity and mortality. As events such as Hurricanes Rita, Katrina, Harvey, Irma, and Maria, Superstorm Sandy in 2012, the 2010 earthquake in Haiti, and the 2011 earthquake and subsequent tsunami in Japan have shown, children and adolescents are often disproportionately affected in a disaster. In 2015, the American Academy of Pediatrics (AAP) published a policy statement that includes recommendations to ensure the health of children who experience disasters.[1]

## OVERVIEW OF LOCAL COMMUNITY, STATE, AND FEDERAL ROLES DURING RESPONSE

Local communities and states have the largest role in disaster preparedness and response; it is the federal government, however, that funds a significant proportion of preparedness activities and drives requirements for readiness. The National Response Framework (NRF), first released in 2008 and followed by the second edition in 2013, provides guiding principles for response preparation by all response entities and provides a unified national response plan for disasters and emergencies from the smallest incident to the largest catastrophe.[2] The second edition adds a focus on the whole community and core capabilities, describing the important role of individuals, families, and households. In 2011, the National Disaster Recovery Framework (NDRF) was released.[3]

The NRF defines roles and structures of entities involved with response; establishes essential processes for requesting and receiving federal assistance; and summarizes key capabilities and emergency support functions (Table 54-1). The emergency support functions most pertinent to medical response include emergency support function 6, which directs the Federal Emergency Management Agency (FEMA) to lead activities relating to mass care, emergency assistance, and human services; emergency support function 8, which directs the US Department of Health and Human Services to lead the public health and medical response; emergency support function 9, which addresses urban search and rescue activities and is led jointly by the US Department of Homeland Security (including FEMA and the US Coast Guard), the Department of the Interior/National Parks Service, and the Department of Defense/US Air Force; and emergency support function 10, which directs the US Environmental Protection Agency (EPA) to coordinate, integrate, and manage the overall federal effort to detect, identify, contain, decontaminate, clean up, dispose of, or minimize discharges of oil or releases of hazardous materials or prevent, mitigate, or minimize the threat of potential releases.[2]

## Table 54-1. Terminology

| ENTITY | RESPONSIBILITY |
|--------|----------------|
| National Response Framework (NRF) | Provides guiding principles for response preparation by all response entities and provides a unified national response plan |
| Federal Emergency Management Agency (FEMA) | Part of the Department of Homeland Security, leads activities relating to mass care, emergency assistance, and human services |
| Incident Command System (ICS) | An organizational framework that guides the application of on-scene disaster management |
| Hospital Incident Command System (HICS) | An incident command system designed for use by hospitals in emergency and nonemergency situations |
| Disaster Medical Assistance Teams (DMAT) | A team of professionals and paraprofessionals organized to provide rapid-response medical services during a disaster |
| ▪ Homeland Security Grants Program<br>▪ Urban Areas Security Initiative (UASI)<br>▪ Metropolitan Medical Response System (MMRS)<br>▪ National Healthcare Preparedness Program | Grants programs to areas for hazard planning and preparedness |

The NDRF was developed to align with the NRF as a guide to promote effective recovery for large scale and catastrophic disasters (Figure 54-1). The focus of the NDRF is on restoring, redeveloping, and revitalizing the health of an affected community and its resources. Like the NRF, the NDRF outlines the role of community members, including individuals and families, and describes the authorities for recovery activities. One of the recovery support functions is Natural and Cultural Resources, coordinated by the Department of the Interior with support from many federal and state agencies and the private sector. The primary function of this recovery support function is to ensure the "ability to protect natural and cultural resources and historical properties through appropriate response and recovery actions...."[3]

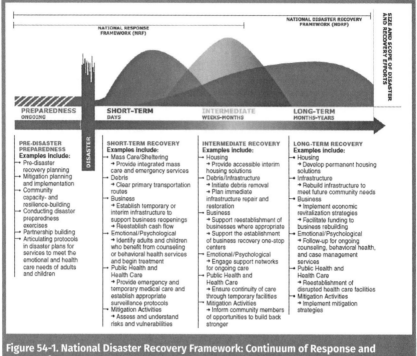

**Figure 54-1. National Disaster Recovery Framework: Continuum of Response and Recovery[3]**

The four phases of the continuum of response and recovery are Preparedness, Short-term Recovery, Intermediate Recovery, and Long-term Recovery. The timing and extent of each phase depends on the nature and severity of the disaster. Preparedness is an ongoing process to ensure that a community has plans and resources in place to respond to an event. Short-term Recovery is the response phase during which search and rescue efforts occur and temporary sheltering and health care are provided. The Intermediate-term Recovery phase takes place in the weeks and months after a disaster when rebuilding of infrastructure begins and reconstitution efforts of the community occur. Long-term Recovery takes place over months and years after a disaster and is when rebuilding infrastructure continues.

Because the needs created by terrorist events and natural disasters are similar, the principle of the "all-hazards approach" serves as the foundation of response to either type of incident. In this approach, public health and emergency management authorities responsible for developing disaster response protocols develop and implement guidelines that can be adapted to human-made disasters, terrorist incidents (which are relatively rare in the United States), or natural disasters (which are inevitable). The development of adaptable and scalable systems promotes efficiency, reduces costs, and may eliminate system redundancy.[4]

Response to disasters begins locally. When a disaster strikes, it is first responders who arrive on the scene to provide an initial assessment to local officials. Such assessments focus on the extent of the incident, the number of casualties, anticipated number of casualties, property damage, and resources needed to treat and transport victims. Local emergency medical services, community health care facilities and providers, and local public health agencies manage medical issues. The local government sets up an emergency operations center and determines whether the incident exceeds or is expected to exceed local capabilities. For incidents beyond local capacity, local officials can request aid from other local governments within the state and from the state government. The Stafford Act provides for federal support of local communities during major disasters. Local communities are responsible for ensuring that any planning or preparation done in anticipation of a disaster response include consideration of the needs of children and families.[5]

The state governor is responsible for activating the state's emergency operations center; the state emergency operations center assesses the extent of the damage and the scope of casualties to determine whether response needs have exceeded state capabilities. If so, the governor then requests aid through the Emergency Management Assistance Compact or through other interstate agreements. The governor can request a presidential declaration, and if the disaster event is antici-pated, such as with a hurricane, the federal government can pre-deploy response assets to the expected disaster area. National-level activities are coordinated by FEMA. When the president declares an emergency or disaster, federal response teams and other resources are deployed, and a joint field office is set up to provide unified coordination of response resources. The US EPA, for example, may be asked to assess and advise on possible exposures to toxic contaminants. A federal medical asset available to an affected area includes Disaster Medical Assistance Teams (DMAT) of the National Medical Disaster System (NMDS).[2] The capacity of NMDS to respond is limited, however, by the amount of time for deployment and set-up as well as the number of teams available.

Before a disaster, the federal government supports a number of state and local preparedness activities. The federal government provides financial resources to state and local governments through grant programs, such as the Homeland Security Grants Program that includes funding through the Urban Areas Security Initiative, the State Homeland Security Program (https://www.fema.gov/homeland-security-grant-program), and Operation Stonegarden (https://www.homelandsecuritygrants.info/GrantDetails.aspx?gid=21875), and to private sector health care institutions through the Hospital Preparedness Program (www.phe.gov/PREPAREDNESS/PLANNING/HPP/Pages/default.aspx). Through these grant programs, the federal government sets requirements and promotes best practices. The federal government also provides guidance to states and territories for disaster preparedness and response activities and funds research on medical countermeasure development, development of detection and response technologies, and best practices. The federal government also stockpiles medications, equipment, and supplies to supplement state and local caches.[6] These stockpiles should, but often do not, have adequate resources for children.[7]

## THE DISASTER CYCLE

Although each disaster is unique because of differences in notice, severity, location, and the socioeconomic conditions and baseline health of the affected population, there are patterns common to all disasters that are described in a disaster cycle model. The disaster cycle occurs in phases. The inter-disaster period occurs between disasters. The prodromal period occurs when a disaster is imminent (eg, a hurricane in the Gulf of Mexico). For some disasters (eg, an earthquake), however, there is no warning but only an impact that varies in length of time depending on the incident. The phase after impact is the rescue phase, during which the actions of first responders are most critical to saving lives. It is during the recovery phase that coordinated efforts bring the population back to its normal state.[8]

Measures to prevent and prepare for disasters occur during the inter-disaster phase. Such measures may include moving people from the vicinity of an active volcano or from areas known to be susceptible to severe flooding. Mitigation measures that aim to reduce the likely impact of a disaster can also occur during this period as well as during other phases. Examples of mitigation measures include applying stringent building codes in earthquake-prone areas, augmenting levees in flood zones, and instituting warning systems for tsunamis.[9]

Successful response depends on adequate training of first responders, prompt institution of incident command, and effective coordination among emergency services, public health authorities, and the health care system. All disasters remain local in scope until the local community becomes overwhelmed. It is critical that local communities undertake robust planning and preparedness activities during the inter-disaster phase to mitigate the effects of disasters. Recovery depends on adequate planning, the baseline resiliency of the community, effective coordination of basic services, and the provision of behavioral health services.

## SPECIAL SUSCEPTIBILITY OF CHILDREN IN DISASTERS

Children have several vulnerabilities during and after disasters. They have physical vulnerabilities because of their size, physiology, and development. Because children are smaller in stature than adults, they often are more vulnerable to injury and drowning in floods and to toxic effects of chemical agents because many of these agents are heavier than air and, therefore, exist in higher concentrations closer to the ground. The same is true for radiation exposure after a radiological-nuclear blast event. Children have a larger ratio of skin surface area to body mass compared with adults and, therefore, may absorb more toxicants per unit of body mass through skin. They have a higher respiratory rate, which increases their exposure to aerosolized or gaseous agents. Children are at increased risk of dehydration because of higher fluid needs. Because children are immature developmentally, they may not have the motor skills to escape a disaster or the judgment to remove themselves from harm.[1] Children are also more curious about their environment and are, therefore, more likely to touch potentially contaminated surfaces and place objects or their fingers in their mouths.[1,10]

Children and adolescents may be separated from their caregivers in a disaster. After Hurricanes Rita and Katrina in 2005, more than 5,000 children were separated from their parents and guardians. Because of the lack of a well-established system for reunification, some of these pediatric victims were separated from their caregivers for as long as 18 months.[11]

Facilities may not have adequate pediatric equipment to care for neonates, infants, and older children or for children with special needs. Resources may not be allocated with children in mind. These and other consequences of disasters have highlighted the importance of including the needs of children and adolescents in disaster planning.[1] Pediatricians must be involved in planning efforts as advisors to local and state officials.[1] Congressional legislation was enacted to ensure that the needs of children and adolescents are met after disasters (eg, the Addressing the Disaster Needs of Children Act of 2007).

## THE PSYCHOSOCIAL NEEDS OF CHILDREN AND ADOLESCENTS DURING AND AFTER DISASTERS

A 2006 Institute of Medicine report on the state of emergency care in the United States concluded that children and adolescents are among those with the highest risk of psychological trauma, including significant behavioral difficulties, after a disaster.[11] Some of these disorders include agoraphobia, separation anxiety, posttraumatic stress disorder, and depression.[12] Risk factors for developing mental health problems include a previous history of mental health issues, direct exposure to the disaster, lower socioeconomic status, loss of a family member, and living a parent who has significant posttraumatic stress reactions.

In the aftermath of a disaster, medical first responders and other health care providers need to provide psychological first aid to children, adolescents, and families. In addition, pediatric and other health care providers need to conduct a brief assessment for the presence of adjustment problems and other risk factors for subsequent difficulties to provide rapid and effective triage for mental health issues.[13,14] The manner in which a child or adolescent reacts to a disaster depends on factors including the nature and extent of the disaster and the child's or adolescent's direct involvement, preexisting vulnerabilities and coping skills, age, and developmental/cognitive level.[14,15] Common immediate reactions in children after a disaster include the following:[16]

- Development of fears
- Development of worries and anxieties
- Sadness and tearfulness
- Regressive behavior
- Social regression
- Difficulty concentrating and focusing
- Physical symptoms, such as headaches or stomach aches
- Exacerbations of underlying disorders (especially stress-induced disorders)

First responders and health care providers have the potential to alleviate some of a child's reactions by initiating psychological first aid, which should be provided broadly to those impacted by the disaster. Psychological first aid is the practice of recognizing and responding to people affected by a disaster to provide help with feelings of stress resulting from their situations.[17]

Immediately after medical stabilization and evaluation, it is recommended that the physician assess the child for adjustment reactions. Psychological first aid includes offering emotional support, providing information and education, encouraging the practice of positive coping, recognizing when more help is needed, and assisting people to obtain this extra help. It is critical to identify children at risk of longer-term mental health issues. These include children who have a family member or friend who has died; who have been exposed to injury, death, or destruction; who perceived at the time of the event that their life was in jeopardy; who have been separated from parents or other caregivers; who have existing mental health problems; and whose parents have difficulty coping. Children with dissociative symptoms, intense grief, extreme cognitive impairment resulting from the disaster with confusion, impaired decision making, and significant somatization also are at higher risk.[13,14]

## EXAMPLES OF DISASTERS

### Climate Change and Impacts on Natural Disasters

The 2014 Synthesis Report issued by the Interagency Panel on Climate Change established by the United Nations Environment Programme and the World Meteorlogical Association states "in recent decades, changes in climate have caused impacts on natural and human systems on all continents and across the oceans. Impacts are due to observed climate change, irrespective of its cause, indicating the sensitivity of natural and human systems to changing climate." The authors also state that the impacts of climate change have included more extreme weather and climate events and "continued emission of greenhouse gases will cause further warming and long-lasting changes in all components of the climate system, increasing the likelihood of severe, pervasive and irreversible impacts for people and ecosystems." More extreme weather conditions have the potential to create more frequent disasters.[18]

## Tornadoes and Hurricanes

Natural disasters can be somewhat predictable because they tend to cluster geographically or temporally. For example, certain geographic regions are more susceptible to tornadoes and hurricanes. During spring 2011, multiple tornadoes in the southern United States killed more than 300 people, and in May 2011, a single tornado killed more than 100 people in Missouri. In recent years, the United States and its neighbor nations also suffered the effects of severe hurricanes, including Superstorm Sandy (2012) and Hurricanes Harvey (2017), Irma (2017), and Maria (2017). These hurricanes were devastating to the infrastructure of affected states and/or territory and uncovered shortcomings in the nation's capabilities to withstand disasters, including the lack of preparedness to care for children and adolescents. Many homes were lost after Hurricane Katrina, and occupants of trailers provided by FEMA and used for temporary housing experienced problems with respiratory illness. Levels of formaldehyde were elevated in some trailers, raising concerns about exposures to residents.[19] The health care infrastructure experienced severe long-term disruptions. Many school buildings were destroyed or damaged so severely that they could not be reoccupied for long periods. Environmental equity issues arose as the hurricane disproportionately affected people living in poverty, who generally occupied the more vulnerable areas within the community. As a result of these problems and others, the lives of children and adolescents were disrupted for months to years, potentially resulting in adverse effects on their development and mental health. In Puerto Rico, power outages remained common even 3 months after Hurricane Maria, leaving hundreds of thousands of US citizens in the dark.[20] Anticipating these effects and developing mitigation measures before, during, and after disasters are key to preventing similar devastation in the future.

## Earthquakes

Earthquakes can be devastating and costly, especially in less wealthy nations that may not have building codes to protect occupants. Mortality can be very high depending on the magnitude and location of the quake. Many children died after the 2008 earthquake in the Sichuan province of China, in part because of a failure to ensure consistent implementation of protective building codes for schools. Earthquakes are a potential problem in many places within the United States, such as California, Idaho, Utah, the Pacific Northwest, and areas in the Midwest. Mitigation measures in earthquake-prone areas include developing and implementing special building codes so that buildings can sustain high forces and remain intact.[21]

Notable earthquakes, such as the 2010 earthquake in Haiti and the 2011 earthquake off the coast of Japan, killed thousands to hundreds of thousands of people and damaged infrastructure, with economic costs well into the billions of dollars.[4] Rescue efforts are complicated by dangers from damage created by the earthquake, difficulties in extricating victims, and possibly running out of time to find victims who can be saved. Most morbidity and mortality from earthquakes results from physical injuries; this includes secondary wound infections and long-term disability. Additional morbidity and mortality may result from radiation leaks, as occurred after the nuclear power plant in Fukushima, Japan, was damaged.

## Floods

Hurricanes Harvey and Maria and the flooding in Bangladesh in 2017 are examples of the devastation that flooding can have on populations. Floods are perhaps the most common of natural disasters, accounting for approximately 30% of disasters worldwide. Twenty-five to 50 million Americans live or work in flood plains, and another 110 million live in coastal areas. Flash floods are especially dangerous to people living in flood-prone zones; most deaths attributable to flash floods are caused by drowning. Floods are otherwise not usually directly associated with loss of life but can cause destruction, disruption, and potentially widespread disease because floodwaters often contain human or animal waste.[22] Floodwater may be contaminated with toxic substances that may have been stored in homes and other sites. Failure to promptly remove water-damaged items after floods can lead to growth of mold in buildings and possible respiratory or chronic disease problems.[23,24] Access to clean drinking water is a major concern after a flood; disinfecting drinking water by boiling or chlorination or by providing alternate sources may be needed.[21]

## Chernobyl, Tokaimura Nuclear Plant, and Fukushima

Children are particularly vulnerable during radiologic and nuclear disasters. Though not common, nuclear disasters have occurred over the last 30 or more years. On April 26, 1986, one of the reactors at the Chernobyl power plant in Ukraine exploded, resulting in a nuclear meltdown that sent massive amounts of radiation into the atmosphere, reportedly more than the fallout from Hiroshima and Nagasaki. Since then, thousands of children have been diagnosed with thyroid cancer, and an almost 20-mile area around the plant remains off-limits.[25] On Sept. 30, 1999, Japan's worst nuclear accident happened in a facility in Tokaimura, a city northeast of Tokyo. Two plant workers died, and hundreds of people were exposed to radiation.[26] The Fukushima nuclear accident was caused by an earthquake and subsequent tsunami. No deaths or cases of radiation sickness resulted from the nuclear accident but 100,000 people were evacuated from their homes. The tsunami inundated about 560 km$^2$ of land, resulting in a death toll of over 19,000 people, including children, and causing much damage to coastal ports and towns with over a million buildings destroyed or partly collapsed.[27]

## Wildfires

Wildfires can occur in nature to manage ecosystems but can become uncontrolled, resulting in air pollution and damage to homes and ecosystems. Forest fires can impact soil, watersheds, animals, and air. Wildfires create carbon emissions that contribute to climate change.[28] Damage to homes and neighborhoods that results in displacement of families disrupts a child's well-being. Moreover, exposure to air pollutants can impact a child's health including increasing his or her risk for asthma exacerbations. A 2015 review found that wildfire smoke was associated with an increased risk of respiratory and cardiovascular diseases and that children, the elderly, and those with underlying chronic diseases are the most susceptible to health effects.[29]

## The World Trade Center

Tens of thousands of children and adolescents living or attending school in or near lower Manhattan were exposed to the World Trade Center disaster in 2001. The atmospheric plume and subsequent collapse of the 2 World Trade Center towers generated thousands of tons of particulate matter containing cement dust, glass fibers, lead, asbestos, polycyclic aromatic hydrocarbons, polychlorinated biphenyls (PCBs), organochlorine pesticides, polychlorinated furans, and dioxins.[30–32] Most studies of World Trade Center-related health effects have been conducted among rescue workers who often were exposed to high levels of debris, dust, fumes, and smoke. The World Trade Center Health Registry, established to evaluate physical and psychological effects of the disaster, also collected information on 3,184 children who were younger than 18 years on September 11, 2001. Many children, especially those exposed to higher amounts of toxicants (eg, the dust cloud), experienced respiratory symptoms immediately after the event.[33] A higher than expected prevalence of asthma was reported in children younger than age 5 years when compared with national estimates.[34] A new diagnosis of asthma in all age groups was higher than expected in children exposed to the dust cloud.[32] In addition, exposure to the disaster was associated with effects on birth outcomes.[35,36] One study examined 187 pregnant women within or near the World Trade Center during or immediately after the attacks. Compared with a group who sustained no exposure, those acutely exposed experienced a twofold increase in the risk of delivering a baby that was small for gestational age. No increases in miscarriages, preterm births, or low birth weight infants were found. The authors suggested that the detrimental effects might have been mediated through exposure to polycyclic aromatic hydrocarbons or particulate matter.[35]

Mental health issues have been identified in children exposed to the World Trade Center disaster. A study of New York City schoolchildren conducted in the first 6 months after the attack found that approximately 1 in 10 children surveyed had symptoms of probable posttraumatic stress disorder (11%), major depressive disorder (8%), separation anxiety disorder (12%), and panic attacks (9%) and that 15% had symptoms of agoraphobia (fear of going outside or taking public transportation).[37–39]

## PREPARING FOR DISASTERS

Pediatricians can help communities prepare for disasters. A pediatric perspective is key when educating emergency and disaster response teams. Many local health departments have established volunteer Medical Reserve Corps units. Medical Reserve Corps units are community-based and function to locally organize and utilize volunteers who want to donate their time and expertise to prepare for and respond to emergencies and promote healthy living throughout the year. Pediatricians can interface with local health departments and emergency operations centers to make sure that the needs of children are considered in community disaster planning. This includes planning for evacuation, sheltering, family reunification, medical needs, mental health, nutrition, and safe return to homes after a disaster. Pediatricians should also ensure that their own practices and institutions are prepared.

Pediatricians have important roles with individual families, providing guidance to help prepare before a disaster as part of preventive health care. This is especially important for families with children and youth with special health care needs and/or who depend on technology. Families with limited proficiency in English may require greater planning efforts. Families living in rural communities and those who live in food deserts, and/or who are geographically, culturally, and economically isolated also require special attention when planning for disasters. These populations may be from indigent farm worker families, Great Plains families, or American Indian lands. The AAP has detailed information about planning for disasters.[1]

The US Food and Drug Administration (FDA) and the Centers for Disease Control and Prevention (CDC) provide guidance aimed at federal agencies and state and local governments responsible for radiation emergencies for the use of KI in radiation emergencies (see Chapter 31). It should be administered as soon as possible in a radiation emergency.

Infectious diseases (eg, leptospirosis, dengue, hepatitis A, typhoid fever, vibriosis, influenza) are common after hurricanes and also occur after other natural disasters. The AAP Web site on natural disasters (https://www.aap.org/en-us/advocacy-and-policy/aap-health-initiatives/Children-and-Disasters/Pages/Natural-Disasters.aspx) and the AAP *Red Book* Online (https://redbook.solutions.aap.org) provide information about infectious diseases. The CDC's Health Action Network also contains useful information (https://emergency.cdc.gov/han).

## SUMMARY

Children are particularly vulnerable to physical and psychological harm from disasters. Pediatric health care providers can educate themselves about disaster preparedness and participate in planning for, managing, and recovering from disasters.

## Frequently Asked Questions

Q  *Where can I find information about preparing my family for a disaster?*

A  Talk to your pediatrician. The American Academy of Pediatrics Disaster Web site has materials that your pediatrician can share with you at www.aap.org/en-us/advocacy-and-policy/aap-health-initiatives/Children-and-Disasters/Pages/Hurricanes-Tornadoes-and-Storms.aspx and www.aap.org/disasters/adjustment. In addition, the Centers for Disease Control and Prevention has a Web site for parents on preparing for disasters at: www.cdc.gov/childrenindisasters/parents.html

## Resources

### American Academy of Pediatrics, Children and Disasters

Web sites: https://www.aap.org/en-us/advocacy-and-policy/aap-health-initiatives/Children-and-Disasters/Pages/default.aspx and www.aap.org/disasters/adjustment. These sites contain information and resources for pediatricians and others who care for children.

### Centers for Disease Control and Prevention (CDC) Emergency Preparedness and Response

Web site: www.bt.cdc.gov

The CDC has a Clinical Outreach and Communication Activity (www.bt.cdc.gov/coca). Clinicians can sign up to receive e-mails, participate in conference calls, and participate in online and other types of training.

## Federal Emergency Management Agency (FEMA)

Web site: www.fema.gov

FEMA operates the Emergency Management Institute (http://training. fema.gov), which provides online and in-person training about the Incident Command System and other topics.

## National Center for Disaster Medicine and Public Health

Web site: http://ncdmph.usuhs.edu/KnowledgeLearning/2013-Learning2. htm

## National Commission on Children and Disasters

Web site: www.childrenanddisasters.acf.hhs.gov

## National Institute of Standards and Technology: Community Resilience Planning Guide

Web site: www.nist.gov/el/resilience/guide.cfm

## Natural Disasters and Weather Emergencies – US Environmental Protection Agency

Web site: www.epa.gov/naturalevents

## State Offices and Agencies of Emergency Management

Web site: www.fema.gov/about/contact/statedr.shtm

## The National Child Traumatic Stress Network

Web site: www.nctsn.org/content/psychological-first-aid

## References

1. American Academy of Pediatrics Disaster Preparedness Advisory Council and Committee on Pediatric Emergency Medicine. Ensuring the health of children in disasters. *Pediatrics.* 2015;136(5):1407–1417. http://pediatrics.aappublications.org/content/pediatrics/ early/2015/10/13/peds.2015-3112.full.pdf. Accessed February 4, 2018

2. Federal Emergency Management Agency. NRF Resource Center. https://www.fema.gov/media-library/assets/documents/117791. Accessed August 6, 2018

3. Federal Emergency Management Agency. National Disaster Recovery Framework. September 2011. http://www.fema.gov/media-library-data/20130726-1820-25045-5325/508_ndrf.pdf. Accessed February 4, 2018

4. Federal Emergency Management Agency. NIMS Resource Center. https://www.fema.gov/ national-incident-management-system. Accessed August 6, 2018

5. Robert T. Stafford Disaster Relief and Emergency Assistance Act, as Amended and Related Authorities. FEMA 592, June 2007. Federal Emergency Management Agency; 2007. http://www. fema.gov/pdf/about/stafford_act.pdf. Accessed February 4, 2018

6. Adirim T. Protecting children during disasters: the federal view. *Clin Pediatr Emerg Med.* 2009;10(3):164–172

7. American Academy of Pediatrics Disaster Preparedness Advisory Council. Medical countermeasures for children in public health emergencies, disasters or terrorism. *Pediatrics*. 2016;137(2):e20154273. http://pediatrics.aappublications.org/content/pediatrics/early/2015/12/31/peds.2015-4273.full.pdf. Accessed February 4, 2018

8. Noji EK. *The Public Health Consequences of Disasters*. New York, NY: Oxford University Press; 1997

9. Waeckerle JF. Disaster planning and response. *N Engl J Med*. 1991;324(12):815–821

10. Institute of Medicine. *Emergency Care for Children: Growing Pains*. National Academies Press; 2007. http://www.nap.edu/catalog.php?record_id=11655. Accessed February 4, 2018

11. American Academy of Pediatrics. Hurricane Katrina, children, and pediatric heroes: hands-on stories by and of our colleagues helping families during the most costly natural disaster in US history. *Pediatrics*. 2006;117(5 Suppl):S355-S460

12. Hoven CW, Duarte CS, Mandell DJ. Children's mental health after disasters: the impact of the World Trade Center attack. *Curr Psychiatr Rep*. 2003;5(2):101–107

13. Schonfeld DJ, Gurwitch RH. Addressing disaster mental health needs of children: practical guidance  for pediatric emergency health care providers. *Clin Pediatr Emerg Med*. 2009;10(3):208–215

14. Schonfeld DJ, Demaria T, American Academy of Pediatrics Disaster Preparedness Advisory Council, Committee on Psychosocial Aspects of Child and Family Health. Providing psychosocial support to children and families in the aftermath of disaster and crisis: a guide for pediatricians. *Pediatrics*. 2015;136(4):e1120–e1130

15. Madrid PA, Grant R, Reilly MJ, Redlener NB. Challenges in meeting immediate emotional needs: short-term impact of a major disaster on children's mental health: building resiliency in the aftermath of Hurricane Katrina. *Pediatrics*. 2006;117(5 Pt 3):S448–S453

16. Schonfeld D, Gurwitch R. Children in disasters. In Elzouki AY, Stapleton FB, Whitley RJ, Oh W, Harfi HA, Nazer H, eds. *Textbook of Clinical Pediatrics*. 2nd ed. New York, NY: Springer-Verlag; 2011:687–698

17. American Red Cross. Foundations of Disaster Mental Health. 2006

18. JPCC, 2014: Climate Change 2014: Synthesis Report. Contribution of Working Groups I, II and III to the Fifth Assessment Report of the Intergovernmental Panel on Climate Change. Pachauri RK, Meyer LA, eds. IPCC, Geneva, Switzerland

19. Centers for Disease Control and Prevention. FEMA-Provided Travel Trailer Study. http://www.cdc.gov/nceh/ehhe/trailerstudy/default.htm. Accessed February 4, 2018

20. USA Today. https://www.usatoday.com/story/news/nation/2017/12/30/puerto-rico-nearly-half-residents-without-power-three-months-after-hurricane-maria/992135001/. Accessed February 4, 2018

21. Agency for Health Care Research and Quality. Pediatric Terrorism and Disaster Preparedness. A Resource for Pediatricians. http://archive.ahrq.gov/research/pedprep/resource.htm. Accessed February 4, 2018

22. Mallett LH, Etzel RA. Flooding: what is the impact on pregnancy and child health? *Disasters*. 2017; doi 10.1111/disa.12256

23. Hajat S, Ebi KL, Kovats S, Meene B, Edwards S, Haines A. The human health consequences of flooding in Europe and the implications for public health: a review of the evidence. *Appl Environ Health Sci Public Health*. 2003;1(1):13–21

24. Janerich DT, Stark AD, Greenwald P, Burnett WS, Jacobson HI, McCusker J. Increased leukemia, lymphoma, and spontaneous abortion in Western New York following a flood disaster. *Public Health Rep*. 1981;96(4):350–356

25. Chernobyl Accident. World Nuclear Association. Updated November 2015. http://www.world-nuclear.org/info/Safety-and-Security/Safety-of-Plants/Chernobyl-Accident/. Accessed February 4, 2018

26. Tokaimura Criticality Accident 1999. World Nuclear Association. Updated October 2013. http://www.world-nuclear.org/info/Safety-and-Security/Safety-of-Plants/Tokaimura-Criticality-Accident/. Accessed February 4, 2018

27. Fukushima Accident. World Nuclear Association. October 2015. http://www.world-nuclear.org/info/safety-and-security/safety-of-plants/fukushima-accident/. Accessed February 4, 2018

28. U.S. Forest Service. Understanding Fire Effects on the Environment. https://www.fs.fed.us/pnw/research/fire/fire-effects.shtml. Accessed February 4, 2018

29. Liu JC, Pereira G, Uhl SA, Bravo MA, Bell ML. A systematic review of the physical health impacts from non-occupational exposure to wildfire smoke. *Environ Res*. 2015;136:120–132

30. Landrigan PJ, Lioy PJ, Thurston G, et al. Health and environmental consequences of the World Trade Center disaster. *Environ Health Perspect*. 2004;112(6):731–739

31. Cone J, Perlman S, Eros-Sarnyai M, et al. Clinical guidelines for children and adolescents exposed to the World Trade Center disaster city health information. New York, NY: New York City Department of Health and Mental Hygiene; 2009:29–40

32. Thomas PA, Brackbill R, Thalji T, et al. Respiratory and other health effects reported in children exposed to the World Trade Center disaster of 11 September 2001. *Environ Health Perspect*. 2008;116(10):1383–1390

33. Berkowitz GS, Wolff MS, Janevic TM, Holzman IR, Yehuda R, Landrigan PJ. The World Trade Center disaster and intrauterine growth restriction. *JAMA*. 2003;290(5):595–596

34. Lederman SA, Rauh V, Weiss L, et al. Effects of the World Trade Center event on birth outcomes among term deliveries at three lower Manhattan hospitals. *Environ Health Perspect*. 2004;112(17):1772–1778

35. Perera FP, Tang D, Rauh V, et al. Relationship between polycyclic aromatic hydrocarbon-DNA adducts and proximity to the World Trade Center and effects on fetal growth. *Environ Health Perspect*. 2005;113(8):1062–1067

36. Perera FP, Tang D, Rauh V, et al. Relationship between polycyclic aromatic hydrocarbon-DNA adducts, environmental tobacco smoke, and child development in the World Trade Center cohort. *Environ Health Perspect*. 2007;115(10):1497–1502

37. Hoven CW, Duarte CS, Lucas CP, et al. Psychopathology among New York City public school children 6 months after September 11. *Arch Gen Psychiatry*. 2005;62(5):545–552

38. Chemtob CM, Nomura Y, Abramovitz RA. Impact of conjoined exposure to the World Trade Center attacks and to other traumatic events on the behavioral problems of preschool children. *Arch Pediatr Adolesc Med*. 2008;162(2):126–133

39. Calderoni ME, Alderman EM, Silver EJ, Bauman LJ. The mental health impact of 9/11 on inner-city high school students 20 miles north of Ground Zero. *J Adolesc Health*. 2006;39(1):57–65

Chapter 55

# Environmental Equity

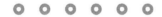

## KEY POINTS

- Children (and others) from lower income and/or minority communities are more likely to be exposed to environmental hazards. Disparities in environmental health are long-standing and persistent.
- "Environmental justice" calls for environmental equity to improve environmental health in lower income and minority communities.
- Focusing on population health and addressing "social determinants of health" (eg, social, economic, and physical conditions) instead of individual-level behavior change approaches will lead to better strategies to eliminate health disparities and achieve health equity.
- Pediatricians have important roles to play by learning about the environmental exposures and related disease affecting patients and communities, becoming involved in medical-legal partnerships, and speaking out on behalf of these children before local, state, and national groups.

## INTRODUCTION

The US Environmental Protection Agency (EPA) defines environmental justice as "the fair treatment and meaningful involvement of all people regardless of race, color, national origin, or income with respect to the development, implementation, and enforcement of environmental laws, regulations, and policies."[1] Advocates argue, however, that environmental justice is more than a governmental statement as previously stated. Rather, environmental justice is a grassroots movement that affirms the fundamental right to political, economic, cultural, and environmental self-determination of all peoples, and other goals as outlined in the 17 Principles of Environmental Justice presented at the First National People of Color Environmental Leadership Summit held in October 1991 in Washington, DC (see www.ejnet.org/ej/principles.html). "Environmental equity" is the recognition of and society's responses to the unequal distribution of environmental hazards, exposures, risks, and impacts by race/ethnicity, social class, age, and gender.[2,3] Responses may include enactment of policies, laws, regulations, and enforcement actions to ameliorate these disparities to achieve environmental justice. Common themes across these many perspectives of environmental equity and environmental justice are health and the protection of the most vulnerable in society.

Children who live in poor or ethnic minority communities frequently suffer disproportionately from the effects of environmental pollution. Children from poor or minority families often live in neighborhoods with poor air quality and occupy homes that are substandard, placing them at risk from exposure to multiple environmental hazards.[4-11] Although these risks are much greater than those experienced by their wealthier counterparts, racial differences often persist across economic strata.[9] In addition, poor communities are relatively powerless compared with their more affluent neighbors and have fewer resources to protect their children from the environmental risks present. Disparities in the burdens of illness and death experienced by minority groups, such as African American, Hispanic, Asian and Pacific Islander, and American Indian/Alaska Native individuals, compared with white individuals and with the US population as a whole, have existed since the government began tracking health outcomes. Research continues to demonstrate that health disparities are produced by environmental (eg, physical, chemical, or biological agents to which individuals are exposed in a multitude of settings, including home, school, and workplace) and social (eg, individual and community level characteristics, such as socioeconomic status, education, psychosocial stress, coping resources, and support systems; residential factors; cultural variables; and institutional and political factors, such as racism and classism) forces.[12] Moreover, environmental justice advocates have encouraged scientists and regulators to view the "environment" holistically, by considering the effects that socioeconomic and other social factors have on exposure to environmental hazards and resulting health outcomes. Eliminating these disparities, differences in health that are closely linked to social, economic, and/or environmental disadvantage, is a major goal of Healthy People 2020, the nation's health agenda for this decade and beyond.[13] Achieving this national health goal will require interventions that address social and physical environmental factors. Public health advocates and local/state health departments are beginning to recognize the connections between physical and social environments. They are focusing more on social determinants of health (eg, poverty and racism)—instead of individual level behavior change approaches—to develop better strategies to eliminate health disparities and achieve health equity.[14,15]

## DISPARITIES IN MORTALITY AND MORBIDITY

Racial and ethnic differences in birth outcomes and the prevalence and severity of many childhood diseases are well recognized. It is postulated that the elevated and/or cumulative exposures to environmental pollutants combined with material deprivation, low social position, structural racism, psychosocial stress, and preexisting health conditions experienced by people of ethnic minorities and low-income populations increase the probability of environmentally induced illness and injury, thereby contributing to observed disparities in health status.[16] Although the specific mechanisms through which social and physical environmental factors interact and produce the differences in morbidity and mortality among racial and ethnic groups are not well understood, there is no doubt that these environmental factors play a role in differences in health outcomes. Social factors may lead to increased sensitivity or vulnerability to the adverse health effects of environmental toxicants such that these social factors act as effect modifiers (eg, enhancing the toxic effects) of exposures to environmental contaminants.[17–22] This is an emerging area of environmental health research.

### Infant Mortality

Infant mortality is generally viewed as good indicator of community health, representing full integration of intrinsic biological factors with environmental and social factors distributed throughout every facet of life.[23] Since the early 1900s, the infant mortality rate in the United States has always been higher for African American and American Indian/Alaska Native infants than for white infants.[24,25] Substantial racial and ethnic disparities continue. Non-Hispanic African American and American Indian/Alaska Native infants have consistently had a higher infant mortality rate than that of any other racial or ethnic groups.[26] For example, in 2014, the mortality rate for non-Hispanic African American infants was 10.9 infant deaths per 1,000 live births and for American Indian/Alaska Native infants was 7.6, both higher than the mortality rate among white, non-Hispanic (4.9), Hispanic (5.0), and Asian/Pacific Islander (3.9) infants.[26] Infant mortality rates also vary within racial and ethnic populations. For example, among Hispanic people in the United States, the infant mortality rate for 2014 ranged from 3.9 deaths per 1,000 live births for infants of Cuban origin to a high of 7.2 per 1,000 live births for Puerto Rican infants.[26] The reasons for the racial disparities are not fully understood. Sudden infant death syndrome (SIDS) is a major contributor to excess infant mortality in nonwhite groups. The rate of deaths from SIDS is higher among Alaska Native, American Indian, and black infants.[27,28] In addition to race/ethnicity, important environmental risk factors for SIDS include prone sleep position, maternal smoking during pregnancy, postnatal exposure to secondhand smoke (SHS), and (possibly) exposure to outdoor air pollution.[29-31]

## Low Birth Weight

Low birth weight is an important predictor of infant morbidity and mortality. African American women are twice as likely as white women to deliver a low birth weight infant, even within the same category of educational attainment (eg, college education).[23,32] Lack of education and low-income status are also associated with low birth weight.[33] Cigarette smoking affects birth weight by causing intrauterine growth retardation.[34,35] These and other risk factors during pregnancy, however, do not adequately account for persistent racial disparities.[33,36] Exposure to environmental contaminants also contributes to the increased risk of having a low birth weight infant. A number of studies have found associations between low birth weight and proximity to landfills and other land-based environmental hazards,[37-40] air pollution,[41-45] and pesticides.[46] Studies[43,46] indicate that interactions of multiple contaminants, including polycyclic aromatic hydrocarbons, pesticides (chlorpyrifos), and SHS are associated with low birth weight, decreased head circumference, and decreased birth length among African American (nonsmoking) women in Harlem. In a study on air pollution and birth outcomes in Connecticut and Massachusetts, researchers found that the risk of low birth weight associated with exposure to fine particle air pollution particulate matter ($PM_{2.5}$) was higher for infants of African American mothers than those of white mothers.[41]

## Asthma

Puerto Rican, African American, and Cuban American children in the United States have a higher prevalence of asthma than do white children.[47] African American children are twice as likely as white children to have asthma.[47] African American individuals younger than age 24 years are 3 to 4 times more likely to be hospitalized for asthma. Asthma is a complex disease with a number of causes. Racial and ethnic differences in the burden of asthma may be related to social and economic status, access to health care, and exposure to environmental triggers.[48] In 2015, approximately 13% of non-Hispanic African American children were reported to currently have asthma, compared with 7% of non-Hispanic white children and 8% of Hispanic children. Disparities exist within the Hispanic population, such that 14% of Puerto Rican children were reported to currently have asthma, compared with 7% of children of Mexican origin.[26]

There are numerous triggers for asthma in the home environment (cockroaches, pesticides, SHS exposure, mites, and molds) and in the urban environment (outdoor air pollution from traffic); these triggers are unequally distributed in a way that affects communities with low socioeconomic status more than others.[49]

## Infant Pulmonary Hemorrhage

Clusters of cases of acute pulmonary hemorrhage have been reported among infants in Cleveland, Chicago, and Detroit.[50-52] Living in a water-damaged, moldy home was a risk factor for acute pulmonary hemorrhage. Most infants in these clusters were African American. It is unlikely that race is a risk factor for acute pulmonary hemorrhage; it is more likely that race is associated with socioeconomic status in these communities.[53] People living in poverty may not have the resources for adequate clean-up of water damage and mold.

## Neurodevelopment

Developmental disabilities have been reported to affect 1 in 6 children in the United States and the rate appears to have increased over time.[54] Most of these disabilities involve neurodevelopmental disorders including learning disabilities, sensory deficits, developmental delays, cerebral palsy, autism, and attention-deficit/hyperactivity disorders (ADHD). These disabilities can have severe consequences: diminished quality of life, reductions in academic achievement, and hyperactive behaviors that can lead to profound consequences for the welfare and productivity of society.[55] A review of data collected in the National Health Interview Survey indicated that a higher prevalence of developmental disabilities was associated with Medicaid insurance coverage, family incomes below poverty level, and low maternal education.[54] These socioeconomic trends were not evident for autism. Growing evidence points to exposures to environmental contaminants, particularly chemicals, as contributors to neurodevelopmental disorders in children. In addition, environmental exposures may disproportionately influence the neurodevelopment of children growing up in disadvantaged environments.[56,57] Project TENDR (Targeting Environmental Neuro-Development Risks), an alliance of more than 50 leading scientists, health professionals, and children's health advocates with expertise on chemicals and brain development, has identified developmental neurotoxicants that should be targets of more aggressive exposure reduction efforts. These include organophosphate (OP) pesticides, polybrominated diphenyl ether (PBDE) flame retardants, combustion-related air pollutants (eg, polycyclic aromatic hydrocarbons [PAHs], nitrogen dioxide [$NO_2$], fine particulate matter), lead, mercury, and polychlorinated biphenyls (PCBs). For a more detailed review of the growing scientific evidence linking toxic environmental chemical exposures to neurodevelopmental disorders, see the 2016 Consensus

Statement by Project TENDR.[58] Social and neighborhood conditions may exert independent influences on neurodevelopment or may confound or moderate the associations between environmental contaminant exposures and neurodevelopment.

## DISPARITIES IN ENVIRONMENTAL EXPOSURES

### Air Pollution Exposure

Indoor air pollution may be caused by SHS, dust mites, molds, and cockroaches. Children of minority populations may experience greater exposure to polluted indoor air.[59,60] They also may live in neighborhoods with substandard outdoor air quality. For example, 50% of all white children in the United States live in counties where the ozone concentrations exceed the national standard, whereas 60% of black children, 67% of Hispanic children, and 66% of Asian or Pacific Islander children live in counties with exceedingly high ozone concentrations. Higher percentages of Hispanic, and Asian or Pacific Islander American children than white children reside in counties in which the air quality exceeds standards for $PM_{2.5}$ (Table 55-1).[61]

### Exposure to Mercury in Fish

Individuals of ethnic minority groups may be exposed to certain chemical contaminants in the food supply because of dietary habits. Individuals from American Indian/Alaska Native, Asian or Pacific Islander American, and subsistence fishing communities may have a much greater health risk from contaminants in fish.[62-66] For example, Burger[63] conducted a survey of fishing behavior and consumption along the New York-New Jersey harbor estuary and found that African American people had the highest consumption rate of locally caught fish; Hispanic people had the second highest rate. White people, more than other groups, engaged in catch and release—they did not eat their catch and had lower consumption rates.[60] American Indian people are also differentially exposed to toxicants because of traditional dietary patterns involving consumption of locally caught fish and game.[65-68] Asian or Pacific Islander American people may consume 10 times more fish and shellfish than the average person in the United States.[69] As a result, Asian or Pacific Islander American children may face more exposure to contaminated seafood than the general population. An analysis of national data found that mercury concentrations among Asian and Pacific Islander American women were statistically higher than those of other racial/ethnic groups.[70] This has implications for children's health because exposure to methylmercury in utero can cause damage to the fetal central nervous system, resulting in impaired cognitive and motor skills.[71] These results were corroborated by a biomonitoring study in New York City showing racial disparities in blood mercury concentrations

## Table 55-1. Percentage of Children Aged 0 to 17 Years Living in Counties with Air Pollutant Concentrations Above the Levels of Current Quality Standards, by Race/Ethnicity, 2016[a]

| POLLUTANT | ALL RACES/ETHNICITIES | WHITE NON-HISPANIC | BLACK NON-HISPANIC | AMERICAN INDIAN/ALASKA NATIVE NON-HISPANIC | ASIAN OR PACIFIC ISLANDER NON-HISPANIC | HISPANIC |
|---|---|---|---|---|---|---|
| Any standard | 62.4 | 55.4 | 65.5 | 39.0 | 73.0 | 74.1 |
| Ozone (8-hour) | 57.8 | 50.6 | 61.1 | 31.8 | 68.0 | 69.7 |
| $PM_{2.5}$ (24-hour) | 21.3 | 15.9 | 20.0 | 16.0 | 28.1 | 32.5 |
| Sulfur dioxide (1-hour) | 3.0 | 3.2 | 5.0 | 2.4 | 2.5 | 1.7 |
| $PM_{2.5}$ (annual) | 3.3 | 1.7 | 1.6 | 2.0 | 3.7 | 7.5 |
| Nitrogen dioxide (1-hour) | 2.0 | 1.6 | 2.8 | 1.1 | 1.4 | 2.5 |
| $PM_{10}$ (24-hour) | 6.7 | 4.5 | 5.3 | 9.5 | 5.7 | 12.1 |
| Carbon monoxide (8-hour) | 0.0 | 0.0 | 0.0 | 0.0 | 0.0 | 0.0 |
| Lead (3-month) | 0.1 | 0.1 | 0.2 | 0.5 | 0.0 | 0.1 |

Abbreviations: $PM_{2.5}$, particulate matter less than 2.5 mcm in aerodynamic diameter; $PM_{10}$, particulate matter less than 10 mcm in aerodynamic diameter.

Source: US Environmental Protection Agency, Office of Air and Radiation, Air Quality System.

[a] The US EPA periodically reviews air quality standards and may change them based on updated scientific findings. Measuring concentrations above the level of a standard is not equivalent to violating the standard. The level of a standard may be exceeded on multiple days before the exceedance is considered a violation of the standard. See the indicator text for additional discussion. The indicator is calculated with reference to the current levels of the air quality standards (with the exception of the new ozone standard issued by the US EPA on October 1, 2015).

among Asian individuals, specifically foreign-born Chinese adults residing in New York City.[72] This study prompted the New York City Department of Health and Mental Hygiene to issue an advisory to health care providers to encourage healthy fish consumption among their patients. However, it is difficult for communities to make decisions about good dietary choices when information is not available regarding mercury concentrations (or other contaminants) in foods, particularly foods sold in specialty shops or ethnic food shops.

## Lead Exposure

Despite recent large decreases in blood lead concentrations, there are persistent racial, ethnic, and income disparities in blood lead concentrations. African American children continue to have higher median and 95th percentile blood lead levels across all income groups. The median blood lead level in African American non-Hispanic children aged 1 to 5 years in 2009 to 2012 was 1.4 mcg/dL, statistically significantly higher than the level of 1.0 mcg/dL in white non-Hispanic children, Mexican-American children, and children of "All Other Races/Ethnicities" (Figure 55-1).[61] An African American child has twice the chance of having a blood lead concentration above the reference

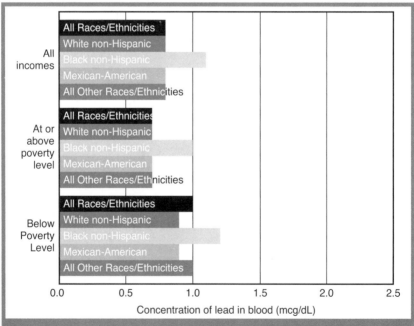

**Figure 55-1. Lead in children aged 1 to 5 years: median concentrations in blood, by race/ethnicity, and family income, 2011-2014**

Source: Centers for Disease Control and Prevention, National Center for Health Statistics and National Center for Environmental Health, National Health and Nutrition Examination Survey. *America's Children and the Environment*, Third Edition, Updated June 2017

level (5 mcg/dL) as does a white child.[73] In the period of 2007 to 2010, blood lead concentrations of 5 mcg/dL or greater in non-Hispanic African American children, non-Hispanic white children, and Mexican American children were 5.6%, 2.4%, and 1.9%, respectively.[73] Lead exposure in disadvantaged populations is thought to be related to older substandard housing (Table 55-2). Although lead-based paints were banned for use in housing in 1978, 38 million housing units in the United States still have lead-based paint and high levels of lead-contaminated dust.[74] Drinking water also can be a source of lead. The decision by government officials in Flint, Michigan, a city of 99,000 people, to switch to a water supply that brought corrosive water from the Flint River into the homes of city residents—56% African American, 40% living below the poverty line—resulted in higher levels of lead in drinking water because the city did not use appropriate corrosion control. A pediatrician drew attention to the city's problem by analyzing the blood lead levels among children living in Flint. The water problem in Flint had a differential effect on immigrant communities (especially, the non-English speaking residents and undocumented people) because of state ID requirements, general distrust, fear, and lack of information in those communities.[75-78]

This event revealed a silent threat to neurodevelopment among children living in lower income and minority communities in older cities—aging and corroding drinking water infrastructure as a source of lead exposure. Use of lead in plumbing material was restricted by law in 1986, but older homes and neighborhoods may still contain lead service lines, lead connections, lead solder, or other lead-based plumbing material. An estimated 3.3 million to 5.6 million lead drinking water service lines are in use; these lines are more prevalent in the metropolitan areas in western, midwestern, and northeastern regions of the United States.[79,80]

Some families use traditional ceramic ware for cooking and food storage, which may have lead in the glazing that can leach into the food. Other sources include ethnic or folk remedies that contain lead, such as "greta," a traditional Mexican laxative, "azarcon," used to treat an upset stomach, and "litargirio," used as a deodorant. Imported makeup, such as "surma" or "kohl," is used primarily by individuals of Asian, African, or Middle Eastern descent. It is also applied to the umbilical stump of newborn infants. Although kohl may be made by hand using recipes that do not contain lead, commercial kohl makeup may have very high lead concentrations and pose a serious threat to human health. One study found that the use of kohl was a potential cause of elevated blood lead concentrations in Saudi school children,[81] suggesting that the cosmetic use of kohl may be a significant source of exposure to lead in children. A blood lead level concentration of 13 mcg/dL found in a Nigerian infant was linked to use of "tiro," an eye cosmetic containing lead.[82] Children can ingest kohl after rubbing their eyes and then licking their fingers.

Table 55-2. Number Sampled and Estimated Percentage of Children Aged 1 to 5 Years With Blood Lead Levels Greater Than or Equal to 5 mcg/dL, by Selected Characteristics—United States, National Health and Nutrition Examination Survey, 1999–2002, 2003–2006, and 2007–2010

| CHARACTERISTIC | 1999–2002 | | | 2003–2006 | | | 2007–2010 | | |
|---|---|---|---|---|---|---|---|---|---|
| | NO. | % | (95% CI) | NO. | % | (95% CI) | NO. | % | (95% CI) |
| **Age of housing** | | | | | | | | | |
| Pre-1950 | 208 | 18.4 | (13.1–24.4) | 242 | 8.8 | (5.3–13.2) | 264 | 5.3 | (1.1–12.6)* |
| 1950–1977 | 341 | 5.3 | (2.9–8.4) | 413 | 2.2 | (0.8–4.3)* | 343 | 1.3 | (0.6–2.4)* |
| 1978 or later | 470 | 2.1 | (0.9–3.7)* | 528 | 1.4 | (0.6–2.4)* | 503 | 0.4 | (0.1–1.0)* |
| Refused/Don't know | 602 | 15 | (10.7–19.9) | 696 | 7.5 | (3.6–12.6) | 543 | 5.1 | (3.3–7.4) |
| **Race/Ethnicity** | | | | | | | | | |
| Black, non-Hispanic | 454 | 18.5 | (13.7–23.8) | 546 | 12.1 | (6.5–19.2) | 338 | 5.6 | (3.3–8.4) |
| Mexican American | 541 | 7.4 | (4.7–10.6) | 611 | 2.6 | (1.1–4.6) | 490 | 1.9 | (0.7–3.7)* |
| White, non-Hispanic | 465 | 7.1 | (3.7–11.5) | 540 | 2.3 | (1.4–3.2) | 536 | 2.4 | (0.7–5.2)* |
| **Poverty income ratio** | | | | | | | | | |
| <1.3 | 817 | 12.9 | (9.5–16.7) | 941 | 8.1 | (5.2–11.6) | 868 | 4.4 | (3.0–6.2) |
| ≥1.3 | 677 | 4.5 | (2.6–6.7) | 852 | 1.6 | (0.7–2.9)* | 642 | 1.2 | (0.1–3.7)* |

Centers for Disease Control and Prevention. Blood lead levels in children aged 1–5 years — United States, 1999–2010. *MMWR Morb Mortal Wkly Rep.* 2013;62(13):245–248

Abbreviation: CI = confidence interval.

*Estimate is statistically unreliable (relative standard error is >30)

Herbal medicine products may also be sources of lead exposure, and their use may vary by ethnic group. In one study, 70 Ayurvedic products from Boston area markets were analyzed (Ayurvedic medicine, or "ayurveda," is a system of health that has been practiced in India for more than 5,000 years). Almost 20% contained lead, ranging from 5 mcg/g to 37,000 mcg/g per sample. Most of these herbal medicine products contain one or more heavy metals that are toxic to adults and children.

## Pesticide Exposure

More than 3 decades ago, surveys reported that levels of dichlorodiphenyltrichloroethane (DDT) and its metabolites (in fat or blood) were higher in black people than in white people.[83] In a community in Florida, DDT and dichlorodiphenyldichloroethylene (DDE, a degradation product of DDT) concentrations in blood were significantly lower in the affluent groups than in the low-income groups, for both black and white people. In comparable income groups, however, black people had higher DDT concentrations than did white people.[83]

Children of farm workers may accompany their parents to fields, live in housing contaminated by direct pesticide spray or drift from nearby fields, and work in the fields themselves.[84,85] Farm workers can bring home pesticides on their shoes, clothes, and skin and then transfer them to their children, food, and home environment. Studies in California and Washington State suggest the potential for higher residential exposure to some pesticides for children of farm workers compared with children of non-farm workers. In a study in Washington State among farm workers in the pome fruit industry (apples and pears), urinary concentrations of dimethyl pesticide metabolites from children of farm workers were significantly correlated with their parents' metabolite concentrations and with house-dust concentrations of the pesticides.[86] The results provide support for a take-home pathway for pesticide exposures among farm worker children.

Concern about disparities in exposures to pesticides extends beyond the farm to impoverished children who live in urban areas. Home pesticide use tends to be more frequent and concentrated in densely populated urban areas. Pesticide use is especially high in multifamily housing with buildings that are in poor repair.[87] In 2004, some 71,000 children in the United States were poisoned by or exposed to household pesticides.[88] There were 15,000 rodenticide exposures involving children aged 6 years and younger. Many of these incidents occurred in cities among low-income minority residents.[88]

Ineffective pest control in low-income urban housing may lead to use of illegal pesticides. For example, in New York City, 9% of all households reported using the pesticide Tempo.[89] Although Tempo is legal to use in agricultural settings, it is not legal to use in homes because residents do not have access to the protective clothing worn and the equipment used by agricultural workers.

Other pesticides that should not be used in homes include "Chinese" chalk and Tres Pasitos, because they contain harmful chemicals that are toxic to people, especially children. To read more about these illegal pesticide products, visit www.epa.gov/opp00001/health/illegalproducts/index.htm.

## Religious and Cultural Practices with Herbs and Dietary Supplements

In certain ethnic groups, religious practices may be potential sources of exposure to environmental contaminants. For example, some Hispanic American people who practice Santeria may sprinkle elemental mercury in the house, possibly resulting in elevated concentrations of mercury in the indoor air (see Chapter 33). Lead and other toxic metals, such as mercury, cadmium, and arsenic, are used in some Latin American and Asian traditional medicines, such as Ayurvedic medicines, that are given to children (see Chapter 32 and Chapter 19). In addition, these metals may be found as contaminants of imported herbs and spices and dietary supplements.[90]

## Exposure to Drinking Water Contaminants

Many small, rural, or low-income neighborhoods do not have access to safe and affordable drinking water supplies. Some water contamination problems may disproportionately affect certain racial or socioeconomic populations. Examples include lead exposure from deteriorating pipes/solder in older homes and fertilizer runoff into rural water supplies. Federal standards for drinking water quality (treatment and monitoring) do not apply to small private systems, many of which are domestic wells. These small private systems serve approximately 43.5 million people in the United States. Many of these systems are in rural and agricultural areas and may be at increased risk from nitrate and fecal contamination as well as from pesticides and other chemicals (eg, arsenic). Water quality data are not routinely collected from private wells; this situation presents a significant limitation to understanding children's exposures.

## Waste Sites

Hazardous waste sites are often located disproportionately in minority neighborhoods. A 1987 report by the United Church of Christ's (UCC) Commission for Racial Justice revealed that 3 of the 5 largest hazardous waste landfills in the United States were in African American or Hispanic neighborhoods and that the mean percentage of residents of minority groups in areas with toxic waste sites was twice that in areas without toxic waste sites.[91] In 1994, in recognition of the disproportionate impact of environmental hazards on low-income communities, the President issued an Executive Order seeking to achieve environmental justice.[92] The UCC report was updated in 2007 and confirmed earlier findings, and also showed that disproportionate sitings of hazardous waste facilities in low-income communities increased.[93] In 2000, in neighborhoods within 3 kilometers (1.8 miles) of commercial hazardous waste facilities, 56% of the residents were minorities, whereas in non-host areas, 30% of the residents were minorities. Thus, percentages of people of minorities as a whole are 1.9 times greater in host neighborhoods than in non-host areas.

## PRACTICAL RECOMMENDATIONS FOR CLINICIANS

Children in poverty face an array of formidable challenges. Environmental health sciences education is an essential tool for achieving environmental equity and protecting children. Pediatricians must work together to protect children, especially those living in low-income or minority communities, from environmental threats to their health.

Advocating for the health and well-being of children from ethnic minority groups requires knowledge of the unique environmental risks of the neighborhood or community, a high index of suspicion for environmental causes of disease, and a willingness to work with local health officials to sort out public health issues and make appropriate referrals. The pediatrician should consider doing the following:

- Build a network to learn about environmental concerns within the community. Meet and establish relationships with the local, county, or state environmental health unit.
- Become involved in medical-legal partnerships.
- Actively learn the history of environmental illness that has affected various ethnic and minority groups within your practice. The special problems may vary between urban and rural settings and between racial and minority groups. Look for patterns of disease and exposures among your patients to help identify areas for policy change. Ask parents and community leaders for their perceptions of environmental exposure and disease.
- Consider local cultural practices that may lead to environmental exposures and risk for illness. These practices may range from subsistence fishing in waters contaminated with PCBs to use of non-Western substances in cooking, home building, and home remedies.
- In taking a history, besides the usual inquiries about use of prescribed and over-the-counter medicines for children and allergies to medicines, specifically ask parents in a culturally sensitive, respectful way, about their use of herbs, dietary supplements, imported spices, religious powders, and ethnic remedies for their children.
- Speak out on behalf of these children before local, state, and national groups. Reframe the debate about health disparities by focusing more on health equity and away from individual behavior as the cause and solution.

## Medical-Legal Partnerships

■ Medical providers and lawyers are the ideal team to help low-income families who face legal problems related to their basic needs, such as housing and income. Medical-legal partners (MLPs) address the social determinants of health that create hardships for vulnerable populations through the integration of free legal services in the health care setting. MLPs currently serve patients at 294 health care institutions in 41 states by providing direct legal services to patients, training and education to health care providers, and a platform for systemic advocacy.

■ See http://medical-legalpartnership.org/ for more information on how to become involved.

### Resources

**American Indian and Alaska Native Health**
Web site: https://americanindianhealth.nlm.nih.gov/

**American Muslim Health Professionals**
Web site: www.amhp.us

**Asian & Pacific Islander American Health Forum**
Web site: www.apiahf.org

**DiversityData, Harvard School of Public Health**
Web site: www.DiversityData.org
This Web site gives information about how people of different racial/ethnic backgrounds live and includes comparative data about housing, neighborhood conditions, residential integration, and education.

**Environmental Justice Resources from Non-governmental Organizations and Academic Research Centers**
Deep South Center for Environmental Justice (DSCEJ)
www.dscej.org
Environmental Justice Project
https://regionalchange.ucdavis.edu/articles/environmental-justice

Working Group on Environmental Justice, Harvard University,
Cambridge, MA
http://ecojustice.net/
Urban Environmental Justice
www.columbia.edu/cu/EJ/index.html
Communities for a Better Environment
www.cbecal.org
Asian Pacific Environmental Network
https://apen4ej.org
Indigenous Environmental Network
www.ienearth.org

## Indian Health Service
Web site: www.ihs.gov

## National Alliance for Hispanic Health
Web site: www.hispanichealth.org

## National Association of County and City Health Officials
*Roots of Health Inequity.* Web site: www.rootsofhealthinequity.org
This course provides an online learning environment from which to explore
root causes of inequity in the distribution of disease, illness, and death.
*Tackling Health Inequities Through Public Health Practice: Theory to Action.*
Hofrichter R, Bhatia R, eds. 2nd ed. New York, NY: Oxford University Press;
2010

## National Center for Medical-Legal Partnership
Web site: http://medical-legalpartnership.org/

## National Center on Minority Health and Health Disparities, National Institutes of Health
Web site: https://www.nimhd.nih.gov

## National Medical Association
Web site: www.nmanet.org

## South Asian Public Health Association
Web site: http://joinsapha.org/

## The Coalition for Asian American Children and Families
Web site: www.cacf.org

## The Raising of America

Web site: www.raisingofamerica.org

*The Raising of America* is a five-part documentary series that explores how a strong start for all our kids can lead to better individual outcomes and a healthier, safer, better educated, and more prosperous and equitable America. The film expands the conversation beyond parenting to include how social conditions, public policies, and racial and economic inequities can impede parental efforts to nurture, care for, and guide their youngest children.

## UNIDOS US

Web site: www.nclr.org

## Unnatural Causes

Web site: www.unnaturalcauses.org

A TV documentary series and public outreach campaign on the causes of socioeconomic racial/ethnic inequities in health.

## US EPA Resources

Visit EPA's Office of Environmental Justice Web site to join their listserv and blog

Web site: https://www.epa.gov/environmentaljustice

EPA's Toxic Release Inventory (TRI) Programs

Web site: https://www.epa.gov/toxics-release-inventory-tri-program

EPA's Environmental Justice Screening and Mapping Tool

Web site: https://www.epa.gov/ejscreen

## References

1. US Environmental Protection Agency 2017 Environmental Justice Web site. https://www.epa.gov/environmentaljustice. Accessed June 4, 2018

2. Northridge ME, Stover GN, Rosenthal JE, Sherard D. Environmental equity and health: understanding complexity and moving forward. *Am J Public Health*. 2003;93(2):209–214

3. US Environmental Protection Agency. 1992. Environmental Equity: Reducing Risk for All Communities. Office of Policy, Planning and Evaluation. Washington, DC. EPA230-R-92008A

4. Powell DL, Stewart V. Children. The unwitting target of environmental injustices. *Pediatr Clin North Am*. 2001;48(5):1291–1305

5. Dilworth-Bart JE, Moore CF. Mercy mercy me: social injustice and the prevention of environmental pollutant exposures among ethnic minority and poor children. *Child Dev*. 2006;77(2):247–265

6. American Lung Association. Urban air pollution and health inequities: a workshop report. *Environ Health Perspect*. 2001;109(Suppl 3):357–474

7. Perera FP, Rauh V, Tsai WY, et al. Effects of transplacental exposure to environmental pollutants on birth outcomes in a multiethnic population. *Environ Health Perspect*. 2003;111 (2):201–205

8. Institute of Medicine. *Toward Environmental Justice: Research, Education, and Health Policy Needs*. Washington, DC: National Academies Press; 1999

9. Morello-Frosch R, Pastor M, Sadd J. Integrating environmental justice and the precautionary principle in research and policy making: the case of ambient air toxics exposures and health risks among schoolchildren in Los Angeles. *Annals AAPSS*. 2002;584:47–68

10. Evans GW, Kantrowitz E. Socioeconomic status and health: the potential role of environmental risk exposures. *Annu Rev Public Health*. 2002;23:303–331

11. Krieger J, Higgins DL. Housing and health: time again for public health action. *Am J Public Health*. 2002;92(5):758–768

12. Gee GC, Payne-Sturges DC. Environmental health disparities: a framework integrating psychosocial and environmental concepts. *Environ Health Perspect*. 2004;112(17):1645–1653

13. US Department of Health and Human Services. *Healthy People 2020. Disparities*. http://healthypeople.gov/2020/about/DisparitiesAbout.aspx. Accessed June 4, 2018

14. National Association of County and City Health Officials. *Tackling Health Inequities Through Public Health Practice: A Handbook for Action*. Washington, DC: National Association of County and City Health Officials; 2006

15. World Health Organization. *Commission on Social Determinants of Health*. Geneva, Switzerland: Interim Statement of the Commission on Social Determinants of Health, World Health Organization; 2007

16. Walker G. *Environmental Justice: Concepts, Evidence and Politics*. New York, NY: Routledge; 2012

17. Rauh VA, Whyatt RM, Garfinkel R, et al. Developmental effects of exposure to environmental tobacco smoke and material hardship among inner-city children. *Neurotoxicol Teratol*. 2004;26(3):373–385

18. Weiss B, Bellinger DC. Social ecology of children's vulnerability to environmental pollutants. *Environ Health Perspect*. 2006;114(10):1479–1485

19. Clougherty JE, Levy JI, Kubzanskyh LD, et al. Synergistic effects of traffic-related air pollution and exposure to violence on urban asthma etiology. *Environ Health Perspect*. 2007;115(8):1140–1146

20. Chari R, Burke TA, White RH, Fox MA. Integrating susceptibility into environmental policy: an analysis of the national ambient air quality standard for lead. *Int J Environ Res Public Health*. 2012;9(4):1077–1096

21. Rossi-George A, Virgolini MB, Weston D, Thiruchelvam M, Cory-Slechta DA. Interactions of lifetime lead exposure and stress: behavioral, neurochemical and HPA axis effects. *Neurotoxicology*. 2011;32(1):83–99

22. Vishnevetsky J, Tang D, Chang HW, et al. Combined effects of prenatal polycyclic aromatic hydrocarbons and material hardship on child IQ. *Neurotoxicol Teratol*. 2015;49:74–80

23. Kington RS, Nickens HW. Racial and ethnic differences in health: recent trends, current patterns, future directions. In: *America Becoming: Racial Trends and Their Consequences*. Washington, DC: National Academy of Sciences; 2003:253–310

24. MacDorman MF, Atkinson JO. Infant mortality statistics from the linked birth/infant death data set—1995 period data. *Mon Vital Stat Rep*. 1998;46(6 Suppl 2):1–22

25. Grossman DC, Baldwin LM, Casey S, Nixon B, Hollow W, Hart LG. Disparities in infant health among American Indians and Alaska Natives in US metropolitan areas. *Pediatrics*. 2002;109(4):627–633

26. Federal Interagency Forum on Child and Family Statistics. *America's Children: Key National Indicators of Well-Being, 2017*. Washington, DC: Federal Interagency Forum on Child and Family Statistics, U.S. Government Printing Office, 2017. https://www.childstats.gov/americaschildren/index.asp. Accessed June 4, 2018

27. Irwin KL, Mannino S, Daling J. Sudden infant death syndrome in Washington State: why are Native American infants at greater risk than white infants? *J Pediatr*. 1992;121(2):242–247

28. Oyen N, Bulterys M, Welty TK, Kraus JF. Sudden unexplained infant deaths among American Indians and whites in North and South Dakota. *Paediatr Perinat Epidemiol.* 1990;4(2):175–183

29. American Academy of Pediatrics Task Force on Infant Positioning and SIDS. *Pediatrics.* 1992;89(2 Pt 1):1120–1126

30. MacDorman MF, Cnattingius S, Hoffman HJ, Kramer MS, Haglund B. Sudden infant death syndrome and smoking in the United States and Sweden. *Am J Epidemiol.* 1997;146(3):249–257

31. Woodruff TJ, Grillo J, Schoendorf KC. The relationship between selected causes of postneonatal infant mortality and particulate air pollution in the United States. *Environ Health Perspect.* 1997;105(6):608–612

32. Montgomery LE, Carter-Pokras O. Health status by social class and/or minority status: implications for environmental equity research. *Toxicol Ind Health.* 1993;9(5):729–773

33. Lu MC, Halfon N. Racial and ethnic disparities in birth outcomes: a life-course perspective. *Matern Child Health J.* 2003;7(1):13–30

34. Kramer MS. Determinants of low birth weight: methodological assessment and meta-analysis. *Bull World Health Organ.* 1987;65(5):663–737

35. Misra DP, Nguyen RH. Environmental tobacco smoke and low birth weight: a hazard in the workplace? *Environ Health Perspect.* 1999;107(Suppl 6):897–904

36. Fuller KE. Low birth-weight infants: the continuing ethnic disparity and the interaction of biology and environment. *Ethn Dis.* 2000;10(3):432–445

37. Baibergenova A, Kudyakov R, Zdeb M, Carpenter DO. Low birth weight and residential proximity to PCB-contaminated waste sites. *Environ Health Perspect.* 2003;111(10):1352–1357

38. Elliott P, Briggs D, Morris S, et al. Risk of adverse birth outcomes in populations living near landfill sites. *BMJ.* 2001;323(7309):363–368

39. Shaw GM, Schulman J, Frisch JD, Cummins SK, Harris JA. Congenital malformations and birthweight in areas with potential environmental contamination. *Arch Environ Health.* 1992;47(2):147–154

40. Vrijheid M. Health effects of residence near hazardous waste landfill sites: a review of epidemiologic literature. *Environ Health Perspect.* 2000;108(Suppl 1):101–112

41. Bell ML, Ebisu K, Belanger K. Ambient air pollution and low birth weight in Connecticut and Massachusetts. *Environ Health Perspect.* 2007;115(7):1118–1124

42. Maisonet M, Bush TJ, Correa A, Jaakkola JJ. Relation between ambient air pollution and low birth weight in the Northeastern United States. *Environ Health Perspect.* 2001;109(Suppl 3):351–356

43. Perera FP, Rauh V, Whyatt RM, et al. Molecular evidence of an interaction between prenatal environmental exposures and birth outcomes in a multiethnic population. *Environ Health Perspect.* 2004;112(5):626–630

44. Rogers JF, Thompson SJ, Addy CL, McKeown RE, Cowen DJ, Decoufle P. Association of very low birth weight with exposures to environmental sulfur dioxide and total suspended particulates. *Am J Epidemiol.* 2000;151(6):602–613

45. Wang X, Ding H, Ryan L, Xu X. Association between air pollution and low birth weight: a community-based study. *Environ Health Perspect.* 1997;105(5):514–520

46. Perera FP, Rauh V, Tsai WY, et al. Effects of transplacental exposure to environmental pollutants on birth outcomes in a multiethnic population. *Environ Health Perspect.* 2003;111(2):201–205

47. Akinbami LJ, Centers for Disease Control and Prevention National Center for Health Statistics. The state of childhood asthma, United States, 1980-2005. *Adv Data.* 2006;(381):1–24

48. Asthma and Allergy Foundation of America and National Pharmaceutical Council. *Ethnic Disparities in the Burden and Treatment of Asthma.* Washington, DC: Asthma and Allergy

Foundation of America; January 2005. http://www.aafa.org/media/Ethnic-Disparities-Burden-Treatment-Asthma-Report.pdf. Accessed June 4, 2018

49. Claudio L, Tulton L, Doucette J, Landrigan PJ. Socioeconomic factors and asthma hospitalization rates in New York City. *J Asthma*. 1999;36(4):343–350

50. Centers for Disease Control and Prevention. Acute pulmonary hemorrhage/hemosiderosis among infants—Cleveland, January 1993–November 1994. *MMWR Morb Mortal Wkly Rep*. 1994;43(48):881–883

51. Centers for Disease Control and Prevention. Acute pulmonary hemorrhage among infants—Chicago, April 1992–November 1994. *MMWR Morb Mortal Wkly Rep*. 1995;44(4):67, 73–74

52. Pappas MD, Sarnaik AP, Meert KL, Hasan RA, Lieh-Lai MW. Idiopathic pulmonary hemorrhage in infancy. Clinical features and management with high frequency ventilation. *Chest*. 1996;110(2):553–555

53. Dearborn DG, Smith PG, Bahms BB, et al. Clinical profile of 30 infants with acute pulmonary hemorrhage in Cleveland. *Pediatrics*. 2002;110(3):627–637

54. Boyle CA, Boulet S, Schieve LA, et al. Trends in the prevalence of developmental disabilities in US children, 1997-2008. *Pediatrics*. 2011;127(6):1034–1042

55. Grandjean P, Landrigan PJ. Neurobehavioural effects of developmental toxicity. *Lancet Neurol*. 2014;13(3):330–338

56. Wright RJ. Moving towards making social toxins mainstream in children's environmental health. *Curr Opin Pediatr*. 2009;21(2):222–229

57. Cory-Slechta DA. Studying toxicants as single chemicals: does this strategy adequately identify neurotoxic risk? *Neurotoxicology*. 2005;26(4):491–510

58. Bennett D, Bellinger DC, Birnbaum LS, et al. Project TENDR: Targeting Environmental Neuro-Developmental Risks. The TENDR Consensus Statement. *Environ Health Perspect* 2016;124(7):A118–A122

59. Sarpong SB, Hamilton RG, Eggleston PA, Adkinson NF Jr. Socioeconomic status and race as risk factors for cockroach allergen exposure and sensitization in children with asthma. *J Allergy Clin Immunol*. 1996;97(6):1393–1401

60. US Environmental Protection Agency. *National Survey on Environmental Management of Asthma and Children's Exposure to Environmental Tobacco Smoke*. Washington, DC: US Environmental Protection Agency; 2004. https://19january2017snapshot.epa.gov/sites/production/files/2013-08/documents/survey_fact_sheet.pdf. Accessed June 4, 2018

61. US Environmental Protection Agency. Biomonitoring. In: *America's Children and the Environment (ACE)*. http://www.epa.gov/ace/ace-biomonitoring. Accessed June 4, 2018

62. Arquette M, Cole M, Cook K, et al. Holistic risk-based environmental decision making: a native perspective. *Environ Health Perspect*. 2002;110(Suppl 2):259–264

63. Burger J. Consumption patterns and why people fish. *Environ Res*. 2002;90(2):125–135

64. Burger J, Gaines KF, Boring CS, et al. Metal levels in fish from the Savannah River: potential hazards to fish and other receptors. *Environ Res*. 2002;89(1):85–97

65. Schell LM, Hubicki LA, DeCaprio AP, et al. Organochlorines, lead, and mercury in Akwesasne Mohawk youth. *Environ Health Perspect*. 2003;111(7):954–961

66. Fitzgerald EF, Hwang SA, Deres DA, Bush B, Cook K, Worswick P. The association between local fish consumption and DDE, mirex, and HCB concentrations in the breast milk of Mohawk women at Akwesasne. *J Expo Anal Environ Epidemiol*. 2001;11(5):381–388

67. Harper BL, Flett B, Harris S, Abeyta C, Kirschner F. The Spokane Tribe's multipathway subsistence exposure scenario and screening level RME. *Risk Anal*. 2002;22(3):513–526

68. Judd NL. Are seafood PCB data sufficient to assess health risk for high seafood consumption groups? *Hum Ecol Risk Assess*. 2003;9(3):691–707

69. Judd NL, Griffith WC, Faustman EM. Consideration of cultural and lifestyle factors in defining susceptible population for environmental disease. *Toxicology.* 2004;198(1-3):121–133

70. Hightower JM, O'Hare A, Hernandez GT. Blood mercury reporting in NHANES: identifying Asian, Pacific Islander, Native American, and multiracial groups. *Environ Health Perspect.* 2006;114(2):173–175

71. US Environmental Protection Agency. *Health Effects of Mercury.* Washington, DC: US Environmental Protection Agency; 2007

72. McKelvey W, Gwynn RC, Jeffery N, et al. A biomonitoring study of lead, cadmium, and mercury in the blood of New York City adults. *Environ Health Perspect.* 2007;115(10):1435–1441

73. Centers for Disease Control and Prevention. Blood lead levels in children aged 1–5 years — United States, 1999–2010. *MMWR Morb Mortal Wkly Rep.* 2013;62(13):245–248

74. Jacobs DE, Clickner RP, Zhou JY, et al. The prevalence of lead-based paint hazards in U.S. housing. *Environ Health Perspect.* 2002;110(10):A599–A606

75. Michigan News. What government owes Flint's poisoned immigrant community. http://www.mlive.com/news/index.ssf/2016/05/what_government_owes_flints_po.html. Accessed June 4, 2018

76. Northwestern Now. Flint's Undocumented Immigrants are Having Trouble Accessing Clean Water. https://news.northwestern.edu/stories/2016/02/opinion-quartz-flint-crisis/. Accessed June 4, 2018

77. National Public Radio. Flint's Undocumented Migrants Hesitate To Request Help During Water Crisis. https://www.npr.org/2016/01/28/464664785/flint-s-undocumented-immigrants-hesitate-to-ask-for-help-during-water-crisis. Accessed June 4, 2018

78. The Flint Water Crisis: Systemic Racism Through the Lens of Flint. http://www.michigan.gov/documents/mdcr/VFlintCrisisRep-F-Edited3-13-17_554317_7.pdf. Accessed June 4, 2018

79. Brown MJ, Margolis S. Lead in drinking water and human blood lead levels in the United States. *MMWR Suppl.* 2012;61(04):1–9

80. Curran R. Flint's Water Crisis Should Raise Alarms for America's Aging Cities. http://fortune.com/2016/01/25/flint-water-crisis-america-aging-cities-lead-pipes/. Accessed June 4, 2018

81. Al-Awamy BH. Evaluation of commonly used tribal and traditional remedies in Saudi Arabia. *Saudi Med J.* 2001;22(12):1065–1068

82. Centers for Disease Control and Prevention. Infant lead poisoning associated with use of tiro, an eye cosmetic from Nigeria—Boston, Massachusetts, 2011. *MMWR Morb Mortal Wkly Rep.* 2012;61(30):574–576

83. Davies JE, Edmundson WF, Raffonelli A, Cassady JC, Morgade C. The role of social class in human pesticide pollution. *Am J Epidemiol.* 1972;96(5):334–341

84. Arcury TA, Grzywacz JG, Barr DB, Tapia J, Chen H, Quandt SA. Pesticide urinary metabolite levels of children in eastern North Carolina farmworker households. *Environ Health Perspect.* 2007;115(8):1254–1260

85. Curwin BD, Hein MJ, Sanderson WT, et al. Pesticide dose estimates for children of Iowa farmers and non-farmers. *Environ Res.* 2007;105(3):307–315

86. Coronado GD, Vigoren EM, Thompson B, Griffith WC, Faustman EM. Organophosphate pesticide exposure and work in pome fruit: evidence for the take-home pesticide pathway. *Environ Health Perspect.* 2006;114(7):999–1006

87. Whyatt RM, Camann DE, Kinney PL, et al. Residential pesticide use during pregnancy among a cohort of urban minority women. *Environ Health Perspect.* 2002;110(5):507–514

88. American Association of Poison Control Centers. 2004 Poison Center Survey. http://www.aapcc.org/. Accessed June 4, 2018

89. New York City Department of Health and Mental Hygiene. Pests can be controlled... safely. *NYC Vital Signs*. 2005;4(3):1–4. http://www1.nyc.gov/assets/doh/downloads/pdf/survey/survey-2005pest.pdf. Accessed June 4, 2018.

90. Posadzki P, Watson L, Ernst E. Contamination and adulteration of herbal medicinal products (HMPs): an overview of systematic reviews. *Eur J Clin Pharmacol*. 2013;69(3):295–307

91. Commission for Racial Justice, United Church of Christ. *Toxic Wastes and Race in the United States: A National Study of the Racial and Socioeconomic Characteristics of Communities with Hazardous Waste Sites*. Cleveland, OH: United Church of Christ; 1987

92. Presidential Executive Order 12898: Federal Actions to Address Environmental Justice in Minority Populations and Low-Income Populations. 59 FR 7629 (1994)

93. Bullard R, Mohai P, Saha R, Wright B. *Toxic Wastes and Race at Twenty: 1987-2007. Grassroots Struggles to Dismantle Environmental Racism in the U.S.* Cleveland, OH: United Church of Christ, Justice and Witness Ministries; 2007

Chapter 56

# Ethical Issues in Environmental Health Research

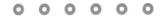

## KEY POINTS

- Regulations and ethical guidelines require that investigators protect the rights and welfare of human subjects who participate in environmental health research.
- Because children are susceptible to harm and exploitation, regulations and guidelines include additional protections for children, which limit the risks to which they may be exposed in research that does not directly benefit them.
- Regulations and guidelines require that investigators obtain consent from parents or guardians for children who participate in environmental health research, and the assent of children who are capable of providing assent.
- Environmental health research that focuses on communities should include provisions to protect the community from harm and solicit the community's input concerning study design and objectives, recruitment, and informed consent.
- Environmental health researchers should consider whether to share individual research results, such as results of laboratory tests, with participants and communities.

## INTRODUCTION

Ethical issues in the conduct of environmental health research on human subjects generally arise from conflicts between protecting the rights and welfare of individuals and promoting the good of society. Although environmental health research can benefit society in important ways, it may expose human research subjects to risks or compromise their rights to autonomy, dignity, and privacy. Because children are especially susceptible to harm and exploitation when they participate in research, they are classified as vulnerable subjects and given additional protections under federal research regulations and ethical guidelines. At the same time, children carry an outsized burden of disease from harmful exposures; therefore, ethical and scientifically sound research is of paramount importance.

This chapter will present some major challenges that investigators must address when conducting environmental health research involving children and offer guidelines for judging the ethical soundness of proposed environmental research protocols involving children. Other sources offer a more complete review of the ethical issues in biomedical research, public health research, and research involving children.[1-3]

## HISTORY

The consideration of ethical issues in medicine can be traced to the time of Hippocrates. Consideration of ethical issues related to biomedical and public health research is, for the most part, a post-World War II phenomenon. The world's first international research ethics guideline, The Nuremberg Code, was adopted in 1949 in response to the morally egregious research conducted by Nazi scientists and physicians on concentration camp prisoners.[4] Although the Nazi experiments helped to raise awareness of the importance of ethics in research with human subjects, the United States did not adopt any comprehensive regulations until the 1970s. The impetus for major policy changes in the United States was the public's growing awareness of unethical or ethically questionable research with human subjects, such as the Tuskegee syphilis study. In that study, federally funded researchers followed 400 African American men with untreated syphilis for several decades without informing them that they were in a research study or telling them about possible treatment for the disease (ie, penicillin) when it became available in the 1940s. Another study that drew considerable scrutiny was the Willowbrook hepatitis experiment in which investigators infected intellectually disabled children at the Willowbrook State School (on Staten Island in New York City) with hepatitis virus that was endemic at the facility to determine whether this would provide them with immunity to the virus.[4]

In 1973, a Congressional committee held hearings on unethical biomedical research conducted in the United States. These hearings led to the passage of the National Research Act (NRA), which authorized federal agencies to develop and revise their human research regulations and established the National Commission for the Protection of Human Subjects of Biomedical and Behavioral Research ("the National Commission").[4-7] In 1977, the National Commission published a report and recommendations that outlined conditions for the ethical conduct of research with children.[8] In 1978, the National Commission published the Belmont Report, titled *Ethical Principles and Guidelines for the Protection of Human Subjects of Research*.[9] This led to a major revision of Title 45, Code of Federal Regulations, Part 46 (45 CFR 46), also known as the Common Rule because it has been adopted in whole or in part by 17 federal agencies.[10] (Note: The Obama Administration announced revisions to the Common Rule on January 19, 2017.[11] Because the Trump Administration has delayed implementation of the revisions until July 19, 2018, this chapter refers to the previous version of the Common Rule. The revisions include expansion of research that is exempt from the Common Rule, additional informed consent requirements, and a mandate for institutions to rely on a single Institutional Review Board (IRB) for review of multisite research. The revisions do not affect the provisions under Subpart D for research involving children.) In 1991, the Common Rule was modified to include special protections for pregnant women, fetuses, neonates, children, and prisoners. Table 56-1 lists allowable categories of research involving children.[12] The Food and Drug Administration (FDA), which oversees research submitted in support of products subject to FDA approval, has regulations similar to the Common Rule's requirements. In addition, the American Academy of Pediatrics and the Academic Pediatric Association have provided recommendations about research involving children.[13-16]

A project undertaken by the staff of the Kennedy Krieger Institute (KKI), a research center associated with Johns Hopkins University in Baltimore, MD, brought concerns about ethical issues in environmental health research involving children to the public's consciousness. The KKI study was designed to compare different methods of lead abatement in homes containing lead paint. The study enrolled families living in homes with lead paint and 2 comparison groups. The first comparison group was composed of families living in houses that had been abated by the city of Baltimore. The second comparison group was composed of families living in houses built after 1978 that were presumably free of lead paint. The comparison group living in houses that had been abated by the city of Baltimore had received the maximum recommended level of lead abatement. Each of 3 experimental groups received different amounts of lead abatement but less than the maximum. The study addressed a significant

## Table 56-1. Allowable Categories of Research Involving Children Under Subpart D: 45 CFR 46 (Common Rule)

| CATEGORY (CFR) | POTENTIAL RISK | POTENTIAL BENEFIT | PARENTAL CONSENT | CHILD ASSENT[a] |
|---|---|---|---|---|
| 46.404 | No greater than minimal | Not necessarily | 1 parent | Yes |
| 46.405 | Justified by potential benefit | Sufficient to justify the risks | 1 parent | Yes |
| | Risk/benefit balance is at least as favorable as that presented by available alternatives | | | |
| 46.406 | Minor increase over minimal risk | No potential for direct benefit | 2 parents | Yes |
| | Intervention or procedure is similar to subject's naturally occurring situations | | | |
| | | Likely to yield generalizable knowledge of vital importance to understanding or ameliorating the condition being studied | | |
| 46.407[b] | | Not otherwise approvable but which 1. has the potential to further the understanding, prevention, or alleviation of a serious problem affecting health or welfare of children; or 2. Follows sound ethical principles | 2 parents | Yes |

Abbreviations: CFR, Code of Federal Regulations.
Adapted from Diekema 2006[12]

[a] Can be waived for children of certain ages if the Institutional Review Board (IRB) determines that the research holds the potential to benefit the child and is only available in the research context, or the child cannot be reasonably consulted.

[b] This category of research also requires that the IRB determine that the research provides a reasonable opportunity to further the understanding, prevention, or alleviation of a serious problem affecting the health and welfare of children, and approval by the secretary of the Department of Health and Human Services.

public health problem because full lead abatement is expensive (as much as $10,000 per home), and landlords might abandon homes if they were required to conduct full lead abatement. Researchers proposed that it was important to learn whether less expensive forms of lead abatement could protect children.

The parents of 2 children in the study filed lawsuits against the researchers and KKI, alleging that parents were not informed in a timely fashion about dangerous levels of lead detected in their children's blood or in the homes. The defendants moved to dismiss the lawsuit on grounds that they did not have legal duties to the research subjects because they did not have relationship with the defendants, such as physician/patient, that created legal duties. After the lower courts ruled in favor of the defendants, the plaintiffs appealed to the Maryland Court of Appeals, which ruled that defendants had legal duties of care to the plaintiffs, including an obligation to inform parents of dangerous lead levels in a timely fashion. The court also found that it was illegal to include children in research that does not offer medical benefits (often called nontherapeutic research). The court later stepped back from this position because it conflicted with federal regulations. The Maryland legislature then passed legislation to allow nontherapeutic research in children.[17-19]

In 2004, another controversy underscored the need for more discussion about ethical issues related to research on children's health and the environment. The US Environmental Protection Agency (EPA) and the Centers for Disease Control and Prevention (CDC) proposed a study known as the Children's Health Environmental Exposure Research Study (CHEERS).[20] The study proposed tracking the use of pesticides and household chemicals by families with young children living in Duvall County, Florida and the impact of those substances on children's health. The study came under severe criticism in the professional and lay press. Some argued that the study improperly targeted poor, minority families and that it encouraged parents to start using pesticides, which would expose children to health risks. Critics also argued that the study was ethically tainted by partial funding from the American Chemistry Council, an industry association that represents pesticide manufacturers and other chemical companies. Ultimately, the study was cancelled and did not begin.

## Regulatory Structure

The Common Rule includes requirements for the ethical conduct of research on humans funded by the federal government (Tables 56-1 and 56-2). The regulations mandate that research be reviewed by an Institutional Review Board (IRB), which is responsible for ensuring that the researcher complies with the regulations. IRBs must include at least 5 members from diverse backgrounds and having the appropriate expertise. At least one IRB member must not be affiliated with the institution and at least one member must not be a scientist. The Common Rule exempts some types of research from IRB review, such as research on de-identified samples or data and some types of survey research. To approve a research protocol that is not exempt from review, an IRB must determine that:[10]

- Risks to participants are minimized;
- Risks posed by research participation are reasonable in relation to potential benefits to the subjects or society via the knowledge expected to be gained;
- Participants are selected equitably;
- Informed consent is obtained and documented appropriately, in accordance with federal, state, and local regulations;
- Measures are taken to protect the privacy and confidentiality of participants; and
- If research involves vulnerable populations, such as children, additional safeguards are implemented.

Guidance for those additional safeguards for children can be found in Subpart D of the Common Rule. Researchers must be more vigilant about risks to which children might be exposed during the research (Table 56-2). The IRB can approve 3 types of pediatric studies: (1) research involving no more than minimal risk to the participants; (2) research involving more than minimal risk but with the prospect of benefits to the participants (eg, medical treatment); and (3) research involving a minor increase over minimal risk that is expected to yield important knowledge about the participants' medical disorders or conditions. Studies that do not fit into the 3 categories cannot be approved by the local IRB and must be referred to federal agencies for further review.[10]

The regulations also mandate that consent for participation must include permission from one or both parents or a guardian and, when age-appropriate, the assent of the child, depending on the nature of the study.[1,21,22] A commonly accepted age of assent is 7 years old. Permission from only 1 parent is sufficient when research does not involve more than minimal risk; if it involves greater than minimal risk, it must present the prospect of direct benefit to the child. Permission from both parents is required for any research that exceeds minimal risk and does not offer the prospect of direct benefit to the participant.[10] The IRB can waive the acquisition of parental signed consent under certain conditions.[10]

Although much public health and environmental health research focuses on or involves communities, the Common Rule does not provide guidance on community involvement in research except to ensure that participants are selected equitably, and the risks and benefits of the research are equitably distributed among the participants. The FDA regulations pertaining to emergency research involving regulated products, however, include a community consultation requirement.[4] (See subsequent discussion of community involvement and oversight.)

| Table 56-2. Guidelines for Judging the Ethical Soundness of Environmental Health Research Protocols Involving Children (Derived From Subpart D: 45 CFR 46) |
| --- |

An appropriate research protocol should consider and disclose the following:

1. The purpose of the research;

2. The expected duration of the child's involvement;

3. A description of procedures to be followed and identification of any experimental procedures;

4. A description of any reasonably foreseeable risks or discomforts to the subject;

5. A description of any reasonably expected benefits to the subject or others;

6. A disclosure of appropriate alternative procedures that may be advantageous to the subject;

7. A description of the extent to which the confidentiality of records will be maintained;

8. An explanation as to whether any compensation is provided or what treatments are available if injury occurs;

9. An explanation of whom to contact with questions about the research;

10. A statement that enrollment is voluntary and that refusal to enroll or to continue to participate, once enrolled, will not result in a loss of benefits the child is otherwise entitled to;

11. Information about the nature of the risk or hazard being studied;

12. Assurance that the subject will be informed of any significant findings discovered during the study that might influence their willingness to continue to participate;

13. Circumstances when the subject may be terminated from the study by the investigator without the consent of the subject; and

14. Although reimbursement of study participants for out-of-pocket expenses is appropriate, care must be taken to ensure that any tokens of appreciation or payments for time and inconvenience are not sufficient to influence a parent's or child's decision to participate or not to participate in the study.

Environmental research often seeks information about early life exposures, including exposures in infancy or in utero. Therefore, enrollment and protection of women who may become pregnant, are pregnant at the time of enrollment, or who become pregnant after enrollment is another issue for IRBs to address. In research involving women who are pregnant, the fetus must not be exposed to more than minimal risk if the research does not offer the woman or the fetus direct benefits.

## THE INSTITUTIONAL REVIEW BOARD

For research projects undertaken in academic institutions, the IRB that reviews the proposal is usually housed in the same institution, which helps to ensure that the IRB considers the local context (such as values, traditions, or beliefs) when reviewing the proposal. In some instances, however, researchers may seek approval from non-local IRBs that are independent of academic institutions. This may be a particularly relevant issue in research involving communities.

The Common Rule defines the responsibilities of the IRB to interpret the federal regulations and apply them to individual research projects. Before research can be conducted, protocols and consent forms must be reviewed and approved by an IRB to ensure compliance with all federal, state, and local laws and regulations. IRBs are responsible for ensuring that research protocols meet specific requirements as described earlier, including that the research is ethical and the protocol will be conducted in a responsible manner. The members of the IRB, in the aggregate, must possess the expertise to evaluate and oversee the research. This includes expertise in child health and in environmental health research for IRBs that review these types of protocols. The typical university-based IRB, which is usually constituted to evaluate university-based research, may not have the appropriate representation to adequately evaluate and oversee environmental health research involving communities. (See subsequent discussion of community advisory boards or environmental health and community review boards.)

## CHILDREN'S INFORMED CONSENT: A SPECIAL CIRCUMSTANCE

The Nuremberg Code states that informed consent is "absolutely essential" to the ethical conduct of research to ensure that the research participant's involvement is not based on "force, fraud, deceit, duress, overreaching, or other ulterior forms of constraint or coercion."[23] Because informed consent is the primary mechanism by which investigators respect the autonomy of research participants, children present a unique challenge because below a certain age, they do not possess the cognitive or emotional maturity needed to make informed decisions. Investigators therefore rely on the proxy judgments of children's parents or legal guardians to offer permission on their behalf, because they assume that parents are in the best position to make choices in line with the child's interests, emerging values, and commitments.

In addition to obtaining parental consent, researchers must procure the child's assent when the IRB deems that the child is capable of providing it based on age, maturity, and psychological development. Assent refers to a "child's voluntary affirmative agreement to participate in research"[10] and, like parental consent, requires the active agreement of the child to participate and not just a failure to object to participation.

The form of assent and information provided will vary depending on the child's maturity. When there is no prospect of direct benefit from participation, children have the right to refuse to participate and to have their dissent respected.

Information collected about children for research purposes may require more than conventional privacy protections, especially for longitudinal studies. Outcomes that may not manifest until years later require long-term data storage and analysis of data, years after a pregnancy is completed or a child is grown. Data cannot be completely de-identified because they will need to be linked with subsequently collected data. Given the gap between data collection periods and children's developing abilities to understand their rights, the privacy rights of children who are participating in longitudinal studies are best protected by viewing parental permission and child assent as ongoing processes that are repeated at appropriate intervals.[24,25] Researchers should allow child participants who reach the age of majority to re-consent or withdraw consent when: (1) the participants are currently enrolled in a study and data and sample collection is ongoing, or (2) when the research is complete but the researchers retain identified samples or data. Child participants who withdraw from research when they reach the age of majority should have the opportunity to have their samples destroyed and data removed from the study, to the extent possible.

## COMMUNITY INVOLVEMENT IN RESEARCH

The primary responsibility of IRBs is to protect individual research participants, but some public health and environmental health research may focus on or significantly impact communities. Such research has the potential to harm as well as help participants, including the members of the community. A community-based project could help a community by generating knowledge that community members can use to promote their own health, or that community representatives could use to leverage government and private resources needed to address health problems in the community. A community-based project could harm a community if it yields information concerning health problems that leads to discrimination, bias, or stigma against community members.[25,26] To protect the community and its members and to consider unique issues that arise when communities are involved in research, some have suggested that investigators work with advisory boards composed of community representatives.[27] Although community approval of a research project should not take the place of the participant's consent, it can play an important role in building the community's trust in the investigators and the research institution. Community advisory boards can enhance research design and implementation by providing investigators with important information concerning community values, traditions, and beliefs that may be relevant to recruitment, publicity, informed consent, protocol and survey development, and publication.[25,26]

An environmental health and community review board combines the fundamental responsibilities and ethical precepts of the traditional IRB with an expanded ethical construct of dignity, veracity, sustainability, and justice and an added focus on community.[26] Dignity incorporates the concept of autonomy with the notion of a right to understand the research and the outcomes of the research. Veracity reflects transparency, indicating that all relevant facts have been revealed, thus allowing the community to make a decision about what is good (beneficence) and what protects them from harm (non-maleficence). Sustainability means that businesses and individuals within the community are likely to thrive as a result of participating in the research. In this context, the notion of justice is expanded to encompass the community and extends beyond the self-interest of an individual or individual business.

## REPORTING RESULTS

Considerable controversy and uncertainty exist about whether to report individual results of environmental contamination or body burden to study subjects. The National Bioethics Advisory Commission[28] recommends disclosing individual results only when the findings have been scientifically validated and confirmed; the findings have significant implications for the subject's health; and a course of action to ameliorate or treat these health issues is readily available. The rationale for this position is that it benefits research subjects by providing them with useful health information and avoids causing them harm or undue concern by sharing results that are false or have uncertain clinical utility.[28] Some ethicists, however, argue that respect for research participants requires investigators to provide individual results to study participants so that they can decide what to do with the information.[28]

Most environmental health researchers and community advocates would agree that results of commonly used clinical tests or biomarkers that conform to the National Bioethics Advisory Commission's criteria, such as blood lead concentration and skin allergy testing, should be reported promptly to families. Most would also agree that laboratories performing tests for biomarkers or environmental indicators should follow quality control procedures designed to ensure that tests results are accurate and reliable. Ideally, the laboratory should have Clinical Laboratory Improvement Amendments (CLIA) certification. Although laboratories that perform clinical tests are required to have CLIA certification, those that test for research purposes are not required to have CLIA certification. There is therefore some debate about whether to share tests results from non–CLIA-certified laboratories with participants.[28]

# References

1. Institute of Medicine, Committee on Clinical Research Involving Children, Board on Health Sciences Policy. *The Ethical Conduct of Research Involving Children*. Field MJ, Behrman RE, eds. Washington, DC: The National Academies Press; 2004

2. Ross LF. *Children in Medical Research: Access Versus Protection (Issues in Biomedical Ethics)*. Oxford, England: Oxford University Press; 2006

3. Kodish E. *Ethics and Research with Children. A Case-Based Approach*. Oxford, England: Oxford University Press; 2005

4. Shamoo AE, Resnik DB. *Responsible Conduct of Research*. 3rd ed. New York, NY: Oxford University Press; 2015

5. Faden RR. Human-subjects research today: final report of the advisory committee on human radiation experiments. *Acad Med*. 1996;71(5):482–483

6. Krugman S. The Willowbrook hepatitis studies revisited: ethical aspects. *Rev Infect Dis*. 1986;8(1):157–162

7. Rothman DJ. Research ethics at Tuskegee and Willowbrook. *Am J Med*. 1984;77(6):A49

8. National Commission for the Protection of Human Subjects of Biomedical and Behavioral Research. Report and Recommendations: Research Involving Children. Washington, DC: National Commission for the Protection of Human Subjects of Biomedical and Behavioral Research; 1977. http://videocast.nih.gov/pdf/ohrp_research_involving_children.pdf. Accessed April 2, 2018

9. National Institutes of Health. Belmont Report on Ethical Principles and Guidelines for the Protection of Human Subjects of Research. Bethesda, MD: National Institutes of Health, Office on Human Subjects Research; 1979. Accessed April 2, 2018

10. Department of Health and Human Services. Federal Policy for the Protection of Human Subjects (45 CFR 46). https://www.hhs.gov/ohrp/regulations-and-policy/regulations/common-rule/index.html. Accessed April 2, 2018

11. Department of Homeland Security; Department of Agriculture; Department of Energy; National Aeronautics and Space Administration; Department of Commerce; Social Security Administration; Agency for International Development; Department of Housing and Urban Development; Department of Labor; Department of Defense; Department of Education; Department of Veterans Affairs; Environmental Protection Agency; Department of Health and Human Services; National Science Foundation; and Department of Transportation. Federal policy for the protection of human subjects. *Fed Regist*. 2017;82(12):7149–7274

12. Diekema DS. Conducting ethical research in pediatrics: a brief historical overview and review of pediatric regulations. *J Pediatr*. 2006;149(1 Suppl):S3–S11

13. American Academy of Pediatrics, Committee on Bioethics. Institutional ethics committees. *Pediatrics*. 2001;107(1):205–209

14. American Academy of Pediatrics, Committee on Bioethics. Informed consent, parental permission, and assent in pediatric practice. *Pediatrics*. 1995;95(2):314–317

15. American Academy of Pediatrics, Committee on Native American Child Health and Committee on Community Health Services. Ethical considerations in research with socially identifiable populations. *Pediatrics*. 2004;113(1 Pt 1):148–151

16. Etzel RA, APA Research Committee. Ambulatory Pediatric Association policy statement: ensuring integrity for research with children. *Ambul Pediatr*. 2005;5(1):3–5

17. Grimes v. Kennedy Krieger Institute. 782 A.2d 807 (2001). 366 Md. 29

18. Phoenix JA. Ethical considerations of research involving minorities, the poorly educated and/or low-income populations. *Neurotoxicol Teratol*. 2002;24(4):475–476

19. Pinder L. Commentary on the Kennedy Krieger Institute lead paint repair and maintenance study. *Neurotoxicol Teratol.* 2002;24(4):477–479

20. Resnik DB, Wing S. Lessons learned from the Children's Environmental Exposure Research Study. *Am J Public Health.* 2007;97(3):414–418

21. American Academy of Pediatrics, Committee on Drugs. Guidelines for the ethical conduct of studies to evaluate drugs in pediatric populations. *Pediatrics.* 1995;95(2):286

22. Wendler D. Protecting subjects who cannot give consent: toward a better standard for "minimal" risks. *Hastings Cent Rep.* 2005;35(5):37–43

23. National Institutes of Health, Office on Human Subjects of Research. Nuremberg Code. https://history.nih.gov/research/downloads/nuremberg.pdf. Accessed April 2, 2018

24. Fisher CB. Privacy and ethics in pediatric environmental health research—part I: genetic and prenatal testing. *Environ Health Perspect.* 2006;114(10):1617–1621

25. Fisher CB. Privacy and ethics in pediatric environmental health research—part II: protecting families and communities. *Environ Health Perspect.* 2006;114(10):1622–1625

26. Gilbert SG. Supplementing the traditional institutional review board with an environmental health and community review board. *Environ Health Perspect.* 2006;114(10):1626–1629

27. Institute of Medicine, Board on Children, Youth, and Families and Behavioral and Social Sciences and Education. *Ethical Considerations for Research on Housing-Related Health Hazards Involving Children.* Lo B, O'Connell ME, eds. Washington, DC: National Academies Press; 2005

28. National Bioethics Advisory Commission. *Research Involving Human Biological Materials: Ethical Issues and Policy Guidance. National Children's Study.* Rockville, MD

# Chapter 57

# Fracking

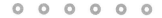

## KEY POINTS

- Fracking (also referred to as "hydraulic fracturing" or "unconventional gas extraction") releases hazardous chemicals into the air and water, some from chemicals used in the process and some from naturally occurring chemicals in the ground.
- The exact nature of many chemicals used to make the hydraulic fracturing fluid is not made public, making it impossible to conduct full risk assessments.
- A growing number of studies show associations between living near unconventional natural gas well sites and adverse health outcomes.

## INTRODUCTION

Shale is a common form of sedimentary rock. Shale that contains oil (ie, oil shale),[1] was formed millions of years ago by deposition of silt and organic debris on lakebeds and sea bottoms. This type of shale contains oil or natural gas in microscopic pockets. The shale is similar to a sponge with tiny pockets holding the gas, except that this sponge is rock hard. Shale containing natural gas can be found in almost half of the states in the United States.[2] Moreover, it is estimated that 17.6 million people live within 1,600 m (<1 mi) of at least one active oil and/or gas well.[3] For those reasons, pediatricians in many parts of the country may get questions about unconventional gas extraction (UGE).

## THE UNCONVENTIONAL GAS EXTRACTION PROCESS

The overall process to recover natural gas from shale rock includes multiple steps (Table 57-1).[4,5]

| Table 57-1. Steps to Recover Natural Gas from Shale Rock |
| --- |

1. Pad construction – leveling of land and other preparation for drilling
2. Drill set-up
3. Drilling
   a. Vertical drilling
   b. Horizontal drilling - When vertical drilling reaches desired depth, the drill turns horizontally and continues drilling for up to a mile or more. This creates what is known as long laterals.
4. Hydraulic fracturing
   a. Water is mixed with chemicals to reduce its viscosity. The product is referred to as "slick water."
   b. The slick water is then mixed with a proppant. This can be sand or some other substance that can wedge into the tiny fractures created in the rock and hold them open. An analogy would be a cardiac stent.
   c. A number of additional chemicals (see Table 57-3) also are mixed with the slick water.
   d. Water + chemicals to reduce viscosity + proppant + other chemicals = hydraulic fracturing fluid (HFF)
   e. The HFF is then pumped underground at extremely high pressure that can exceed 9,000 lbs/in$^2$ (632.8 kg/cm$^2$) into the shale to break open the small pockets of gas.
   f. Hydraulic fracturing fluid and gas return to the surface.
      i. The material that returns to the surface is known as flow-back water.
      ii. Flow-back water contains not only the chemicals sent down the pipe but also chemicals that became dissolved in the HFF, such as brine and radon.
      iii. Gas and water are separated.
         1. Gas is compressed and piped or trucked off-site for distribution.
         2. Gas may be flared or burned on-site.
         3. Gas may be vented into the atmosphere.
         4. Water may be reprocessed and reused.
         5. Water may be stored in pits on-site (not as common now as 5 to 10 years ago).
         6. Water may be trucked off-site for processing.
   g. Wells are usually fracked multiple times.
5. Well decommissioning – occurs months to years later depending on the well
6. Land restoration – years later

Figure 57-1 illustrates the UGE water cycle.

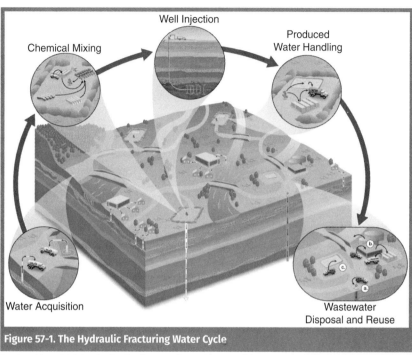

**Figure 57-1. The Hydraulic Fracturing Water Cycle**

Reprinted from *EPA's Study of Hydraulic Fracturing and Its Potential Impact on Drinking Water Resources.*
https://www.epa.gov/hfstudy/hydraulic-fracturing-water-cycle.

## PUBLIC HEALTH CONCERNS IN UNCONVENTIONAL GAS EXTRACTION

Although each step in the UGE process may have health consequences, public health concerns arise from pad construction, drilling, hydraulic fracturing, natural gas extraction, and gas processing stages. Drill set-up, well decommissioning, and land restoration have potential adverse health impacts for workers but generally not for the public.

### Air Pollution

Air pollution occurs during every stage of UGE. Chemicals emitted into the air or formed as a result of chemical reactions in the air vary from place to place because different chemicals are used in the fracking fluid; different chemicals return from underground in flow-back and produced water (water that returns once the well is producing gas); the composition of the gas extracted varies; and chemicals vary as different stages in the process occur. Chemicals in the air may vary in the same place at the same part in the process on a day-to-day basis.[6] In an analysis of all chemicals used in UGE processes, 37% were found

| Table 57-2. Emissions Occurring in Conjunction With Natural Gas Facilities |
|---|
| Acetaldehyde |
| Benzene |
| Butadiene |
| CO (carbon monoxide) |
| 1,3, carbon disulfide |
| Carbon tetrachloride |
| Ethyl benzene |
| Formaldehyde |
| *n*-Hexane |
| NOx (oxides of nitrogen) |
| PM$_{2.5}$ (particulate matter less than 2.5 microns) |
| PM$_{10}$ (particulate matter less than 10 microns) |
| SOx (oxides of sulfur) |
| Toluene |
| Tetrachloroethylene |
| 2,2,4-trimethylpentane |
| Trimethyl pentene |
| VOCs (volatile organic compounds) |
| Xylenes (isomers and mixtures) |

Adapted from Brown et al[6]

to be volatile and therefore able to aerosolize.[7] Of these volatile chemicals, 81% were known central nervous system toxicants.[7] Table 57-2 lists possible emissions from natural gas facilities.

During site preparation, heavy equipment is used to clear and prepare the well pad site and to create new roads. These vehicles and diesel generators produce emissions, and there is increased coarse particulate matter and dust from new roads and increased truck traffic on roads. During the drilling phase, diesel generators operate around the clock to power the drill, lights, and other equipment. Trucks continue to bring supplies to the well site. These generators and trucks contribute to diesel-associated air pollution. Analysis of materials from a well explosion prior to the fracking process of the well revealed 22 chemicals used in the drilling process of which 100% had adverse respiratory effects.[8] The period after fracking, when gas starts to come back to the surface, is the highest period of air pollution,[9] with air pollutants such as methane, hydrogen sulfide, and volatile organic compounds (VOCs) coming back to the surface in flow-back water. Venting (releasing gas to the atmosphere), and flaring (burning gas at the well as waste)—where they occur—also contribute to air pollution. Other equipment and the gas pipelines themselves release methane and other VOCs that can contribute to the formation of ozone.

## Air Pollution from Diesel Engines and Truck Traffic

Thousands of truck trips are necessary to establish a pad, set up the drilling equipment, bring workers and supplies to the pad, drill and frack the well, and remove waste from the pad. Trucks are used to bring large quantities of water from the source to the well pad. It is estimated that between 1 and 10 million gallons (3.78 and 37.8 million liters) of water are required to frack a well a single time. Thousands of tons of sand must be trucked in. One analysis commissioned by the New York State Department of Environmental Conservation estimated that approximately 1,975 round trips with heavy-load trucks and 1,420 round trips with light trucks took place for each horizontal well with high-volume hydraulic fracturing.[10] Materials to construct the well, such as pipe segments that can be 31 to 48 feet (9.4 to 14.6 m) long, also must be brought to the pad. If a well is 7,000 feet (2.1 km) deep and extends one mile laterally, almost 260 segments each measuring 48 feet (14.6 m) are required.

The large volume of truck traffic creates dust and particulate matter. For people who live along haul routes, this truck traffic increases diesel exhaust, noise, and vibration, and creates safety risks. Traffic also increases from a larger population of workers who commute to and from pads. A health impact assessment in Battlement Mesa, Colorado, estimated that traffic would increase by 40 to 280 truck trips per day per pad, and that 120 to 150 additional workers would commute to the well pads.[11]

Diesel exhaust includes carbon dioxide, oxygen, carbon monoxide, nitrogen compounds, sulfur compounds, low molecular weight hydrocarbons, formaldehyde, acetaldehyde, acrolein, benzene, 1-3 butadiene, and polycyclic aromatic hydrocarbons (PAHs). Diesel exhaust particulates include PAHs, sulfates, nitrates, metals, organic chemicals, and trace elements. PAHs are carcinogenic and cause respiratory problems.[12] Much of the particulate matter in diesel exhaust is at the $PM_{2.5}$ (also known as fine particulate) level. $PM_{2.5}$ particles are small enough to bypass many of the body's protective mechanisms to enter further into the lungs than $PM_{10}$ (also known as coarse particles). $PM_{2.5}$ particles are small enough to enter directly into the bloodstream and are considered more hazardous than $PM_{10}$ particles. Diesel exhaust is recognized as a human carcinogen.[13-16] One study found high PAH levels in the ambient air near UGE sites.[8] Samples taken closer to wells had higher PAH levels. PAH levels closest to natural gas activity "were an order of magnitude higher than levels previously reported in rural areas."

## Air Pollution from Extraction

Release of hazardous air pollutants (HAPs), methane, and VOCs can occur at any stage of exploration. During production, release can occur through venting (ie, intentional release of the gas to the atmosphere) or through flashing or flaring (ie, burning the gas at the top of a pipe in the open air). During storage and transportation, there can be fugitive emissions.[17] Most VOC emissions during extraction come during the well completion phase. Trucks, pneumatic controllers, and drill rigs also are significant sources.[18] Many pieces of industrial equipment—including diesel trucks, diesel engines, drilling rigs, power generators, phase separators, dehydrators, storage tanks, compressors, and pipelines—are needed during UGE. Each can be a source of methane, VOCs, nitrogen oxides, particulate matter, and other gases.[18] Methane coming up from the well is not pure but is a mixture of methane and other VOCs and HAPs. Once methane is recovered and moved through tanks, pumps, pneumatics, and pipelines, all components leak to some degree, or vent by design as with pneumatic controllers, and thereby contribute to air pollution. Even during the use phase of methane, natural gas continues to leak from pipes and storage containers. Recently, in Boston, Massachusetts, 3,356 methane leaks exceeding 2.5 parts per million (ppm)[19] (a level of 2.5 ppm is higher than the normal background level of methane) were identified; in Washington, DC, 5,893 methane leaks above 2.5 ppm were identified.[20]

### Air Pollution from Flaring

Flaring (burning of methane and other gases not captured for commercial sale) is done at the top of the stack in the open air. Federal regulations limit flaring but there are instances in which it is still allowed.[21] Emissions from this incomplete combustion include VOCs, carbon monoxide, particulate matter, sulfur dioxide, nitrogen dioxide,[22] hydrogen sulfide, acetaldehyde, acrolein, benzene, ethylbenzene, formaldehyde, hexane, naphthalene, propylene, toluene, and xylenes.[23]

### Air Pollution from Compressor Stations and Dehydrators

Compressor stations, which are fueled by gas coming directly from the ground (ie, unrefined natural gas) are another significant source of emissions that include diesel exhausts, VOCs, oxides of nitrogen and sulfur, carbon monoxide, carbon dioxide, and ozone. Dehydrators may leak glycol, water, and other compounds in the liquid phase of the flow-back material benzene, toluene, ethylbenzene, and xylene.[24]

### Air Pollution from Sand

Sand, usually consisting of silicon dioxide (also known as silica), is used as a proppant, or a wedge, to hold open the fractures in the shale to allow the gas to escape. When sand is mined, transported, or used at the drill site before wetting, it can become aerosolized, presenting a hazard to the miners and workers on the pad. Aerosolized sand is a known cause of silicosis.[25] Studies have not been conducted to determine whether sand used at the drill site poses any health threat to individuals away from the pad site.

### Air Pollution from Hazardous Air Pollutants and Volatile Organic Compounds

Hazardous air pollutants, methane, and other VOCs are leaked into the air intentionally and unintentionally. Leakage begins once flow-back starts and continues from wellheads, compressor stations, storage facilities, and pipelines. Debate exists about the amount of gas leaked throughout the supply chain. One study estimated that between 3.6% and 7.9% of the lifetime production of a shale gas well is vented or leaked to the atmosphere.[26] The US Environmental Protection Agency (EPA) estimates that just 1.5% of the lifetime production of gas produced is lost.[27]

Methane is the main component of the gas released from the ground following hydraulic fracturing. The gas also contains chemicals, such as benzene, that must be separated from methane before being transported through pipelines for use in businesses and homes for purposes such as cooking and heating. Although there are no studies examining the relationship between benzene exposure from UGE and adverse health outcomes, studies examined child health outcomes after perinatal exposure to benzene from Texas petroleum refineries. Studies using the Texas birth defects registry found associations between a woman's estimated exposure to benzene during pregnancy and an increased likelihood of having children with neural tube defects (NTDs) and the two most common types of leukemia (acute lymphocytic leukemia and acute myeloid leukemia).[28,29] Various US and international agencies consider benzene to be a human carcinogen.[30–32] McKenzie et al[33] found an association between maternal residence in proximity to UGE sites and congenital heart defects and possibly NTDs in offspring. A study in France assessed perinatal exposure to benzene in women who wore monitors to collect data on their personal benzene exposure. Women with the most exposure to automobile and truck traffic near their homes were more likely to have children with smaller growth parameters than women who were less exposed to traffic near their homes.[34]

McKenzie et al[9] performed a human health risk assessment of air emissions to quantify the risk of non-cancer and cancer outcomes. Exposure was estimated for residents who lived less than half a mile from well pads and residents who lived more than a half mile away. Exposure was determined with ambient air samples around well pads and categorized as "during the well completion phase," "when at least one well was undergoing uncontrolled flow-back emissions," and "not during the completion phase." High exposure during the completion phase was estimated to create the greatest risk as a result of higher exposure levels to several hydrocarbons.[5] Residents who lived less than a half mile (0.8 km) from a well had an elevated risk of both non-cancer and cancer outcomes. The elevated risk for cancer was found to be 6 in 1 million for residents living less than half a mile (0.8 km) from the well, and 10 in 1 million for residents living more than half a mile (0.8 km) from the well, both above the US EPA target of acceptable cancer risk of 1 in a million.[9] The authors noted that benzene was a major component of the elevated cancer risk.

Macey et al[35] found markedly elevated levels of multiple air pollutants in samples from Arkansas, Colorado, Ohio, Pennsylvania, and Wyoming. Many samples that showed elevated benzene levels were collected on residential property close to well pads (30 to 350 yards [27 to 320 m]). The study authors stated that "[t]he results suggest that existing regulatory setback distances from wells to residences may not be adequate to reduce human health risks."[35]

Models created for the New York State *Draft Supplementary General Environmental Impact Statement*[22] indicate that particulate matter will be dispersed over long distances. To meet National Ambient Air Quality Standards (NAAQS), receptor distance had to be greater than 80 m for $PM_{10}$ and 500 m for $PM_{2.5}$. Colburn et al[36] found many VOCs in air samples gathered at a residence 1.1 km from UGE facilities and where there was no nearby industrial activity.

### Air Pollution from Ozone

Unconventional gas extraction processes create an environment in which there are multiple precursors to ozone formation. Ozone is formed when oxides of nitrogen, which can come from diesel exhaust, and VOCs interact with sunlight. Ground-level ozone is a lung irritant. Health effects associated with ozone include shortness of breath, coughing, and exacerbation of chronic lung diseases such as asthma.[37] Damage to the lungs continues even when symptoms have dissipated.

Exposure to ozone during childhood not only exacerbates asthma, but also can lead to new onset of asthma[38] as well as permanently impact lung function. The Children's Health Study examined lung function of 3,677 children aged 10 to 18 years to determine the role of air pollution in lung development.[39] Children living within 500 meters of a freeway had less lung function compared with counterparts living 1,500 or more meters from a freeway.[39] Everyone loses some lung function with age; in children with decreased lung function, chronic lung diseases may be more likely to develop when they become adults.

In general, ozone levels in metropolitan areas are higher in the summer. In the Upper Green River basin of Wyoming, Field et al[40] found that high levels of ozone were produced in the winter. In 2012, the Upper Green River basin was designated a non-attainment zone for the NAAQS for ozone. Three contributing factors—combustion/traffic, fugitive natural gas, and fugitive condensate—were identified. In a study of air pollution in southwestern Pennsylvania, researchers found that UGE contributed high quantities of VOCs to the atmosphere, enough to make compliance with ozone standards more difficult.[41]

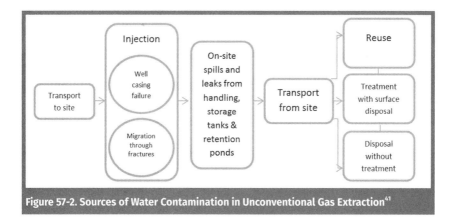

**Figure 57-2. Sources of Water Contamination in Unconventional Gas Extraction[41]**

## Water Pollution

Figure 57-2 describes areas within the UGE process in which water contamination may occur. During the drilling or injection process, well casing failure may occur, and gas or water can migrate through fractures. On the well pad, water contamination can occur because of spills or leaks from storage or movement of drilling mud, frack fluid, produced water, chemicals, and fluid held onsite in tanks or containment ponds.

### Methane and Other Substances in Water

Well-documented episodes of migration of natural gas into drinking water have been found in Pennsylvania and Texas. Researchers sampled Pennsylvania wells and demonstrated that proximity to a well increases the risk of having methane and other VOCs in well water.[42] Samples analyzed from 141 drinking water wells showed that methane concentrations in drinking water wells from homes less than 1 km from natural gas wells (59 of 141) were 6 times higher on average than concentrations from homes farther away. Ethane and propane concentrations also were higher in drinking water of homes near natural gas wells; for example, ethane concentrations were 23 times higher on average for homes less than 1 km from a gas well.[43] Analysis of carbon isotopes from methane in these wells showed that the methane was made thousands of years ago and therefore was more likely to come from shale gas, as opposed to newer methane, which can occur with decomposing organic material. The causes of gas migration and stray gas are well known, but the risk of this migration process is difficult to predict because of differing geology and drilling practices.[44] An analysis of the aquifer serving at least 3 homes in Bradford County, Pennsylvania, showed contamination with multiple chemicals associated with drilling and fracturing fluids.[43–45] Well water in aquifers over Barnett shale in Texas was found to contain arsenic, selenium, strontium, and total dissolved solids at levels greater than the water maximum contaminant level (MCL) set by the US EPA, and more than in wells not located over Barnett shale.[44–46]

### Hydraulic Fracturing Fluid in Water

Hydraulic fracturing fluid is a mixture of substances pumped underground at very high pressure to break up the gas-containing shale. In most instances, the primary component of the hydraulic fracturing fluid is water. Other components include a proppant, a substance such as sand used to prop open the tiny fractures, and various chemicals such as those listed in Table 57-3. Brine solutions, radon, and other chemicals that normally occur underground become dissolved in or mixed with the hydraulic fracturing fluid and return to the surface in the form of flow-back water. The hydraulic fracturing fluid and material added from underground have the potential to contaminate ground or surface waters and thereby expose humans.

The composition of hydraulic fracturing fluid can vary widely depending on a number of factors. Hydraulic fracturing fluids have many components including surfactants, acids, gelling agents, biocides, proppants, bactericides, corrosion inhibitors, stabilizers, and friction reducers.[47] Colburn et al[7] identified 632 chemicals used in the drilling, fracking, processing, and transport processes; this number only represents the chemicals in products with listed Chemical Abstract Service (CAS) numbers. The same study found that for 407 of the 944 products identified (43%), there was essentially no available information about product composition.[7] A study from Pennsylvania found 181 unique chemicals (81% of total chemicals) with CAS numbers and 19% proprietary chemicals (without CAS numbers).[48] Data collected by the Minority Staff of the Committee on Energy and Commerce of the US House of Representatives in 2011, based on data submitted by the 14 leading oil and gas service companies, revealed the use of more than 2,500 hydraulic fracturing products containing 750 chemicals and other components.[47] From the limited information available, it is evident that many substances used in hydraulic fracturing fluid are toxic, including some that are known carcinogens or endocrine disrupting chemicals.

Kassotis et al[49] studied potential endocrine disrupting characteristics of chemicals added to hydraulic fracturing fluid. Groundwater and surface water samples were collected from areas with much UGE activity and compared with water collected from areas with less or no UGE activity. Groundwater and surface water samples had varying degrees of estrogenic, anti-estrogenic, or anti-androgenic activity in test assays, generally with higher activities in samples collected from UGE areas with higher activity. Not all differences were statistically significant.

Companies are not required to disclose the contents of their products, and listing "proprietary ingredients" is an acceptable description. As a result, the full range of chemicals that can be incorporated into hydraulic fracturing fluid has never been publicly revealed. This makes it nearly impossible to determine the possible exposures to workers and individuals in nearby communities. This situation is untenable for first responders, emergency and primary care providers, poison control centers, pediatric environmental health specialty units, occupational medicine providers, and other health care providers. Appropriate emergency planning is also impossible as are accurate diagnostic and therapeutic decisions about exposed individuals. Table 57-3 lists hydraulic fracturing fluid additives and their purposes.

| Table 57-3. Hydraulic Fracturing Fluid Additives, Their Purpose, and Examples[7,50] | | |
|---|---|---|
| **ADDITIVE TYPE** | **USES** | **MAIN COMPONENTS** |
| Acid | Removes near well damage, cleans out the wellbore, dissolves minerals, initiates cracks in rock | Hydrochloric acid |
| Biocide | Controls bacterial growth | Glutaraldehyde, 2,2-dibromo-3-nitrilopropionamide (DBNPA) |
| Breaker | Delays breakdown of the gelling agent | Ammonium persulfate |
| Corrosion inhibitor | Prevents corrosion of pipes | N,N-dimethyl formamide |
| Crosslinker | Maintains fluid viscosity as temperature increases | Borate salts |
| Friction reducers | Decreases pumping friction | Polyacrylamide, petroleum distillate |
| Gelling agents | Improves proppant placement | Guar gum, hydroxyethyl cellulose |
| Potassium chloride | Creates a brine carrier fluid | Potassium chloride |
| Oxygen scavenger | Prevents corrosion of well tubulars | Ammonium bisulfite |
| pH adjusting agent | Adjusts pH of fluid to maintain effectiveness of other components | Sodium carbonate, carbonate |
| Scale inhibitor | Prevents scale deposits in the pipe | Ethylene glycol |
| Surfactant | Winterizing agent | Isopropanol, ethanol, 2-butoxyethanol |

## Normally Occurring Underground Toxic Substances in Water

When water, sand, and chemicals are injected into the drill hole, some water stays underground but as much as 90% is estimated to return to the surface during extraction. In addition to the materials injected into water, other materials return with the fracturing fluid, including radioactive material, salts of manganese, chlorides, sodium, bromides, and heavy metals such as lead and arsenic.[44] "Flow-back" water refers to the water that returns during the fracking process; "produced" water returns once the well is producing gas and continues to return throughout the life of the well. Materials that would otherwise be stored in the rock and do not have a pathway of exposure to humans are released and come back with fracturing fluids. In the Marcellus shale area of Pennsylvania, as much as 200 tons of salt per well can return in flow-back water.[44] Naturally occurring radioactive material (NORM) is radiation underground in geographic formations that becomes "technologically enhanced naturally occurring radioactive material" (TENORM) when it is disturbed and has the potential to expose humans.[51] Radionuclides in natural gas wastes include radon, [226]radium, and [228]radium, and radionuclides of potassium, strontium, lead, thallium, bismuth, and thorium. Radium in flow-back and produced water often incorporates into solids formed during wastewater treatment, thereby producing low-level radioactive waste.

Casey et al[52] showed a statistically significant upward trend in residential basement radon levels from 2004 to 2012 in Pennsylvania counties, with higher levels in counties having 100 wells or more drilled for UGE production versus counties with none, with the highest levels in the Reading Prong, a section of Pennsylvania with high bedrock uranium concentrations.

## Wastewater

Up to 90% of the water injected during the hydraulic fracturing phase (flow-back water) returns to the surface. Water also continues to return to the surface throughout the life of the well (produced water). Although the use of pits is becoming less common, waste from the well pad is sometimes stored in pits (also called containment ponds) before being trucked off-site. Pits can contain flow-back and produced water, drilling mud, brine, hydraulic fracturing fluids, and cuttings (ie, metal, rock, other shavings produced by the drill bit).[51] If pits are not properly lined, some of this water can seep out. In heavy rains, pit contents can breach or overflow the walls.[41]

Reports from pits in New Mexico identified 40 chemicals and metals in evaporation pits; 98% of the chemicals were listed under the US EPA's Comprehensive Environmental Response, Compensation, and Liability Act (CERCLA) (Superfund) list and 73% under the Emergency Planning and Community Right-to-Know Act (EPCRA) reportable toxic chemicals.[7]

Under anaerobic conditions that exist in the pits, hydrogen sulfide, methyl mercaptan, dimethyl sulfide, and dimethyl disulfide can be generated.[44] Some organic material naturally aerosolizes when stored in the pits and contributes to local air pollution. In some cases, aerators are used to increase how much water is aerosolized, thus dramatically increasing the amount of material released into the air. Pits with aerators can also pollute soil and crops downwind from the pit, creating the potential for secondary exposure by ingestion.[51]

## POPULATION HEALTH IMPACTS

Unconventional gas extraction may cause more subtle changes in community health. A health impact assessment done in Battlement Mesa, Colorado[9,11] found that UGE activities create community-wide impacts, including an increased transient worker population and decreased use of public outdoor areas. The assessment also found increased rates of crime and sexually transmitted diseases (STDs). Although crime rates and STDs cannot be directly correlated with UGE activities, they are nonetheless community changes that coincided with the introduction of UGE. Other identified health impacts include increased collisions, reduced physical activity, increased stress, decline of social cohesion, and strain on community resources, such as health care and housing because of the influx of workers.

### Mental Health

When fully set up, well pad operations often run 24 hours a day near homes, schools, and public areas, creating unhealthy noise levels for the surrounding area. In their review of potential health impacts of UGE, the Maryland Institute for Applied Environmental Health[53] stated that increased noise levels are expected during all phases of development and production. They rated noise as having a moderately high probability of negatively impacting public health.

Although human health outcomes from noise exposure caused by UGE are unknown, long-term exposure to environmental noise in other industries is associated with multiple adverse health outcomes, including stress and annoyance, sleep disturbances, hypertension, and cardiovascular disease. Some groups, including children, are more susceptible to environmental noise (see Chapter 35).

A community study found that the predominant stressor for citizens impacted by shale gas drilling in Pennsylvania was a concern for their health.[54] Most people interviewed felt that their health concerns were largely ignored; the most common health complaint was stress. Stressors may include exposure to odors, such as from the rotten egg smell of hydrogen sulfide released by UGE operations. In communities in which UGE are located, views on whether UGE is beneficial for a community are often polarized, creating disputes and stress among neighbors.

## Birth Outcome Studies

Hill,[55] the first investigator to examine the relationship between maternal proximity to well operations and infant health, compared exposed mothers (those living near active wells) with mothers living near wells under permit but not yet developed. An association was found between exposure to shale gas development and increased incidence of low birth weight and small for gestational age babies (25% and 18% increased risk, respectively).

McKenzie et al[33] examined the relationship between living near Colorado gas wells and the incidence of birth defects, preterm birth, and fetal growth abnormalities. At the time of the study, a larger amount of natural gas in Colorado came from conventional wells. Two exposure groups were formed for births in rural Colorado between 1996 and 2009: those persons living near zero wells within 10 miles (16 km), and those living near 1 or more wells within 10 miles (16 km). Women with 1 or more wells within 10 miles (16 km) were then categorized into 3 groups of increasing number of wells within 10 miles (16 km). Women in the highest exposure group, with more than 125 wells per mile (1.6 km), had an elevated risk of having children born with congenital heart disease (CHD) (odds ratio [OR] 1.3; CI: 1.2 to 1.5) and NTDs (OR 2.0; CI: 1.0 to 3.9). A relationship was seen between increased risk for both CHD and NTD and living near more wells. The authors discussed established associations between exposure to chemicals such as benzene and solvents, and to air pollutants, as risk factors for CHDs and NTDs.

A community-based participatory research study of residents in Pennsylvania examined self-reported symptoms of residents who lived in close proximity to well pads (less than 1,500 feet [0.46 km]) and farther away (more than 1,500 feet [0.46 km]).[56] Residents who lived closer to the wells reported more health symptoms including increased fatigue, nasal and throat irritation, sinus problems, shortness of breath, headaches, and sleep disturbance.[56] One-time water and air monitoring samples measured in a subset of participants found that reported symptoms were similar to the health effects of chemicals found in air and water monitoring tests.

A retrospective assessment of the possible association between childhood cancer and UGE in Pennsylvania showed no increase in childhood cancers after UGE commenced.[57] The study, however, took place during a time when fracking was relatively uncommon and did not include sufficient lag-time to allow for the development of most childhood cancers.[58]

Using electronic health records from the Geisinger health system in Pennsylvania, Casey et al[59] performed a retrospective review of births in the Geisinger system from January 2009 to January 2013. The data were linked to information on UGE from Pennsylvania governmental databases. The authors linked the distance from the maternal residence to wells in the vicinity and the status of those wells. After results were adjusted for covariates, the most exposed group had a greater likelihood of having a preterm birth (OR 1.4; CI = 1.0 to 1.9). There were no associations of activity with Apgar score, small for gestational age birth, or term birth weight (after adjustment for year of birth). This study involved many births over a long period of time but lacked direct exposure measurements.

Jemielita et al[60] examined inpatient hospitalizations in Bradford and Susquehanna Counties in Pennsylvania (which had UGE) and in Wayne County, which had comparable demographic characteristics but no UGE. Increases in living in counties with active wells generally were associated with increases in inpatient hospitalization rates.The authors did not stratify their findings by age, but because most inpatient hospitalizations in the United States occur among adults,[61] their results likely reflect predominantly adult admissions.

Rabinowitz et al[62] performed a cross-sectional, random sample survey of the self-reported health of residents who had ground-fed water wells in the vicinity of natural gas extraction wells. Individuals living in homes less than 1 kilometer from a gas well had more health complaints than those living more than 2 kilometers away. Complaints included skin and upper respiratory problems.

Rasmussen et al,[63] using records from the Geisinger health system and a measure of well proximity and activity, looked at prescriptions of new oral corticosteroids for asthma, emergency visits for asthma, and hospitalizations for asthma. The authors found a statistically significant association between asthma exacerbations and the measure of unconventional natural gas exploration. Living closer to more wells, or wells that are more active, increased an individual's likelihood of an asthma exacerbation 1.5 to 4 times. The largest increase in asthma exacerbations was associated with wells in the production phase.

## PUBLIC POLICY ISSUES

Policy issues related to UGE are complicated, even relative to other environmental health issues. This makes potential advocacy by pediatricians onerous because appropriate targeting of the advocacy is difficult to accomplish. It is often unclear whether it is better for advocates to work with the federal government, or state or local governments.

The 2005 Federal Energy Policy Act exempted many of the processes of UGE from the Safe Drinking Water Act. Various aspects of UGE are also exempt from the following federal laws: the Clean Air Act, the Clean Water Act, the National Environmental Policy Act, the Resource Conservation and Recovery Act, the Emergency Planning and Community Right-to-Know Act, and the

Comprehensive Environmental Response, Compensation, and Liability Act (Superfund).[64] Conversely, in 2014, New York State banned UGE. Maryland and Vermont also issued bans. Other states and local governments have weighed in on UGE in other ways. Since 2017 there have been many attempts to curtail regulations related to UGE.[65]

Pediatricians can be advocates for protecting children and families from the health hazards associated with UGE. Their involvement could start with a discussion with the local chapter of the American Academy of Pediatrics (AAP) to determine the status of UGE state and local legislation and regulation. A discussion with the AAP Office of Federal Affairs can provide an update on the status of federal legislation and regulation about UGE.

## CONCLUSION

Many toxic chemicals are used or derived from the UGE process. There are known or plausible routes of exposure of those chemicals to humans. Numerous research studies have found associations between UGE activities and adverse human health outcomes. Therefore, to protect the health of children and all people against the known and the still undiscovered hazards of unconventional natural gas extraction, the practice should be banned by law or regulation until ample evidence demonstrates that it can be done without jeopardizing the health of communities in which it occurs, particularly through its potential to contaminate water supplies. Much more attention also should be given to natural gas infrastructure, including pipelines, to limit leaks that contribute to greenhouse gas accumulation and worsening climate change.

## Resources

### Pediatric Environmental Health Specialty Units (PEHSUs)
Web site: www.pehsu.net

### Physicians, Scientists & Engineers for Healthy Energy
Maintains one of the most comprehensive datasets on the health impacts of UGE.
Web site: https://www.psehealthyenergy.org

## Frequently Asked Questions

Q   *A drilling company wants to drill immediately next to the playground of my child's school. What should I do?*

A   Unconventional gas extraction is associated with many health risks. You therefore may want to raise your voice about this proposed well development. The AAP can provide scientific information that may be helpful.

Q   *The water from our family well has become contaminated as the result of a spill of "fracking fluid" at a nearby well site. What should we do?*

A   It is prudent to use bottled water for all drinking, cooking, and tooth brushing until it can be determined if the well is contaminated. The state health department should be able to test your water or direct you to where the testing should be done. Consult with your state health department to determine whether it is safe to bathe in the water.

## References

1. Argonne National Laboratory. About Oil Shale. http://ostseis.anl.gov/guide/oilshale/. Accessed June 17, 2018

2. US Energy Information Administration. 2015. US Shale Oil and Natural Gas Map, Lower 48 States. https://www.eia.gov/oil_gas/rpd/shale_gas.pdf. Accessed June 17, 2018

3. Czolowski ED, Santoro RL, Srebotnjak T, Shonkoff SBC. Toward consistent methodology to quantify populations in proximity to oil and gas development: a national spatial analysis and review. *Environ Health Perspect.* 2017;125(8):86004

4. US Department of Energy. How is Shale Gas Produced? https://energy.gov/sites/prod/files/2013/04/f0/how_is_shale_gas_produced.pdf. Accessed June 17, 2018

5. US Environmental Protection Agency. The Process of Unconventional Natural Gas Production. https://www.epa.gov/uog/process-unconventional-natural-gas-production. Accessed June 17, 2018

6. Brown DR, Lewis C, Weinberger BI. Human exposure to unconventional natural gas development: a public health demonstration of periodic high exposure to chemical mixtures in ambient air. *J Environ Science Health A Tox Hazard Subst Environ Eng.* 2015;50(5):460–472

7. Colborn T, Kwiatkowski C, Schultz K, Bachran M. Natural gas operations from a public health perspective. *Hum Ecol Risk Assess.* 2011;17(5):1039–1056

8. Paulik LB, Donald CE, Smith BW, et al. Impact of natural gas extraction on PAH levels in ambient air. *Environ Sci Technol.* 2015;49(8):5203–5210

9. McKenzie LM, Witter RZ, Newman LS, Adgate JL. Human health risk assessment of air emissions from development of unconventional natural gas resources. *Sci Total Environ.* 2012;424:79–87

10. ALL Consulting. NY DEC SGEIS Information Requests: New York Department of Environmental Conservation. 2010

11. Witter RZ, McKenzie L, Stinson KE, Scott K, Newman LS, Adgate J. The use of health impact assessment for a community undergoing natural gas development. *Am J Public Health.* 2013;103(6):1002–1010

12. US Environmental Protection Agency. Development of a Relative Potency Factor (RPF) Approach for Polycyclic Aromatic Hydrocarbon (PAH) Mixtures. Washington, DC: Integrated Risk Information Systems (IRIS); 2010

13. Benbrahim-Tallaa L, Baan RA, Grosse Y, et al. Carcinogenicity of diesel-engine and gasoline-engine exhausts and some nitroarenes. *Lancet Oncol.* 2012;13(7):663–664

14. Attfield MD, Schleiff PL, Lubin JH, et al. The diesel exhaust in miners study: a cohort mortality study with emphasis on lung cancer. *J Natl Cancer Inst.* 2012;104(11):869–883

15. Attfield MD, Schleiff PL, Lubin JH, et al. Erratum: The diesel exhaust in miners study: a cohort mortality study with emphasis on lung cancer. *J Natl Cancer Inst.* 2014;106(8):1–4

16. International Agency for Research on Cancer Working Group on the Evaluation of Carcinogenic Risks to Humans. Diesel and gasoline exhausts and some nitorareanes. Lyon, France. 2012

17. Gilman JB, Lerner BM, Kuster WC, de Gouw JA. Source signature of volatile organic compounds from oil and natural gas operations in northeastern Colorado. *Environ Sci Technol.* 2013;47(3):1297–1305

18. Roy AA, Adams PJ, Robinson AL. Air pollutant emissions from the development, production, and processing of Marcellus shale natural gas. *J Air Waste Manag Assoc.* 2014;64(1):19–37

19. Phillips NG, Ackley R, Crosson E, et al. Natural gas leaks in Boston. *Mineralogical Magazine.* 2012;76(6):2229

20. Jackson RB, Down A, Phillips NG, et al. Natural gas pipeline leaks across Washington, DC. *Environ Sci Technol.* 2014;48(3):2051–2058

21. Observer-Reporter: Green County. Consol to Flare Test Well in Greene County. January 9, 2016. https://observer-reporter.com/news/localnews/consol-to-flare-test-well-in-greene-county/article_2795d9f5-d492-5267-a357-e9f5ec11df01.html. Accessed June 17, 2018

22. New York State Department of Environmental Conservation. Revised Draft Supplemental General Environmental Impact Statement on the Oil, Gas and Solution Mining Regulatory Program. September 2011. http://www.dec.ny.gov/data/dmn/rdsgeisfull0911.pdf. Accessed June 17, 2018

23. US Environmental Protection Agency. Report to Congress on Hydrogen Sulfide Air Emissions Associated with the Extraction of Oil and Natural Gas. October 1993. https://nepis.epa.gov/Exe/ZyPDF.cgi/00002WG3.PDF?Dockey=00002WG3.PDF. Accessed June 17, 2018

24. Brandt AR, Heath GA, Kort EA, et al. Methane leaks from North American natural gas systems. *Science.* 2014;343(6172):733–735

25. Liu YW, Steenland K, Rong Y, et al. Exposure-response analysis and risk assessment for lung cancer in relationship to silica exposure: a 44-year cohort study of 34,018 workers. *Am J Epidemiol.* 2013;178(9):1424–1433

26. Howarth RW, Ingraffea A, Engelder T. Natural gas: Should fracking stop? *Nature.* 2011;477(7364):271–275

27. US Environmental Protection Agency. Inventory of U.S. greenhouse gas emissions and sinks: 1990-2013. Tech. Rep. EPA 430-R-15-004. April 2015

28. Lupo PJ, Symanski E, Waller DK, et al. Maternal exposure to ambient levels of benzene and neural tube defects among offspring: Texas, 1999-2004. *Environ Health Perspect.* 2011;119(3): 397–402

29. Whitworth KW, Symanski E, Coker AL. Childhood lymphohematopoietic cancer incidence and hazardous air pollutants in Southeast Texas, 1995-2004. *Environmental Health Perspect.* 2008;116(11):1576–1580

30. National Toxicology Program. Report on Carcinogens, 14th ed. Benzene. CAS No. 71-43-2. https://ntp.niehs.nih.gov/ntp/roc/content/profiles/benzene.pdf. Accessed June 17, 2018

31. International Agency for Research on Cancer (IARC) Monographs on the Evaluation of Carcinogenic Risks to Humans. Benzene. http://monographs.iarc.fr/ENG/Monographs/vol100F/mono100F-24.pdf. Accessed June 17, 2018

32. US Environmental Protection Agency. Integrated Risk Information System (IRIS). Benzene. CASRN 71-43-2. https://cfpub.epa.gov/ncea/iris2/chemicalLanding.cfm?substance_nmbr=276. Accessed June 17, 2018

33. McKenzie LM, Guo R, Witter RZ, Savitz DA, Newman LS, Adgate JL: Birth outcomes and maternal residential proximity to natural gas development in rural Colorado. *Environ Health Perspect.* 2014;122(4):412–417

34. Slama R, Thiebaugeorges O, Goua V, et al. Maternal personal exposure to airborne benzene and intrauterine growth. *Environ Health Perspect.* 2009;117(8):1313–1321

35. Macey GP, Breech R, Chernaik M, et al. Air concentrations of volatile compounds near oil and gas production: a community-based exploratory study. *Environ Health.* 2014;13:82

36. Colborn T, Schultz K, Herrick L, Kwiatkowski C. An exploratory study of air quality near natural gas operations. *Human Ecol Risk Assess.* 2014;20:86–105

37. US Environmental Protection Agency. Health Effects of Ozone Pollution. https://www.epa.gov/ozone-pollution/health-effects-ozone-pollution.html. Accessed July 13, 2018

38. Searing D, Rabinovitch N. Environmental pollution and lung effects in children. *Curr Opinion Pediatr.* 2011;23(3):314–318

39. Gauderman WJ, Vora H, McConnell R, et al. Effect of exposure to traffic on lung development from 10 to 18 years of age: a cohort study. *Lancet.* 2007;369(9561):571–577

40. Field RA, Soltis J, McCarthy MC, Murphy S, Montague DC. Influence of oil and gas field operations on spatial and temporal distributions of atmospheric non-methane hydrocarbons and their effect on ozone formation in winter. *Atmos Chem Phys.* 2015;15:3527–3542

41. Rozell DJ, Reaven SJ. Water pollution risk associated with natural gas extraction from the Marcellus shale. *Risk Anal.* 2012;32(8):1382–1393

42. Osborn SG, Vengosh A, Warner NR, Jackson RB. Methane contamination of drinking water accompanying gas-well drilling and hydraulic fracturing. *Proc Natl Acad Sci U S A.* 2011;108(20):8172–8176

43. Jackson RB, Vengosh A, Darrah TH, et al. Increased stray gas abundance in a subset of drinking water wells near Marcellus shale gas extraction. *Proc Natl Acad Sci U S A.* 2013;110(28):11250–11255

44. Vidic RD, Brantley SL, Vandenbossche JM, Yoxtheimer D, Abad JD. Impact of shale gas development on regional water quality. *Science.* 2013;340(6134):1235009

45. Llewellyn GT, Dorman F, Westland JL, et al. Evaluating a groundwater supply contamination incident attributed to Marcellus Shale gas development. *Proc Natl Acad Sci U S A.* 2015;112(20):6325–6330

46. Fontenot BE, Hunt LR, Hildenbrand ZL, et al. An evaluation of water quality in private drinking water wells near natural gas extraction sites in the Barnett Shale formation. *Environ Sci Tech.* 2013;47(17):10032–10040

47. Minority Staff, Committee on Energy & Commerce, US House of Representatives. 2011. Chemicals Used in Hydraulic Fracturing. http://frackinginsider.wp.lexblogs.com/wp-content/uploads/sites/179/2011/05/EandC-Dems-fracking-report-2011.pdf. Accessed June 17, 201848.

48. Skytruth. Fracking Chemical Database. http://frack.skytruth.org/fracking-chemical-database. Accessed June 17, 2018

49. Kassotis CD, Tillitt DE, Davis JW, Hormann AM, Nagel SC. Estrogen and androgen receptor activities of hydraulic fracturing chemicals and surface and ground water in a drilling-dense region. *Endocrinology.* 2014;155(3):897–907

50. US Government Accountability Office. Oil and Gas: Information on Shale Resources, Development, and Environmental and Public Health Risks (GAO-12-732). Washington, DC: Government Accountability Office; 2012

51. Rich AL, Crosby EC. Analysis of reserve pit sludge from unconventional natural gas hydraulic fracturing and drilling operations for the presence of technologically enhanced naturally occurring radioactive material (TENORM). *New Solut.* 2013;23(1):117–135

52. Casey JA, Ogburn EL, Rasmussen SG, et al. Predictors of indoor radon concentrations in Pennsylvania, 1989–2013. *Environ Health Perspect.* 2015;123(11):1130–1137

53. Maryland Institute for Applied Environmental Health. Potential Public Health Impacts of Natural Gas Development and Production in the Marcellus Shale in Western Maryland. 2014. http://www.marcellushealth.org/final-report.html. Accessed June 17, 2018

54. Ferrar KJ, Kriesky J, Christen CL, et al. Assessment and longitudinal analysis of health impacts and stressors perceived to result from unconventional shale gas development in the Marcellus shale region. *Int J Occup Environ Health.* 2013;19(2):104–112

55. Hill E. Shale Gas Development and Infant Health: Evidence from Pennsylvania. Working paper. 2013. http://publications.dyson.cornell.edu/research/researchpdf/wp/2012/Cornell-Dyson-wp1212.pdf. Accessed June 17, 2018

56. Steinzor N, Subra W, Sumi L. Investigating links between shale gas development and health impacts through a community survey project in Pennsylvania. *New Solut.* 2013;23(1):55–83

57. Fryzek J, Pastula S, Jiang X, Garabrant DH. Childhood cancer incidence in Pennsylvania counties in relation to living in counties with hydraulic fracturing sites. *J Occup Environ Med.* 2013;55(7):796–801

58. Goldstein BD, Malone S. Obfuscation does not provide comfort: response to the article by Fryzek et al on hydraulic fracturing and childhood cancer. *J Occup Environ Med.* 2013;55:1376–1378

59. Casey JA, Savitz DA, Rasmussen SG, et al. Unconventional natural gas development and birth outcomes in Pennsylvania, USA. *Epidemiology.* 2016;27(2):163–172

60. Jemielita T, Gerton GL, Neidell M, et al. Unconventional gas and oil drilling is associated with increased hospital utilization rates. *PLoS One.* 2015;10(7):e0131093

61. Agency for Healthcare Research and Quality. Care of Children and Adolescents in U.S. Hospitals. http://archive.ahrq.gov/data/hcup/factbk4/factbk4.htm. Accessed June 17, 2018

62. Rabinowitz PM, Slizovskly IB, Lamers V, et al. Proximity to natural gas wells and reported health status: results of a household survey in Washington County, Pennsylvania. *Environ Health Perspect.* 2015;123(1):21–26

63. Rasmussen SG, Ogburn EL, McCormack M, et al. Association between unconventional natural gas development in the Marcellus Shale and asthma exacerbations. *JAMA Intern Med.* 2016;176(9):1334–1343

64. Sinding K, Raichel D, Krois J. How fracturing shale for gas affects us and our worlds. In: Finkel ML, ed. *The Human and Environmental Impacts of Fracking.* Santa Barbara, CA: ABC-CLIO, LLC; 2015:131–153

65. Concerned Health Professionals of New York & Physicians for Social Responsibility. Compendium of scientific, medical, and media findings demonstrating risks and harms of fracking (unconventional gas and oil extraction, 5th ed. http://concernedhealthny.org/compendium/. Accessed June 17, 2018

Chapter 58

# Global Climate Change

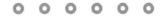

## KEY POINTS

- There is broad consensus that our warming climate results mainly from human activity.
- Children are among the most vulnerable to health effects and other adverse effects of climate change.
- Pediatricians can adopt mitigation and adaptation strategies in response to climate change.

## INTRODUCTION

Weather describes atmospheric conditions over weeks, days, and hours. Climate describes weather conditions averaged over months and longer. Although the Earth's climate has been stable for most of modern human history, it is now changing. Each of the last 3 decades has been successively warmer than any preceding decade since 1850. The globally averaged temperature (combined land and ocean surface) increased 0.85°C (0.65°C to 1.06°C) between 1850 and 2012. Much of this increased heat has been absorbed by the ocean.[1] In the United States, the average temperature has increased by approximately 0.83°C since record keeping began in 1895, most of which has occurred since approximately 1970.[2] The warmest year ever recorded in the 137-year record was 2016, marking it as the third consecutive year of record global warmth.[3] The second warmest year on record was 2015, and the third warmest was 2017.

There is broad consensus that rising global temperature is primarily a result of increasing concentrations of human-generated greenhouse gases, primarily carbon dioxide ($CO_2$), over the last century.[4,5] Atmospheric $CO_2$ has increased from approximately 280 parts per million (ppm) before the industrial revolution to greater than 400 ppm in 2017, a level last reached approximately 3 million years ago.[6] This increase is primarily a result of fossil fuel emissions and secondarily a result of deforestation that reduces carbon storage.[1] Approximately half of the total $CO_2$ increase has occurred in the last 40 years.[7]

The Earth's climate has changed naturally throughout its history. The last ice age ended only about 14,000 years ago, when the global surface temperature was about 5°C lower than it is today. Over the following approximately 5,000 years, the Earth's temperature gradually warmed and then stabilized. It is in this stable climate that modern human civilization developed. About 100 years ago, human activities caused a rapid increase in $CO_2$ and other greenhouse gas concentrations in the atmosphere, causing global temperature to rapidly increase (Figure 58-1).[2] The heat-trapping nature of $CO_2$ and other gases has been recognized since the 1800s[8] and can be demonstrated by simple experiments. It has been agreed by 99.94% of publishing scientists[9] and virtually every relevant scientific organization in the world[4,5,10,11] that increasing greenhouse gases are the major driver of current climate change rather than natural factors that caused changes in the Earth's past.

Warming of the planet is associated with shrinkage of glaciers across the world, decreasing mass of ice sheets in Greenland and the Antarctic, and diminished spring snow cover in the Northern Hemisphere. The frost-free season has increased in every region of the United States, with increases ranging from 6 to 19 days.

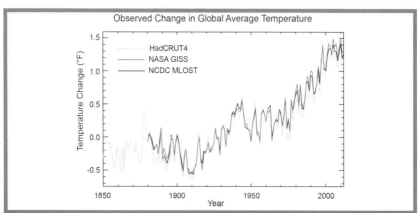

**Figure 58-1. Three different global surface temperature records all show increasing trends over the last century. The lines show annual differences in temperature relative to the 1901-1960 average. Differences among data sets, because of choices in data selection, analysis, and averaging techniques, do not affect the conclusion that global surface temperatures are increasing.**

Source: National Climate Assessment[2]
Abbreviations: HadCRUT4, Data from Met Office Handley Center, UK and Climatic Research Unit, University of East Anglia, UK (http://dx.doi.org/10.1029/2011JD017187); NASA GISS, GISTEMP dataset from NASA's Goddard Institute for Space Studies (http://data.giss.nasa.gov/gistemp/); NCDC MLOST, NOAA dataset (https://www.ncdc.noaa.gov/data-access/marineocean-data/mlost).

The global sea level has risen by approximately 8 inches (20.3 cm) since 1880, and the rate of rise has accelerated. It is projected to rise another 1 to 4 feet (30.5 cm to 1.2 m) by the year 2100.[2] Regions experience varying relative sea level rise because of local changes in land movement or coastal circulation patterns.[12]

Warmer air has greater capacitance for water vapor than cooler air, contributing to an increase in heavy precipitation events in many regions, including the United States. Increases have been greatest in the Midwest and Northeast. Conversely, prolonged record high temperatures have been associated with droughts, particularly in the Southwestern United States.[2]

More frequent and or/prolonged heat waves are affecting many regions, whereas the number of extreme cold waves in the United States is the lowest since record keeping began.[2] Other forms of severe weather, such as hurricanes in the North Atlantic, have increased in intensity since 1970, although causality remains uncertain.[1] From 2000 through 2009, 3 times as many natural disasters occurred than from the period of 1980 through 1989. Deforestation, environmental degradation, urbanization, and intensified climate variables also have contributed to an increased scale of natural disasters.[13] Wildfire frequency, duration, and severity in North American forests have increased.[14]

Climate change is occurring, and some continued changes are inevitable because of past and present emissions. However, projected levels of global warming, sea ice shrinkage, and sea level rise by the mid-21st century vary greatly for different greenhouse gas emission scenarios (Figure 58-2). Limiting temperature rise to 2°C above preindustrial times has been envisioned by the

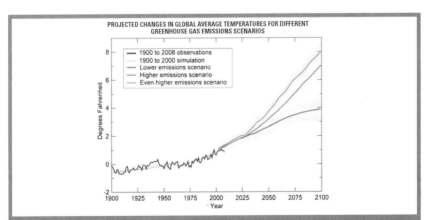

**Figure 58-2. Scientists have modeled future temperature changes based on a variety of greenhouse gas emissions scenarios. Each scenario is based on a set of assumptions about population trends, economic development, and technology—all of which affect the amount of greenhouse gases emitted over time. The figure shows the best estimate (solid line) and likely range (shaded area) of how much temperature will have changed at different points in time relative to the 1960 to 1979 average for emissions scenarios cited.**

Source: Centers for Disease Control and Prevention[15]

Intergovernmental Panel on Climate Change (IPCC) as a goal to prevent the most damaging consequences on humans, food systems, and ecosystems.[16] Higher future emission levels will result in more warming and, thus, more severe effects on the natural world, human society, and health.[2]

## CLIMATE CHANGE-ASSOCIATED HEALTH EFFECTS IN CHILDREN

Major determinants of human health are being affected by observed changes in temperature, precipitation patterns, sea level, and extreme weather events. Children's immature physiology and metabolism; incomplete development; higher exposure to air, food, and water per unit of body weight; unique behavior patterns; and dependence on caregivers place them at a much higher risk of climate-related health burdens than adults.[17] It is estimated that 88% of the existing global burden of disease attributable to climate change occurs in children aged younger than 5 years in both industrialized and developing countries.[18] Children in the world's poorest regions, where the disease burden is already disproportionately high, are at greatest risk from climate change.[19]

Climate change is affecting the health of children today through increased heat stress, decreased air quality, altered disease patterns of some climate-sensitive infections, physical and mental health effects of extreme weather events, and food insecurity in vulnerable regions. At present, the global health burden attributable to climate change is poorly quantified compared with other health stressors.[14] Over the 21st century, however, it is expected that the negative health effects will increase.

Climate change effects on human health have been categorized as primary, secondary, and tertiary. Although the primary effects are easiest to detect, many significant effects will occur through climatic influences on environmental systems and social conditions. Broad societal impacts of unchecked climate change have the potential for the most far-reaching effects and can be categorized as tertiary.[20,21]

## Primary

Children are at direct risk of injury or death as a result of extreme weather events, including severe storms, floods, and wildfires. Children's unique health, behavioral, and psychosocial needs place them at unique risk from these events.[22] Extreme weather events place children at risk of injury,[23] loss of or separation from caregivers,[22] exposure to infectious diseases,[24] and mental health consequences, including posttraumatic stress disorder (PTSD), depression, and adjustment disorder.[25] Devastation of homes, schools, and neighborhoods as result of disasters can cause irrevocable harm to children's physiologic and cognitive development.[26]

In 2017, Hurricane Harvey hit Houston, Texas. This event impacted up to 3 million children, caused over 34,000 people to take refuge in shelters, and caused over 1 million children not to start school on time.[27] Following Hurricanes Katrina and Rita in 2005, more than 5,000 children were separated from their families and the last missing child was reunited with her family after 6 months.[22] Between 200,000 and 300,000 children were evacuated and temporarily or permanently relocated.[28]

Children displaced by Hurricane Katrina experienced an average of 3 moves per child. Some experts believe that a child requires 4 to 6 months for academic recovery following a move that results in a change in schools.[21] In the year following Hurricane Katrina, displaced students in Louisiana public schools performed worse, on average, in all subjects and grades compared with other students.[21] Displaced students experienced problems related to attendance, academic performance, behavior, and mental health.[22] In 1 study, 11.5% of children and adolescents experienced serious emotional disturbances that persisted 3 years after the hurricane compared with an estimated 4.2% prevalence before the hurricane.[29] Another study found PTSD symptoms in 46% of 4th through 6th graders 33 months after Hurricane Katrina.[30]

Increased severity and duration of heat waves put children at direct risk of heat illness. Numerous studies in diverse countries have shown an increase in child morbidity and mortality during extreme heat events.[31] Infants younger than 1 year[32,33] and high school athletes[34,35] appear to be at particularly increased risk of heat-related illness. The Centers for Disease Control and Prevention (CDC) reported heat illness as a leading cause of death and disability in high school athletes, with a national estimate of 9,237 illnesses annually; football players were at highest risk.[34] This risk appears to be increasing. Between 1997 and 2006, emergency department (ED) visits for heat illness increased 133.5%, according to 1 study.[36] The number of deaths from heat stroke per 100,000 American football players increased after the mid-1990s. Increased minimum apparent temperatures are thought to have contributed to this increase, particularly because more than one half of the deaths occurred in the morning.[37]

## Secondary

Climate change alters the environmental systems on which humans rely and causes shifts in ecosystems and diseases of animals, crops, and natural systems. Air quality is reduced through temperature-associated elevations in ground-level ozone concentration.[38] Ozone concentrations in the United States have been projected to increase by 5% to 10% between now and the 2050s because of climate change alone.[39] Climate change-associated increases in ground-level ozone may result in increased visits to the ED for children with asthma, with 1 study showing an increase of 5% to 10% in New York City by 2020.[38]

Rising global temperature and atmospheric $CO_2$ concentrations have been associated with increased length and severity of the pollen allergy season.[40,41]

In North America, delayed first frost and lengthening of the frost-free period has been associated with a lengthening of the ragweed pollen season by 13 to 27 days since 1995, with greater increases in higher latitudes.[40] Ragweed and grass pollen production have been shown to increase in response to increased levels of $CO_2$.[42,43] Average US pollen counts increased by more than 40% in the 2000s relative to the 1990s.[44] Longer and more severe allergy seasons exacerbate respiratory diseases, such as asthma, in children.[45]

Wildfire smoke contains hundreds of chemicals, many of which are harmful to human health. These include particulate matter, carbon monoxide, and ozone precursors, all of which can exacerbate children's respiratory diseases, including asthma.[46]

Climate influences the behavior, development, and mortality of a wide range of living organisms,[47,48] some of which have the potential to cause infection in children. It is difficult, however, to precisely determine the effects of climate change on infectious diseases because of the confounding contributions of economic development and land use, changing ecosystems, international travel, and commerce.[49] Currently, climate warming has been identified as contributing to the northern expansion of Lyme disease in North America.[50] Earlier onset of the Lyme disease season has been correlated with more warm days (greater than 10°C) during the first 5 months of the year.[51] Higher temperatures have a positive effect on mosquito populations, survival, range, disease transmission season, and replication of some viruses within the mosquito.[52,53] These factors may contribute to the global spread of mosquito-borne diseases, including dengue, chikungunya, and Zika.

In general, cases of bacterial gastroenteritis, including *Salmonella*, *Campylobacter*, *Escherichia coli*, *Cryptosporidium*, and *Shigella*, increase when temperatures are higher although patterns vary by organism and location.[54–57] Concern has been expressed that these infections may increase because of rising global temperatures. Heavy precipitation and drought events have been associated with increased gastrointestinal illness resulting from disruption and contamination of water systems.[58–60] It has therefore been projected that the burden of childhood diarrheal illness will increase, particularly in Asia and sub-Saharan Africa, where the disease risk is already high.[61] Concern has also been expressed about climate links to other infections, including coccidioidomycosis[62] and amebic meningoencephalitis.[63] Further investigation into climatic influences on infectious diseases is needed.

Altered agricultural conditions, including extreme heat, increased water demands, and increased severe weather events, will affect food availability and cost, particularly in vulnerable regions where child undernutrition is already a major threat.[64] An additional 95,000 child deaths caused by malnutrition and an additional 7.5 million moderate or severely growth-stunted children have been projected for the year 2030 compared with a future with no climate change.[61] Decreased protein, iron, and zinc content of certain major crops has been demonstrated for plants grown under increased $CO_2$ conditions,[65,66] carrying significant implications for child nutrition.

## Tertiary

Children's biological and cognitive development occurs within the context of stable families, schools, neighborhoods, and communities. The social foundations of children's mental and physical health and well-being are threatened by unchecked climate change, through effects of sea level rise and decreased biologic diversity on the economic viability of agricultural, tourism, and indigenous communities; water scarcity and famine; disruption of power and supply chains; mass migrations; decreased global stability;[67] and potentially increased violent conflict.[68] These effects will likely be greatest for communities already experiencing socioeconomic disadvantage.[69]

## SOLUTIONS TO CLIMATE CHANGE THROUGH MITIGATION AND ADAPTATION STRATEGIES

Mitigation strategies strive to limit climate change effects through reductions in greenhouse gas emissions. Reducing energy consumption and waste; decreasing reliance on carbon-intensive fuels including coal, oil, and gas; increasing use of renewable energy sources, such as wind and solar; and incorporating low carbon footprint building design, transportation, and food supply systems are all necessary to minimize planetary warming attributable to carbon pollution. Such a paradigm shift in production and consumption of energy presents an opportunity for major innovation, job creation, and significant, immediate associated health benefits.[70] A low-carbon economy can promote increased physical activity, decreased air pollution, and reduced red meat consumption, all of which benefit health. Protection of child health, safety, and security underlies the American Academy of Pediatrics' (AAP) support of national and international initiatives to reduce greenhouse gas emissions and mitigate further planetary warming. These include AAP's support for the US Environmental Protection Agency's Clean Power Plan[71,72] and the Paris Climate Agreement, an agreement within the United Nations Framework Convention on Climate Change to mitigate global warming from which President Donald Trump withdrew the United States in 2017.[73]

Adaptation strategies involve developing policies that increase preparedness for current and anticipated climate-associated changes. Such diverse policies include early warning systems for extreme weather events, physical protection against such events, hospital and health system preparedness, anticipating power and supply chain disruptions, improving surveillance of climate-associated infectious diseases, developing climate-resistant crops, and enhancing community resilience.[74] Strategies also include educating health

## Table 58-1. Responding to Climate Change: What Pediatricians Can Do

**IN YOUR PRACTICE**
**Adaptation**
- Maximize immunizations
- Educate families on preparedness for:
  1. excessive heat, using http://emergency.cdc.gov/disasters/extremeheat/index. asp as a guide
  2. reduced air quality, using https://www.airnow.gov as a reference for local air quality
  3. extreme weather events, using https://www.ready.gov as a reference
  4. vector-borne illness, using www.cdc.gov/ncezid/dvbd/index.html as a guide
- Identify and report unusual diseases or disease patterns
- Refer to AAP *Red Book* for management of infectious diseases at https://redbook. solutions.aap.org/
- Support medical education opportunities on climate-associated health risks

**Mitigation**
- "Green" your office and hospital; helpful references include:
  1. The American College of Physicians "Greening the Physician Office" at https:// www.acponline.org/system/files/documents/advocacy/advocacy_in_action/ climate_change_toolkit/greening_the_physician_office.pdf
  2. Practice Greenhealth (https://practicegreenhealth.org)
  3. HealthCare Without Harm (https://noharm.org)
  4. MyGreenDoctor (www.mygreendoctor.org)
- Institute policies to reward coworkers who bike/walk/carpool/use public transportation
- Reduce waste and recycle
- Engage medical students and residents in advocacy for the planet
- Offer expert testimony, speak at hearings, write op-eds on health threats from climate change
- Post and distribute educational materials about the relationship between climate change and child health, and actions that reduce climate change
- Acknowledge that pediatricians are generally perceived as trusted experts and that modeling sustainable lifestyles impacts coworkers and patients

**WORKING WITH LOCAL PUBLIC HEALTH OFFICIALS**
- Engage in disaster preparedness and response planning
- Develop low toxicity approaches to insect and toxic plant control
- Augment surveillance of climate-related infectious diseases

**IN YOUR COMMUNITY/REGION**
- Engage your state AAP chapter on climate change and child health and related advocacy
- Advocate for greener energy power sources
- Serve as an expert resource for public officials
- Engage in education on climate change at schools, community centers and places of worship
- Support local, organic agriculture, green space and pedestrian-centered communities
- Engage in community readiness planning for extreme events

Abbreviation: AAP, American Academy of Pediatrics

care providers and vulnerable patients about climate-associated health risks, such as managing chronic diseases during periods of extreme heat or poor air quality.

## STRATEGIES FOR PEDIATRICIANS AND THE HEALTH SECTOR

As advocates for children, pediatricians have a critical role to play in the societal response to climate change. Table 58-1 provides recommendations to pediatricians to help achieve this goal.

### Frequently Asked Questions

Q   *What impact can individual actions have on a problem as overwhelming as global climate change?*

A   Carbon dioxide emissions come from creating electricity to power homes and businesses and driving vehicles. Collectively, changes made to reduce individual carbon emissions through energy conservation and efficiency not only will have global impact but also are a necessary part of effective greenhouse gas mitigation strategies. Individuals also can speak out to peers and policy makers to increase awareness about the health impacts of climate change, and exercise influence through the media, consumer choices, and voting.

Q   *What practical actions can pediatricians take to fight climate change?*

A   The table "Responding to Climate Change" and the AAP policy statement "Global Climate Change and Child Health"[75] contain concrete actions and recommendations for pediatricians. Pediatricians and other pediatric health care professionals can work to reduce emissions in their personal and professional lives, support policy changes to prepare for and lessen future climate change, and work with local and regional public health officials to develop strong, locally relevant adaptive strategies to minimize the health consequences from climate change.[76,77]

Q   *How should considerations about climate change be incorporated into pediatric practice?*

A   Every parent can do something every day to protect their children against dangerous climate change. For example, parents and children can increase walking and biking, reduce waste production, and support clean energy utilization. Families should understand how to access, interpret, and use local air quality indices, daily pollen counts, and heat advisories. Families should also be encouraged to develop disaster response plans for the extreme weather events and weather disasters likely to occur in their locale. Pediatricians should remember that as health care providers they serve as important lifestyle role models and the choices they make can educate and impact the behavior of others.

Q   *How much time do we have before it is too late to do anything about climate change or avoid catastrophic climate change?*

A   Although the effects of climate change are already being felt across the world, the magnitude of the effects of future changes depends on our ability to substantially reduce greenhouse gas emissions and implement adaptation strategies within the ensuing decades.[7]

Q   *Why should pediatricians be involved in climate change issues?*

A   Pediatricians speak for children, a vulnerable and politically powerless constituency. Children cannot take the individual and political actions needed to ensure a safe climate for the future in which they will live and raise their own families. The history of pediatrics is one of advocacy for the rights and health of children; working to mitigate and adapt to climate change is consistent with that history.

## Resources

### Climate Change Science

Intergovernmental Panel on Climate Change www.ipcc.ch

NASA Global Climate Change http://climate.nasa.gov

National Academy of Sciences http://nas-sites.org/americasclimatechoices/

NOAA Climate www.noaa.gov/climate.html

The Lancet health and climate change www.thelancet.com/climate-and-health

US EPA, Climate Change Indicators in the United States www3.epa.gov/climatechange/science/indicators/index.html

US Global Change Research Program www.globalchange.gov/what-we-do/assessment

### Climate Change Solutions

A Human Health Perspective on Climate Change www.niehs.nih.gov/health/materials/a_human_health_perspective_on_climate_change_full_report_508.pdf

American Academy of Pediatrics www.aap.org/climatechange

American College of Physicians Climate Change Toolkit https://www.acponline.org/advocacy/advocacy-in-action/climate-change-toolkit; CDC Climate and Health www.cdc.gov/climateandhealth/default.htm

Children's Environmental Health Network http://cehn.org

Health Care Without Harm https://noharm.org

Mom's Clean Air Force www.momscleanairforce.org

My Green Doctor www.mygreendoctor.org

Practice Greenhealth https://practicegreenhealth.org

# References

1. Intergovernmental Panel on Climate Change. Summary for policymakers. In: *Climate Change 2013: The Physical Science Basis. Contribution of working group I to the fifth assessment report of the intergovernmental panel on climate change*. 2013

2. Melillo JM, Richmond TC, Yohe GW, eds. *Climate Change Impacts in the United States: The Third National Climate Assessment*. U.S. Global Change Research Program. 2014

3. National Oceanographic and Atmospheric Administration. National Centers for Environmental Information. State of the Climate: Global Climate Report for Annual 2016. https://www.ncdc.noaa.gov/sotc/global/201613. Accessed June 22, 2018

4. Oreskes N. Beyond the ivory tower: the scientific consensus on climate change. *Science*. 2004;306(5702):1686

5. Anderegg WR, Prall JW, Harold J, Schneider SH. Expert credibility in climate change. *Proc Natl Acad Sci USA*. 2010;107(27):12107–12109

6. Monastersky R. Global carbon dioxide levels near worrisome milestone. *Nature*. 2013;497(7447):13–14

7. Intergovernmental Panel on Climate Change. Summary for policymakers. In: *Climate Change 2014: Mitigation of Climate Change. Contribution of working group III to the fifth assessment report of the intergovernmental panel on climate change*. 2014

8. Arrhenius S. On the influence of carbonic acid in the air upon the temperature of the ground. *Philosophical Magazine and Journal of the Sciences*. 1896;5(41):237–276

9. Powell JL. The consensus on anthropogenic global warming matters. *Bulletin of Science, Technology & Society*. 2016;36(3):157–163

10. Doran PT, Zimmerman MK. Examining the scientific consensus on climate change. *Eos*. 2009;90(3):22–23

11. Molina M, McCarthy J, Wall D, et al. *What We Know: The Reality, Risks, and Response to Climate Change*. Washington, DC: American Association for the Advancement of Science; 2014. http://whatweknow.aaas.org/wp-content/uploads/2014/07/whatweknow_website.pdf. Accessed June 22, 2018

12. US Environmental Protection Agency. Climate Change Indicators in the United States, 2014. 3rd ed. EPA-430-R-14-004

13. Leaning J, Guha-Sapir D. Natural disasters, armed conflict, and public health. *N Engl J Med*. 2013;369(19):1836–1842

14. Intergovernmental Panel on Climate Change. *Climate Change 2014: Impacts, Adaptation, and Vulnerability. Part A: Global and Sectoral Aspects*. New York, NY: Cambridge University Press; 2014

15. Climate Change and Extreme Heat Events. http://www.cdc.gov/climateandhealth/pubs/ClimateChangeandExtremeHeatEvents.pdf. Accessed June 22, 2018

16. Swaminathan MS, Kesavan PC. Agricultural research in an era of climate change. *Agriculture Research*. 2012;1(1):3–11

17. Sheffield PE, Landrigan PJ. Global climate change and children's health: threats and strategies for prevention. *Environ Health Perspect*. 2011;119(3):291–298

18. Zhang Y, Bi P, Hiller JE. Climate change and disability-adjusted life years. *J Environ Health*. 2007;70(3):32–36

19. Haines A, Kovats RS, Campbell-Lendrum D, Corvalan C. Climate change and human health: Impacts, vulnerability, and mitigation. *Lancet*. 2006;367(9528):2101–2109

20. Butler CD, Harley D. Primary, secondary and tertiary effects of eco-climatic change: the medical response. *Postgrad Med J*. 2010;86(1014):230–234

21. McMichael AJ. Globalization, climate change, and human health. *N Engl J Med.* 2013;368(14):1335–1343

22. National Commission on Children and Disasters, ed. 2010 Report to the President and Congress. Rockville, MD: Agency for Healthcare Research and Quality; 2010; No. AHRQ Publication No. 10-M037. http://archive.ahrq.gov/prep/nccdreport/nccdreport.pdf. Accessed June 22, 2018

23. Miranda DS, Choonara I. Hurricanes and child health: lessons from Cuba. *Arch Dis Child.* 2011;96(4):328–329

24. Ivers LC, Ryan ET. Infectious diseases of severe weather-related and flood-related natural disasters. *Curr Opin Infect Dis.* 2006;19(5):408–414

25. Goldmann E, Galea S. Mental health consequences of disasters. *Annu Rev Public Health.* 2014;35:169–183

26. Noffsinger MA, Pfefferbaum B, Pfefferbaum RL, Sherrib K, Norris FH. The burden of disaster: part I. Challenges and opportunities within a child's social ecology. *Int J Emerg Ment Health.* 2012;14(1):3–13

27. Pacheco SE. Hurricane Harvey and climate change: the need for policy to protect children. *Pediatr Res.* 2018;83(1-1):9–10

28. Drury SS, Scheeringa MS, Zeanah CH. The traumatic impact of Hurricane Katrina on children in New Orleans. *Child Adolesc Psychiatr Clin N Am.* 2008;17(3):685–702

29. McLaughlin KA, Fairbank JA, Gruber MJ, et al. Trends in serious emotional disturbance among youths exposed to Hurricane Katrina. *J Am Acad Child Adolesc Psychiatry.* 2010;49(10):990–1000

30. Moore KW, Varela RE. Correlates of long-term posttraumatic stress symptoms in children following Hurricane Katrina. *Child Psychiatry Hum Dev.* 2010;41(2):239–250

31. Xu Z, Etzel RA, Su H, Huang C, Guo Y, Tong S. Impact of ambient temperature on children's health: a systematic review. *Environ Res.* 2012;117:120–131

32. Basu R, Ostro BD. A multicounty analysis identifying the populations vulnerable to mortality associated with high ambient temperature in California. *Am J Epidemiol.* 2008;168(6):632–637

33. Deschenes O, Greenstone M. Climate Change, Mortality, and Adaptation: Evidence from Annual Fluctuations in Weather in the US. Washington, DC: National Bureau of Economic Research; 2007. http://www.nber.org/papers/w13178. Accessed June 22, 2018

34. Centers for Disease Control and Prevention. Heat illness among high school athletes—United States, 2005-2009. *MMWR Morb Mortal Wkly Rep.* 2010;59(32):1009–1013

35. Gottschalk AW, Andrish JT. Epidemiology of sports injury in pediatric athletes. *Sports Med Arthrosc Rev.* 2011;19(1):2–6

36. Nelson NG, Collins CL, Comstock RD, McKenzie LB. Exertional heat-related injuries treated in emergency departments in the U.S., 1997-2006. *Am J Prev Med.* 2011;40(1):54–60

37. Grundstein AJ, Ramseyer C, Zhao F, et al. A retrospective analysis of American football hyperthermia deaths in the United States. *Int J Biometeorol.* 2012;56(1):11–20

38. Sheffield PE, Knowlton K, Carr JL, Kinney PL. Modeling of regional climate change effects on ground-level ozone and childhood asthma. *Am J Prev Med.* 2011;41(3):251–257

39. Kinney PL. Climate change, air quality, and human health. *Am J Prev Med.* 2008;35(5):459–467

40. Ziska L, Knowlton K, Rogers C, et al. Recent warming by latitude associated with increased length of ragweed pollen season in central North America. *Proc Natl Acad Sci U S A.* 2011;108(10):4248–4251

41. Ziska LH, Caulfield FA. Rising carbon dioxide and pollen production of common ragweed, a known allergy-inducing species: implications for public health. *Aust J Plant Physiol.* 2000;27:893–898

42. Singer BD, Ziska LH, Frenz DA, Gebhard DE, Straka JG. Increasing Amb a 1 content in common ragweed (ambrosia artemisiifolia) pollen as a function of rising atmospheric CO2 concentration. *Functional Plant Biology*. 2005;32(7):667–670

43. Albertine JM, Manning WJ, DaCosta M, Stinson KA, Muilenberg ML, Rogers CA. Projected carbon dioxide to increase grass pollen and allergen exposure despite higher ozone levels. *PLoS One*. 2014;9(11):e111712

44. Zhang Y, Bielory L, Mi Z, Cai T, Robock A, Georgopoulos P. Allergenic pollen season variations in the past two decades under changing climate in the United States. *Glob Chang Biol*. 2015;21(4):1581–1589

45. Anenberg SC, Weinberger KR, Roman H, et al. Impacts of oak pollen on allergic asthma in the United States and potential influence of future climate change. *GeoHealth*. 2017;1(3):80–92

46. Delfino RJ, Brummel S, Wu J, et al. The relationship of respiratory and cardiovascular hospital admissions to the southern California wildfires of 2003. *Occup Environ Med*. 2009;66(3):189–197

47. Altizer S, Ostfeld RS, Johnson PT, Kutz S, Harvell CD. Climate change and infectious diseases: from evidence to a predictive framework. *Science*. 2013;341(6145):514–519

48. Parmesan C, Yohe G. A globally coherent fingerprint of climate change impacts across natural systems. *Nature*. 2003;421(6918):37–42

49. Institute of Medicine. Microbial Threats to Health: Emergence, Detection, and Response. 2003. https://www.nap.edu/catalog/10636/microbial-threats-to-health-emergence-detection-and-response. Accessed July 17, 2018

50. Ogden NH, Radojevic M, Wu X, Duvvuri VR, Leighton PA, Wu J. Estimated effects of projected climate change on the basic reproductive number of the Lyme disease vector ixodes scapularis. *Environ Health Perspect*. 2014;122(6):631–638

51. Moore SM, Eisen RJ, Monaghan A, Mead P. Meteorological influences on the seasonality of Lyme disease in the United States. *Am J Trop Med Hyg*. 2014;90(3):486–496

52. Anyamba A, Small JL, Britch SC, et al. Recent weather extremes and impacts on agricultural production and vector-borne disease outbreak patterns. *PLoS One*. 2014;9(3):e92538

53. Sirisena PD, Noordeen F. Evolution of dengue in Sri Lanka-changes in the virus, vector, and climate. *Int J Infect Dis*. 2014;19:6–12

54. Fleury M, Charron DF, Holt JD, Allen OB, Maarouf AR. A time series analysis of the relationship of ambient temperature and common bacterial enteric infections in two Canadian provinces. *Int J Biometeorol*. 2006;50(6):385–391

55. Britton E, Hales S, Venugopal K, Baker MG. Positive association between ambient temperature and salmonellosis notifications in New Zealand, 1965-2006. *Aust N Z J Public Health*. 2010;34(2):126–129

56. Naumova EN, Jagai JS, Matyas B, DeMaria A,Jr, MacNeill IB, Griffiths JK. Seasonality in six enterically transmitted diseases and ambient temperature. *Epidemiol Infect*. 2007;135(2):281–292

57. Hu W, Mengersen K, Fu SY, Tong S. The use of ZIP and CART to model cryptosporidiosis in relation to climatic variables. *Int J Biometeorol*. 2010;54(4):433–440

58. Nichols G, Lane C, Asgari N, Verlander NQ, Charlett A. Rainfall and outbreaks of drinking water related disease and in England and Wales. *J Water Health*. 2009;7(1):1–8

59. Cann KF, Thomas DR, Salmon RL, Wyn-Jones AP, Kay D. Extreme water-related weather events and waterborne disease. *Epidemiol Infect*. 2013;141(4):671–686

60. Curriero FC, Patz JA, Rose JB, Lele S. The association between extreme precipitation and waterborne disease outbreaks in the United States, 1948-1994. *Am J Public Health*. 2001;91(8):1194–1199

61. Hales S, Kovats S, Lloyd S, Campbell-Lendru D. *Quantitative Risk Assessment of the Effects of Climate Change on Selected Causes of Death, 2030s and 2050s.* Vol 2014. Geneva, Switzerland: World Health Organization; 2014:1–128. http://www.who.int/globalchange/publications/quantitative-risk-assessment/en/. Accessed June 22, 2018

62. Centers for Disease Control and Prevention. Increase in reported coccidioidomycosis—United States, 1998-2011. *MMWR Morb Mortal Wkly Rep.* 2013;62(12):217–221

63. Kemble SK, Lynfield R, DeVries AS, et al. Fatal Naegleria fowleri infection acquired in Minnesota: possible expanded range of a deadly thermophilic organism. *Clin Infect Dis.* 2012;54(6):805–809

64. Lloyd SJ, Kovats RS, Chalabi Z. Climate change, crop yields, and undernutrition: development of a model to quantify the impact of climate scenarios on child undernutrition. *Environ Health Perspect.* 2011;119(12):1817–1823

65. Taub DR, Miller B, Allen H. Effects of elevated CO2 on the protein concentration of food crops: a meta-analysis. *Global Change Biol.* 2008;14(3):565–575

66. Myers SS, Zanobetti A, Kloog I, et al. Increasing CO2 threatens human nutrition. *Nature.* 2014;510(7503):139–142

67. CNA Military Advisory Board. *National Security and the Accelerating Risks of Climate Change.* Alexandria, VA: CNA Corporation; 2014. https://www.cna.org/cna_files/pdf/MAB_5-8-14.pdf. Accessed June 23, 2018

68. Hsiang SM, Burke M, Miguel E. Quantifying the influence of climate on human conflict. *Science.* 2013;341(6151):1235367

69. Fritze JG, Blashki GA, Burke S, Wiseman J. Hope, despair and transformation: climate change and the promotion of mental health and wellbeing. *Int J Ment Health Syst.* 2008;2(1):13

70. Haines A, McMichael AJ, Smith KR, et al. Public health benefits of strategies to reduce greenhouse-gas emissions: overview and implications for policy makers. *Lancet.* 2009;374(9707):2104–2114

71. Perrin JM. American Academy of Pediatrics Statement on EPA Action to Regulate Carbon Emissions. American Academy of Pediatrics Website. https://www.aap.org/en-us/about-the-aap/aap-press-room/Pages/AAP-Statement-on-EPA-Action-to-Regulate-Carbon-Emissions.aspx. Accessed June 24, 2018

72. Stein F. American Academy of Pediatrics Statement on Executive Order Halting Clean Power Plan. American Academy of Pediatrics Web site. https://www.aap.org/en-us/about-the-aap/aap-press-room/Pages/CPPExecutiveOrder.aspx. Accessed June 24, 2018

73. Stein F. American Academy of Pediatrics Statement on Withdrawal from Paris Climate Agreement. American Academy of Pediatrics Web site. https://www.aap.org/en-us/about-the-aap/aap-press-room/pages/AAP-Statement-on-Withdrawal-from-Paris-Climate-Agreement.aspx. Accessed June 24, 2018

74. McMichael AJ, Lindgren E. Climate change: present and future risks to health, and necessary responses. *J Intern Med.* 2011;270(5):401–413

75. American Academy of Pediatrics Council on Environmental Health. Global climate change and children's health. *Pediatrics.* 2015;136(5):992–997

76. Frumkin H, Hess J, Luber G, Malilay J, McGeehin M. Climate change: the public health response. *Am J Public Health.* 2008;98(3):435–445

77. Jackson R, Shields KN. Preparing the U.S. health community for climate change. *Annu Rev Public Health.* 2008;29:57–73

Chapter 59

# Green Offices and Practice Sustainability

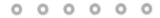

## KEY POINTS

- Pediatricians have important roles as advocates and practice managers in reducing the negative environmental impact of health care operations.
- The environmental performance of health care facilities can be improved in ways that include increasing energy efficiency, reducing waste, and purchasing environmentally preferable products.
- Improving environmental performance in health care benefits patients, staff, and surrounding communities, and can reduce practices' and hospitals' operating costs.

## INTRODUCTION

The delivery of health care services creates environmental conditions that have impacts on human health. These impacts can affect occupants of health care facilities and surrounding communities, and can also have more far-reaching, even global, effects. For example, the health care sector accounts for 10% of US greenhouse gas emissions,[1] contributing to global climate change.

"Greening" refers to the concept of sustainability in health care operations—ie, integrating of environmental as well as social and economic considerations into all aspects of practice operations. Improving the environmental performance of hospitals and practice operations can benefit the health of patients, staff, and the broader community, and provides opportunities to save costs and operate more efficiently. Because of the significant purchasing power of the health care sector, and its platform for advocacy, the growing health care sustainability movement can have a transformative influence on supply chain practices and governmental policies and regulations, a potential that is already being realized. In this way, adopting sustainable operating practices in health care can have far-reaching positive impacts on environmental health nationally and globally.

Because environmental burdens such as air pollution, chemical exposures, and climate change disproportionately impact children, pediatricians should understand that advocating for greening their practice or hospital operations benefits the health of their patients. Although many environmentally preferable operating practices, such as energy efficiency and waste reduction, are cost saving, they may require up-front investment of resources to change established practices or to purchase equipment. Legislative and regulatory policies that provide financial incentives for these investments, and policies that support appropriate payment for services rendered, can help to ensure that pediatricians and other health care leaders have the resources to successfully improve the environmental performance of their practices and hospitals.

Opportunities to improve the environmental performance of medical offices and hospitals fall into several categories summarized below. It is beneficial to engage multiple team members and colleagues, across disciplines, in evaluating environmental performance, setting and prioritizing goals for improvement, tracking and reporting progress, and communicating the practice's or department's environmental commitment to patients, visitors, and others. This collaborative approach can take place within the context of existing operations or leadership meetings, or by creating a sustainability committee or "green team." Engaged and committed leadership provides support and accountability to these efforts and is critical to improving sustainability in health care environments.

## ENERGY AND TRANSPORTATION

The burning of fossil fuels to generate energy used to power buildings, equipment, and vehicles results in air and water pollution that cause direct human health effects; greenhouse gas emissions that contribute to climate change; and is associated with harms to workers and local environments through extraction and processing. A draft World Health Organization (WHO) report used data from the US Environmental Protection Agency (EPA) to estimate that $600 million in health care costs annually are attributable to the increased respiratory disease burden associated with energy use in the health care sector.[2] Improving energy efficiency of health care facilities, using renewable energy sources, and encouraging carpooling and multimodal transportation have significant environmental and health benefits.

---

### US EPA Energy Star Program

The US EPA Energy Star Program was established in 1992, and includes, in partnership with many public and private organizations, a suite of technical tools and resources that guide individuals and organizations in implementing energy efficient operating practices. The Energy Star program includes a labeling system for appliances that identifies and rates energy efficient products. It also includes the Portfolio Manager, an online tool that allows tracking and benchmarking of a building's energy and water consumption, setting targets for energy performance to help inform building design and operations, and earning recognition for energy efficient buildings.
https://www.energystar.gov/

---

## Energy Efficiency

The health care sector is among the most energy-intensive industries in the United States. Moreover, the average commercial building in the United States wastes 30% of the energy it uses.[3] Energy efficiency improvements in ambulatory and hospital environments can save significant operating costs.[4]

The following energy efficiency measures are common to most successful energy management programs, and are applicable in medical office and hospital buildings:

### Tracking and Benchmarking

Measuring and tracking trends in energy use and cost are critical to identifying opportunities to improve efficiency and evaluating the effectiveness of energy efficiency investments. Using a standard, no-cost tool such as the US EPA's Energy Star Portfolio Manager[5] allows weather normalization (that permits tracking of energy performance that accounts for variability in weather), benchmarking energy performance against similar buildings, and estimating savings in energy use and cost from planned efficiency projects.

### Building Envelope

Ensuring adequate insulation and appropriate window glazing and shading on buildings can be one of the most effective ways to improve energy performance, with a rapid return on investment.

## Lighting

On average, in US commercial buildings, lighting accounts for about 25% of energy consumption.[6] Retrofitting inefficient fluorescent lights (optimally, to LED models) and adding occupancy sensors are investments that result in returns from saved energy costs ( from reduced energy use for the lights themselves and reduced need for cooling because of less heat coming from the lights). Another benefit to retrofitting is avoiding labor costs needed to maintain and change bulbs, especially in buildings with extended hours, including those in health care. Internal and external lighting retrofits should be considered.

## Heating, Ventilation, and Air Conditioning

Heating, ventilation, and air conditioning (HVAC) accounts for about 30% of energy used in US commercial buildings.[7] Optimizing the building envelope and increasing the efficiency of lighting and equipment reduce heating and cooling loads (referring to the amount of energy required to heat and cool a building). Reducing these loads can allow use of a smaller HVAC system, with significant energy efficiency benefits. In addition, using efficient HVAC equipment and ensuring appropriate settings are often cost-effective opportunities to improve energy performance. Steps to ensure appropriate HVAC settings depend on the type of HVAC system in place. These measures include employing programmable thermostats that permit minimizing heating and cooling during hours of low occupancy, ensuring appropriate temperature settings, and ensuring ventilation with outside air that meets but does not exceed code or regulatory requirements.

## Energy Efficient Appliances

Purchasing Energy Star-certified appliances and equipment and EPEAT- (Electronic Product Environmental Assessment Tool) certified computers can significantly improve building energy performance. Computer power

---

### EPEAT (Electronic Product Environmental Assessment Tool)

EPEAT is a global environmental rating program for electronics established in 2003, when the US EPA convened a stakeholder process to launch EPEAT. This rating program addresses the environmental impact of electronics throughout their life cycle, including design, production, use, and disposal.
www.epeat.net

management (turning computers off or placing them into standby/sleep mode during low-use periods) can yield significant energy use and cost savings—according to Energy Star, an estimated $40 per computer per year.[8] Installing technology that automates shutting down, or shifting to sleep mode after a defined period of time without use, can help to achieve power management goals.

### Retro-commissioning

Retro-commissioning refers to the process of improving efficiency of a building's equipment and systems. This process addresses problems that can arise when a building ages or experiences changes in its use over time. Engaging a professional commissioning agent to ensure that mechanical, electrical, controls, and other building systems are functioning optimally reduces energy use by an average of 15% in a typical commercial building.[9] This typically represents a modest investment that pays back, on average, in less than 1 year.[8]

### Behavior Change

Engaging and educating workplace staff to become more aware of energy use can save an average of 10% on energy use and cost in a typical commercial building and is essentially free of cost to implement.[10] Energy awareness is demonstrated by behaviors such as turning off lights and reducing plug loads.

### Renewable Energy

Investing in renewable energy, such as solar, geothermal, or wind, can help to mitigate the environmental impact of building operations. In many regions, rebates and incentives can help defray the cost of these investments. The most critical and cost-effective component of energy management, however, is to optimize energy efficiency. Hospitals and ambulatory facilities across the country have demonstrated success in incorporating renewable energy sources in their operations.[11]

### Transportation

Motor vehicles contribute to air pollution and climate change—about half of the toxic air pollution emissions in the United States—is from vehicles.[12] Alternatives to single-occupant car transportation can directly benefit the health of individuals who use more active modes of transportation. Medical practices and hospitals can encourage carpooling and multimodal transportation by providing incentives, such as preferred parking for carpoolers, subsidized transit passes, and wellness "points" for walking, biking, or taking public transportation to work, and supporting engagement activities such as the National Bike Challenge.

## Water

Stewardship of water resources in medical practices or hospital environments includes use of water-saving fixtures, management of stormwater, and green landscaping practices.

Using US EPA WaterSense certified fixtures is one way to use less water; WaterSense certified fixtures use up to 20% less water than conventional fixtures without sacrificing performance.[13] Water saving also results in energy saving: energy is used to heat water, and to pump and purify it. Water use and costs can be tracked and managed using the US EPA Energy Star Portfolio Manager tool.

Stormwater management and green landscaping practices are other examples of water stewardship initiatives with health benefits. When large precipitation events occur, water rushing from non-porous surfaces, such as parking lots, can overwhelm storm drains, resulting in overflow of untreated water, including raw sewage, into the water system. Stormwater management systems delay, capture, store, treat, or infiltrate stormwater runoff. Examples include rain barrels, porous pavement, and bioretention systems (landscaping features designed to slow stormwater runoff, remove pollutants, and then allow infiltration of treated water into native soil or direction to nearby drains).

Green landscaping practices limit the use of chemical pesticides, herbicides, and fertilizers, which decreases human exposure to these chemicals in and around the landscape, and also prevents chemical runoff into waterways.

## Waste

Health care buildings produce a large volume of waste, including disposable medical devices, regulated medical waste, and typical office waste. Most waste produced in hospitals and medical office buildings is typical office and food waste, and most of this is recyclable and compostable.[14]

Landfills contribute to air and water pollution through off-gassing and leaching. Approximately 50% of landfill gas is methane,[15] a potent greenhouse gas that contributes to climate change. Reducing landfill waste therefore has many environmental benefits.

Regulated and hazardous waste streams are expensive to process, and have higher environmental impacts because they are often transported and require energy-intensive processing, such as autoclaving or incinerating. Commonly, much of the waste in health care settings placed in regulated waste receptacles is not truly regulated waste, but simply regular trash or recyclable materials placed there inappropriately[16] because of lack of staff awareness or lack of conveniently placed appropriate receptacles. Reducing inappropriate placement of nonregulated waste into regulated receptacles can save significant costs and reduce environmental impact.

Implementing practices to reduce the production of waste, reduce inappropriate placement of nonregulated waste into regulated waste containers, and divert nonregulated waste from landfills by recycling and composting can save costs through avoiding waste hauling and tipping fees, and through rebates for some recyclable materials. Recycling and composting programs that are visible and require users to sort waste into appropriate receptacles are good ways to engage and educate patients and staff.

### Environmentally Preferable Purchasing

Environmentally preferable purchasing (EPP) practices include minimizing waste (by limiting packaging or using fewer disposable products), specifying energy and water efficient products, avoiding chemicals of concern, supporting the local economy by preferentially purchasing local products and services, and purchasing healthy and sustainably sourced food. An EPP policy can help to codify and prioritize purchasing goals.[17] When comparing products for their environmental attributes, it is useful to consider their impact across their life cycle, from production, to use, to eventual disposal.

Several EPP topics are worth highlighting as potential priorities in medical practice and hospital environments because they directly impact the health of building occupants and represent targeted areas for focused, measurable, and achievable change. These topics are listed here and in the following section on Green Building and Operations. People in the United States, on average, spend 87% of their time indoors.[18] Purchasing and operating practices that promote healthier indoor environments, such as improved indoor air quality, directly benefit health.

### Healthy Interiors

Paints containing low or zero volatile organic compounds (VOCs) can protect indoor air quality. When purchasing furniture and furnishings, the following chemicals should be avoided if possible: formaldehyde, perfluoroalkyl and polyfluoroalkyl substances, antimicrobial agents, polyvinyl chloride, and all flame retardants. These chemicals do not confer any proven benefits, but all cause harm in one or more phases of their life cycle. Furniture and furnishings free of these chemicals are well established in the marketplace. Fire codes in specific localities should be verified, but in general, chemical flame retardant-free furniture is typically allowable in fully sprinklered buildings.

Interior materials that can be cleaned and maintained without the use of potentially toxic cleaning chemicals are also preferred.

### Healthier Food

Food purchasing is an essential component of EPP practice for hospital environments and practices where food is served. EPP food purchasing practices tend to align well with goals to improve the nutritional quality and healthfulness of food services. For example, beef production is associated with a large environmental impact.[19] In parallel, heart-healthy nutrition includes limiting red meat intake, and preferring plant-based protein, poultry, and fish.[20] Purchasing less red meat for health care food services by controlling portion sizes or adjusting menu options can save costs, improve healthfulness of offerings, and reduce environmental impact.

Most antibiotics in the United States are used in animal agriculture for non-therapeutic purposes (such as growth promotion), contributing to antibiotic resistance in human pathogens.[21] Therefore, purchasing animal products produced without non-therapeutic antibiotics is an important component of antibiotic stewardship. Discussing meat sourcing options that promote responsible antibiotic use with nutrition services vendors or food distributors serving specific offices and hospitals is important to develop specific goals. Health care institutions across the country are beginning to commit to purchasing meat produced without the use of non-therapeutic antibiotics, and these commitments have collective power in motivating systemic change toward more judicious use of antibiotics in animal agriculture.[22]

Serving healthier beverages (such as non-sugared beverages) and using filtered tap water instead of bottled water when possible, are examples of environmentally preferable food purchasing practices that benefit health. Plastic bottles have negative environmental impacts in every phase of their life cycle. Fossil fuels are used for their manufacture and transport, their use results in increased landfill waste, and they are a significant source of pollution in waterways.

Targeting the purchase of locally sourced food (typically defined in health care as within 250 miles of a facility) and third-party certified food items such as "USDA Certified Organic" or "Marine Stewardship Council Certified" may also be included in environmentally preferable food purchasing goals.[23]

Minimizing waste from packaging and disposable serviceware and reducing food waste are additional opportunities for reducing the environmental impact of health care food services. The US EPA's Food Recovery Hierarchy is a tool that can help develop food waste reduction goals (Figure 59-1).[24]

**Medical Products**

Considering use of reusable products instead of disposable ones can reduce environmental impacts and save costs. When purchasing medical products, it is prudent to consider the total cost of ownership and life cycle impacts, including exposure to possibly harmful chemicals. One example of a chemical of concern is the phthalate di(2-ethylhexyl)phthalate (DEHP), a plasticizer added to medical products made from polyvinyl chloride (PVC) to soften them. DEHP can leach from the product into patients.[25] In animal studies, DEHP has been shown to cause male reproductive toxicity and other effects and is a suspected endocrine disruptor in humans.[26] Because of the potentially

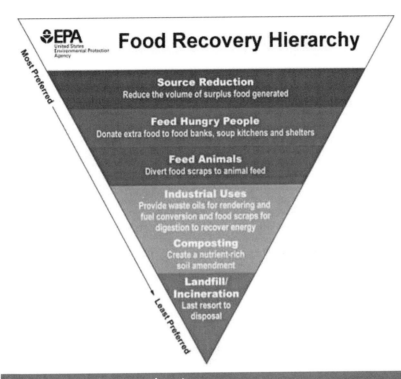

**Figure 59-1. The Food Recovery Hierarchy**

significant exposure of neonatal intensive care unit (NICU) babies to DEHP, a growing number of NICUs are turning to DEHP-free medical equipment.[27] (See Chapter 41).

## Green Building and Operations

### Construction and Renovation

New construction and renovation activities create opportunities to optimize environmental performance of practices and hospitals. Planners can construct high-performance green health care buildings at minimum to no additional up-front cost. This can be accomplished by specifying goals for sustainable design and construction (using, for example, the US Green Building Council's Leadership in Energy and Environmental Design [LEED] certification program),[28] prioritizing goals (such as optimizing energy efficiency or indoor air quality) from the earliest stages of design, and taking an integrated approach to executing sustainable design goals.[29] Because these buildings are designed to operate efficiently, they may save costs over the lifetime of their operation and result in safer, healthier, more comfortable environments for working and healing.

## Green Cleaning

Green cleaning practices employ fewer and less toxic chemicals for cleaning and minimize waste of chemicals and disposable equipment. These practices improve indoor air quality while maintaining cleaning standards.[30] Green cleaning strategies include using steam-based cleaners and application-specific cleaning policies, such as specifying that disinfectant cleaners are used only when disinfection is required. GreenSeal and EcoLogo are examples of third-party verification systems used to evaluate whether non-disinfectant cleaners are nontoxic.

Work-related asthma associated with exposure to cleaning products is most prevalent in health care settings, with housekeeping and nursing staff most likely to be affected.[31] Greener cleaning practices directly benefit these front-line staff, as well as patients.

## Green Landscaping and Integrated Pest Management

Sustainable landscaping practices emphasize limiting chemical use, managing stormwater, and saving water used for irrigation, thus creating healthier and more cost-effective external building environments.

Integrated Pest Management (IPM) refers to a multi-pronged strategy for pest prevention and the judicious use of chemical pesticides.[32] Inspection, monitoring, and reporting are undertaken to identify opportunities to mechanically or structurally prevent or control pests, limit the preventive application of chemical pesticides, and reserve pesticide use for targeted situations. IPM can reduce chemical pesticide exposure for workers, staff, and patients.

## EDUCATION

Maximizing opportunities to communicate about and promote environmental initiatives can educate and inspire patients and staff. Opportunities include placing signs on waste receptacles to explain the process and rationale behind landfill diversion, communicating in food service areas about the benefits of sustainable and healthy food purchasing, creating public dashboards to celebrate energy efficiency, and observing events such as Earth Day or National Food Day. Patients and staff may be inspired to adopt sustainable practices at home: improving indoor air quality and decreasing chemical exposures through green cleaning and landscaping, increasing healthy and sustainable food procurement, and choosing active transportation modalities.

## CONCLUSION

Opportunities to improve the environmental performance of medical practices and hospital operations can save costs and improve the health of staff, patients, and the surrounding community, and can have national and global health impacts. Transformation in purchasing, food services, and building design

## Summary of Opportunities to Improve Environmental Performance of Health Care Buildings

- Improve energy efficiency
- Consider incorporating renewable energy sources
- Support efficient transportation practices
  - o Support alternatives to single-occupant car commuting for staff and visitors
  - o When applicable, support efficient delivery routes of purchased goods and laboratory samples
- Optimize water efficiency
- Reduce waste
- Purchase environmentally preferable products and services
  - o Food service operations can prefer sustainable food sources and reduce waste
  - o Minimize use of chemicals of concern in building materials, cleaning, and landscaping
- Educate staff, patients, and community about the hospital's or practice's environmentally preferable operating practices, and their benefits

and operation can have far-reaching impacts that result in healthier and more sustainable practices throughout the supply chain. These effects can educate and inspire staff, patients, and community members. Pediatricians should embrace improvements to the environmental performance of their practices as powerful opportunities to advocate for the health of children and families.

## Frequently Asked Questions

Q  *Pediatricians are trained to provide clinical care. What role do they have in "greening" practice or hospital operations?*

A  Many pediatricians run their practices and therefore have opportunities to directly influence the environmental performance of practice operations. Employed pediatricians can be powerful advocates within their organizations to recommend increasing energy efficiency, environmentally responsible waste management, and environmentally preferable purchasing including safer chemicals and healthier food. Pediatricians can make a case for incorporating environmental stewardship into practice and hospital operations by explaining the health benefits—including for children—of adopting these practices.

Q   *Can the improvement of the environmental performance of a single practice or hospital really have much impact?*

A   The collective impact of improving energy efficiency, managing waste, and implementing environmentally preferable purchasing extends beyond the walls of a single practice or hospital. Staff and patients may adopt certain practices at home and educate friends and family. A growing number of medical practices, hospitals, and health systems are adopting environmentally responsible operating practices with far-reaching impacts. For example, the growing demand for antibiotic-free meat and eggs is transforming the food supply chain toward healthier animal husbandry practices. The growing demand for furniture and furnishings free of chemicals of concern is resulting in a growing and more diverse supply, and lower cost, of these products.

Q   *Do environmental initiatives in hospital and practice operations compete with other needs that require investment of time and resources?*

A   Environmentally responsible operating practices align with core strategic priorities and values in a typical practice or hospital setting, including efficiency, quality, and safety. These practices can typically be integrated into existing organizational structures but do require a shared focus and support from leadership, with accountability for performance metrics, to become embedded in an organization, especially if the organization is just getting started with these practices. When environmental considerations are embedded with social and economic considerations in all aspects of a practice or hospital's culture, values, mission, and operations, improving environmental performance is well integrated into the organization and does not necessarily require additional staff or resources. In fact, these initiatives can save organizations costs, year over year.

## References

1.  Eckelman MJ, Sherman J. Environmental impacts of the U.S. health care system and effects on public health. *PLoS One.* 2016;11(6):e0157014

2.  World Health Organization. Healthy hospitals, healthy planet, healthy people: Addressing climate change in health care settings. 2009. http://www.who.int/globalchange/publications/healthcare_settings/en/. Accessed May 28, 2018

3.  US Environmental Protection Agency. A Better Building. A Better Bottom Line. A Better World. http://www.energystar.gov/ia/partners/publications/pubdocs/C+I_brochure.pdf?442a-1e83. Accessed May 28, 2018

4.  Kaplan S, Sadler B, Little K, Franz C, Orris P. Can Sustainable Hospitals Help Bend the Health Care Cost Curve? The Commonwealth Fund, November 2012

5. Energy Star Portfolio Manager. https://www.energystar.gov/buildings/facility-owners-and-managers/existing-buildings/use-portfolio-manager. Accessed May 28, 2018

6. US Department of Energy. Energy efficiency trends in residential and commercial buildings. August 2010. http://apps1.eere.energy.gov/buildings/publications/pdfs/corporate/building_trends_2010.pdf. Accessed May 28, 2018

7. US Department of Energy. Office of Energy Efficiency & Renewable Energy. Energy Savings Potential and RD&D Opportunities for Commercial Building HVAC Systems. https://www.energy.gov/sites/prod/files/2017/12/f46/bto-DOE-Comm-HVAC-Report-12-21-17.pdf. Accessed May 28, 2018

8. US Energy Star Program. Save Energy. https://www.energystar.gov/buildings/facility-owners-and-managers/existing-buildings/save-energy/put-computers-sleep. Accessed May 28, 2018

9. US Environmental Protection Agency. State and Local Climate Program Rules of Thumb. https://www.epa.gov/sites/production/files/2016-03/documents/table_rules_of_thumb.pdf. Accessed July 1, 2018

10. US Environmental Protection Agency. Improve Energy Use in Commercial Buildings. https://www.energystar.gov/buildings/about-us/how-can-we-help-you/improve-building-and-plant-performance/improve-energy-use-commercial. Accessed May 28, 2018

11. Cohen G. How Health Care Can Lead the Way on Renewable Energy. *Health Progress (Journal of the Catholic Health Association of the United States).* May-June 2016. https://www.chausa.org/publications/health-progress/article/may-june-2016/how-health-care-can-lead-the-way-on-renewable-energy. Accessed May 28, 2018

12. US Environmental Protection Agency. The Plain English Guide to the Clean Air Act. https://www.epa.gov/clean-air-act-overview/plain-english-guide-clean-air-act. Accessed May 28, 2018

13. US Environmental Protection Agency. WaterSense, an EPA Partnership Program. https://www.epa.gov/watersense. Accessed May 28, 2018

14. Healthcare Without Harm. Waste Minimization, Segregation, and Recycling in Hospitals. https://noharm-uscanada.org/sites/default/files/documents-files/2386/Waste_Min_Seg_Recyc_in_Hosp.pdf. Accessed May 28, 2018

15. US Environmental Protection Agency. Inventory of Greenhouse Gas Emissions and Sinks: 1990-2014. April 15, 2016. EPA 430-R-16-002. https://www.epa.gov/sites/production/files/2016-04/documents/us-ghg-inventory-2016-main-text.pdf. Accessed May 28, 2018

16. Healthier Hospitals: A Practice Greenhealth Program. Case Study: Less Waste Challenge, Regulated Medical Waste Reduction. https://practicegreenhealth.org/sites/default/files/upload-files/case_studies/st._marys_regional_medical_center.pdf. Accessed May 28, 2018

17. Practice Greenhealth. EPP Specifications and Resources Guide. https://practicegreenhealth.org/sites/default/files/upload-files/epp_specifications_and_resources_guide.pdf. Accessed May 28, 2018

18. Klepeis NE, Nelson WC, Ott WR, et al. The National Human Activity Pattern Survey (NHAPS): a resource for assessing exposure to environmental pollutants. *J Expo Anal Environ Epidemiol.* 2001;11(3):231–252

19. Eishel G, Shepon A, Makov T, Milo R. Land, irrigation water, greenhouse gas, and reactive nitrogen burdens of meat, eggs, and dairy production in the United States. *Proc Natl Acad Sci U S A.* 2014;111(33):11996–12001

20. American Heart Association. Eat More Chicken, Fish, and Beans. http://www.heart.org/HEARTORG/HealthyLiving/HealthyEating/Nutrition/Eat-More-Chicken-Fish-and-Beans_UCM_320278_Article.jsp#.VqroiPkrLIU. Accessed May 28, 2018

21. Paulson JA, Zaoutis TE, American Academy of Pediatrics Council on Environmental Health and Committee on Infectious Diseases. Nontherapeutic use of antimicrobial agents in animal agriculture: implications for pediatrics. *Pediatrics.* 2015;136(6):e1670–e1677

22. Health Care Without Harm. Clinician Champions in Comprehensive Antibiotic Stewardship. https://noharm-uscanada.org/CCCAS. Accessed May 28, 2018

23. Healthier Hospitals. Healthier Food. http://healthierhospitals.org/hhi-challenges/healthier-food. Accessed May 28, 2018

24. US Environmental Protection Agency. Sustainable Management of Food. https://www.epa.gov/sustainable-management-food/food-recovery-hierarchy. Accessed May 28, 2018

25. Calafat AM, Needham LL, Silva MJ, Lambert G. Exposure to di-(2-ethylhexyl) phthalate among premature neonates in a neonatal intensive care unit. *Pediatrics*. 2014;113(5):e429–e434

26. National Toxicology Program. US Department of Health and Human Services. NTP-CERHR Monograph on the Potential Human Reproductive and Developmental Effects of di-(2-ethylhexyl) phthalate (DEHP). https://noharm-uscanada.org/sites/default/files/documents-files/111/NTP-CERHR_DEHP_Monograph.pdf. Accessed May 28, 2018

27. Health Care Without Harm. Case Study: PVC and DEHP in Neonatal Intensive Care Units - Kaiser Permanente. https://noharm-uscanada.org/documents/case-study-pvc-and-dehp-neonatal-intensive-care-units-kaiser-permanente. Accessed May 28, 2018

28. US Green Building Council. LEED. http://www.usgbc.org/leed. Accessed May 28, 2018

29. Langdon D. Cost of Green Revisited: Reexamining the Feasibility and Cost Impact of Sustainable Design in the Light of Increased Market Adoption. http://sustainability.ucr.edu/docs/leed-cost-of-green.pdf. Accessed May 28, 2018

30. Quan X, Joseph A, Jelen M. Green Cleaning in Healthcare: Current Practices and Questions for Future Research. https://noharm-uscanada.org/sites/default/files/documents-files/65/Green_Cleaning_in_Healthcare.pdf. Accessed May 28, 2018

31. Rosenman KD, Reilly MJ, Schill DP, et al. Cleaning products and work-related asthma. *J Occup Environ Med*. 2003;45(5):556–563

32. US Environmental Protection Agency. Integrated Pest Management in Buildings. https://www.epa.gov/managing-pests-schools/integrated-pest-management-buildings. Accessed May 28, 2018

# Chapter 60

# Idiopathic Environmental Intolerance

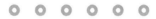

## KEY POINTS

- Idiopathic environmental intolerance (IEI) is a controversial condition most commonly seen in adults.
- IEI is defined as an acquired, chronic disorder characterized by recurrent symptoms occurring in response to low doses of chemically unrelated compounds.
- A thorough history and complete physical are needed for children whose parents believe they may have IEI.
- There are no proven clinical tests to diagnose IEI, and no evidence-based therapies.

## INTRODUCTION

Idiopathic environmental intolerance (IEI) (also known as "toxicant-induced loss of tolerance [TILT]," "environmental illness," or "multiple chemical sensitivity") is a highly controversial condition. There is overlap between the syndrome and other ill-defined conditions, such as fibromyalgia, chronic fatigue syndrome, and sick building syndrome. Although it most commonly is seen in adults, conditions attributed to IEI are reported to occur in children and adolescents.[1,2] To respond to parental concerns, pediatricians should be familiar with the condition.

Idiopathic environmental intolerance has been defined as an acquired, chronic disorder characterized by recurrent symptoms, referable to multiple organ systems, occurring reproducibly in response to exposure to many chemically unrelated compounds (or other environmental entities, such as electromagnetic radiation) at doses far below those established in the general population to cause harmful effects.[3,4] No single clinical test is diagnostic for defining which patients have the IEI syndrome; the symptoms generally improve when the incitants are removed. In contradistinction to sick building syndrome, symptoms are not associated with a single physical environment but can occur anywhere.

## CLINICAL SYMPTOMS

Exposure to low levels of a wide variety of chemically unrelated substances elicits a myriad of complaints in people with IEI. Adults with this condition often can recall an initial sensitizing exposure to an overpowering chemical, often occurring in the workplace. Symptoms can involve any organ system and commonly include fatigue, gastrointestinal problems, joint and muscle pains, rashes or other skin problems, and upper respiratory tract complaints. Most patients have neurologic or neuropsychological effects (ie, "mental fog" or impaired cognition, confusion, headaches, memory loss, paresthesias, irritability, and depression) as prominent features of the syndrome. Other features include malaise, dizziness, burning sensations, and breathlessness. In children and adolescents, hyperactivity and attention deficits or poor school performance have been cited by some as developmental consequences of IEI.[5]

Symptoms can wax and wane unpredictably over time; sensitivity expands from a single "inciting" chemical to a wide variety of unrelated substances. Pesticides, fragrances in perfumes, aftershaves or other household products, copy machine emissions, latex, food dyes and additives, cigarette smoke, formaldehyde, nylon fabrics, rayon material, and gases released from new carpets are substances commonly implicated in IEI.[6] Some people complain of foul odors (cacosmia) from chemicals or perfumes as triggers for their symptoms. The olfactory nerve mediates odor perception, while branches of the trigeminal nerve perceive irritation and pungency for taste and smell. Odor seems to be a prominent factor in precipitating the symptoms and serves as an important warning for the presence of toxic exposures. Some investigators argue that an explanation of the role of odor is a necessary component of any model of the causes of IEI.

Reportedly, symptoms also can migrate from one target organ system to another over time (switching). The progressive nature of symptoms, experienced after smaller and smaller doses of precipitants, the olfactory warning of offending odors, and the progressive restrictions on the patient's activities and habitable environments often characterize this condition.

## EPIDEMIOLOGY

One major difficulty in studying the epidemiology of IEI is the lack of a case definition agreed on by the medical and scientific community. Many published reports consist of case series or the clinical experiences of referral practices; none describe affected children. Small surveys have estimated the prevalence rates of self-reported IEI among adults to be approximately 12%,[7,8] although one subspecialty-based study (allergy, otolaryngology, occupational medicine) found an overall prevalence rate ranging from 5% to 27% of referrals.[9] None of these studies included children, and all are potentially confounded by the subjective, varying definition of the syndrome.

## HISTORICAL BACKGROUND

The late Theron Randolph, an allergist from Chicago, first described multiple chemical sensitivity during the 1950s.[10] He believed that traditional allergists defined "sensitivity" too narrowly by limiting it exclusively to antibody-antigen reactions. He hypothesized that foods and chemicals might cause other derangements of the immune system. Increasing exposure to petroleum products, pesticides, synthetic textiles, and food additives in modern life were identified as responsible for his patients' health problems, which included mental and behavioral disturbances, as well as rhinitis, headache, and asthma. A group of physicians, often called "clinical ecologists," who supported Dr Randolph's concept of environmental illness, founded the American Academy of Environmental Medicine.

In several position papers, traditional medical organizations have questioned the scientific basis of this syndrome. The American Academy of Allergy, Asthma and Immunology asserted that there were no adequate studies to support the theories of the clinical ecologists and, in 1986, issued a position statement stating that the diagnostic and therapeutic principles of clinical ecology were based on unproven methods.[11] Similarly, the American College of Physicians in 1989 and the American Medical Association in 1992 criticized clinical ecology.[12,13] A position statement by the American College of Occupational and Environmental Medicine in 1999 called for more research into the "phenomenon" of multiple chemical sensitivity.[14]

## PROPOSED CAUSATIVE MECHANISMS

A number of different models have been proposed to explain IEI. A model of immunologic dysfunction postulates that chemicals may damage the immune system so that it no longer functions normally. However, no clinical laboratory, other than those associated with clinical ecologists, has found consistent immune abnormalities in patients with IEI.[15]

Some have proposed that altered activity of receptors, such as the vanilloid and/or N-methyl-D-aspartate receptors, in the central and peripheral nervous systems underlie the reactions to xenobiotics experienced by persons with IEI.[16] However some well-controlled, blinded studies in adults have found no physiological differences between patients with IEI and controls in response to chemical challenges.[17] Another theory of causation involves the impaired metabolism of toxic chemicals, such that altered biotransformations lead to idiosyncratic toxic effects of common substances. One study found genotypic differences in a group of women with IEI versus controls in homozygous active CYP2D6 and rapid NAT2 enzyme systems. Gene-gene interactions between both enzymes predicted a substantially elevated risk in group membership.[18]

Investigators also have proposed a classic conditioned response to odor as an explanation for IEI. After an initial traumatic exposure to a strong-smelling odor, subsequent exposure may cause a conditioned response to much lower concentrations of the chemical. This conditioned response may be accompanied by varying degrees of "stimulus generalization" to the development of symptoms in response to other strong odors. Some researchers have suggested that an extreme form of this response be called an "odor-triggered panic attack."[19]

Affective disorders, somatoform disorders, and anxiety are the most frequent psychological conditions used to explain IEI.[20] People in whom IEI develops have a high degree of preexisting psychiatric morbidity and a tendency toward somatization.[21] These findings suggest that psychological factors, although not necessarily causative, may predispose some people to the development of a generalized chemical sensitivity. Comorbidities, such as posttraumatic stress disorder or childhood physical or sexual abuse or school refusal syndrome, also may have roles as underlying determinants of vulnerability to the development of IEI.[22]

The limbic-olfactory model provides a speculative biological explanation for affective and cognitive symptoms. The model depends on the anatomic links between the olfactory nerve, the limbic system, and other regions of the brain. Subconvulsive kindling (the ability of a subthreshold electrical or chemical stimulus to cause a response) and time-dependent sensitization are central nervous system constructs that provide a mechanism by which low-level chemical exposures can be amplified and produce symptoms referable to multiple organ systems.[23] One Japanese research team has performed case-control studies of adults that support a finding of alterations in cerebral blood flow after olfactory stimulation in patients with multiple chemical sensitivities when compared with controls.[24,25] Other proposed causes, such as "neuropathic" porphyria[26] or hypersensitization to yeast, have been discredited. There are scant research studies of IEI in children.

## CLINICAL EVALUATION OF A CHILD BELIEVED TO HAVE ENVIRONMENTAL SENSITIVITY

The pediatrician should approach the evaluation of a child whose parents believe that IEI is the cause of the child's symptoms in the same manner as any other problem: with a thorough history, a physical examination, and a methodical workup. Table 60-1 offers some diagnostic criteria that, although not studied systematically, may be applicable to children and adolescents. By using the history and selecting appropriate clinical tests, the pediatrician should first rule in or rule out conditions that are part of the differential diagnosis. Other diseases to consider are those with symptoms that are nonspecific and

---

**Table 60-1. Diagnostic Elements of Idiopathic Environmental Illness in Children[a]**

**Nature of Incitants Provoking a Response**
- Responses to offending environmental toxicants occur at levels of exposure below the 2.5th percentile for responses in the general population.
- Child responds to multiple substances that are unrelated chemically. The symptoms are not confined to one environment (eg, only "sick" buildings).

**Biological Plausibility, Identifiable Exposure**
- Symptoms are reproducible with exposure with reasonable consistency.
- Symptoms resolve after removal of incitant exposures.
- An identifiable exposure preceded the onset of the problem.

**Characteristics of Responses**
- Adverse responses affect more than one body system.
- Primary complaints include neuropsychological symptoms.
- The child exhibits altered sensitivity to odor.
- The disorder is chronic.

**Diagnosis**
- No single, accepted test of physiological function correlates with the symptoms.

**Subjective Responses and Ameliorative Actions of Affected Children**
- The caregivers and/or child perceive the child's response as unpleasant.
- The family has sought professional advice.
- The individual's caregivers believe he or she has a disorder.
- The family takes action to avoid exposures to symptom-inducing chemicals or other environmental incitants.

---

[a]Modified from Nethercott JR, Davidoff LL, Curbow B, Abbey H. Multiple chemical sensitivities syndrome: toward a working case definition. *Arch Environ Health.* 1993;48(1):19–26

inconstant, including Lyme disease, Munchausen by proxy, or psychosocial problems such as school refusal syndrome. The assessment should be directed toward the inclusion or exclusion of other diagnoses, such as asthma, migraine, allergies, chronic urticaria, hereditary angioedema, or an autoimmune disease. Specific environmental causes of systemic illness should be considered. Carbon monoxide poisoning, for example, can produce generalized complaints, such as headache, fatigue, dizziness, nausea, lethargy, and confusion. Chronic poisoning with heavy metals, such as mercury, arsenic, thallium, selenium, or lead, can sometimes result in behavioral symptoms and appetite disturbances.

Chronic or seasonal upper respiratory tract symptoms and wheezing suggest the possibility that the child has allergies and asthma, respectively. Although rhinorrhea, nasal obstruction, and sneezing would suggest an allergic etiology, children and adolescents may present with fatigue and irritability because of sleep disorders, perhaps induced by upper airway obstruction. Allergic stigmata found on physical examination, supported with appropriate laboratory studies, skin testing, and in cases of suspected reactive airway disease, pulmonary function tests, will suggest a diagnosis. Headache and dizziness, common complaints in IEI, are sometimes seen in children and adolescents with sinus disease or familial migraine.

Psychiatric disorders in parents and/or children, dysfunctional family dynamics, or child abuse and neglect must be considered in the evaluation of children or adolescents presenting for assessment of IEI. A positive family history for psychiatric diagnoses and treatment may be common in these patients. For some families, the illness may serve as a coping strategy or a more socially acceptable medical condition within which to express depressive symptoms. Children or adolescents may be attracted to the attention they gain when they are in the dependency role of patient or there may be issues in the family underlying a school refusal syndrome.

## DIAGNOSTIC METHODS

No laboratory tests are diagnostic, although several unproven tests have been proposed. For example, the use of positron emission tomography and single-photon emission computed tomography scans has not been standardized or validated and is not recommended. Diagnostic provocation-neutralization tests with different chemicals ("desensitization" routines of frequent injections or sublingual or dermal application of incitants), advocated by clinical ecologists, have been repudiated as being without scientific basis or validity and may cause harm themselves. The American College of Physicians reviewed 15 studies of provocation-neutralization testing performed by clinical ecologists and criticized the introduction of bias, lack of controls, and their uniformly poor methodologic designs.[12]

Testing of hair, blood, urine, or other tissues to screen for environmental chemicals generally is not helpful. When appropriate, laboratory testing to rule in or rule out other diagnoses or underlying medical conditions should be performed. Testing should be performed only at laboratories that adhere to the guidelines for quality control and laboratory operations established by the Clinical Laboratory Improvement Amendments (CLIA) of 1988.

## TREATMENT

The demands of adult patients with IEI on health care professionals, their high use of health care resources, and their dissatisfaction with proffered advice, especially if that advice suggests psychological counseling as a management option, are frustrating for the patient and practitioner alike. Adult patients with IEI are high-frequency users of medical facilities and suffer a considerable amount of functional disability because of their complaints and the strategies they must use to get through the day. Parental overuse of care services for their child can also be challenging to pediatricians, who must nevertheless continue to offer their availability and support in the best interests of the child.

Proposed therapies, none of which are evidence-based or recommended, include restricted, rotating diets, provocation-neutralization, and the use of saunas for chemical detoxification. Patients with IEI seek out a variety of treatments, not only from physicians but also clinical ecologists, naturopaths, homeopaths, and other practitioners. Clinical ecologists and others may recommend herbs, oxygen, oral nystatin, and minerals to treat their patients by improving their "tolerance" of the environment, although a scientific basis for such treatments is lacking. Some postulate that sufferers of IEI have deficits of essential cofactors or enzymes necessary for chemical detoxification; they prescribe dietary supplements, herbs, antioxidants, and vitamins to repair such theoretical deficiencies. None of these therapies is supported by credible scientific studies.

Some therapies used hold special risks for children and adolescents, and their use should be discouraged. Parents should be warned against potentially harmful and expensive remedies, such as chelation, gamma globulin injections, catharsis, or "sweat therapies," because there is little scientific evidence that these are effective for treatment. Chelation can cause death from hypocalcemia, neurologic damage, and other adverse events (see Chapter 50). Severely restricted diets may not supply the essential protein, minerals, vitamins, and other nutrients needed for a growing body. Desensitization remedies and products containing multiple herbs, dietary supplements, and/ or megavitamins may be especially harmful to children and adolescents who are still developing. Children may have limited capacity to detoxify certain herbs, minerals, hormones, and dietary supplements through the liver and kidneys, with a consequent higher risk of toxic reactions. They may experience allergic reactions to such substances as well as those used in "desensitization" routines.

Many patients restrict their activities and reconstruct their habitats so that they can avoid those environmental agents causing symptoms, essentially living in a relatively chemical-free environment. There are known sensitizing chemicals in some household products, such as paraphenylenediamine found in hair dyes and henna-based temporary tattoos,[28,29] colors (eg, tartrazine, azo dyes, amaranth), flavorings (eg, ethylvanilline, monosodium glutamate), antioxidants (eg, butylated hydroxytoluene) and other preservatives and additives (eg, benzoic acid, xanthum gum, sodium benzoate, sulphites) in foods,[2,30] and some common chemicals used as fragrances in a range of products from detergents to toothpaste to moisturizers. Avoidance of such compounds when purchasing household items is an important strategy pursued by affected families. A word of caution: some "fragrance-free" home products actually contain chemicals to mask the natural odor of the shampoo or sunscreen; other "fragrance-free" products still use preservatives, such as benzyl alcohol.[31]

Some adults use barrier clothing such as special masks, gloves, coveralls, and even self-contained breathing apparatus in the attempt to avoid chemical triggers. The disability in adults is such that they often isolate themselves from others socially and cannot hold a job. Children and adolescents who cannot attend school or develop normal peer relationships because of IEI would be similarly disabled. These children should be managed in consultation with a social worker or other mental health professional.

Newer inventories show promise for standardizing the diagnosis and measuring the impact and severity of IEI.[32] Biopsychological modalities of management, including biofeedback, electrophysiological monitoring, coping strategies, cognitive-behavioral therapy, family-centered therapy, and behavioral modification (psychological deconditioning) techniques, are worth investigating in children.[33] Addressing directly any parental mistrust and hostility to allopathic medicine is important. Offering to work with families should extend to collaboration with school systems, social services, and other community-based agencies in helping families cope with the condition.

## CONCLUSION

Examining a child purported to have IEI is a challenge for the pediatrician who is faced with treating the child's health as it fits into the family's belief system. Exploring the basis for the beliefs and keeping an open mind to the different values that underlie them will allow effective and compassionate use of the pediatrician's medical knowledge and skills.

## Frequently Asked Questions

Q *I have been told that my child has a short attention span and that he frequently is inattentive in class. The teacher has suggested psychological testing. My child is fine at home. Could these problems be related to chemical exposure at school?*

A A thorough evaluation of the child's difficulty and appropriate testing are initial steps in dealing with this problem. Sources of potential environmental contamination cited in schools include cleaning agents, art supplies (eg, glues, markers, aerosol sprays), pesticides, and diesel exhaust fumes from school buses. Dust and molds also are sources of indoor air pollution. Symptoms in one setting only (the school) may suggest an environmental etiology. Often, when queried, other students and teachers in a school with poor indoor air quality or other environmental hazards will report similar health complaints. While performing such a thorough evaluation, pediatricians also should keep in mind that parental anxieties about learning and behavior problems might be displaced toward concerns about chemical exposures in the school.

Q *My child is being made sick by the chemicals that she is exposed to in school. Can you, as my pediatrician, intervene and help me decrease my child's exposure to chemicals in the school?*

A Parents often ask pediatricians to write a letter supporting the child's withdrawal from some activity or area in the school. In these instances, the pediatrician should be open-minded but careful about fostering negative associations between the child and the child's environment. A thorough history and physical examination of the child, with attention to finding or excluding other medical diagnoses, is an essential first step. Another issue raised by this question is less obvious but of crucial importance in considering the problem of chemical sensitivity in children. It usually is the parent who attributes the child's symptoms to chemical exposures in various environments, and the parent may have fixed beliefs about the causal relationship in their advocacy for their child. Although there might sometimes be a temporal relationship between the exposure and symptoms, the association may or may not be causal. The pediatrician can be proactive in working closely with both the parents and school officials toward an assessment of the school environment and an educational solution that serves the best interests of the child. A regional pediatric environmental health specialty unit and local and/or state health department officials may be of assistance as additional resources to the pediatrician, the school, and the family.

Q   *What do I need to do to my home to prevent my child from being exposed to chemicals that might be toxic?*

A   It is important for parents to understand that their child's exposure to chemicals is cumulative: the sum of inhalation, ingestion, and dermal exposures. Parents should be encouraged to consider all activities and situations in which their child might be exposed. The home may be a source of environmental exposures (see Chapter 5). The school environment may be a source of additional exposures to chemicals (see Chapter 11). One common environmental exposure is to secondhand tobacco smoke—thus, one of the most important things parents can do is to eliminate their child's exposure to secondhand tobacco smoke. Parents should also know that "thirdhand" tobacco smoke[34]—the smoke residue remaining on items such as clothing and furniture—may be irritating. Parents who smoke should be encouraged to quit. Smoking should be prohibited inside the home and smokers should change their clothes and wash their hands before interacting with a child. The substitution of environmentally friendly alternatives for household solvents, cleaners, pesticides, and other chemicals are prudent measures that all families can adopt.

## References

1.  Woolf A. A 4-year-old girl with manifestations of multiple chemical sensitivities. *Environ Health Perspect*. 2000;108(12):1219–1223

2.  Inomata N, Osuna H, Fujita H, Ogawa T, Ikezawa Z. Multiple chemical sensitivities following intolerance to azo dye in sweets in a 5-year-old girl. *Allergol Int*. 2006;55(2):203–205

3.  Cullen MR. The worker with multiple chemical sensitivities: an overview. *Occup Med*. 1987;2(4):655–661

4.  Multiple chemical sensitivity: a 1999 consensus. *Arch Environ Health*. 1999;54(3):147–149

5.  Kidd PM. Attention deficit/hyperactivity disorder (ADHD) in children: rationale for its integrative management. *Altern Med Rev*. 2000;5(5):402–428

6.  Hu H, Stern A, Rotnitzky A, Schlesinger L, Proctor S, Wolfe J. Development of a brief questionnaire for screening for multiple chemical sensitivity syndrome. *Toxicol Ind Health*. 1999;15(6):582–588

7.  Kreutzer R, Neutra RR, Lashuay N. Prevalence of people reporting sensitivities to chemicals in a population-based survey. *Am J Epidemiol*. 1999;150(1):1–12

8.  Meggs WJ, Dunn KA, Bloch RM, Goodman PE, Davidoff AL. Prevalence and nature of allergy and chemical sensitivity in a general population. *Arch Environ Health*. 1996;51(4):275–282

9.  Kutsogiannis DJ, Davidoff AL. A multiple center study of multiple chemical sensitivity syndrome. *Arch Environ Health*. 2001;56(3):196–207

10. Randolph TG. Sensitivity to petroleum including its derivatives and antecedents. *J Lab Clin Med*. 1952;40:931–932

11. Executive Committee of the American Academy of Allergy and Immunology. Clinical ecology. *J Allergy Clin Immunol*. 1986;78(2):269–271

12. American College of Physicians. Clinical ecology. *Ann Intern Med*. 1989;111(2):168–178

13. Council on Scientific Affairs, American Medical Association. Clinical ecology. *JAMA*. 1992;268(24):3465–3467

14. American College of Occupational and Environmental Medicine. ACOEM position statement. Multiple chemical sensitivities: idiopathic environmental intolerance. *J Occup Environ Med.* 1999;41(11):940–942

15. Simon GE, Daniell W, Stockbridge H, Claypoole K, Rosenstock L. Immunologic, psychological, and neuropsychological factors in multiple chemical sensitivity. A controlled study. *Ann Intern Med.* 1993;119(2):97–103

16. Pall ML, Anderson JH. The vanilloid receptor as a putative target of diverse chemicals in multiple chemical sensitivity. *Arch Environ Health.* 2004;59(7):363–369

17. Dantoft TM, Skovbjerg S, Andersson L, et al. Inflammatory mediator profiling of n-butanol exposed upper airways in individuals with multiple chemical sensitivity. *PLoS One.* 2015;10(11):e0143534

18. McKeown-Eyssen G, Baines C, Cole DE, et al. Case-control study of genotypes in multiple chemical sensitivity: CYP2D6, NAT1, NAT2, PON1, PON2 and MTHFR. *Int J Epidemiol.* 2004;33(5):971–978

19. Staudenmayer H. Multiple chemical sensitivities or idiopathic environmental intolerances: psychophysiologic foundation of knowledge for a psychogenic explanation. *J Allergy Clin Immunol.* 1997;99(4):434–437

20. Terr AI. Environmental illness. A clinical review of 50 cases. *Arch Intern Med.* 1986;146(1): 145–149

21. Black DW, Rathe A, Goldstein RB. Environmental illness. A controlled study of 26 subjects with "20th century disease." *JAMA.* 1990;264(24):3166–3170

22. Black DW, Okiishi C, Gable J, Schlosser S. Psychiatric illness in the first-degree relatives of persons reporting multiple chemical sensitivities. *Toxicol Ind Health.* 1999;15(3-4):410–414

23. Ross PM, Whyser J, Covello VT, et al. Olfaction and symptoms in the multiple chemical sensitivities syndrome. *Prev Med.* 1999;28(5):467–480

24. Azuma K, Uchiyama I, Takano H, et al. Changes in cerebral blood flow during olfactory stimulation in patients with multiple chemical sensitivity: a multi-channel near-infrared spectroscopic study. *PloS One.* 2013;8(11):e80567

25. Azuma K, Uchiyama I, Tanigawa M, et al. Assessment of cerebral blood flow in patients with multiple chemical sensitivity using near-infrared spectroscopy – recovery after olfactory stimulation: a case-control study. *Environ Health Prev Med.* 2015;20(3):185–194

26. Ellefson RD, Ford RE. The porphyrias: characteristics and laboratory tests. *Regul Toxicol Pharmacol.* 1996;24(1 Pt 2):S119–S125

27. Nethercott JR, Davidoff LL, Curbow B, Abbey H. Multiple chemical sensitivities syndrome: toward a working case definition. *Arch Environ Health.* 1993;48(1):19–26

28. Sosted H, Johansen JD, Andersen KE, Menne T. Severe allergic hair dye reactions in 8 children. *Contact Dermatitis.* 2006;54(2):87–91

29. Marcoux D, Couture-Trudel PM, Riboulet-Delmas G, Sasseville D. Sensitization to parapheylenediamine from a streetside temporary tattoo. *Pediatr Dermatol.* 2002;19(6): 498–502

30. Madsen C. Prevalence of food additive intolerance. *Hum Exp Toxicol.* 1994;13(6):393–399

31. Scheinman PL. The foul-side of fragrance-free products: what every clinician should know about managing patients with fragrance allergy. *J Am Acad Dermatol.* 1999;41(6):1020–1024

32. Miller CS, Prihoda TJ. The Environmental Exposure and Sensitivity Inventory (EESI): a standardized approach for measuring chemical intolerances for research and clinical applications. *Toxicol Ind Health.* 1999;15(3-4):370–385

33. Spyker DA. Multiple chemical sensitivities—syndrome and solution. *J Toxicol Clin Toxicol.* 1995;33(2):95–99

34. Winickoff JP, Friebely J, Tanski SE, et al. Beliefs about the health effects of "thirdhand" smoke and home smoking bans. *Pediatrics.* 2009;123(1):e74–e79

# Chapter 61

# Methamphetamine Laboratories

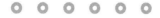

## KEY POINTS

- Illicit manufacture of methamphetamine may occur in homes where children live.
- Children from these homes may need evaluation and treatment for acute chemical exposures.
- These children need evaluation and treatment for abuse and neglect.
- Residues of methamphetamine and other chemicals may persist at former sites and pose a hazard to future occupants.

## INTRODUCTION

Amphetamines and methamphetamines are stimulants that affect the central and the sympathetic nervous systems. Methamphetamine (the chemical name for which is desoxyephedrine) is the $N$-methyl homologue of amphetamine. Although Mexican drug trafficking organizations have become the primary methamphetamine manufacturers and suppliers, illicit methamphetamine ("meth") manufacturing can occur on a smaller scale in homes in which children live, potentially exposing them to toxic chemicals. Children living at a clandestine methamphetamine laboratory site may be subjected to fires and explosions. They are at risk of unintentional ingestion of methamphetamine with resulting toxicities. Their caregivers' hazardous lifestyles may also include the presence of firearms, pornography, and other social problems. Homes may be substandard, may lack plumbing, and may have code violations with hazardous conditions. Children often are witnesses to violence and often suffer abuse and neglect and lack of food. Thus, when these children are removed from methamphetamine laboratory sites, their care is coordinated among medical, social work, and law enforcement professionals. Pediatricians may be asked to do a medical evaluation of children from such homes or of parents who use methamphetamine and are rendered unable to care for their children.

Amphetamine was first synthesized in 1887, but it was not tested in animal models until 1910. It was first commercially available in 1931 as the nasal spray Benzedrine, a racemic *d,l* form of amphetamine. The first amphetamine tablet appeared in 1937 and was used to treat narcolepsy. Because of its euphoric, stimulating, and appetite-suppressing effects, amphetamine became widely used during the 1930s and 1940s and was used by foreign armies in World War II.[1]

Methamphetamine was first synthesized in 1919 by a Japanese chemist. In the late 1970s, biker gangs began to manufacture methamphetamine, primarily using the phenyl-2-propanone (P2P) method. Manufacturing via another method, ephedrine reduction, began to occur in trailer parks and mobile homes and was more commonly found in rural areas. In the rural United States, makeshift "mom and pop" laboratories produce relatively small amounts of methamphetamine. The domestic clandestine laboratories produce methamphetamine on a smaller scale using diverted products that contain precursor chemicals and may include pseudoephedrine obtained illegally. Laboratories capable of producing more than 10 pounds of methamphetamine ("superlaboratories") are more common in California, are controlled by California- and Mexico-based criminal groups, and use different precursor chemicals.[2] The market for methamphetamine has been sustained by drug-trafficking organizations. Mexico is now the primary source for methamphetamine, and large-scale methamphetamine production is increasing in Canada. To avoid law enforcement officials, laboratories are mobile. A single batch of methamphetamine may be produced in several stages, with each stage occurring at a different location. Laboratories can be active, in the process of active chemical reactions; set-up, ready for manufacture but having no chemical reactions; boxed, stored for transit; or former laboratories, from which all reaction vessels have been removed.[3]

Methamphetamine exists as a powder resembling granulated crystals or as a rock form called "ice," the smokable version that came into use in the 1980s. Methamphetamine can be heated to form a vapor that is smoked, snorted, orally ingested, or injected. The "rush" results from the release of high levels of dopamine into the brain, which is almost instantaneous if methamphetamine is smoked or injected, occurs after about 5 minutes if it is snorted, and occurs after about 20 minutes if orally ingested.[4]

The major action of amphetamines is to cause the release of monoamines from storage sites in axon terminals, increasing the concentration of these amines in the synaptic cleft. Amphetamines are taken into the neurons, enter the neurotransmitter storage vesicles, and block the transport of dopamine into these vesicles. This action results in intracellular and extravesicular accumulation of dopamine. The dopamine may undergo oxidation, producing toxic, reactive chemicals such as oxygen radicals, peroxides, and hydroxyquinones. Amphetamines also cause the release of serotonin and norepinephrine.[5] Methamphetamine inhibits the reuptake of norepinephrine, dopamine, and serotonin into the presynaptic terminals, which causes postsynaptic hyperstimulation of alpha-1 and beta-1 receptors.[6]

The primary site of metabolism is in the liver by aromatic hydroxylation, $N$-methylation (to form the metabolite amphetamine), and deamination. Acidic urine enhances excretion, leading to a shorter half-life, while basic urine slows excretion and prolongs half-life.[7] The elimination half-life varies from 12 to 34 hours.

## CHEMICALS INVOLVED IN MANUFACTURE

Clandestine manufacturing methods ("cooks") generally start with pseudoephedrine (prior to 2005) or phenylacetic acid as the precursor and require the combination and addition of several other household chemicals as reagents. These chemicals include acids, bases, and organic solvents as well as lithium, red phosphorus, or iodine, depending on the method of synthesis. The older amalgam method started with phenylacetic acid to generate phenyl-2-propanone. Lead acetate was used in one of the first steps. Methylamine and mercuric chloride were used in the second step to generate methamphetamine.[8] This method may result in mercury and lead contamination at the cook site.[9]

After phenyl-2-propanone became a scheduled drug, production methods involved the chemical reduction of ephedrine or pseudoephedrine to produce methamphetamine chloride. There are 3 different processes commonly used to accomplish this reduction. Two of these processes (red phosphorus and hypophosphorous acid) are similar in their use of phosphorus and iodine. The third process is the Birch reduction, or anhydrous ammonia method, commonly found in agricultural communities where anhydrous ammonia is used as a fertilizer. All 3 methods utilize hydrogen chloride gas that is typically generated using sulfuric acid and sodium chloride (rock salt) to precipitate methamphetamine hydrochloride. The classes of chemicals used to produce methamphetamine by the previously listed processes and their major adverse effects are listed in Table 61-1. After the passage of the Combat Methamphetamine Epidemic Act in 2005, which restricted the public's access to pseudoephedrine, the number of new methamphetamine users dropped. However, this decline was short lived because illicit methamphetamine manufacturers began using the phenyl-2-propanone method once again, resulting in rising numbers of new users since 2012.[10] In addition, pseudoephedrine imports have fed continued methamphetamine manufacturing.

A complete list of chemicals used in methamphetamine manufacture may be found in the Drug Enforcement Agency's *"Guidelines for Law Enforcement for the Cleanup of Clandestine Drug Laboratories."*[11] The Drug Enforcement Agency estimates that for every pound of methamphetamine manufactured, 5 to 6 pounds of toxic waste may be generated, largely within the structure and surrounding environment. This number does not account for the contamination of other water sources downstream from the methamphetamine sites.[12] Hundreds of chemicals have been found in methamphetamine laboratories that have little or nothing to do with methamphetamine production. This may be the result of confusion over look-alike/sound-alike names, ignorance of what is useful for manufacture, or manufacture of other products (eg, drugs, explosives). First responders should use caution when entering these "facilities," and clinicians caring for children living in these facilities should be aware that children may have been exposed to numerous chemicals.

Methamphetamine-related chemical incidents with injured persons increased from less than 5% in 2008 to 10% in 2012.[13] Explosions, while uncommon, can occur from the misuse of flammable chemicals in the manufacturing process. The most commonly reported injuries are respiratory irritation, chemical and thermal burns, and eye irritation. Most injuries are sustained by the general public followed by law enforcement officials. Exposed children face threats in addition to their health and safety.

## Table 61-1. Chemical Components of Methamphetamine Laboratories and Risks

| CHEMICAL CLASS | ROUTE OF EXPOSURE | ADVERSE EFFECTS |
|---|---|---|
| Anhydrous ammonia | Inhalation | Eye, nose, throat irritation, dyspnea, wheezing, chest pain, pulmonary edema |
| | Dermal | Skin burns, vesiculation, frostbite[14] |
| Acids and bases | Inhalation | Pneumonitis, pulmonary edema |
| | Dermal | Caustic burns |
| | Ingestion | Gastric perforation, esophageal burns with later strictures, nausea, vomiting |
| Solvents | Inhalation and ingestion<br>Inhalation | Liver and kidney damage, bone marrow suppression, headache<br>Respiratory irritation, central nervous system depression or excitation, aspiration[15] |
| Iodine | Inhalation | Respiratory distress, mucus membrane irritation[16] |
| | Ingestion | Corrosive gastritis |
| Phosphorus | Ingestion | Gastrointestinal tract irritation, liver damage, oliguria |
| Red phosphorus | | Caustic burns |
| Potential: phosphine gas | Inhalation | Ocular irritation, nausea, vomiting, fatigue, chest pain, headache, fatal respiratory effects, seizures, coma[17] |

## ROUTES OF EXPOSURE

Exposure to methamphetamine, the chemicals used in its production, and the chemical by-products is commonly by inhalation or dermal contact. Adolescents may intentionally abuse methamphetamine. Children may unintentionally ingest methamphetamine manufactured in drug laboratories.

## SOURCES OF EXPOSURE

Children may be exposed through primary or secondary sources, depending on the status of the laboratory. An active or recently active laboratory poses hazards, primarily from inhalation. Once these primary sources are removed, secondary sources include solvent spills and upholstered furniture, drapes, carpet, and wallboard that have absorbed solvent vapors and volatile contaminants. These chemicals may be rereleased during cleanup. Nonvolatile compounds, such as the hydrochloride salt of methamphetamine, are possible skin contaminants.[18] In one study, investigators sampled former clandestine laboratory sites immediately after entry by law enforcement personnel. Controlled cooks were performed in these inactive laboratories to simulate exposures during illicit methamphetamine manufacturing and to identify chemicals that were present. Methamphetamine was detected on multiple surfaces, including refrigerators, microwaves, and ceiling fans. Methamphetamine was detected on surfaces after experimental cooks via the anhydrous ammonia, red phosphorus, and hypophosphorous methods.[19] The median methamphetamine particle diameter was less than 0.1 mcm, a respirable size that may penetrate the lungs and bloodstream. Sequential sampling up to 24 hours after simulated red phosphorus cooks in a 1-story home yielded higher levels of airborne methamphetamine with increasing activity, such as walking and vacuuming. This may represent probable resuspension from contaminated surfaces.[20] Surface iodine was detected after red phosphorus and hypophosphorous cooks. Hydrochloric acid was released during all cook methods, with extraction phase levels close to the "Immediately Dangerous to Life and Health" level of 50 parts per million (ppm) as defined by the National Institute for Occupational Safety and Health. Ammonia was detected after an experimental anhydrous cook.

Products of passive exposure to methamphetamine were assessed via simulating single and multiple sessions of smoking varying amounts of methamphetamine in a hotel room. Study authors assumed that a person smoking methamphetamine would absorb 67% to 90% of the drug.[2] They found that an average smoke of approximately 100 mg of methamphetamine results in airborne methamphetamine concentrations from 37 to 123 mcg/m$^3$. These levels likely result in surface deposition levels approaching 0.07 mcg/100 cm$^2$ in the vicinity of the smoke. As more smoking occurs, levels may exceed 5 mcg/100 cm$^2$.

These studies highlight the risk of exposure to methamphetamine or other chemicals during and after an active cook, passive smoking, or inhabiting a former cook site.

## SYSTEMS AFFECTED

The lungs, central nervous system, and skin are most affected.

## CLINICAL EFFECTS

### Acute Effects

The most significant health risk related to methamphetamine production is acute injury secondary to massive chemical exposure via inhalation and contact with the skin and eyes. Thus, when a clandestine laboratory is raided, team members wear special protective gear, including a self-contained breathing apparatus and chemical-resistant suits, gloves, and boots. Most exposures reported from clandestine laboratory incidents were from inhalation. These were reported in adult first responders who were not wearing proper personal protective equipment, such as respirators.[3,13] Data specific to children's exposures via inhalation and dermal contact are very limited.

Pediatric exposures result primarily from acute poisoning from unintentional methamphetamine ingestions while children are in the care of the users or when they are left alone in the home. Children found in methamphetamine homes are usually taken to an emergency department for evaluation even if they are asymptomatic because of protocols established by local emergency medical services. Despite the lack of symptoms, urine drug screens are obtained to assess for the presence of methamphetamine. In some jurisdictions, laws mandate finding drugs in urine samples before further child abuse charges can be filed. In other jurisdictions, evidence of drug use or manufacture in the home is enough to criminally charge an adult. In child protection proceedings, it is not uniformly required that a child has a positive drug screen to bring forth a report/finding of child maltreatment. Scene investigation is sufficient in some jurisdictions to prove that exposure in the home has occurred.

Several case series have shown that if symptoms are present, central nervous and cardiovascular system effects predominate. In a larger case series, the most common presenting symptom was agitation. In a series of children younger than 6 years reported to the California Poison Control Center, 82% presented with agitation.[22] In a series of patients with an average age of 19 months, 89% presented with crying.[23] Other central nervous system findings included irritability, seizures, or abnormal movements.[24] Cardiovascular findings were tachycardia and hypertension. Other organ systems may be affected (Table 61-2). In one 14-year-old patient, multisystem organ failure and secondary hyperthermia developed after intentional abuse of methamphetamine.[25]

| Table 61-2. Reported Signs and Symptoms of Acute Methamphetamine Ingestion in Children[6,22,25-29] | |
|---|---|
| SYSTEM | FINDINGS |
| Central nervous: mental status | Irritability<br>Agitation<br>Inconsolability with and without crying<br>Hyperactivity<br>Delirium |
| Central nervous: movement | Ataxia<br>Constant movement<br>Seizure<br>Flailing movements of head, neck, and extremities<br>Involuntary side-to-side head turning |
| Ocular | Roving eye movements<br>Cortical blindness |
| Central and peripheral nervous | Hyperthermia |
| Cardiovascular | Tachycardia<br>Hypertension<br>Myocarditis |
| Gastrointestinal tract | Vomiting<br>Esophagitis |
| Respiratory tract | Respiratory distress<br>Hypoxia |
| Musculoskeletal | Rhabdomyolysis |
| Cutaneous/orofacial | Burns of lips, tongue |
| Metabolic | Decreased serum bicarbonate<br>Hyperkalemia<br>Hepatic and renal failure |

## Chronic Exposure

Historically, methamphetamine use has primarily occurred among adults, but epidemiological studies, while small in numbers, have shown that the demographic profile has widened to include adolescents.[30] Adolescents in treatment for methamphetamine abuse are more likely to have a psychiatric history or a family history of substance abuse, and higher rates of depression and suicidal ideation. Psychological and behavioral symptoms may continue after methamphetamine use has ceased perhaps, in part, because of the drug's effects on an immature brain, and because of other issues.

Chronic methamphetamine use in adult users may result in anxiety, confusion, insomnia, mood disturbances, and violent behavior. Adult users also may display psychotic symptoms such as paranoia, visual and auditory hallucinations, and delusions, such as the sensation of insects crawling under the skin. Repetitive motor activity, weight loss, and severe dental problems may occur.[31] Choreoathetoid movement disorders, acute and chronic cardiomyopathy, acute aortic dissections, arterial aneurysms, pulmonary hypertension, hepatocellular damage, and acute renal failure have been reported.[32] No data are available about the health risks of longer-term exposures among children living in currently or previously contaminated home settings.

## MANAGEMENT OF CHILDREN EXPOSED TO METHAMPHETAMINE LABORATORIES

Children removed from methamphetamine laboratories require comprehensive medical, social work, developmental, and psychological evaluations. An evaluation for abuse includes attention to possible physical, sexual, and emotional abuse. An evaluation for neglect includes assessing the child's medical, dental, and educational needs as well as basic needs for food, clothing, and shelter. Many children who have lived in drug-endangered environments have experienced or witnessed multiple forms of trauma. As a result, many will benefit from assessment for trauma-focused therapy if they are developmentally able to participate.

The National Alliance for Drug Endangered Children, established in 2000, authored the national protocol for the medical evaluation of children found in drug laboratories, along with reference fact sheets (available at www.nationaldec. org).[33] Management of these children involves decontamination, medical evaluation, and toxicologic evaluation. In all cases of children removed from the home of a methamphetamine laboratory, law enforcement and child protection service collaboration is mandatory to ensure the welfare of the child. If law enforcement officials suspect that a child is present prior to assessing the home, child protection services should be notified and be available at the time of the search.

### Decontamination

Full decontamination according to standard protocols is indicated (if the child is medically stable) when there has been significant chemical exposure, such as in an explosion or fire. Basic life support measures take precedence over decontamination. Rescuers should take measures to avoid injury to themselves. In cases with significant chemical exposure (as evidenced by a chemical smell on the person or by clothes with chemical stains), the child should have the chemicals removed at the scene by removing clothes. These clothes are then given to law enforcement agents.

Clothes should be removed in a supervised and sensitive environment. Clothing or robes used to cover the child for transport from the scene should be seasonally appropriate and made from a breathable type of fabric. Occlusive or non-breathable coverings (such as plastic) should be avoided because this can increase the transdermal absorption of drugs and chemicals present on the child's skin prior to bathing.

The child should be cleansed with running water and soap when this can be done without causing trauma. An asymptomatic child who is removed from a laboratory and has no signs of obvious chemical contamination is unlikely to present a significant danger to other individuals. The child's clothing should be removed as soon as it is reasonably safe. Although it is unlikely that significant amounts of methamphetamine or other chemicals will be transferred from clothing, a cloth may be placed over vehicle seats for further protection. Toys and objects should be left at the home.[34]

## Medical Evaluation

A child must be transported to the closest emergency department if there has been an explosion at the laboratory site or if the child has respiratory distress, burns, lethargy, or somnolence. Decontamination may be required on-site or during transportation. The emergent evaluation suggested by the National Alliance for Drug Endangered Children national protocol focuses on the child's respiratory and neurologic status along with the usual assessments of temperature, blood pressure, respiration, and pulse. It is not necessary to transport asymptomatic children to an emergency department. Instead, it is recommended that clinicians provide an assessment and find the child a medical home within 72 hours of removal from the home. The child should have a thorough physical examination including a detailed head-to-toe skin examination. At that time, the child also should also be assessed for nutritional and developmental deficiencies, and for physical and emotional neglect.

## Toxicologic Evaluation

The authority over drug laboratory and federal drug testing programs resides with the Division of Workplace Programs in the Substance Abuse and Mental Health Services Administration (SAMHSA), which is part of the US Department of Health and Human Services. The treatment of the child in an emergency department setting, however, is directed by the attending physician.

If necessary, examination of the urine is the preferred method to detect acute exposure to methamphetamine. Obtaining this sample is at the discretion of the treating physician, and the decision to obtain it in an asymptomatic child should occur after a discussion among law enforcement officials, child protective services personnel, and medical personnel. When toxicologic evaluation is performed, high false-negative rates may occur with immunoassays because they may not detect small concentrations found in children; false-positive results can occur from other substances with similar chemical structure. For example, use of cough and cold medications can result in a false-positive result for amphetamines. The referring laboratory should be informed that the specimen comes from a child. Any sample with a drug detected should be sent for confirmatory testing by gas chromatography-mass spectrometry.[35] A negative test indicates that if a drug was present at the time of collection, the level was lower than the limit of detection. A negative test does not mean that the child was never exposed to methamphetamine. Thus, the situation in which the child was found should be the primary consideration.

If a urine sample is obtained, it is best obtained within 8 to 12 hours of removal from the laboratory site. The commonly used initial screening test for amphetamines (methamphetamine and amphetamine) is an immunoassay with a commonly used federal workplace cutoff of 1,000 nanograms (ng)/mL that was lowered by SAMHSA to 500 ng/mL in 2010.

Isomer resolution by further toxicologic analysis can distinguish between the *l*–isomer and the *d*-isomer more commonly found in illicit preparations.[36]

Testing of hair for drugs is used in some jurisdictions to detect methamphetamine exposure because hair has a longer window of detection. Depending on the methodology of the laboratory, a positive hair drug test could reflect either exposure from environmental contamination of the outer surface of the hair shaft by drug residue or systemic exposure from ingestion or inhalation of the drug picked up by the hair follicle from the circulation and then growing out in the shaft of the hair.[37] Despite the inability of some tests to distinguish between what has been deposited in the hair from external contaminants and drugs acquired through systemic exposure, the underlying issue is that the child was in an environment in which methamphetamine was present.

## TREATMENT OF ACUTE METHAMPHETAMINE TOXICITY

Because there is no antidote for methamphetamine, treatment of methamphetamine toxicity in children is based on symptoms and should be managed in consultation with a pediatric toxicologist or poison control center. Agitation in pediatric patients hospitalized in an intensive care unit was successfully treated with parenteral benzodiazepines, alone or in combination with haloperidol.[23] A monitored setting is recommended because haloperidol use has been associated with prolongation of the QT interval. Haloperidol is not recommended if children have seizures.

## REMEDIATION

Methamphetamine residues may be found at former makeshift laboratory sites and may pose risks to future residents. Remediation standards are usually legislated and vary by state. Several state regulations regarding methamphetamine contamination of residences are based on the detection limit of methamphetamine and not on the chemicals that were present in the manufacturing process. The State of Colorado assessed several states' technology-based cleanup standards for their health-protectiveness,[9] and then selected 0.5 mg/100 cm$^2$ as the final clean up standard for methamphetamine residues. The California Environmental Protection Agency published 2 research papers addressing remediation.[18,38] The first attempted to identify a subchronic daily reference dose of methamphetamine. The subchronic daily reference dose is an estimate of daily exposure for a subchronic duration (up to 10% of a lifespan) that will not have deleterious effects in the general population, including sensitive subpopulations such as children, during a lifetime (www.epa.gov/IRIS/help_gloss.htm#s). The methodology described in the paper results in a subchronic daily reference dose of 0.3 mcg/kg/day.[38] The second paper uses the daily reference dose established in the first paper to suggest a risk-based cleanup standard of 1.5 mcg/100 cm$^2$.[18] The State of Washington Department of Health has published information about remediation (www.doh.wa.gov/ehp/ts/CDL). At the federal level, the Methamphetamine Remediation Research Act of 2007, Public Law No. 110-143, provides for establishing voluntary guidelines based on scientific knowledge for the remediation of former methamphetamine laboratories. The Act also addresses the need for research on the effects of methamphetamine on former residents, particularly children.

## REGULATION

The Controlled Substance Act of 1970 regulated the manufacture of methamphetamine, restricting its availability. The Federal Chemical Diversion and Trafficking Act of 1988 placed phenyl-2-propanone and other chemicals on the controlled-substance list, making it more difficult to obtain precursors for the phenyl-2-propanone method. In 2006, the federal Combat Methamphetamine Epidemic Act of 2005 took effect to regulate the sale of pseudoephedrine. Provisions include limiting, in grams, the retail sale of pseudoephedrine, ephedrine, and phenylpropanolamine; specifying placement of these compounds behind the counter; and establishing the recording of sales in logbooks. Individual states have added requirements such as a prescription requirement for pseudoephedrine products. These actions, along with sustained law enforcement pressure, have decreased domestic methamphetamine production. These actions have also led to a resurgence of the phenyl-2-propanone method and the use of higher potency methamphetamine from outside the United States. Smaller clandestine laboratories persist, resulting in harm to children and emergency responders; 9,338 methamphetamine clandestine laboratory incidents were reported in 2014.[39]

Children removed from methamphetamine laboratories or from parents who are chronic users of methamphetamine may be considered neglected because of supervision, environmental, or physical features of the home (depending on state-specific statutes). Children who have been living with parents who have substance abuse issues are at risk for events that could adversely impact their health and safety because of the effects that substance abuse has on the parent's ability to provide appropriate care. These could include, but are not limited to, sexual abuse, physical abuse, and neglect of the child's supervision or basic care needs. Several states have established their own Alliances for Drug Endangered Children (www.nationaldec.org/statesites. html). Pediatricians can provide a medical home for these children and help to coordinate and advocate for services needed.

## Frequently Asked Questions

Q  *What are the long-term effects when children live in a methamphetamine manufacturing environment?*

A  There is no long-term information available. Neglect by caregivers appears to be the primary concern, and a complete developmental assessment is indicated. Studies have shown that although drug-exposed children can exhibit concerning behaviors and disordered sleep, the more pronounced cause is the environment in which they live and not the drug.

Q  *How can I find out if the home I moved into was a former clandestine laboratory?*

A  The Drug Enforcement Administration (DEA) maintains a list of former clandestine laboratories. It can be accessed at www.usdoj.gov/dea/ seizures/index.html.

Q  *What should I do to have my children evaluated if I find my home was a former site?*

A  Few studies have documented that exposure to former methamphetamine sites results in symptoms that can be attributed to the manufacturing of methamphetamine. If a child is symptomatic, a comprehensive pediatric health assessment is indicated. Referrals to specialists should be based on symptoms. If the home is on the DEA database, local agencies should be contacted to verify that proper remediation was completed. If the home is a previously unknown methamphetamine site, environmental testing could be done to assess for contamination.

## Resources For Professionals

### Decontamination
http://health.utah.gov/meth/Pages/DeconDiscussion.html

### Drug Enforcement Agency 2017 National Drug Threat Assessment
https://www.dea.gov/docs/DIR-040-17_2017-NDTA.pdf

## Drug Enforcement Agency: Guidelines for Law Enforcement for the Cleanup of Clandestine Drug Laboratories

https://www.dea.gov/resources/img/redbook.pdf

### Legislation

National Alliance for Model State Drug Laws (NAMSDL)

www.namsdl.org

### Management

American Association for Poison Control Centers

(800) 222-1222

### Pediatric Environmental Health Specialty Units

http://pehsu.net

## Resources For Parents

### National Alliance for Drug Endangered Children

Web site: www.nationaldec.org

Parents can contact them directly with questions. Frequently asked questions can also be accessed at www.nationaldec.org/resourcecenter/faqs.html.

## References

1. Beebe DK, Walley E. Smokable methamphetamine ("ice"): an old drug in a different form. *Am Fam Physician*. 1995;51(2):449–453

2. United States Department of Justice, National Drug Intelligence Center. *Methamphetamine Drug Threat Assessment*. Johnstown, PA: US Department of Justice; March 2005. Document ID No. 2005-Q0317-009

3. Burgess JL, Barnhart S, Checkowar H. Investigating clandestine drug laboratories: adverse medical effects in law enforcement personnel. *Am J Ind Med*. 1996;30(4):488–494

4. Rawson RA, Gonzalez R, Brethen P. Treatment of methamphetamine use disorders: an update. *J Subst Abuse Treat*. 2002;23(2):145–150

5. Sadock BJ, Sadock V, eds. *Kaplan and Sadock's Comprehensive Textbook of Psychiatry*. 8th ed. Philadelphia, PA: Lippincott Williams and Wilkins; 2005:1191–1192

6. Ruha AM, Yarema MC. Pharmacologic treatment of acute pediatric methamphetamine toxicity. *Pediatr Emerg Care*. 2006;22(12):782–785

7. Huestis MA, Cone EJ. Methamphetamine disposition in oral fluid, plasma, and urine. *Ann N Y Acad Sci*. 2007;1098:104–121

8. Burgess JL, Chandler D. Clandestine drug laboratories. In: Greenburg MI, ed. *Occupational, Industrial and Environmental Toxicology*. 2nd ed. Philadelphia, PA: Mosby; 2003:746–764

9. Hammon TL, Griffin S. Support for selection of a methamphetamine cleanup standard in Colorado. *Regul Toxicol Pharmacol*. 2007;48(1):102–114

10. Courtney KE, Ray LA. Methamphetamine: an update on epidemiology, pharmacology, clinical phenomenology, and treatment literature. *Drug Alcohol Depend*. 2014;143:11–21

11. US Drug Enforcement Administration. *Guidelines for Law Enforcement for the Cleanup of Clandestine Drug Laboratories.* https://www.dea.gov/resources/img/redbook.pdf. Accessed February 11, 2018

12. Kates LN, Knapp CW, Keenan HE. Acute and chronic environmental effects of clandestine methamphetamine waste. *Sci Total Environ.* 2014;493:781–788

13. Melnikova N, Orr MF, Wu J, Christensen B. Injuries from methamphetamine-related chemical incidents – five states, 2011-2012. *MMWR Morb Mortal Wkly Rep.* 2015;64(33):909–912

14. Centers for Disease Control and Prevention. Anhydrous ammonia thefts and releases associated with illicit methamphetamine production 16 states, January 2000-June 2004. *MMWR Morb Mortal Wkly Rep.* 2005;54(14):359–361

15. Amdur MO, Klassen CD, Doull J, Casarett LJ, eds. *Casarett and Doull's Toxicology: The Basic Science of Poisons.* 4th ed. New York, NY: Pergammon Press; 1991

16. Oishi, SM, West KM, Stuntz S. *Drug Endangered Children Health and Safety Manual.* Los Angeles, CA: The Drug Endangered Children Resource Center; 2000

17. Lineberry TW, Bostwick JM. Methamphetamine abuse: a perfect storm of complications. *Mayo Clin Proc.* 2006;81(1):77–84

18. Salocks CB. *Assessment of Children's Exposure to Surface Methamphetamine Residues in Former Clandestine Methamphetamine Labs, and Identification of a Risk-Based Cleanup Standard for Surface Methamphetamine Contamination.* Sacramento, CA: California Environmental Protection Agency; 2009. https://oehha.ca.gov/media/downloads/crnr/exposureanalysis022709.pdf. Accessed February 11, 2018

19. Martyny JW, Arbuckle SL, McCammon CS Jr, et al. Chemical exposures associated with clandestine methamphetamine laboratories. *J Chem Health Safety.* 2007;14(4):40–52

20. VanDyke M, Erb N, Arbuckle S, Martyny J. A 24-hour study to investigate persistent chemical exposures associated with clandestine methamphetamine laboratories. *J Occup Environ Hyg.* 2009;6(2):82–89

21. Martyny J, Arbuckle SL, McCammon CS, Erb N, Van Dyke M. Methamphetamine contamination on environmental surfaces caused by simulated smoking of methamphetamine. *J Chem Health Safety.* 2008;15(5):25–31

22. Matteucci MJ, Auten JD, Crowley B, Combs D, Clark RF. Methamphetamine exposures in young children. *Pediatr Emerg Care.* 2007;23(9):638–640

23. Ruha AM, Yarema MC. Pharmacologic treatment of acute pediatric methamphetamine toxicity. *Pediatr Emerg Care.* 2006;22(12):782–785

24. Hassanian-Moghaddam H, Ranjbar M, Farnaghi F, Zamani N, Alizadeh AM, Sarjami S. Stimulant toxicity in children: a retrospective study on 147 patients. *Pediatr Crit Care Med.* 2015;16(8):e290–e296

25. Prosser JM, Naim M, Helfaer M. A 14 year old girl with agitation and hyperthermia. *Pediatr Emerg Care.* 2006;22(9):676–679

26. Gospe SM Jr. Transient cortical blindness in an infant exposed to methamphetamine. *Ann Emerg Med.* 1995;26(3):380–382

27. Nagorka AR, Bergensen PS. Infant methamphetamine toxicity posing as scorpion envenomation. *Pediatr Emerg Care.* 1998;14(5):350–351

28. Farst K. Methamphetamine exposure presenting as caustic ingestions in children. *Ann Emerg Med.* 2007;49(3):341–343

29. Horton KD, Berkowitz Z, Kaye W. The acute health consequences to children exposed to hazardous substances used in illicit methamphetamine production, 1996 to 2000. *J Child Health.* 2003;1:99–108

30. Buck JM, Siegel JA. The effects of adolescent methamphetamine exposure. *Front Neurosci.* 2015;9:151

31. National Institute on Drug Abuse. Research Report Series: *Methamphetamine Abuse and Addiction.* Bethesda, MD: National Institute on Drug Abuse; April 1998; Reprinted January 2002; Revised September 2006. NIH Publication No. 06-4210

32. Albertson TE, Derlet RW, Van Hoozen BE. Methamphetamine and the expanding complications of amphetamines. *West J Med.* 1999;170(4):214–219

33. National Alliance for Drug Endangered Children. Medical Evaluation of Children Removed from Clandestine Labs. http://www.nationaldec.org/resourcecenter/faq.html#. Accessed February 12, 2018

34. National Alliance for Drug Endangered Children. How to Care for Children Removed from a Drug Endangered Environment. http://www.nationaldec.org/resourcecenter/faq.html#. Accessed February 12, 2018

35. Moeller KE, Kissack JC, Atayee RS, Lee KC. Clinical interpretation of urine drug tests: what clinicians need to know about urine drug screens. *Mayo Clin Proc.* 2017;92:774–796

36. Dasgupta A, ed. *Critical Issues in Alcohol and Drugs of Abuse Testing.* Washington, DC: American Association for Clinical Chemistry Press; 2009

37. White RM. Drugs in hair. Part I. Metabolisms of major drug classes. *Forensic Sci Rev.* 2017;29(1):23–55

38. Salocks C. Development of a Reference Dose (RfD) for Methamphetamine. Sacramento, CA: California Environmental Protection Agency, Office of Environmental Health Hazard Assessment, Integrated Risk Assessment Branch; 2007. http://www.oehha.ca.gov/public_info/public/kids/meth022609.html. Accessed February 12, 2018

39. U.S. Drug Enforcement Administration. Methamphetamine Lab Incidents, 2004-2014. https://www.dea.gov/resource-center/meth-lab-maps.shtml. Accessed February 12, 2018

Chapter 62

# Obesity

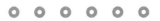

## KEY POINTS

- Although unchanged over the last decade, obesity rates have increased in recent years and are more prevalent at younger ages and in certain racial and ethnic groups.
- The "obesogen hypothesis" refers to the potential for environmental exposures at critical windows of child development (or later in life) to alter growth and ultimately increase the risk for obesity.
- The socioecological model provides a broad framework for understanding child, family, and community factors that influence childhood obesity.
- Programs and policies that support healthy lifestyles and healthy communities are important public health strategies for addressing the childhood obesity epidemic.
- Pediatricians can help to prevent and manage childhood obesity by assessing weight status and discussing recommendations for diet, including breast feeding early in infancy, and activity, with patients and families.

## INTRODUCTION

Obesity in children aged 2 years and older is defined as a body mass index (BMI) at or above the sex-specific 95th percentile on the BMI-for-age growth charts of the US Centers for Disease Control and Prevention (CDC). Severe obesity is defined as a BMI at or above 120% of the sex-specific 95th percentile on the BMI-for-age growth charts of the CDC.[1] A more widely accepted classification of obesity has been defined using the "Class System": Class 1 (95th to 120th percentile), Class 2 (120th to 140th percentile), and Class 3 (greater than 140th percentile). Generally, Class 2 and 3 are considered severe.[2] The prevalence of childhood obesity has increased in recent decades although it is unchanged over the past decade. In a nationally representative study of US children and adolescents aged 2 to 19 years, the prevalence of obesity (Class 1) in 2015 to 2016 was 18.5%, and the prevalence of severe obesity was nearly 8%.[3]

Significant disparities exist in childhood obesity, with higher rates among non-Hispanic black, Hispanic, American Indian/Alaska Native, and Native Hawaiian/Pacific Islander youth compared with non-Hispanic white youth. In addition, higher rates of obesity occur among youth in households headed by individuals with a high school degree or less compared with households headed by individuals with more than a high school degree.[3-6]

Obesity is a critical public health issue because of its many associated medical and social consequences. Obesity in childhood often persists into adulthood with associated increased morbidity and mortality, particularly in non-Hispanic blacks, Hispanics, American Indian/Alaska Native, and Native Hawaiian/Pacific Islander people.[7,8] Obesity-related comorbidities including hypertension, dyslipidemia, insulin resistance, impaired glucose metabolism, obstructive sleep apnea, fatty liver disease, depression, and psychosocial complications have become more common in childhood.[9] Even children who are modestly overweight/obese have an adverse cardiovascular risk profile.[10]

Childhood obesity is now recognized as a major contributor to increasing health care expenditures. The direct cost of obesity from medical care expenses is estimated to be as much as $147 billion per year for adults and $14.3 billion per year for children, with additional costs attributed to factors such as lost productivity.[11] For these reasons, it is important to prevent childhood obesity, and to identify overweight and obese children as early as possible so they can begin treatment to attain and maintain a healthy weight.[9] Obesity in childhood has been strongly associated with increased rates of early death in adults.[12] Children today may be the first generation to have a shorter life span than the preceding generation. One study found that children in the highest quartile of BMI were more than twice as likely to die before age 55 compared with children in the lowest quartile.[2]

## ENVIRONMENTAL CHEMICAL FACTORS AND OBESITY

### Obesogens

Endocrine disrupting chemicals (EDCs; also known as endocrine disruptors or endocrine disrupters) can alter hormones and lead to a variety of diseases. Some EDCs are "obesogens" and "diabetogens" that can promote adipogenesis resulting in weight gain and increasing the risk for obesity and diabetes mellitus when exposure occurs at critical windows of child development (or later in life).[13] Candidate obesogens include dioxins and dioxin-like compounds, organochlorine pesticides, perfluoroalkyl and polyfluoroalkyl substances (PFAS) (eg, perfluorooctanoic acid [PFOA]), polybrominated diphenyl ethers (PBDEs), phthalates, bisphenol A (BPA), lead, and air pollutants including cigarette smoke and diesel exhaust (see Chapter 29).[13]

The potential mechanisms of action by which EDCs are implicated in alteration of growth and development include disruption of (1) glucose and lipid metabolism, (2) adipogenesis, and (3) thyroid function. Cross-sectional studies primarily among adults and some children implicated EDCs in the development of obesity, diabetes mellitus, and cardiovascular disease.[14,15] For example, studies of phthalates (ie, plasticizers used in certain consumer products and personal care products) found associations with obesity among Chinese and non-Hispanic black children. Not all studies of phthalates, however, have shown consistent associations with childhood obesity.[16] Population-based studies of obesogens have demonstrated far-reaching health consequences of obesity, such as metabolic syndrome, cardiovascular disease, diabetes mellitus, and non-alcoholic fatty liver disease.[13,18–25]

Research has increasingly focused on the interactions between obesogenic chemicals and other environmental, genetic, and lifestyle factors. Exposure to obesogenic chemicals has the potential to magnify existing health disparities. The same neighborhoods that have a high prevalence of chronic childhood conditions (eg, asthma, obesity) often are the neighborhoods that carry a disproportionate burden of environmental exposures (eg, increased siting of diesel bus depots in urban minority neighborhoods). Even if the contribution of environmental exposures to obesity is small, the potential benefits of interventions aimed at reducing environmental exposures in the context of healthy environments and healthy communities could be large because of the high prevalence of obesity and its significant medical, social, and economic costs.

Given the global challenges of climate change and air pollution, strategies that address these environmental challenges as well as obesity have potentially combined benefits. Promoting sustainable energy, sustainable food sources, and public transportation networks that encourage active transport while reducing carbon footprints can have benefits for the health of individuals, the population, and the environmental impact on the planet.[23–25]

## The Socioecological Model of Obesity

The ecological model provides a broad framework for understanding child, family, and community mediators and moderators of childhood obesity.[26] Emerging research in children's environmental health has gone beyond individual risk factors to consider a broader context. The ecological systems theory, specific to childhood obesity, examines the child's setting with regard to

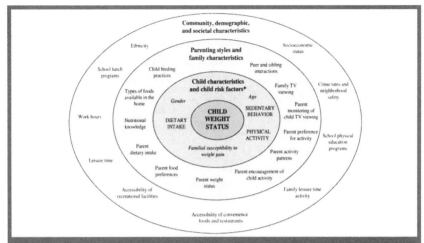

**Figure 62-1. Ecological model of predictors of childhood overweight.**[26] **Child risk factors (in uppercase lettering) refer to behaviors associated with development of overweight. Characteristics of the child (in italic lettering) interact with child risk factors and contextual factors to influence the development of overweight (ie, moderator variables).**

parenting styles, family characteristics, and broader community, demographic, and societal characteristics. School lunch programs, work hours, public transportation, availability of green spaces, and access to health-promoting resources are examples of broader environmental factors that can affect children's growth and development (Figure 62-1).

As depicted in the ecological model, many community environmental factors—such as living in lower-income neighborhoods with limited access to healthy foods and safe outdoor play spaces—are associated with a higher risk of obesity. Therefore, policy and environmental interventions will likely have the largest impact on reducing childhood obesity rates (Table 62-1).[27]

## RECOMMENDATIONS TO PEDIATRICIANS

The American Academy of Pediatrics (AAP) 2007 Expert Committee publication *Recommendations Regarding the Prevention, Assessment, and Treatment of Child and Adolescent Overweight and Obesity: Summary Report*[9] advises clinicians to support school and community programs that help prevent obesity through local, state, or national advocacy. The Institute of Medicine reports on obesity prevention provide a model for school policies and other community-based initiatives.[28,29] These reports make recommendations that, when efforts are combined, can improve the health and well-being of all children.

## Table 62-1. Examples of Environmental Strategies for Preventing Childhood Obesity[27]

| SCOPE | |
|---|---|
| Site-specific | Banks, stores, professionals give incentives to children that do not contribute to unhealthful habits or energy imbalance (examples: stickers instead of candy or cookies)[c]<br>Corner stores and quick marts offer low fat/sugar snacks, fruits, and vegetables[b]<br>Entertainment venues offer healthful options, water; allow outside (home-packed) foods[b]<br>Point-of-decision prompts (elevator versus stairs initiatives; menu, cafeteria, or buffet signage and prompts)[a] |
| Local | Establish shared-use agreements for physical activity space and equipment[b]<br>Promote ways to allow active transport to and from school (bike lanes and racks, crossing guards, group walks to school)[b]<br>Emphasize maintaining or re-establishing time for recess, physical activity, physical education[b]<br>Support school and community gardens, partnerships with local farmers[c]<br>Access to safe, free drinking water in recreation environments[b] |
| State | Subsidies for schools/childcare sites that provide healthy foods[a]<br>Incentives for grocers in rural or urban areas[c]<br>Mechanism for small vendors (farmers' markets) to take Supplemental Nutrition Assistance Program (SNAP) (food stamps) cards[c]<br>Medicaid coverage for all medical services including dietician services and preventive counseling[c]<br>Support for increasing sites and access for recreation[a] |
| National | Healthy and Hunger Free Kids Act, including standards for meals in school (eg, the National School Lunch Program)[a]<br>Changes to WIC food package and SNAP policies[a]<br>Changes to SNAP-Ed guidance for educational programs[a]<br>Menu labeling for restaurants[b]<br>Laws addressing advertising to children[c]<br>Food and beverage industry incentives[c] |
| International | Published guidelines for member states for population-level strategies for obesity prevention across settings.[30] |

Abbreviations: WIC, Women, Infants, and Children
[a] Evidence or existing systematic review to support.
[b] Emerging strategy but more data needed.
[c] Sample policy change needing pilot data and further study.

Recommendations for pediatricians include

1. Encouraging a healthy diet early in life. This includes encouraging breast feeding because it may have a role in attenuation of obesity in early childhood. Introducing unique and healthy fruits and vegetables early in life can lead to better choices as children grow.

2. Ensuring that children are not at risk for food insecurity using the AAP Screening for Food Insecurity Tool.[31]

3. Advocating for policies related to maintenance of safe neighborhoods that encourage physical activity, and availability of healthy foods and beverages in childcare settings, schools, and communities.

4. Encouraging families to voice their concerns through parent-teacher organizations or school board meetings or directly to principals, teachers, and after-care program directors.

5. Working with school administrators to ensure adequate physical education and recess periods and establishing nutritional standards for all foods served in schools, including foods from vending machines.

6. Advocating for the establishment and maintenance of safe parks and recreation centers, and increasing availability of public transit systems.[32]

7. Discussing the use of incentives so that child care and school programs can promote more outdoor time and less screen time.[33]

8. Advocating for the availability of healthy, low-cost foods at local grocery stores and restaurants consistent with the cultures of the community they serve.

Efforts have been made to encourage children to eat fresh fruits and vegetables instead of processed foods known to be sources of environmental chemicals that may impact growth and development.[34] Many groups are working to reprogram existing resources, such as green spaces and trails, to ensure that children are actually using them. For example, the University of Southern California has examined the benefits of urban parks on children's health.[35] Research of this kind provides evidence that helps to promote policies that shape healthy communities and enhance children's well-being. Clinicians can help with these strategies by screening for social determinants of health and making referrals to community nutrition and activity programs.[36]

## SUMMARY

The pediatric obesity epidemic has profound medical and societal consequences. Pediatricians and other clinicians can play critical roles in mitigating the impact of obesity. Obesity rates have recently increased above baseline, although not in all sociodemographic groups.[3] Ongoing research is examining environmental obesogens. Reducing exposure to obesogens and eating a healthier diet may have a significant effect on reducing childhood obesity and related adverse health outcomes.

Public health initiatives may further improve access to healthy and affordable foods and more opportunities for physical activity where children live and play. Efforts have been made to bring together diverse stakeholders to think about health policy frameworks and how to work together to design healthy communities and promote a culture of health.

Early prevention is a key factor in promoting healthy lifestyles for children and adults. It is recommended that pediatricians regularly assess whether children and adolescents have a healthy weight or are overweight or obese, discuss recommendations for healthy diet and increased activity, and make treatment plans as indicated. These steps can be taken on annual well child or well adolescent visits and at other times as appropriate.[9]

## Frequently Asked Questions

Q  *I am concerned about my son's weight. He continues to gain weight despite my efforts to help him eat healthier. I have heard news stories about chemicals in the food supply (eg, bisphenol A lining cans, phthalates in food packaging) and wonder if there is more I can do to make healthy food choices. What should I do?*

A  The primary dietary interventions to prevent and treat obesity focus on eliminating sugar-sweetened beverages and increasing daily consumption of a variety of fruits and vegetables. Other strategies include reducing intake of high-calorie/high-fat foods, decreasing the frequency of eating food outside the home, encouraging portion control, eating breakfast daily, encouraging family meals and healthy snacks, and consuming whole grains, lean proteins, and water. To reduce a child's exposure to chemicals in foods, choose fresh foods over processed foods. Consideration can be given to choosing organic foods when possible, especially for foods that a child consumes frequently that may be high in pesticides. Readily available guides can help families identify conventional (nonorganic) foods that are low in pesticides. One such resource is the Environmental Working Group's Annual listing of the Clean Fifteen and Dirty Dozen (conventional fruits and vegetables either lowest or highest in pesticides).[37] The most important recommendation is to encourage children to eat a variety of foods, especially fruits and vegetables (organic or nonorganic—see https://www.choosemyplate.gov/ten-tips) and to drink mostly water.

Resources include:
- Environmental Working Group. EWGs 2017 Shopper's Guide to Pesticides in Produce
  https://www.ewg.org/foodnews/dirty_dozen_list.php#.WmY2SrynGUk
- Pediatric Environmental Health Specialty Units. Consumer Guide: Phthalates and Bisphenol
  www.pehsu.net/_Library/facts/bpapatients_factsheet03-2014.pdf

- US Department of Agriculture MyPlate Tip Sheets
  https://www.choosemyplate.gov/ten-tips

Q   *I have been told my child is obese. I am worried about the lack of fresh, affordable fruits and vegetables in my neighborhood and also worry about my child's safety while playing in local parks. What can I do?*

A   It is important to remember that children should receive their fruits and vegetables in any form that is available. Frozen and canned (without endocrine disrupting chemical liners) can be good alternatives when fresh produce is not accessible. I can refer you to your local WIC program and local food bank. Other local resources may be available.[36] Free or low-cost physical activity resources, such as after school programs and summer camps, may be available and can significantly increase the amount of time your child spends outdoors and in active play. Local public health agencies and community-based organizations often have information on additional resources for children. You may want to voice your concerns at local community board meetings or Parent-Teacher Association meetings or by calling or writing to your local government representatives. The American Academy of Pediatrics has information for parents and caregivers (www.healthychildren.org).

Resources:
- WIC
  https://www.fns.usda.gov/wic/women-infants-and-children-wic
- SNAP
  https://www.fns.usda.gov/snap/
  supplemental-nutrition-assistance-program-snap
- Children and Nature Infographic
  https://www.neefusa.org/resource/children-and-nature-infographic
- Children and Urban Parks Infographic http://envhealthcenters.usc.edu/
  infographics/infographic-childrens-health-urban-parks
- Farmers Markets Search
  https://www.ams.usda.gov/local-food-directories/farmersmarkets

## Resources

### Centers for Disease Control and Prevention
Web site: https://www.cdc.gov/obesity/childhood/causes.html

### Endocrine Society 2nd Scientific Statement on EDCs Executive Summary
Web site: https://academic.oup.com/edrv/article/36/6/593/2354738/
Executive-Summary-to-EDC-2-The-Endocrine-Society-s

**National Institute of Environmental Health Sciences**

Web site: https://www.niehs.nih.gov/health/topics/agents/endocrine

**National Toxicology Program**

Web site: https://ehp.niehs.nih.gov/1104597/

**Robert Wood Johnson Foundation: Culture of Health**

Web site: https://www.rwjf.org/en/our-focus-areas/focus-areas/healthy-communities.html

**US Environmental Protection Agency: America's Children and the Environment**

Web site: https://www.epa.gov/sites/production/files/2015-06/documents/health-obesity.pdf

**World Health Organization**

Web site: www.who.int/ceh/risks/cehemerging2/en/

## References

1. Centers for Disease Control and Prevention. CDC Growth Charts. 2000.
2. Skinner AC, Skelton JA. Prevalence and trends in obesity and severe obesity among children in the United States, 1999-2012. *JAMA Pediatr.* 2014;168(6):561–566
3. Skinner AC, Ravanbakht SN, Skelton JA, Perrin EM, Armstrong SC. Prevalence of obesity and severe obesity in US children, 1999-2016. *Pediatrics.* 2018;141:e20173459
4. Segal LM, Rayburn J, Bock SE. The State of Obesity: 2017. Trust for America's Health; 2017. https://stateofobesity.org/files/stateofobesity2017.pdf. Accessed July 16, 2018
5. Overweight and Obesity Among American Indian and Alaskan Native Youths. Leadership for Healthy Communities, Robert Wood Johnson Foundation; 2010. http://aztribaltransportation.org/htp/pdf/101012_Overweight_Obesity.pdf. Accessed July 16, 2018
6. Native Hawaiian and Pacific Islander Health Disparities. Asian and Pacific Islander American Health Forum 2010. https://www.apiahf.org/wp-content/uploads/2011/02/NHPI_Report08a_2010-1.pdf. Accessed July 16, 2018
7. Inge TH, King WC, Jenkins TM, et al. The effect of obesity in adolescence on adult health status. *Pediatrics.* 2013;132(6):1098–1104
8. Obesity and Overweight Fact Sheet: World Health Organization; 2017. http://www.who.int/mediacentre/factsheets/fs311/en/. Accessed July 16, 2018
9. Barlow SE. Expert committee recommendations regarding the prevention, assessment, and treatment of child and adolescent overweight and obesity: summary report. *Pediatrics.* 2007;120(Suppl 4):S164–S192
10. Wright N, Wales J. Assessment and management of severely obese children and adolescents. *Arch Dis Child.* 2016;101(12):1161–1167
11. Hammond RA, Levine R. The economic impact of obesity in the United States. *Diabetes Metab Syndr Obes.* 2010;3:285–295

12. Franks PW, Hanson RL, Knowler WC, Sievers ML, Bennett PH, Looker HC. Childhood obesity, other cardiovascular risk factors, and premature death. *N Engl J Med*. 2010;362(6):485–493

13. La Merrill M, Birnbaum LS. Childhood obesity and environmental chemicals. *Mt Sinai J Med*. 2011;78(1):22–48

14. Lang IA, Galloway TS, Scarlett A, et al. Association of urinary bisphenol A concentration with medical disorders and laboratory abnormalities in adults. *JAMA*. 2008;300(11):1303–1310

15. Trasande L, Attina TM, Blustein J. Association between urinary bisphenol A concentration and obesity prevalence in children and adolescents. *JAMA*. 2012;308(11):1113–1121

16. Darbre PD. Endocrine disrupters and obesity. *Curr Obes Rep*. 2017;6(1):18–27

17. Gore AC, Chappell VA, Fenton SE, et al. EDC-2: The Endocrine Society's Second Scientific Statement on Endocrine-Disrupting Chemicals. *Endocr Rev*. 2015;36(6):E1–E150

18. Khalil N, Chen A, Lee M. Endocrine disruptive compounds and cardio-metabolic risk factors in children. *Curr Opin Pharmacol*. 2014;19:120–124

19. Braun JM. Early-life exposure to EDCs: role in childhood obesity and neurodevelopment. *Nat Rev Endocrinol*. 2017;13(3):161–173

20. Alderete TL, Song AY, Bastain T, et al. Prenatal traffic-related air pollution exposures, cord blood adipokines and infant weight. *Pediatr Obes*. 2018;13(6):348–356

21. McConnell R, Shen E, Gilliland FD, et al. A longitudinal cohort study of body mass index and childhood exposure to secondhand tobacco smoke and air pollution: the Southern California Children's Health Study. *Environ Health Perspect*. 2015;123(4):360–366

22. Kim HW, Kam S, Lee DH. Synergistic interaction between polycyclic aromatic hydrocarbons and environmental tobacco smoke on the risk of obesity in children and adolescents: the U.S. National Health and Nutrition Examination Survey 2003-2008. *Environ Res*. 2014;135:354–360

23. An R, Ji M, Zhang S. Global warming and obesity: a systematic review. *Obes Rev*. 2018;19(2):150–163

24. Bhatnagar A. Environmental determinants of cardiovascular disease. *Circ Res*. 2017;121(2):162–180

25. Blauw LL, Aziz NA, Tannemaat MR, et al. Diabetes incidence and glucose intolerance prevalence increase with higher outdoor temperature. *BMJ Open Diabetes Res Care*. 2017;5(1):e000317

26. Davison KK, Birch LL. Childhood overweight: a contextual model and recommendations for future research. *Obes Rev*. 2001;2(3):159–171

27. Brown CL, Halvorson EE, Cohen GM, Lazorick S, Skelton JA. Addressing childhood obesity: opportunities for prevention. *Pediatr Clin North Am*. 2015;62(5):1241–1261

28. Koplan JP, Liverman CT, Kraak VI, Committee on Prevention of Obesity in Children and Youth. Preventing childhood obesity: health in the balance: executive summary. *J Am Diet Assoc*. 2005;105(1):131–138

29. McGuire S. Institute of Medicine. Accelerating progress in obesity prevention: solving the weight of the nation. Washington, DC: the National Academies Press; 2012. *Adv Nutr*. 2012;3(5):708–709

30. World Health Organization. Population-based approaches to childhood obesity prevention. 2012. http://www.who.int/dietphysicalactivity/childhood/approaches/en/. Accessed September 10, 2018

31. American Academy of Pediatrics Council on Community Pediatrics, Committee on Nutrition. Promoting food security for all children. *Pediatrics*. 2015;136(5):e1431–e1438

32. MacDonald JM, Stokes RJ, Cohen DA, Kofner A, Ridgeway GK. The effect of light rail transit on body mass index and physical activity. *Am J Prev Med*. 2010;39(2):105–112

33. Audubon Education Supporting Conservation through Education: National Audubon Society. http://www.audubon.org/conservation/education. Accessed July 16, 2018

34. Toxic Chemicals in our Food System. Washington, DC: Physicians for Social Responsibility. http://www.psr.org/assets/pdfs/toxic-chemicals-in-our-food.pdf. Accessed July 16, 2018

35. Infographic: Children's Health & Urban Parks: University of Southern California. http://envhealthcenters.usc.edu/infographics/infographic-childrens-health-urban-parks. Accessed July 16, 2018

36. Garg A, Toy S, Tripodis Y, Silverstein M, Freeman E. Addressing social determinants of health at well child care visits: a cluster RCT. *Pediatrics*. 2015;135(2):e296–e304

37. Environmental Working Group's 2018 Shopper's Guide to Pesticides in Produce: Environmental Working Group; 2018. https://www.ewg.org/foodnews/summary.php. Accessed July 16, 2018

Chapter 63

# Environmental Health Advocacy

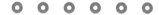

*"It is not enough, however, to work at the individual bedside in the hospital. In the near or dim future, the pediatrician is to sit in and control school boards, health departments, and legislatures. He is a legitimate advisor to the judge and jury, and a seat for the physician in the councils of the republic is what the people have a right to demand."*

—Abraham Jacobi, MD

**KEY POINTS**

- Advocacy is an essential part of a pediatrician's role.
- Pediatric environmental health advocacy efforts occur at individual, community, state, and federal levels.
- The Washington DC office of the American Academy of Pediatrics and state chapters are important resources for advocacy efforts.

**INTRODUCTION**

A pediatrician's role in environmental health—encouraging children's activities in health-promoting outdoor spaces and protecting children from environmental hazards—does not end at the office door. Advocacy work at all levels is an essential component of pediatric environmental health promotion and is critical to reducing and preventing children's exposure to environmental hazards. By the nature of their training and expertise, pediatricians are uniquely qualified to provide greater context and meaning to debates over pressing environmental issues. Pediatricians' input is critical to ensuring that the needs of children and adolescents are met when key policy decisions are made. This chapter outlines the need for pediatricians to advocate about environmental health issues; the kinds of advocacy work in which pediatricians can engage to achieve changes in public policy; the importance of consistent, coordinated messages about environmental health; and key tools and resources available for effective advocacy work.

The nation urgently requires pediatricians to engage in environmental health issues. Children are uniquely vulnerable to environmental harms, and these harms potentially affect every aspect of a child's present and future health and well-being. Since the 1970s, state and federal legislators have enacted and revised landmark legislation addressing clean air, clean water, chemicals, pesticides, product safety, and other key environmental health issues.[1] When developing and applying laws and regulations, policy makers often require and seek technical guidance from stakeholder groups–including pediatricians. Pediatricians possess the knowledge and first-hand experience that can help close gaps in environmental policies that allow toxic exposures to continue, and to aid in the development of new policies as novel threats to child health emerge. Pediatricians may be among the first to recognize new or emerging threats, such as in Flint, Michigan, in 2014 when a switch to a new water supply resulted in leaching of lead into water and a public health crisis.[2]

Advocacy and the practice of pediatrics have always been intrinsically connected.[3–5] Advocacy is such an integral part of pediatric practice that it is included as a component of pediatric residency training. Advocacy also is central to the mission of many nongovernmental organizations and professional organizations, such as the American Academy of Pediatrics (AAP).

## LEVELS OF PEDIATRIC ADVOCACY

The AAP has identified 4 levels of pediatric advocacy work.[6] *Individual advocacy* involves direct care and resources provided to patients and families every day. An example of individual advocacy is calling an insurance company or contacting a social service agency about abating a health hazard in the home that is exacerbating a child's asthma. Many pediatricians engage in advocacy efforts for individual patients; these efforts often are the first steps in broader efforts at the community, state, and federal levels.

*Community advocacy* builds on and reaches beyond individual advocacy in that it affects children within the community. A community can be defined geographically (as in a neighborhood, school district, or city) or culturally (as an ethnic or racial group or religious cluster). Community advocacy takes into consideration the environmental and social factors influencing child health and addresses ways in which pediatricians can work with community partners to address issues that affect their patients.

*State advocacy* efforts focus primarily on the state legislative process. State legislatures play increasingly important roles in health policy and are prolific sources of new laws and regulations; as a whole, the nation's approximately 7,380 state legislators consider more than 150,000 bills every year.[7] Although legislatures are the primary focus of advocacy on the state level, there are also advocacy opportunities with the state executive branch through the governor's office, with state agencies and regulatory activities, through the budget process, and through the judicial branch. Working through AAP chapters and in coalitions with other groups, pediatricians have had major effects on environmental health issues in their states. Issues include improving indoor air quality by eliminating secondhand smoke exposure, improving outdoor air quality by limiting emissions of pollutants, promoting screening for lead poisoning, decreasing skin cancer risk by banning minors from tanning in salons, and many others.

*Federal advocacy* involves national environmental health issues. For dozens of years, pediatricians have advocated at the federal level about clean air, food safety, lead poisoning prevention, toxic chemicals in children's products and commerce, global climate change, and other environmental issues that affect children's health.[8] The AAP Washington Office leads the Academy federal policy and advocacy agenda, serving as the AAP voice to advance child health priorities via federal legislation, regulations and, occasionally, the courts. AAP staff provide technical and strategic assistance for expert pediatricians who testify at congressional hearings, work with pediatricians to use media and social media to share federal policy priorities for children, and conduct advocacy trainings to teach pediatricians to effectively work with the federal government to advance an issue.

A pediatrician may feel that to become involved in advocacy, he or she must know everything about an issue and about the political or legislative process. The clinical skills a clinician already possesses, however, are similar to those needed to be an effective advocate—the ability to translate complex scientific and medical concepts into simple language, to diagnose a problem, and to outline a course of treatment. Advocacy may begin as soon as a particular problem is identified. The next step is to bring awareness of the issue to decision makers and others who can help generate a solution. Although one does need a basic understanding of the legislative and policy process (available from AAP resources[6]), two of the most important attributes needed for success are enthusiasm and a willingness to speak out on behalf of children. The AAP Washington Office is designed to provide detailed strategy and knowledge so that pediatricians have the support they need to use their expertise to influence the policy process.

Coordination is key to the success of any advocacy effort. By working with and through their AAP chapters, pediatricians can take full advantage of the resources and information available from state chapters and coalition partners. Additional resources are AAP Policy Statements, Technical Reports, and Clinical Reports.

Broadening support with diverse coalitions of issue stakeholders, either through gaining the participation of other pediatricians in efforts or by seeking the partnership of other organizations that share similar goals and priorities, is critical to a successful advocacy effort. This broad base of support will demonstrate to community leaders and elected officials that many people care about pediatric environmental health issues and that those people are taking action to create change.

Pediatricians often use media to promote advocacy efforts. The 4 types of advocacy can be enhanced by using media to spotlight issues through activities such as letters to the editor, op-ed pieces, news stories, or obtaining editorial support. These media stories can then be sent to congressional offices as additional ways to draw their attention to the issue. Social media has played an important role in amplifying the reach of media coverage and other advocacy messages, and in facilitating diverse engagements among different audiences, driving traffic to resources and sharing live-streaming information from advocacy meetings and events. In addition to proactively creating and promoting positive child health messages, it is equally important to counter inaccurate information about pediatric environmental health topics. The media and social media can help pediatricians provide wide-reaching platforms to reach large audiences with accurate medical information.

When working on pediatric environmental health issues, it may be hard to imagine that others would not support a pediatrician's efforts, or even oppose them. However, pediatricians' advocacy priorities for resources and funding will nearly always compete with those of other groups, or reflect different points of view. It is often helpful to bring evidence-based arguments to the table to underscore the importance of the particular issue as decision makers consider positions of differing interests. In addition, it is critical to support evidence-based arguments with compelling anecdotes that help personalize and frame an advocacy issue for legislators and the press.

The success of pediatric environmental advocacy ultimately rests with the volunteer efforts of individual pediatricians. The AAP, along with many of its state chapters, has lobbyists and other public policy and communications staff who help to shape laws and regulations on behalf of children. The work of professional staff alone is not enough. The unique perspective and credibility of pediatricians is critical in helping create the social and political change needed to make lasting advancements in pediatric environmental health policy.[9]

For more information on advocacy by pediatricians and how pediatricians can influence child health policy, please see the *AAP Advocacy Guide*.[6]

## Resources

**American Academy of Pediatrics**

Department of Federal Affairs

http://federaladvocacy.aap.org/ (AAP member login required)

Division of State Government Affairs

www.aap.org/stateadvocacy

Chapter and District Information

https://www.aap.org/en-us/about-the-aap/chapters-and-districts/
Pages/chapters-and-districts.aspx

**Congressional**

Thomas: Legislative Information on the Internet

http://thomas.loc.gov

US House of Representatives

https://www.house.gov/

US Senate

https://www.senate.gov/

**Federal**

White House

www.whitehouse.gov

Regulations issued by Federal Agencies

https://www.regulations.gov/

**State**

Council of State Governments

www.csg.org

National Association of Counties

www.naco.org

National Conference of State Legislatures

www.ncsl.org

National Governors Association

www.nga.org

National Association of State and Territorial Health Officials

www.astho.org

National Association of County and City Health Officials

www.naccho.org

State environmental agencies

www.epa.gov/epahome/state.htm

# References

1. US Environmental Protection Agency. Milestones in EPA and Environmental History. https://www.epa.gov/history. Accessed February 2, 2018
2. National Public Radio. Lead-Laced Water In Flint: A Step-By-Step Look At The Makings Of A Crisis. http://www.npr.org/sections/thetwo-way/2016/04/20/465545378/lead-laced-water-in-flint-a-step-by-step-look-at-the-makings-of-a-crisis. April 20, 2016. Accessed February 2, 2018
3. Gruen RL, Campbell EG, Blumenthal D. Public roles of US physicians: community participation, political involvement, and collective advocacy. *JAMA*. 2006;296(20):2467–2475
4. Rushton FE Jr, American Academy of Pediatrics Committee on Community Health Services. The pediatrician's role in community pediatrics. *Pediatrics*. 2005;115(4):1092–1094
5. American Academy of Pediatrics Council on Community Pediatrics. Poverty and child health in the United States. *Pediatrics*. 2016;137(4):e20160339
6. American Academy of Pediatrics. *AAP Advocacy Guide*. https://www.aap.org/en-us/my-aap/advocacy/state-government-affairs/Pages/AAP-Advocacy-Guide.aspx (AAP member log-in required). Accessed February 28, 2018
7. Council of State Governments. *The Book of the States 2016*. Lexington, KY: Council of State Governments; 2016. http://knowledgecenter.csg.org/kc/category/content-type/bos-2016. Accessed February 2, 2018
8. Goldman L, Falk H, Landrigan PJ, Balk SJ, Reigart JR, Etzel RA. Environmental pediatrics and its impact on government health policy. *Pediatrics*. 2004;113(4 Suppl):1146–1157
9. American Academy of Pediatrics, Council on Community Pediatrics and Committee on Native American Child Health. Policy statement—health equity and children's rights. *Pediatrics*. 2010;125(4):838–849

Chapter 64

# Precautionary Principle

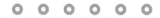

## KEY POINTS

- The Precautionary Principle holds that where there are threats of serious or irreversible damage, lack of full scientific certainty shall not be used as a reason for postponing cost-effective measures to prevent environmental degradation.
- This principle provides justification for public policy actions in situations of scientific complexity, uncertainty, and incomplete information.
- Rather than asking how much exposure to a potentially toxic substance is tolerable, precaution asks how exposures can be prevented through application of alternative technologies.

## INTRODUCTION

One of the central challenges in environmental health is determining how best to set environmental and chemical management policies and standards that protect health in the constantly changing context of complexity, incomplete information, and scientific uncertainty. The more science probes the health effects of interactions between genes and environmental exposures (environmental exposures in this context can be biological, chemical and/or physical, internal, and/or external), the more complex, interdependent, and subtle becomes our understanding of the cause-and-effect relationships of disease (and health). Reductionist, one-cause/one-effect models of disease—reinforced by germ theory—break down. The traditional approach to setting an environmental standard for a particular chemical has been to identify a limit of exposure below which the statistical likelihood of specific adverse health outcomes is minimized. In such analyses, the chemical is examined individually—that is, without consideration of exposures to other chemicals that may potentiate or reduce effects of exposures.

For some well-understood environmental health threats (eg, mercury, dioxins, radon), traditional quantitative human health risk assessment (see Chapter 65) is a powerful tool that can successfully protect health. For most environmental exposures, however, the level of knowledge of toxicology, human exposure, and interactions is insufficient to permit definitive decision making to protect health. The rapidly changing organ systems of the growing and developing child further challenge this inherently resource-intensive approach to controlling environmental health risks. In response to this, a broader approach, sometimes called the "Precautionary Principle" (also known as the "precautionary approach" or "precaution"), has been increasingly invoked as an alternative.

## PRECAUTION: BACKGROUND AND DEFINITIONS

Precaution is an old weapon of public health. When Dr. John Snow removed the handle to the Broad Street pump in 1854 and stopped the cholera epidemic in London without identifying the causal organism, this was a precautionary action, albeit taking place after significant exposures and consequences had been demonstrated. When the US Congress inserted the Delaney Clause into the Food, Drug and Cosmetics Act in 1957, banning animal carcinogens from the human food chain, this was a precautionary action.[1] Precaution is also a core component of both preventive medicine and disease management. In public health, precaution is analogous to primary prevention (eg, neonatal screening and childhood immunizations). In clinical medicine, it is reflected in the classical medical maxim, "First, do no harm."

The concept of precaution was first incorporated into environmental law as the *Vorsorgeprinzip* (foresight or precautionary principle) in the German Clean Air Act of 1974. Since then, it has been specified in numerous international agreements, treaties, and laws (Table 64-1). This principle, applicable to the environment, was most famously articulated in Principle 15 of the 1992 Rio Declaration on Environment and Development: "In order to protect the environment, the precautionary approach shall be widely applied by States according to their capabilities. Where there are threats of serious or irreversible damage, lack of full scientific certainty shall not be used as a reason for postponing cost-effective measures to prevent environmental degradation."[2]

| Table 64-1. Some International Agreements Invoking Precaution[3] |
|---|
| ■ Montreal Protocol on Substances that Deplete the Ozone Layer, 1987 |
| ■ Third North Sea Conference, 1990 |
| ■ The Rio Declaration on Environment and Development, 1992 |
| ■ United Nations Framework Convention on Climate Change, 1992 |
| ■ Treaty of European Union (Maastricht Treaty), 1992 |
| ■ Kyoto Protocol, 1997 (linked to the United Nations Framework Convention on Climate Change) |
| ■ Cartagena Protocol on Biosafety, 2000 |
| ■ Stockholm Convention on Persistent Organic Pollutants, 2001 |
| ■ Paris Climate Accord, 2015 |

Since the Rio Declaration, environmental health professionals and advocates have increasingly sought to integrate precaution into policy. Although no specific definition has been universally accepted, a good working definition has been proposed by the European Environment Agency (EEA):

The Precautionary Principle provides justification for public policy actions in situations of scientific complexity, uncertainty and ignorance, where there may be a need to act in order to avoid, or reduce, potentially serious or irreversible threats to health or the environment, using an appropriate level of scientific evidence, and taking into account the likely pros and cons of action or inaction.[3]

This working definition importantly identifies that public policy action to protect health and/or the environment is the purpose of applying precaution, that the setting requiring precaution is one of imperfect information, and that the consequences of both action and inaction should be considered. In other words, when there is scientific evidence of potential serious harm from environmental exposure(s), preventive or protective action should not need to await acquisition of knowledge that is comprehensive, detailed, and/or mechanistic. Instead, the Precautionary Principle is a process that takes preventive action in the face of incomplete information, shifting the burden of proof to those advocating for risky action, exploring a wide range of alternative actions to achieve given goals, and broadening the discussion to include the public and not just regulatory agencies and the industries being regulated. The concept is logical, but the application is controversial.[4,5]

One major cause of controversy involves conflicting opinions about the stage at which the Precautionary Principle should be applied in the risk assessment, risk management, risk communication continuum (see Chapter 65). Some experts advocate applying it throughout the process, but others insist that it should be used only in risk management after risk is calculated using strict, quantitative procedures. A second category of disagreement is whether the Precautionary Principle can or does represent a reproducible, standardized process of decision making; a general approach and process; or more properly, a philosophical stance that determines how risk is evaluated and decisions are made. Finally, some experts tend to consider standard risk assessment apart from and in opposition to the Precautionary Principle in philosophy and approach, and others consider them as a unified approach, applicable differently depending on the question or risk under consideration and the quality and quantity of the evidence available.[6] These debates are the subject of scores of scholarly articles and numerous books, the details of which are beyond the scope of this chapter. Discussed below is a brief outline of 2 extreme positions to introduce some dimensions of the debate. This is followed by a discussion of how and why the Precautionary Principle is inherently important to children's health using the historical example of leaded gasoline.

## QUANTITATIVE RISK ASSESSMENT

US federal agencies have commonly applied a quantitative approach to risk assessment using a standardized 4-stage system including hazard identification, dose-response assessment, exposure assessment, and risk characterization. The outcome of this process is a probability statement of what proportion of a specified population will be expected to develop an adverse health condition from a specific level of exposure. This estimate then forms the basis for decisions made by risk managers and policy makers to determine public environmental health policy, often on the narrow question of how much exposure to a specific agent or stressor can be tolerated without excess illness. This approach has been criticized as being generally conducted with little public input, requiring great amounts of data, being built on default assumptions that may not be accurate, placing the burden of proof of harm on the regulatory agencies, and inadequately dealing with uncertainty, data gaps, and ignorance.

## CONTRASTING POLICY APPROACHES

A common oversimplification of the contrasting approaches is summed up as follows: risk assessment assumes a stressor, chemical, or technology is "innocent until proven guilty" whereas the Precautionary Principle assumes it is "guilty until proven innocent." Barrett and Raffensperger[7] compare dimensions of 2 idealized models that correspond to the strict separation of quantitative risk assessment (based in mechanistic science) and the Precautionary

Principle (based on precautionary science). Two of these dimensions, Error and Authority, are reviewed here to help illustrate the contrasting positions.

The contrasting approaches to error (ie, assumptions used in statistical calculations) differ in the trade-off between type I (false-positive) and type II (false-negative) errors.[8] Standard risk assessment methods tend to minimize type I errors, whereas the precautionary approach seeks to minimize type II errors. Rarely can both types of errors be minimized simultaneously. Traditionally, scientific research seeks to minimize type I errors. Because scientific knowledge builds iteratively, identifying a false positive as a true positive and building more research on an incorrect assumption would lead to both faulty science and wasted resources. In the context of medicine, however, it is often desirable to accept more false positives to avoid false negatives. For example, given that a safe, inexpensive, and reliable screening test is available to identify a curable but potentially fatal disease at a preclinical stage, most clinicians would agree that it is better to err in the direction of over-identifying individuals who potentially have the disease (increase type I errors) so as not to miss people who may die without treatment (minimize type II errors). Thus, the precautionary principle is analogous to a highly sensitive screening test, which will have some false positives. Strong proponents of standard environmental health risk assessment would argue that it is preferable to avoid false positives. Strong proponents of precaution would argue in favor of minimizing false negatives.

A second dimension often used to separate the 2 approaches is differing definitions of authority. Authority refers to who is qualified or entrusted to determine risk. Under the strict definition of risk assessment, it is an applied, quantitative scientific method conducted by scientists and validated by independent scientific review. The approach seeks to eliminate social or ethical considerations, avoid bias, and produce an objective, value-free, quantitative prediction of risk usually with a quantitative expression of statistical uncertainty. The questions and processes are defined and specified by scientists and are usually narrow in scope as is consistent with best scientific practices. Under the precautionary approach, open-ended dialogue, multidisciplinary participation, qualitative and quantitative inputs, and public review are used to incorporate the larger social and ethical context and definitions of risk. The expression of risk may be qualitative, narrative, and/or quantitative.

## PRECAUTIONARY PRINCIPLE AND RISK ASSESSMENT INTEGRATED

Rather than viewing standard risk assessment and the Precautionary Principle as distinct and at odds, they can be seen as parts of an integrated strategy available to describe and minimize risks from environmental stressors.[4] Depending on the conditions and questions, one approach might be more

## Table 64-2. Characteristics of Hazards and Preferred Regulatory Approach

| EMPHASIZE PRECAUTIONARY PRINCIPLE | EMPHASIZE QUANTITATIVE RISK ASSESSMENT |
|---|---|
| Manmade | Naturally occurring |
| Novel/not yet introduced | Established/already in the environment |
| Serious toxicity | Minor toxicity |
| Irreversible toxicity | Reversible toxicity |
| Very potent | Less potent |
| Dispersible (ubiquitous distribution) | Nondispersible (finite distribution) |
| Persistent | Transient |
| Bioaccumulative | Does not bioaccumulate |
| Nonessential use | Critical use |
| No threshold of toxicity | Threshold of toxicity |
| Large scale (eg, global) | Small scale (eg, occupational) |
| Harmful to immature systems | Not harmful to immature systems |
| Transgenerational effects | No transgenerational effects |
| Alternatives exist | No alternatives exist |
| Large uncertainty in data | Small uncertainty in data |

appropriate than the other (Table 64-2). Almost always, information about basic questions of toxicity and exposure will be incomplete and imperfect. Ideally, environmental health policy makers would utilize the full spectrum of tools and inputs to develop the most health protective laws and regulations using a unified approach that is flexible, iterative, and includes quantitative and qualitative inputs.

## CHILDREN'S ENVIRONMENTAL HEALTH ISSUES AND PRECAUTION

For many children's environmental health issues, policy emphasizing a precautionary approach is most logical.[9,10] The traditional quantitative risk assessment approach is inherently time- and data-intensive, especially so for the many life stages of children's exposures and vulnerabilities (see Chapter 3). Information on developmental, reproductive, and transgenerational toxicity is incomplete or absent for many environmental exposures. Traditional dose-response analysis fails to adequately consider exposures during critical periods of development. These issues create large data gaps and uncertainties in the inputs required for traditional quantitative human health risk assessment. In addition, children's exposures are, in general, involuntary, and children will inherit the environmental, health, and social consequences of decisions made during their formative years. Inclusion of a precautionary approach to controlling environmental health risks is ideal for protecting their future well-being and that of future generations.

## HISTORICAL CASE STUDY—TETRAETHYL LEAD IN GASOLINE

The history of childhood lead poisoning offers clear illustrations of what can happen when precaution is ignored.[11-13] In the 1920s, tetraethyl lead was identified as a cheap and effective antiknock agent for internal combustion engines and added to gasoline. Unlike the lead oxides used in paints, tetraethyl lead is absorbed through the skin. After a series of fatal incidents with researchers and production workers, the Surgeon General of the United States Public Health Service declared a moratorium on "ethyl" production in 1925 and convened a group of experts to assess the situation. The ethyl producers argued for lifting the moratorium to maintain industrial progress, but doctors and public advocates articulated a precautionary message. In response, the Surgeon General appointed an advisory panel of 7 physicians and scientists and gave them 7 months to conduct research and report their findings. The panel completed a single case-control study of 252 gas station employees and chauffeurs that failed to find a statistically significant correlation between use of ethyl gas additives and elevation of blood and stool lead concentrations. The panel stressed that this study was not definitive, and that longer experience and differing populations were needed in the evaluation.[12] Disregarding this warning, the Surgeon General lifted the moratorium, and leaded gas became ubiquitous, resulting in inhalational lead exposure of the entire population, including infants and children.

From 1950 to 1990, information about the dangers of lead poisoning in children exploded. Data began to accumulate on the long-term morbidity of acute lead poisoning in children. The "threshold" level for public health action fell as the special vulnerabilities of children were more precisely documented.[14] The differences in absorption, distribution, and metabolism of lead in infants and children compared with adults were identified, and the long-term, chronic toxicities, particularly to the central nervous system, were described. Even during this period, however, there were loud voices arguing that lead exposure without acute poisoning was of no significance, and lead continued to be used in many products. A growing body of evidence, however, documented the adverse neurodevelopmental effects of even low lead levels. Lead in gasoline finally fell to regulation and was banned from gasoline because of the need to comply with the Clean Air Act of 1970, which required manufacturers to apply catalytic converters to automobile internal combustion engines to reduce the emissions of hydrocarbons, oxides of nitrogen, and carbon monoxide. The removal of lead from gasoline was prompted by the need to protect the catalytic converter from being destroyed by lead.[15] A large proportion of the eventual phasedown of lead in gasoline was attributable to the decreasing share of leaded gasoline that resulted from the transition to cars with catalytic converters. Phasing out lead in gasoline however, provided a "natural experiment" that resulted in dramatic declines in population lead concentrations.[16] It took almost a century to develop the comprehensive data on childhood lead toxicity; earlier full application of the Precautionary Principle could have prevented inhalation exposure and damage to generations of children.

## APPLYING THE PRECAUTIONARY PRINCIPLE

Despite the increasing endorsement of the Precautionary Principle in international treaties and national and state laws, there remains a lack of clarity on how it should be applied.[17] General agreement exists on 4 central components:[18]

- taking preventive action in the context of scientific uncertainty;
- shifting the burden of proof of safety to those who advocate a potentially risky action;
- exploring a comprehensive set of alternative actions to achieve desired goals; and
- enlarging the decision-making process to include the public and other stakeholders.

Tools of precaution include but are not limited to developing clean production processes that eliminate toxic materials and create toxic waste, substituting nontoxic or less toxic materials and/or components, promoting regulatory reform and overhaul that incorporate strong principles of precaution, restricting or minimizing use of toxic substances, and instituting total bans. Critical to the transition to precaution is reframing the questions asked about environmental exposures. For example, rather than asking how much exposure to a potentially toxic substance is tolerable, precaution asks how exposures can be prevented through application of alternative technologies.

Large initiatives in precaution are underway in the European Union (EU) under the Registration, Evaluation, Authorisation and Restriction of Chemicals (EU REACH) program and in states such as California and Massachusetts that have instituted strict toxic chemical laws. These initiatives and others, along with the widening dialogue on precaution involving multiple stakeholders, are the kinds of processes that will help to clarify and develop consensus regarding the practical application of the Precautionary Principle in environmental health policy into the future.

## Frequently Asked Questions

Q  *Does the Precautionary Principle stifle innovation?*

A  Because the Precautionary Principle explicitly requires exploring alternative technologies and solutions by experts and the public, it can enhance innovation. For example, developing renewable, clean energy to satisfy increased energy demands would be preferred over creating more coal-fired power plants. Using biodegradable, nontoxic, non-heavy metal-containing pigments would be preferred over older pigments containing known carcinogens and heavy metals.

Q  *Isn't the Precautionary Principle "anti-scientific?"*

A  Seen as an overall, broad approach to risk characterization and risk management, the precautionary approach encompasses all traditional quantitative risk assessment and also explicitly recognizes uncertainty, knowledge gaps, ignorance, and alternatives. This can be interpreted as being more scientifically rigorous because unknown factors are highlighted, and analyzing these unknown factors is part of decision-making, developing ongoing research questions, and searching for additional solutions.

Q  *Why do pediatricians need to know about the Precautionary Principle?*

A  Children's special vulnerabilities to environmental harms make application of the Precautionary Principle particularly important. Pediatricians have a tradition of child health advocacy, and the Precautionary Principle is an important preventive tool.

Q  *Will applying the Precautionary Principle always result in bans?*

A  There are many precautionary tools available, including bans and restricted use, substitution, redesign, and improved materials management. Some bans, such as banning lead from gasoline, paint, and children's toys and jewelry, are appropriate. In other situations, restrictions or substitutions may be sufficient.

## References

1.  Harrendoes P, Gee D, MacGarvin M, et al, eds. *Late Lessons from Early Warnings: The Precautionary Principle 1986-2000.* Environmental Issue Report No 22. Luxembourg: European Environment Agency, Office of Official Publications for the European Communities; 2001

2.  United Nations Environment Program. Rio Declaration on Environment and Development. http://www.un.org/documents/ga/conf151/aconf15126-1annex1.htm. Accessed June 14, 2018

3. Gee D. Late lessons from early warnings; toward realism and precaution with endocrine-disrupting substances. *Environ Health Perspect.* 2006;114(Suppl 1):152–160

4. Stirling A. Risk, precaution and science: towards a more productive policy debate. *EMBO Rep.* 2007;8(4):309–315

5. Peterson M. The Precautionary Principle should not be used as a basis for decision-making. *EMBO Rep.* 2007;8(4):305–308

6. Silbergeld EK. Commentary: the role of toxicology in prevention and precaution. *Int J Occcup Med Environ Health.* 2004;17(1):91–102

7. Barrett K, Raffensperger C. Precautionary Science. In: Raffensperger C, ed. *Protecting Public Health and the Environment: Implementing the Precautionary Principle.* Covelo, CA: Island Press; 1999:51–70

8. Gee D. Establishing evidence for early action: the prevention of reproductive and developmental harm. *Basic Clin Pharmacol Toxicol.* 2008;102(2):257–266

9. Tickner JA, Hoppin P. Children's environmental health: a case study in implementing the Precautionary Principle. *Int J Occup Environ Health.* 2000;6(4):281–288

10. Jaronsinska D, Gee D. Children's environmental health and the precautionary principle. *Int J Hyg Environ Health.* 2007;210(5):541–546

11. Warren C. *Brush with Death: A Social History of Lead Poisoning.* Baltimore, MD: The Johns Hopkins University Press; 2000

12. English PC. *Old Paint: A Medical History of Childhood Lead-Paint Poisoning in the United States to 1980.* New Brunswick, NJ: Rutgers University Press; 2001

13. Berney B. Round and round it goes: the epidemiology of childhood lead poisoning, 1950-1990. In: Kroll-Smith S, Brown P, Gunter VJ, eds. *Illness and the Environment: A Reader in Contested Medicine.* New York, NY: New York University Press; 2000:215–257

14. Agency for Toxic Substances and Disease Registry Case Studies in Environmental Medicine. Lead Toxicity. https://www.atsdr.cdc.gov/csem/lead/docs/CSEM-Lead_toxicity_508.pdf. Accessed June 14, 2018

15. Newell RG, Rogers K. The U.S. Experience with the Phasedown of Lead in Gasoline. Resources for the Future Discussion Paper (2003) Resources for the Future. http://web.mit.edu/ckolstad/www/Newell.pdf. Accessed April 30, 2018

16. Centers for Disease Control and Prevention. Update: blood lead levels—United States, 1991-1994. *MMWR Morb Mortal Wkly Rep.* 1997;46(7):141–144

17. Lokke S. The Precautionary Principle and chemical regulation: past achievements and future possibilities. *Environ Sci Pollut Res Int.* 2006;13(15):342–349

18. Kriebel D, Tickner J, Epstein P, et al. The Precautionary Principle in environmental science. *Environ Health Perspect.* 2001;109(9):871–876

# Chapter 65

# Risk Assessment, Risk Management, and Risk Communication

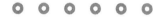

## KEY POINTS

- The systematic framework of risk assessment, risk management, and risk communication is used by public health officials to assess environmental health risks, manage these risks, and share knowledge and recommendations about a potential environmental health risk for individual patients, or in a larger public health context, such as for a community.
- Pediatricians may need to assess or communicate about environmental health risks in practice, to the media, or to local institutions. They therefore should be familiar with the systematic framework.
- Pediatricians should use the 3 principles of risk communication in practice: addressing risk perception, establishing trust, and reducing cognitive attenuation. Pediatricians can follow the 7 cardinal rules of risk communication to create a dialogue and use message maps to construct concise messaging.

## INTRODUCTION

Pediatricians may need to assess or communicate potential environmental health risks to families or institutions for which they work. Examples might be contamination of a community's well water with nitrates, or mold in a school building that contributes to respiratory symptoms and ill health. Public health officials and toxicologists have a systematic framework for approaching these issues. Hospitals and clinic management teams may employ these methods to make decisions in clinical settings. For example, a water leak might arise, creating the question of whether the leak is significant enough to justify shutting down a floor because of the risk of nosocomial infection, or whether other remediation steps would suffice.

The systematic framework approach that public health officials use to address these questions is a 3-part process that includes risk assessment, risk management, and risk communication. This framework was developed to create a standardized, comprehensive process to address complex questions. The 3 pieces exist to separate stakeholder value judgments and policy influences from the initial scientific assessment.[1] The process can be performed formally at the federal level or informally at the local level. Pediatricians can benefit from and play a role in any step of this process. Pediatricians often informally perform risk assessment or risk communication through counseling in local clinical settings.

Risk assessment is the characterization of the potential adverse health effects of exposures to environmental hazards, such as chemicals, the built environment, and climate factors. Risk assessments include several elements. The first is a description of the environmental hazard. A hazard is an agent that has the potential to cause harm to humans, property, or the environment. Risk is defined as the probability that exposure to a hazard will lead to a negative consequence. This is followed by characterizing a dose-response relationship between the hazard and an adverse health outcome. The next step involves characterizing the extent of the exposure in the population followed by the final piece that predicts the extent of health effects in humans under given conditions of exposure. Based on these data, judgments are made about the overall magnitude of the public health problem. Some uncertainty is inherent in the calculations made in all risk assessments.

Risk management is the process of evaluating approaches to regulate or mitigate environmental risks. Public agencies use the results of risk assessment to guide this process. Considering scientific uncertainties and cost-benefit scenarios is part of this step. This process often results in different possible approaches to address the problem and involves a value judgment to make a final management decision. Pediatricians may play a role in this process by contributing ideas about local management policies.

Risk communication may be of the greatest interest to pediatricians. Risk communication involves transmitting information about the risk, potential for health impacts, and how to control exposures. Pediatricians often perform risk communication in daily practice. For example, pediatricians often talk to families about the increased risk of asthma exacerbations if the child is exposed to secondhand smoke or pets. In the larger context of environmental hazards, counseling may be more complicated because there is sometimes uncertainty about the risks and how to mitigate or control them. Using a set of risk communication rules and creating effective messaging are keys to successful risk communication.

It is useful for pediatricians and other health care professionals to be familiar with risk assessment, risk management, and risk communication approaches applicable to environmental contaminants. Pediatricians may be involved in these activities as community advisors, advocates, and practitioners. This chapter gives descriptions of each of the steps in the systematic framework and explains how each applies to practice. The chapter also provides tools for risk communication in the clinical setting.

## RISK ASSESSMENT

The first step in risk assessment is defining the question to be answered. This includes identifying potentially relevant exposures and establishing their sources in the child's environment. Once defined, further information regarding exposure and the potential for adverse health effects should be sought. Public health and regulatory bodies with responsibility for evaluating environmental health risks often follow established protocols designed to study a particular type of substance or condition. In 1983, the National Research Council proposed a 4-step risk assessment paradigm, which consists of (1) hazard identification; (2) dose-response assessment; (3) exposure assessment; and (4) risk characterization.[1] These concepts continue to be employed in modern regulatory and nonregulatory settings. This model was designed primarily to evaluate chemicals. It relies on scientific studies to identify health outcomes (often referred to as "endpoints"), evaluate dose-response relationships, characterize exposures, and determine population-level risks associated with these exposures. The broader potential of this model will also be discussed in this chapter.

Risk assessors, in general, examine the effects of chemical toxicants/carcinogens on populations using quantitative methods and statistical paradigms to apply or establish governmental regulations and guidelines. Clinicians may use this process in a less formal way for environmental agents, chemical and nonchemical. Clinicians usually focus on risks to individuals or small groups using a qualitative approach, applying a "best fit" diagnosis for many different environmental hazards. Table 65-1 compares and contrasts the formal process and the process as it may be practiced by clinicians.

## Table 65-1. Risk Assessment as Performed by Risk Assessors and Clinicians

| RISK ASSESSMENT STEP | QUESTIONS ASKED BY RISK ASSESSOR | QUESTIONS ASKED BY CLINICIAN |
|---|---|---|
| Hazard assessment | What are the chemicals of concern, and what kind of harm are they known or suspected to cause? Which chemicals will we focus on? | What information do we have about an environmental problem, what chemicals or other agents were involved, and what sources of information are there? |
| Dose-response assessment | What effects are seen in animals or humans at different exposure levels? What are the doses at which cancerous and non-cancerous effects occur? Is there a threshold below which no effect is expected? | What information is available from a literature review, or consultation with experts? How do the levels at which effects have been demonstrated compare with levels in the patient or community? Are these levels higher than regulatory limits? |
| Exposure assessment | What are the sources and duration of exposures? How many people are exposed? What do the monitoring or modeling data predict about the range of doses in the population? | Is there a chance that the patient may be coming in contact with (breathing, touching, ingesting, etc) this exposure source? How often and for how long? Is the source highly contaminated or only slightly contaminated? |
| Risk characterization | Given the above, what are the human impacts of current exposures? What is the population risk? Are there sensitive subpopulations? How confident are we in this analysis? | Are regulations based on effects in the fetus or child? Is there reason to be concerned that this patient or children in general may be at greater risk than adults from exposure to this chemical or agent? |
| Risk communication | Is the information understandable and relevant to the audience? Does it respond to public concerns? What are the limitations in this assessment? | Have I listened to the concerns presented, responded with compassion, and helped identify information needed and credible sources for obtaining it? What additional steps are needed? |

Modified from: Miller and Solomon.[2]

## Step 1: Hazard Identification

Hazard identification is a qualitative step that involves identifying and review-ing data to help elucidate health concerns and endpoints that may be associ-ated with exposure to a substance. To determine causality between exposures and health effects, the US Environmental Protection Agency (EPA) and other authoritative health and regulatory bodies employ "weight of evidence" classi-fication schemes based on their reviews of existing evidence.[3] The standard scheme assigns the highest confidence to epidemiologic studies, followed (in descending order) by studies of laboratory animals, in vitro studies, and structure-activity relationships (predicting a chemical's possible activity on the basis of knowledge of its chemical structure). Other schemes rank animal and human evidence separately and combine ratings for each to create an overall hazard risk. A hazard causes no risk if there is no exposure to that hazard.

## Step 2: Dose-response Assessment

Dose-response assessment seeks to determine the relationship between the magnitude of the dose and the occurrence or lack of occurrence of health effects. Dose-response information for chemicals usually is derived from experimental studies of toxicity in animals. Epidemiologic studies also may provide information on the relationship between exposure variations and health outcomes in people. In regulatory settings, to generate a useful dose-response curve, sophisticated toxicologic studies, extrapolation schemes, and pharmacokinetic modeling are used with the goal of finding the maximal safe exposure of an individual to a specific chemical. Study designs and interpreta-tion of data vary according to the health endpoint of concern. For example, carcinogens are considered to be "nonthreshold" hazards. That is, there is no exposure level below which a carcinogen is considered "safe." Therefore, rather than seeking a threshold effect, researchers expose groups of animals to several high doses of the toxicant, and the resulting data are fit into a simple linear model extrapolated to zero. The assumption of a linear dose-response relation-ship has been challenged by recent data showing nonlinear relationships, such as U-shaped curves, that illustrate other responses to varying doses. These data are important because toxicologic studies in animals often do not assess low doses; if an effect only exists at a low dose, it may be missed using a traditional linear dose-response model.

## Step 3: Exposure Assessment

Exposure assessment is used to determine the likely human exposures to the hazard identified. To be most informative, it must accurately characterize all important sources of a particular toxicant or other substance in the environ-ment (eg, groundwater, surface water, air, soil, food, human milk), and quantify exposures (eg, mcg/L in drinking water, mcg/g in soil). Realistic exposure scenarios must be considered to identify at-risk populations or subpopulations, duration of exposure, routes of exposure, timing of exposure, and types of substances. In recent years, efforts to improve exposure assessment for children have been increasing. Children's physiological and behavioral characteristics greatly influence their exposures and often make them different from adults' exposures.[3] Understanding these differences is important in order to accurately evaluate the hazards to children from environmental pollutants or conditions. Biomarkers, such as urinary or blood concentrations of substances or their metabolites, have been increasingly used to more accurately determine exposure. Biomarkers in exposed populations complement exposure assessment on the basis of measurements in environmental media.[2]

## Step 4: Risk Characterization

The last step of risk assessment—risk characterization—involves the synthesis of the dose-response and exposure assessments. Results often are expressed as the maximum acceptable exposure that ensures that the health of an exposed population is protected, or as the number of people likely to be affected at a certain level of exposure.

For carcinogens, risk is typically characterized as the number of excess cancers that may occur in a population following continuous, low-dose exposure at a specific average level over a 70-year lifetime. Risk is generally considered to be acceptable if the exposure results in an increase of less than 1 excess cancer per 1 million ($10^{-6}$) people exposed over a lifetime. Because children have increased biological vulnerability, the US EPA established guidelines that weigh exposures during infancy, childhood, or adolescence more heavily when data specific to these life-stages are not available.[4]

Noncarcinogens with presumed thresholds for adverse health effects are evaluated by comparing the estimated exposure, on the basis of exposure assessment, with the acceptable exposure level defined by the dose-response data. In general, extrapolation from testing of toxicity in animals is required to determine a reference dose (used by US EPA) or an acceptable daily intake (used by the Food and Drug Administration). If these values are not exceeded over a lifetime, there should be no unacceptable effects in exposed humans. To determine what level of exposure to a chemical is likely to be safe in humans, risk assessors use the most reliable animal or human data at which no adverse effects were observed (NOAEL) or the lowest level at which adverse effects were observed (LOAEL). These values are then divided by uncertainty or safety factors to account for the various extrapolations required (Table 65-2). Safety or uncertainty factors usually are multiples of 10, an arbitrary multiplier, but may be applied as some fraction of 10 depending on the quality of data available. Use of an additional safety factor has been considered in recent years to

| Table 65-2. Extrapolation from Animal Toxicity Data to Reference Dose[a] (RfD) |||
|---|---|---|
| $$RfD = \frac{NOAEL \text{ or } LOAEL}{UF_1 \times UF_{2...}}$$ |||
| **EXAMPLES OF UNCERTAINTY FACTORS** |||
| 10 x || Human variability |
| 10 x || Extrapolation from animals to humans |
| 10 x || Use of LOAEL instead of NOAEL |
| 10 x || Increased child susceptibility |
| 0.1–10 x || Modifying factor |

Adapted from National Library of Medicine.[5]

Abbreviations: LOAEL, lowest observed adverse effect level; NOAEL, no observed adverse effect level; RfD, reference dose; UF, uncertainty factor.

[a] Reference doses are calculated by the US EPA. Similar measures include Acceptable Daily Intake (used by the Food and Drug Administration; the same calculation is performed, but modifying factors are not used) and Minimal Risk Levels (calculated by the Agency for Toxic Substances and Disease Registry for non-cancer endpoints).

account for the potential increased susceptibility of children when data on early life exposures are inadequate.

The formal output of this 4-step risk assessment process is an expression of risk, most commonly quantified as the proportion (or probability) of a specific population (or populations) exposed to a toxicant at a particular level that will express a particular health effect related to that exposure. The less formal application of these concepts by clinicians can provide a method for addressing environmental health concerns of their patients or communities.

After more than 2 decades of experience with the process of risk assessment of chemicals by the US EPA, several shortcomings have been revealed. In 2008, the National Academy of Sciences published *Science and Decisions, Advancing Risk Assessment,*[3] a report that evaluated the current process of risk assessment and the causes for decision-making gridlock. A major cause is uncertainty, an inherent property of scientific data, that leads to multiple interpretations. The National Academy of Sciences' recommendations to the US EPA focused on enhancing collaborative involvement throughout the risk assessment process, further defining the scope of risk assessment, providing guidelines for use when data are lacking, and expanding application of the process to nonchemical agents and stressors.

While regulators grapple with the formal processes, the core concepts remain a useful framework for clinicians. Better characterization of the environmental sources of concern can be obtained by reviewing the scientific and medical literature and investigating the child's environment, either from the health history or from on-site investigation by trained environmental assessors. Governmental agencies, such as the US EPA, regional EPA offices, the Agency for Toxic Substances and Disease Registry, the Consumer Product Safety Commission, the Centers for Disease Control and Prevention, the Food Safety and Inspection Service, and others also may have relevant information. For well-characterized exposures, dose-response relationships may be relatively well defined, permitting crude exposure estimates using estimations based on established facts about the exposure, the environmental history, and the medical history. This information can then be compiled, and a determination of potential risks versus benefits of continued exposure versus mitigation can be developed. At times, the appropriate therapeutic and mitigation decisions will be obvious, such as removing all sources of lead from the environment of a child with an elevated blood lead level.[6] At other times, however, the answer may not be clear cut—for example, recommending removal of carpeting in the bedroom of a child with dust mite sensitivity and asthma when the head of household has just lost a job and the family cannot afford to pay for the removal.

## RISK MANAGEMENT

Public agencies (federal, state, and local) responsible for minimizing environmental health risks review the results of commissioned risk assessments and, when possible, enact and amend regulations to reduce such health risks through an ongoing iterative process. Examples include banning hazardous substances from products and tightening controls on levels of emissions allowed. Considering scientific uncertainties, risk-benefit relationships and cost-benefit relationships are part of this process. A pediatrician can play a role in risk management for organizations and communities as well as for individual patients. A pediatrician may help to set policies for hospital and outpatient care on the basis of risk assessment data collected in-house or by public agencies. One example is the mandated use of soap and water or alcohol-based hand sanitizers for hand cleansing to reduce the risk of spreading highly infectious or aggressive microbial agents, such as methicillin-resistant *Staphylococcus aureus*. A number of schools have taken action in their cafeterias to manage the availability of foods high in fat and calories to combat obesity in their students. Pediatricians may play important roles as advocates for changes in policies such as these.

When pediatricians and others address concerns about environmental factors, they may find that the evidence base that informs risk characterization for children is inadequate.[7] Taking precautionary measures when there is an environmental threat is welcomed by many individuals and communities, especially when adequate data are not available. The Precautionary Principle is discussed in greater detail in Chapter 64.

## RISK COMMUNICATION

Risk communication can be defined as a process of informing people about the nature, magnitude, significance, and control of potential hazards to their person, property, or community. The exchange goes both ways. Parents frequently ask questions about the potential health effects of environmental exposures. Pediatricians often need to discuss environmental health risks and interventions with patients or parents and sometimes with representatives of the family, such as attorneys. At other times, they may need to address larger audiences, such as parent groups, colleagues, and governmental agencies. Communities and environmental advocacy groups often are in need of physicians with a clinical background to advise them about the potential health implications of various situations and exposures and identify paths of action. Clinicians generally hold positions of trust and high credibility within their communities and, thus, may serve as knowledgeable intermediaries between affected communities and other parties.

Risk communication is built upon 3 theoretical principles: risk perception, trust determination, and cognitive attenuation. These principles provide insight into the ways audiences form perceptions about the risk, establish trust, process information, and ultimately make decisions about risks.[8]

Risk communication is not a "one size fits all" procedure. The characteristics of the audience, the nature of the environmental hazard, the qualifications of the presenter, the social context of the risk, and other factors determine the risk message perceived ("risk perception") by the audience (Table 65-3).

When people are highly concerned, anxious, or fearful, they want to know that the person they are speaking with cares about them. Trust develops by demonstrating 4 qualities

- Care and empathy;
- Honesty and openness;
- Dedication and commitment; and
- Competence and expertise.

Active listening, removing physical barriers between the clinician and the audience, mirroring (identifying similarities between clinician and audience), and residing in the neighborhood enhance trustworthiness. Cognitive attenuation refers to the "mental noise" that interferes with the ability to process information. This can be accentuated by fear, anxiety, or high levels of concern.

Effective communication addresses the needs of the various components of the audience. The audience may be composed of people from different backgrounds. The clinician should aim to know the background and

## Table 65-3. Some Factors Related to Decreased or Increased Perception of Risk[2]

| DECREASES PERCEIVED RISK | INCREASES PERCEIVED RISK |
| --- | --- |
| **Hazard Factors** | |
| Familiar | Unfamiliar |
| Not catastrophic | Catastrophic or catastrophic potential |
| Natural | Synthetic |
| Adults affected | Fetuses or children affected |
| Non-dreaded effect | Dreaded effect (cancer, birth defects) |
| Voluntary | Involuntary |
| **Personal Factors** | |
| Male gender | Female gender |
| White race | Nonwhite race |
| Scientist | Nonscientist |
| Employed by industry or government | Employed by academic institutions |
| **Social and Ethical Factors** | |
| Trust in the risk communicator | Mistrust |
| Trust in the risk imposer (polluter) | Mistrust |
| Equal distribution of risk and benefits | Unfair or unequal distribution of risks and benefits |
| No perception of preexisting problem | Perception of unfair burden of cumulative risk in the community |

educational level of the audience and what information would be of greatest use to these individuals. Involving the audience in the decision-making process as much as possible can decrease mistrust and fear. The process can begin by assessing the answers to these questions: What are the personal characteristics of audience members? What are their concerns? What are the relevant social and ethical factors? It is important for the clinician to know about the nature of the hazard being discussed. Is it natural or man-made? Catastrophic or not? Adults or children affected? Awareness of how these factors influence the audience's perception of the risk and addressing those that can be addressed ultimately will determine the success or failure of the risk communication. When possible, it is advisable to develop alternatives to public hearings through meetings with smaller numbers of people who are more vulnerable to potential harmful effects. Small group or individual conversations are more conducive to an effective exchange of information with highly affected or concerned people.

Suggestions for developing a message for communicating risk have been published.[7] Adhering to the "rule of 3" is important because people can only process 2 or 3 bits of information at a time, and they have a natural ability to remember triplets. In practical terms, this means developing no more than 3 key messages, with 3 supporting facts for each key message (Figure 65-1). Message maps are frameworks in which the 3 key messages can be organized to communicate with an audience. Typically the first key message explains the exposure of concern, the second message explains the potential health effects or clinical management issues, and the third message provides action steps for physicians and families.

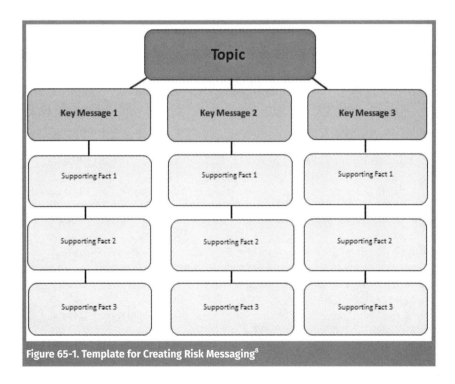

**Figure 65-1. Template for Creating Risk Messaging**[8]

These messages can come in the form of a brochure, handout, newsletter, or any other means that is appropriate for the audience. It is also important to avoid "negative amplification," the concept whereby people give greater weight and attend more to negative information than positive. Presenting more positive information than negative can be effective, as is avoiding sentences with negative words, such as "no," "not," and "never." Research demonstrates that individuals who are experiencing high levels of concern, anxiety, or fear, whether caused by real or perceived threats, demonstrate "cognitive attenuation." Only a narrow window exists for communicating information when cognitive attenuation is present. Risk communication messaging can help address this important window for information. Lastly, keeping the message simple and using straightforward language and clear terminology helps the audience to more clearly understand messages. Face-to-face communication is always preferred. Table 65-4 lists principles that aid in establishing trust, decreasing cognitive attenuation, and communicating effectively.

## A Pediatrician's Role in Addressing Risk

Pediatricians may have many opportunities to apply risk principles when addressing environmental health concerns from patients and their communities. These are extensions of routine pediatric practice. For example, when evaluating a child with asthma, the components of risk assessment can be used: (1) defining the question—are there environmental factors that are making the patient's asthma worse? (2) understanding the scientific evidence

---

### Table 65-4. Seven Cardinal Rules of Risk Communication[9]

1. Accept and involve the public as a partner—your goal is an exchange of information, not to diffuse public concerns or convince the public of your point of view.

2. Plan carefully and evaluate your efforts—conform your interaction to the nature of subject matter, the nature of the audience, and your goals.

3. Listen to the public's specific concerns—trust, credibility, competence, fairness, and empathy are more important to your audience than statistics and detail.

4. Be honest, frank, and open—it is hard to regain credibility and trust once they have been lost.

5. Work with other credible sources—conflicts and disagreements among risk communicators create problems communicating with the audience.

6. Meet the needs of the media—they are frequently more interested in politics, simplicity, and danger than risk, complexity, and safety.

7. Speak clearly and with compassion—don't forget to acknowledge the tragedy of human injury or environmental contamination.

base that links exposure to environmental triggers with asthma status and control; (3) taking an environmental history to identify the presence and extent of environmental triggers in the child's everyday environments; (4) developing a management plan that includes reducing exposure to relevant environmental triggers and possibly desensitizing the child to these triggers; and (5) educating the patient and family regarding the role of these factors in the child's asthma. All of this can be delivered in a dialogue engaging the parent and using terminology and a level of language that the parent and child (if appropriate) can understand.

Beyond interacting with individual patients and families, it is likely that a pediatrician will have numerous opportunities to use the 7 cardinal rules of risk communication (see Table 65-4) and other communication skills discussed in this chapter. Interacting with the media, public health professionals, and environmental agencies; contributing to health care policy; and providing community education are opportunities to assess, manage, and communicate risk in different ways.

For the community, the media is critical in getting the story out. The pediatrician should be proactive in contacting the media with accurate health information, correcting misinformation, promoting appropriate caution, and allaying fears.[8] These activities involve media skills that can be learned.

## SUMMARY

Faced with an environmental or health risk, the process of risk assessment, risk management, and risk communication can be used as a unit or as individual components to evaluate, manage, and share knowledge and recommendations about the potential risk at the level of an individual patient encounter or in a larger public health context, such as a community. Although this process is most often associated with the evaluation of chemicals, it lends itself to many other environmental agents, conditions, and stressors.

Risk management, as a regulatory and policy tool, aims to eliminate or at least control sources of exposures. The same approach to eliminating or mitigating sources of exposures of concern can be applied in environmental risk management for individual patients and families.

Risk communication should be based on the needs, beliefs, and knowledge base of the audience. The venue for delivering the message should be as appropriate as possible to be certain that 2-way communication is achieved and all parties understand one another. Careful consideration should be given to the social context in which the public perceives the risk because this can distort the public's perception.

# References

1. Committee on the Institutional Means for Assessment of Risks to Public Health and National Research Council, Commission on Life Sciences. *Risk Assessment in the Federal Government: Managing the Process.* Washington, DC: National Academies Press; 1983

2. Miller M, Solomon G. Environmental risk communication for the clinician. *Pediatrics.* 2003;112(1 Pt 2):211–217

3. Committee on Improving Risk Analysis Approaches Used by the US Environmental Protection Agency, National Research Council. *Science and Decisions: Advancing Risk Assessment.* Washington, DC: National Academies Press; 2008

4. US Environmental Protection Agency. *Child-Specific Exposure Factors Handbook.* Washington, DC: US Environmental Protection Agency; 2008

5. US National Library of Medicine. 6. Risk assessment. In: *Toxicology Tutor.* Washington, DC: US Department of Health and Human Services. http://toxtutor.nlm.nih.gov. Accessed June 19, 2018

6. State of California Environmental Protection Agency, Air Resources Board. *Lead Risk Management Activities.* http://www.arb.ca.gov/toxics/lead/lead.htm. Accessed June 19, 2018

7. Anderson ME, Kirkland KH, Guidotti TL, Rose C. A case study of tire crumb use on playgrounds: risk analysis and communication when major clinical knowledge gaps exist. *Environ Health Perspect.* 2006;114(1):1–3

8. Galvez MP, Peters R, Graber N, Forman J. Effective risk communication in children's environmental health: lessons learned from 9/11. *Pediatr Clin North Am.* 2007;54(1):33–46

9. Covello V, Allen F. *Seven Cardinal Rules of Risk Communication.* Washington, DC: US Environmental Protection Agency, Office of Policy Analysis; 1992

Chapter 66

# Chemicals and Chemicals Regulation

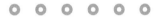

## KEY POINTS

- Tens of thousands of manufactured chemicals—many produced in enormous quantities—have entered US commerce and the environment over the past decades.
- Most of these chemicals have not been adequately tested for safety or toxicity, and fewer still have been tested for developmental toxicity in fetuses, infants, and children.
- Fetuses, infants, and children often are more susceptible than adults to adverse effects of chemicals and can be injured by chemicals at very low exposure levels.
- Recent federal legislation has resulted in improvements in chemical regulation, but many chemicals in wide use are known to pose risks to children's health; much work is needed to ensure that infants, children, and others are protected from the hazardous effects of chemicals.

## INTRODUCTION

Chemicals are substances that are manufactured, processed, or used in commerce. The term "chemicals" includes a wide spectrum of substances including metals, inorganic chemicals, and organic chemicals. Chemicals can be classified by their properties or their uses.

## CHEMICAL PROPERTIES

Chemicals have specific physico-chemical properties, such as molecular size, solubility, and half-life, that can determine their persistence in the environment and their potential for accumulation in biological systems including humans. Chemicals also exhibit potentially harmful characteristics (eg, ability to ignite, explode, corrode, etc).

Toxicity, the potential to harm people, plants, and animals, is the chemical's inherent ability to cause a specific toxic effect. Any substance, even water, may cause toxic effects if ingested or inhaled in excessive quantities. Therefore, assessment of the risk posed by a substance involves consideration of dose as well as toxicity. Toxicity is assessed in the context of the time frame of exposure associated with an adverse effect. Acute toxicity occurs when adverse effects are caused by a single or very short-term exposure, for example, an unintentional ingestion of iron tablets. Chronic toxicity occurs when a chemical exposure causes harmful effects with continuous or repeated exposure over an extended period of time (eg, cancer caused by tobacco smoking). Subchronic toxicity occurs in between these periods: effects are caused with exposure over more than 1 year but less than a lifetime. Toxicity leading to cancer is called carcinogenicity. Almost any organ system can be a target of a toxic substance. Just as dosing and response to pharmaceuticals are highly age-dependent, so is toxicity. These age-specific differences are known as "critical windows of susceptibility" (see Chapter 3). There are various dose-response curves, many of which are monotonic (higher doses confer greater hazards). In some situations, however, there are non-monotonic responses (greater responses at lower doses) when, for example, higher doses are required to trigger metabolism and detoxification of a chemical.

Persistence refers to the length of time a substance stays in the environment without breaking down to other chemicals. A substance may persist for less than a second or indefinitely. So-called persistent chemicals remain in the environment for longer periods of time than nonpersistent chemicals, usually weeks or years. Persistence per se is not a negative characteristic. It poses a problem only when it is coupled with toxicity or other forms of environmental harm. Many chemicals are persistent in water, especially groundwater. Fewer chemicals persist in air. Sunlight, as well as oxygen and other constituents of outdoor air, can cause some chemicals to break down. Metals and certain inorganic and organic chemicals are able to persist in air for long periods of time, and thus can travel long distances from their source. This is why certain metals and organic chemicals are found in remote locations, such as the Arctic and Antarctic, far away from the chemical source areas where such substances have been manufactured and used.

Degradation in the environment is an important physico-chemical process that breaks down chemicals to other substances. Photodegradation by sunlight, biodegradation by bacteria, and oxidation by oxygen can cause some less persistent chemicals to break down. The breakdown products can be more or less toxic, depending on the final product. Many organic products eventually degrade to carbon dioxide and water.

Some chemicals have properties that make them bioaccumulative; that is, they accumulate in the tissues of living species. Chemicals that are bioaccumulative often show a pattern of higher and higher concentrations in tissues of organisms, ascending the food chain from plants and plant-eating species to carnivores, including humans.

Chemicals with a combination of persistent, bioaccumulative, and toxic (PBT) properties are of particular concern. Once released to the environment, they can travel far from their source, remain in the environment for long periods of time, and increase in concentration as they move up the food chain. Some well-known PBT chemicals include dioxins and furans, lead, mercury, polychlorinated biphenyls (PCBs), and hexachlorobenzene (see Chapter 37).

## CHEMICAL USES

A distinction generally is made between chemicals on the basis of intended use and whether or not the production of the substance is by design or occurs unintentionally. Types of chemical uses include

- Food additives are substances in food that are added deliberately to change flavor, color, consistency, or other attributes of food. In the United States, these also include substances added inadvertently via migration of substances from packaging.

- Pharmaceuticals have medicinal properties and are marketed for health benefits. These include ingredients added for other useful properties, such as appropriate drug delivery and preservation. They also include medical antimicrobial agents.

- Pesticides are substances or mixtures formulated for preventing, controlling, repelling, or mitigating pests including animals, plants and fungi. Categories include insecticides for killing insects, herbicides for controlling weeds, fungicides for controlling fungi (eg, on fresh produce), industrial antimicrobial agents and drinking water treatment agents, and rodenticides used to kill rodents. Pesticides are frequently used in agriculture, industry, by municipalities, in institutions such as schools and hospitals, and in the home. As regulated, safety reviews consider not only the pesticide active ingredients but also inert ingredients ("inerts") used as vehicles and additives, as well as manufacturing byproducts. For example, the highly toxic dioxin (2,3,7,8-TCDD) was formed as a byproduct in the manufacture of the herbicide, 2,4,5-T ("Agent Orange") and accounted for most of the toxicity of that chemical.

- Combustion byproducts are formed when chemicals are heated or burned. The most common combustion products of organic substances are carbon dioxide and water, but other more toxic substances, such as carbon monoxide, may be formed. Minute quantities of dioxins and furans can be created during incineration (eg, backyard burning). Even smaller amounts are produced in forest fires; these are not included in pollutant registries. The common pollutants that create smog and air pollution, such as ozone, nitrogen oxides, sulfur dioxides, and certain volatile organic compounds (VOCs) and particulates, are also formed in the burning of fossil fuels, known as combustion. Combustion can also contribute to the formation of greenhouse gases, such as carbon dioxide and nitrous oxide. Breakdown byproducts, like combustion byproducts, are formed when chemicals degrade in the environment via natural weathering processes or biodegradation by microorganisms.

- A toxicant is a chemical substance with the potential to cause toxicity. Toxins are naturally formed toxic substances that may occur as contaminants in food (eg, aflatoxin), water (eg, domoic acid), or air (satratoxin).

- Industrial chemicals are developed or manufactured for use in industrial operations or research by industry, government, or academia. In the legal and regulatory context, they do not include the chemicals with uses listed previously (food additives, pharmaceuticals, pesticides, combustion and breakdown products, and toxins). They do include metals as well as polymers and organic chemicals. Many industrial chemicals, such as windshield washer fluids and household chemicals, also are used in consumer products. Industrial chemicals include fuels used to generate energy and manufacturing byproducts generated as a consequence of a manufacturing process. Byproducts of manufacture can be more toxic than the intended product of manufacture.

## CHEMICAL MANAGEMENT

A revolution in materials sciences occurred in the 20th century and more than 140,000 new chemicals were produced during this time. Expansion in chemical manufacture began in Germany and Switzerland in the late 19th century with the identification of chemical elements and a series of fundamental discoveries that laid the groundwork for the ability to synthesize (or break apart) known or new compounds. This revolution subsequently spread globally and resulted in an enormous growth in industrial and consumer use of chemicals and materials derived from chemicals. Global chemical production continues to grow at a rate of 3% to 4 % annually, and two thirds of global manufacture now takes place in low- and middle-income countries where safeguards often are scant and the public health infrastructure is weak. In addition to synthetic chemicals, production and use of metals and inorganic chemicals also have increased along a similar trajectory. The increase in volume and numbers of chemicals in commerce during the 20th century created the need for government intervention to ensure that chemicals were being used safely. Today, the chemical industry is undergoing a new revolution with the increased production of specialty chemicals (eg, detergent enzymes) using genetically modified microbes and nanotechnology.

Children are most likely to be exposed to the 3,000 to 5,000 chemicals that are produced in largest volumes and incorporated into tens of thousands of consumer products. The US Environmental Protection Agency (EPA) terms these "high production volume" (HPV) chemicals. HPV chemicals have become widely disseminated in the environment and are detected today in the most remote reaches of the planet. The National Biomonitoring Survey conducted on an ongoing basis by the Centers for Disease Control and Prevention routinely detects several hundred manufactured chemicals in the bodies of virtually all Americans.

In the United States and in most countries worldwide, there are two approaches to the regulatory management of chemicals: media-specific approaches that seek to decrease or eliminate exposures from specific substances in specific media, and comprehensive approaches that address the entire lifecycle of a chemical or a chemical process. Examples of media-specific statutes that address chemical safety in the United States are shown in Table 66-1.

In the United States and globally, regulation of chemicals had lagged significantly behind the growth and development of the chemical industry. Until 1976, there were no laws in the United States specifically related to the introduction of chemicals into commerce and the control of the hazards of existing chemicals. The basic structure of the domestic laws of the United States with respect to chemicals was established in 1972 for pesticides (the Federal Insecticide, Fungicide and Rodenticide Act [FIFRA])[18] and in 1976 for industrial chemicals (the Toxic Substances Control Act [TSCA]).[19] Up to that point, regulation of chemicals was limited to food additives, cosmetics, and pharmaceuticals by the Food and Drug Administration (FDA) and pesticides (initially by the US Department of Agriculture and the FDA, and in 1972 by the newly created US EPA). By 1976, it is estimated that there were 60,000 chemical substances in commerce in the United States; the government, however, did not have an inventory of chemicals manufactured and imported into the United States. In 1988, Congress amended and strengthened the FIFRA. In 1986, Congress enacted the Emergency Preparedness and Community Right to Know Act (EPCRA), thereby establishing the Toxic Release Inventory (TRI) for tracking the releases and transfers of chemicals from industry.[20] In 1990, Congress adopted the Pollution Prevention Act (PPA).[21]

## Table 66-1. Media-specific Statutes that Address Chemical Safety in the United States

| AGENCY, STATUTE, DATE | STANDARD (BASIS)[a] | WEB LINK |
|---|---|---|
| Consumer Product Safety Commission, Consumer Products Safety Act, 1972[1] | Consumer Products: Controlled Hazardous Substances and Articles (H)[b] | https://www.cpsc.gov/Regulations-Laws--Standards/Statutes/Summary-List/Consumer-Product-Safety-Act[2] |
| US Environmental Protection Agency (EPA), Clean Air Act, 1990[3] | Air: Hazardous Air Pollutants Standards, HAPS (T) | https://www.epa.gov/laws-regulations/summary-clean-air-act[4] |
| US EPA, Clean Water Act, 1972[5] | Water: National Pollutant Discharge Elimination System, NPDES, Permits (T) | https://www.epa.gov/laws-regulations/summary-clean-water-act[6] |
| US EPA, Food Quality Protection Act, 1996[7] | Food: Tolerances (H) | https://www.epa.gov/laws-regulations/summary-food-quality-protection-act[8] |
| US EPA, Resource Conservation and Recovery Act, 1984[9] | Waste: Listing as a Hazardous Waste (H)[b] | https://www.epa.gov/laws-regulations/summary-resource-conservation-and-recovery-act[10] |
| US EPA, Safe Drinking Water Act, 1996[11] | Drinking Water: Maximum Contaminant Level, MCL (T) | https://www.epa.gov/laws-regulations/summary-safe-drinking-water-act[12] |
| US Food and Drug Administration (FDA), Federal Food Drug and Cosmetics Act Cosmetics, 1938 Food Additives, 1958[13,14] | Cosmetics: Very few specifically managed chemicals and adulterants (H); no prior reviews or approvals Food Additives: Tolerances (H or Exempt[c]) | https://www.fda.gov/RegulatoryInformation/LawsEnforcedbyFDA/FederalFoodDrugandCosmeticActFDCAct/default.htm[15] |
| US Occupational Safety and Health Administration, Occupational Safety and Health Act, 1970[16] | Workplaces: Permissible Exposure Limit, PEL (T)[d] | https://www.osha.gov/pls/oshaweb/owadisp.show_document?p_table=oshact&p_id=2743[17] |

[a] T = Technology Based, ie, based on availability and/or feasibility of technology approaches to monitoring and/or control or H = Health Based, ie, based solely on health and/or environmental protection considerations

[b] Also for other reasons, eg, explosivity, corrosivity, ignitability

[c] Under the Federal Food Drug and Cosmetics Act there are 2 categories of exempt substances: (1) those that were determined to be safe before the 1958 amendments and (2) those considered to be "Generally Recognized as Safe" (GRAS) based on extensive use before 1958

[d] Usually over a given time period, and as a time weighted average (TWA), eg, an 8-hour TWA

From the start, the TSCA covered all chemicals not already regulated as food additives, drugs, cosmetics, and pesticides. The TSCA also contained specific requirements to regulate PCBs. Over the years, the TSCA was amended to specifically regulate asbestos (1986, Title II) and radon (1988, Title III). In 1992, Congress amended the TSCA to specifically regulate lead in housing. Asbestos, PCBs, and lead are referred to collectively by the US EPA as "national program" chemicals; the radon program is located in the US EPA's Office of Air and Radiation.

The Voluntary Children's Chemical Exposure Program (VCCEP) was the only child-specific initiative created under the TSCA. The VCCEP was initiated in 1998 with the goal of designing a process to assess and report on the safety of chemicals to children. The US EPA concluded that the VCCEP was unsuccessful in 2011 and discontinued the program but recommended that the US EPA design and implement a new process to assess the safety of chemicals to children.[22]

As shown in Table 66-2, the TSCA, the Food Quality Protection Act (FQPA), and the Federal Food, Drug, and Cosmetic Act (FFDCA) (for drugs) have similar provisions relating to areas that need to be addressed in comprehensive management of chemicals.

The FIFRA was amended most recently in 1996 in an omnibus statute, the Food Quality Protection Act,[7] that amended pesticide regulation both under the FIFRA and the FFDCA (see Chapter 40).

In 2011, the American Academy of Pediatrics (AAP) issued a statement on chemicals management policy that called for a number of fundamental changes in the TSCA.[24] As stated by the AAP at the time, the law had not effectively protected children and pregnant women, as well as the general population, from harmful chemicals. Specifically, it was noted that the US EPA was not required to account for vulnerabilities of children, and that only a handful of existing chemicals on the market ever had been regulated. The AAP was concerned about the lack of regulation of existing chemicals on the market and about the lack of premarket testing of new chemicals. The AAP recommended an overhaul of existing chemicals regulation to:

- Require consideration of a wide range of consequences of chemical use for children and their families.
- Adopt policies at all levels of government that would
  — Base chemical regulation on scientific evidence and promote the substitution of less hazardous chemicals;
  — Require the same level of evidence for existing and new chemicals;
  — Provide the US EPA with authority to require evidence that chemicals are demonstrated to be safe for pregnant women and children;
  — Base decisions on chemical hazards, uses, and exposures;

## Table 66-2. Features of Comprehensive Chemical Laws

| LIFE CYCLE | TSCA[19] | FQPA[7] | FFDCA (DRUGS)[23] |
|---|---|---|---|
| Safety standard | Unreasonable risk | Unreasonable risk<br>Reasonable certainty of no harm (tolerance) | "Substantial evidence" of drug safety and efficacy |
| Protection of children | Infants, children, pregnant women | Additional 10× factor for children for food tolerances | Best Pharmaceuticals for Children Act (2002) |
| Research and development uses | Section 5: Premanufacture Notification (PMN) for New Chemicals | Section 5: Pesticide Experimental Use Permits | Investigational New Drug (IND) application prior to clinical testing |
| Commercialization and scaling up production | Section 5: Significant New Use Rule (optional) | Section 3: Pesticide Registration | New Drug Application (NDA) for first use. Health care providers can use drugs "off label" |
| Ability to require testing and other information generation | Section 4: Where risks or exposures of concern are found | Section 3: Pesticide Registration and Registration Review | Phase I and Phase II testing requirements |
| Ability to manage hazards | Section 6: Chemical Management | Section 3: Pesticide Registration | Drug labels for consumers and health care providers; black box warnings |
| Control products on the market | Section 8: Chemical Inventory | Section 3(g): Requires Pesticide Registration Review (reassessment) periodically | Postmarket surveillance |

| | | | |
|---|---|---|---|
| Control import of chemicals into United States | Section 13: Importers must certify that chemicals comply with TSCA | Section 17: Pesticides imported into the United States must comply with US law | Prohibits import of unapproved drugs into the United States |
| Report risks of injury or to health | Section 8(e): Requires reports from those who manufacture, process, or distribute in commerce | Section 6(a)(2): Requires reports from pesticide registrants of any new information or incidents of harmful effects | Required of product manufacturers. Voluntary for health care practitioners and patients |
| Worker exposures (in production, formulation, use, and disposal) | Section 9: US EPA must forward a report to OSHA of any unreasonable risks related to worker health and safety | Section 6: Product specific restrictions Section 25(a): General Worker Protection Standards under US EPA authority to regulate pesticide risks | FDA Good Manufacturing Practices not designed to protect workers. Worker hazards are under OSHA |
| Consumer exposures (in product use) | Section 9: US EPA must forward a report to CPSC of any unreasonable risks related to worker health and safety | Section 6: Product specific restrictions | Product specific information on labels; black box warnings |
| Waste (emissions, disposal, recycling, reuse) | Section 9: US EPA must use RCRA if under TSCA it identifies unreasonable risks related to wastes | Section 19: Regulation of storage, disposal, transportation, and recall | Regulated by US EPA under RCRA |
| Authority of states | Balancing of federal and state authorities | Section 24: States may not permit any use prohibited by FIFRA and may not impose different requirements for labeling and packaging | FDA has jurisdiction for premarket approval of drugs and drug labels |

Abbreviations: CPSC, Consumer Product Safety Commission; FDA, Food and Drug Administration; FFDCA, Federal Food, Drug, and Cosmetic Act; FIFRA, Federal Insecticide, Fungicide and Rodenticide Act; FQPA, Food Quality Protection Act; OSHA, Occupational Safety and Health Act; RCRA, Resource Conservation and Recovery Act; TSCA, Toxic Substances Control Act; US EPA, US Environmental Protection Agency.

— Require chemicals to meet public health safety standards;
— Require postmarket safety monitoring;
— Require methods for biomonitoring of all chemicals that are marketed; and
— Require that companies develop a health communication document for each chemical on the market.

- Provide the US EPA with a simpler process for requiring additional testing of chemicals.
- Expand federal biomonitoring programs.
- Increase federal funding for research about the health effects of chemicals.
- Adopt federal policies that promote development of greener chemicals to replace existing chemicals of concern.

The 2016 TSCA amendments, known as the Frank R. Lautenberg Chemical Safety for the 21st Century Act[25] (the Lautenberg Act), strengthened the TSCA in several ways and for the first time required the US EPA to specifically assess health threats to children, pregnant women, and other vulnerable populations. Industrial chemicals are broken down into subcategories as follows: "existing" chemicals (those grandfathered by the TSCA); national program chemicals (existing chemicals that have specific requirements set by the US Congress); and "new" chemicals (chemicals manufactured post-TSCA). Table 66-3 summarizes the major features of the TSCA as amended in 2016. The Lautenberg Act addressed many of the AAP's policy recommendations, with the exception of requiring biomonitoring methods and health communications documents; expanding federal biomonitoring programs; and increasing federal funding for research on chemicals' health effects. As such, the Lautenberg Act represented meaningful progress over prior toxic chemicals regulation. The Lautenberg Act amended the original TSCA to require a health-based safety standard. The Act also included references to vulnerable populations (because of elevated chemical exposures or heightened susceptibility to their effects), including infants, children, and pregnant women, and required that restrictions imposed on chemicals be sufficient to ensure the protection of such vulnerable populations. The Lautenberg Act also struck the "Catch 22" posed by the original TSCA, which required that the US EPA first show potential risk or high release or exposure to require testing of a chemical. The Act required new chemicals to meet the safety standard prior to being marketed and required the US EPA to conduct a review of existing chemicals.

In establishing these standards, the Lautenberg Act also preempted state chemical management laws. State laws that impose restrictions that are stricter than a federal requirement or that conflict in other ways with federal requirements, are preempted. States can still act on a chemical to address a different health or environmental concern than the US EPA considers under the Lautenberg Act (eg, VOC restrictions to address ozone formation). The Lautenberg Act also included important exceptions to its preemption of state laws: Any state action taken on a chemical before April 22, 2016, or taken under a law in effect on August 31, 2003, remains in place regardless of US EPA action. In addition, California's Proposition 65 and Massachusetts' Toxics Use Reduction Act are excluded from the scope of preemption.

| Table 66-3. Frank R. Lautenberg Chemical Safety for the 21st Century Act of 2016 | |
|---|---|
| **STATUTE (JUNE 22, 2016)** | **PUBLIC LAW No: 114-182** |
| **Existing Chemicals** | Provisions |
| Chemical Assessments | Prioritization<br>US EPA to establish a risk-based process to prioritize chemicals for assessment<br>○ High priority–the chemical *may* present an unreasonable risk of injury to health or the environment due to potential hazard and route of exposure, including to susceptible subpopulations<br>○ Low priority–the chemical use *does not* meet the standard for high priority |
| | Risk Evaluations<br>High-priority designation triggers a requirement and deadline for US EPA to complete a risk evaluation on that chemical to determine its safety<br>Low-priority designation does not require further action, although the chemical can move to high priority based on new information<br>Assessment pipeline<br>○ First 180 days–US EPA must have 10 ongoing risk evaluations<br>○ Within 3.5 years–US EPA must have 20 ongoing risk evaluations |
| | New Risk-based Safety Standard<br>Chemicals are evaluated against a new risk-based safety standard to determine whether a chemical use poses an "unreasonable risk"<br>Risk evaluation excludes consideration of costs or non-risk factors<br>Must consider risks to populations with elevated chemical exposures or heightened susceptibility; such populations may include (but are not limited to) infants, children, pregnant women, workers, the elderly |

*(continued)*

## Table 66-3. Frank R. Lautenberg Chemical Safety for the 21st Century Act of 2016 (*continued*)

| STATUTE (JUNE 22, 2016) | PUBLIC LAW No: 114-182 |
|---|---|
| | Action to Address Unreasonable Risks<br>When unreasonable risks are identified, the US EPA must take final risk management action within 2 years, or 4 years if extension needed<br>Restrictions imposed must be sufficient to ensure protection of susceptible and highly exposed populations<br>Costs and availability of alternatives considered when determining appropriate action to address risks but the US EPA is no longer required to select the "least burdensome" option<br>Action, including bans and phase-outs, must begin as quickly as possible but no later than 5 years after the final regulation |
| | Manufacturer-requested Assessments<br>Manufacturers can request that the US EPA evaluate specific chemicals, and pay the associated costs as follows:<br>○ If on the TSCA Workplan, manufacturers pay 50% of costs<br>○ If not on the TSCA Workplan, manufacturers pay 100% of costs<br>These assessments must account for between 25% to 50% of the number of ongoing risk evaluations for high-priority chemicals, but do not count toward the minimum 20 ongoing risk evaluation requirements |
| Chemical Testing Authority | Expands authority to obtain testing information for prioritizing or conducting risk evaluations on a chemical and expedites the process with new order and consent agreement authorities<br>Promotes the use of non-animal alternative testing methodologies |
| Persistent, Bioaccumulative, and Toxic (PBT) Chemicals | New fast-track process to address certain PBT chemicals on the TSCA Workplan<br>Risk evaluation not needed, only use and exposure to chemical needed<br>Action to reduce exposure to extent practicable must be proposed no later than 3 years after the new law and finalized 18 months later |

## Table 66-3. Frank R. Lautenberg Chemical Safety for the 21st Century Act of 2016 (*continued*)

| STATUTE (JUNE 22, 2016) | PUBLIC LAW No: 114-182 |
|---|---|
| **NEW CHEMICALS** | |
| Premarket Review of New Chemicals | New requirement that the US EPA must make an affirmative finding on the safety of a new chemical or significant new use of an existing chemical before it is allowed into the marketplace<br>The US EPA can still take a range of actions to address potential concerns including ban, limitations, and additional testing on the chemical |
| Confidential Business Information | Establishes new substantiation requirements for certain types of confidentiality claims from companies<br>Requires that the US EPA review and make determinations on all new confidentiality claims for the identity of chemicals and a subset of other types of confidentiality claims<br>The US EPA must review past confidentiality claims for chemical identity to determine if still warranted |
| Source of Sustained Funding | Allows the US EPA to collect up to $25 million annually in user fees from chemical manufacturers and processors when they<br>○ Submit test data for US EPA review<br>○ Submit a premanufacture notice for a new chemical or a notice of new use<br>○ Manufacture or process a chemical substance that is the subject of a risk evaluation; or<br>○ Request that the US EPA conduct a chemical risk evaluation<br>New fees will defray costs for new chemical reviews and a range of TSCA implementation activities for existing chemicals |
| **FEDERAL-STATE PARTNERSHIP** | |
| Preservation of State Laws | States can continue to act on any chemical, or particular uses or risks from a chemical, that the US EPA has not yet addressed<br>Existing state requirements (prior to April 22, 2016) are grandfathered in<br>Existing and new state requirements under state laws in effect on August 31, 2003, are preserved<br>Preserves states' environmental authorities related to air, water, waste disposal, and treatment<br>States and federal government can co-enforce identical regulations |

(*continued*)

| Table 66-3. Frank R. Lautenberg Chemical Safety for the 21st Century Act of 2016 (*continued*) | |
| --- | --- |
| STATUTE (JUNE 22, 2016) | PUBLIC LAW No. 114-182 |
| Preemption of State Laws | State action on a chemical is preempted when<br>○ US EPA finds (through a risk evaluation) that the chemical is safe, or<br>○ US EPA takes final action to address the chemical's risks<br>State action on a chemical is temporarily "paused" when the US EPA's risk evaluation on the chemical is underway, but lifted when the US EPA<br>○ completes the risk evaluation, or<br>○ misses the deadline to complete the risk evaluation |
| Exemptions | States can apply for waivers from both general and "pause" preemption<br>If certain conditions are met, the US EPA *may* grant an exemption from general preemption, and *must* grant an exemption from pause preemption |
| **Mercury Export and Disposal** | Amends requirements of the Mercury Export Ban Act (MEBA) and addresses the Department of Energy's (DOE) responsibility to designate a long-term storage facility<br>If the facility is not operational by 1/1/2020, the DOE must accept title to and pay for permitting and storage costs for mercury accumulated in accordance with MEBA prior to that date<br>Requires that the US EPA create an inventory of supply, use, and trade of mercury and mercury compounds; and prohibits export of certain mercury compounds |

Abbreviations: TSCA, Toxic Substances Control Act; US EPA, US Environmental Protection Agency.

The Lautenberg Act does not include postmarketing surveillance of the effects of a chemical, and the US EPA was not given the authority and means to remove a chemical if postmarketing surveillance indicates that it no longer meets the standard for being released to the market. Fidelity in implementation and enforcement of the Lautenberg Act by the US EPA remains the critical challenge. The scientific and public health community has raised concerns that the US EPA regulations implementing the Act ignore significant health risks posed by TSCA-covered chemicals, especially those affecting pregnant women, infants, and children.[26] In April 2018, the AAP joined an amicus brief challenging US EPA implementation of 2 Lautenberg Act rules.

## Frequently Asked Questions

Q   *What are some ways to prevent children from being exposed to chemicals?*

A   Prevent unintentional ingestions of toxic materials. When it is necessary to use such products, store them out of the reach of young children. Products that are not sold in child-resistant containers are likely to be particularly hazardous. Do not store them in alternative containers, make sure the containers are completely capped during storage, and keep them out of reach. If an unintentional ingestion of a hazardous chemical is suspected, call 9-1-1 and/or immediately take your child to the nearest emergency department for evaluation and possible treatment. For other known or possible ingestions, you may also call the poison control center or (if present) the number on the container to receive any instructions on first aid and whether the child needs to be seen at the emergency department for further evaluation and treatment. The poison control center can be reached at 800-222-1222.

Whenever possible, avoid products that are more toxic. Household tasks that involve chemicals, including refinishing, paint stripping, painting, automotive work, home hobby work involving lead or solvents, and other tasks that use products that may contain chemicals, should be done when young children are not in the house, using adequate ventilation before children return to the home (or garage). The California Proposition 65 warning label (https://oehha.ca.gov/proposition-65) is a valid indicator of products that should be kept out of the reach of young children and which, for the sake of caution, should not be used around them.[27]

Children need safe places to play. Do not allow children to play in industrial sites, either occupied or abandoned. Some of these have been identified as Superfund sites, but even sites not identified as such may have contaminated soil and air.

Be mindful that chemicals in occupational environments may be brought home on clothing and skin by parents, thus creating the potential for hazards to children. When possible, workers in such occupations should shower and change before coming home. When these actions are not possible, avoid contact before showering and changing clothes and shoes at home, and do not launder work clothes with children's clothing, bedding, and other items.

Q   *How can I avoid chemicals when I clean my home?*

A   There are numerous sources of information about household chemicals. The US EPA produced an excellent, user-friendly guide for parents and families that facilitates a room-by-room assessment and provides common sense advice for safer alternatives: https://www.epa.gov/sites/production/files/2014-06/documents/lesson2_handout.pdf.[28] In addition, the National Library of Medicine has a Household Products Database that is useful: https://householdproducts.nlm.nih.gov.[29]

## Resources

### Children's Environmental Health Network
Developed a series of "Eco-Healthy Child Care Fact Sheets" that are available for a number of chemicals and products (eg, art supplies, furniture and carpets, plastics and plastic toys) that are often found in both childcare and household environments.
Web site: http://cehn.org/our-work/eco-healthy-child-care/ehcc-factsheets[30]

### Consumer Products Safety Commission
Developed a guide to the identification of safe arts and crafts products.
Web site: https://www.cpsc.gov/PageFiles/112284/5015.pdf[31]

### Environmental Working Group
Produced consumer guides to sunscreens, insect repellents, and cosmetics, including in each of these a number of products specifically marketed for children.
Web sites: https://www.ewg.org/sunscreen/#.WoCGISOZMWo[32] https://www.ewg.org/research/ewgs-guide-bug-repellents#.WoCGeiOZMWo[33] https://www.ewg.org/skindeep#.WoCGlCOZMWo[34]

### Moms Clean Air Force
Provides a number of resources on toxic chemicals including "School Air Facts," a guide to clean air in schools, a "Healthier Classroom Checklist" for teachers, and a user-friendly guide to the "Toxics Under Review" by the US EPA.
Web sites: www.momscleanairforce.org/school-air-facts[35] https://cdn.momscleanairforce.org/wp-content/uploads/classroom_checklist-2-1.pdf[36] www.momscleanairforce.org/toxics-under-review[37]

### National Library of Medicine
A useful Environmental and Toxicology site that provides useful peer reviewed information about chemicals.
Web site: http://sis.nlm.nih.gov/enviro.html[38]
Web site: https://toxnet.nlm.nih.gov/newtoxnet/lactmed.htm[39]

**Pediatric Environmental Health Specialty Unit network**

Published a number of fact sheets on prevention of chemical exposures, specifically, on lead, trichloroethylene, phthalates and Bisphenol A, formaldehyde, and arsenic.

Web site: https://www.pehsu.net/public_facts.html[40]

## References

1. Consumer Product Safety Act, 86 15 U.S.C., §2051 et seq. (1972). https://www.cpsc.gov/PageFiles/105435/cpsa.pdf. Accessed September 3, 2018

2. Consumer Product Safety Commission. Consumer Product Safety Act Summary. 2018. https://www.cpsc.gov/Regulations-Laws--Standards/Statutes. Accessed July 13, 2018

3. Clean Air Act Amendments of 1990, USC, §7401 et seq. (1990)

4. US Environmental Protection Agency. Summary of the Clean Air Act. 2018. https://www.epa.gov/laws-regulations/summary-clean-air-act. Accessed June 20, 2018

5. Clean Water Act of 1972 (1972)

6. US Environmental Protection Agency. Summary of the Clean Water Act. 2018. https://www.epa.gov/laws-regulations/summary-clean-water-act. Accessed June 20, 2018

7. Food Quality Protection Act of 1996, USC (1996)

8. US Environmental Protection Agency. Summary of the Food Quality Protection Act. 2018. https://www.epa.gov/laws-regulations/summary-food-quality-protection-act. Accessed June 20, 2018

9. Resource Conservation and Recovery Act of 1976, (1976)

10. US Environmental Protection Agency. Summary of the Resource Conservaton and Recovery Act. 2018. https://www.epa.gov/laws-regulations/summary-resource-conservation-and-recovery-act. Accessed June 20, 2018

11. Safe Drinking Water Act, USC, §103 (1996)

12. US Environmental Protection Agency. Summary of the Safe Drinking Water Act. 2018. https://www.epa.gov/laws-regulations/summary-safe-drinking-water-act. Accessed June 20, 2018

13. Federal Food Drug and Cosmetics Act Subtitle 4: Cosmetics, (1938)

14. Federal Food Drug and Cosmetics Act Chapter IV: Food, (1958)

15. Food and Drug Administration. Federal Food, Drug, and Cosmetic Act (FD&C Act). 2018. https://www.fda.gov/RegulatoryInformation/LawsEnforcedbyFDA/FederalFoodDrugandCosmeticActFDCAct/default.htm. Accessed June 20, 2018

16. Occupational Safety and Health Act of 1970, (1970)

17. Occupational Safety and Health Administration. OSH Act of 1970. 2018. https://www.osha.gov/pls/oshaweb/owadisp.show_document?p_table=oshact&p_id=2743. Accessed June 20, 2018

18. Federal Insecticide, Fungicide, and Rodenticide Act, (1996)

19. Toxic Substances Control Act, USC, §2601 et seq. (1976). https://www.epa.gov/laws-regulations/summary-toxic-substances-control-act. Accessed September 3, 2018

20. Emergency Planning & Community Right-To-Know Act (EPCRA), 42 (1986). https://www.epa.gov/epcra. Accessed September 3, 2018

21. Pollution Prevention Act (PPA), U.S.C. (1990). https://www.epa.gov/laws-regulations/summary-pollution-prevention-act. Accessed September 3, 2018

22. US Environmental Protection Agency. EPA's Voluntary Chemical Evaluation Program Did Not Achieve Children's Health Protection Goals. https://www.epa.gov/sites/production/files/2015-09/documents/20110721-11-p-0379.pdf. Accessed June 20, 2018

23. Federal Food Drug and Cosmetics Act Chapter V: Drugs and Devices, (2017)

24. American Academy of Pediatrics Council on Environmental Health. Chemical-management policy: prioritizing children's health. *Pediatrics*. 2011;127(5):983–990

25. US Environmental Protection Agency. Lautenberg Chemical Safety for the 21st Century Act. 2018. https://www.epa.gov/assessing-and-managing-chemicals-under-tsca/frank-r-lautenberg-chemical-safety-21st-century-act+&cd=1&hl=en&ct=clnk&gl=us. Accessed September 3, 2018

26. Case No.17-72260. Safer Chemicals, Healthy Families et al., Petitioners, vs. U.S. Environmental Protections Agency, Respondents, Brief of Amici The American Academy of Pediatrics, the American College of Obstetricians and Gynecologists, and the American Public Health Association in support of Petitioners. https://www.apha.org/-/media/files/pdf/advocacy/testimonyandcomments/180423_schf_v_epa_tsca_health_amicus.ashx?la=en&hash=677D59D2CAFCE43447C0CB21386530D3558B01EC. Accessed September 3, 2018

27. State of California. Office of Environmental Health Hazard Assessment. Proposition 65. 2018. https://oehha.ca.gov/proposition-65. Accessed June 20, 2018

28. US Environmental Protection Agency. Household Hazards Hunt. 2014. https://www.epa.gov/sites/production/files/2014-06/documents/lesson2_handout.pdf. Accessed June 20, 2018

29. National Library of Medicine. National Institutes of Health. Household Products Database: Health & Safety Information on Household Products. 2017. https://householdproducts.nlm.nih.gov. Accessed June 20, 2018

30. Children's Environmental Health Network. Eco-Healthy Child Care Fact Sheets. 2018. http://cehn.org/our-work/eco-healthy-child-care/ehcc-factsheets/. Accessed June 20, 2018

31. Consumer Product Safety Commission. Art and Craft Safety Guide. Vol Pub. No. 5015. Bethesda, MD: CPSC; 2005

32. Environmental Working Group. EWG's Guide to Sunscreens. 2018. https://www.ewg.org/sunscreen/#.WoCGISOZMWo. Accessed June 20, 2018

33. Environmental Working Group. EWG's Guide to Bug Repellants in the Age of Zika. 2016. https://www.ewg.org/research/ewgs-guide-bug-repellents#.WrGsgmaZMWp. Accessed June 20, 2018

34. Environmental Working Group. EWG's Skin Deep Cosmetics Database. 2018. https://www.ewg.org/skindeep/#.WrGs-GaZMWp. Accessed June 20, 2018

35. Moms Clean Air Force. School Air Quality: Why We Need Healthy Schools. 2018. http://www.momscleanairforce.org/school-air-facts/. Accessed June 20, 2018

36. Moms Clean Air Force. The Healthier Classroom Checklist: Environmental Health Guidance for Teachers. 2018. https://cdn.momscleanairforce.org/wp-content/uploads/classroom_checklist-2-1.pdf. Accessed June 20, 2018

37. Moms Clean Air Force. Toxics Under Review. 2018. http://www.momscleanairforce.org/toxics-under-review/. Accessed June 20, 2018

38. National Library of Medicine. National Institutes of Health. Environmental Health & Toxicology. 2010. https://sis.nlm.nih.gov/enviro.html. Accessed June 20, 2018

39. National Library of Medicine. National Institutes of Health. Lactmed: A Toxnet Database. 2018. https://toxnet.nlm.nih.gov/newtoxnet/lactmed.htm. Accessed June 20, 2018

40. Pediatric Environmental Health Specialty Units. PEHSU National Resources for Families and Communities. 2018. https://www.pehsu.net/public_facts.html. Accessed June 20, 2018

Appendix A

# Pediatric Environmental Health Specialty Units (PEHSUs)

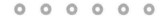

United States Pediatric Environmental Health Specialty Units (PEHSUs) are regional, academic center-based, and publicly supported resources that fulfill several well-defined needs:

- to provide educational resources to pediatric and reproductive health care and public health professionals,
- to train health care students, residents, and providers in the principles of pediatric and reproductive environmental health,
- to provide high quality consultative and referral medical services for children, their families, health professionals, public health officials, and communities.

## HISTORY

In the 1990s, it was recognized that a new level of expertise was needed to address and prevent environmentally related chronic childhood diseases. Pediatricians and other child health clinicians were increasingly called on to provide guidance to families about the environmental risks that their children face daily in their homes, child care settings, schools, and other sites in their communities. Yet the training of health care professionals often did not include many environmental topics, and most health care providers had a limited understanding of the environmental origins and/or exacerbations of disease and how these might pose preventable hazards for families. A 1995 Institute of Medicine report pointed out a crucial need to improve the education of students, trainees, and clinicians regarding environmental health issues affecting their patients and families.[1]

In April 1997, Executive Order 13045, the "Protection of Children from Environmental Health Risks and Safety Risks," was signed by President William Clinton.[2] It charged federal agencies, including the US Environmental Protection Agency (EPA), to consider and address special environmental risks to children. The order led to the creation of the Office of Children's Health Protection (OCHP) within the US EPA. At the same time, leaders in the OCHP and the Agency for Toxic Substances & Disease Registry (ATSDR) fostered the concept that health professionals, trained in the principles of pediatric environmental health and readily available through a network of easily accessible units, could serve as vital resources for public health officials and policymakers, pediatric health care providers, and the general public. As a result, the Pediatric Environmental Health Specialty Units (PEHSUs) were established by the ATSDR in 1999, in conjunction with the US EPA's Superfund Office. The first 3 PEHSUs were founded in Boston, Seattle, and New York City; another 8 PEHSUs were added over the following 3 to 4 years. Funding for PEHSUs continues to be provided principally by the US EPA Office of Children's Health Protection and the ATSDR, with some additional funding from state and local sources, as well as grants from nonprofit organizations.

From the outset, PEHSUs had a vision of a healthier world for children through the provision of expanded educational outreach, consultative, and referral clinical services, using their expertise in pediatric environmental health to benefit the public, public health personnel, and primary care providers. Most recently, PEHSUs have added reproductive environmental risks for women of reproductive age and pregnant and lactating women as additional topics to be addressed through the provision of expertise and education.

PEHSUs have achieved remarkable success during their first 15 years of operation. Between 2001 and 2014, PEHSU personnel provided information and consultative services to 300,000 health professionals, 62,000 trainees, 324,000 members of the public, and 18,000 public health personnel at the federal, state, and/or local levels: a total of over 700,000 outreach contacts.[3] During this period, the top 5 reasons for contacting a PEHSU included: childhood lead poisoning, exposure to fungi and molds, environmental contamination with phthalates and bisphenol A, incidental exposures to pesticides, and environmental contamination with forms of mercury.[3]

## MISSION

The original PEHSU mission was: (1) to provide pediatric and environmental health education to health care providers, health profession students, and others; (2) to offer consultation to health care professionals, parents, and others regarding environmental health exposures and medical interventions that might be needed for pediatric age groups; and (3) to provide referrals to specialized medical resources when necessary. Over the ensuing years, the PEHSU Network has adapted to other newly defined environmental concerns, such as the need for a higher level of pediatrician involvement and to include a greater focus on reproductive and pre-pregnancy concerns, working collaboratively with specialists in obstetrics, gynecology, and maternal-fetal medicine. PEHSUs have adapted to meet newly defined issues and educational needs in pediatric environmental health, including goals within 6 themes: outdoor air quality, surface and ground water quality, toxic substances and hazardous wastes, homes and communities, infrastructure and surveillance, and global environmental health, as discussed in *Healthy People 2020 Objectives for Healthy Homes and Healthy Communities.*[4]

## PEHSU OPERATIONS AND PRODUCTIVITY

### Clinical Consultation

PEHSUs are staffed by pediatric environmental health experts with previous training in pediatric or reproductive medicine and environmental and clinical toxicology, who provide access to clinical consultation services. To reduce barriers, PEHSUs offer toll-free telephone access and have Internet-based Web sites with a central site at www.pehsu.net.[5] PEHSUs enjoy close partnerships with federal agencies, tribal leaders, state and local health departments, nonprofit organizations (such as the American Academy of Pediatrics and the American College of Medical Toxicology), and regional collaborations with Poison Control Centers throughout the country.

### Community Outreach

PEHSU staff attend health fairs, hold public forums, and participate in community meetings. PEHSUs engage in a variety of community-based activities that serve the needs of both health professionals and the general public. They can respond to inquiries with clinical information regarding health impacts of specific environmental toxicants and can collaborate with other agencies and community leaders to facilitate an early response to public health issues.

### Training of Health Professionals

PEHSUs provide physician and nursing education and training opportunities and seek to build manpower capacity with expertise in reproductive and pediatric environmental health. PEHSU faculty teach students, residents, fellows, and pediatric health care providers in practice. PEHSUs have made progress in addressing the lack of medical expertise in environmental health by developing a new specialty within pediatric medicine. New competencies have been adopted in the fellowship training of physicians who learn the complexities of environmental health and can offer technical assistance to community practitioners.[6] Graduates of these fellowships have gone on to productive careers and have been instrumental in staffing some of the PEHSUs, as noted in a 5-year follow-up report of fellowship alumni.[7]

## Health Professional Continuing Education

In addition, the PEHSUs work to educate local clinicians on pediatric environmental health topics. PEHSUs offer a variety of venues for engaging in health professional educational outreach activities, including grand rounds, seminars, workshops, webinars, widely distributed fact sheets on specific environmental topics, eLearning modules, and a robust Web page.

## Locations

*[NOTE: Information in this section was abstracted from the Web site: www. pehsu.net (reference 4) accessed on February 27, 2018.]*

There are 10 PEHSUs and 1 satellite PEHSU in the United States, covering the entire population, including services to citizens in Puerto Rico and the US Virgin Islands. Two others, in Canada and Mexico, are not funded by the US EPA or ATSDR.

**REGION 1**

**Service area: Connecticut, Maine, Massachusetts, New Hampshire, Rhode Island, and Vermont**

New England Pediatric Environmental Health Specialty Unit: Boston, MA

*Academic Affiliation:* Harvard Medical School and Harvard T.H. Chan School of Public Health

*Hospital Affiliation:* Boston Children's Hospital and Cambridge Hospital

Contact Information

Phone: (617) 355-8177

Toll Free: (888) CHILD14 or (888) 244-5314

Web site: www.childrenshospital.org/pehc

**REGION 2**

**Service area: New Jersey, New York, Puerto Rico, and US Virgin Islands**

Region 2 PEHSU: New York, NY

*Academic Affiliation:* Mount Sinai School of Medicine: Department of Pediatrics. Department of Community and Preventive Medicine

*Hospital Affiliation:* Mount Sinai Medical Center
Contact Information
Toll Free: (866) 265-6201
E-mail: pehsu@mountsinai.org
Web site: http://icahn.mssm.edu/research/programs/
    pediatric-environmental-health-specialty-unit

**REGION 3**
**Service area: Delaware, Maryland, Pennsylvania, Virginia, Washington DC, West Virginia**
Mid-Atlantic Center for Children's Health & the Environment Pediatric
    Environmental Health Specialty Unit: Washington, DC
*Academic Affiliation:* Georgetown University
*Hospital Affiliation:* Georgetown University Medical Center
Contact Information
Phone: (202) 687-2330
Toll Free: (866) 622-2431
Web site: http://kidsandenvironment.georgetown.edu

**REGION 4**
**Service area: Alabama, Florida, Georgia, Kentucky, Mississippi, North Carolina, South Carolina, Tennessee**
Southeast Pediatric Environmental Health Specialty Unit: Atlanta, GA
*Academic Affiliation:* Emory University Department of Pediatrics
*Hospital Affiliation:* Children's Healthcare of Atlanta – Egleston Children's
    Hospital and Hughes Spalding Children's Hospital
Contact Information
Phone: (404) 727-9428
Toll Free: (877) 33PEHSU or (877) 337-3478
E-mail: sepehsu@emory.edu
Web site: www.pediatrics.emory.edu/centers/pehsu/index.html

**REGION 5**
**Service area: Illinois, Indiana, Michigan, Minnesota, Ohio, Wisconsin**
Great Lakes Centers' Pediatric Environmental Health Specialty Unit:
    Chicago, IL
*Academic Affiliation:* University of Illinois at Chicago, School of Public Health
*Hospital Affiliation:* Stroger Hospital of Cook County
Contact Information
Phone: (312) 864-5526
Toll Free: (866) 967-7337
E-mail: ChildrensEnviro@uic.edu
Web site: www.uic.edu/sph/glakes/childrenshealth/index.htm

**Satellite location: Cincinnati, OH**
*Academic Affiliation:* University of Cincinnati
*Hospital Affiliation:* Cincinnati Children's Hospital & Medical Center
Contact Information
Phone: (513) 803-3688
Toll Free: (866) 967-7337
Web site: www.cincinnatichildrens.org/service/e/environmental-health/
  default/

## REGION 6

**Service area: Arkansas, Louisiana, New Mexico, Oklahoma, Texas**
Southwest Center for Pediatric Environmental Health: El Paso, TX
*Academic Affiliation:* Texas Tech University Health Sciences Center - Paul L.
  Foster School of Medicine
*Hospital Affiliation:* University Medical Center of El Paso & El Paso Children's
  Hospital
Contact Information
Phone: (915) 534-3807
Toll Free: (888) 901-5665
E-mail: swcpeh@ttuhsc.edu
Web site: http://swcpeh.org

## REGION 7

**Service area: Iowa, Kansas, Missouri, Nebraska**
Mid-America Pediatric Environmental Health Specialty Unit: Kansas City, MO
*Academic Affiliation:* University of Missouri-Kansas City School of Medicine
*Hospital Affiliation:* Children's Mercy Hospitals and Clinics
Contact Information
Phone: (913) 588-6638
Toll Free: (800) 421-9916
E-mail: mapehsu@cmh.edu
Web site: www.childrensmercy.org/mapehsu

## REGION 8

**Service area: Colorado, Montana, North Dakota, South Dakota, Utah,
Wyoming**
Rocky Mountain Pediatric Environmental Health Specialty Unit: Denver, CO
*Academic Affiliation:* University of Colorado Health Sciences Center
*Hospital Affiliation:* Denver Health and Hospitals Authority and the Rocky
  Mountain Poison and Drug Center
Contact Information
Toll Free: (877) 800-5554
Web site: www.rmrpehsu.org

**REGION 9**

**Service area: Arizona, California, Hawaii, Nevada**

Western States PEHSU: San Francisco, CA

*Academic Affiliation*: University of California at San Francisco

*Hospital Affiliation:* University of California San Francisco Medical Center

Contact Information

Phone: (415) 206-4083

Toll Free: 866-UC-PEHSU or (866) 827-3478

E-mail: pehsu@ucsf.edu

Web site: http://coeh.berkeley.edu/ucpehsu/

**REGION 10**

**Service area: Alaska, Idaho, Oregon, Washington**

Northwest Pediatric Environmental Health Specialty Unit: Seattle, WA

*Academic Affiliation:* University of Washington: Department of Occupational
and Environmental Health Sciences, Occupational and Environmental
Medicine Program, Department of Pediatrics

*Hospital Affiliation:* University of Washington Medical Center; Harborview
Medical Center; Children's Hospital and Regional Medical Center

Contact Information

Toll Free: 1-877-KID-CHEM or (877) 543-2436

E-mail: pehsu@u.washington.edu

Web site: http://depts.washington.edu/pehsu

## Global

The PEHSU model developed in the United States has been studied by many
countries throughout the world. Health officials in Canada and Mexico have
established PEHSUs. In Canada, the PEHSU is in the Child Health Clinic at
Misericordia Community Hospital in Edmonton, Alberta. In Mexico the PEHSU
is part of the Unidad Pediatrica Ambiental at the National Institute for Public
Health and the Morelos Children's Hospital in Cuenevaca. The World Health
Organization (WHO) has previously affirmed its position of advocacy for the
protection of children from environmental threats to their health.[8] The WHO
has described the creation of children's environmental health units. Health
officials in Argentina, the Republic of Korea, Uruguay, Spain, and Chile have
developed children's environmental health units.[9–11]

## References

1. Executive Order 13045. The Protection of Children from Environmental Health Risks and
   Safety Risks. Federal Register (19885), Vol 62, No. 78, April 23, 1997
2. Pope AM, Rall DP, eds. Committee on Curriculum Development, Institute of Medicine (IOM):
   *Environmental Medicine: Integrating a Missing Element into Medical Education.* Washington,
   DC: National Academy Press; 1995

3. Woolf AD, Sibrizzi C, Kirkland K. Pediatric environmental health specialty units: an analysis of operations. *Acad Pediatr.* 2016;16(1):25–33

4. National PEHSU Network. www.pehsu.net. Accessed February 27, 2018

5. U.S. Department of Health & Human Services (2013). Healthy People 2020 Topics and Objectives. http://www.healthypeople.gov/2020/TopicsObjectives2020/. Accessed February 27, 2018

6. Etzel RA, Crain EF, Gitterman BA, Oberg C, Scheidt P, Landrigan PJ. Pediatric environmental health competencies for specialists. *Amb Pediatr.* 2003;3:60–63

7. Landrigan PJ, Woolf AD, Gitterman B, et al. The ambulatory pediatric association fellowship in pediatric environmental health: a 5-year assessment. *Environ Health Persp.* 2007;115(10):1383–1387

8. World Health Organization. *Children in the New Millenium: Environmental Impact on Health.* Geneva, Switzerland: WHO; 2003

9. Ortega Garcia JA, Ferris i Tortajada J, Claudio Morales L, Berbel Rornero O. Pediatric environmental health specialty units in Europe: from theory to practice. *An Pediatr (Barc).* 2005;63(2):143–151

10. Paris E, Bettini M, Molina H, Mieres JJ, Bravo V, Rios JC. The relevance of environmental health and the scope of pediatric environmental health specialty units. *Rev Med Chil.* 2009;137(1):101–105

11. Oh JK, Lee SI. The Environmental Health Centre. 2009. Third WHO International Conference on Children's Health and the Environment, Busan, Korea www.ceh2009.org/ accessed 1 July 2018.

12. World Health Organization. Children's Environmental Health Units. Geneva, Switzerland: WHO; 2010. http://www.who.int/ceh/publications/units/en/. Accessed February 27, 2018

# Resources for Pediatric Environmental Health

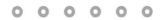

The American Academy of Pediatrics has not reviewed the material on these Web sites. Inclusion in this list does not imply endorsement.

The material in this Appendix is organized as follows:

- US Federal & State Governments
- Non-US Government (including World Health Organization)
- Non-Governmental Organizations
- Pediatric Environmental Health Specialty Units

| ORGANIZATION | CONTACT INFORMATION |
|---|---|
| **US FEDERAL & STATE GOVERNMENTS** | |
| **US FEDERAL GOVERNMENT** | |
| **Agency for Toxic Substances and Disease Registry (ATSDR)**<br>US Department of Health and Human Services (DHHS)<br>1600 Clifton Rd NE; Mail Stop E-28<br>Atlanta, GA 30333 | Web site: www.atsdr.cdc.gov<br>Information Center Clearinghouse:<br>Phone: 404-639-6360<br>Emergency Response Branch Phone:<br>  404-639-0615 |
| ■ ATSDR GATHER (Geographic Analysis Tool for Health and Environmental Research) | Web site: http://gis.cdc.gov |

*(continued)*

| ORGANIZATION | CONTACT INFORMATION |
|---|---|
| **US FEDERAL & STATE GOVERNMENTS** | |
| ■ ATSDR Toxicological Profiles | Web site: www.atsdr.cdc.gov/toxprofiles/index.asp |
| ■ ATSDR Regional Offices | Web site: www.atsdr.cdc.gov/dro |
| ■ ATSDR Pediatric Environmental Health Toolkit Training Module | Web site: https://www.atsdr.cdc.gov/emes/health_professionals/pediatrics.html |
| **National Center for Environmental Health (NCEH)**<br>Centers for Disease Control & Prevention<br>4770 Buford Hwy, NE<br>Mail Stop F-28<br>Atlanta, GA 30341-3724 | Web site: www.cdc.gov/nceh<br>E-mail: ncehinfo@cdc.gov<br>NCEH Health Line: 888-232-6789 |
| ■ NCEH Asthma Program | Web site: https://www.cdc.gov/nceh/information/asthma.htm |
| ■ NCEH Lead Poisoning Prevention Program | Web site: www.cdc.gov/nceh/lead |
| ■ National Report on Human Exposure to Environmental Chemicals | Web site: www.cdc.gov/exposurereport |
| **National Institute for Occupational Safety and Health (NIOSH)** | Web site: www.cdc.gov/niosh/homepage.html<br>E-mail: cdcinfo@cdc.gov<br>Phone: 800-35-NIOSH<br>800-356-4674 |
| ■ NIOSH Young Worker Safety and Health | Web site: www.cdc.gov/niosh/topics/youth |
| **Consumer Product Safety Commission**<br>4340 East West Hwy<br>Bethesda, MD 20814 | Web site: www.cpsc.gov<br>Phone: 800-638-2772<br>Fax: 301-504-0124 |
| **US Environmental Protection Agency (EPA)**<br>1200 Pennsylvania Ave NW<br>Washington, DC 20460 | Web site: www.epa.gov<br>Administrative Phone: 202-272-0167 |
| ■ EPA Office of Children's Health Protection | Web site: http://yosemite.epa.gov/ochp/ochpweb.nsf/content/homepage.htm<br>Office of Child Health Protection Phone: 202-564-2188 |

| ORGANIZATION | CONTACT INFORMATION |
|---|---|
| **US FEDERAL & STATE GOVERNMENTS** | |
| ▪ EPA Office of Pesticide Programs | Web site: www.epa.gov/pesticides<br>Office of Pesticide Programs Phone:<br>703-305-5017<br>National Pesticides Hotline: 800-222-1222 |
| ▪ EPA Office of Air and Radiation | Office main Web site: www.epa.gov/oar<br>Indoor Air Web site: www.epa.gov/iaq<br>Indoor Air Quality Information<br>Clearinghouse Phone: 800-438-4318<br>Tools for Schools Program Web site: www.<br>epa.gov/iaq/schools/index.html<br>Air Now–ground-level ozone Web site:<br>www.epa.gov/airnow<br>The Healthy School Environments<br>Assessment Tool (HealthySEATv2)<br>Web site: www.epa.gov/schools/<br>healthyseat/index.html |
| ▪ EPA Endocrine Disruptor Screening Program | Web site: www.epa.gov/scipoly/oscpendo |
| ▪ EPA Children's Environmental Health Research Centers | Web site: www.epa.gov/ncer/<br>childrenscenters/newsroom/archive.<br>html<br>Health Research Initiative |
| ▪ EPA Chemical Emergency Preparedness and Prevention | Web site: www.epa.gov/<br>region5superfund/cepps<br>Chemical Spills Emergency Hotline:<br>800-424-8802<br>Hazardous Waste/Community Right to<br>Know Hotline: 800-424-9346 |
| ▪ EPA Office of Water | Web site: www.epa.gov/water/index.html<br>Safe Drinking Water Hotline:<br>800-426-4791<br>Drinking Water Advisories Web site: www.<br>epa.gov/waterscience/drinking<br>Fish Consumption Advisories Web site:<br>www.epa.gov/ost/fish |
| ▪ EPA Office of Pollution Prevention & Toxics | Web site: www.epa.gov/opptintr/index.<br>html<br>Toxic Substances Control Act (TSCA)<br>Information Line: 202-554-1404 |
| ▪ EPA Toxics Release Inventory Program | Web site: www.epa.gov/tri |

*(continued)*

| ORGANIZATION | CONTACT INFORMATION |
|---|---|
| **US FEDERAL & STATE GOVERNMENTS** | |
| ▪ EPA Children's Environmental Health Resource, Toxicity and Exposure Assessment for Children's Health (TEACH) | Web site: https://archive.epa.gov/ region5/teach/web/html/index.html |
| ▪ EPA–America's Children & the Environment | Web site: https://www.epa.gov/ace |
| ▪ EPA Sun Safety | Web site: https://www.epa.gov/sunsafety |
| ▪ EPA Healthy Schools, Healthy Kids | Web site: https://www.epa.gov/schools |
| ▪ EPA Health Research Grants | Web site: https://www.epa.gov/research-grants/health-research-grants |
| **Food & Drug Administration** 10903 New Hampshire Avenue Silver Spring, MD 20993 | Web site: www.fda.gov/ Phone: 1-888-INFO-FDA (1-888-463-6332) |
| ▪ Center for Food Safety and Applied Nutrition (CFSAN) Food and Drug Administration (FDA) 5100 Paint Branch Parkway College Park, MD 20740-3835 | Web site: www.cfsan.fda.gov Phone: 888-SAFEFOOD |
| ▪ Food Safety: Gateway to Government Food Safety Information | Web site: www.FoodSafety.gov |
| ▪ Center for Tobacco Products (CTP) | Web site: www.fda.gov/TobaccoProducts/ default.htm E-mail: AskCTP@fda.hhs.gov Phone: 1-877-287-1373 |
| **National Institute of Environmental Health Sciences (NIEHS)** US DHHS PO Box 12233 Research Triangle Park, NC 27709 | Web site: www.niehs.nih.gov Phone: 919-541-1919 |
| ▪ The Environmental Genome Project | Web site: www.niehs.nih.gov/research/ supported/programs/egp |
| ▪ NIEHS Children's Environmental Health Research Initiative | Web site: www.niehs.nih.gov/research/ supported/centers/prevention/index. cfm |
| ▪ National Toxicology Program | Web site: http://ntp-server.niehs.nih.gov |

| ORGANIZATION | CONTACT INFORMATION |
|---|---|
| **US FEDERAL & STATE GOVERNMENTS** | |
| ▪ Center for the Evaluation of Risks to Human Reproduction | Web site: http://cerhr.niehs.nih.gov |
| ▪ Environmental Health Perspectives — Children's Health Pages | Web site: http://ehp03.niehs.nih.gov/home.action<br>Web site: https://ehp.niehs.nih.gov/childrens-health/ |
| ▪ NIEHS Superfund Research Program | https://www.niehs.nih.gov/research/supported/centers/srp/index.cfm |
| **National Cancer Institute (NCI)**<br>US Department of Health and Human Services<br>National Institutes of Health (NIH)<br>9000 Rockville Pike<br>Bethesda, MD 20892 | Web site: www.nci.nih.gov<br>Surveillance, Epidemiology and End Results (SEER) Program Web site: http://seer.cancer.gov<br>Phone: 800-4-CANCER |
| **National Quit-smoking Hotline**<br>1-800-QUIT-NOW | Web site: http://1800quitnow.cancer.gov<br>Phone: 1-800-QUIT-NOW |
| **National Library of Medicine, Environmental Health & Toxicology** | Web site: http://sis.nlm.nih.gov/enviro.html |
| ▪ TOXNET | Web site: http://toxnet.nlm.nih.gov |
| ▪ Drugs and Lactation Database (LactMed) | Web site: http://toxnet.nlm.nih.gov/cgi-bin/sis/htmlgen?LACT |
| ▪ Tox Town | Web site: https://toxtown.nlm.nih.gov/ |
| **Office of Healthy Homes and Lead Hazard Control**<br>US Department of Housing & Urban Development<br>451 7th St SW<br>Washington, DC 20410 | Web site: www.hud.gov/offices/lead |
| **US Department of Agriculture**<br>Food Safety and Inspection Service<br>Food Safety Education Office<br>1400 Independence Ave, SW<br>Washington, DC 20250 | Web site: www.fsis.usda.gov<br>E-mail: fsis.webmaster@usda.gov<br>Phone: 301-504-9605 |
| **US Global Change Research Program**<br>Suite 250<br>1717 Pennsylvania Ave, NW<br>Washington, DC 20006 | Web site: www.climatescience.gov<br>Phone: 202-223-6262 |

*(continued)*

| ORGANIZATION | CONTACT INFORMATION |
|---|---|
| **US FEDERAL & STATE GOVERNMENTS** | |
| **STATE AGENCIES** | |
| List of state health and environmental agencies with links to Web sites | Web site: https://www.epa.gov/home/health-and-environmental-agencies-us-states-and-territories |
| **California Electric and Magnetic Fields (EMF) Program**<br>1515 Clay St, Suite 1700<br>Oakland, CA 94612 | Web site: www.dhs.ca.gov/ehib/emf |
| **California Environmental Protection Agency**<br>1001 I Street<br>P.O. Box 2815<br>Sacramento, CA 95812-2815 | Web site: www.calepa.ca.gov |
| **New York State Centers of Excellence in Children's Environmental Health** | Web site: www.nysceceh.org/ |
| **NON-US GOVERNMENT** | |
| **European Union information on Environmental Health** | Web site: http://europa.eu/pol/env/index_en.htm |
| **Registration, Evaluation, Authorisation and Restriction of Chemicals (REACH)** | Web site: http://ec.europa.eu/environment/chemicals/reach/reach_intro.htm |
| **Canadian Association of Physicians for the Environment**<br>208-145 Spruce St<br>Ottawa, ON K1R 6P1 Canada | Web site: www.cape.ca/children.html<br>E-mail: info@cape.ca<br>Phone: 613-235-2273 |
| **Canadian Institute of Child Health**<br>384 Bank St, Suite 300<br>Ottawa, ON K2P 1Y4 Canada | Web site: www.cich.ca<br>E-mail: cich@cich.ca<br>Phone: 613-230-8838 |
| **Canadian Partnership for Children's Health and Environment (CPCHE)**<br>215 Spadina Avenue, Suite 130<br>Toronto, Ontario, Canada<br>M5T 2C7 | Web site: www.healthyenvironmentforkids.ca/english<br>E-mail: info@healthyenvironmentforkids.ca<br>Phone: 819-458-3750 |
| **World Health Organization (WHO) Public Health, Environmental and Social Determinants of Health** | Web site: www.who.int/phe/en |

| ORGANIZATION | CONTACT INFORMATION |
|---|---|
| **NON-US GOVERNMENT** | |
| ■ WHO Environmental Health Information | Web site: www.who.int/topics/environmental_health/en |
| ■ Global Initiative on Children's Environmental Health Indicators | Web site: www.who.int/ceh/indicators/en |
| ■ Children's Environmental Health | Web site: www.who.int/ceh/en |
| ■ Training Package for Health Care Providers | Web site: www.who.int/ceh/capacity/trainpackage/en/ |
| ■ Children's Environment and Health Action Plan for Europe | Web site: www.euro.who.int/__data/assets/pdf_file/0006/78639/E83338.pdf |
| ■ WHO collaborating centres for children's environmental health | Web site: www.who.int/ceh/ceh_ccnetwork/en/<br>Web site: https://www.niehs.nih.gov/research/programs/geh/partnerships/network/index.cfm |
| ■ WHO water specific information | Web site: www.who.int/water_sanitation_health |
| ■ WHO chemical specific information | Web site: www.who.int/pcs |
| ■ WHO information about ionizing radiation | Web site: www.who.int/ionizing_radiation/en |
| ■ WHO information about air quality and health | Web site: www.who.int/mediacentre/factsheets/fs313/en |
| ■ WHO information about ultraviolet radiation | Web site: www.who.int/peh-uv |
| ■ WHO information about electromagnetic fields | Web site: www.who.int/peh-emf/en |
| ■ WHO information about occupational health | Web site: www.who.int/oeh/index.html |
| ■ Intergovernmental Panel on Climate Change (IPCC) | Web site: www.ipcc.ch/index.htm |
| **NON-GOVERNMENTAL ORGANIZATIONS** | |
| **Alliance for Healthy Homes**<br>50 F St NW, Suite 300<br>Washington, DC 20002 | Web site: www.afhh.org/index.htm<br>E-mail: afhh@afhh.org<br>Phone: 202-347-7610 |

*(continued)*

| ORGANIZATION | CONTACT INFORMATION |
|---|---|
| **NON-GOVERNMENTAL ORGANIZATIONS** | |
| **American Academy of Pediatrics**<br>Julius B. Richmond Center of Excellence<br>345 Park Blvd.<br>Itasca, IL 60143 | Web site: http://aap.org/richmondcenter<br>Phone: 800-433-9016 |
| **American Association of Poison Control<br>Centers**<br>3201 New Mexico Ave NW<br>Suite 310<br>Washington, DC 20016 | Web site: www.aapcc.org<br>Phone: 202-362-7217 |
| **American Cancer Society**<br>1599 Clifton Rd NE<br>Atlanta, GA 30329 | Web site: www.cancer.org<br>Phone: 404-320-3333 or 800-ACS-2345 |
| **American College of Medical Toxicology**<br>10645 N. Tatum Blvd, Suite 200-111<br>Phoenix, AZ 85028 | Web site: www.acmt.net<br>Phone: 844-226-8333 |
| **American Lung Association**<br>61 Broadway<br>6th Floor<br>New York, NY 10016 | Web site: www.lungusa.org<br>Phone: 800-LUNG-USA |
| **American Public Health Association**<br>800 I St NW<br>Washington, DC 20001 | Web site: www.apha.org<br>Phone: 202-777-2742 |
| **Association of State and Territorial<br>Health Officials (ASTHO)** | Web site: www.astho.org/?template=<br>environment.html |
| **Asthma and Allergy Foundation of<br>America**<br>1233 20th St NW<br>Suite 402<br>Washington, DC 20005 | Web site: www.aafa.org<br>Phone: 202-466-7643 |
| **Beyond Pesticides**<br>701 E St SE, #200<br>Washington, DC 20003 | Web site: www.beyondpesticides.org<br>E-mail: info@beyondpesticides.org<br>Phone: 202-543-5450 |
| **Center for Health, Environment and<br>Justice**<br>PO Box 6806<br>Falls Church, VA 22040 | Web site: www.chej.org<br>E-mail: chej@chej.org<br>Phone: 703-237-2249 |
| ■ Child Proofing Our Communities<br>Campaign | Web site: www.childproofing.org<br>E-mail: childproofing@chej.org<br>Phone: 703-237-2249, Ext 21 |

| ORGANIZATION | CONTACT INFORMATION |
|---|---|
| **NON-GOVERNMENTAL ORGANIZATIONS** | |
| **Children's Environmental Health Institute**<br>PO Box 50342<br>Austin, TX 78763-0342 | Web site: www.cehi.org<br>E-mail: janie.fields@cehi.org<br>Phone: 512-567-7405 |
| **Children's Environmental Health Network**<br>110 Maryland Ave NE, Suite 511<br>Washington, DC 20002 | Web site: www.cehn.org<br>E-mail: cehn@cehn.org<br>Phone: 202-543-4033 |
| **Commonweal**<br>PO Box 316<br>Bolinas, CA 94924 | Web site: www.commonweal.org<br>E-mail: commonweal@commonweal.org<br>Phone: 415-868-0970 |
| **Earth Portal** | Web site: www.earthportal.org |
| **EMR Network**<br>PO Box 5<br>Charlotte, VT 05445 | Web site: www.emrnetwork.org/index.htm<br>E-mail: info@emrnetwork.org<br>Phone: 978-371-3035 |
| **Encyclopedia of the Earth** | Web site: www.eoearth.org |
| **Environmental Defense**<br>257 Park Ave S<br>New York, NY 10010 | Web site: www.environmentaldefense.org<br>Phone: 212-505-2100 |
| ■ Scorecard | Web site: http://scorecard.org |
| **Environmental Justice Resource Center at Clark Atlanta University**<br>223 James P Brawley Dr SW<br>Atlanta, GA 30314 | Web site: www.ejrc.cau.edu<br>Phone: 404-880-6911 |
| **Environmental Working Group**<br>1436 U St NW<br>Suite 100<br>Washington, DC 20009 | Web site: www.ewg.org |
| **EXTOXNET InfoBase** | Web site: http://ace.ace.orst.edu/info/extoxnet |
| **Farm*A*Syst**<br>303 Hiram Smith Hall<br>1545 Observatory Dr<br>Madison, WI 53706-1289 | Web site: www.uwex.edu/farmasyst<br>E-mail: farmasys@uwex.edu<br>Phone: 608-262-0024 |
| **FoodNews** | Web site: www.foodnews.org |

*(continued)*

| ORGANIZATION | CONTACT INFORMATION |
|---|---|
| **NON-GOVERNMENTAL ORGANIZATIONS** | |
| **Health Care Without Harm**<br>1755 S St NW, Suite 6B<br>Washington, DC 20009 | Web site: www.noharm.org<br>E-mail: info@hcwh.org<br>Phone: 202-234-0091 |
| **Healthy Schools Network, Inc.**<br>773 Madison Ave<br>Albany, NY 12208 | Web site: www.healthyschools.org<br>E-mail: info@healthyschools.org<br>Phone: 518-462-0632 |
| **Home*A*Syst Program**<br>303 Hiram Smith Hall<br>1545 Observatory Dr<br>Madison, WI 53706 | Web site: www.uwex.edu/homeasyst<br>E-mail: homeasys@uwex.edu<br>Phone: 608-262-0024 |
| **Institute for Agriculture and Trade Policy**<br>2105 1st Ave S<br>Minneapolis, MN 55404 | Web site: www.iatp.org<br>Phone: 612-870-0453 |
| **International Network for Children's Health, Environment and Safety** | Web site: www.inchesnetwork.org/index.html |
| **International Society for Children's Health & the Environment** | Web site: www.ische.ca |
| **Learning Disabilities Association of America**<br>4156 Library Rd<br>Pittsburgh, PA 15234-1349 | Web site: www.ldanatl.org<br>E-mail: info@ldaamerica.org<br>Phone: 412-341-1515; 412-341-8077 |
| **March of Dimes Birth Defects Foundation**<br>1275 Mamaroneck Ave<br>White Plains, NY 10605 | Web site: www.modimes.org<br>Phone: 914-428-7100<br>Fax: 914-428-8203 |
| **Allergy & Asthma Network Mothers of Asthmatics**<br>2751 Prosperity Ave, Suite 150<br>Fairfax, VA 22031 | Web site: www.aanma.org<br>Phone: 800-878-4403 |
| **Moms Clean Air Force** | Web site: www.momscleanairforce.org |
| **National Association of County and City Health Officials**<br>1201 Eye St NW, Suite 400<br>Washington, DC 20005 | Web site: www.naccho.org<br>Phone: 202-783-5550 |

| ORGANIZATION | CONTACT INFORMATION |
|---|---|
| **NON-GOVERNMENTAL ORGANIZATIONS** | |
| **National Center for Healthy Housing**<br>10227 Wincopin Circle, Suite 100<br>Columbia, MD 21044 | Web site: www.centerforhealthyhousing.<br>org/index.htm<br>Phone: 410-992-0712 |
| **National Council on Skin Cancer Prevention** | Web site: www.skincancerprevention.org |
| **National Environmental Education Foundation**<br>4301 Connecticut Avenue NW, Suite 160<br>Washington, DC 20008 | Web site: www.neefusa.org<br>Phone: 202-833-2933 |
| **National Lead Information Center**<br>422 S Clinton Ave<br>Rochester, NY 14620 | Web site: www.epa.gov/lead/nlic.htm<br>Phone: 800-424-LEAD (5323) |
| **National Pesticide Information Center** | Web site: http://npic.orst.edu |
| **National Safety Council, Environmental Health and Safety**<br>1025 Connecticut Ave NW, Suite 1200<br>Washington, DC 20036 | Web site: www.nsc.org/safety_home/<br>Resources/Pages/EnvironmentalHealth<br>andSafety.aspx |
| ■ National Safety Council, Environmental Health Center, Indoor Air Quality | Web site: www.nsc.org/news_resources/<br>Resources/Documents/Indoor_Air_<br>Quality.pdf |
| **Natural Resources Defense Council**<br>40 West 20th St<br>New York, NY 10011 | Web site: www.nrdc.org<br>E-mail: nrdcinfo@nrdc.org<br>Phone: 212-727-2700 |
| **North American Commission for Environmental Cooperation**<br>393, rue St-Jacques Oust<br>Bureau 200<br>Montréal, QC H2Y 1N9 Canada | Web site: www.cec.org/Page.asp?PageID=<br>1115&AA_SiteLanguageID=1<br>E-mail: info@ccemtl.org<br>Phone: 514-350-4300 |
| **Organization of Teratology Information Specialists** | Web site: www.otispregnancy.org |
| **Our Stolen Future** | Web site: www.ourstolenfuture.org/index.<br>htm |
| **Pediatric Environmental Health Clinic**<br>Misericordia Child Health Centre<br>Edmonton, AB Canada | E-mail: occdoc@connect.ab.ca<br>Phone: 780-930-5731 |

*(continued)*

| ORGANIZATION | CONTACT INFORMATION |
|---|---|
| **NON-GOVERNMENTAL ORGANIZATIONS** | |
| **Physicians for Social Responsibility**<br>1875 Connecticut Ave NW<br>Suite 1012<br>Washington, DC, 20009 | Web site: www.psr.org<br>E-mail: psrnatl@psr.org<br>Phone: 202-667-4260 |
| ■ Pediatric Environmental Health Toolkit | Web site: www.psr.org/resources/<br>pediatric-toolkit.html |
| **School Integrated Pest Management** | Web site: http://schoolipm.ifas.ufl.edu |
| **Smoke Free Homes** | Web site: www.kidslivesmokefree.org |
| **Teratology Society**<br>1821 Michael Faraday Dr<br>Suite 300<br>Reston, VA 20190 | Web site: http://www.teratology.org<br>E-mail: tshq@teratology.org<br>Phone: 703-438-3104 |
| **Tulane/Xavier Center for<br>  Bioenvironmental Research**<br>1430 Tulane Ave, SL-3<br>New Orleans, LA 70112 | Web site: www.cbr.tulane.edu<br>E-mail: cbr@tulane.edu<br>Phone: 504-585-6910 |
| **University of Minnesota**<br>Environmental Health & Safety Program<br>W-140 Bayton Health Service<br>410 Church St SE<br>Minneapolis, MN 55455x | Web site: www.dehs.umn.edu<br>E-mail: dehs@tc.umn.edu |
| **Centers for Children's Environmental<br>  Health & Disease Prevention Research** | Web site: www.niehs.nih.gov/research/<br>supported/centers/prevention/<br>grantees/index.cfm |
| ■ Children's Environmental Health<br>and Disease Prevention Center at<br>Dartmouth | Web site: www.dartmouth.edu/<br>~childrenshealth/index.html |
| ■ Columbia University Mailman School<br>of Public Health | Web site: http://cpmcnet.columbia.edu/<br>dept/sph/ccceh/index.html |
| ■ Duke University Neurodevelopment<br>and Improving Children's Health<br>following ETS exposure | Web site: www.niehs.nih.gov/research/<br>supported/centers/prevention/<br>grantees/duke/index.cfm |
| ■ Emory University Center for Children's<br>Health, the Environment, the<br>Microbiome, and Metabolomics | Web site: www.nursing.emory.edu/<br>c-chem2/index.html |

| ORGANIZATION | CONTACT INFORMATION |
|---|---|
| **NON-GOVERNMENTAL ORGANIZATIONS** | |
| ■ Johns Hopkins University Center for Childhood Asthma in the Urban Environment | Web site: https://projectreporter.nih.gov/ project_info_description.cfm?aid=898 9734&icde=26719324&ddparam=&dd value=&ddsub=&cr=2&csb=default &cs=ASC |
| ■ National Jewish Health Environmental Determinants of Airway Disease in Children | Web site: www.nationaljewish.org/ professionals/research/programs-depts/genetics-therapeutics/research/ childrens-environmental-health/ |
| ■ UC Berkeley/Stanford Children's Environmental Health Center | Web site: http://chaps.berkeley.edu/ |
| ■ University of California at Berkeley Center for Environmental Research and Children's Health | Web site: http://cerch.org/ |
| ■ University of California at Berkeley Center for Integrative Research on Childhood Leukemia and the Environment | Web site: http://circle.berkeley.edu/ |
| ■ University of California, Davis The Center for Children's Environmental Health and Disease Prevention | Web site: www.ucdmc.ucdavis.edu/ mindinstitute/research/cceh/index.html |
| ■ The University of California San Francisco Pregnancy Exposures to Environmental Chemicals Children's Center | Web site: http://prhe.ucsf.edu/prhe/ maternalfetalexposure.html |
| ■ Northeastern University Center for Research on Early Childhood Exposure and Development in Puerto Rico | Web site: www.coe.neu.edu/orgs/center-research-early-childhood-exposure-and-development-puerto-rico-crece |
| ■ Southern California Children's Environmental Health Center | Web site: http://hydra.usc.edu/cehc/ index.html |
| ■ University of Michigan Children's Environmental Health Center | Web site: https://sph.umich.edu/cehc/ |

(*continued*)

| ORGANIZATION | CONTACT INFORMATION |
|---|---|
| **PEDIATRIC ENVIRONMENTAL HEALTH SPECIALTY UNITS (PEHSUs)** | |
| **Pediatric Environmental Health Specialty Units (PEHSUs)** | Web site: www.pehsu.net<br>(Includes links to all PEHSUs) |
| **New England Pediatric Environmental Health Specialty Unit - Boston, MA**<br>*Academic Affiliation:* Harvard Medical School and Harvard School of Public Health<br>*Hospital Affiliation:* Children's Hospital Boston and Cambridge Hospital<br>**Connecticut, Maine, Massachusetts, New Hampshire, Rhode Island, and Vermont** | Phone: 617-355-8177<br>Toll Free: (888) CHILD14 or 888-244-5314<br>Web site: www.childrenshospital.org/pehc |
| **The Pediatric Environmental Health Specialty Unit Region 2, Serving: New Jersey, New York, Puerto Rico, and the US Virgin Islands**<br>*Academic Affiliation:* Icahn School of Medicine at Mount Sinai, Department of Preventive Medicine<br>*Hospital Affiliation:* The Mount Sinai Hospital<br>**New Jersey, New York, Puerto Rico, and US Virgin Islands** | Phone: 866-265-6201<br>E-mail: PEHSU@mountsinai.org<br>Web site: http://icahn.mssm.edu/research/programs/pediatric-environmental-health-specialty-unit |
| **Mid-Atlantic Center for Children's Health & the Environment Pediatric Environmental Health Specialty Unit - Washington, DC**<br>*Academic Affiliation:* Georgetown University<br>*Hospital Affiliation:* Georgetown University Medical Center<br>**Delaware, Maryland, Pennsylvania, Virginia, Washington DC, West Virginia** | Phone: 202-687-2330<br>Toll Free: 866-622-2431<br>Web site: http://kidsandenvironment.georgetown.edu |
| **Southeast Pediatric Environmental Health Specialty Unit - Atlanta, GA**<br>*Academic Affiliation:* Emory University Department of Pediatrics<br>*Hospital Affiliation:* Children's Healthcare of Atlanta – Egleston Children's Hospital and Hughes Spalding Children's Hospital<br>**Alabama, Florida, Georgia, Kentucky, Mississippi, North Carolina, South Carolina, Tennessee** | Phone: 404-727-9428<br>Toll Free: (877) 33PEHSU or 877-337-3478<br>E-mail: sepehsu@emory.edu<br>Web site: www.pediatrics.emory.edu/centers/pehsu/index.html |

| ORGANIZATION | CONTACT INFORMATION |
|---|---|
| **PEDIATRIC ENVIRONMENTAL HEALTH SPECIALTY UNITS (PEHSUs)** | |
| **Great Lakes Centers' Pediatric Environmental Health Specialty Unit - Chicago, IL** *Academic Affiliation:* University of Illinois at Chicago, School of Public Health *Hospital Affiliation:* Stroger Hospital of Cook County **Illinois, Indiana, Michigan, Minnesota, Ohio, Wisconsin** | Phone: 312-864-5526 Toll Free: 866-967-7337 E-mail: ChildrensEnviro@uic.edu Web site: http://publichealth.uic.edu/ great-lakes/childrens-health |
| **Southwest Center for Pediatric Environmental Health - El Paso, TX** *Academic Affiliation:* Texas Tech University Health Sciences Center - Paul L. Foster School of Medicine *Hospital Affiliation:* University Medical Center of El Paso & El Paso Children's Hospital **Arkansas, Louisiana, New Mexico, Oklahoma, Texas** | Phone: 915-534-3807 Toll Free: 888-901-5665 E-mail: swcpeh@ttuhsc.edu Web site: http://swcpeh.org |
| **Mid-America Pediatric Environmental Health Specialty Unit - Kansas City, MO** *Academic Affiliation:* University of Missouri-Kansas City School of Medicine *Hospital Affiliation:* Children's Mercy Hospitals and Clinics **Iowa, Kansas, Missouri, Nebraska** | Phone: 913-588-6638 Toll Free: 800-421-9916 E-mail: mapehsu@cmh.edu Web site: www.childrensmercy.org/ mapehsu |
| **Rocky Mountain Pediatric Environmental Health Specialty Unit - Denver, CO** *Academic Affiliation:* University of Colorado Health Sciences Center *Hospital Affiliation:* Denver Health and Hospitals Authority and the Rocky Mountain Poison and Drug Center **Colorado, Montana, North Dakota, South Dakota, Utah, Wyoming** | Toll Free: 877-800-5554 Web site: www.rmrpehsu.org |

*(continued)*

| ORGANIZATION | CONTACT INFORMATION |
|---|---|
| **PEDIATRIC ENVIRONMENTAL HEALTH SPECIALTY UNITS (PEHSUs)** | |
| **Western States Pediatric Environmental Health Specialty Unit- San Francisco, CA** <br> *Academic Affiliation:* University of California at San Francisco <br> *Hospital Affiliation:* University of California San Francisco Medical Center <br> **Arizona, California, Hawaii, Nevada** | Phone: 415-206-4083 <br> Toll Free: 866-UC-PEHSU or 866-827-3478 <br> E-mail: pehsu@ucsf.edu <br> Web site: http://wspehsu.ucsf.edu/ |
| **Northwest Pediatric Environmental Health Specialty Unit - Seattle, WA** <br> *Academic Affiliation:* University of Washington: Department of Occupational and Environmental Health Sciences, Occupational and Environmental Medicine Program, Department of Pediatrics <br> *Hospital Affiliation:* University of Washington Medical Center; Harborview Medical Center; Children's Hospital and Regional Medical Center <br> **Alaska, Idaho, Oregon, Washington** | Toll Free: 1-877-KID-CHEM or 877-543-2436 <br> E-mail: pehsu@u.washington.edu <br> Web site: http://depts.washington.edu/ pehsu |

# Curricula for Environmental Education and Environmental Health Science Education in Primary and Secondary Schools

○ ○ ○ ○ ○ ○

At the first major international conference on the environment, the United Nations Conference on the Human Environment in Stockholm, Sweden, in 1972, countries recommended the establishment of "an international program in environmental education, interdisciplinary in approach, in school and out of school, encompassing all levels of education and directed toward the general public, in particular the ordinary citizen living in rural and urban areas, youth and adult alike, with a view to educating him as to the simple steps he might take, within his means, to manage and control his environment."[1]

Four years later, at the Belgrade Conference, the following goal of environmental education was proposed: "The goal of environmental education is to develop a world population that is aware of, and concerned about the environment and its associated problems, and which has the knowledge, skills, attitudes, motivation and commitment to work individually and collectively toward solution of current problems and the prevention of new ones."[2] This goal is still widely used today.

Environmental education should begin early and continue through high school. Children who receive environmental education may be able to prevent environmental exposures through community involvement and through personal health choices. As adults, these children should be better prepared to participate in the political process as informed and environmentally literate citizens. Many countries in Europe and the Americas have taken on the challenge of environmental education. In Europe, the GREEEN network was established in 2014 to bring together European organizations with a common interest in environmental education.[3] This chapter will focus primarily on environmental education in the United States.

In the United States, a number of excellent environmental education curricula have been developed by the North American Association for Environmental Education, a network of people working in the field of environmental education in the United States and 55 other countries. In 1996, the National Project for Environmental Education published *Excellence in Environmental Education—Guidelines for Learning (K–12)*; the Guidelines were most recently updated in 2010.[4] More than 1,000 practitioners and scholars developed the Guidelines through a critique and consensus process.

Environmental health science education has been an emerging area of study and curriculum development since the mid-1990s. Within the school system, environmental health can play a valuable role in bridging the gap between traditional environmental education and health education. Too often, students see environmental health as health of the environment and may not consider how the environment can affect their health. To address this educational need and to incorporate health into the environment picture, many novel and engaging environmental health education curricular materials have been created to align with the Next Generation Science Standards.[5] These standards were grounded in a framework for K–12 science education that identified the key scientific ideas and practices all students should learn by the end of high school.[6] On this basis, problem-based and integrated environmental health curricula were created, implemented, and evaluated.[7] Research shows a variety of positive outcomes for teachers who implement and for students who are exposed to problem-based and integrated curricula (https://www.niehs.nih.gov/research/supported/translational/ehsic/highlights/index.cfm).

As evidenced by various projects, the most successful environmental and environmental health science education programs result from combining excellent curricula with the efforts of enthusiastic individuals (teachers, parents, and administrators) at the local level. These programs can provide primary and secondary school students with sufficient knowledge to participate in activities that will help to improve the environmental health knowledge and overall health of their communities, including their families. Curricula relevant to communities might include topics such as global climate change and its effects on children's health, sun safety, drinking water contaminants, the causes and effects of outdoor air pollution, and the importance of avoiding secondhand smoke.[8]

Clinicians can stimulate and strengthen environmental health education efforts in schools through volunteer activities in the classroom, school health programs, and technical partnerships with local school boards and state departments of education. Classroom volunteer work can include assisting teachers in designing and executing hands-on environmental science and environmental health activities that actively link human health to the state of the physical environment. Within the tradition of school health is the concept of the healthy school environment. Clinicians can help local schools identify ways in which the school environment can be made healthier. A first step might involve evaluating the school facility for any environmental, health, and safety issues. The Model School Environmental Health Program developed by the US Environmental Protection Agency may be a helpful tool.[9]

On the basis of that evaluation, a school might choose to address a specific agent or toxicant. For example, a clinician could help to develop a plan for the school to reduce pesticide use, or work with students and faculty to ensure that the school is in compliance with state and federal health and safety regulations. Clinicians can participate in PTA activities and teacher training on environmental health issues pertinent to their community, drawing examples from their practices. Clinicians located at universities might approach their education departments to learn about ongoing or planned work in the area of environmental health science education and determine whether partnership opportunities exist. Finally, they can work with the district or state department of education to help systematically introduce environmental health education. Increasingly, states are creating offices of environmental education within departments of education to stimulate preservice and in-service teacher training as well as to include environmental sciences in K–12 curricula. Clinicians can add insight and expertise to this process by stimulating discussion about the links between the environment and human health.

## Environmental Education Curricula and Resources

### *General Environmental Education*

1. Project Learning Tree, 1111 19th St NW, Suite 780, Washington, DC 20036, phone: 202-463-2462, Internet: https://www.plt.org/curriculum-offerings/. Project Learning Tree uses the forest and trees as a "window on the world" to increase students' understanding of our complex environment, stimulate critical and creative thinking, develop the ability to make informed decisions on environmental issues, and instill the confidence and commitment to take responsible action on behalf of the environment (K–12).

2. Project WILD, 5555 Morningside Dr, Suite 212, Houston, TX 77005, phone: 713-520-1936, Internet: www.projectwild.org/resources.htm. The *Project WILD K–12 Activity Guide* focuses on wildlife and habitat, and the *Project*

*WILD Aquatic Education Activity Guide* emphasizes aquatic wildlife and aquatic ecosystems. The guides are organized thematically and are designed for integration into existing courses of study.

3. Project WET, 1001 West Oak, Suite 210, Bozeman, MT 59715, phone: 406-585-2236 or toll-free at 866-337-5486, Internet: www.projectwet.org/what-we-do. The goal of Project WET is to promote awareness, appreciation, knowledge, and stewardship of water resources through the development and dissemination of classroom-ready teaching aids and the establishment of state and internationally sponsored programs (K–12).

4. North American Association for Environmental Education, 2000 P St, NW, Suite 540, Washington, DC 20036, phone: 202-419-0412, Internet: https://naaee.org/. NAAEE is an association that represents professional environmental educators. Two projects are noteworthy regarding curricula. First, *eePRO* provides an array of information about teaching and curricula resources https://naaee.org/. Second, the *National Project for Excellence in Environmental Education* has developed national guidelines for materials, K–12 students, educators, and nonformal programs. https://naaee.org/eepro/resources/ee-wisconsin. Of particular importance are the Environmental Education Materials: Guidelines for Excellence and the Excellence in Environmental Education: Guidelines for Learning (K–12). The Materials Guidelines are a set of recommendations for developing and selecting environmental education materials to ensure quality. The Learner Guidelines set a standard for high-quality environmental education based on what an environmentally literate person should know and be able to do in grades K–12. http://resources.spaces3.com/89c197bf-e630-42b0-ad9a-91f0bc55c72d.pdf

5. The Expanding Capacity in Environmental Education Project—EECapacity—provides opportunities for professionals and volunteers to join in discussions about their environment and their communities, share success stories of where environmental education has made a difference, and learn about successful practices from across the globe. By providing these opportunities for individuals working in environmental education, youth and community development, resource management, and related fields, it is possible to build on and expand the critical role environmental education plays in fostering healthy environments and communities. A major part of the research component is housed in Cornell University's Civic Ecology Lab, which will document how diverse groups of educators, given opportunities to share practices and ideas, develop innovative environmental education practices. In addition, the North American Association for Environmental Education and other partners are working on how to develop a research to practice component that will

Appendix C: Curricula for Environmental Education and Environmental Health Science Education
in Primary and Secondary Schools

1183

help environmental education professionals everywhere understand how research supports practice. (www.eecapacity.net/about-us/)

6. US Environmental Protection Agency, Office of Environmental Education, 1200 Pennsylvania Avenue, NW, Room 1426, Washington, DC 20460, phone: 202-564-0443, Internet: www.epa.gov/enviroed. The Office implements the National Environmental Education Act of 1990. One program funded by this office is the Environmental Education and Training Partnership (EETAP), which provides training and support to teachers and other education professionals (www.eetap.org). EETAP has developed many resources for educators such as "Meeting Standards Naturally"—a CD-ROM that includes curriculum activities that demonstrate how environmental lessons can support grade level education standards. Other EPA environmental education resources include Web sites designed for children (www.epa.gov/kids), middle school students (www.epa.gov/students), high school students (www.epa.gov/highschool), and teachers (www.epa.gov/teachers).

7. US Environmental Protection Agency, Office of Children's Health Protection, 1200 Pennsylvania Avenue, NW, Room 1144, Washington, DC 20460, phone: 202-564-2188, Internet: https://www.epa.gov/children/. The Office has produced a Student Curriculum *Recipes for Healthy Kids and a Healthy Environment* (https://www.epa.gov/children/student-curriculum). This 9-lesson program was designed to excite children aged 9 to 13 about environmental health and empower them to take steps in their everyday lives to improve the environment for their community and reduce their environmental risk.

8. National Environmental Education Foundation, 4301 Connecticut Avenue, NW, Suite 160, Washington, DC 20008, Internet: https://www.neefusa.org/. NEEF is a private, nonprofit organization chartered by Congress under the National Environmental Education Act of 1990 to advance environmental knowledge. NEEF's National Environmental Education Week program provides references to environmental education and environmental health education curricula as well as resources and tools for health care providers. In 2015, NEEF published Environmental Literacy in the United States: An Agenda for 21st Century Leadership.[10]

9. California Department of Education, Office of Environmental Education, 1430 N St, Sacramento, CA 95814, Internet: www.cde.ca.gov/pd/ca/sc/oeeintrod.asp. This office has reviewed and rated hundreds of environmental education curricula (K–12) and published them in a compendium.

10. The Earth Science Communications Team at the National Aeronautics and Space Administration (NASA) Jet Propulsion Laboratory at the California Institute of Technology has a Web site for children called *Climate Kids* (https://climatekids.nasa.gov/).

11. The National Oceanographic and Atmospheric Administration (NOAA) has developed a series of short documentaries called "Young Voices for the Planet" that champions and publicizes inspirational, authentic, and positive youth-led models of success. They bring the films and programs directly to educators and youth through museums and science centers, such as the American Museum of Natural History in New York City, and other institutions. The films are also available subtitled in Spanish. The films help teachers to teach about climate change by acting as an antidote to fear. The Young Voices for the Planet films break through barriers of fear and "motivated avoidance" so people can take action (https://www.climate.gov/teaching/climate-youth-engagement/case-studies/young-voices-planet-film-series).

### Environmental Health Science Education

1. The National Institute of Environmental Health Sciences (NIEHS), Division of Extramural Research and Training, PO Box 12233 (MD-EC21), Research Triangle Park, NC 27709, phone: 919-541-7733. Education outreach is a key mechanism for achieving the mission of the National Institute of Environmental Health Sciences. The Environmental Health Science Education Web site provides educators, students, and scientists with easy access to reliable tools, resources, and classroom materials. Available in English and Spanish, it is designed to increase awareness of the link between the environment and human health (www.niehs.nih.gov/health/scied/index.cfm and https://www.niehs.nih.gov/health/scied/teachers/educacion/index.cfm).

The NIEHS supported the development of standards-based curricular materials that integrate environmental health sciences within a variety of subject areas (eg, biology, geography, history, math, civics, art). More than 81 materials were created by 9 projects. These materials can be found at: https://www.niehs.nih.gov/health/scied/teachers/index.cfm.

The NIEHS also released Climate Change and Human Health lesson plans in 2016. These materials are intended to promote student discovery and learning about the complex interactions between climate change, the environment, and human health. Using content from the US Global Change Research Program's 2016 report, *The Impacts of Climate Change on Human Health in the United States: A Scientific Assessment*, students are prompted to describe the impacts of changing climatic conditions on human health with emphasis on vulnerable populations and apply systems thinking to create a visual model of the health implications arising from climate change.[5,11] Students also consider the benefits of climate mitigation

Appendix C: Curricula for Environmental Education and Environmental Health Science Education
in Primary and Secondary Schools

1185

on human health and are thus introduced to the concept of co-benefits. Students are invited to identify and evaluate adaptation strategies that are protective of human health. To provide a solutions focus to the module, a culminating activity is offered that enables students to engage with local, state, or regional data and the US Climate Resilience Toolkit to evaluate climate adaptation and mitigation strategies. If desired, students can plan a resilience building project to address a climate change-related human health impact relevant to their local community. https://www.niehs.nih.gov/health/scied/teachers/cchh/index.cfm.

2. University of Medicine and Dentistry of the New Jersey School of Public Health. ToxRAP and SUC2ES2 (Students Understanding Critical Connections between the Environment, Society and Self). http://web.sph.rutgers.edu/toxrweb/index.html. Using a curriculum development model, teachers, scientists, and education specialists worked collaboratively to develop 3 curriculum guides. In this innovative, 3-part curricular series, students become health hazard detectives to cooperatively investigate environmental health hazards and their impact on human health. By applying an environmental health risk assessment framework, students learn how to state a health problem, investigate hazards and people who may be exposed, and identify hazard-control methods. A detective theme helps students to study air contaminants and learn the principles of toxicology and the process of risk assessment.

3. Baylor College of Medicine Center for Educational Outreach. My World and My World and Me. Developed by teams of educators, scientists, and health specialists at Baylor College of Medicine, My World (https://www.bcm.edu/education/programs/educational-outreach/curriculum-materials) and My World and Me educational materials provide students and teachers with knowledge of the environment and its relationship to human health.

   BioEd Online: www.bioedonline.org/. BioEd Online is an online educational resource for educators, students, and parents, sponsored by the Baylor College of Medicine and developed under the guidance of an expert editorial board. BioEd Online utilizes state-of-the-art technology to give instant access to reliable, cutting-edge information and educational tools for biology and related subjects. The goal is to provide useful, accurate, and current information and materials that build on and enhance the skills and knowledge of science educators.

4. Bowling Green State University, Project EXCITE: Environmental Health Science Exploration Through Cross-Disciplinary & Investigative Team Experiences: www.bgsu.edu/colleges/edhd/programs/excite. Project EXCITE engages students in learning experiences across disciplinary areas using

locally relevant environmental health science topics. The project reflects current thinking about effective teaching and learning and is aligned with national and state education goals. Project EXCITE emphasizes critical thinking and problem-solving skills, interdisciplinary connections, collaborative learning, and the use of technology. Students investigate local environmental health science issues, explain fundamental understandings of concepts, and apply the knowledge and skills generated to improve performance on standardized achievement tests.

5. Maryland Public Television. EnviroHealth Connections: www.thinkport. org/classroom/connections/default.tp. The curricular materials developed for this project include lesson plans, videos, and online interactive activities. They are disseminated to teachers throughout Maryland and beyond on the EnviroHealth Connections (http://envirohealth.thinkport.org). The Connections Web site hosts more than 60 classroom-tested lesson plans aligned to state standards. Additional materials include a teacher discussion board, PowerPoint presentations by researchers at the Johns Hopkins Bloomberg School of Public Health, and links to other high-quality resources. Also accessible through the Web site is Meet the Experts: Environmental Health, an interactive question and answer activity that features 13 professionals whose careers center on environmental health. Students learn what these individuals studied in school; how and why they began their careers; and how their environmental health work affects our lives.

6. Oregon State University. Hydroville Curriculum Project: www.hydroville. org. The Hydroville Curriculum Project has created problem-based curricula for high school students focusing on environmental health science. The problems occur in the fictitious town of Hydroville, which has to contend with 1 of 3 environmental health scenarios: a pesticide spill, a problem with air quality at a local middle school, and a water quality problem. The Hydroville curricula are based on real-life case studies and use real data. The town of Hydroville could be a town anywhere in America. Students work in teams to solve environmental health problems. This integrated curriculum promotes teamwork, critical thinking, subject integration, and problem-solving. Oregon State University provides additional environmental health science education resources for K–12 education at http://ehsc.oregonstate.edu.

7. Texas A&M University System. Partnership for Environmental Education and Rural Health (PEER): http://peer.tamu.edu. The Partnership for Environmental Education and Rural Health is a program for rural middle school students and teachers. The program aims to improve student enthusiasm for learning, increase overall academic performance of students, and encourage teachers throughout the state across all subject areas to use

environmental health science topics to motivate students and help them relate science instruction to real-world situations.

8. The University of Miami Coral Gables. Atmospheric and Marine-Based Interdisciplinary Environmental Health Training (AMBIENT): http://yyy. rsmas.miami.edu/groups/ambient/. The AMBIENT Project is a systemic approach to environmental health science education. Focused around the 4 themes of air, water, soil, and food, a health-science problem-based learning approach is delivered by trained educators to the ethnically diverse population of high school students in Miami-Dade County. The AMBIENT curriculum modules consist of segments. Some can be taught independently and others are meant to be used together in a certain order. All modules begin with a Teacher's Guide, which contains the basic information necessary to knowledgeably lead class discussions and guide students' research efforts.

9. The University of Rochester. My Environment, My Health, My Choices: https://www.urmc.rochester.edu/life-sciences-learning-center/lessons. aspx. My Environment, My Health, My Choices is an environmental health curriculum development project sponsored by the University of Rochester's Environmental Health Sciences Center. The project involves teachers from the greater Rochester, New York area (as well as throughout New York State) who create environmental health curriculum units with the support of University of Rochester faculty. The curriculum units focus on specific environmental health questions or problems of local, regional, or national concern. Such problems include water pollution caused by farm runoff, links between air pollution and asthma, and the health effects linked to pesticides.

10. The University of Washington, Integrated Environmental Health Middle School Project: https://depts.washington.edu/ceeh/downloads/HEART_ Manual.pdf. The Integrated Environmental Health Middle School Project (IEHMSP) introduces middle school teachers and students in Washington State and New Mexico to environmental health sciences and facilitates interdisciplinary teaching across the middle school curriculum. The IEHMSP has developed a multitiered model of integrated and contextualized learning. Project materials have been used by school districts across Washington State and in New Mexico. Additional resources are offered for K–12 Classroom Outreach at http://depts.washington.edu/ceeh/ educators/k12-resources.html.

11. The WGBH Educational Foundation has developed a Web site on Climate and Human Health that describes impacts on airway diseases, developmental disorders, mental health disorders, vectorborne diseases, and waterborne diseases. https://www.pbslearningmedia.org/asset/envh10_int_cchealth/

## Healthy School Environments Resources

US Environmental Protection Agency, Indoor Environments Division, Office of Air and Radiation, 1200 Pennsylvania Avenue, NW, MC 1131-G, Washington, DC 20460, phone: 202-564-3284, Internet: www.epa.gov/schools/. The US EPA has developed a 1-stop location for information and links to school environmental health issues and resources. US EPA and non-EPA on-line resources are available to assist facility managers, school administrators, architects, design engineers, school nurses, parents, teachers, and staff in addressing environmental health issues in schools. The Web site includes links to the EPA's Tools For Schools resources (https://www.epa.gov/iaq-schools), 3T's for Reducing Lead in Drinking Water in Schools, and the School Flag program, as well as many other tools and resources for schools. The EPA's Model School Environmental Health Program provides a set of key actions to assist schools and school districts in implementing and sustaining environmental health programs (https://www.epa.gov/schools/eh-guidelines-model-program). The model program provides links and resources to US EPA and non-EPA tools to help schools establish or enhance a school environmental health program.

## References

1. United Nations. Report of the United Nations Conference on the Human Environment. 1972. http://www.un-documents.net/aconf48-14r1.pdf. Accessed January 22, 2018
2. UNESCO-UNEP. 1976. The Belgrade Charter. *Connect: UNESCO-UNEP Environmental Education Newsletter,* Vol. 1(1):1–2. https://naaee.org/sites/default/files/153391eb.pdf. Accessed January 22, 2018
3. GREEEN Network. http://greeen-eu.net/about-greeen/. Accessed January 22, 2018
4. North American Association for Environmental Education. *Excellence in Environmental Education—Guidelines for Learning (K–12).* 2010. http://resources.spaces3.com/89c197bf-e630-42b0-ad9a-91f0bc55c72d.pdf. Accessed January 22, 2018
5. Next Generation Science Standards: For States by States. http://www.nextgenscience.org/. Accessed January 22, 2018
6. National Academies of Science. A Framework for K-12 Science Education: Practices, Crosscutting Concepts, and Core Ideas. 2012. https://www.nap.edu/catalog/13165/a-framework-for-k-12-science-education-practices-crosscutting-concepts. Accessed January 22, 2018
7. National Institute of Environmental Health Sciences. Environmental Health Science Education. https://www.niehs.nih.gov/health/scied/index.cfm. Accessed January 22, 2018. Web site: https://www.niehs.nih.gov/health/scied/teachers/educacion/index.cfm. Accessed January 22, 2018
8. Hursh DW, Martina CA. Teaching Environmental Health to Children: An Interdisciplinary Approach. New York, NY: Springer; 2011
9. Environmental Protection Agency. Model School Environmental Health Program. https://www.epa.gov/schools/eh-guidelines-model-program. Accessed January 22, 2018
10. National Environmental Education Foundation. Environmental Literacy in the United States: An Agenda for 21st Century Leadership. https://naaee.org/eepro/resources/environmental-literacy-united-states. Accessed January 22, 2018
11. US Global Change Research Program. *The Impacts of Climate Change on Human Health in the United States: A Scientific Assessment.* 2016. https://health2016.globalchange.gov/. Accessed January 22, 2018

Appendix D

# AAP Policy Statements, Technical Reports, and Clinical Reports Authored by the Council on Environmental Health

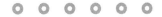

Please visit the American Academy of Pediatrics (AAP) public online policy site for updated information and access to COEH-authored AAP policy documents: http://pediatrics.aappublications.org/collection/council-environmental-health

## CURRENT STATEMENTS

### Food Additives and Child Health
Policy Statement: *Pediatrics*, Vol. 142, No. 2, e20181408, August 2018
Technical Report: *Pediatrics*, Vol. 142, No. 2, e20181410, August 2018

### Indoor Environmental Control Practices and Asthma Management
*Pediatrics*, Vol. 138, No. 5, e20162589, November 2016

### Prevention of Childhood Lead Toxicity
*Pediatrics*, Vol. 138, No. 1, e20161493, July 2016

### Nontherapeutic Use of Antimicrobial Agents in Animal Agriculture: Implications for Pediatrics
*Pediatrics*, Vol. 136, No. 6, e1670–e1677, December 2015

### Global Climate Change and Children's Health
Policy Statement: *Pediatrics*, Vol. 136, No. 5, 992–997, November 2015
Technical Report: *Pediatrics*, Vol. 136, No. 5, e1468–e1484, November 2015

**Iodine Deficiency, Pollutant Chemicals, and the Thyroid: New Information on an Old Problem**

*Pediatrics*, Vol. 133, No. 6, 1163–1166, June 2014

**Pesticide Exposure in Children**

Policy Statement: *Pediatrics*, Vol. 130, No. 6, e1757–e1763, December 2012
Technical Report: *Pediatrics*, Vol. 130, No. 6, e1765–e1788, December 2012

**Organic Foods: Health and Environmental Advantages and Disadvantages**

*Pediatrics*, Vol. 130, No. 5, e1406–e1415, November 2012

**Chemical-Management Policy: Prioritizing Children's Health**

*Pediatrics*, Vol. 127, No. 5, 983–990, May 2011

**Ultraviolet Radiation: A Hazard to Children and Adolescents**

Policy Statement: *Pediatrics*, Vol. 127, No. 3, 588–597, March 2011
Technical Report: *Pediatrics*, Vol. 127, No. 3, e791–e817, March 2011

**Drinking Water from Private Wells and Risks to Children**

Policy Statement: *Pediatrics*, Vol. 123, No. 6, 1599–1605, June 2009
Technical Report: *Pediatrics*, Vol. 123, No. 6, e1123–e1137, June 2009

**The Built Environment: Designing Communities to Promote Physical Activity in Children**

*Pediatrics*, Vol. 123, No. 6, 1591–1598, June 2009

**Spectrum of Noninfectious Health Effects from Molds**

Policy Statement: *Pediatrics*, Vol. 118, No. 6, 2582–2586, December 2006
Technical Report: *Pediatrics*, Vol. 118, No. 6, e1909–e1926, December 2006

**Chemical-Biological Terrorism and Its Impact on Children**

*Pediatrics*, Vol. 118, No. 3, 1267–1278, September 2006

**Infant Methemoglobinemia: The Role of Dietary Nitrate in Food and Water**

*Pediatrics*, Vol. 116, No. 3, 784–786, September 2005

**Ambient Air Pollution: Health Hazards to Children**

*Pediatrics*, Vol. 114, No. 6, 1699–1707, December 2004

**Radiation Disasters and Children**

*Pediatrics*, Vol. 111, No. 6, 1455–1466, June 2003

## RETIRED STATEMENTS

**Secondhand and Prenatal Tobacco Smoke Exposure**
*Pediatrics*, Vol. 124, No. 5, e1017–e1044, November 2009
Retired November 2017

**Lead Exposure in Children: Prevention, Detection, and Management**
*Pediatrics*, Vol. 116, No. 4, 1036–1046, October 2005
Retired July 2016

**Nontherapeutic Use of Antimicrobial Agents in Animal Agriculture: Implications for Pediatrics**
*Pediatrics*, Vol. 114, No. 3, 862–868, September 2004
Retired December 2015

**Global Climate Change and Children's Health**
Policy Statement: *Pediatrics*, Vol. 120, No. 5, 1149–1152, November 2007
Technical Report: *Pediatrics*, Vol. 120, No. 5, e1359–e1367, November 2007
Retired November 2015

**Tobacco Use: A Pediatric Disease**
*Pediatrics*, Vol. 124, No. 5, 1474–1487, November 2009
Retired November 2015

**Mercury in the Environment: Implications for Pediatricians**
*Pediatrics*, Vol. 108, No. 1, 197–205, July 2001
Retired April 2012

**Pediatric Exposure and Potential Toxicity of Phthalate Plasticizers**
*Pediatrics*, Vol. 111, No. 6, 1467–1474, June 2003
Retired January 2011

**Irradiation of Food**
*Pediatrics*, Vol. 106, No. 6, 1505–1510, December 2000
Retired October 2004

**Chemical-Biological Terrorism and Its Impact on Children: A Subject Review**
*Pediatrics*, Vol. 105, No. 3, 662–670, March 2000
Retired September 2006

**Thimerosal in Vaccines—An Interim Report to Clinicians**
*Pediatrics*, Vol. 104, No. 3, 570–574, September 1999
Retired November 2002

## Ultraviolet Light: A Hazard to Children
*Pediatrics*, Vol. 104, No. 2, 328–333, August 1999
Retired March 2011

## Screening for Elevated Blood Lead Levels
*Pediatrics*, Vol. 101, No. 6, 1072–1078, June 1998
Retired October 2005

## Risk of Ionizing Radiation Exposure to Children: A Subject Review
*Pediatrics*, Vol. 101, No. 4, 717–719, April 1998
Retired April 2002

## Toxic Effects of Indoor Molds
*Pediatrics*, Vol. 101, No. 4, 712–714, April 1998
Retired December 2006

## Noise: A Hazard to the Fetus and Newborn
*Pediatrics*, Vol. 100, No. 4, 724–727, October 1997
Retired April 2006

## Environmental Tobacco Smoke: A Hazard to Children
*Pediatrics*, Vol. 99, No. 4, 639–642, April 1997
Retired November 2009

## Hazards of Child Labor
*Pediatrics*, Vol. 95, No. 2, 311–313, February 1995
Retired January 2005

## PCBs in Breast Milk
*Pediatrics*, Vol. 94, No. 1, 122–123, July 1994
Retired February 2001

## Use of Chloral Hydrate for Sedation in Children
*Pediatrics*, Vol. 92, No. 3, 471–473, September 1993
Retired February 2000

## Lead Poisoning: From Screening to Primary Prevention
*Pediatrics*, Vol. 92, No. 1, 176–183, July 1993
Retired June 1998

## Ambient Air Pollution: Respiratory Hazards to Children
*Pediatrics*, Vol. 91, No. 6, 1210–1213, June 1993
Retired December 2004

### Radon Exposure: A Hazard to Children
*Pediatrics*, Vol. 83, No. 5, 799–802, May 1989
Retired February 2001

### Childhood Lead Poisoning
*Pediatrics*, Vol. 79, No. 3, 457–465, March 1987
Retired October 1993

### Asbestos Exposure in Schools
*Pediatrics*, Vol. 79, No. 2, 301–305, February 1987
Retired February 2001

### Involuntary Smoking: A Hazard to Children
*Pediatrics*, Vol. 77, No. 5, 755–757, May 1986
Retired April 1997

### Smokeless Tobacco — A Carcinogenic Hazard to Children
*Pediatrics*, Vol. 76, No. 6, 1009–1011, December 1985
Retired February 2001

### Special Susceptibility of Children to Radiation Effects
*Pediatrics*, Vol. 72, No. 6, 809, December 1983
Retired April 1998

### Environmental Consequences of Tobacco Smoking: Implications for Public Policies that Affect the Health of Children
*Pediatrics*, Vol. 70, No. 2, 314–315, August 1982
Retired February 1987

### National Standard for Airborne Lead
*Pediatrics*, Vol. 62, No. 6, 1070–1071, December 1978
Retired February 1987

### PCBs in Breast Milk
*Pediatrics*, Vol. 62, No. 3, 407, September 1978
Retired September 1994

### Infant Radiant Warmers
*Pediatrics*, Vol. 61, No. 1, 113–114, January 1978
Retired June 1995

### Hyperthermia from Malfunctioning Radiant Heaters
*Pediatrics*, Vol. 59, No. 6, 1041–1042, June 1977
Retired February 1987

**Carcinogens in Drinking Water**
*Pediatrics*, Vol. 57, No. 4, 462–464, April 1976
Retired February 1987

**Effects of Cigarette Smoking on the Fetus and Child**
*Pediatrics*, Vol. 57, No. 3, 411–413, March 1976
Retired September 1994

**Noise Pollution: Neonatal Aspects**
*Pediatrics*, Vol. 54, No. 4, 476–478, October 1974
Retired October 1997

**Animal Feedlots**
*Pediatrics*, Vol. 51, No. 3, 582–592, March 1973
Retired September 1994

**Lead Content of Paint Applied to Surfaces Accessible to Young Children**
*Pediatrics*, Vol. 49, No. 6, 918–921, June 1972
Retired February 1987

**Pediatric Problems Related to Deteriorated Housing**
*Pediatrics*, Vol. 49, No. 4, 627, April 1972
Retired February 1987

**Earthenware Containers: A Potential Source of Acute Lead Poisoning**
Newsletter, Vol. 22, No. 13, 4, August 15, 1971
Retired February 1987

**Neurotoxicity from Hexachlorophene**
Newsletter, Vol. 22, No. 7, 4, May 1971
Retired February 1987

**Acute and Chronic Childhood Lead Poisoning**
*Pediatrics*, Vol. 47, No. 5, 950–951, May 1971
Retired November 1986

**Pediatric Aspects of Air Pollution**
*Pediatrics*, Vol. 46, No. 4, 637–639, October 1970
Retired February 1987

**More on Radioactive Fallout**
Newsletter Supplement, Vol. 21, No. 8, April 15, 1970
Retired February 1987

**Smoking and Children: A Pediatric Viewpoint**
*Pediatrics*, Vol. 44, No. 5, Part 1, 757–759, November 1969
Retired February 1987

**Present Status of Water Pollution Control**
*Pediatrics*, Vol. 34, No. 3, 431–440, September 1964
Retired February 1987

**Hazards of Radioactive Fallout**
*Pediatrics*, Vol. 29, No. 5, 845–847, May 1962
Retired February 1995

**Statement on the Use of Diagnostic X-Ray**
*Pediatrics*, Vol. 28, No. 4, 676–677, October 1961
Retired February 1987

## PEDIATRICS SUPPLEMENTS

**A Partnership to Establish an Environmental Safety Net for Children**
Supplement to *Pediatrics*, Vol. 112, No. 1, Part II, July 2003

**The Susceptibility of the Fetus and Child to Chemical Pollutants**
Supplement to *Pediatrics*, Vol. 53, No. 5, Part II, May 1974

**Conference on the Pediatric Significance of Peacetime Radioactive Fallout**
Supplement to *Pediatrics*, Vol. 41, No. 1, Part II, January 1968

# Chairs of the AAP Council on Environmental Health

## Committee on Radiation Hazards and Epidemiology of Malformations

Robert A. Aldrich, MD; 1957–1961

In 1961, the committee was split in 2: a short-lived Committee on Malformations and the Committee on Environmental Hazards.

## Committee on Environmental Hazards

Lee E. Farr, MD; 1961–1967

Paul F. Wehrle, MD; 1967–1973

Robert W. Miller, MD, DrPH; 1973–1979

Laurence Finberg, MD; 1979–1980

In 1979, the AAP established the Committee on Genetics with Charles Scriver, MD, as chair. In 1980, the AAP combined this committee with the Committee on Environmental Hazards to form the:

## Committee on Genetics & Environmental Hazards

Laurence Finberg, MD; Cochair, 1980–1983

Charles Scriver, MD; Cochair, 1980–1983

In 1983, the 2 committees were separated again.

## Committee on Environmental Hazards

Philip J. Landrigan, MD, MSc; 1983–1987

Richard J. Jackson, MD, MPH; 1987–1991

In 1991, the committee was renamed the Committee on Environmental Health.

## Committee on Environmental Health

J. Routt Reigart, MD; 1991–1995
Ruth A. Etzel, MD, PhD; 1995–1999
Sophie J. Balk, MD; 1999–2003
Michael W. Shannon, MD, MPH; 2003–2007

## Council on Environmental Health

Helen J. Binns, MD, MPH; 2007–2011
In 2009, the committee adopted the AAP's "Council" format.
Jerome A. Paulson, MD; 2011–2015
Jennifer A. Lowry, MD; 2015–2019

# Appendix F

# Selected Abbreviations

○ ○ ○ ○ ○ ○

| | |
|---|---|
| 2,4-D | 2,4-dichlorophenoxyacetic acid |
| 2-PAM | pralidoxime |
| 4-MBC | 4-methyl-benzylidene camphor |
| ACE | angiotensin-converting enzyme |
| AChE | acetylcholinesterase |
| AAP | American Academy of Pediatrics |
| ALARA | as low as reasonably achievable |
| AP | Approved Product |
| ACMI | Art & Creative Materials Institute |
| ACS | American Cancer Society |
| ADHD | attention-deficit/hyperactivity disorder |
| AHERA | Asbestos Hazard Emergency Response Act |
| AI | adequate intake |
| AQI | Air Quality Index |
| ASD | autism spectrum disorder |
| ASTM D4236 | American Society for Testing and Materials Standard (art materials) |
| AT | ataxia-telangiectasia |
| ATSDR | Agency for Toxic Substances and Disease Registry |
| BAL | British anti-lewisite (2,3-dimercatopropanol, dimercaprol) |
| BBP | butyl benzyl phthalate |
| BLL | blood lead level |
| BP-3 | benzophenone-3 |
| BPA | bisphenol A |
| $c$-decaBDE | $c$-decabrominated diphenyl ether |
| $c$-octaBDE | $c$-octabrominated diphenyl ether |
| $c$-pentaBDE | $c$-pentabrominated diphenyl ether |
| $CaNa_2EDTA$ | edetate disodium calcium |

| | |
|---|---|
| CCA | chromated copper arsenate |
| CDC | Centers for Disease Control and Prevention |
| CEHAPE | Children's Environment and Health Action Plan for Europe |
| CERCLA | Comprehensive Environmental Response, Compensation, and Liability Act |
| CFC | chlorofluorocarbon |
| CFL | compact fluorescent light |
| CFOI | Census of Fatal Occupational Injuries |
| CFR | Code of Federal Regulations |
| CFU | colony forming unit |
| CHEAR | Children's Health Exposure Analysis Resource |
| CHEERS | Children's Environmental Exposure Research Study |
| CLIA | Clinical Laboratory Improvement Amendments |
| $ClO_4^-$ | perchlorate |
| CO | carbon monoxide |
| $CO_2$ | carbon dioxide |
| COHb | carboxyhemoglobin |
| CNS | central nervous system |
| CP | Certified Product |
| CPSC | Consumer Product Safety Commission |
| CPT | Current Procedural Terminology |
| CT | computed tomography |
| DALY | disability-adjusted life year |
| dB | decibel |
| dBA | decibels weighted by the A scale |
| DBP | dibutyl phthalate |
| DDE | dichlorodiphenyldichloroethylene |
| DDT | dichlorodiphenyltrichloroethane |
| DEET | *N,N*-diethyl-m-toluamide, also known as *N,N*-diethyl-3-methyl-benzamide |
| DEHP | di(2-ethylhexyl) phthalate |
| DEP | diethyl phthalate |
| DES | diethylstilbestrol |
| DHA | dihydroxyacetone |
| DHA | docosahexaenoic acid |
| DHHS | Department of Health and Human Services |
| DIDP | di-isodecyl phthalate |
| DINP | di-isononyl phthalate |
| DMP | dimethyl phthalate |
| DMPS | 2,3-dimercaptopropane-1-sulfonate (dimaval) |
| DMSA | dimercaptosuccinic acid (succimer) |
| DnBP | di-*n*-butyl phthalate |

| | |
|---|---|
| DNL | day-night average sound level |
| DnOP | di-*n*-octylphthalate |
| DOP | dioctyl phthalate |
| DSHEA | Dietary Supplement Health and Education Act |
| *DSM-V* | *Diagnostic and Statistical Manual of Mental Disorders, Fifth Edition* |
| ED | emergency department |
| EEA | European Environment Agency |
| EEG | electroencephalogram |
| EHR | electronic health record |
| EMF | electric and magnetic fields |
| EMLAP | Environmental Microbiology Laboratory Accreditation Program |
| EPA | eicosapentaenoic acid |
| EPA | US Environmental Protection Agency |
| eV | electron volts |
| FEMA | Federal Emergency Management Agency |
| $FEV_1$ | forced expiratory volume in 1 second |
| FLSA | Fair Labor Standards Act |
| FDA | US Food and Drug Administration |
| FQPA | Food Quality Protection Act |
| FSIS | Food Safety and Inspection Service |
| GABA | gamma-aminobutyric acid |
| GIS | geographic information system |
| Gy | gray |
| G6PD | glucose-6-phosphate dehydrogenase |
| HBV | hepatitis B virus |
| HDL | high-density lipoprotein |
| HDPE | high-density polyethylene |
| HEPA | high-efficiency particulate air |
| HL | Health Label (Non-Toxic) |
| HPV | high production volume |
| HPV | human papilloma virus |
| $H_2SO_4$ | sulfuric acid |
| HUD | US Department of Housing and Urban Development |
| HVAC | heating, ventilation, and air conditioning |
| Hz | hertz |
| IAQ | indoor air quality |
| IARC | International Agency for Research on Cancer |
| ICD-9-CM | International Classification of Diseases, Ninth Revision, Clinical Modification |
| IFCS | Intergovernmental Forum on Chemical Safety |

| | |
|---|---|
| Ig | immunoglobulin |
| IPCC | Intergovernmental Panel on Climate Change |
| IPM | integrated pest management |
| IRB | institutional review board |
| J | joule |
| kGy | kilogray |
| KI | potassium iodide |
| kV | kilovolt |
| Leq24 | 24-hour equivalent noise exposure |
| LOAEL | lowest observable adverse effect level |
| mcg | micrograms |
| MCL | maximum contaminant level |
| mcm | micrometers |
| MCV | mean corpuscular volume |
| MEHP | mono(2-ethylhexyl) phthalate |
| MERV | minimum efficiency reporting value |
| MHz | megahertz |
| MMA | methyl methacrylate |
| MMR | measles-mumps-rubella |
| MMT | methylcyclopentadienyl manganese tricarbonyl |
| MRA/MRI | magnetic resonance angiogram/magnetic resonance imaging |
| mrem | millirem |
| MRSA | methicillin-resistant *Staphylococcus aureus* |
| MSG | monosodium glutamate |
| mSv | millisievert |
| MTBE | methyl tertiary butyl ether |
| Na$_2$EDTA | edetate disodium |
| NAAQS | National Ambient Air Quality Standards |
| NAS | National Academy of Sciences |
| NCI | National Cancer Institute |
| NEISS-Work | National Electronic Injury Surveillance System occupational supplement |
| NHANES | National Health and Nutrition Examination Survey |
| NIEHS | National Institute of Environmental Health Sciences |
| NIHL | noise-induced hearing loss |
| NIOSH | National Institute for Occupational Safety and Health |
| NITS | noise-induced threshold shift |
| nm | nanometer |
| NMP | *N*-methyl-2-pyrrolidone |
| NMSC | nonmelanoma skin cancer |
| NO$_2$ | nitrogen dioxide |
| NO$_3$-N | nitrate-nitrogen |

| | |
|---|---|
| NOAEL | no observable adverse effect level |
| NOC | $N$-nitroso compound |
| NPL | National Priorities List |
| NRC | National Research Council |
| NRC | Nuclear Regulatory Commission |
| NSAID | nonsteroidal anti-inflammatory drug |
| NTD | neural tube defect |
| NTP | National Toxicology Program |
| OEHHA | California Office of Environmental Health Hazard Assessment |
| OMC | octyl methoxycinnamate |
| OSHA | Occupational Safety and Health Administration |
| Pa | pascal |
| PABA | para amino benzoic acid |
| PAH | polycyclic aromatic hydrocarbon |
| PBB | polybrominated biphenyl |
| PBDE | polybrominated diphenyl ether |
| PC | polycarbonate |
| PCB | polychlorinated biphenyl |
| PCDD | polychlorinated dibenzodioxin |
| PCDF | polychlorinated dibenzofuran |
| pCi | picocurie |
| PEHSU | Pediatric Environmental Health Specialty Unit |
| PFAS | perfluoroalkyl and polyfluoroalkyl substances |
| PFOA | perfluorooctanoic acid |
| PFOS | perfluorooctane sulfonate |
| PKU | phenylketonuria |
| $PM_{10}$ | particles with aerodynamic diameter smaller than 10 mcm |
| $PM_{2.5}$ | particles with aerodynamic diameter smaller than 2.5 mcm |
| $PM_{1.0}$ | particles with aerodynamic diameter smaller than 1 mcm |
| POP | persistent organic pollutant |
| PP | polypropylene |
| ppb | parts per billion |
| ppm | parts per million |
| ppt | parts per trillion |
| PTS | persistent toxic substance |
| PVC | polyvinyl chloride |
| rad | radiation absorbed dose |
| RAST | radioallergosorbent test |
| REACH | Registration, Evaluation, Authorisation and Restriction of Chemicals |
| RBE | relative biological effectiveness |
| RCRA | Resource Conservation and Recovery Act |

| RDW | red cell distribution width |
| rem | roentgen equivalent man |
| RfD | reference dose |
| SAICM | Strategic Approach to International Chemicals Management |
| SAMHSA | Substance Abuse and Mental Health Services Administration |
| SARA | Superfund Amendments and Reauthorization Act |
| SARS | severe acute respiratory syndrome |
| SDS | Safety Data Sheet |
| SIDS | sudden infant death syndrome |
| SHS | secondhand smoke |
| $SO_2$ | sulfur dioxide |
| SPF | sun protection factor |
| SPL | sound pressure level |
| Sv | sievert |
| T-2 | trichothecene mycotoxin |
| $T_4$ | thyroxine |
| TCDD | 2,3,7,8 tetrachlorodibenzo-$p$-dioxin |
| TEQ | toxic equivalent |
| TSH | thyroid stimulating hormone |
| TNF-$\alpha$ | tumor necrosis factor-alpha |
| TRI | Toxics Release Inventory |
| TSCA | Toxic Substances Control Act |
| UL | Underwriters Laboratories |
| UN | United Nations |
| UNEP | United Nations Environment Programme |
| UPF | ultraviolet protection factor |
| USDA | US Department of Agriculture |
| UVA | ultraviolet A |
| UVB | ultraviolet B |
| UVC | ultraviolet C |
| UVR | ultraviolet radiation |
| VEE | Venezuelan equine encephalitis |
| VOC | volatile organic compound |
| WHO | World Health Organization |
| WTO | World Trade Organization |
| XRF | x-ray fluorescence |
| YRBSS | Youth Risk Behavior Surveillance System |
| YTS | Youth Tobacco Survey |

# Index

○ ○ ○ ○ ○ ○

*Note: Numbers in italics indicate figures or tables.*